# Shoulder Surgery

## PRINCIPLES *and* PROCEDURES

# Shoulder Surgery

## PRINCIPLES *and* PROCEDURES

**Frederick A. Matsen III, MD**
Professor and Chairman
Department of Orthopaedics and Sports Medicine
University of Washington School of Medicine
Seattle, Washington

**Steven B. Lippitt, MD**
Northeast Ohio Orthopaedic Associates
Associate Professor of Orthopaedic Surgery
Northeastern Ohio Universities College of Medicine
Akron, Ohio

**Susan E. DeBartolo**
Managing Editor
Department of Orthopaedics and Sports Medicine
University of Washington School of Medicine
Seattle, Washington

**SAUNDERS**
An imprint of Elsevier

**Saunders**
*An Imprint of Elsevier*

The Curtis Center
Independence Square West
Philadelphia, Pennsylvania 19106

ISBN 0-7216-9598-1

**SHOULDER SURGERY: Principles and Procedures**


**NOTICE**

Surgery is an ever-changing field. Standard safety precautions must be followed but as new research and clinical experience broaden our knowledge, changes in treatment and drug therapy may become necessary or appropriate. Readers are advised to check the most current product information provided by the manufacturer of each drug to be administered to verify the recommended dose, the method and duration of administration, and contraindications. It is the responsibility of the treating physician, relying on experience and knowledge of the patient, to determine dosages and the best treatment for each individual patient. Neither the publisher nor the author assumes any liability for any injury and/or damage to persons or property arising from this publication.

The Publisher

**Library of Congress Cataloging-in-Publication Data**

Matsen, Frederick A.
Shoulder surgery: principles and procedures/Frederick A. Matsen III, Steven B. Lippitt.—1st ed.
p. ; cm.
ISBN 0-7216-9598-1
1. Shoulder—Surgery. 2. Shoulder joint—Surgery.
[DNLM: 1. Shoulder Joint—surgery. WE 810 M434s 2004] I. Lippitt, Steven B. II. Title.
RD557.5 .M387 2004
617.5'72059—dc21 2003042440

*Publishing Director, Surgery*: Richard Lampert
*Developmental Editor*: Heather Krehling
*Publishing Services Manager*: Tina Rebane
*Project Manager*: Mary Anne Folcher

K/MY
Printed in the United States of America.
Last digit is the print number: 9 8 7 6 5 4 3 2 1

*We dedicate our work to our loving families, Joellen, Corey, and Scott Lippitt and Anne, Susanna, Erick, and Laura Jane Matsen. Their love and encouragement are essential to all we have done and will do.*

# FOREWORD

In the United States I have noticed that every year or so there is a new textbook on the shoulder—basic shoulder texts, comprehensive shoulder texts, and texts dealing with complications of shoulder problems. At a recent shoulder conference in Germany, I visited a bookseller's booth and saw eight new shoulder texts that had been written in various languages. For these reasons I can say that the "Age of the Shoulder" is certainly with us.

The two authors of this text, which deals with the principles and procedures of shoulder surgery, are internationally recognized as shoulder experts. Dr. Matsen, the long-standing Chairman of the Department of Orthopaedic Surgery at the University of Washington School of Medicine in Seattle, is and has been a champion in the field of orthopaedic surgery. His Shoulder Service has successfully educated 22 shoulder surgeons who are practicing in the United States and internationally. Steve Lippitt, MD, following his orthopaedic residency, spent two years working with Rick Matsen in Seattle and now has an established shoulder practice in Akron, Ohio.

Rick and Steve have combined their talents both as teachers and Steve as a superb illustrationist. Together they have given us a wonderful and concise atlas of the basic principles and rationale for treating shoulder problems and procedures.

*Charles A. Rockwood, Jr., MD*

# PREFACE

This book is dedicated to those who are in awe of the shoulder's mechanics and who are challenged by the opportunity to reconstruct this joint when it goes awry. Here we illustrate some of the mechanical principles that guide our understanding of the joint as well as the surgical procedures that have, in our hands, proved effective in restoring the shoulder's function.

Our contention is that excellence of clinical result depends on an accurate assessment of the mechanics of the clinical problem and expert execution of a surgery appropriate for the mechanical derangement. The procedures described herein have been developed from more than 30 years of close observation, not only of the clinical results of our own practice but also of a careful analysis of well over 1000 patients who have come to us for help after the surgical procedures of others have failed. It is through consideration of these failures that we have learned what does not work—lessons fully as important as learning what does work.

*Warning:* Shoulder surgery is not for all patients with shoulder symptoms. The fact that a patient has shoulder pain does not mean that an operation can make it better. Distress is not, of itself, an indication for surgery.

*Warning:* This book does not concern itself with the discussion of open versus arthroscopic approaches. The nature of the approach should not change either the indications for or the mechanical principles underlying a procedure. We present what our experience has proved to be the most robust, effective, dependable, and durable surgical approaches to the major mechanical problems of the shoulder. However, because each patient is an individual, each procedure needs to be modified to meet the specific situation encountered with each patient's shoulder.

*Warning:* These shoulder surgeries are not for all surgeons. Those who practice this art on a regular basis are best suited to help individuals with mechanical problems of the shoulder. As in painting, sculpture, or playing the violin, it matters who holds the brush, the chisel, the bow, or the scalpel. The surgeon is the method!

In each section of this book, we provide some of the principles that underlie the procedures we use. This is for two reasons: (1) We believe that if a surgeon knows why a step is important, he or she will be in the best position to accomplish it well. (2) Some of these procedures are different than those historically used; thus, provision of their rationale is necessary to support their use.

We hope you enjoy using this book as much as we did putting it together.

Happy Shouldering!

Frederick A. Matsen III, MD
Steven B. Lippitt, MD

# ACKNOWLEDGMENTS

There are so many who have helped us build the knowledge in this book. First, we would like to acknowledge our partner and teacher, Douglas T. Harryman II, who passed away on his forty-sixth Birthday. Not only did he provide the highest level of inspiration and analysis, but he and his wife Kevin were also mainstays of the shoulder fellowship at the University of Washington.

Next we would acknowledge our unbelievable succession of shoulder fellows. The 22 individuals listed in the Appendix to this text have brought fresh vision, insight, and energy to the pursuit of the clinical and basic research that has become the groundwork of this book. They, along with John Sidles (our physicist partner), Kevin Smith, and our residents have challenged every idea and application. As we encouraged them to be critical, they practiced their art on us with vigor.

We have had so many great teachers, nationally and internationally. We would particularly recognize Charles Neer, Charles Rockwood, and Bob Cofield. While ideas differ somewhat among us, there is no difference in our pursuit of the best treatment for patients with shoulder disorders.

Without our patients we would not have had the experience on which to practice the art and science of shoulder surgery. So many allowed us to partner with them as we sought greater understanding and developed new innovations in management. They along with Sarah Jackins, our shoulder therapist, keep us in contact with reality.

The key person who made this project happen is Susan DeBartolo. Her relentless dedication to excellence at every level and her work nights and weekends created a very special book.

# CONTENTS

# PART I

# GENERAL PRINCIPLES

CHAPTER 1

# Principles of Patient Selection

*"Good judgment comes from experience, experience comes from bad judgment (hopefully not one's own)."*

As a senior professor once said, "The fact that you know how to do a procedure is not, of itself, an indication for doing it." Much of orthopaedic education is in "skills labs" and "learning centers," where the focus is on an element of technique, such as how to insert implants in plastic models. Although models may represent bones, a plastic humerus clamped to a table does not represent the situation of a real humerus surrounded by important soft tissues. No laboratory can represent the complexities of clinical surgery: matching a well-defined mechanical problem in a living patient with a surgeon who has the experience to manage it safely and effectively. Often an even greater challenge is to determine the role the identified mechanical problem plays in the overall health and function of the patient. So, to rephrase the professor's comment, "The fact that a patient has a condition is not, of itself, an indication for operating on it."

It is useful to group patients with shoulder problems into three categories. Category A includes those patients whose problems can be attributed to a mechanical cause and for which we have a mechanical solution. A common example is recurrent anterior glenohumeral instability after a traumatic anterior dislocation. Category B includes those patients whose problems have a known basis but for which we do not have a mechanical solution. An example might be weakness due to brachial neuritis. Category C includes those patients with problems for which we cannot find a definite medical basis. Examples could include generalized arm pain after an automobile accident or dissatisfaction with a rating of permanent partial disability.

When considering a patient for surgery, we find a general health inventory to be of great value. We are on the lookout for medical conditions or medications that might increase the perioperative risk. We probe the results of previous surgeries and are encouraged when the patient is proud of the benefit he or she received from procedures on other joints. We are concerned when patients smoke, because this habit compromises soft tissue and bone healing as well as respiratory health. We worry when patients are on narcotic medications before surgery, suggesting that pain, rather than mechanics, may be the problem. We obtain a preoperative Short Form-36 on all of our patients because our research has shown that patients who show good preoperative mental, social, and physical health on this questionnaire do better with surgery than those who score substantially below age- and gender-matched control subjects. Patients who do well after shoulder surgery typically have good scores on the physical and social function, general and mental health, and vitality scales. We also ask all of our patients to complete a preoperative inventory of common shoulder functions: the Simple Shoulder Test (see **Table 2–1**). This inventory informs us of some of the important functional deficits the patient is perceiving. These functional deficits are the target of our treatment. In this regard, we recognize that patients who answer "yes" to all

12 questions may have little room for improvement after shoulder surgery, and patients who answer "no" to all 12 questions may have factors complicating their disability other than mechanical ones.

The informed consent discussion plays a major role in patient selection as well. Patients who are unwilling to listen to the fact that infection, nerve and blood vessel injury, stiffness, weakness, instability, pain, and the need for revision surgery are all possible outcomes of any surgery are often not good surgical candidates. Patients who understand their condition, who know and accept the risks, and who understand their critical role in preoperative preparation and postoperative recovery have a greater chance of doing well.

The final, and perhaps the most important, consideration in patient selection is the question of the "fit" of the patient, the problem, the physician, and the procedure. The fact that a surgeon 1000 miles away has published "good" results with a procedure does not necessarily relate to my patient and me. Thus, it is prudent to ask, "Am I the right person to do this procedure for this mechanical condition in this patient at this time?" and "Since 'the surgeon is the method,' am I the right surgeon?"

CHAPTER 2

# Principles of Evaluation

We do shoulder surgery because we want to improve our patients' comfort and function over the preoperative state. Although we can gain an impression that our patients have benefited from our surgeries, it is difficult to determine which types of patients having what problems are improved by which of our own procedures and by how much. It is obvious that our personal skills, approaches, patient selection, and postoperative management are not the same as those represented in the published literature by other surgeons. We need data that relate to our own practices.

To know whether a specific treatment made a difference, it is essential that the status of the patient before treatment (the "ingo") and after treatment (the "outcome") are quantitated using the same tool. In this way, the postoperative–preoperative difference is obtained by simple subtraction. If only the outcome of treatment is known, the efficacy of the treatment cannot be known. Thus, the routine measurement of ingo becomes a matter of great importance: unless these data are collected before treatment, it is virtually impossible to collect them in a reliable way later.

Because we are all getting increasingly busy, ingo and outcome data are ideally collected in a way that is minimally intrusive to our practice. Since a major reason for measuring the difference we make is to communicate this information to our patients, the data need to be expressible in terms patients can readily understand, rather than in terms of medical metrics (such as range of motion, foot-pounds of torque, or scores on a grading system). In this regard, patients are most likely to be interested in information regarding changes in function, comfort, and well-being. Fortunately, the most direct way to obtain this information is also the most efficient in the context of a busy office practice: patient self-assessment. Because patient self-assessment questionnaires can be completed at home and mailed or e-mailed to the office, they have the additional advantage of not requiring the patient to return to the office every time outcome data are needed.

Various shoulder evaluation systems are available, but many are time consuming and expensive to implement, which reduces the practicality of their use in everyday practice. Furthermore, the results of these evaluation systems are usually expressed in terms of a "score" that has little meaning to a prospective patient. Our experience indicates that a simple 12-item functional inventory, the Simple Shoulder Test, provides a valid, practical, and meaningful tool that allows the patient to assess the functional status of his or her shoulder before and sequentially after treatment (**Table 2–1**). Not only does patient self-assessment save the time of the office staff, it also ensures that the data directly reflect the view of the patient, rather than having the information interpreted by others. When collected in this way, the data on functional improvement following a procedure are easily shared with prospective patients considering that procedure. Furthermore, with these data in hand, we can learn of our own personal efficacy and can use this information on an ongoing basis to progressively fine-tune our practice. If our results with a given procedure fall short of expectations, we can seek additional information on how to do it better, or we can stop doing the procedure. If we find that a certain procedure works well in our hands for certain patients, but not for others, we can use this information to select prospectively the best surgical candidates.

**Table 2–1**

**The Simple Shoulder Test**

Please answer each of the questions about your left/right shoulder by circling "yes" or "no" beside each one.

| | | |
|---|---|---|
| 1. Is your shoulder comfortable with your arm at rest by your side? | yes | no |
| 2. Does your shoulder allow you to sleep comfortably? | yes | no |
| 3. Can you reach the small of your back to tuck in your shirt with your hand? | yes | no |
| 4. Can you place your hand behind your head with the elbow straight out to the side? | yes | no |
| 5. Can you place a coin on a shelf at the level of your shoulder without bending your elbow? | yes | no |
| 6. Can you lift 1 pound (a full pint container) to the level of your shoulder without bending your elbow? | yes | no |
| 7. Can you lift 8 pounds (a full gallon container) to the level of the top of your head without bending your elbow? | yes | no |
| 8. Can you carry 20 pounds (a bag of potatoes) at your side with the affected extremity? | yes | no |
| 9. Do you think you can toss a softball underhand 10 yards with the affected extremity? | yes | no |
| 10. Do you think you can throw a softball overhand 20 yards with the affected extremity? | yes | no |
| 11. Can you wash the back of your opposite shoulder with the affected extremity? | yes | no |
| 12. Would your shoulder allow you to work full-time at your regular job? | yes | no |

As an example of the utility of the Simple Shoulder Test, **Table 2–2** shows the changes in the number of shoulder functions performable by 102 individuals with osteoarthritis 30 to 60 months after total shoulder arthroplasty. It shows not only the chances of each function being regained after shoulder arthroplasty in our hands but also the chances of each function being lost, if it was present before surgery. This information is both important to and understandable by the patient.

**Table 2–2**

**Simple Shoulder Test: Total Shoulder Arthroplasty for Glenohumeral Degenerative Joint Disease**

| | Preoperative State, *n* | | Percent Change from Preoperatative State | | Statistical Significance |
|---|---|---|---|---|---|
| | *No* | *Yes* | *Yes→No* | *No→Yes* | |
| 1. Arm comfortable at side? | 31 | 71 | 6 | 100 | <.01 |
| 2. Sleep comfortably? | 93 | 9 | 0 | 87 | <.01 |
| 3. Tuck in shirt? | 77 | 25 | 12 | 84 | <.01 |
| 4. Hand behind head? | 74 | 28 | 7 | 90 | <.01 |
| 5. Place a coin on a shelf? | 43 | 59 | 5 | 91 | <.01 |
| 6. Lift 1 pound to shoulder level? | 54 | 48 | 8 | 91 | <.01 |
| 7. Lift 8 pounds to shoulder level? | 86 | 16 | 19 | 69 | <.01 |
| 8. Carry 20 pounds at side? | 34 | 68 | 4 | 59 | <.01 |
| 9. Toss softball 20 yards underhand? | 50 | 52 | 0 | 2 | n.s. |
| 10. Toss softball 20 yards overhand? | 98 | 4 | 25 | 59 | <.01 |
| 11. Wash back of opposite shoulder? | 94 | 8 | 12 | 77 | <.01 |
| 12. Work full-time regular job? | 63 | 39 | 5 | 64 | <.01 |

CHAPTER 3

# Principles of Glenohumeral Radiology

Lots of shoulder radiographs are taken, and it is interesting how many are done poorly. When we are shown cases from other institutions, the radiographs are often accompanied by the apology "we can't get good plain films because . . ." In some regards, a bad shoulder radiograph is worse than none at all. For example, an anteroposterior (AP) view taken in the plane of the body may not reveal a posterior fracture dislocation, falsely reassuring the observer that "nothing is wrong" (**Fig. 3–1**).

Although computed tomographic scanning can provide information on glenohumeral bony anatomy, we find that properly taken plain radiographs usually provide all the bony imaging necessary for the presurgical decision making, surgical planning, and patient education.

It is of great value to standardize a series of three glenohumeral radiographic views and series. The purpose of these three views is (1) to see the glenohumeral joint from two orthogonal perspectives, (2) to evaluate the bony anatomy of the glenoid and humeral joint surfaces, and (3) to allow for magnification-corrected templating of the proximal humerus. Two other views are used to evaluate the glenohumeral relationship and to evaluate the posterolateral humeral head and the anteromedial glenoid lip.

The five views we use most commonly are the following:

1. *AP in the scapular plane*—an AP view of the glenohumeral joint with the film in the plane of the scapula and with the forearm rotated 30 degrees external to the line of the beam. This view reveals the radiographic joint space with the arm in adduction and the contour of the humerus and glenoid (**Fig. 3–2**).

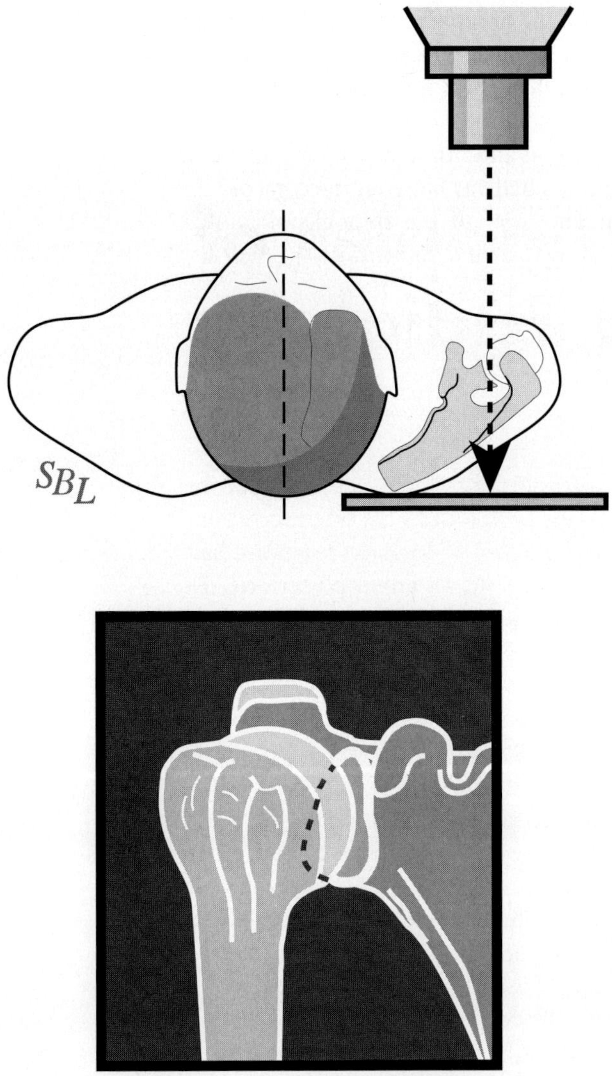


**Figure 3–1. Anteroposterior x-ray in the plane of the body**
An anteroposterior view in the coronal plane of the body is of limited use in the evaluation of the glenohumeral joint, the joint space, or the relationship of the humeral head to the glenoid fossa.

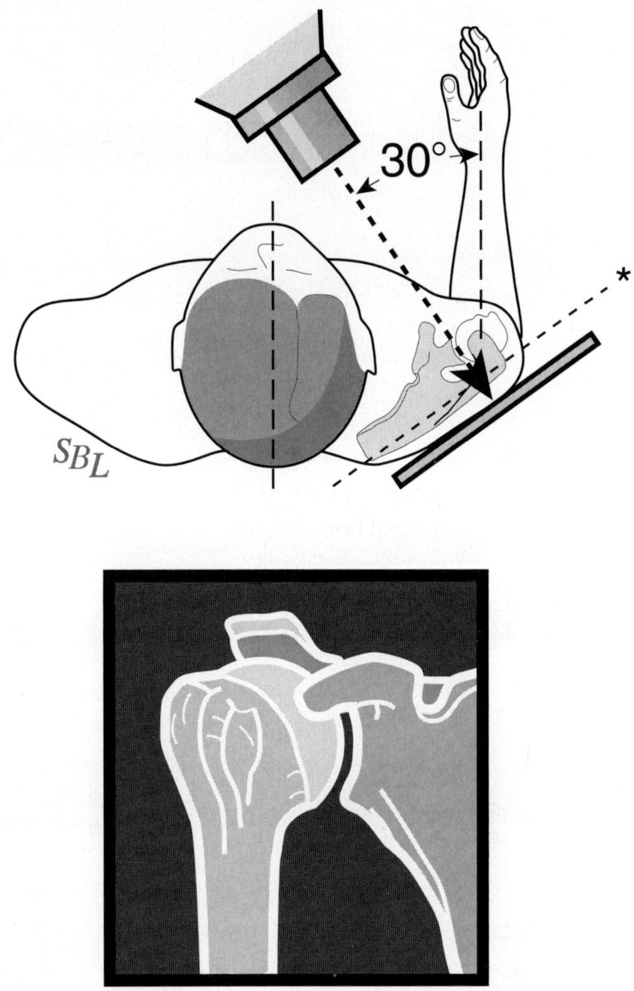


**Figure 3–2. Anteroposterior x-ray in the plane of the scapula**
An anteroposterior view in the plane of the scapula reveals the glenohumeral joint space and demonstrates whether the humeral head has a normal relationship to the glenoid fossa. It is most easily taken by positioning the patient's scapula flat on the cassette and then passing the x-ray beam at right angles to the film, aiming at the coracoid process. (From Rockwood CA, Matsen FA [eds]: The Shoulder, 2nd ed. Philadelphia: WB Saunders, 1998, p. 650.)

2. *Axillary view*—an axillary view projection with the film perpendicular to the plane of the scapula and the glenohumeral joint in a mid-range position. It may be convenient to have the patient hold on to an IV pole to help hold this position. This view reveals the radiographic joint space with the arm in a mid-range position as well as the contour and orientation of the glenoid and humeral articular surfaces. In a properly taken film, the glenoid is projected halfway between the coracoid tip and the posterior angle of the acromion. The "eye" of the spinoglenoid notch should be visible (**Fig. 3–3**).

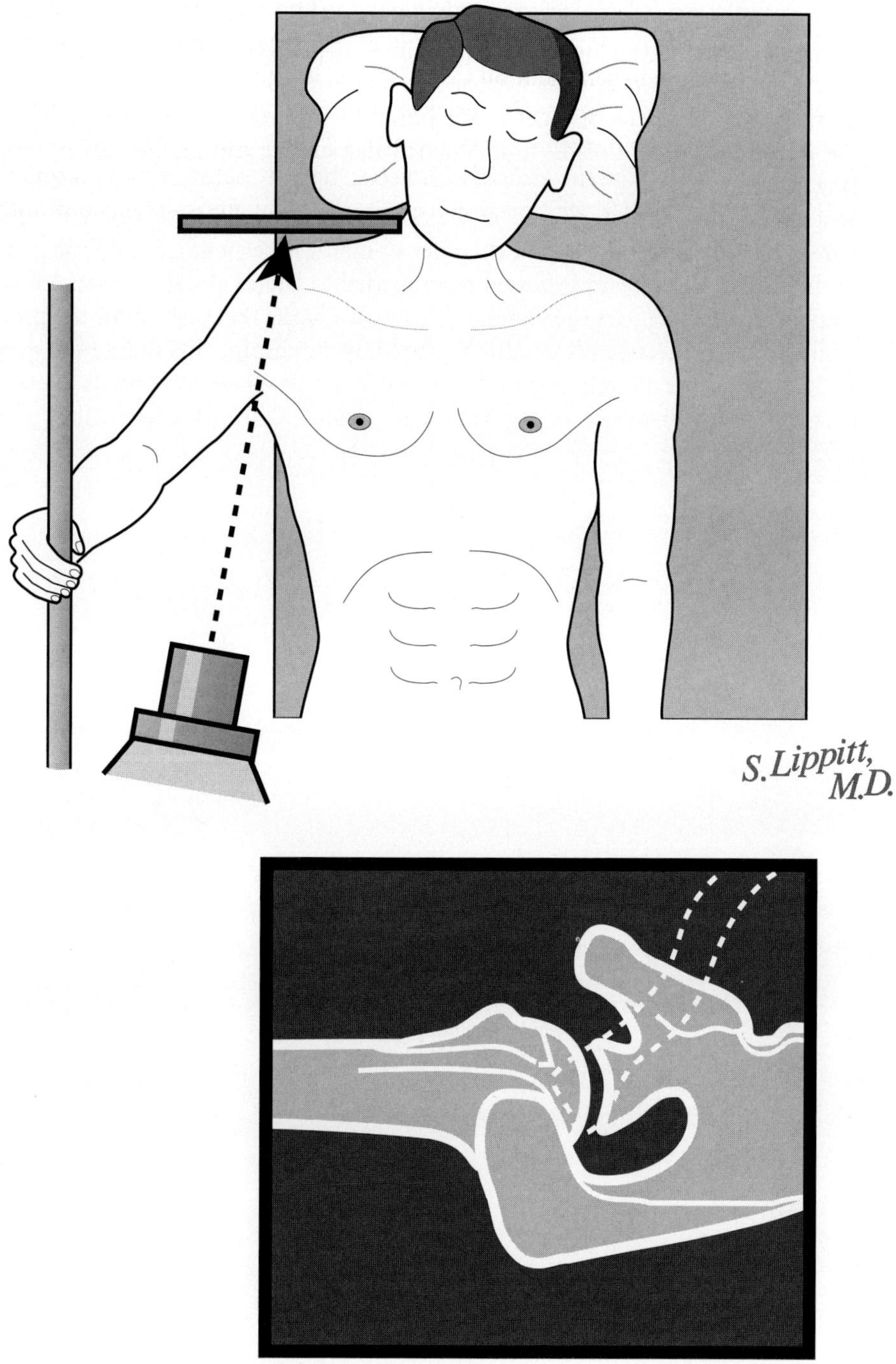


**Figure 3–3. Axillary x-ray**

An axillary x-ray reveals the glenohumeral joint space and the anteroposterior position of the humeral head and glenoid fossa. It is obtained by having the patient's arm in abduction (for example, holding on to an IV pole), the cassette on the superior aspect of the shoulder, and the x-ray beam passing up the axilla, aiming at the coracoid. (From Rockwood CA, Matsen FA [eds]: The Shoulder, 2nd ed. Philadelphia: WB Saunders, 1998, p. 651.)

3. *Templating view*—an AP view of the humerus with the forearm rotated 30 degrees external to the line of the beam, in 45 degrees of abduction, and with a 10 cm magnification marker attached to the arm so that it is parallel to the humerus and the same distance as the humerus from the film. This view shows the size and alignment of the humeral articular surface and the medullary canal **(Fig. 3–4)**.
4. *Scapular lateral*—the lateral view in the plane of the scapula. In this view, the cassette is placed against the lateral shoulder so that it is perpendicular to the plane of the scapula. The beam is passed from medial to lateral along the plane of the scapula and centered on the glenoid. This view reveals the position of the proximal humerus in relationship to the Y created by the coming together of the spine of the scapula, the acromion, and the body of the scapula. It also reveals the contour of the undersurface of the bony component of the coracoacromial arch **(Fig. 3–5)**.

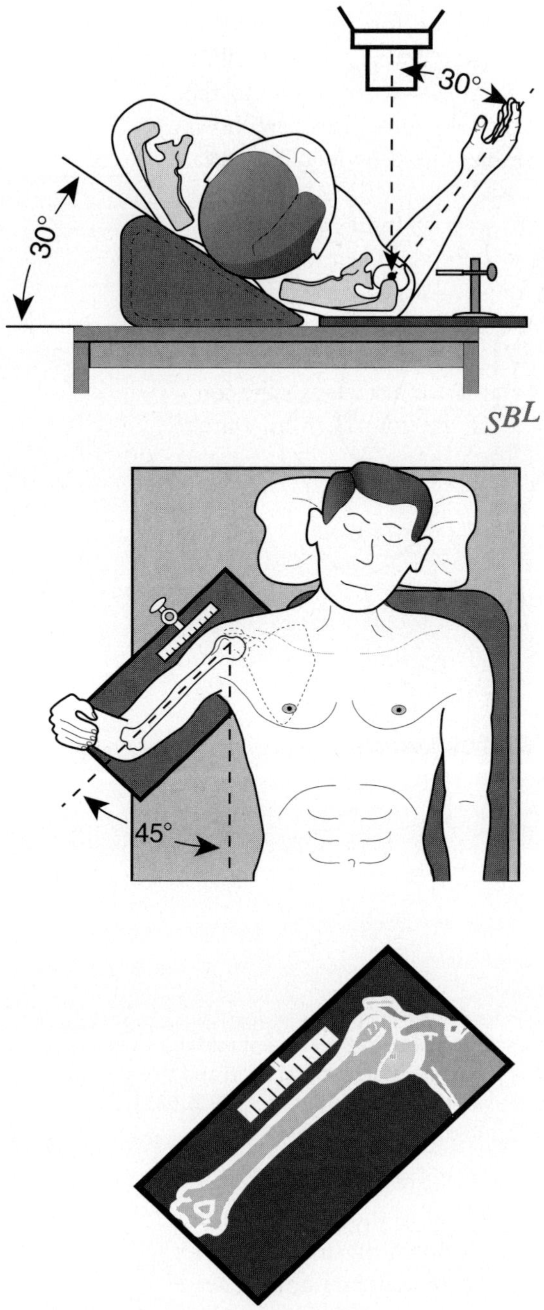


**Figure 3–4. Humeral templating view**
The humeral templating view shows the humeral shaft with the humeral head and neck in maximal profile. It is obtained by having the flexed forearm externally rotated with respect to the x-ray beam. A calibrated marker helps correct for magnification in templating. (From Matsen FA, Lippitt SB, Sidles JA, et al [eds]: Practical Evaluation and Management of the Shoulder. Philadelphia: WB Saunders, 1994, p. 160.)

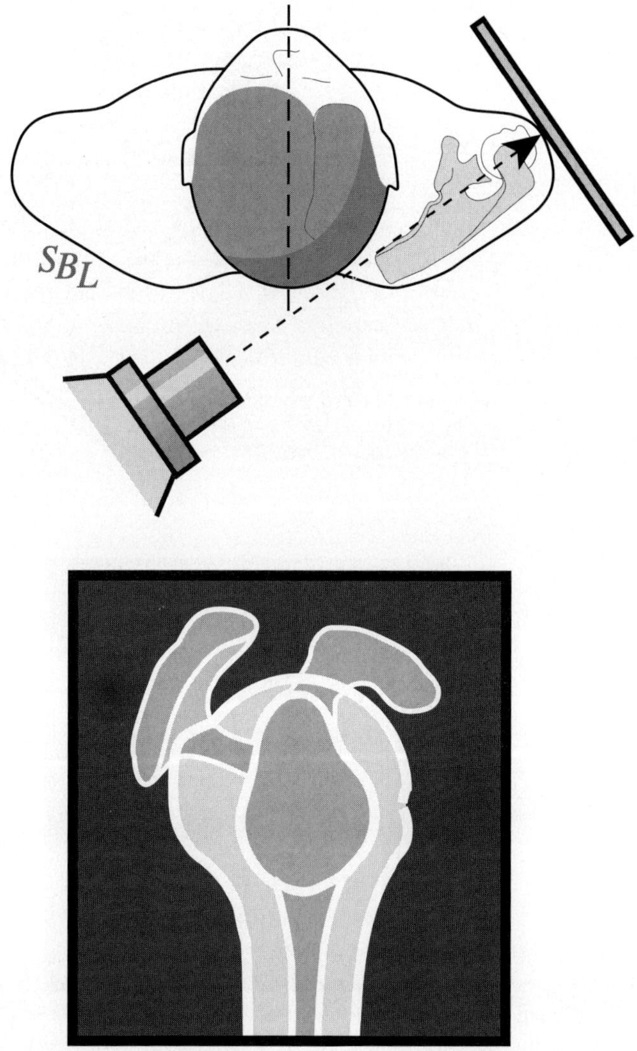


**Figure 3–5. Scapular lateral view**
The shoulder is placed against the radiographic cassette so that the scapular spine is perpendicular to it. The x-ray beam is passed parallel to the scapular spine and centered on the intersection of the coracoid process, the acromion process, and the plane of the scapular body. This intersection lies in the glenoid fossa. The humeral head should lie centered at this intersection. (From Matsen FA, Lippitt SB, Sidles JA, et al [eds]: Practical Evaluation and Management of the Shoulder. Philadelphia: WB Saunders, 1994, p. 159.)

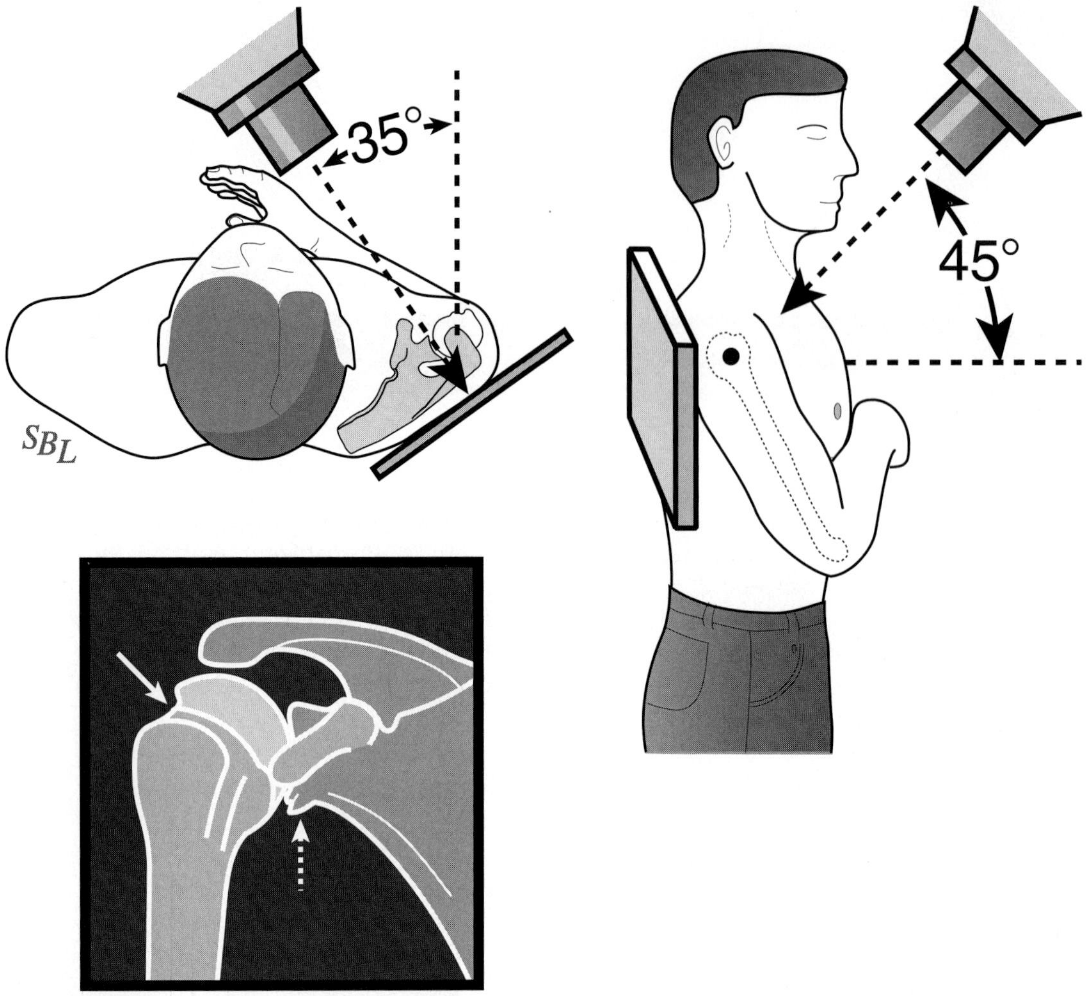


**Figure 3–6. Apical oblique view**

The shoulder is positioned as for an anteroposterior view in the plane of the scapula (see Fig. 3–2) except that the x-ray beam is angled inferiorly at an angle of 45 degrees. This reveals the contour of the posterolateral humeral head and the anteroinferior glenoid. (From Rockwood CA, Matsen FA [eds]: The Shoulder, 2nd ed. Philadelphia: WB Saunders, 1998, p. 685.)

5. *Apical oblique*—This view is taken in a manner identical to the AP view in the plane of the scapula except that the beam is angled down at an angle of 45 degrees. In this view, the beam passes tangent to the posterolateral humeral head and to the anteroinferior glenoid lip, showing any possible defects related to traumatic anterior instability **(Fig. 3–6)**.

Established sets of these five views can be used for specific problem-oriented approaches to shoulder radiography:

1. *General shoulder series*:
   AP in the scapular plane
   Axillary view
   Scapular lateral
2. *Instability series:*
   AP in the scapular plane
   Axillary view
   Scapular lateral
   Apical oblique
3. *Rotator cuff series*:
   AP in the scapular plane
   Axillary view
   Scapular lateral
4. *Arthritis series:*
   AP in the scapular plane
   Axillary view
   Templating view
5. *Initial trauma series:*
   AP in the scapular plane
   Axillary view
   Scapular lateral

CHAPTER 4

# Principles of Surgical Preparation

On the day of surgery, we once again review the patient's general health, medications, and allergies. Before the patient is premedicated, we ask the patient to mark the side and site of his or her procedure with a marking pen. As the patient enters the operating room, we check to be sure that the consent form has been signed, the radiographs are available and hung on the view box where they can be seen by the surgeon during the case, the preoperative note is posted, and all evidence confirms the procedure and the site and side where it is to be performed. This is especially important when patients are examined supine and operated on in the prone position.

The templating of the procedure is verified to preview the type, size, and fit of the implants of potential applicability to the case.

The procedure is reviewed with the nursing staff to ensure the availability of the instruments, power tools, supplies, and possible implants.

We do not routinely use urinary catheters during surgery. The exception is when the procedure is likely to take longer than 3 hours or when there is potential concern about the patient's hemodynamic stability.

If the procedure is to be performed with the patient in the supine position, the anesthetic process is completed and the examination under anesthesia (EUA) is performed with the patient on the operating table. The EUA includes the range of motion in elevation, external rotation at the side, cross-body adduction, and internal and external rotation with the arm in 90 degrees of abduction. These values are written on a whiteboard in the operating room and transcribed into the chart along with the results of the anterior and posterior load and shift tests.

If the procedure is to be performed with the patient in the prone position, the EUA is performed with the patient supine on the stretcher before the patient is transferred to the operating table.

In either position, the patient is positioned flat on the operating table so that the position of the thorax is defined; no bumps are placed under the shoulder. The patient is positioned with the glenohumeral joint at the edge of the operating table so that the arm can be moved without impairment. The patient's body and head are secured to the operating table. The table is positioned in the operating room so that all the lights can be brought to bear on the intended surgical field.

If laminar flow is used, the patient is positioned so that the air path moves up the body from the feet to the shoulder. Unscrubbed personnel are not allowed to walk or stand between the air source and the patient.

At this time, all doors to the operating room are locked except the one nearest the anesthesiologist. Unnecessary traffic and conversation are eliminated so that sterility is maximized and attention focused on the procedure at hand. The lights and TV monitors are positioned before the preparation is begun so that any dust dislodged from them during positioning does not affect the patient.

In most cases, prophylactic antibiotics are administered at the start of the preparation of the skin. Antibiotics are withheld in revision cases or in cases with previous open injury until the surgeon has had the opportunity to collect fluid and tissue for Gram stain, culture, and frozen section.

The immediate area of the skin incision is shaved. The axilla is not shaved. Loose hair is removed.

In all procedures, the forequarter is prepped anteriorly and posteriorly, including the entire arm. We routinely use an iodine solution unless the patient has an iodine allergy. A sterile drape is placed beneath the shoulder girdle, ensuring that the preparation solution has not pooled beneath the patient.

After the body has been draped, a tubular stockinet is placed over the hand, forearm, and arm up to the mid-humerus. The skin incision is marked. A sterile, counted, $4 \times 4$ sponge is placed in the axilla. A transparent adhesive drape is carefully placed over the marked skin so that the skin is not distorted. This drape completes the coverage of the skin and connects the drapes covering the body and head to the stockinet, avoiding the need for towel clips that may interfere with intraoperative radiographs. A fluid-catching drape is attached below the shoulder to collect blood and irrigation fluids draining from the surgical field.

We use a horizontal bar secured to two IV poles to hold the drapes up off the head of the patient and to allow easy inspection of the head by the anesthesiologist. It is high enough to separate the nonsterile activities of the anesthesiologist from the surgical field, but low enough to allow the anesthesiologist to look over to see the surgical field. This bar is slanted so that there is room for one member of the surgical team cephalad to the shoulder, one lateral to it, and one in the axillary position. Usually the surgeon is in the axillary position, the first assistant in the cephalad position, and the second assistant in the lateral position. Slanting the bar in this way allows the anesthesiologist access to the contralateral arm and head.

The scrub nurse stands opposite the surgeon. The instrument and implant trays are at the patient's feet and behind the nurse.

CHAPTER 5

# Principles of Post-surgical Rehabilitation

## PATIENT EQUALS THERAPIST

Our patient-centric philosophy begins with putting the patient in charge of the decision to have surgery and concludes with putting the patient in charge of his or her own postsurgical rehabilitation and follow-up.

Instruction regarding rehabilitation begins even before the patient has decided to have surgery, in that if he or she does not feel ready to accept responsibility for the rehabilitation, the patient may need to reconsider undergoing the procedure. The goal is to emphasize the partnership between patient and surgeon and that each needs to fulfill his or her respective role.

Thus, in our presurgical information packet, we describe to the patient the required activities and limitations at different stages after the procedure and ensure that the patient is confident in his or her ability to fulfill the program. In this way we seek to avoid surprising patients with new information and expectations after surgery and give them assurance that they are moving along a predefined path. When each step in the recovery proceeds according to expectation, the patient's confidence is maintained at the highest level. For example, if the need for a cane in the contralateral hand for ambulation after an iliac crest graft for anterior glenoid lip deficiency is reviewed preoperatively with patients, they are not surprised that walking is painful without a cane immediately after surgery. The same can be said for continuous passive motion, wound drains, and restrictions on lifting, driving, and working.

We explain before surgery that patients will be their own therapists—they will be shown their exercises in the hospital and have the responsibility of performing them multiple times each day during the healing period. Because many of our patients live long distances from our center, we explain that we cannot rely on local therapists to conduct the rehabilitation in the way that is needed; by putting the patient in charge of the exercise program, we can minimize the risk of errors in rehabilitation. Most often, postoperative programs consist of a very small set of easy routines requiring minimal equipment. All these programs begin on either the day of surgery or the first day after surgery. We show patients how to measure their own forward elevation, external rotation, internal rotation, and cross-body adduction so that they can inform us of their postoperative progress. We teach them what we mean by the different degrees of elevation and rotation. We teach them the difference between "active" exercise, which the patient performs under control of the operated shoulder, using the other arm only for assistance as necessary, and "passive" exercise, in which the operated shoulder is powered by the opposite arm or a friend or family member.

Here we list some of the exercises we commonly use after shoulder surgery.

1. *The 90–0 active program*: Used after repairs for anterior instability, the patient begins on the first postoperative day to elevate the arm to 90 degrees and externally rotate to 0 degrees. These exercises can be performed actively or passively using the opposite hand **(Fig. 5–1)**.

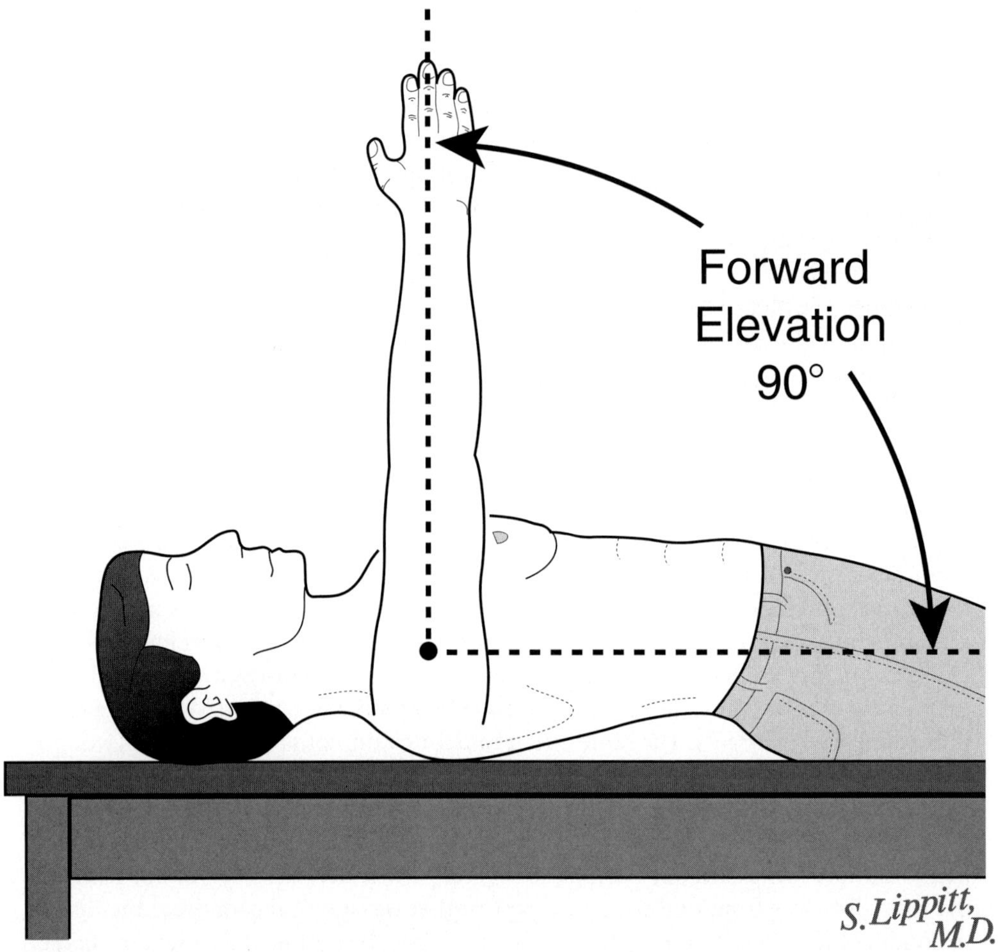


A

**Figure 5–1. The 90-0 active program**
We use this program for the first 2 weeks after an instability repair. The patient actively or passively flexes the arm to 90 degrees (**A, B**) and externally rotates it to 0 degrees (**C, D**).

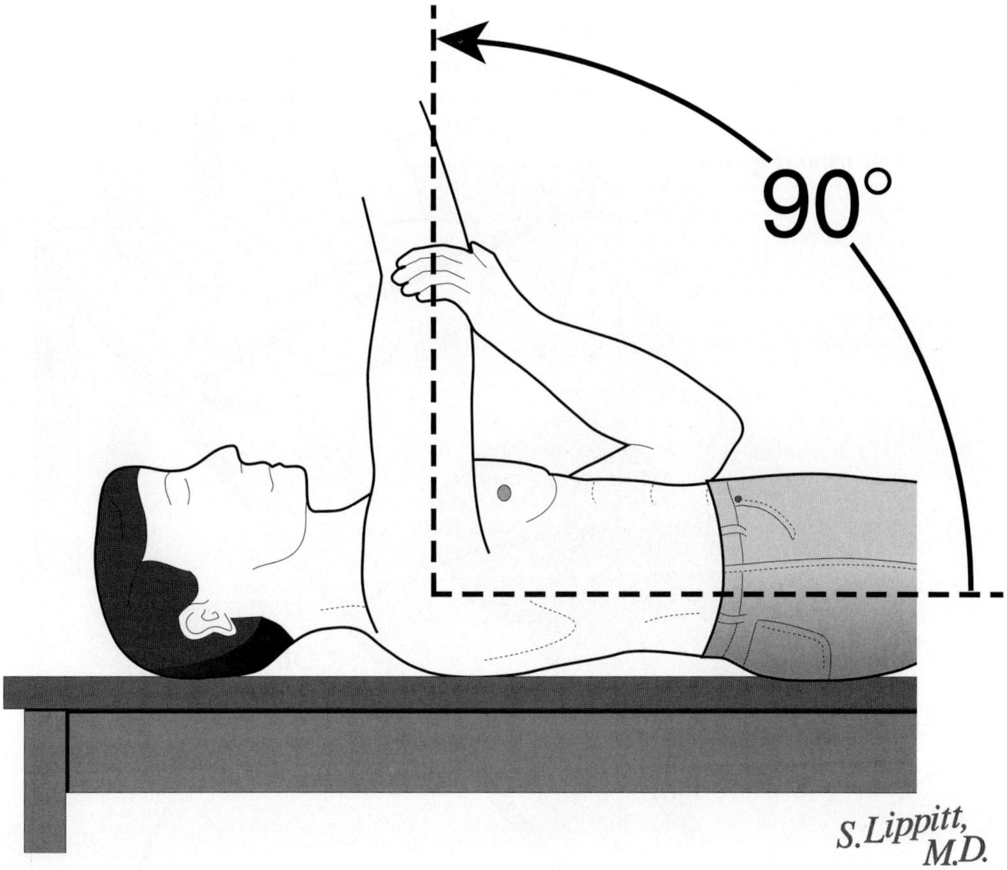


B

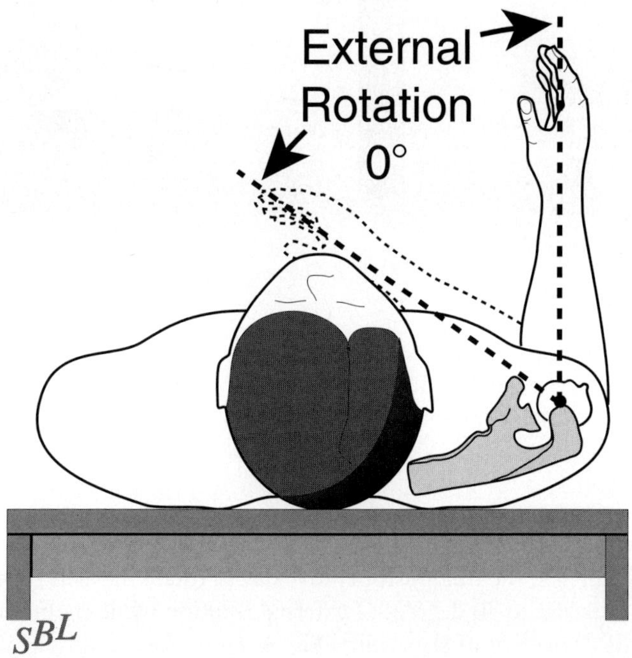


C

**Figure 5–1.** *Continued*

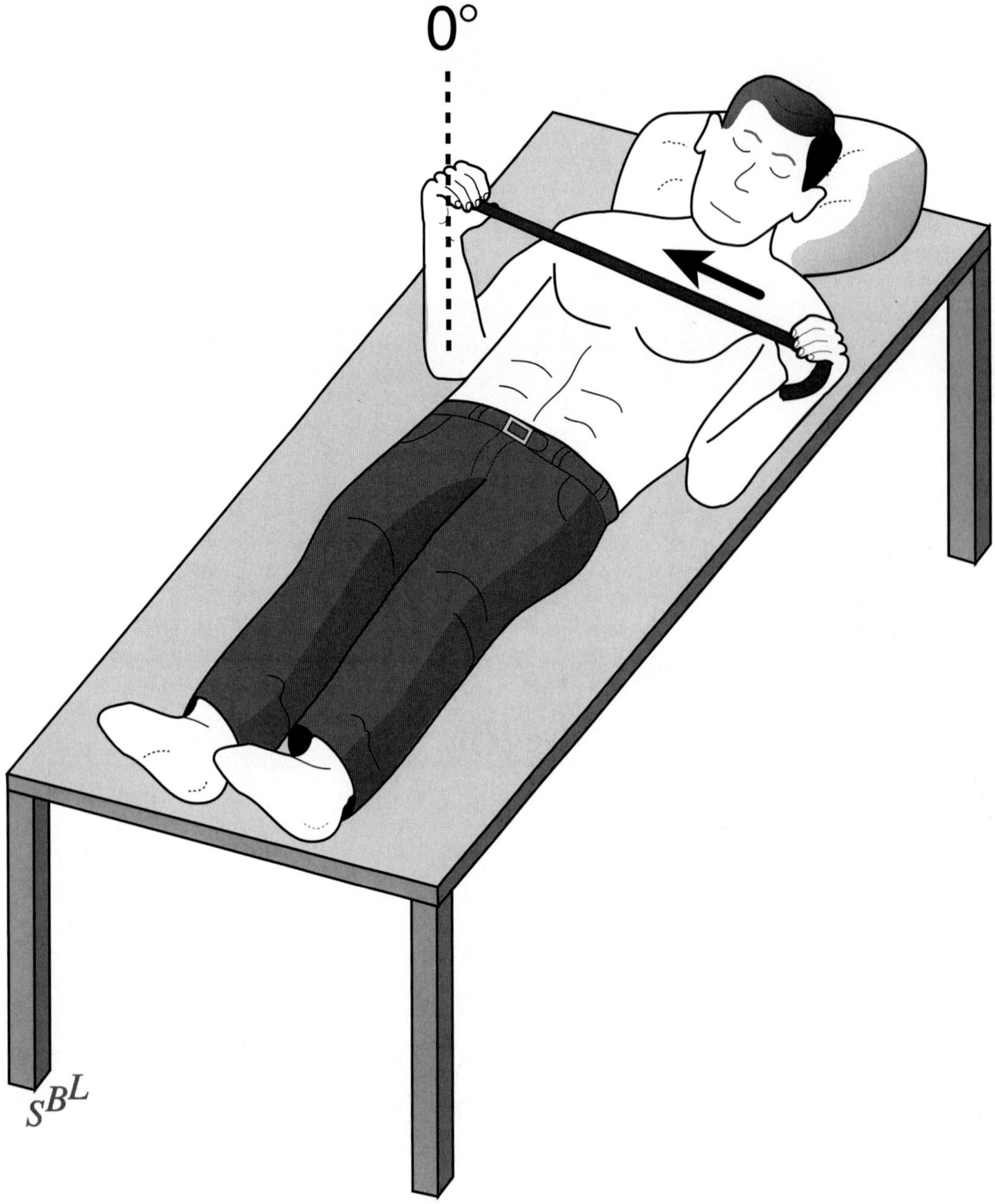


D

**Figure 5–1.** *Continued*

2. *The 0–40–40 active program*: Used after repairs for posterior instability, the patient begins on the first postoperative day to rotate the arm from 40 degrees of internal rotation to 40 degrees of external rotation while maintaining the elbow at the side (0 degrees of elevation) **(Fig. 5–2)**.
3. *The 140–40 active program*: Used after shoulder arthroplasty, the patient begins on the first postoperative day to elevate the arm to 140 degrees and externally rotate it to 40 degrees **(Fig. 5–3)**.

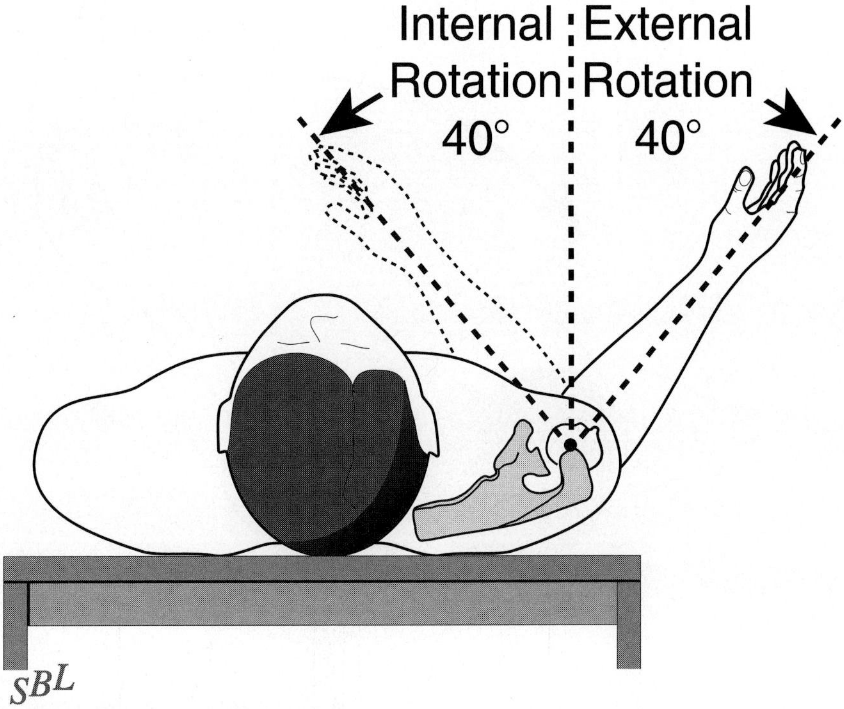


**Figure 5–2. The 0-40-40 program**
We use this program for the first 4 to 6 weeks after a posterior repair. The elbow is kept at the side while the arm is internally and externally rotated by 40 degrees each.

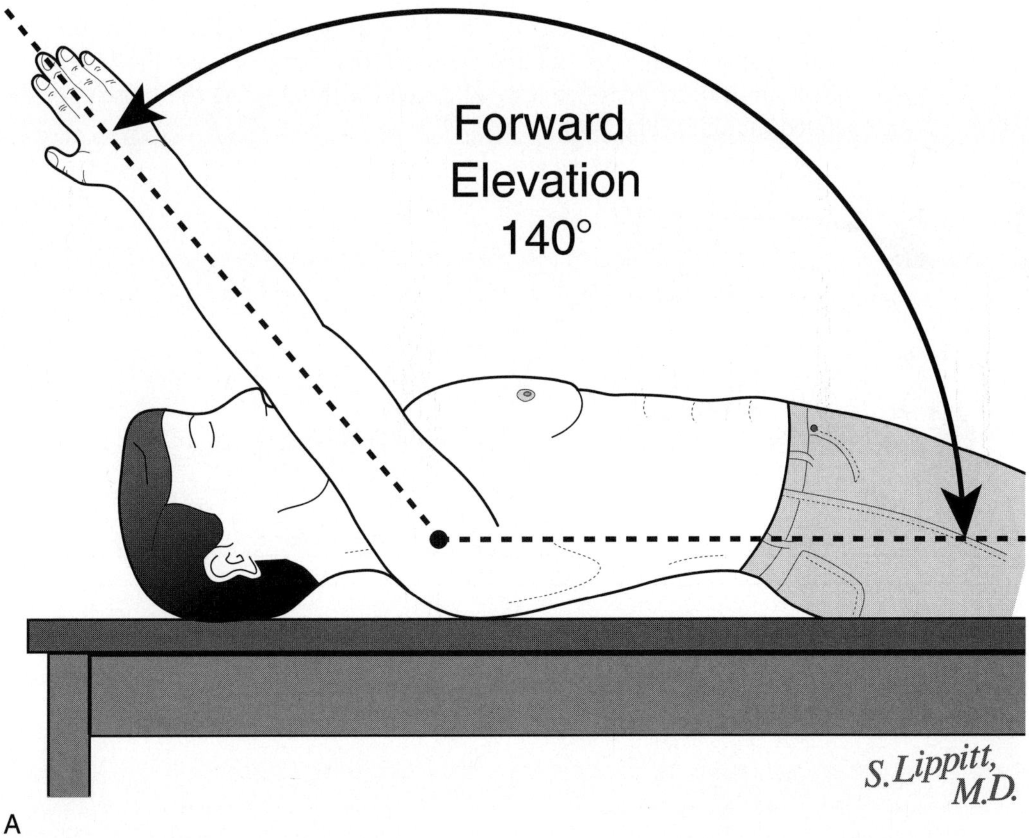


A

**Figure 5–3. The 140-40 active program**
We use this program after shoulder arthroplasty and other procedures in which the rotator cuff is not in need of protection. The patient actively flexes the arm to 140 degrees (**A**) and externally rotates it to 40 degrees (**B**).

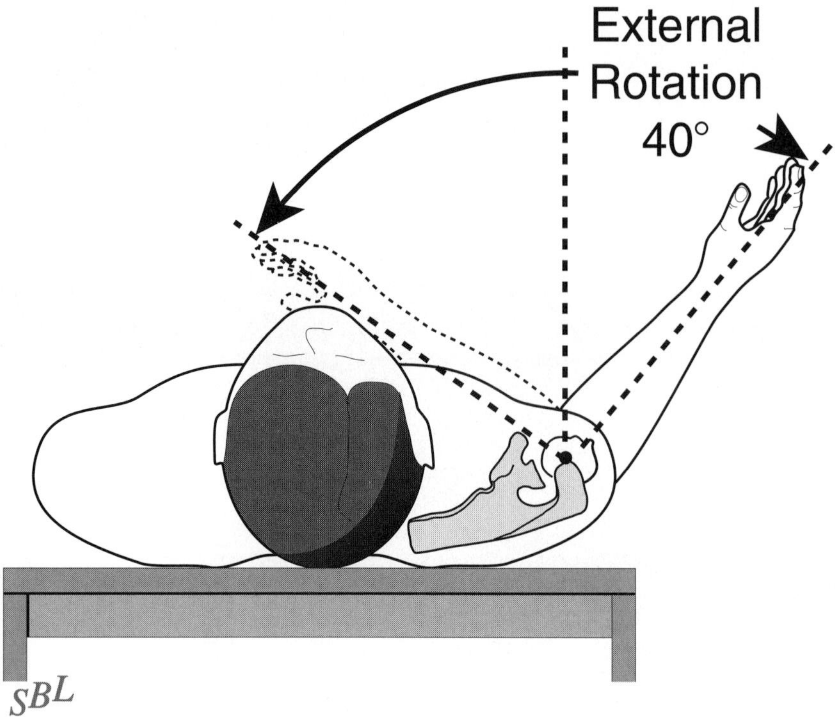


B

**Figure 5–3.** *Continued*

4. *The 140–40 passive program*: Used after rotator cuff repairs and secure fracture fixation, the patient begins on the first postoperative day to elevate the arm to 140 degrees and externally rotate it to 40 degrees without using the muscles of the operated shoulder (**Fig. 5–4**).

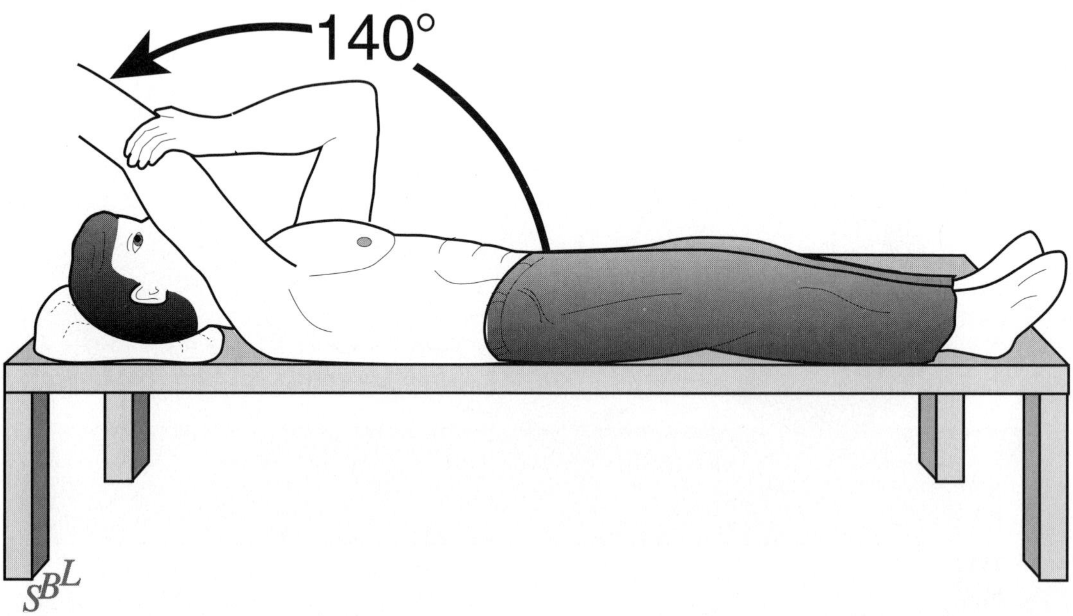


A

**Figure 5–4. The 140-40 passive program**

We use this program after cuff repair in which the rotator cuff is in need of protection. The patient passively flexes the arm to 140 degrees (**A**) and externally rotates it to 40 degrees (**B**). (Modified from Matsen FA, Lippitt SB, Sidles JA, et al [eds]: Practical Evaluation and Management of the Shoulder. Philadelphia: WB Saunders, 1994, p. 47.)

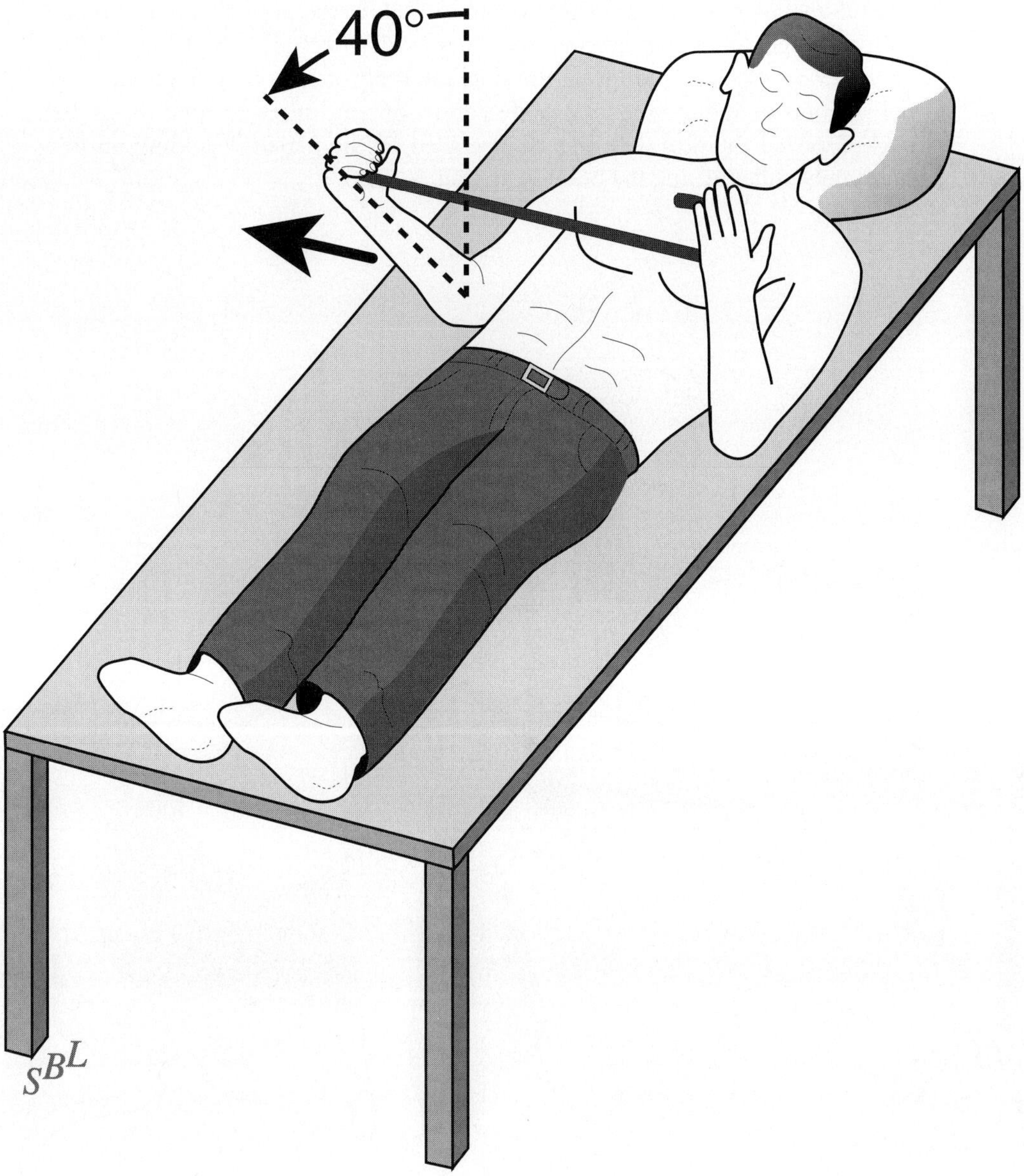


B

**Figure 5–4.** *Continued*

5. *The full-motion program*: Used after open surgical release, smooth and move, and cuff curettage, the patient begins stretching in all directions on the day of surgery: flexion, external motion at the side, external rotation in abduction, internal rotation in abduction, cross-body adduction, and internal rotation up the back. External rotation may also be stretched by the patient's holding on to a doorknob while turning the body away **(Fig. 5–5)**.

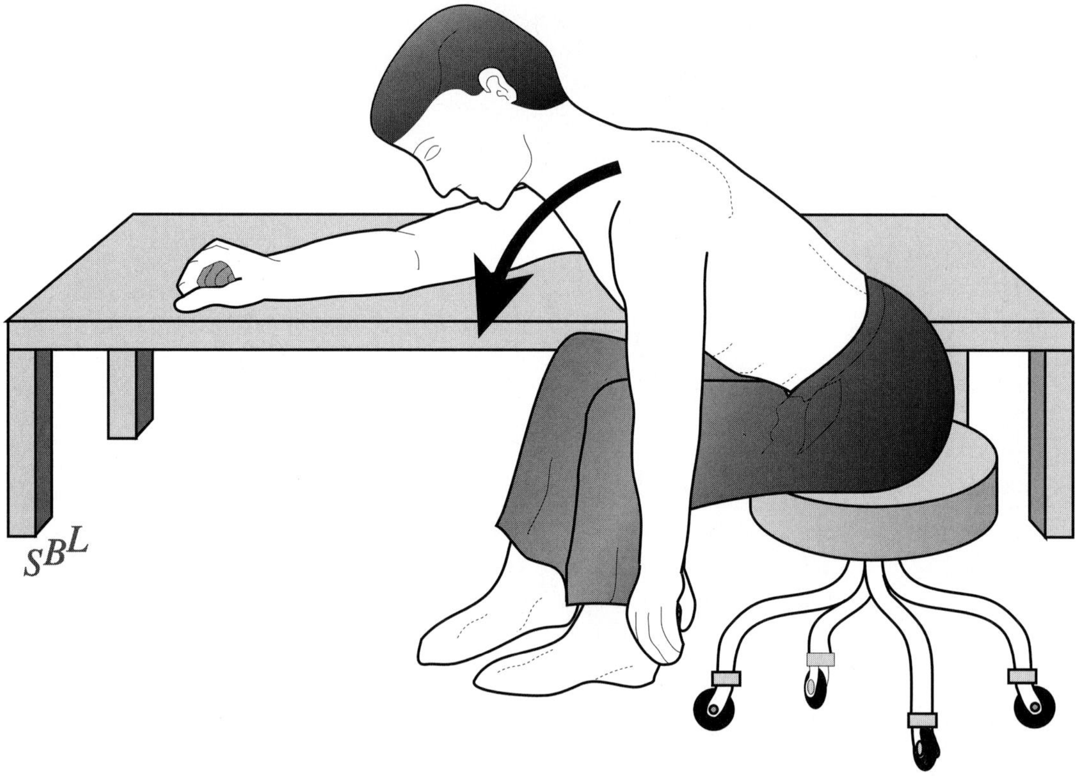


A

**Figure 5–5. The full-motion program**

**A,** The forward lean. We use this exercise to gain the final 30 degrees of forward elevation. The patient places the arm on a table and slides it forward while sliding the stool backward and leaning forward. The stretch is sustained for 1 minute.

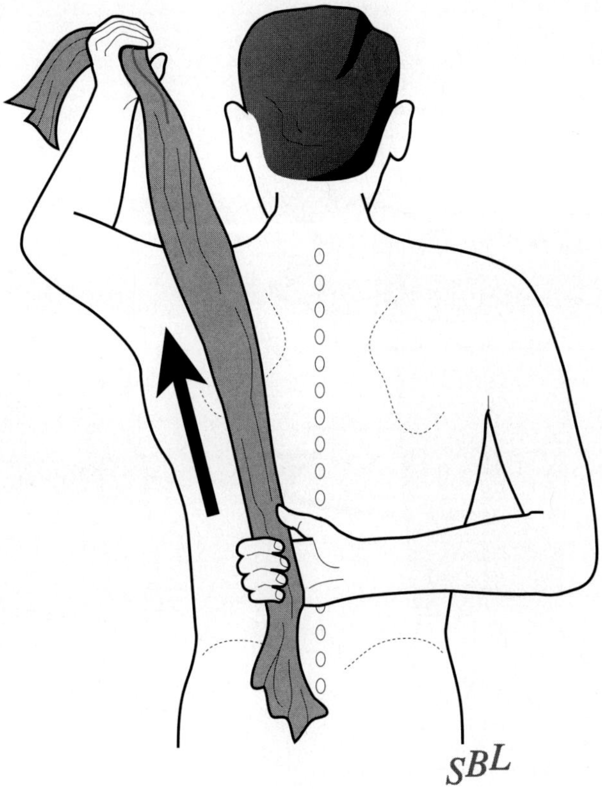


B

**Figure 5–5. The full-motion program—***Continued*
**B,** Internal rotation up the back. We use this exercise to gain reach up the back. The patient's sound arm pulls the affected arm up the back, using a towel.

*Continued*

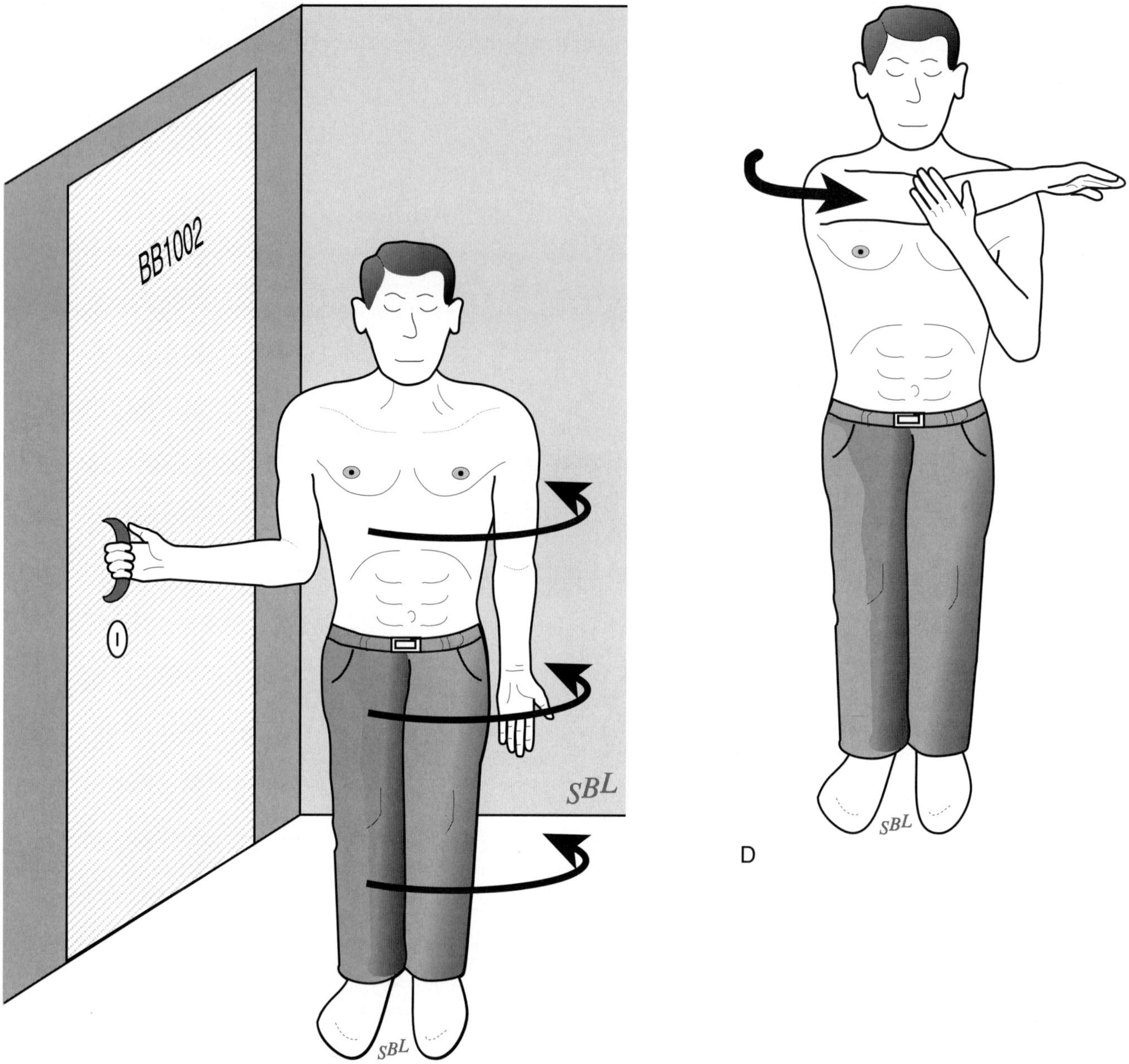


C

**Figure 5–5. The full-motion program**—*Continued*
**C,** External rotation against a fixed object. While holding the elbow at the side and at 90 degrees of flexion, the patient grasps a fixed object such as a doorknob. The patient then turns the body away so that a gentle external rotation stretch is applied to the shoulder. **D,** Cross-body adduction. The posterior capsule can be stretched by adducting the arm across the body. (Modified from Matsen FA, Lippitt SB, Sidles JA, et al [eds]: Practical Evaluation and Management of the Shoulder. Philadelphia: WB Saunders, 1994, p. 49.)

Certain strengthening exercises are useful for shoulder rehabilitation. These include strengthening of the external rotators, the internal rotators, the trapezius, and the forward elevators.

1. *Internal rotator strengthening*: The internal rotators are strengthened by the patient's flexing the elbow to 90 degrees and rotating the humerus toward the body against isometric resistance or the resistance of elastic tubing or weights **(Fig. 5–6)**.

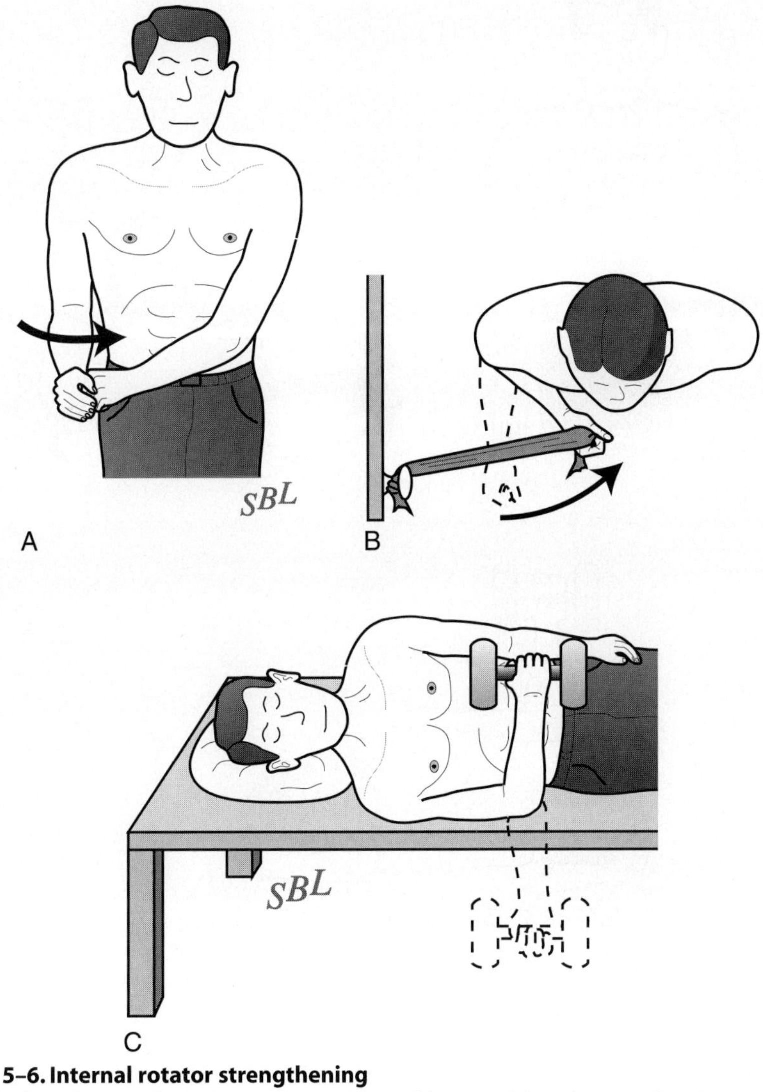


**Figure 5–6. Internal rotator strengthening**

The muscles of internal rotation are strengthened by exercising them against isometric resistance, against elastic tubing, and against weights. (From Matsen FA, Lippitt SB, Sidles JA, et al [eds]: Practical Evaluation and Management of the Shoulder. Philadelphia: WB Saunders, 1994, p. 86.)

2. *External rotator strengthening*: The external rotators are strengthened by the patient's flexing the elbow to 90 degrees and rotating the humerus away from the body against isometric resistance or the resistance of elastic tubing or weights **(Fig. 5–7)**.

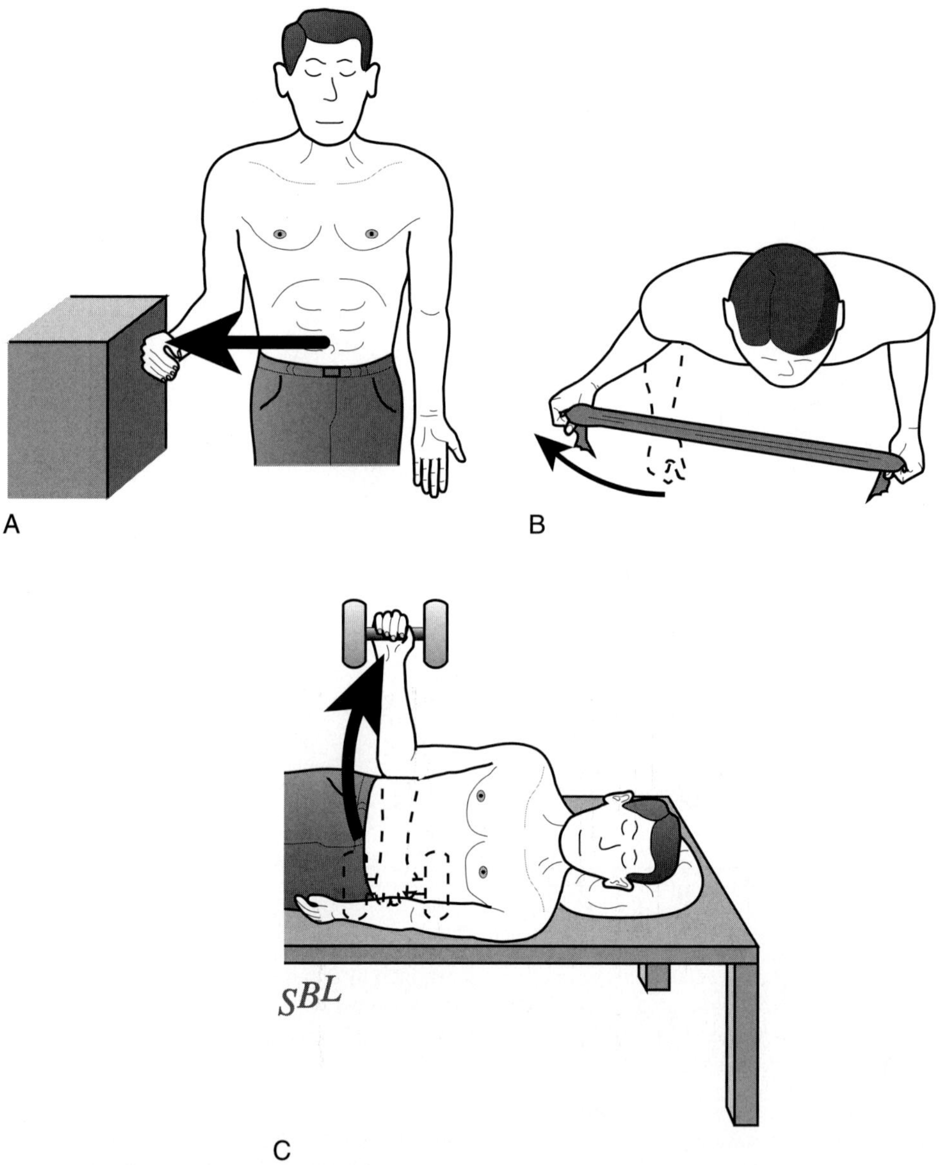


**Figure 5–7. External rotator strengthening**
The muscles of external rotation are strengthened by exercising them against isometric resistance, against elastic tubing, and against weights. (From Matsen FA, Lippitt SB, Sidles JA, et al [eds]: Practical Evaluation and Management of the Shoulder. Philadelphia: WB Saunders, 1994, p. 86.)

3. *Trapezius strengthening*: The trapezius is strengthened by the patient's shrugging the shoulder upward while holding a weight in the hand **(Fig. 5–8)**.

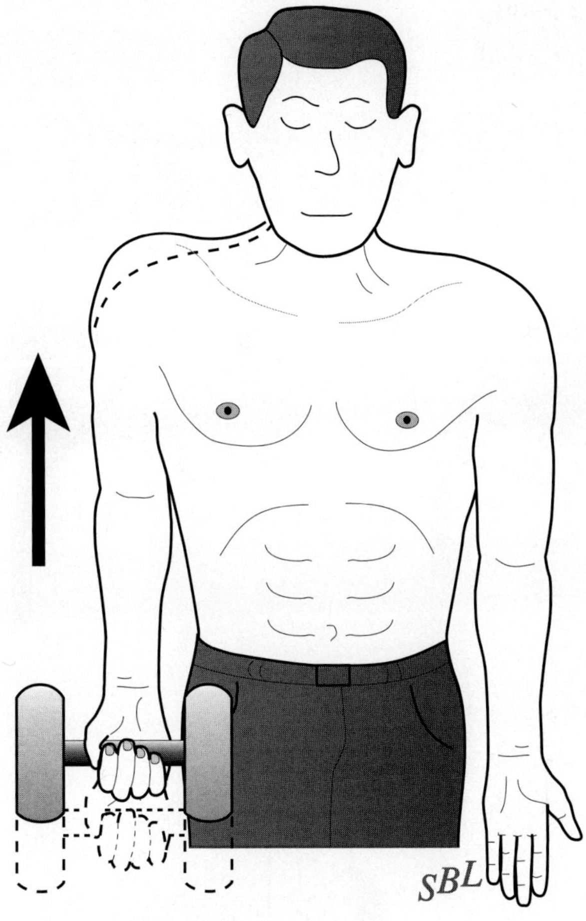


**Figure 5–8. Trapezius strengthening**
The trapezius is strengthened by the patient's shrugging the shoulders upward while a weight is held in the hand. (From Matsen FA, Lippitt SB, Sidles JA, et al [eds]: Practical Evaluation and Management of the Shoulder. Philadelphia: WB Saunders, 1994, p. 87.)

4. *Flexion strengthening*: The progressive tilting supine press is a key exercise for building the integrated strength of forward elevation (**Fig. 5–9**). In the first phase, the patient lies supine with the hands close together on a towel or a light stick. Both hands are pressed up toward the ceiling, finishing by protraction of the scapula off the table. In phase two, the hands are progressively separated, allowing them to act more independently. In phase three, one hand presses alone. In phase four, weight is added to the hand in small increments until the weight totals 2 pounds. In phase five, the back of the table (or lawn chair or recliner) is progressively raised until the patient is in the sitting position. Each phase is continued until 20 repetitions can be performed easily before the patient advances to the next phase. At the end of each press, the scapula is always protracted (**Fig. 5–10**).

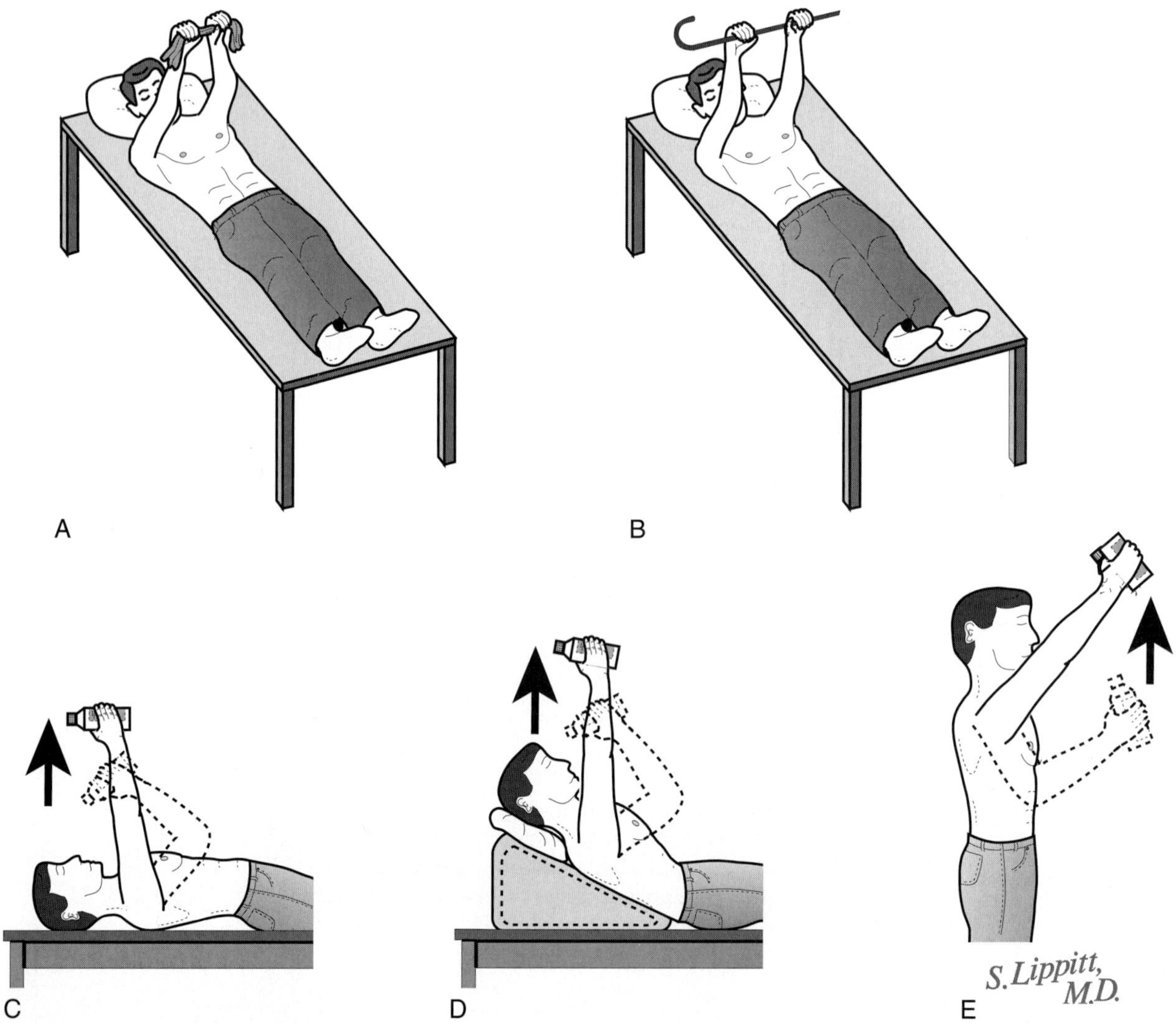


**Figure 5–9. The progressive tilting supine press**
Integrated forward elevation is developed by a series of exercises that can be progressed in small increments. First, two hands are placed close to each other on a towel or a light stick and both hands are pressed upward toward the ceiling while the patient is in the supine position (**A**). Next, the same exercise is repeated with the arms progressively farther apart (**B**). Next, the arm does the supine press unassisted. Next, small amounts of weight are added to the hand until 2 pounds can be pressed upward for 20 times (**C**). Then the patient's back is elevated slightly while the weight is pressed vertically upward (**D**). The amount of elevation is increased when 2 pounds can be pressed upward 20 times. The progression is continued until the exercise can be performed with the back in a vertical position (**E**). (Modified from Matsen FA, Lippitt SB, Sidles JA, et al [eds]: Practical Evaluation and Management of the Shoulder. Philadelphia: WB Saunders, 1994, p. 131.)

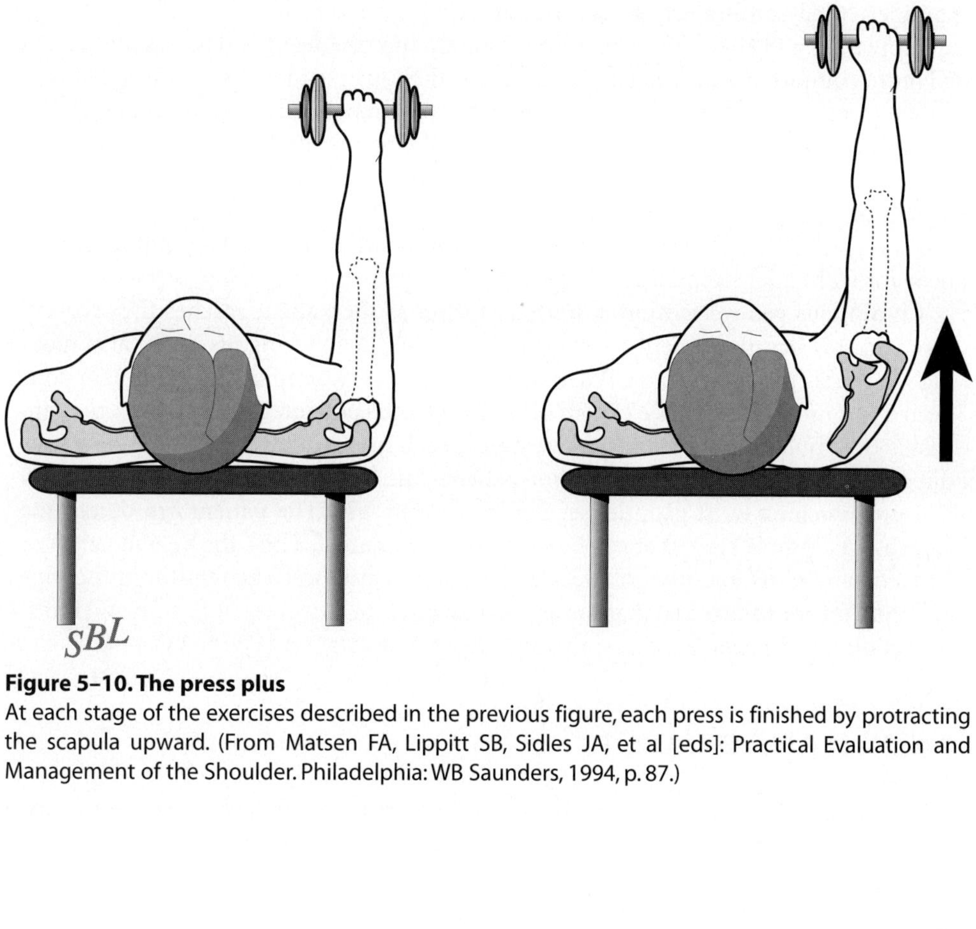


**Figure 5–10. The press plus**
At each stage of the exercises described in the previous figure, each press is finished by protracting the scapula upward. (From Matsen FA, Lippitt SB, Sidles JA, et al [eds]: Practical Evaluation and Management of the Shoulder. Philadelphia: WB Saunders, 1994, p. 87.)

## CONTINUOUS PASSIVE MOTION

Our understanding of the body's response to injury is that multipotential stem cells activated at the surgical site begin immediately after surgery to differentiate into fibroblasts, serosal cells, chondroblasts, or osteoblasts. Furthermore, one of the most important influences over this differentiation is the mechanical environment at the site of repair. Thus, it is important that we create the optimal environment for the desired differentiation immediately after the surgery. For many procedures, the optimal mechanical environment is one in which the humeroscapular motion interface is moved, preventing scar from bridging from the proximal humerus to the overlying deltoid, coraco-acromial arch, and coracoid muscles. It seems that if motion at this interface is delayed, even for a day, the establishment of full, smooth motion is more difficult for the patient. On the other hand, if motion is instituted immediately and continued for the first 36 hours after surgery, it is rarely lost. For these reasons, we have routinely used continuous passive motion (CPM) for the first day and a half after arthroplasties and after cuff surgery. Interestingly, most patients find their shoulders to be more comfortable during CPM than when their arm is in a sling. This is particularly the case for rotator cuff repairs, after which the repaired cuff tendons are relaxed by flexion and external rotation (in contrast to being put under tension by the sling position of adduction and internal rotation). It is also of interest that the incremental benefit of CPM seems to taper off after the first 36 hours, by which time the patient can conduct his or her own motion program unassisted. Thus, we have not found the need for CPM after hospital discharge.

Continuous passive motion is started as soon as the patient reaches the recovery room. In this way, the patient recovers from the anesthetic seeing his or her arm moving—a reassuring sight. The CPM unit we use is a very simple adjustable cam connected to a motor that can be turned off and on by the patient. The rope from the cam passes over pulleys on a standard overhead bed frame so that a vertical pull results directly over the shoulder of the supine patient. The rope is connected to the hand by a Velcro-fastening wrist gauntlet secured by a safety pin. The patient can detach the rope using a simple clasp that can be operated one-handed. Thus, the patient can start and stop and hook and unhook the CPM without assistance. The tension in the rope and the cam are adjusted so that the arm is moved from 0 degrees of flexion and internal rotation to 90 degrees of flexion and 0 degrees of rotation (**Fig. 5–11**).

## PAIN MANAGEMENT

It is essential that patients know preoperatively that shoulder surgery hurts for the first 36 hours afterward. The knowledge that pain is expected helps them "steel" themselves for this period. In patients who have not used significant amounts of pain medications or alcohol before surgery, problems with discomfort and the need for narcotic medications are rare after the first week. Patients who are taking substantial narcotics at the time they present for surgery can expect to have more of a challenge with postoperative comfort. In these situations, we ask patients preoperatively to make arrangements with their primary care physician or another practitioner for their pain management, and we delegate this responsibility after the first 2 weeks.

We often perform shoulder surgery under a brachial plexus block anesthetic. This provides excellent surgical anesthesia that often lasts for 8 to 12 hours after surgery. It is critical, however, to warn patients that as the block wears off, the shoulder may become suddenly painful. The block usually wears off from the lower to the upper aspect of the plexus. Thus, we suggest that as soon as patients can actively move their fingers, they should begin taking oral pain medication, working to stay ahead of the pain. Often we use patient-controlled analgesia because, once again, it gives the patient

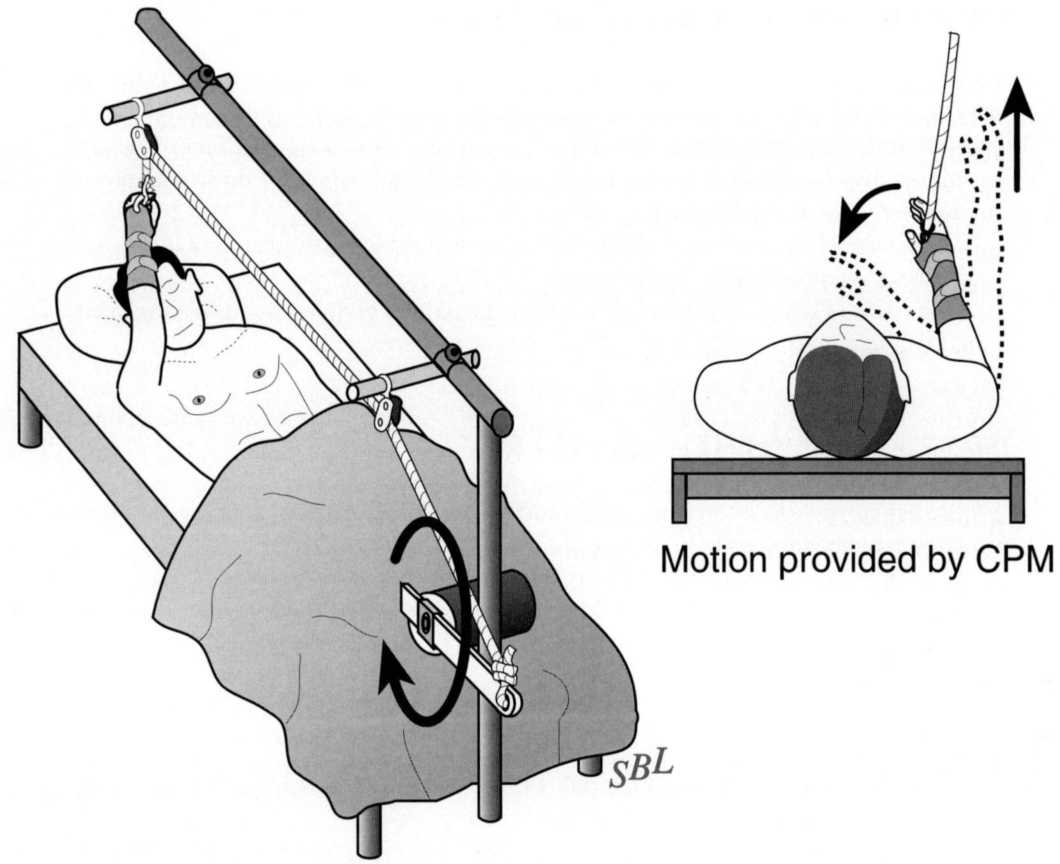


**Figure 5–11. Continuous passive motion**

Continuous passive motion (CPM) is used after most surgeries other than glenohumeral arthrodesis and instability repairs. The motion desired is from internal rotation with the arm on the abdomen and the elbow at the side to neutral rotation with the arm in 90 degrees of elevation. Cycle time is slow to allow the muscles the chance to relax. The CPM is initiated in the recovery room immediately after surgery. (From Matsen FA, Lippitt SB, Sidles JA, et al [eds]: Practical Evaluation and Management of the Shoulder. Philadelphia: WB Saunders, 1994, p. 50.)

control over his or her situation. It is believed that patients use less narcotics when they know it is immediately available to them.

The advent of injectable nonsteroidal anti-inflammatory medications offers an adjunct to postoperative pain management. These can be helpful after arthroplasty or smooth-and-move procedures. We avoid them in cases involving a healing risk, such as cuff repairs and fracture fixation as well as in elderly individuals or those with bleeding tendencies or renal dysfunction.

We have avoided the use of catheters left in the wound for the infusion of local anesthetics because of the risk of infection.

At the time of discharge, our goal is to have the patient taking only simple oral analgesics and to eliminate narcotics by 2 weeks after surgery.

## TUBES AND OTHER DEVICES

Sequential compression devices and thromboembolic prevention stockings are used until the patient is fully and actively ambulatory.

Wound drains are generally removed after 36 hours.

The intravenous line is removed after 36 hours of perioperative antibiotics have been administered and after it is determined that there is no need for transfusion of blood products.

# PART II

# MOBILITY

CHAPTER 6

# Principles of Glenohumeral Mobility

## CONCEPTS

The evaluation and management of the stiff shoulder requires understanding of motion and laxity. We will begin with some definitions.

### Glenohumeral Translation and Rotation

The *translational laxity* of the glenohumeral joint in a specified direction is the distance the humeral head can be translated from an initial position centered in the glenoid socket **(Fig. 6–1)**. The translational laxity is determined by (1) the length of the capsule and ligaments constraining the translation and (2) the position and orientation of the humeral head at the start of the translation. At one extreme, if the ligament is already under tension when the translation is attempted, no further translation is possible in the direction limited by the ligament. On the other hand, if the shoulder is positioned so that the ligament has slack, translation should be possible. The translational laxity of the normal shoulder is normally greater than 1 centimeter in all directions when the glenohumeral joint is in mid-range positions. This translation is both normal and essential to the mobility of the glenohumeral joint.

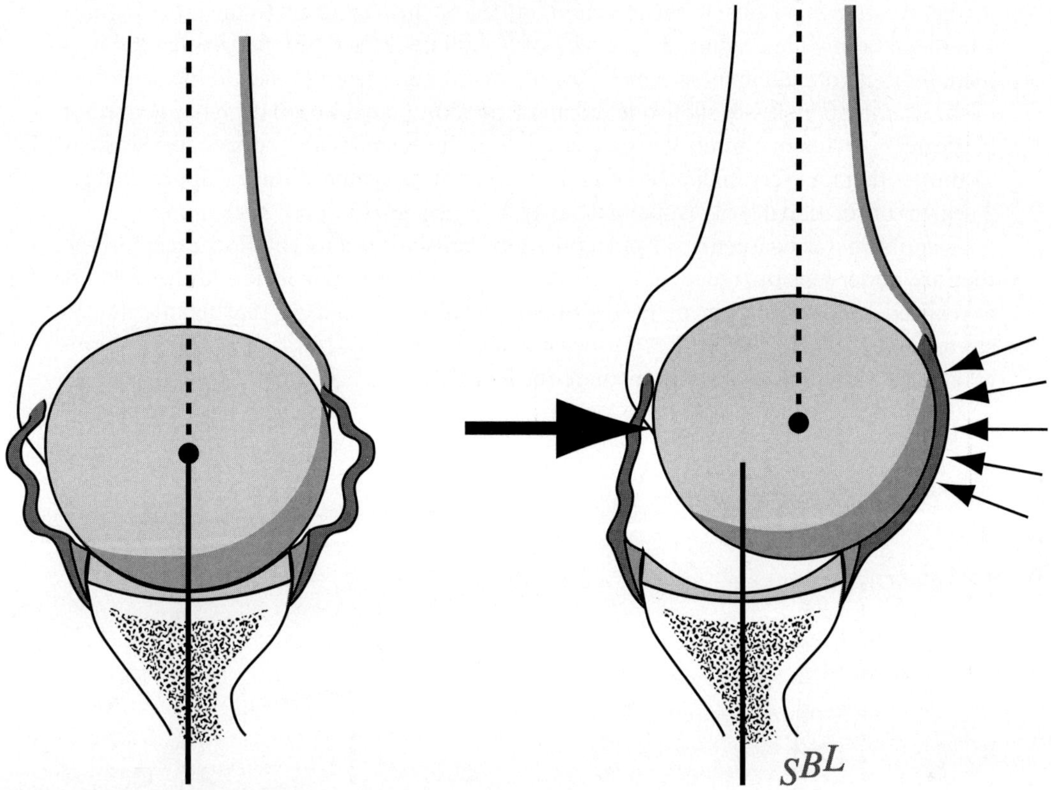


**Figure 6–1. Translational laxity**

The translational laxity is the distance the humeral head can be moved in a specified direction from its centered position in the glenoid. The translational laxity is affected by the starting position and orientation of the humerus. (Modified from Rockwood CA, Matsen FA [eds]: The Shoulder, 2nd ed. Philadelphia: WB Saunders, 1998, p. 631.)

The *rotational laxity* of the glenohumeral joint in a specified direction is the angle through which the humeral head can be rotated from an initial position centered in the glenoid socket **(Fig. 6–2)**. The rotational laxity is determined by (1) the length of the capsule and ligaments constraining the rotation, (2) the position and orientation of the humeral head at the start of the rotation, and (3) the radius of curvature of the humeral head. At one extreme, if the ligament is already under tension when the rotation is attempted, no further rotation is possible in the direction limited by the ligament. On the other hand, if a humeral head with a radius of curvature of R millimeters is positioned so that the ligament limiting rotation in the specified direction has R millimeters of slack at the beginning of the examination, it will allow one radian of rotation (equal to 360 degrees / $(2 \times \pi)$ or 57 degrees. A rule of thumb for an average-sized humeral head (radius approximately 25 mm) is that for every millimeter of slack of the limiting ligament, there is approximately 2 degrees of rotational laxity (rotational laxity $\cong$ 57 degrees/25 mm $\times$ slack in mm).

Glenohumeral ligaments do not constrain translation and rotation except when they are under tension. Once the ligaments come under tension, little additional laxity is realized by deformation of the ligament (a rule of thumb is that ligaments can stretch only 10% beyond their resting length). Many important shoulder functions take place in the range of motion where the ligaments are lax.

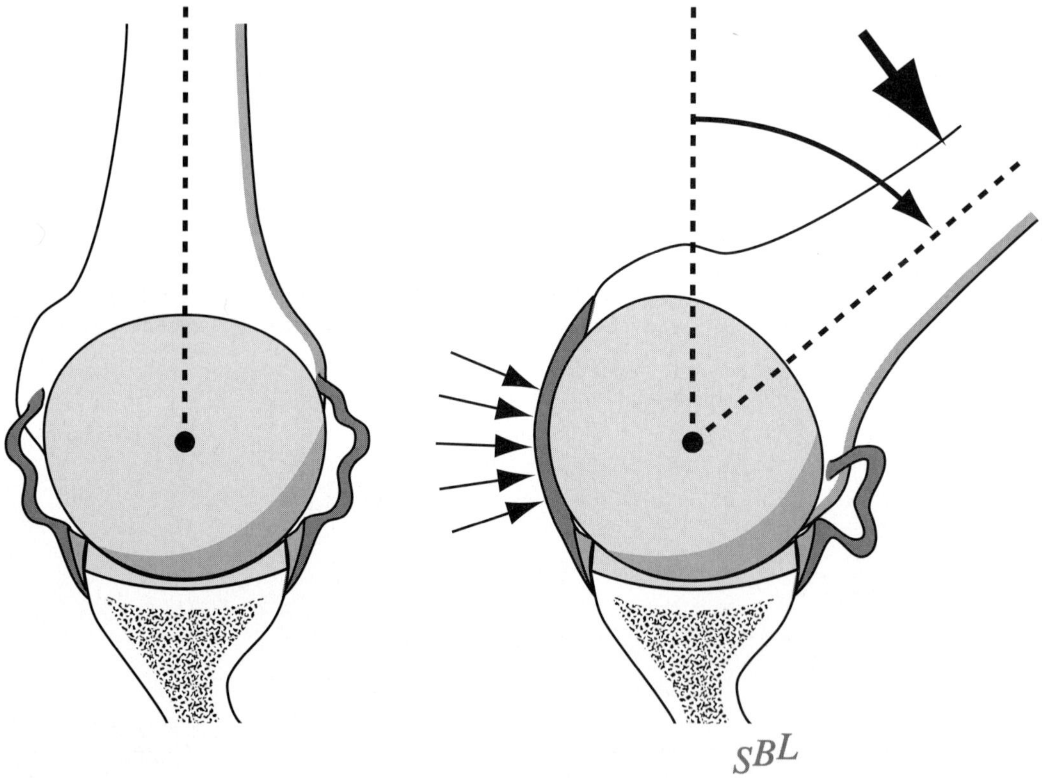


A

**Figure 6–2. Rotational laxity**

**A,** Rotational laxity. The rotational laxity is the angle the humeral head can be rotated in a specified direction from a specified starting position while remaining centered in the glenoid. The rotational laxity is affected by the starting position and orientation of the humerus. (Modified from Rockwood CA, Matsen FA [eds]: The Shoulder, 2nd ed. Philadelphia: WB Saunders, 1998, p. 632.)

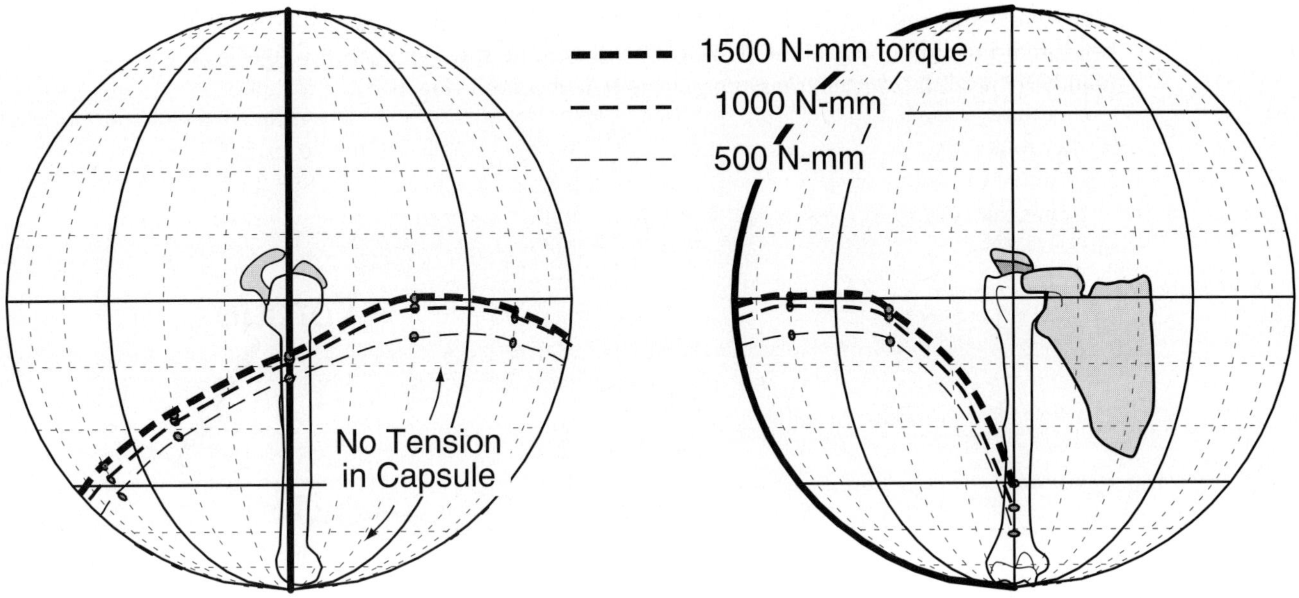


B

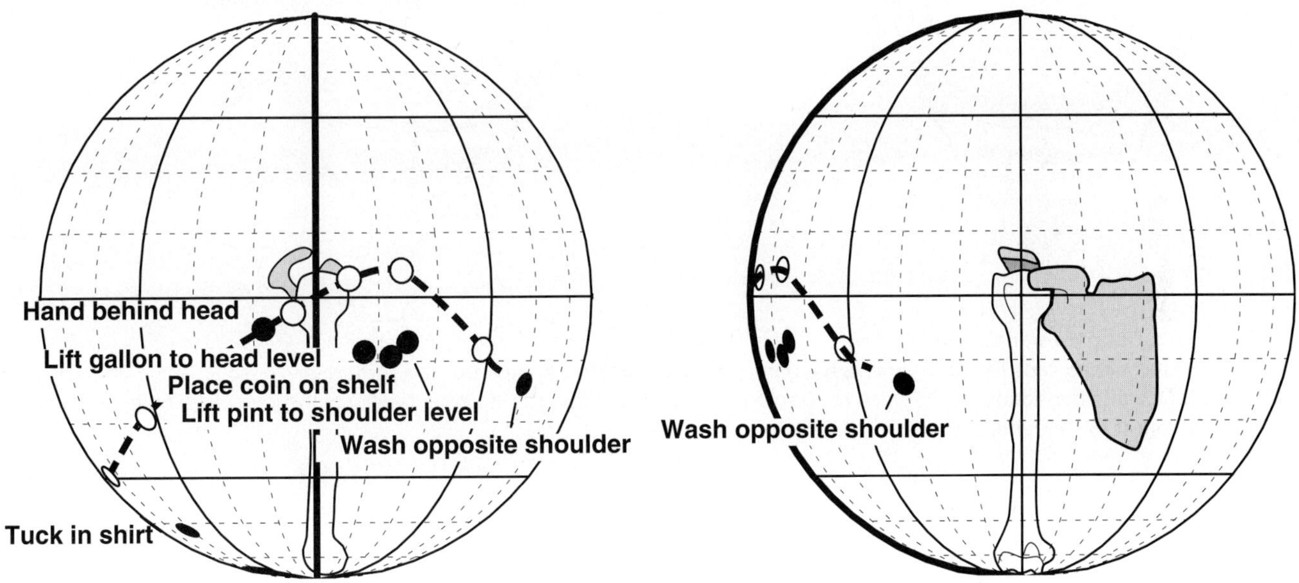


C

**Figure 6–2. Rotational laxity—***Continued*
**B,** Tension-free zone. This diagram shows the torque that has to be applied to the glenohumeral joint to achieve different glenohumeral positions. It is a global representation centered on the center of glenohumeral rotation and oriented with respect to the plane of the scapula. It shows that the great preponderance of glenohumeral motion is in the zone where there is no tension in the glenohumeral capsule and ligaments. (From Matsen FA, Lippitt SB, Sidles JA, et al [eds]: Practical Evaluation and Management of the Shoulder. Philadelphia: WB Saunders, 1994, p 75.) **C,** Activities of daily living. This global diagram shows that the preponderance of shoulder functions are performed in positions in which there is minimal tension in the glenohumeral ligaments and capsule. (From Matsen FA, Lippitt SB, Sidles JA, et al [eds]: Practical Evaluation and Management of the Shoulder. Philadelphia: WB Saunders, 1994, p. 32.)

At the extreme of rotation when a ligament comes under tension, the force exerted by the ligament can be resolved into (1) a compressive component parallel to the glenoid center line and (2) an orthogonal displacing component forcing the humeral head in a direction opposite the tight ligament. Forcing rotation against a tight ligament may result in *obligate translation* of the humeral head **(Fig. 6–3)**.

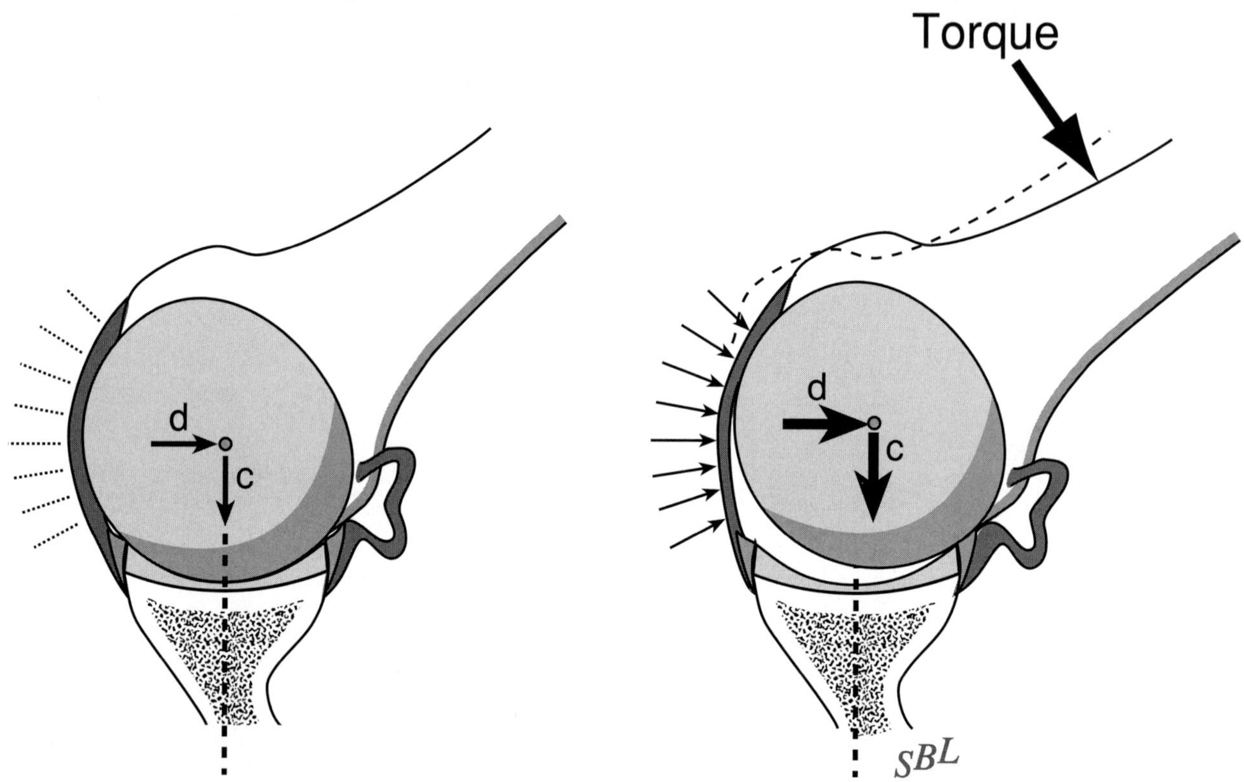


**Figure 6–3. Obligate translation**
Once the restraining capsule and ligaments are tight, forcing further rotation produces a compressive load (c) and a displacing force (d). Obligate translation results when the displacing force overcomes the intrinsic stability of the joint. Such obligate translation occurs at the extreme of rotation in normal glenohumeral joints.

Ligaments can become functionally shortened in conditions such as idiopathic frozen shoulder, diabetes, and post-traumatic adhesions and after surgical procedures, such as capsulorrhaphy for shoulder instability. When ligaments become shortened, they can limit the range of glenohumeral rotation and translation (**Fig. 6–4**). Exerting a large torque against strong, tight ligaments can result in a major compressive force at

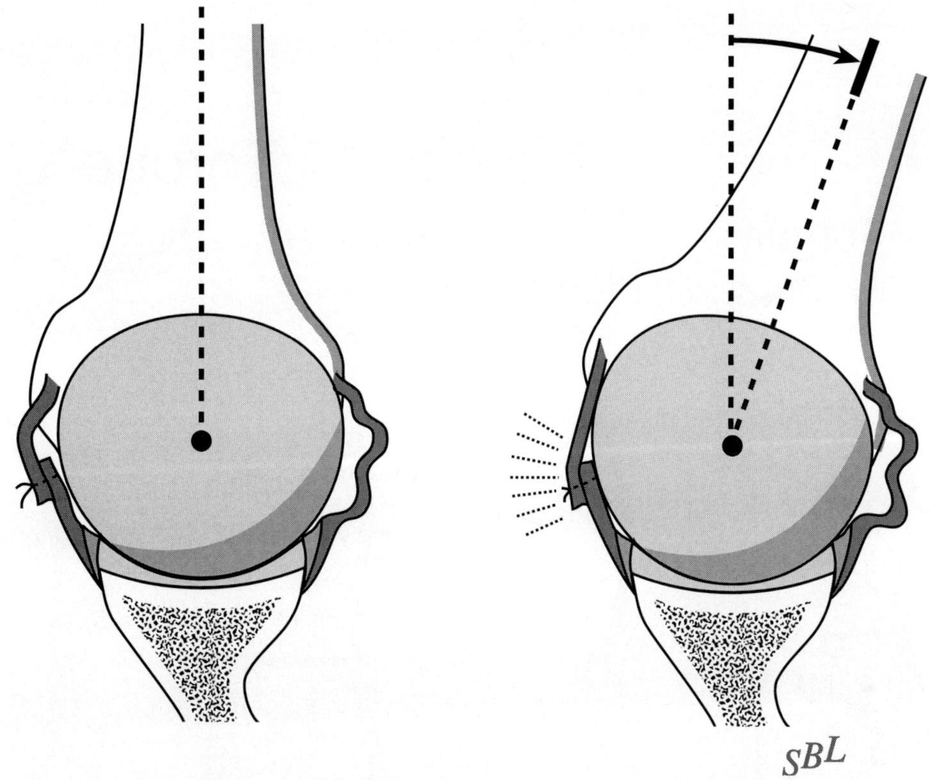

**Figure 6–4. Ligament shortening limits rotation**
If the capsule and ligaments on one side of the joint are shortened, they limit the rotation of the humerus in the direction opposite the tight structures.

the glenohumeral joint, which could damage the joint surface or underlying bone (**Fig. 6–5**). A large torque can also produce a significant amount of obligate translation of the humeral head on the glenoid, potentially damaging the glenoid rim (**Fig. 6–6**). A small force applied a distance away from the joint can produce such a large torque (**Fig. 6–7**). These factors are particularly relevant when vigorous physical therapy or manipulations under anesthesia are used in the management of stiff shoulders. The progressive loss of the labrum, then the articular cartilage, and even the bone of the glenoid lip from obligate translation may result in the condition known as *capsulorrhaphy arthropathy.*

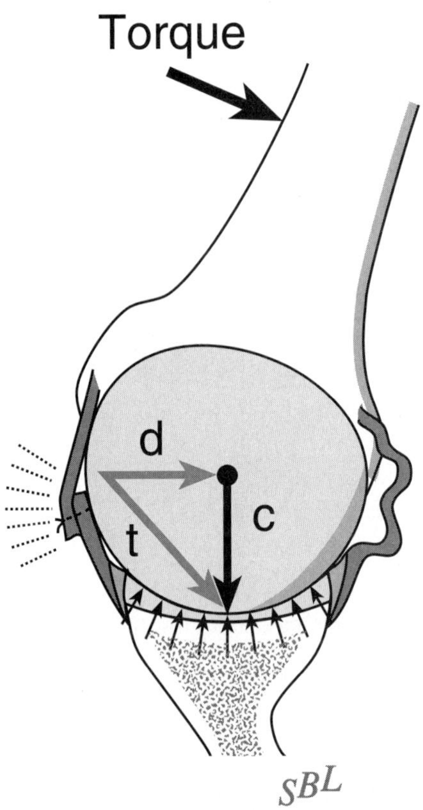


**Figure 6–5. Ligament shortening can cause increased joint pressure**
If the capsule and ligaments on one side of the joint are shortened, applying torque against them may increase the compressive load (c) applied to the joint surface. This increased joint pressure may damage the joint surface.

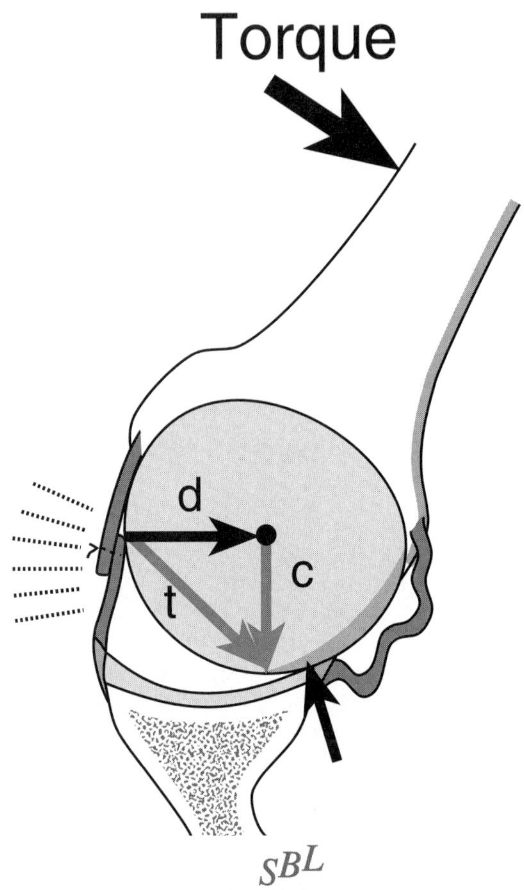


**Figure 6–6. Ligament shortening can cause premature obligate translation**
If the capsule and ligaments on one side of the joint are shortened, applying torque against them may cause obligate translation to occur in functional positions of the joint. This translation may compromise the lip of the joint (*arrow*), destabilizing the joint in the direction opposite the tight structures.

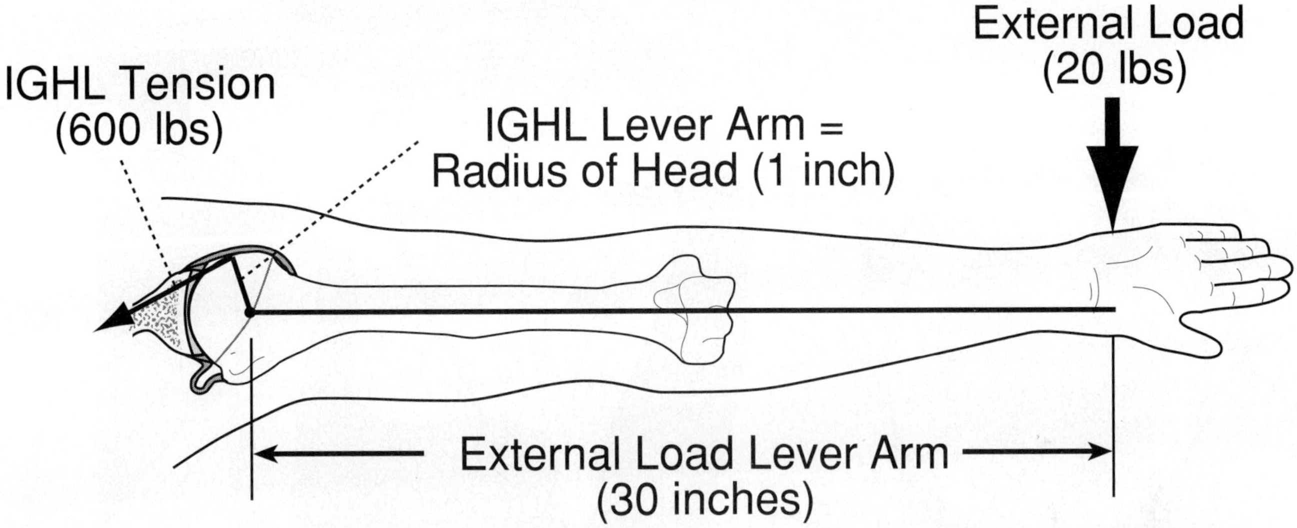


**Figure 6–7. Leverage**
The glenohumeral ligaments must work through a short moment arm equal to the radius of the humeral head (R). A force exerted at the end of the arm has a very long moment arm (E). As a result, the tension in the restraining ligaments (T) is magnified by the ratio of E/R. In this example, the tension in the inferior glenohumeral ligament (IGHL) is equal to the external load (B) multiplied by E/R. If the distance from the center of the humeral head to the point of application of the force is 40 inches and the radius of the head is 1 inch, the tension in the IGHL is 40 times the applied force. (Modified from Matsen FA, Lippitt SB, Sidles JA, et al [eds]: Practical Evaluation and Management of the Shoulder. Philadelphia: WB Saunders, 1994, p. 97.)

## Humeroscapular Motion

It is apparent that for every degree of rotation taking place at the glenohumeral joint, an equal amount of rotation must also take place at the articulation known as the *humeroscapular motion interface* (**Figs. 6–8** and **6–9**). Anatomically, this articular interface has a proximal humeral convexity—the rotator cuff, long head tendon of the biceps, and proximal humerus—and a coracoacromial concavity—the deltoid, acromion, coracoacromial ligament, coracoid, and coracoid muscles. The center of the glenoid concavity, the center of the coracoacromial concavity, the center of the proximal humeral concavity, and the center of the humeral head are superimposed in normal shoulder movement (**Fig. 6–10**).

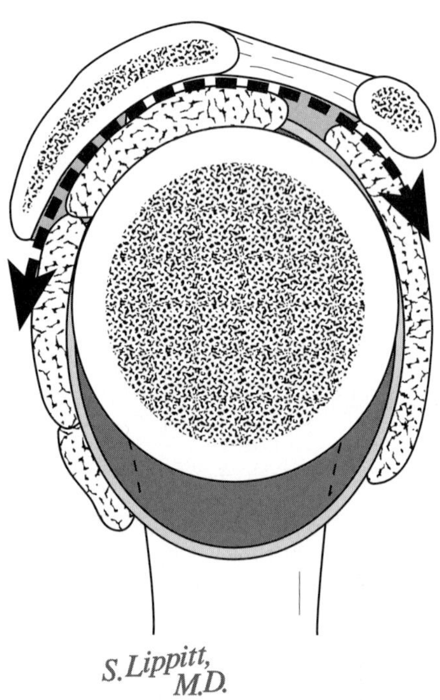


**Figure 6–8. The humeroscapular motion interface beneath the coracoacromial arch**
The external surface of the rotator cuff articulates with the undersurface of the coracoacromial arch. This articulation is part of the humeroscapular motion interface. Smooth, unrestrained movement at this interface is required for normal shoulder function. (From Rockwood CA, Matsen FA [eds]: The Shoulder, 2nd ed. Philadelphia: WB Saunders, 1998, p. 618.)

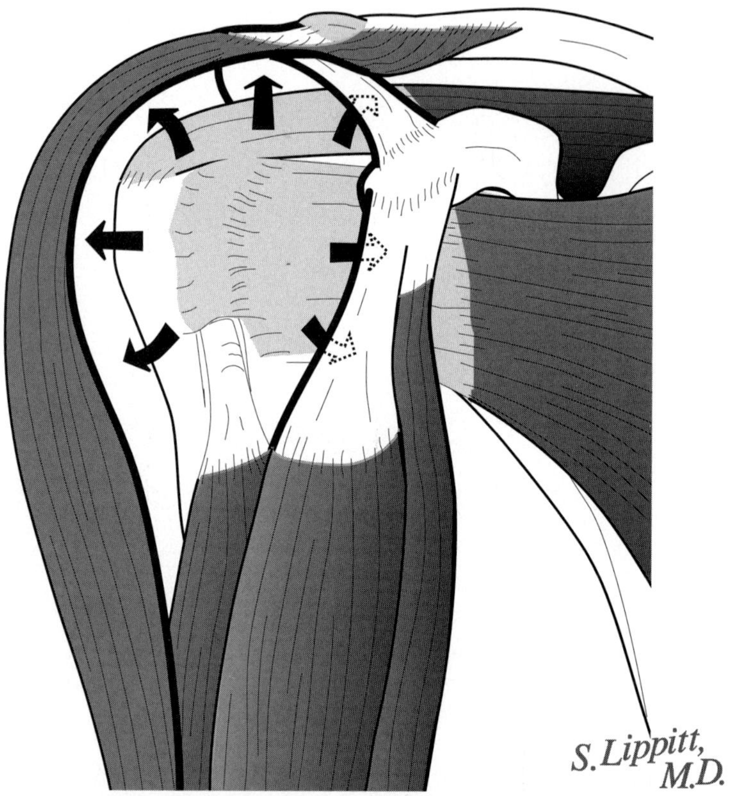


**Figure 6–9. The humeroscapular motion interface**
The humeroscapular motion interface is the set of gliding surfaces between the proximal humerus covered by the rotator cuff tendons on one hand and the overlying structures attached to the scapula, including the deltoid, the acromion, the coracoacromial ligament, the coracoid, and the tendons of the coracoid muscles on the other. Approximately 4 cm of motion takes place at this interface during normal shoulder movement. (From Matsen FA, Lippitt SB, Sidles JA, et al [eds]: Practical Evaluation and Management of the Shoulder. Philadelphia: WB Saunders, 1994, p. 34.)

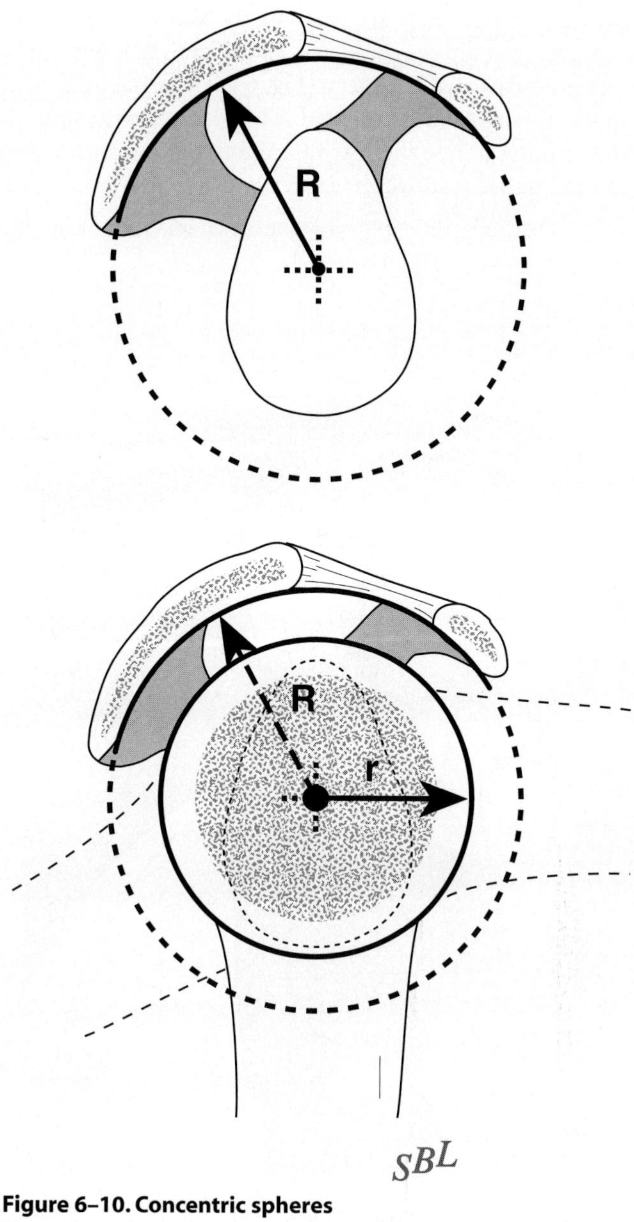


**Figure 6–10. Concentric spheres**

The spherical proximal humeral convexity is formed by the tuberosities and the superficial surface of the rotator cuff tendons. It has a radius of *R* and articulates with the undersurface of the coracoacromial arch. The spherical humeral articular surface has a radius of *r* and articulates with the glenoid. The difference between these two radii is made up by the height of the tuberosities and the thickness of the cuff tendons. The centers of these two spheres and the concavities with which they articulate must be superimposed in normal shoulder function. These two mating spheres enable the shoulder to have both great mobility and stability. (Modified from Rockwood CA, Matsen FA [eds]: The Shoulder, 2nd ed. Philadelphia: WB Saunders, 1998, p. 764.)

Limited range of motion can be caused by capsular contracture and adhesions in the humeroscapular motion interface (**Fig. 6–11**). Spot welds or scarring across the humeroscapular motion interface can restrict the range of glenohumeral rotation (**Fig. 6–12**). Such scarring and adhesions are particularly likely to occur after previous surgery or injury causing bleeding around the shoulder. They seem to be particularly common after acromioplasty, cuff surgery (**Fig. 6–13**), or fracture surgery when early postoperative motion was not implemented. These adhesions can be quite thick and strong, so that attempting to lyse them with a manipulation can require a substantial amount of force that may jeopardize the integrity of the humerus or cuff.

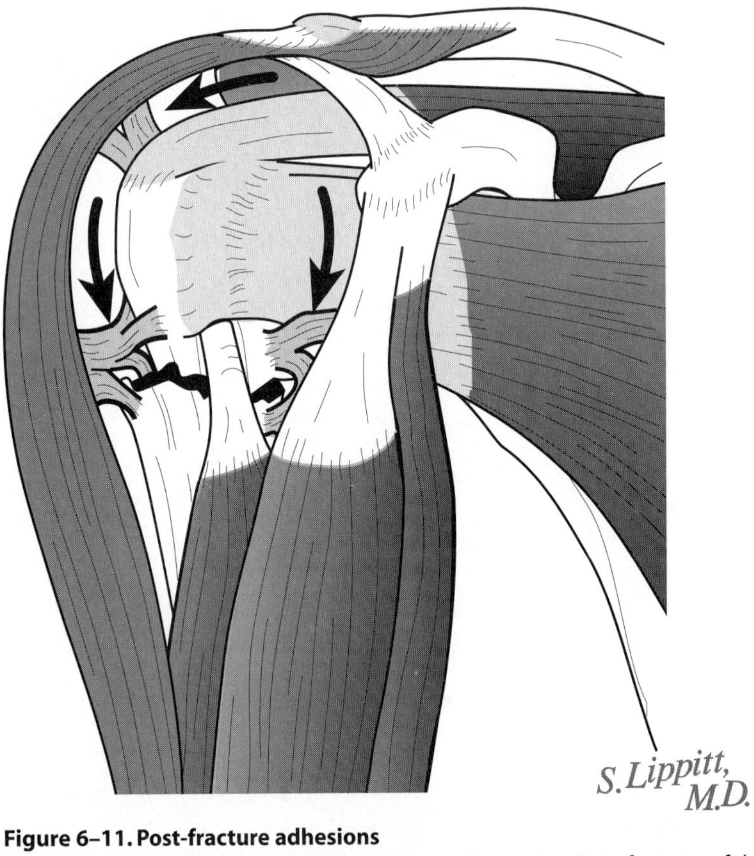


**Figure 6–11. Post-fracture adhesions**
Motion-limiting adhesions in the humeroscapular motion interface may follow a fracture, such as the subtuberous fracture shown here.

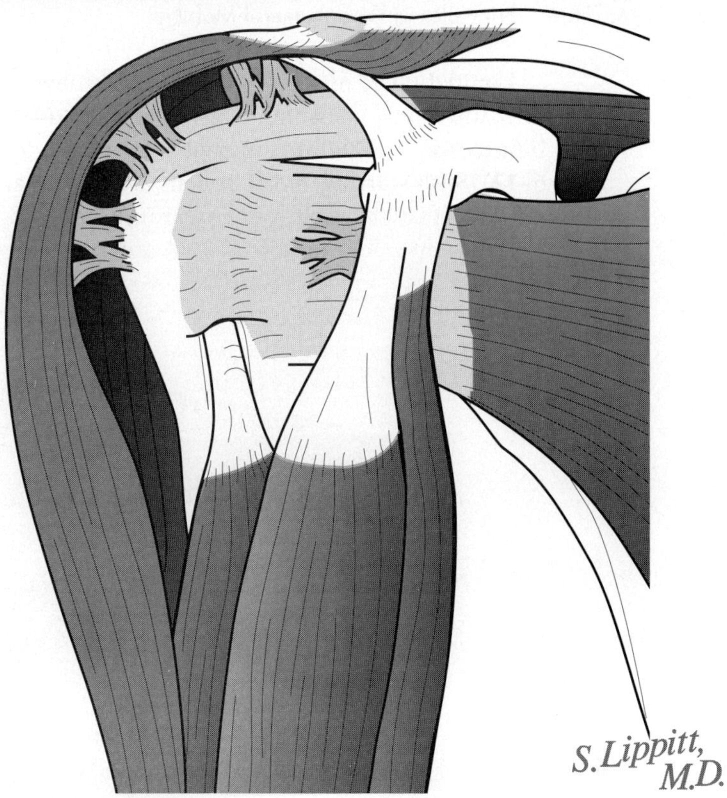


**Figure 6–12. Spot welds**
Adhesions from the external to the internal surface of the humeroscapular motion interface can restrict the range and smoothness of motion.

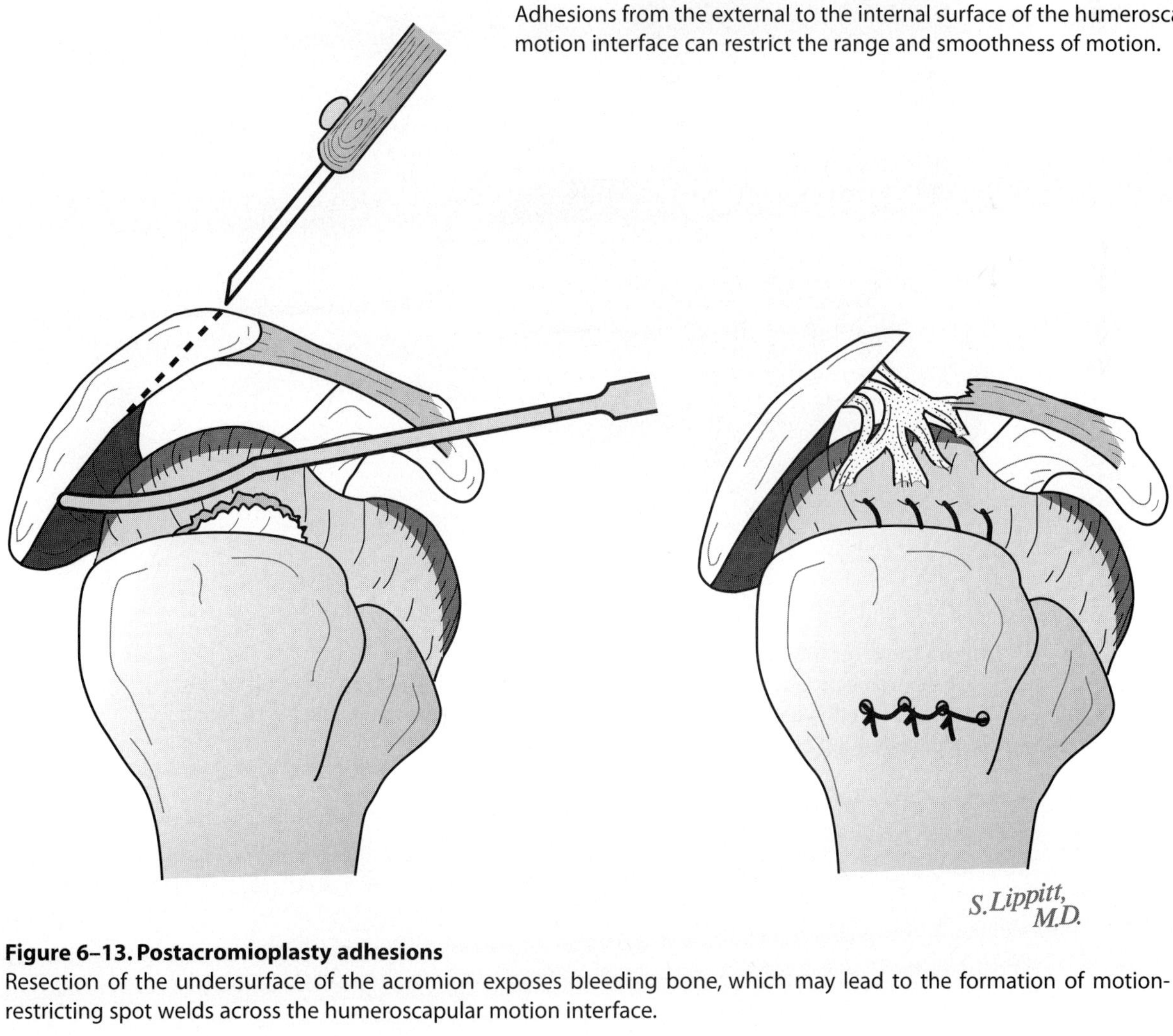


**Figure 6–13. Postacromioplasty adhesions**
Resection of the undersurface of the acromion exposes bleeding bone, which may lead to the formation of motion-restricting spot welds across the humeroscapular motion interface.

Glenohumeral rotation can also be limited by contact between the edge of the tuberosities and the edge of the glenoid—a phenomenon known as *internal abutment* (**Fig. 6–14**). Osteophytes, malunited fracture fragments, and heterotopic bone can block rotation of the humerus by creating unnatural contact with the glenoid (**Figs. 6–15, 6–16,** and **6–17**).

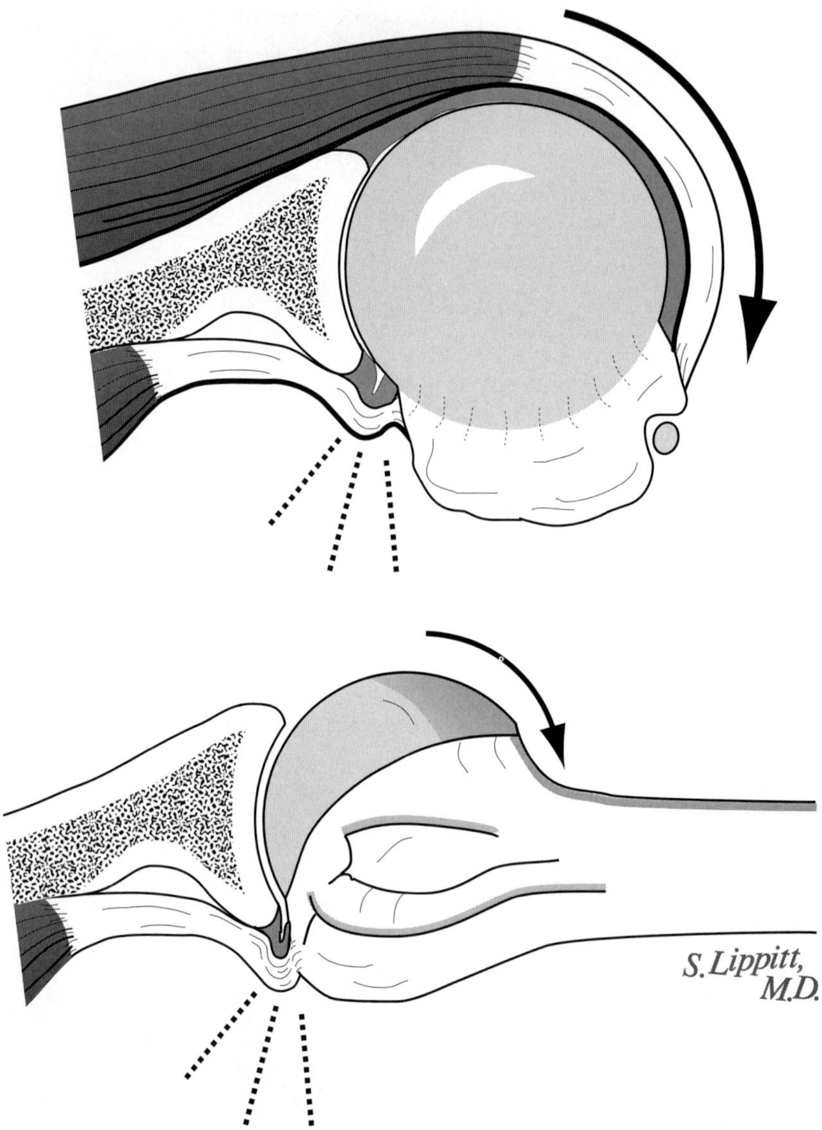


**Figure 6–14. Internal abutment**
At the extreme of rotation, the rim of the glenoid abuts against the insertion of the rotator cuff tendon to the tuberosity. (Modified from Rockwood CA, Matsen FA [eds]: The Shoulder, 2nd ed. Philadelphia: WB Saunders, 1998, p. 770.)

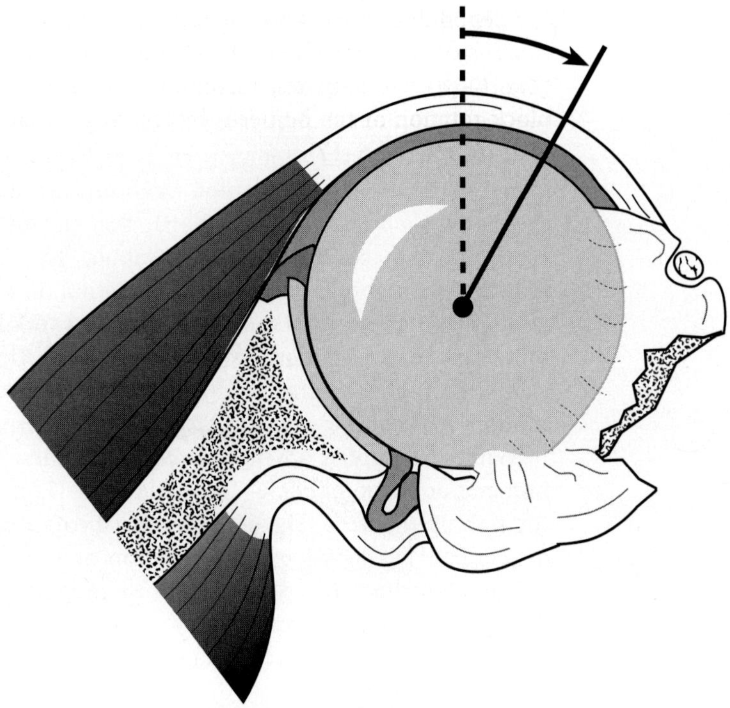

**Figure 6–16. Posteriorly displaced tuberosity**
A malunited tuberosity may abut the glenoid lip, limiting the range of rotation.

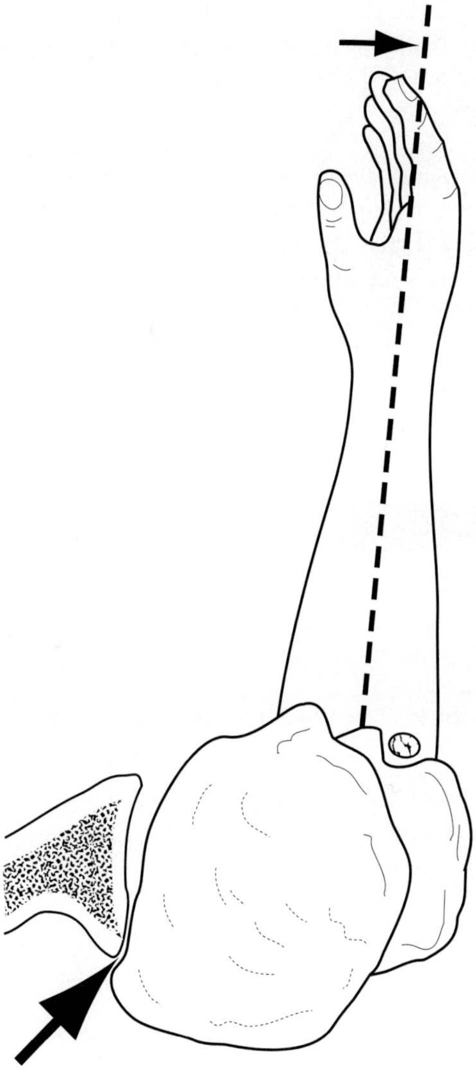

**Figure 6–15. Blocking osteophytes**
A humeral osteophyte may abut the glenoid lip, limiting the range of rotation.

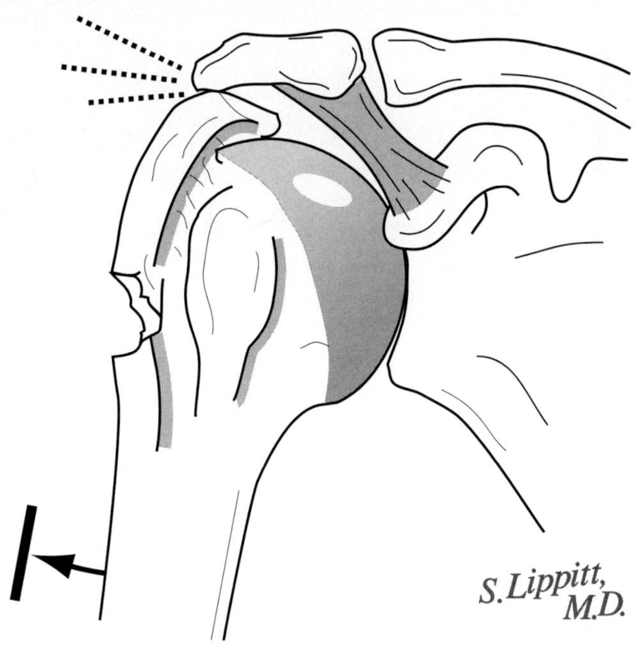


**Figure 6–17. Superiorly displaced tuberosity**
A malunited tuberosity may abut the acromion, limiting the range of abduction.

## CLINICAL CONSIDERATIONS

Tight shoulders are not only stiff but also often painful, especially at night. Frequently patients with tight shoulders are more comfortable sitting up than lying down.

In examining stiff shoulders, it is important to quantitate *glenohumeral* motion. Whereas traditional examination methods measure the motion of the arm relative to the body (*humerothoracic* motion), the glenohumeral examination measures the motion of the arm relative to the scapula. This is most easily accomplished by first reducing the scapula to its anatomic position on the chest wall (i.e., to a position similar to that of the normal shoulder) and gently holding it there with one hand while the other hand moves the arm in the desired directions. Scapulothoracic reduction and stabilization are required to maintain the glenoid in a defined position so that the motion of the humerus relative to it can be determined.

While the scapula is held secured to the chest wall, the rotational range of glenohumeral adduction (**Fig. 6–18**), abduction (**Fig. 6–19**), flexion (**Fig. 6–20**), internal rotation up the back (**Fig. 6–21**), external rotation at the side (**Fig. 6–22**), cross-body movement (**Fig. 6–23**), external rotation in abduction (**Fig. 6–24**), and internal rotation in abduction (**Fig. 6–25**) can be quantitated. These motions give the examiner a good feel for the rotational laxity of the humerus relative to the scapula. Selective examination of the different components of the capsule can reveal the parts that are tight (**Table 6–1**).

**Table 6–1**

**Relation of Motion Limitation to Location of Capsular Tightness**

| Limitation of this motion | Suggests tightness of this part of the capsule |
|---|---|
| External rotation at the side | Anterior superior and coracohumeral ligament |
| Internal rotation at the side | Posterior superior |
| External rotation in abduction | Anterior inferior |
| Internal rotation in abduction | Posterior inferior |
| Cross-body movement | Posterior |
| Flexion | Posterior inferior |
| Abduction | Inferior |
| Adduction | Superior |

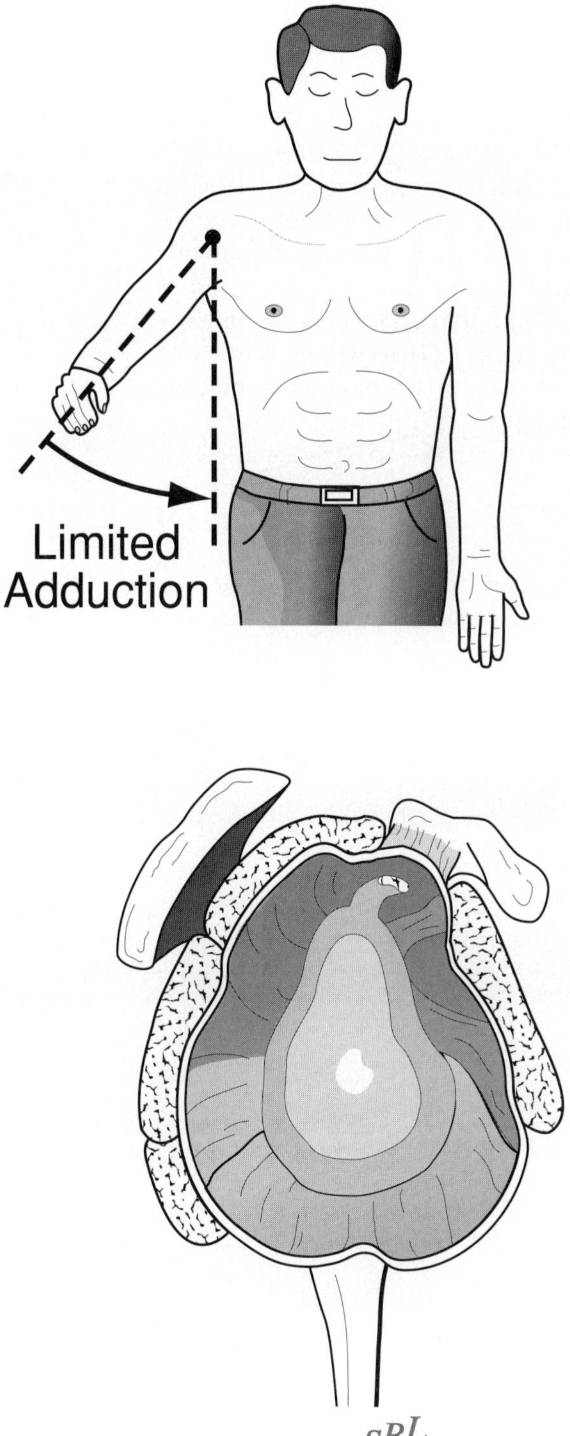


**Figure 6–18. Limited adduction**
Tightness of the superior capsule can limit glenohumeral adduction.

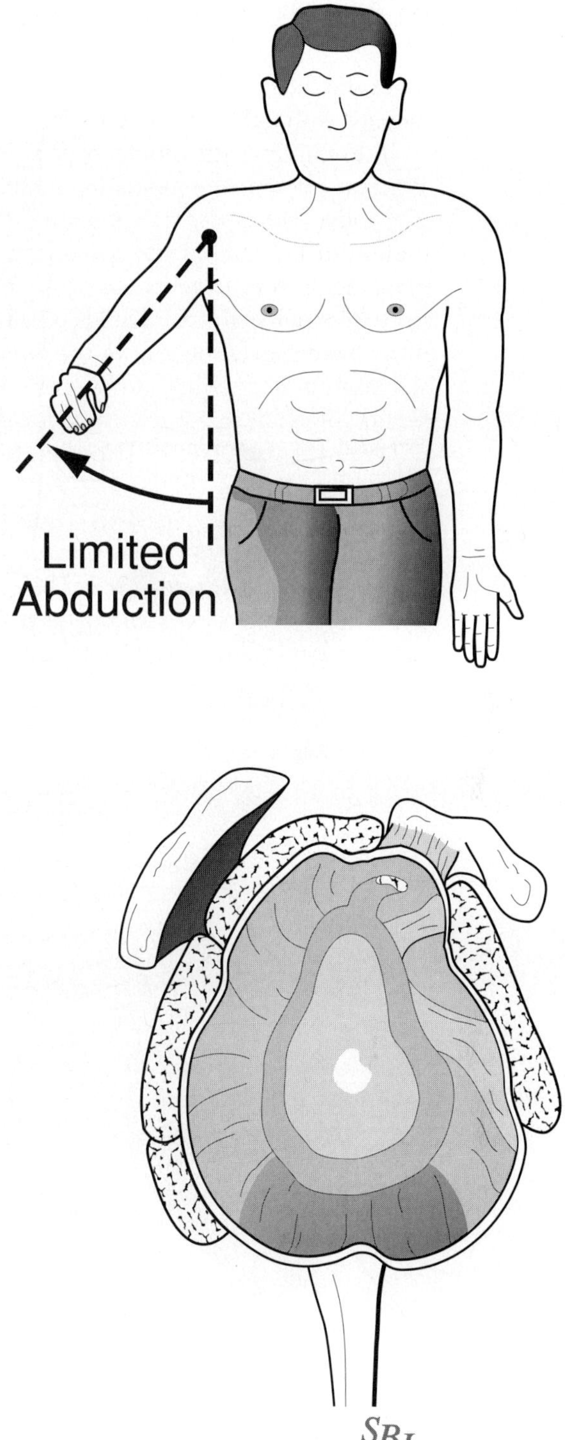


**Figure 6–19. Limited abduction**
Tightness of the inferior capsule can limit glenohumeral abduction.

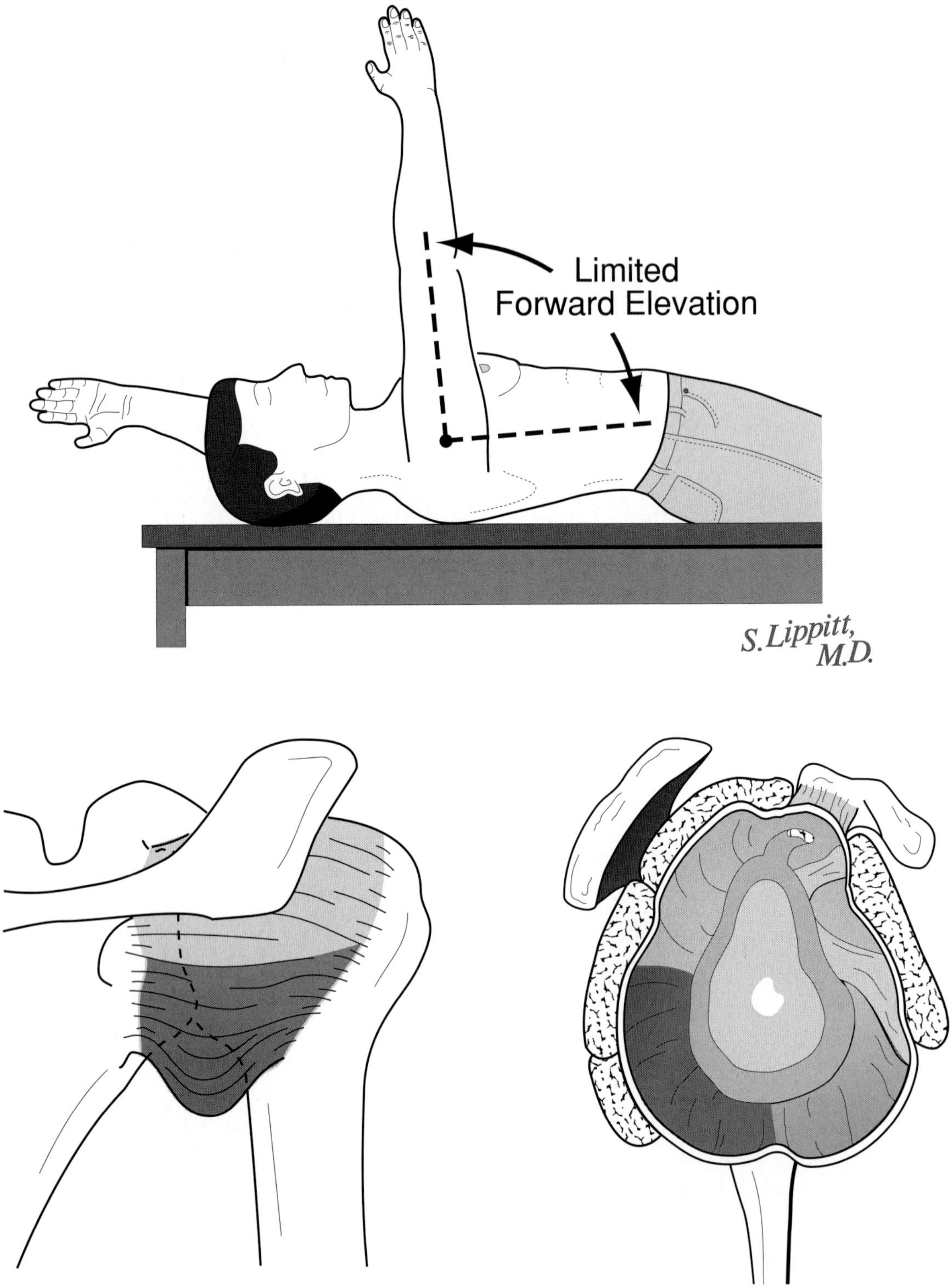


**Figure 6–20. Limited forward elevation**
Tightness of the posteroinferior capsule can limit glenohumeral forward elevation, also known as flexion.

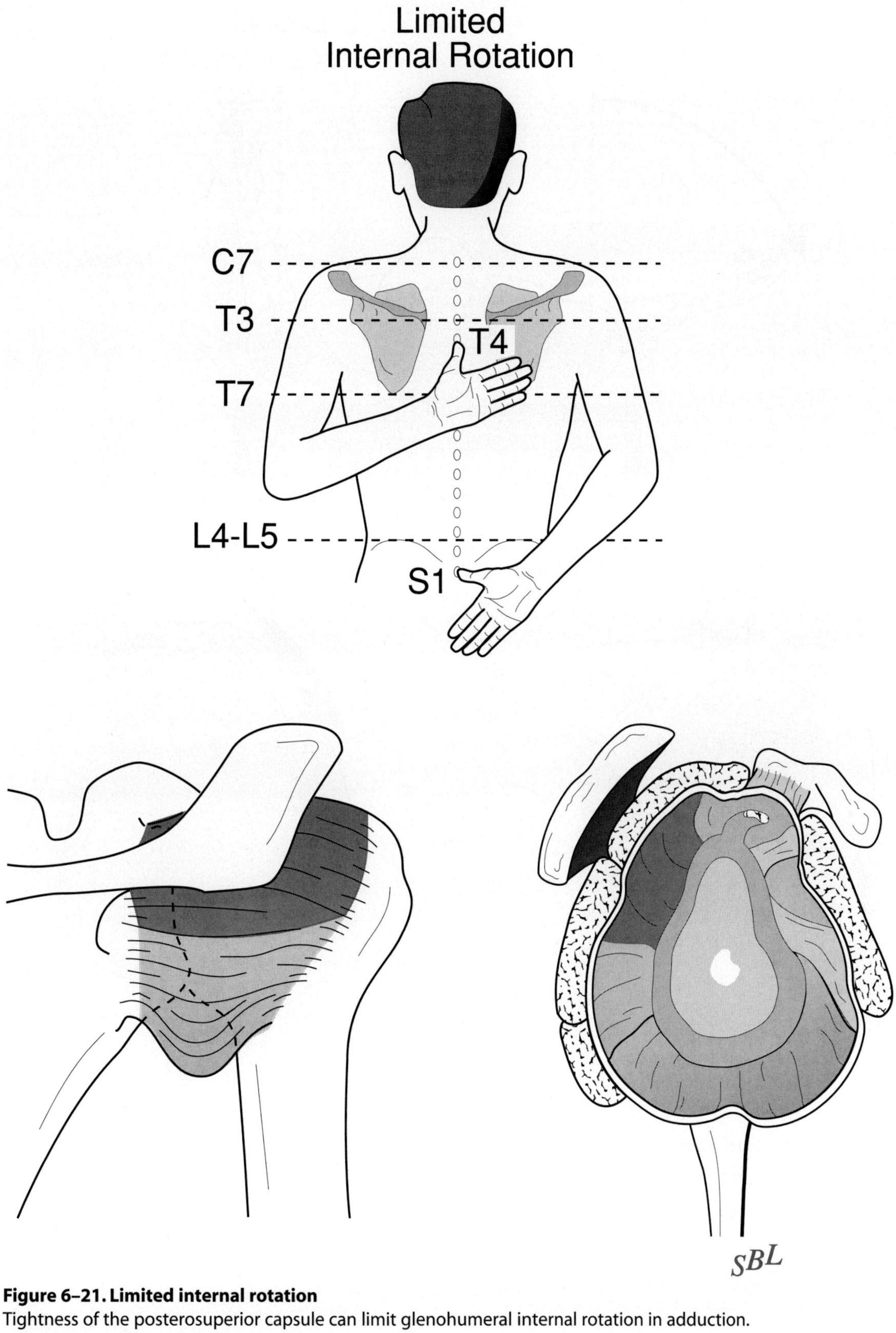


**Figure 6–21. Limited internal rotation**
Tightness of the posterosuperior capsule can limit glenohumeral internal rotation in adduction.

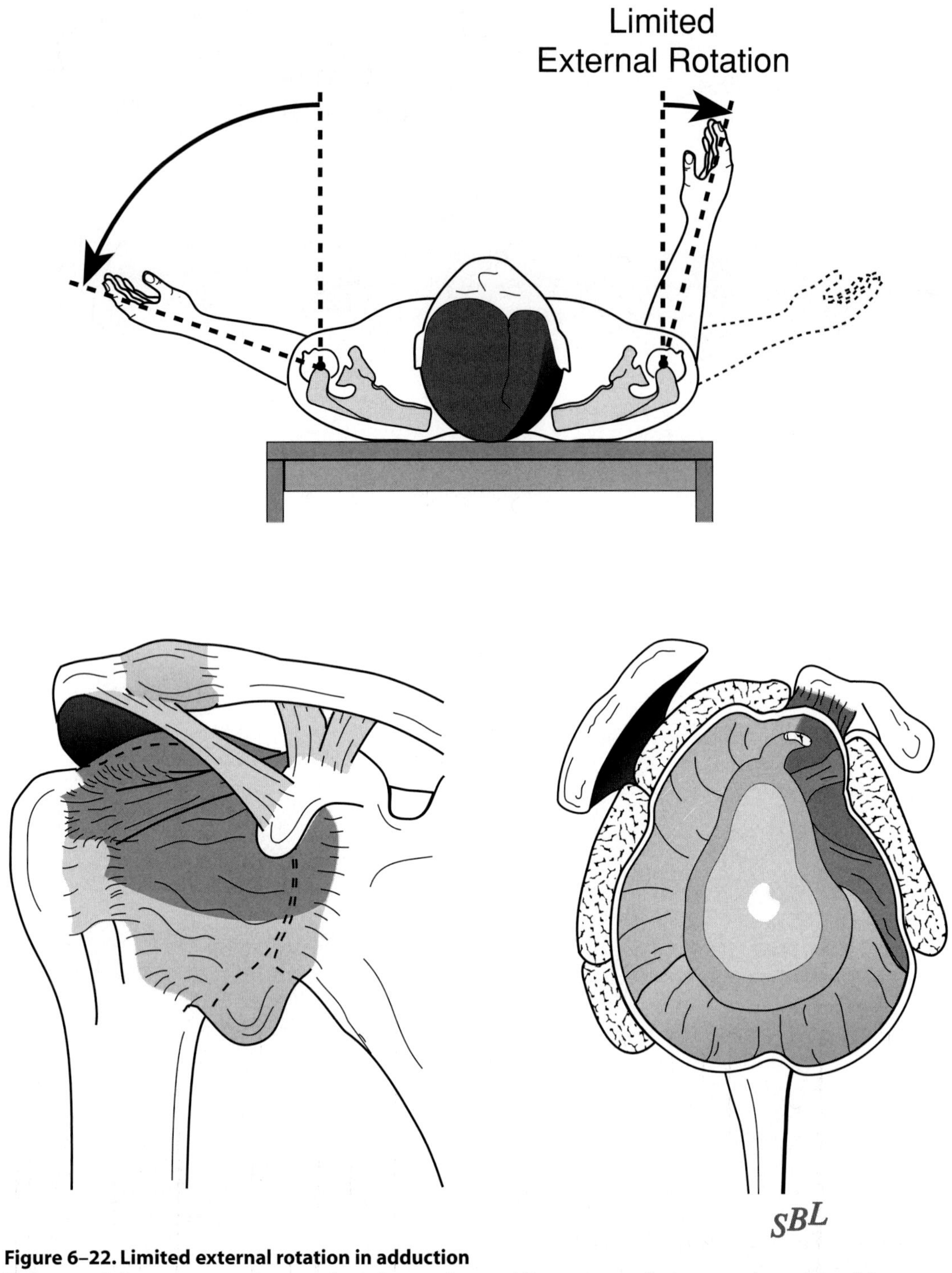


**Figure 6–22. Limited external rotation in adduction**
Tightness of the anterosuperior capsule and coracohumeral ligament can limit external rotation of the arm at the side.

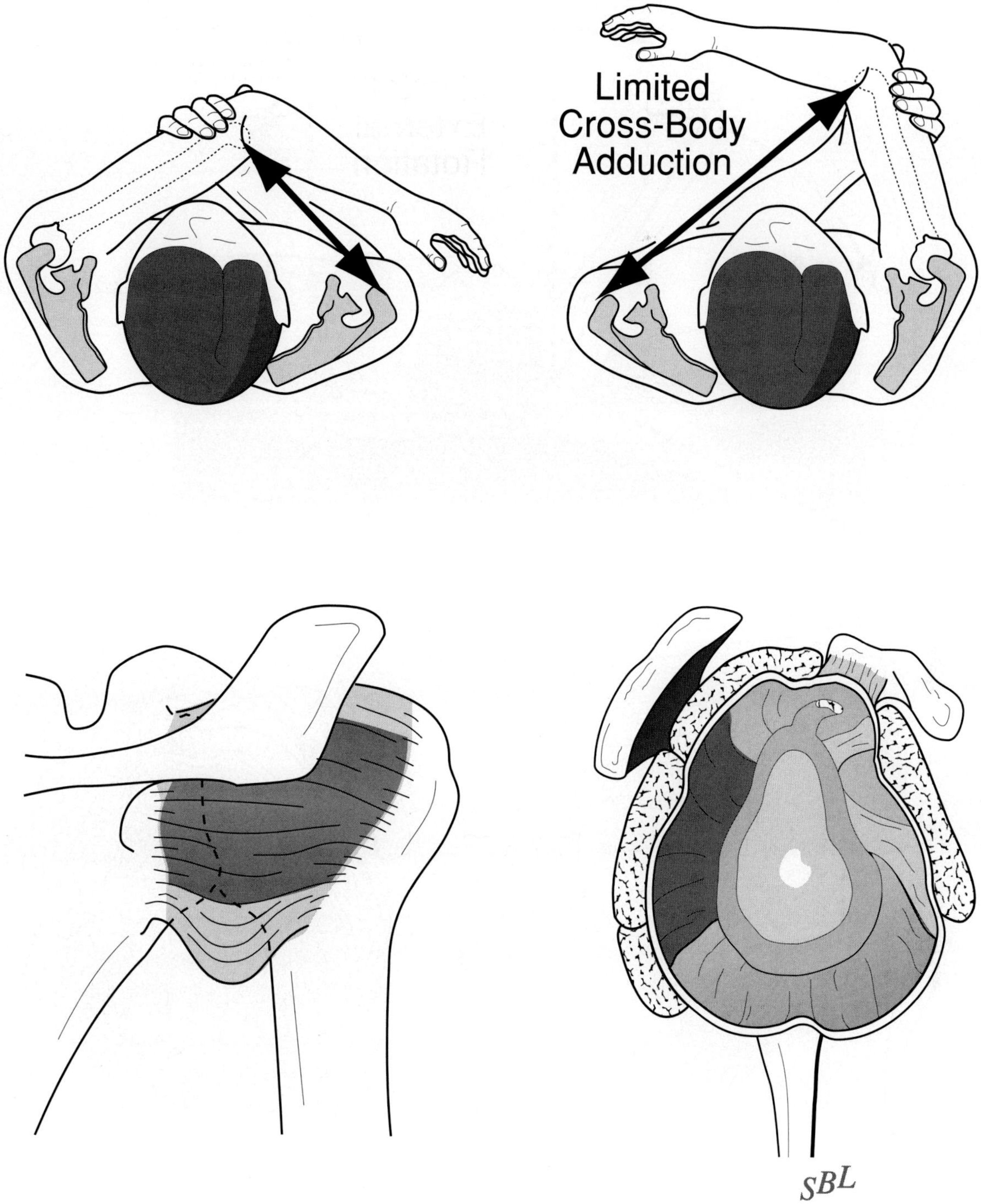


**Figure 6–23. Limited cross-body adduction**
Tightness of the posterior capsule can limit adduction of the arm across the body.

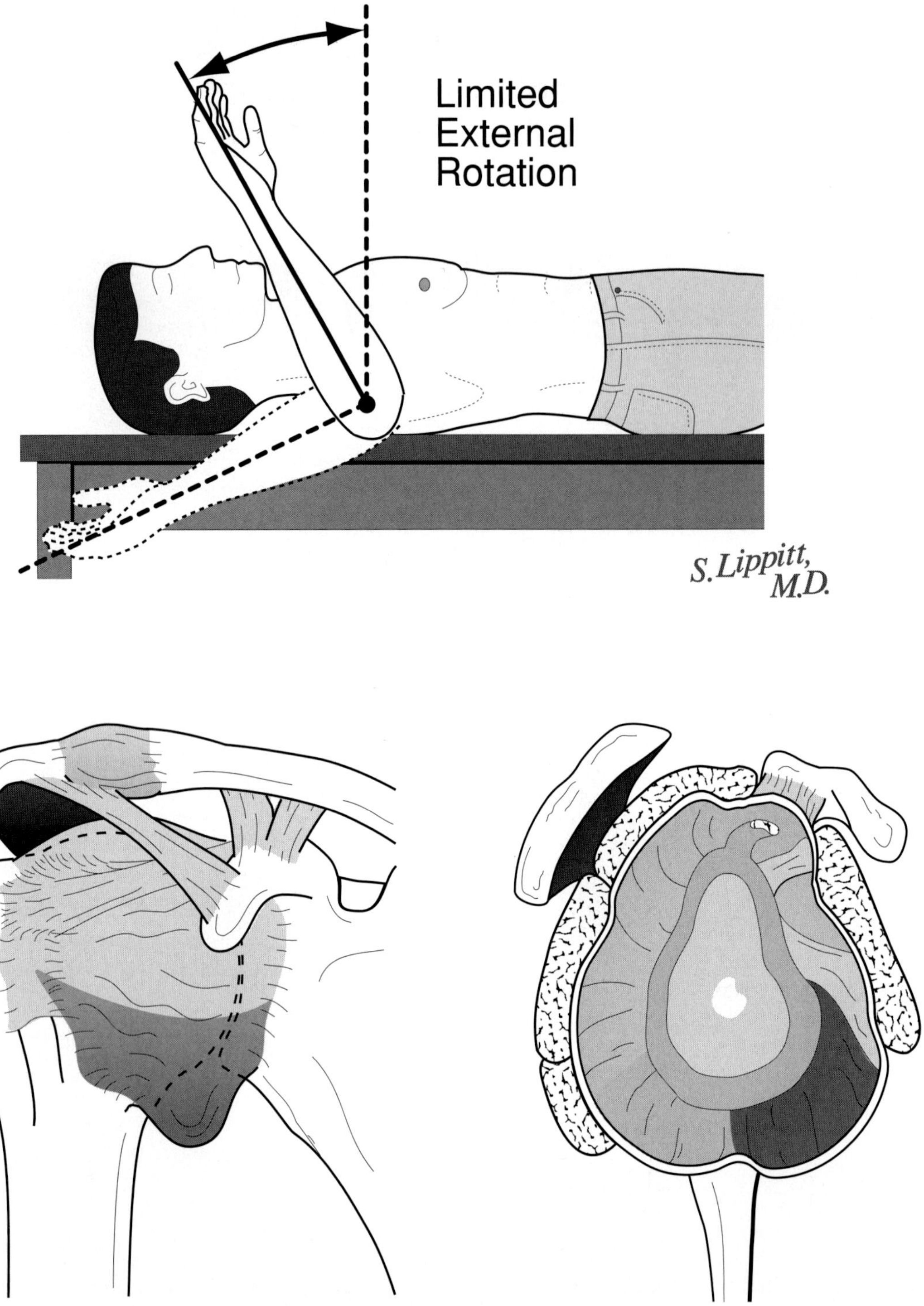


**Figure 6–24. Limited external rotation in abduction**
Tightness of the anteroinferior capsule can limit external rotation of the abducted arm.

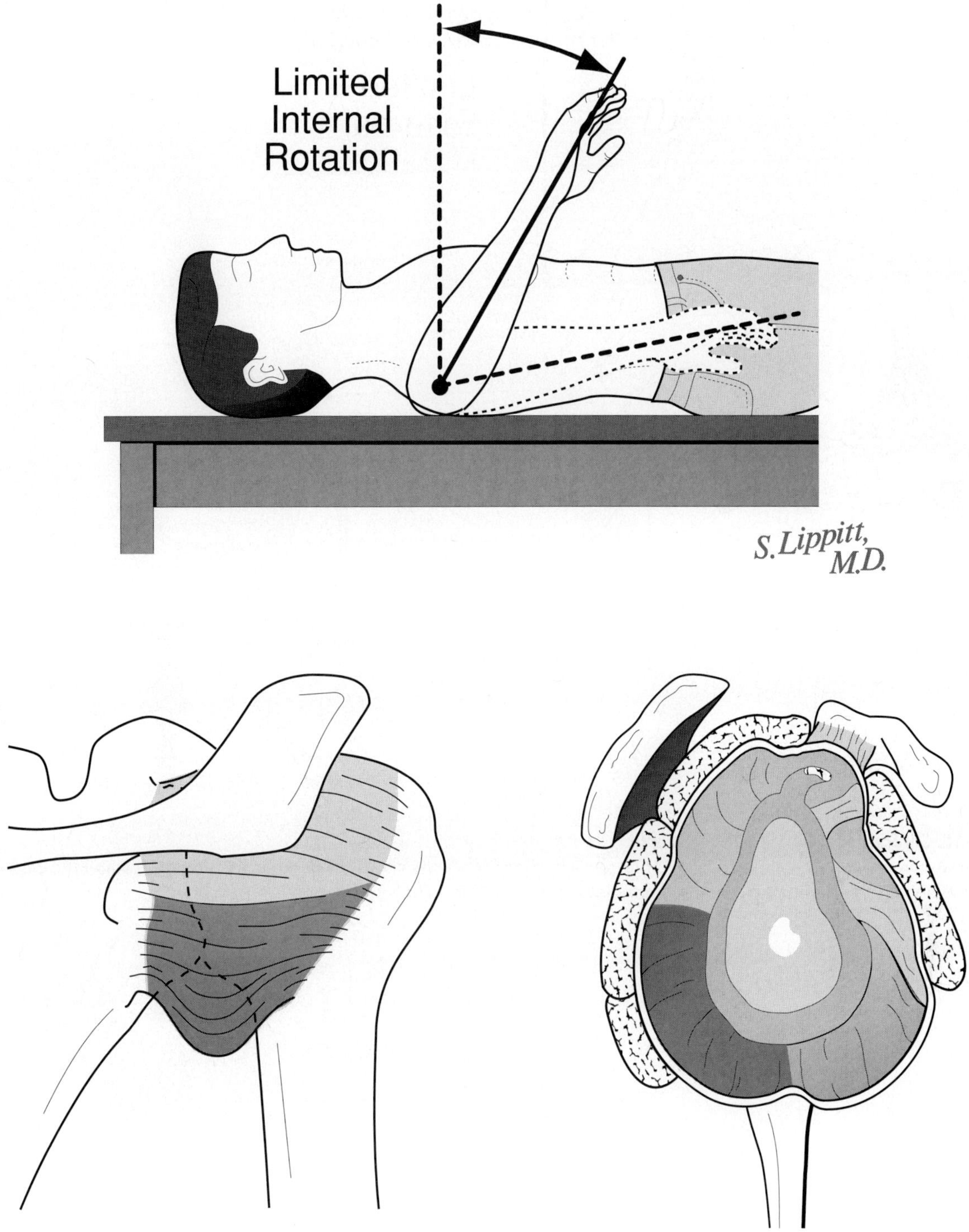


**Figure 6–25. Limited internal rotation in abduction**
Tightness of the posteroinferior capsule can limit internal rotation of the abducted arm.

The translational laxity of the glenohumeral joint can be quantitated by gently pressing the humeral head anteriorly, posteriorly, and inferiorly relative to the glenoid **(Fig. 6–26)**.

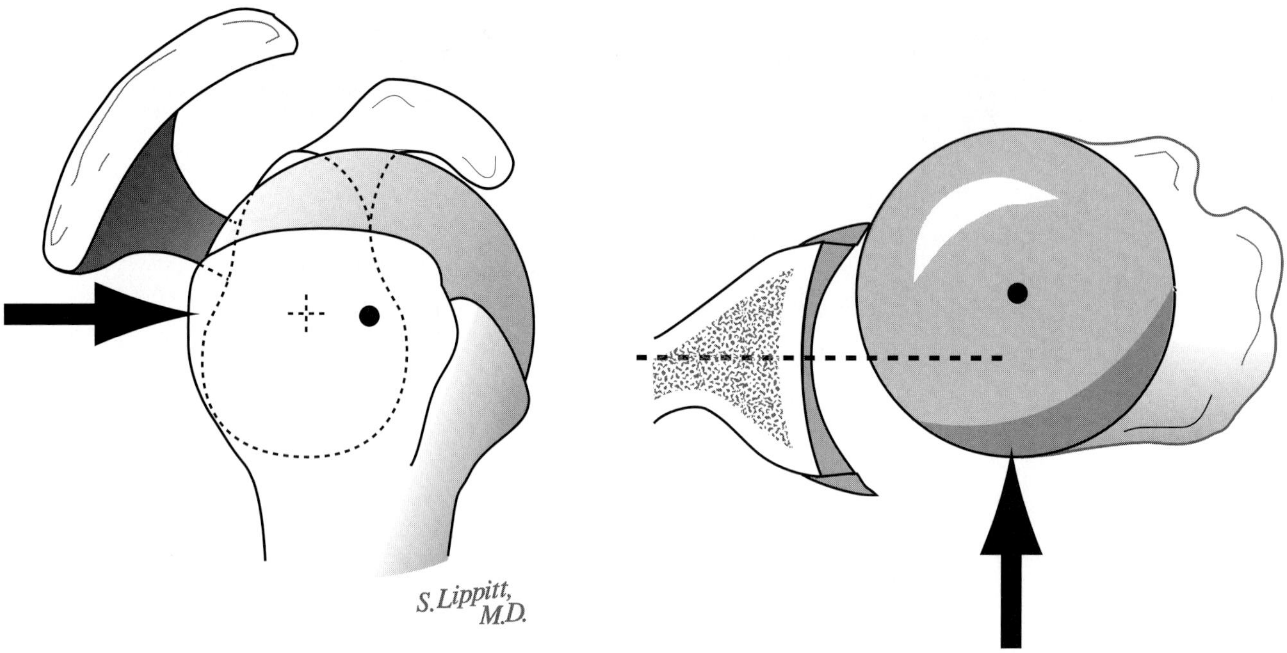


A

**Figure 6–26. Clinical tests for translational laxity**

**A,** The anterior drawer test. The humeral head is grasped with one of the examiner's hands while the scapula is stabilized with the other. The humeral head is translated to its anterior endpoint while the extent of this translation is noted.

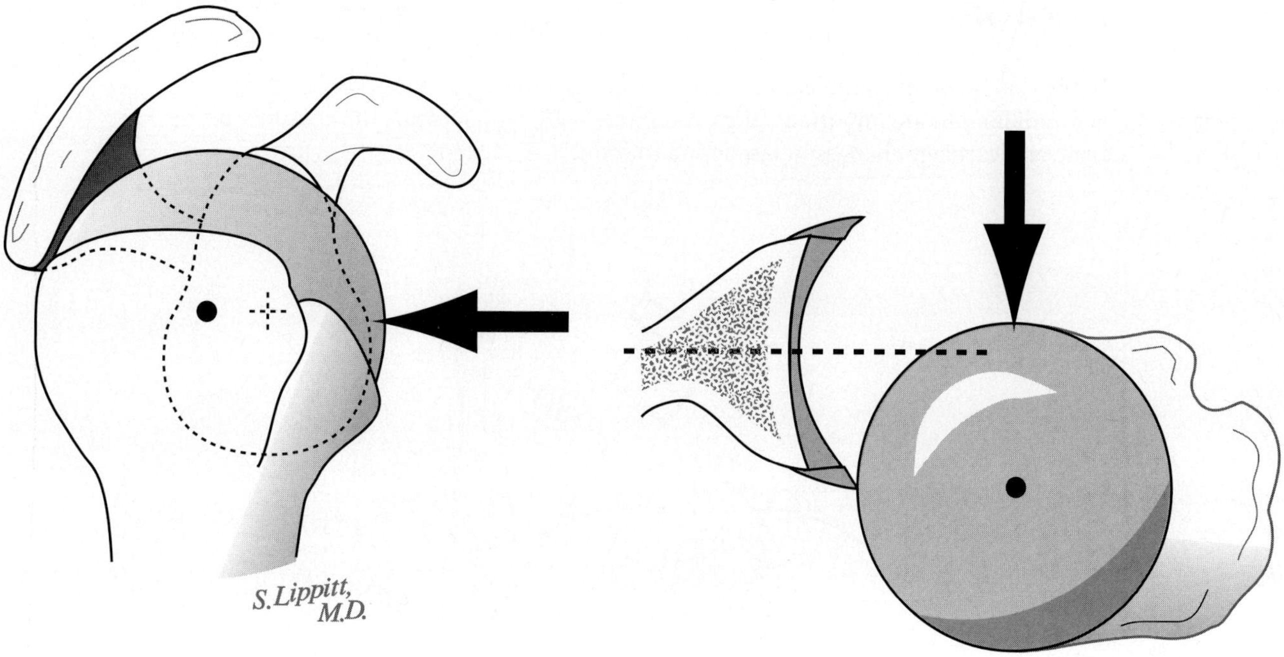


B

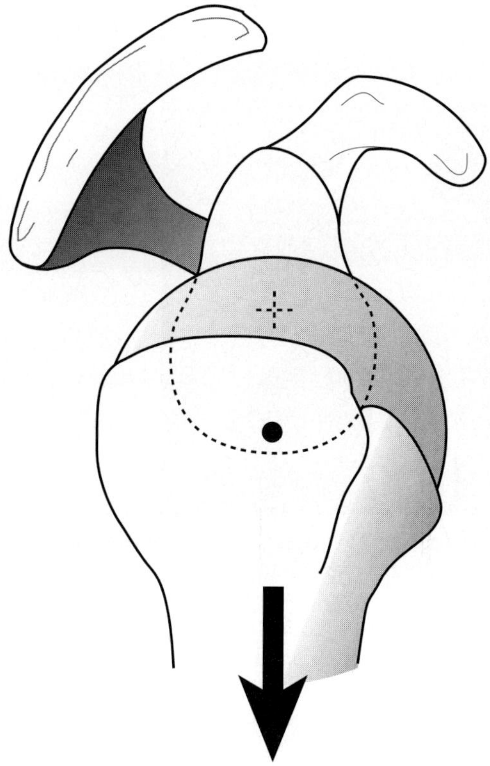

C

**Figure 6–26. Clinical tests for translational laxity**—*Continued*

**B,** The posterior drawer test. The humeral head is grasped with one of the examiner's hands while the scapula is stabilized with the other. The humeral head is translated to its posterior endpoint while the extent of this translation is noted. **C,** The sulcus test. The arm is grasped with one of the examiner's hands while the scapula is stabilized with the other. The humeral head is translated to its inferior endpoint while the extent of this translation is noted. For each of these tests, maximal translation is observed if the patient's muscles are relaxed and if the starting position is in the midrange of motion.

## IMAGING

In the evaluation of shoulders with limited range of motion, anteroposterior and axillary radiographs are important (**Figs. 6–27** and **6–28**) to determine the possible role of bone and cartilage changes in restricting motion.

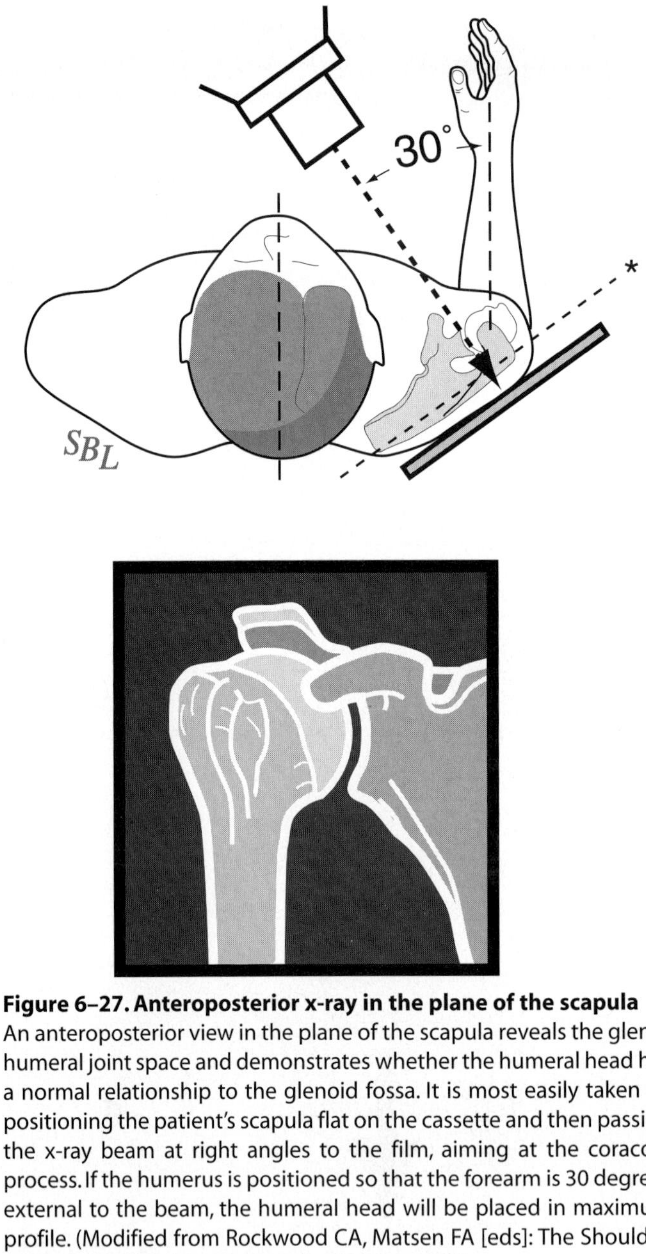


**Figure 6–27. Anteroposterior x-ray in the plane of the scapula**
An anteroposterior view in the plane of the scapula reveals the glenohumeral joint space and demonstrates whether the humeral head has a normal relationship to the glenoid fossa. It is most easily taken by positioning the patient's scapula flat on the cassette and then passing the x-ray beam at right angles to the film, aiming at the coracoid process. If the humerus is positioned so that the forearm is 30 degrees external to the beam, the humeral head will be placed in maximum profile. (Modified from Rockwood CA, Matsen FA [eds]: The Shoulder, 2nd ed. Philadelphia: WB Saunders, 1998, p. 650.)

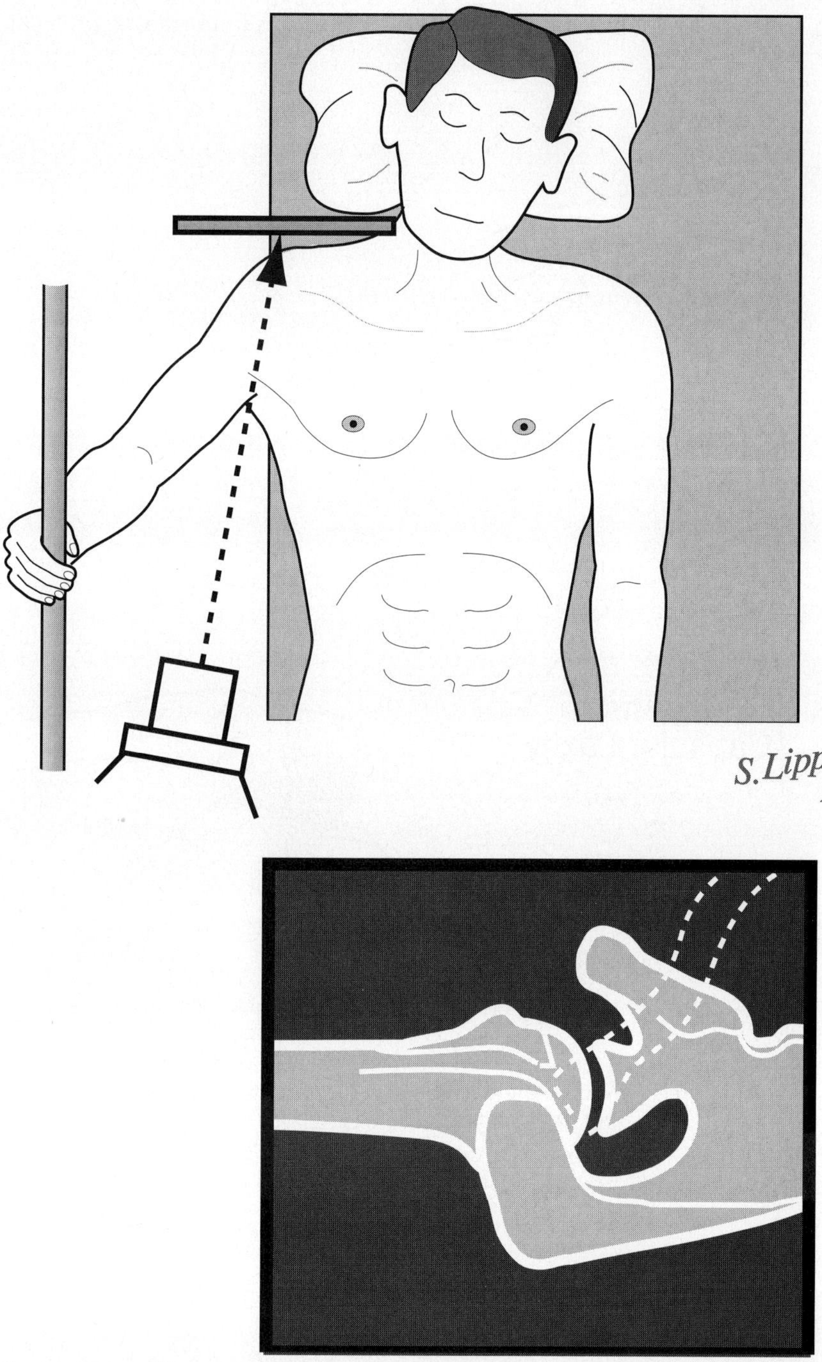


**Figure 6–28. Axillary x-ray**

An axillary x-ray reveals the glenohumeral joint space and the anteroposterior position of the humeral head and glenoid fossa. It is obtained by having the patient's arm in abduction (for example, holding on to an IV pole), the cassette on the superior aspect of the shoulder, and the x-ray beam passing up the axilla, aiming at the coracoid. (Modified from Rockwood CA, Matsen FA [eds]: The Shoulder, 2nd ed. Philadelphia: WB Saunders, 1998, p. 651.)

## SURGICAL CONSIDERATIONS

One of the common limiting structures is the coracohumeral ligament running from the coracoid to the bicipital groove (**Fig. 6–29**). It is most easily released from the coracoid, ensuring that both the supraspinatus and the subscapularis are not tethered to the coracoid process (**Fig. 6–30**). In considering the surgical release of tight ligaments and capsule, it is important to recognize that these structures are best released peripheral to the glenoid labrum (**Fig. 6–31**), preserving the contribution of the labrum to glenohumeral stability. In the process of capsular release, it is important to protect the

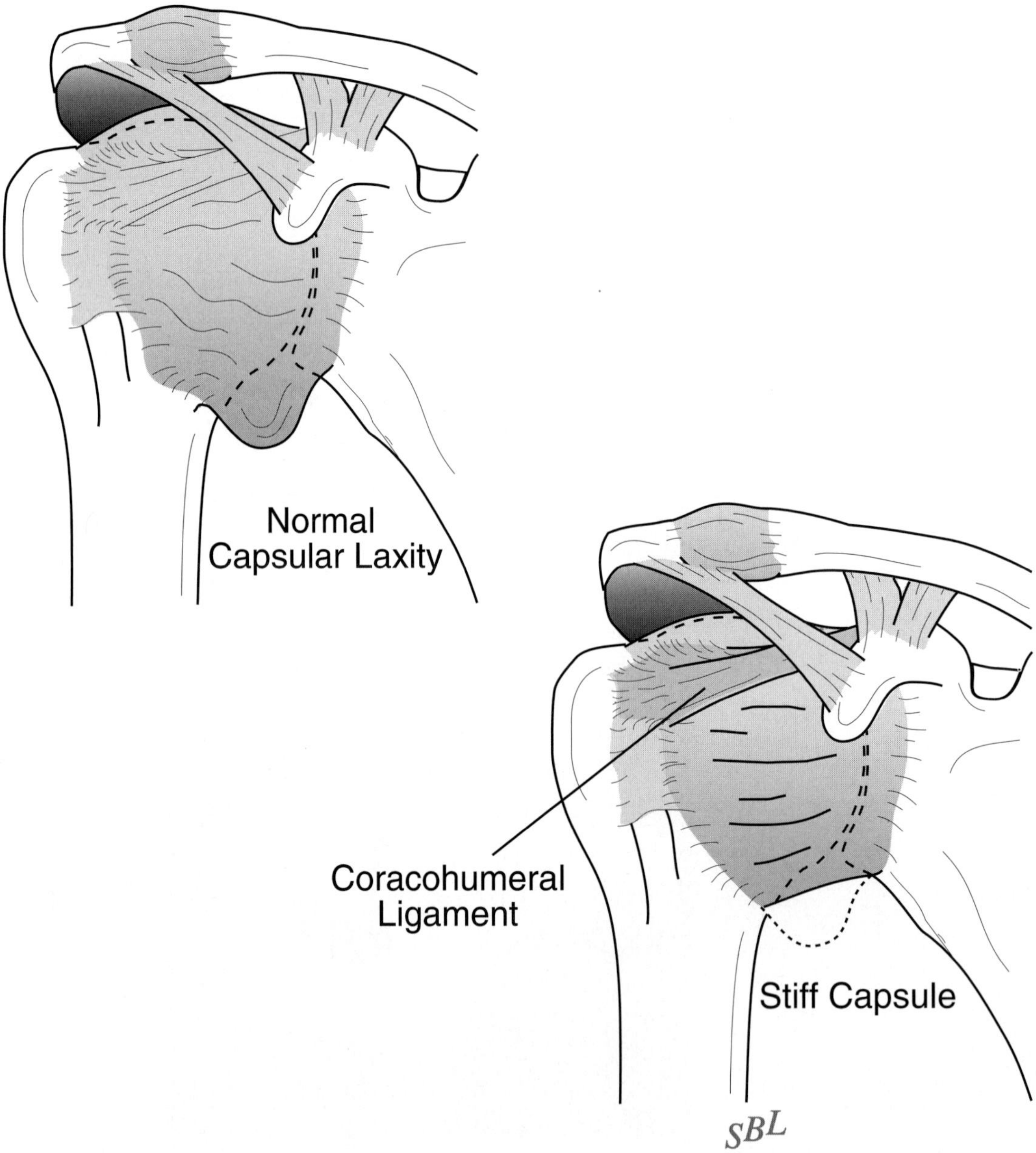


**Figure 6–29. The stiff glenohumeral joint**
Stiffness of the glenohumeral joint is commonly related to contracture of the coracohumeral ligament and obliteration of the axillary recess.

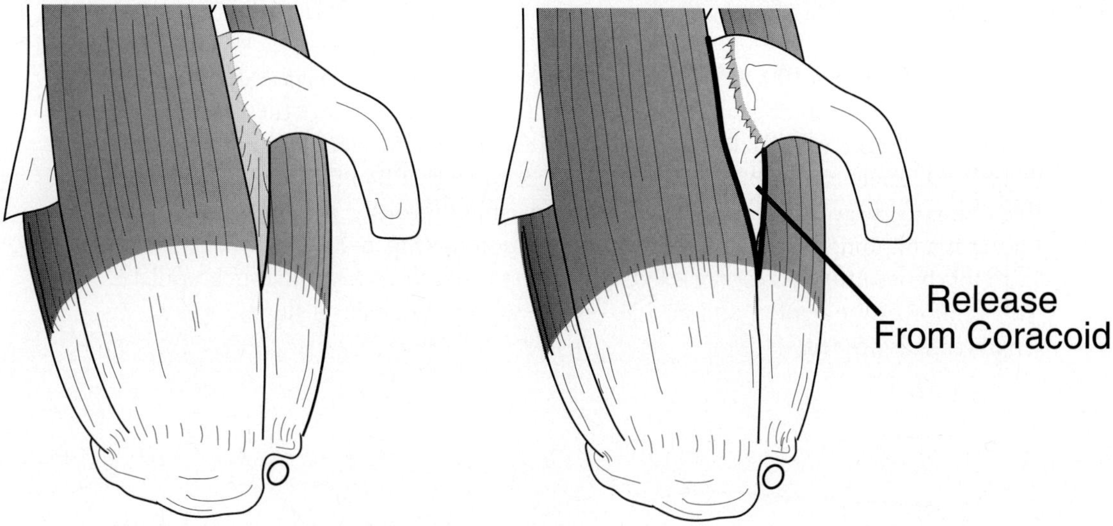


**Figure 6–30. Release of the coracohumeral ligament**
The coracohumeral ligament is released from the base of the coracoid process, allowing the subscapularis and supraspinatus unrestricted gliding past the coracoid. (Modified from Matsen FA, Lippitt SB, Sidles JA, et al [eds]: Practical Evaluation and Management of the Shoulder. Philadelphia: WB Saunders, 1994, p. 138.)

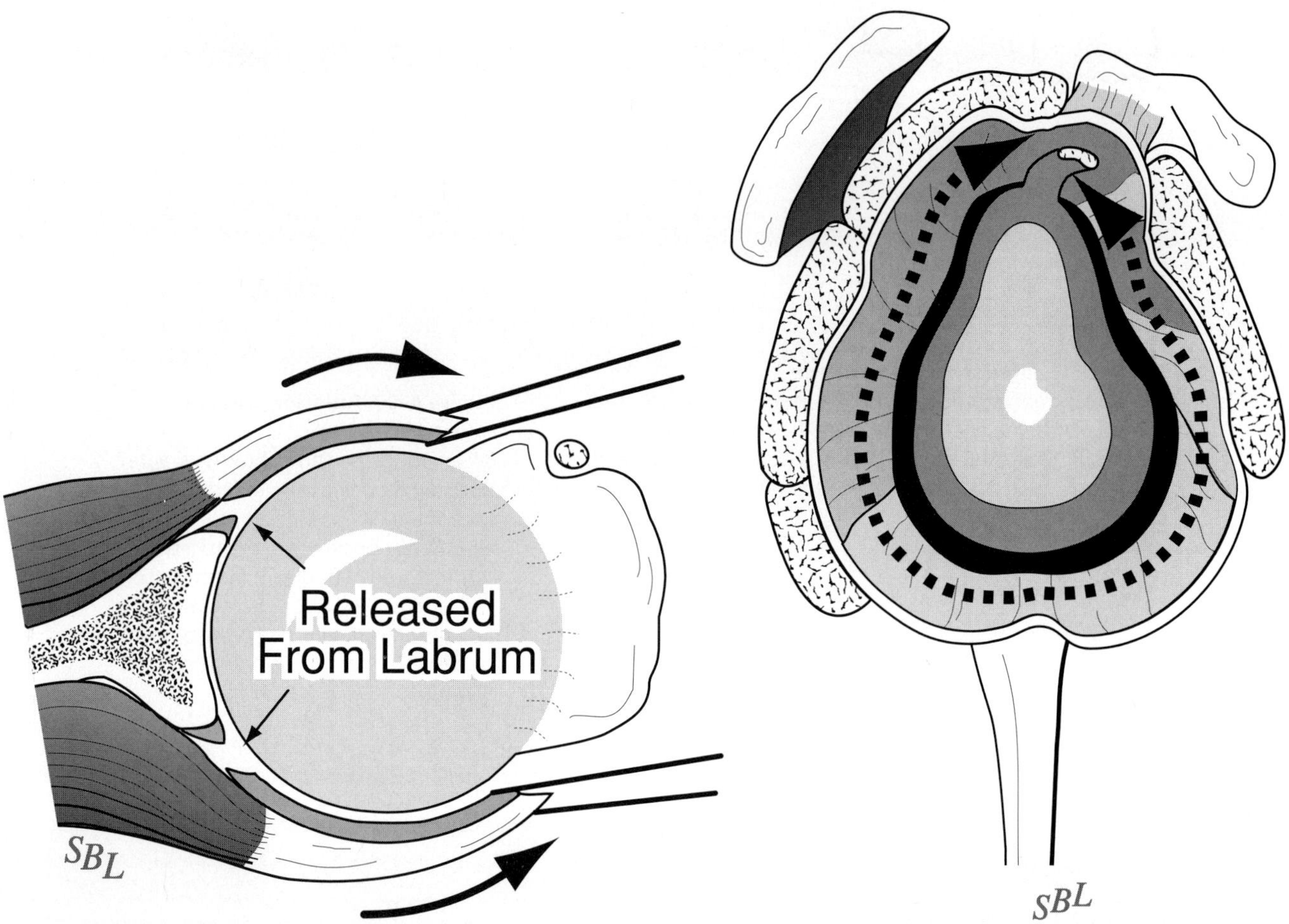


**Figure 6–31. Circumferential capsular release**
The capsule can be released circumferentially around the glenoid, leaving the glenoid labrum intact so that the glenoid concavity is not compromised. (Modified from Matsen FA, Lippitt SB, Sidles JA, et al [eds]: Practical Evaluation and Management of the Shoulder. Philadelphia: WB Saunders, 1994, p. 138; and from Rockwood CA, Matsen FA [eds]: The Shoulder, 2nd ed. Philadelphia: WB Saunders, 1998, p. 811.)

axillary nerve (**Fig. 6–32**). If the tightness is only anterior, the release can stop just beyond 190 degrees on the face of the glenoid (**Fig. 6–33**). If the tightness is also posterior, the release must be taken a full 360 degrees around the glenoid. In exposing the posterior capsule, it is helpful to twist the retractor so that its inferior surface pushes the humerus away from the glenoid and to simultaneously internally rotate the humerus a bit to tighten the capsule for easy sectioning (**Fig. 6–34**).

In this procedure, the capsule is left applied to the deep surface of the subscapularis. This reinforces the tendon and also leaves the capsule in position in case a Z-plasty lengthening is needed.

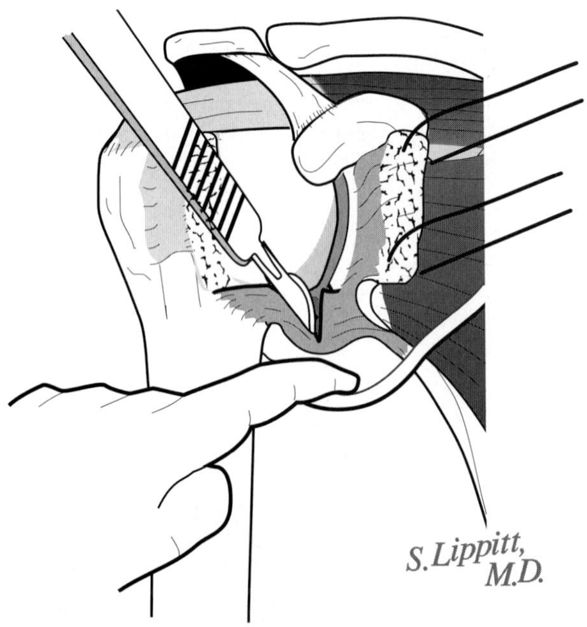


**Figure 6–32. Inferior capsular release**
The axillary nerve is identified and protected during the release of the inferior capsule. (Modified from Matsen FA, Lippitt SB, Sidles JA, et al [eds]: Practical Evaluation and Management of the Shoulder. Philadelphia: WB Saunders, 1994, p. 205.)

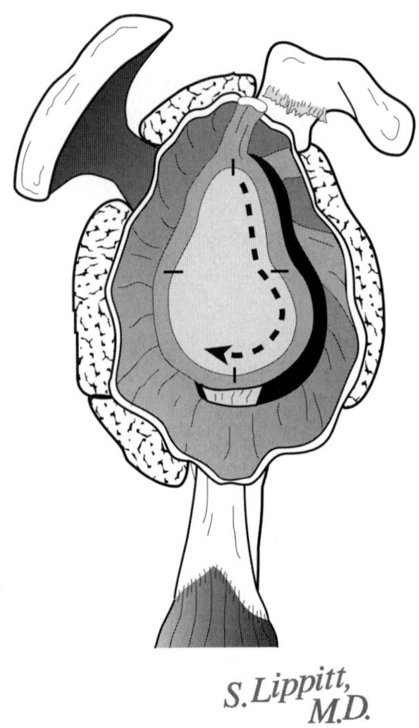


**Figure 6–33. Anterior capsular release**
When the capsular tightness is anterior only, the release is carried from the root of the biceps tendon superiorly to a point just posterior to the triceps origin inferiorly. (Modified from Matsen FA, Lippitt SB, Sidles JA, et al [eds]: Practical Evaluation and Management of the Shoulder. Philadelphia: WB Saunders, 1994, p. 205.)

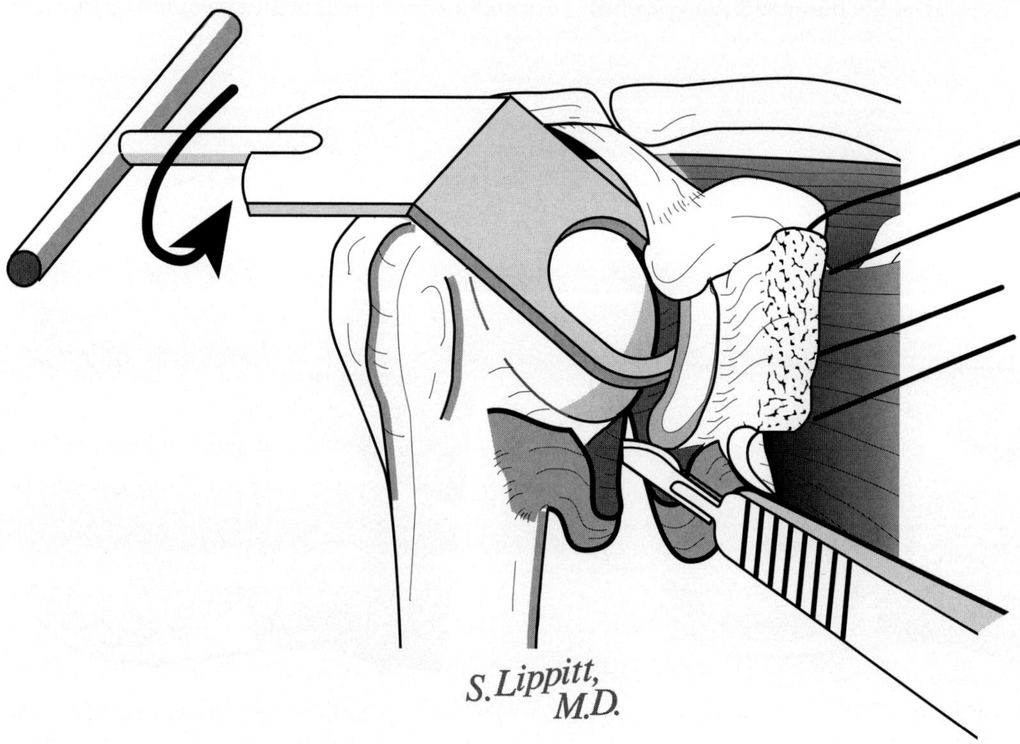


**Figure 6–34. Posterior capsular release**

The capsular release can be continued around the glenoid posteriorly. Exposure of the posterior capsule is facilitated by exerting a twist on the humeral head retractor so that the inferior capsule is placed under tension. (Modified from Matsen FA, Lippitt SB, Sidles JA, et al [eds]: Practical Evaluation and Management of the Shoulder. Philadelphia: WB Saunders, 1994, p. 209.)

Before closure of the surgical incision, the range of motion can be verified and compared with that of the normal shoulder. The capsular releases are not repaired. Only the mobilized and released subscapularis is sutured back to its insertion. In rare cases, for example those in which there has been a previous subscapularis tightening procedure, a Z-plasty lengthening may be considered **(Fig. 6–35)**. An indication for this lengthening is when direct reattachment of the subscapularis tendon would limit external rotation excessively. In this procedure, the capsule is dissected from the deep surface of the subscapularis from medial to lateral, leaving it attached laterally. Flipping the capsule laterally and then approximating it to the tissue at the lesser tuberosity lengthens the tendon. External rotation is increased by approximately a number of degrees equal to the lengthening in millimeters multiplied by 57 degrees divided by the radius of curvature of the humeral head in millimeters. Thus, if the radius of the humeral head is 25 mm, each millimeter of lengthening would increase external rotation by about 2 degrees (57 degrees/25 mm × 1 mm of lengthening).

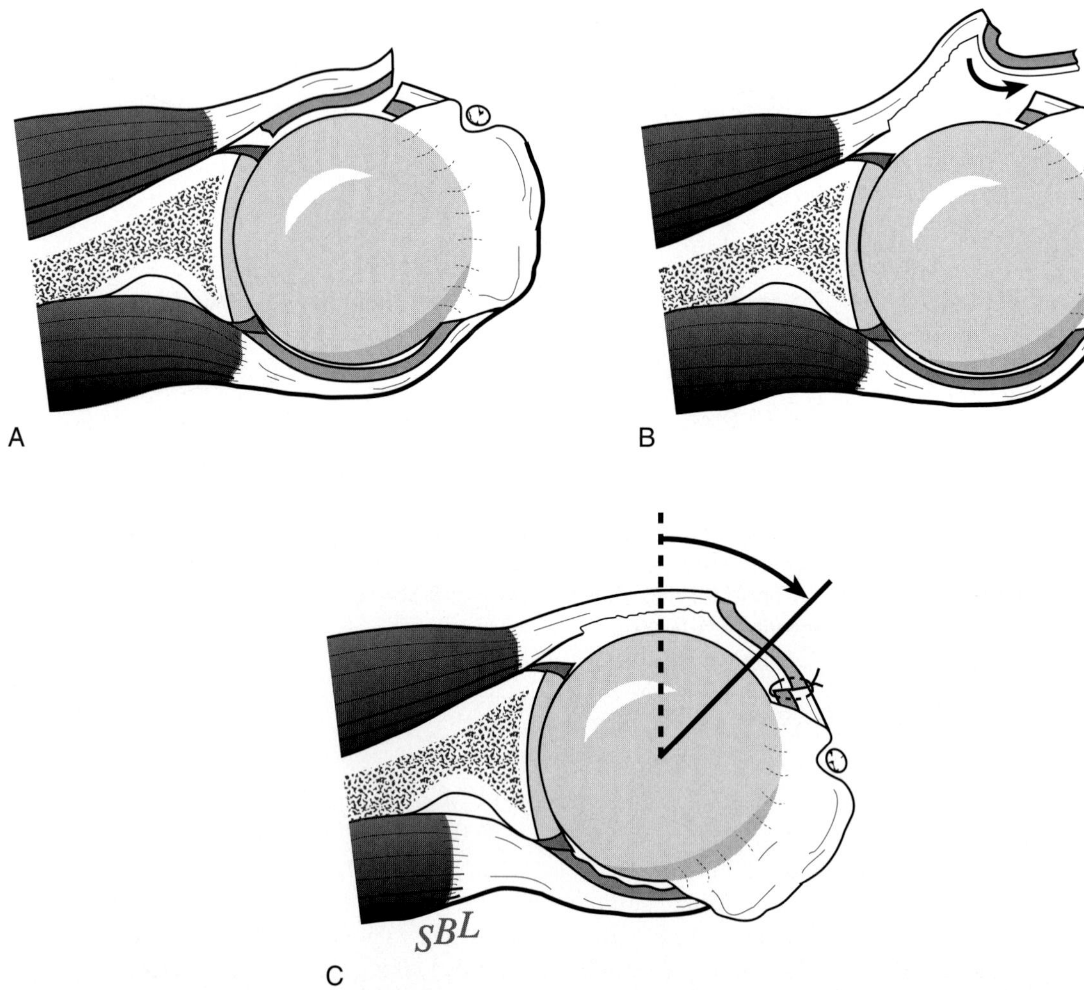


**Figure 6–35. Subscapularis lengthening**
The subscapularis tendon can be lengthened by dissecting the capsule from its deep surface, leaving it attached laterally. Flipping the capsule laterally lengthens the tendon, allowing greater external rotation.

CHAPTER 7

# Procedure: Surgical Release of Stiff Shoulder

***Diagnosis***

***Idiopathic frozen shoulder 726.0***
***Diabetic stiff shoulder 718.41***
***Post-traumatic shoulder stiffness 718.41***
***Postsurgical shoulder stiffness 718.41***

***Surgical Procedure***

***Open surgical release of stiff shoulder CPT CODE 23020***

## INDICATIONS

The patient has limited glenohumeral motion, seriously compromising his or her comfort and function. The stiffness has not responded to nonoperative management, including a supervised home stretching program. The anteroposterior and axillary radiographs show a normal glenohumeral joint space, no evidence of locked dislocation, no osteophytes, no heterotopic bone, and no other explanation for the joint stiffness.

Knowing the alternatives as well as the risks of infection, neurovascular injury, recurrent stiffness, pain, weakness, instability, and the need for revision surgery, as well as anesthetic complications, the patient desires to proceed with the above-described procedure. The patient understands that the purpose of the procedure is to increase glenohumeral laxity. The patient recognizes that this procedure cannot be expected to fully restore normal comfort and function to the shoulder. And lastly, the patient understands his or her critical role in postsurgical rehabilitation.

## FINDINGS

Examination under anesthesia indicates that glenohumeral motion is restricted in internal and external rotation at the side, in internal and external rotation in abduction, in cross-body adduction, and in flexion.

Surgical findings include adhesions in the humeroscapular motion interface, especially between the subscapularis and the coracoid muscles. The undersurface of the coracoacromial arch is smooth. The rotator cuff is intact. The capsule is contracted, limiting the range of motion. The glenohumeral joint surfaces are normal.

## OPERATION

Under satisfactory anesthesia, the patient is placed in a low beach chair position with the glenohumeral joint at the edge of the operating table (**Fig. 7–1**). The entire forequarter is carefully prepped and draped in the usual sterile fashion with the arm free to be moved. The shoulder is approached through a standard deltopectoral incision along a line connecting the mid-clavicle to the mid-lateral humerus at the deltoid tubercle (**Fig. 7–2**).

The shoulder is released in four successive steps until the desired range of motion is achieved.

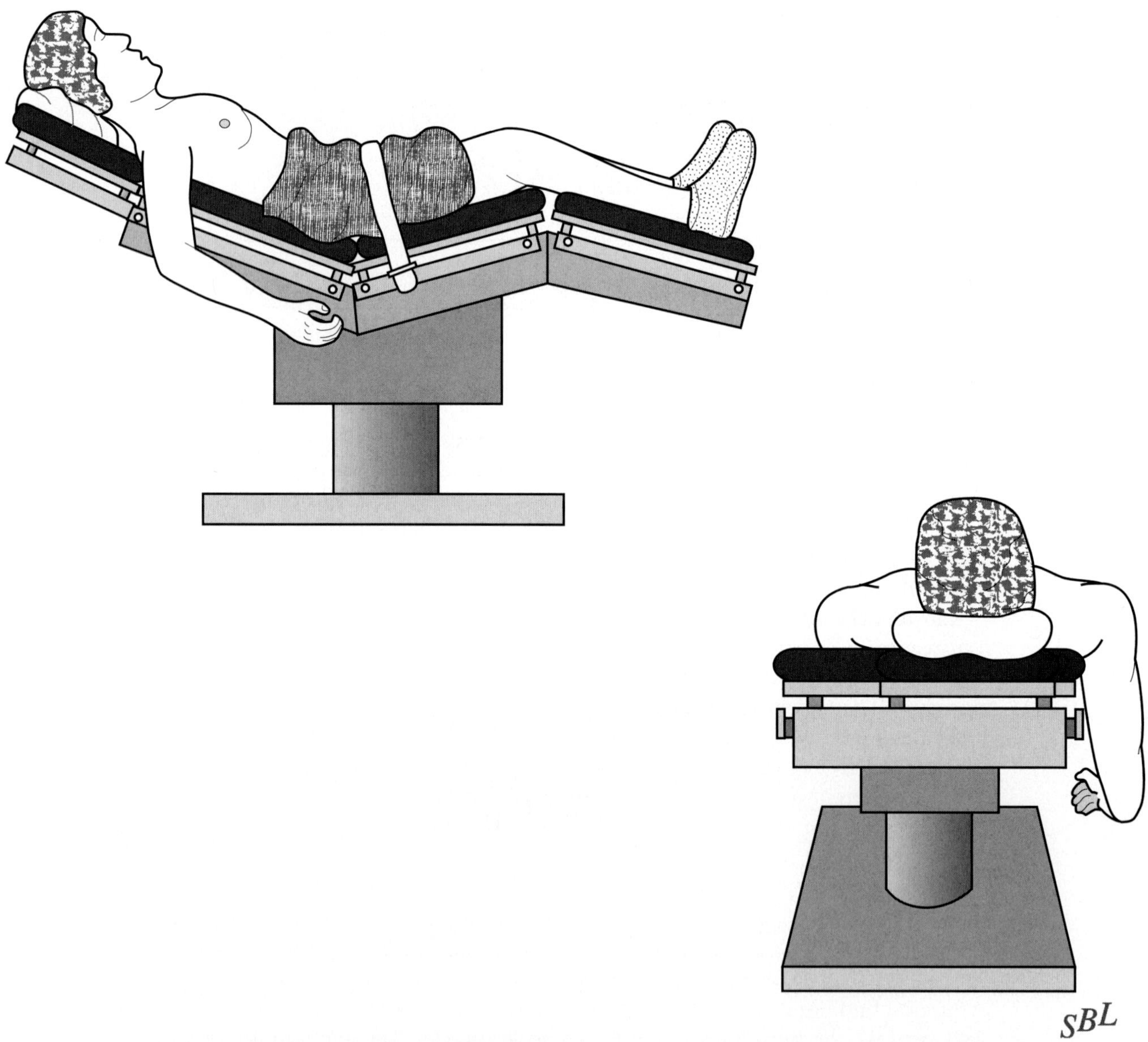


**Figure 7–1. The beach chair position for surgery**
The patient is placed in a comfortable position, as in a beach chair, with the thorax angled 30 degrees above the horizontal. The neck is in neutral position. The glenohumeral joint is at the edge of the table, and the arm is completely free. Compressive stockings (not shown here) are applied to the legs. This position allows the skin preparation to be applied to the entire shoulder girdle and arm.

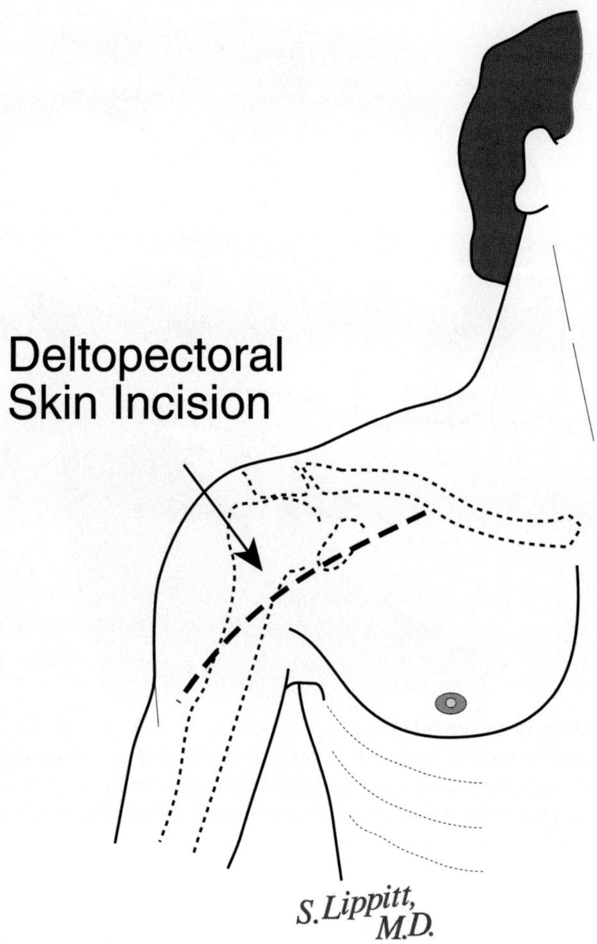


**Figure 7–2. The skin incision**
The skin incision overlies the deltopectoral groove and the tip of the coracoid process from mid-clavicle to mid-humerus. It is well away from the axilla. (From Matsen FA, Lippitt SB, Sidles JA, et al [eds]: Practical Evaluation and Management of the Shoulder. Philadelphia: WB Saunders, 1994, p. 202.)

## Stage 1

The adhesions in the humeroscapular motion interface are resected, leaving smooth surfaces on its concave and convex sides. Particular attention is paid to releasing the adhesions between the coracoid muscles and the subscapularis. The axillary nerve is identified medially as it runs across the subscapularis and laterally as it exits the quadrilateral space; it is protected throughout the case. To verify the completeness of the humeroscapular motion interface, an index finger is passed from the nerve medially, under the coracoacromial arch, and to the nerve posteriorly: a "nerve-to-nerve" release (**Fig. 7–3**).

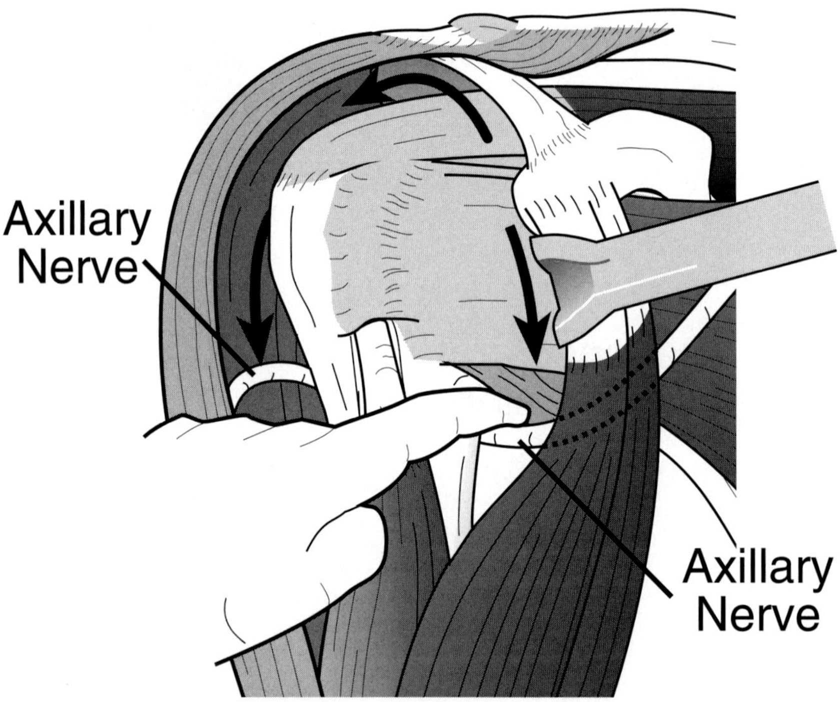


**Figure 7–3. Nerve-to-nerve release**
The humeroscapular motion interface is freed of all adhesions from the axillary nerve medially, underneath the coracoacromial arch, to the axillary nerve laterally. (Modified from Matsen FA, Lippitt SB, Sidles JA, et al [eds]: Practical Evaluation and Management of the Shoulder. Philadelphia: WB Saunders, 1994, p. 138.)

### Stage 2

The coracohumeral ligament is released from the coracoid process so that the subscapularis and supraspinatus can pass smoothly by the coracoid process (**Fig. 7–4**).

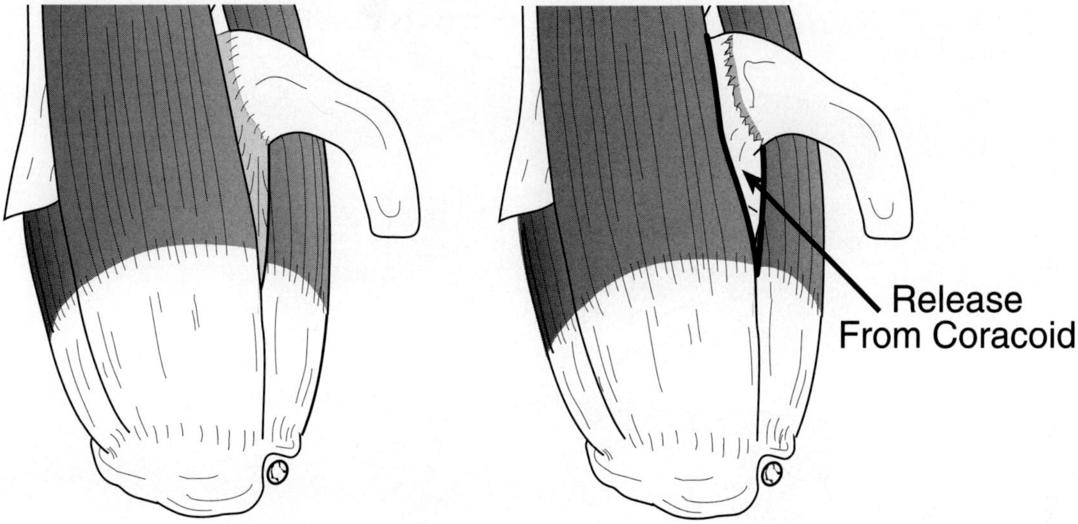


**Figure 7–4. Release of the coracohumeral ligament**
The coracohumeral ligament is completely released from the coracoid, allowing the subscapularis and the supraspinatus to glide by the coracoid.

### Stage 3

The subscapularis and subjacent capsule are incised near their insertion to the lesser tuberosity (**Fig. 7–5**). A 360-degree subscapularis release is performed, successively incising the superior, middle, and inferior glenohumeral ligaments (**Fig. 7–6**).

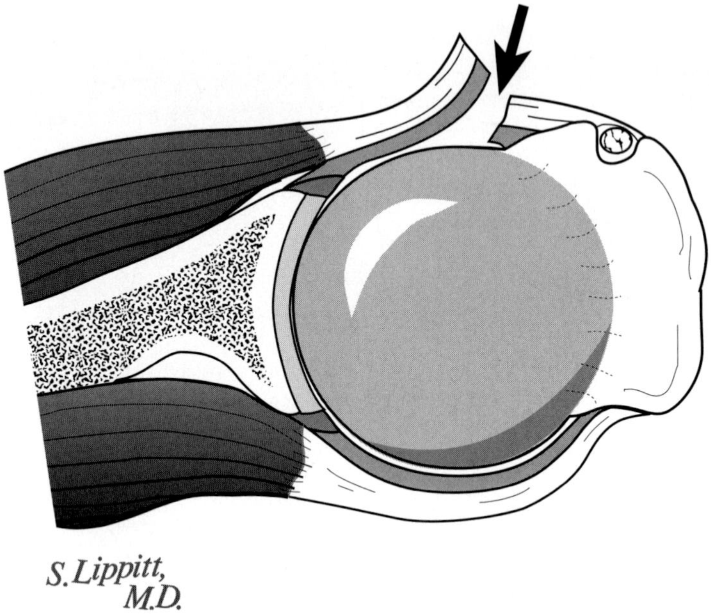


**Figure 7–5. Subscapularis incision**
The subscapularis tendon and subjacent capsule are incised near their insertion to the lesser tuberosity.

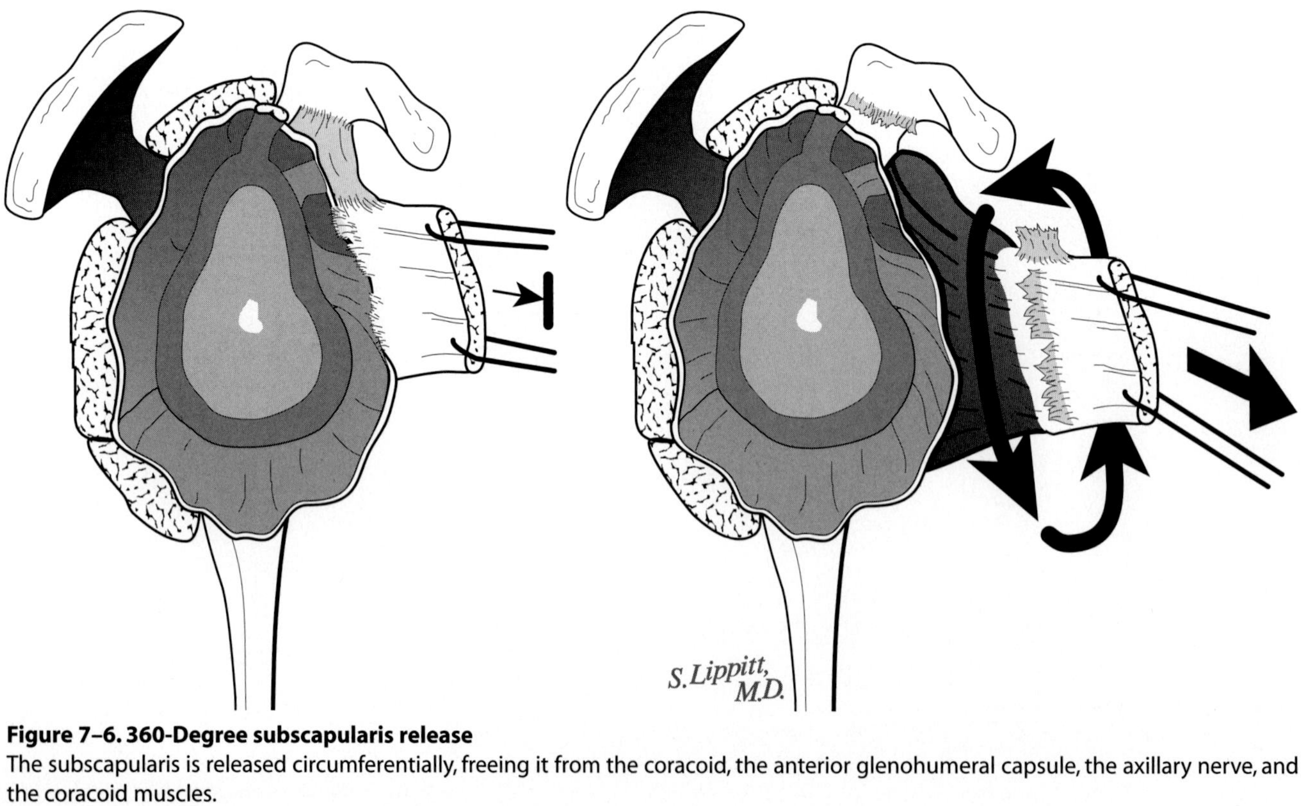


**Figure 7–6. 360-Degree subscapularis release**
The subscapularis is released circumferentially, freeing it from the coracoid, the anterior glenohumeral capsule, the axillary nerve, and the coracoid muscles.

## Stage 4

The glenohumeral capsule is incised just lateral to the labrum, starting anterosuperiorly and continuing around the glenoid until full motion is achieved. The labrum is left intact to the bony glenoid to preserve the glenoid concavity (**Figs. 7–7, 7–8, 7–9, and 7–10**).

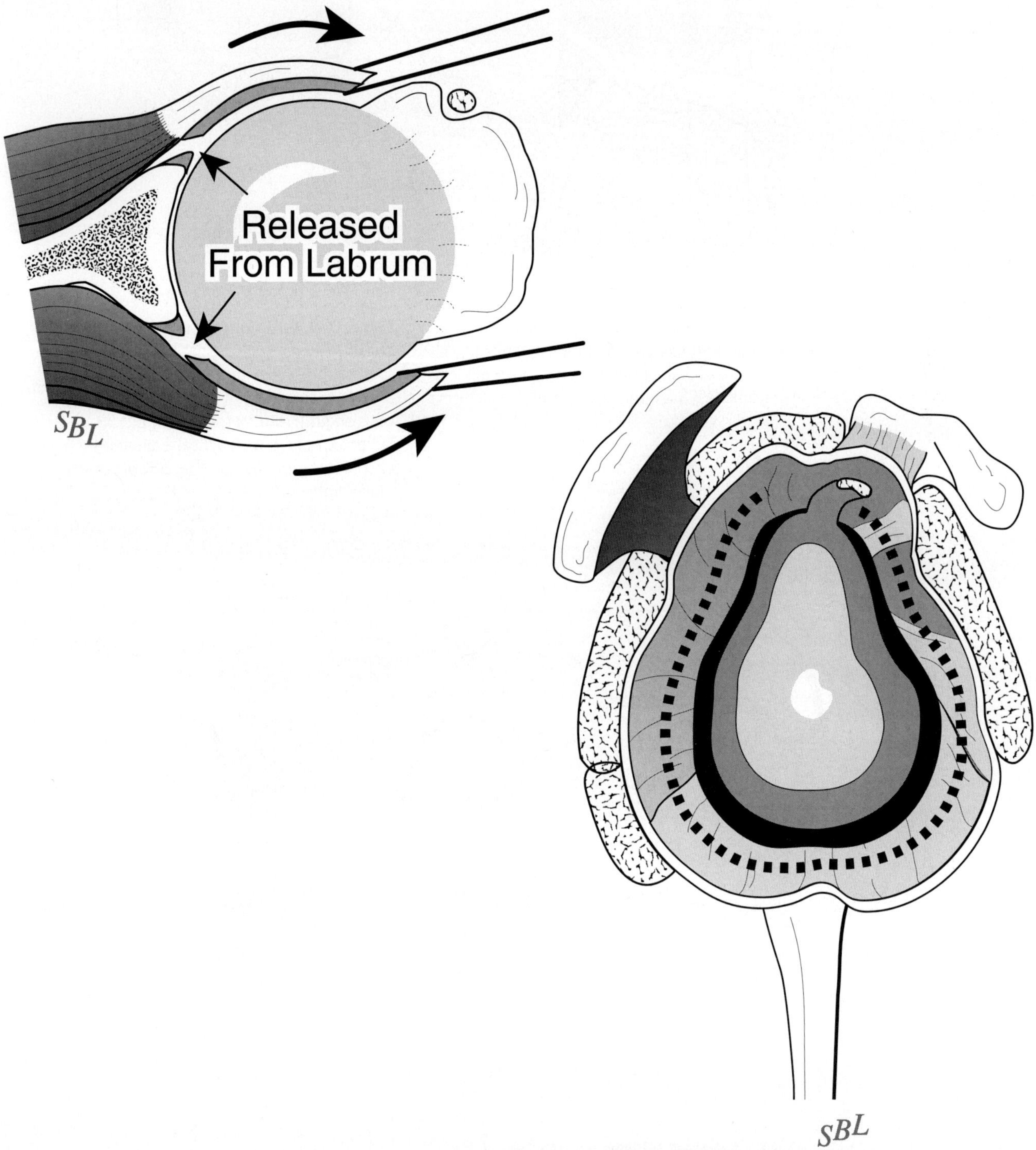


**Figure 7–7. Extralabral capsular release**
The capsule is incised from the glenoid labrum so that motion is restored without compromising the intrinsic stability of the glenoid fossa. (Modified from Matsen FA, Lippitt SB, Sidles JA, et al [eds]: Practical Evaluation and Management of the Shoulder. Philadelphia: WB Saunders, 1994, p. 138; and from Rockwood CA, Matsen FA [eds]: The Shoulder, 2nd ed. Philadelphia: WB Saunders, 1998, p. 811.)

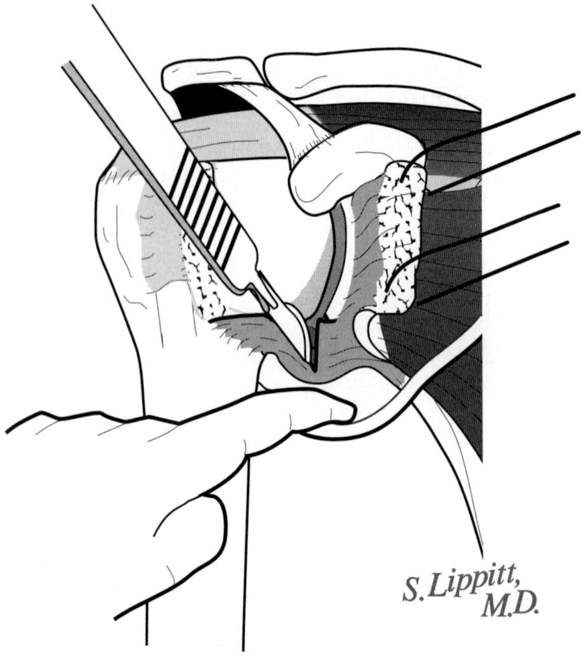


**Figure 7–8. Inferior capsular release**
The inferior capsule is released under direct vision while the axillary nerve is protected. (Modified from Matsen FA, Lippitt SB, Sidles JA, et al [eds]: Practical Evaluation and Management of the Shoulder. Philadelphia: WB Saunders, 1994, p. 205.)

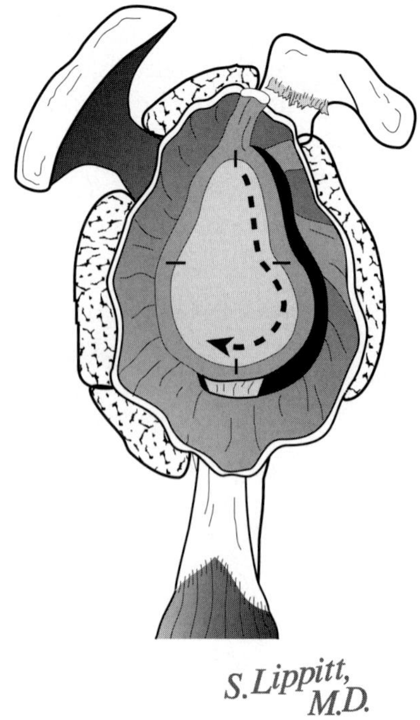


**Figure 7–9. Anterior capsular release**
The anterior capsule is released from the root of the biceps around the glenoid anteriorly to the point just past the triceps origin. (From Matsen FA, Lippitt SB, Sidles JA, et al [eds]: Practical Evaluation and Management of the Shoulder. Philadelphia: WB Saunders, 1994, p. 205.)

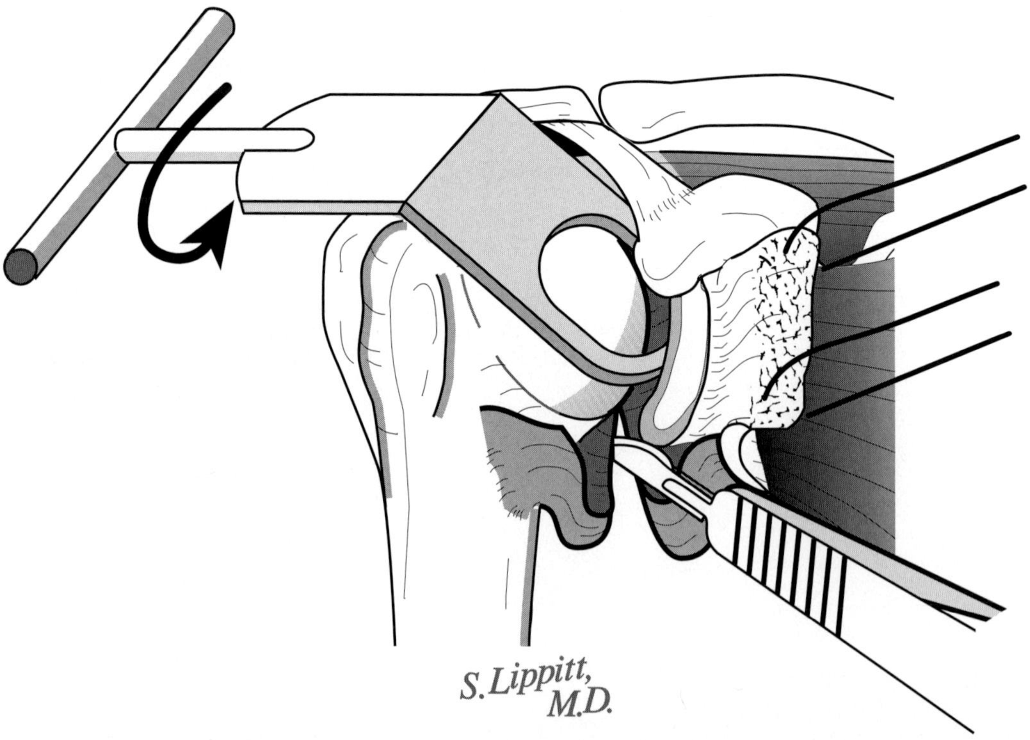


**Figure 7–10. Posterior capsular release**
The posterior capsular release is accomplished under direct vision. The capsule is exposed and put under tension by twisting the inferior aspect of the humeral head retractor away from the glenoid. (Modified from Matsen FA, Lippitt SB, Sidles JA, et al [eds]: Practical Evaluation and Management of the Shoulder. Philadelphia: WB Saunders, 1994, p. 205.)

After these releases, the glenohumeral range of motion includes at least 40 degrees of external rotation, with the subscapularis approximated to its intended reattachment site (**Fig. 7–11**), 60 degrees of internal rotation with the arm in 90 degrees of abduction (**Fig. 7–12**), and 140 degrees of flexion (**Fig. 7–13**).

The joint is carefully inspected to ensure that no cartilaginous or bony irregularities restrict the range of glenohumeral motion.

The wound is thoroughly irrigated. The subscapularis is securely repaired using six sutures of #2 braided nonabsorbable suture. This secure repair allows immediate postoperative motion to be conducted without concern about disrupting the reattachment.

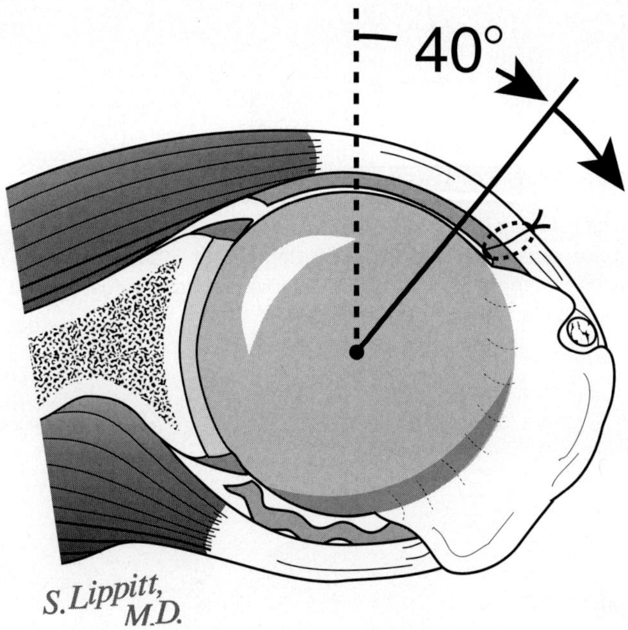


**Figure 7–11. External rotation of 40 degrees**
The subscapularis is repaired, ensuring that the humerus can be easily externally rotated to at least 40 degrees. (Modified from Matsen FA, Lippitt SB, Sidles JA, et al [eds]: Practical Evaluation and Management of the Shoulder. Philadelphia: WB Saunders, 1994, p. 50.)

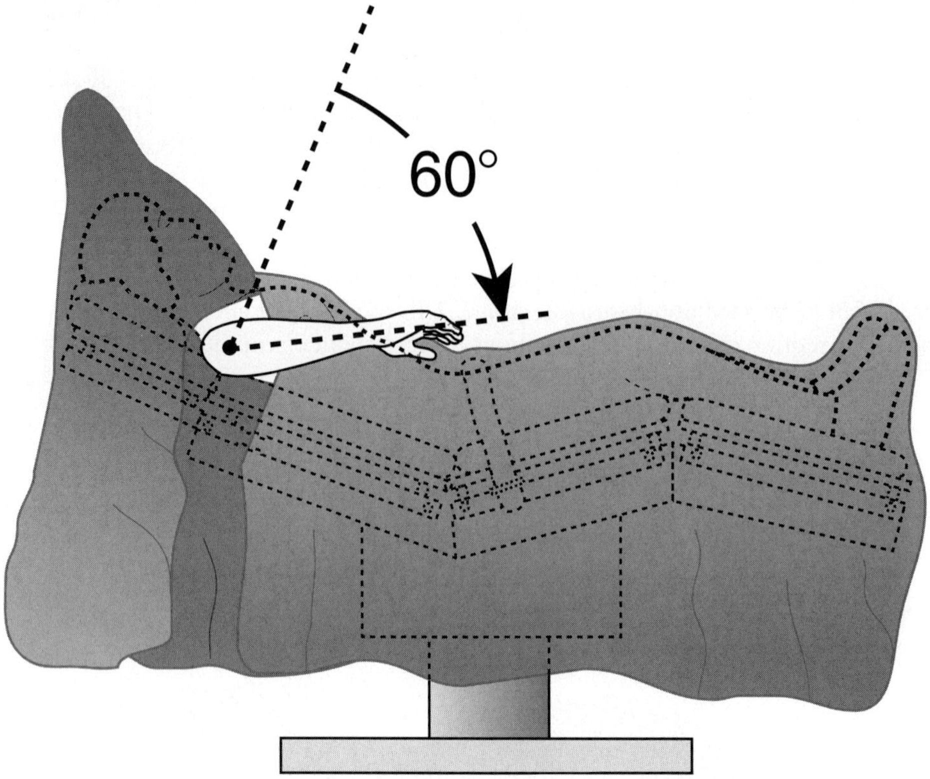


**Figure 7–12. Internal rotation in abduction of 60 degrees**
The released posterior capsule should allow 60 degrees of internal rotation in abduction. (Modified from Matsen FA, Lippitt SB, Sidles JA, et al [eds]: Practical Evaluation and Management of the Shoulder. Philadelphia: WB Saunders, 1994, p. 46.)

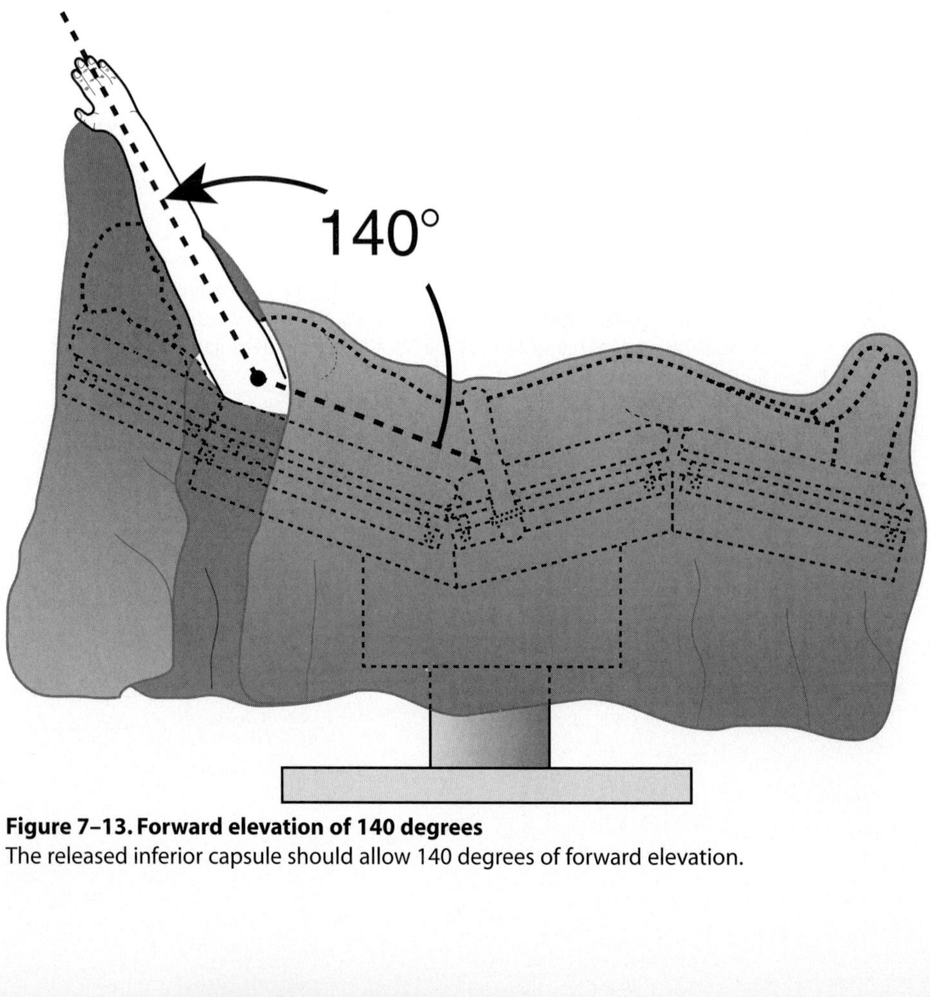


**Figure 7–13. Forward elevation of 140 degrees**
The released inferior capsule should allow 140 degrees of forward elevation.

The wound is again irrigated and closed in layers. Dry sterile dressings are applied, and the patient is returned to the recovery room with the arm in continuous passive motion (**Fig. 7–14**).

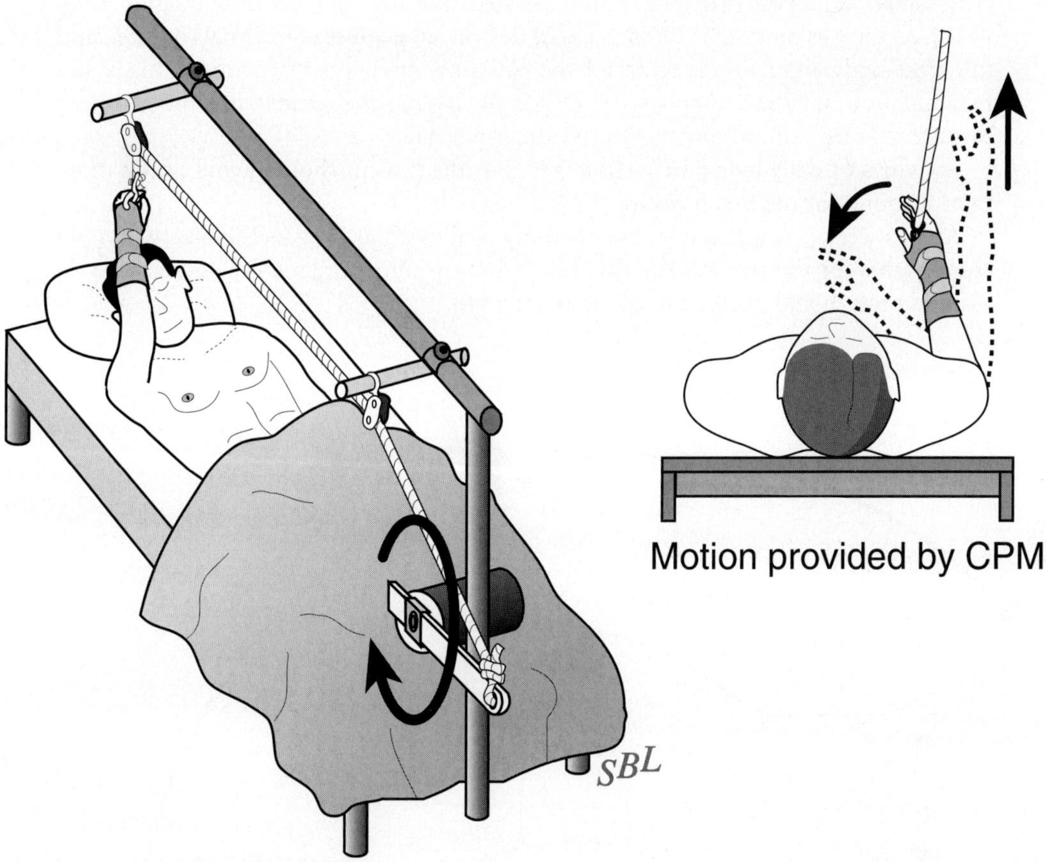


**Figure 7–14. Continuous passive motion**
Continuous passive motion is started immediately after surgery and continued for 36 hours when the patient is in bed. The range of motion is from adduction and internal rotation across the abdomen to 90 degrees of flexion and neutral rotation. (From Matsen FA, Lippitt SB, Sidles JA, et al [eds]: Practical Evaluation and Management of the Shoulder. Philadelphia: WB Saunders, 1994, p. 50.)

## POSTOPERATIVE PLAN

Continuous passive motion is continued while the patient is in bed for the first 36 hours after surgery. It is removed when the patient is in a chair or ambulating.

On the day of surgery, the patient begins the full motion program with flexion to 140 degrees (**Fig. 7–15**), assisted external rotation to 40 degrees (**Fig. 7–16**), assisted cross-body adduction (**Fig. 7–17**), and assisted internal rotation in abduction (**Fig. 7–18**). As soon as motion of 140 degrees of flexion, 40 degrees of external rotation, and full cross-body adduction is achieved, the patient is discharged to continue his or her rehabilitation at home. Emphasis is placed on having the patient put the shoulder through its range of motion at least five times per day.

Activities of daily living are encouraged, but the patient should avoid lifting more than 1 pound for the first 6 weeks.

After 6 weeks, progressively more activity is allowed as long as these activities are comfortable for the patient. For the first 3 months after surgery, the emphasis is on assisted motion and comfort rather than strength.

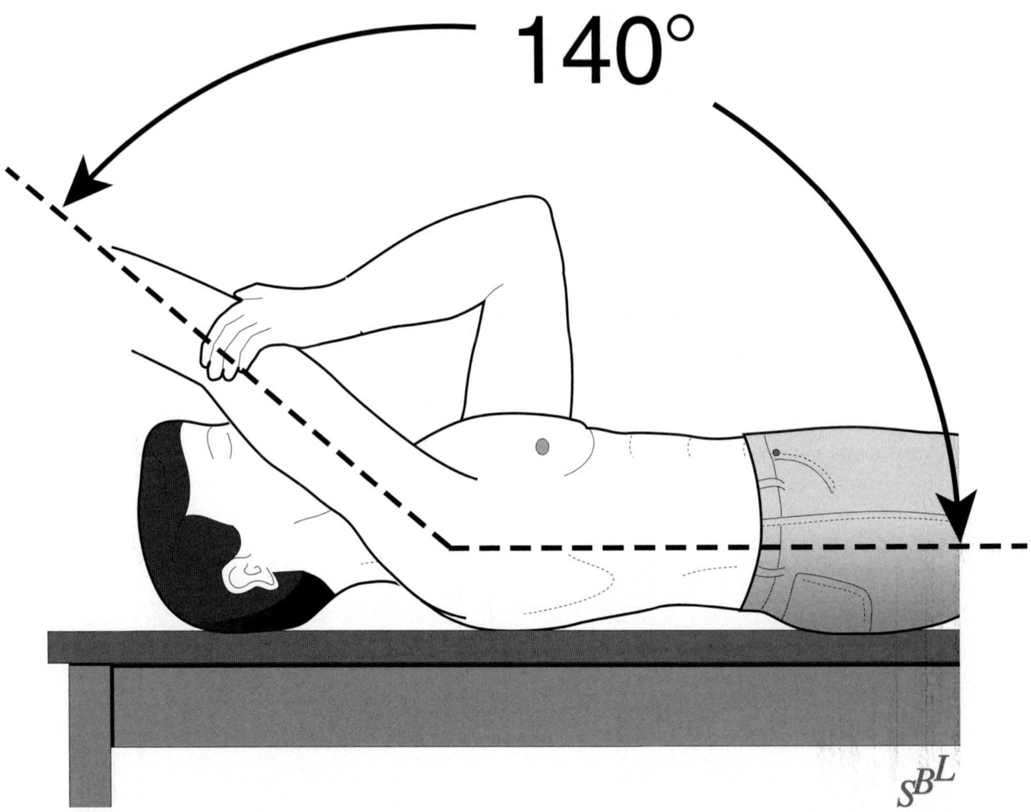


**Figure 7–15. Assisted forward elevation**
The sound arm helps the operated arm to 140 degrees of forward elevation. (Modified from Matsen FA, Lippitt SB, Sidles JA, et al [eds]: Practical Evaluation and Management of the Shoulder. Philadelphia: WB Saunders, 1994, p. 46.)

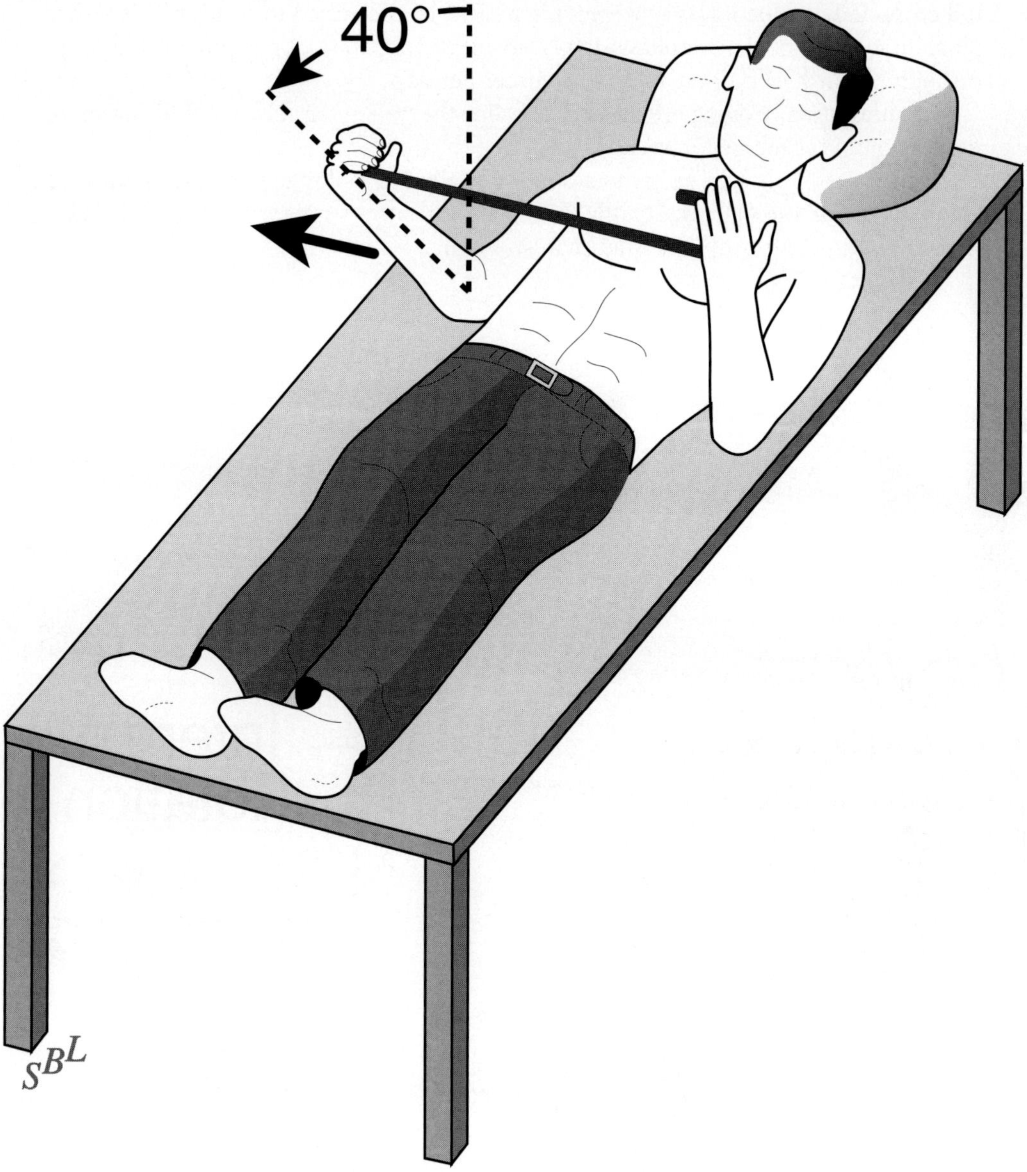


**Figure 7–16. Assisted external elevation**
The sound arm helps the operated arm to 40 degrees of external rotation using a cane or yardstick. Each elbow should be held in a position of 90 degrees of flexion. (Modified from Matsen FA, Lippitt SB, Sidles JA, et al [eds]: Practical Evaluation and Management of the Shoulder. Philadelphia: WB Saunders, 1994, p. 47.)

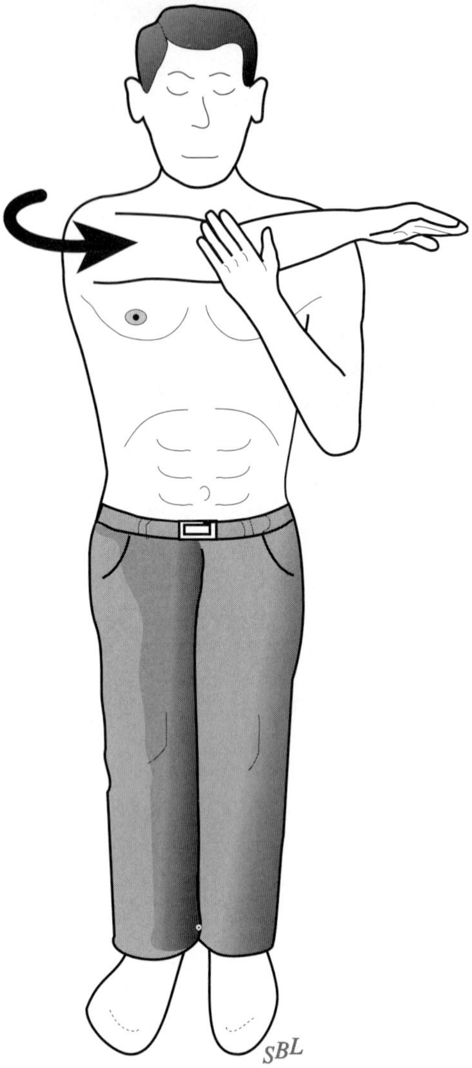


**Figure 7–17. Assisted cross-body adduction**
The sound arm draws the operated arm across the body to the point where it matches the normal arm. (Modified from Matsen FA, Lippitt SB, Sidles JA, et al [eds]: Practical Evaluation and Management of the Shoulder. Philadelphia: WB Saunders, 1994, p. 47.)

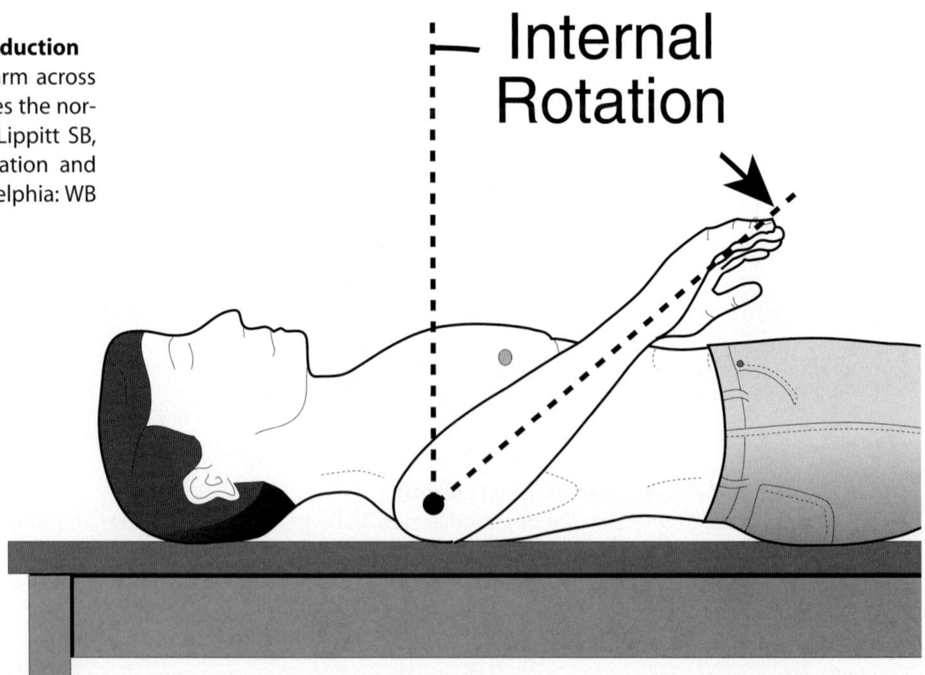


**Figure 7–18. Internal rotation in abduction**
The abducted arm is passively internally rotated to stretch the posterior capsule. (From Rockwood CA, Matsen FA [eds]: The Shoulder, 2nd ed. Philadelphia: WB Saunders, 1998, p. 1083.)

# PART III

# STABILITY

CHAPTER 8

# Principles of Glenohumeral Stability

## CONCEPTS

Ideally, a glenohumeral joint will enjoy a wide range of rotation and still remain precisely centered within the socket. As was detailed in the section on Principles of Glenohumeral Mobility, translational and rotational laxity of the glenohumeral joint are related: because of the relatively flat glenoid socket, the joint capable of rotation can also be translated. In this section, we will clarify how the lax joint can also be stable.

### A Ball within a Ball

Glenohumeral *stability* is the ability to center the humeral head on the articular surface of the scapula. The *center of rotation of the humeral head* is the center of the spherical convexity that best fits its articular surface (**Fig. 8–1**). The tuberosities and the rotator cuff establish another spherical convexity, the *proximal humeral convexity*, the radius of which is equal to the radius of the humeral head plus the thickness of the cuff tendons (which is the same as the height of the tuberosities) (**Fig. 8–2**). The *center of rotation of the glenoid* is the center of the spherical concavity that best fits the glenoid articular surface (**Fig. 8–3**). The *center of rotation of the coracoacromial arch* is the center of the spherical concavity that best fits the underside of the coracoacromial arch (**Fig. 8–4**). In normal shoulder function, the spherical humeral articular surface articulates with the spherical concavity of the glenoid while the proximal humeral convexity articulates with the spherical concavity of the coracoacromial arch (**Fig. 8–4**)—two concentric spherical articulations. The shoulder joint is stable when the centers of these four spheres remain coincident with each other while the upper extremity carries out its activities.

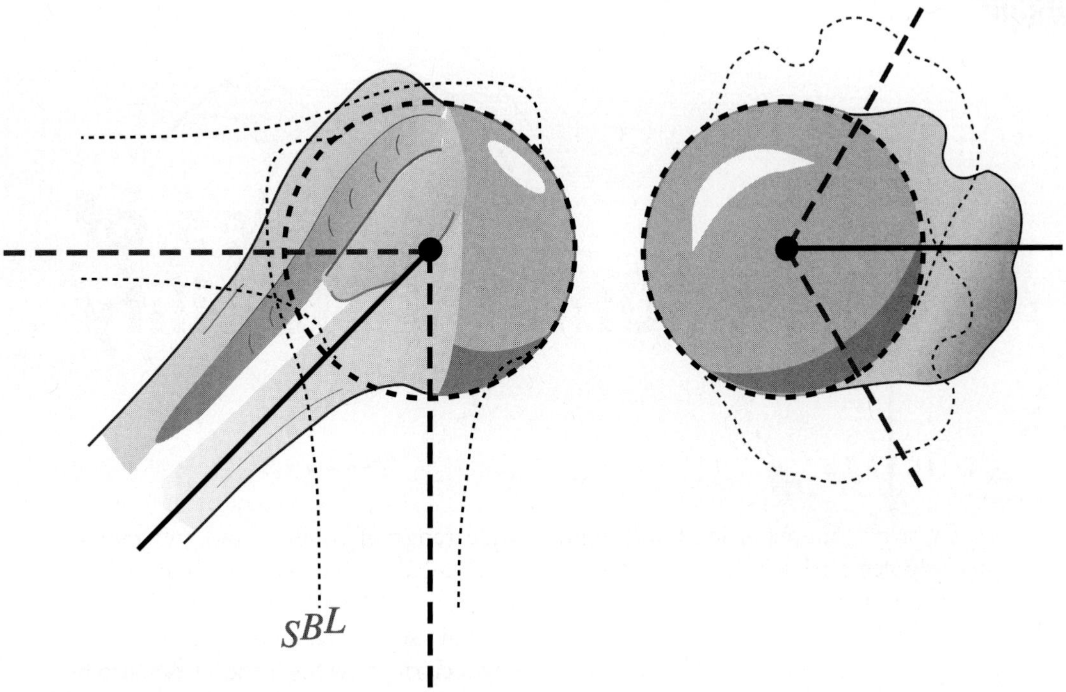


**Figure 8–1. The humeral articular convexity**
The rotational center of the humeral articular surface is the center of the sphere that best fits the articular surface (the articular surface sphere).

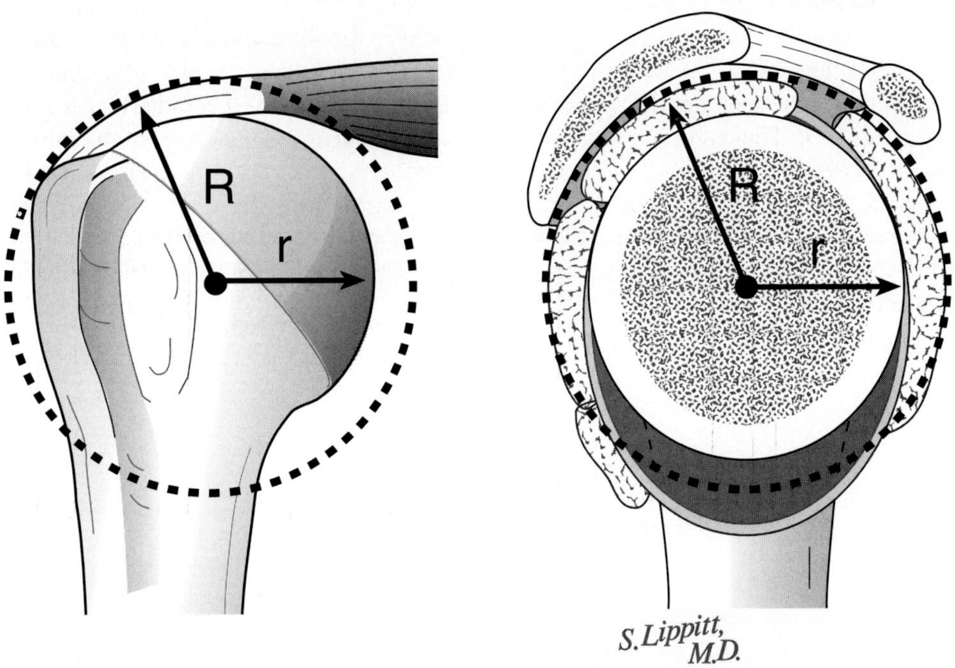


**Figure 8–2. The proximal humeral convexity**
The rotational center of the proximal humeral convexity is the center of the sphere that best fits the tuberosities and the cuff tendons near their insertion. The radius of the proximal humeral convexity (R) should be equal to the radius of the humeral articular surface sphere (r) plus the thickness of the rotator cuff tendons.

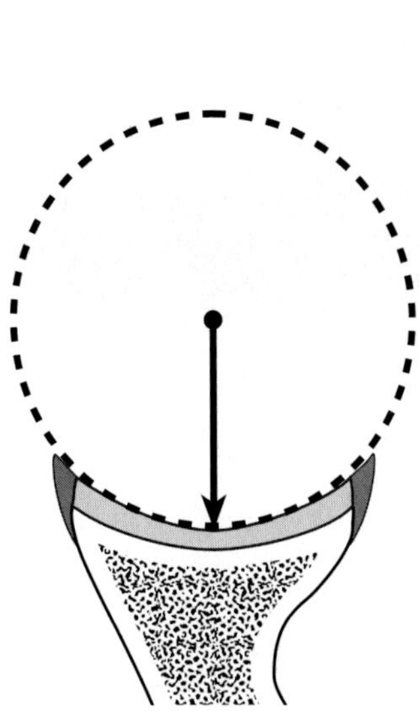

**Figure 8–3. The glenoid concavity**
The center of rotation of the glenoid is the center of the spherical concavity that best fits the glenoid articular surface.

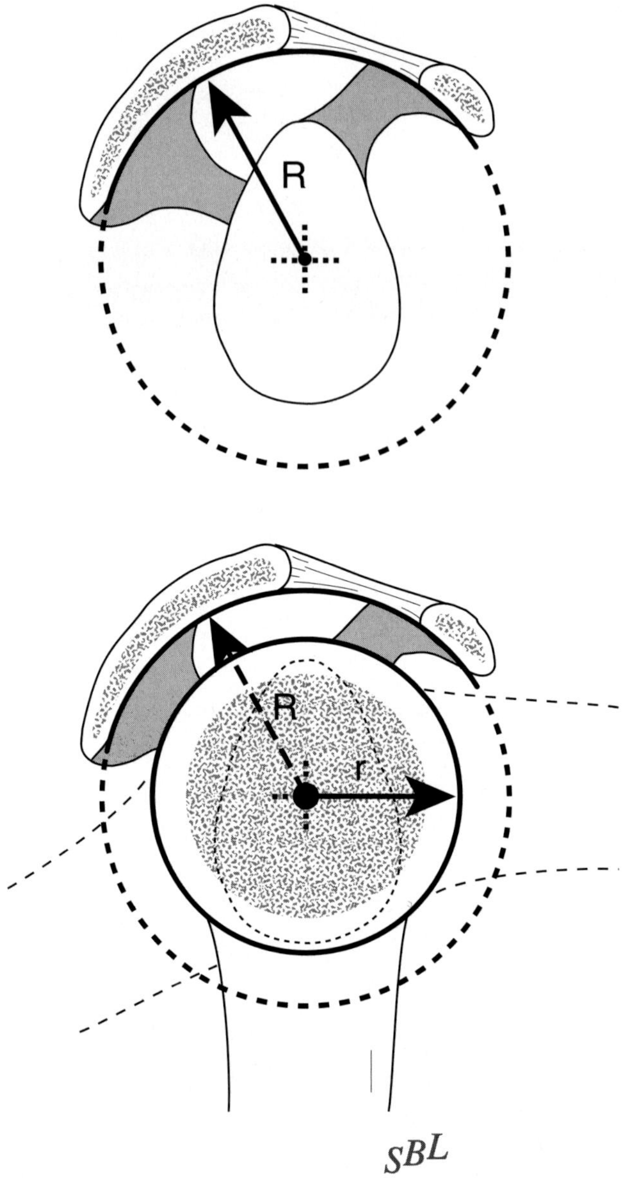


**Figure 8–4. The coracoacromial concavity**
The center of the coracoacromial concavity is the center of the sphere that best fits the concave undersurface of the coracoacromial arch. (From Rockwood CA, Matsen FA [eds]: The Shoulder, 2nd ed. Philadelphia: WB Saunders, 1998, p. 764.)

This double articular system provides support for substantial forces directed medially or superiorly, or both. The combination of a spherical concavity and a force pressing the spherical convexity into it centers the convexity by the concavity compression mechanism, like pressing a baseball into a catcher's mitt or pressing a golf ball into a golf tee. Compression of the ball into the socket prevents translation away from the centered position (**Fig. 8–5**).

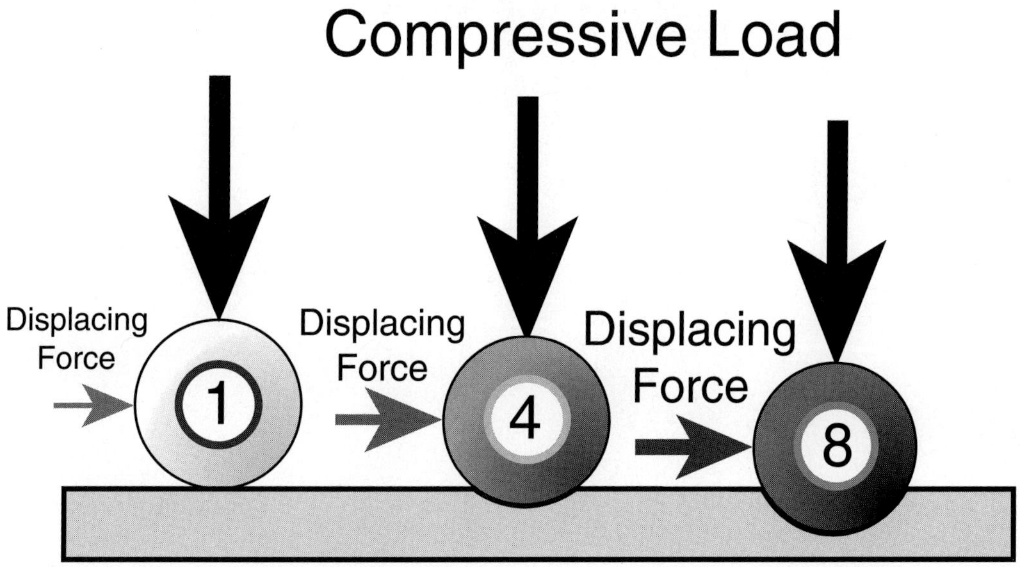


**Figure 8–5. Concavity and compression**
In the absence of a concavity, only a minimal translational force is required to displace the sphere. As the concavity becomes deeper, a greater displacing force is required for a given compressive load.

The deltoid is the major compressor into the coracoacromial arch concavity, while the rotator cuff is the major compressor into the glenoid concavity (**Figs. 8–6** and **8–7**).

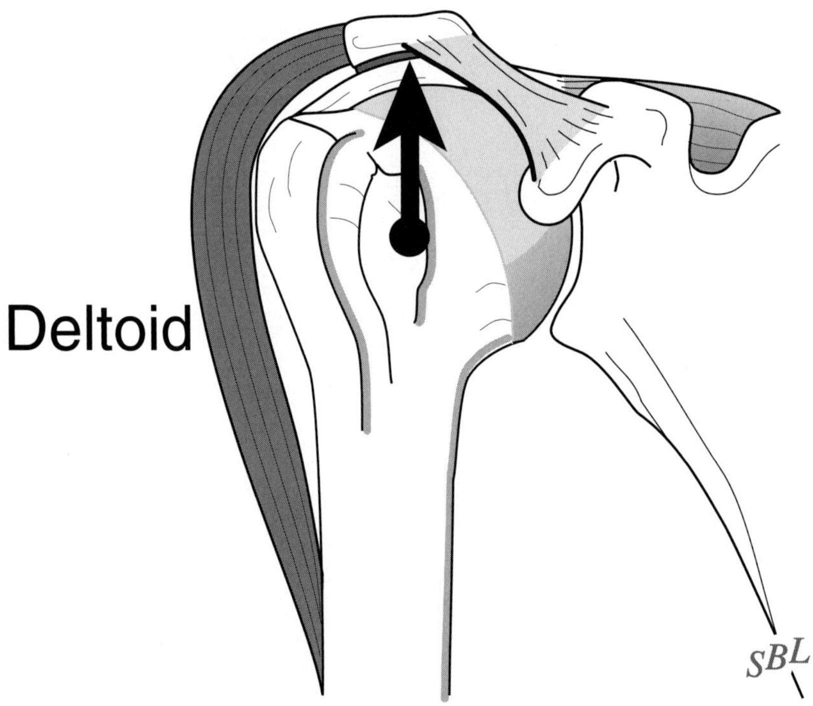


**Figure 8–6. Compression into the coracoacromial concavity**
The deltoid compresses the proximal humeral convexity into the coracoacromial concavity.

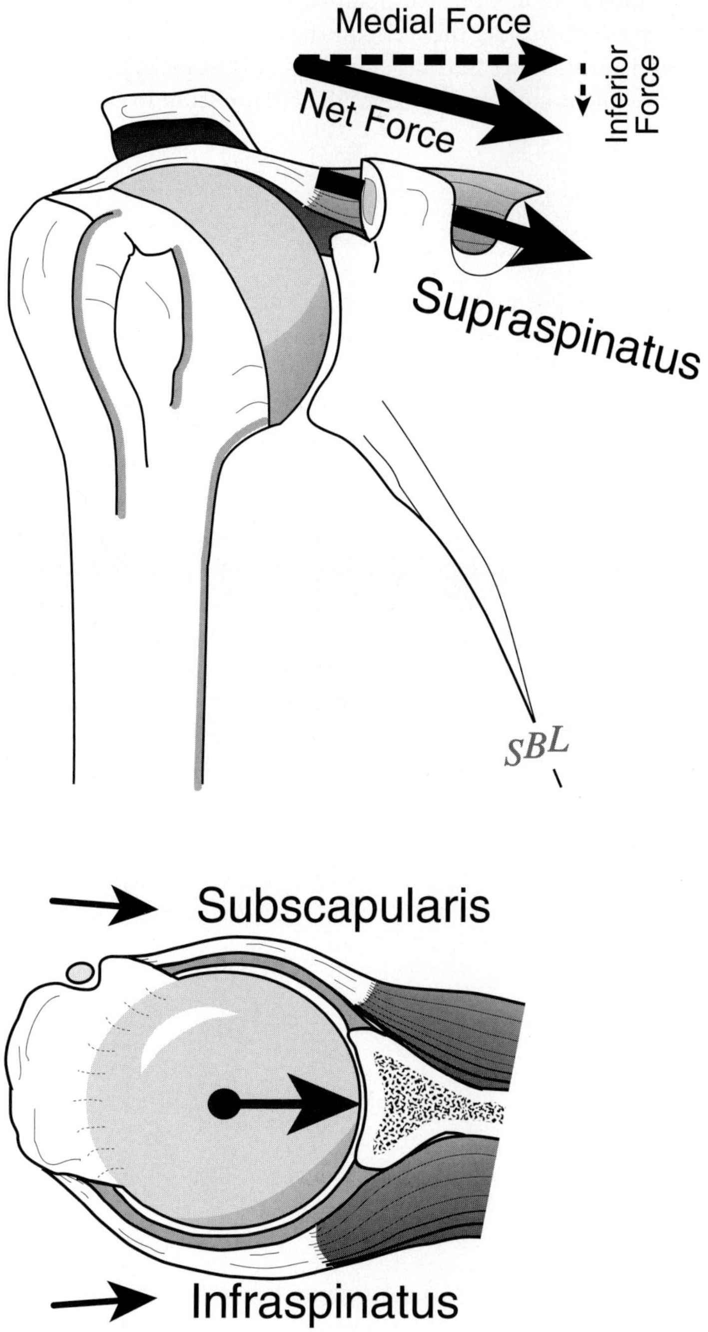


**Figure 8–7. Compression into the glenoid concavity**
The rotator cuff compresses the humeral articular convexity into the glenoid concavity. (Modified from Matsen FA, Lippitt SB, Sidles JA, et al [eds]: Practical Evaluation and Management of the Shoulder. Philadelphia: WB Saunders, 1994, p. 70; and from Rockwood CA, Matsen FA [eds]: The Shoulder, 2nd ed. Philadelphia: WB Saunders, 1998, p. 638.)

## The Load and Shift Tests

The efficacy of the concavity compression stabilization mechanism for a glenoid can be demonstrated in the living (or cadaveric) shoulder by (1) noting the anterior, posterior, and inferior translational laxity of the relaxed shoulder in the mid-range of glenohumeral motion (anterior and posterior drawer and sulcus tests) and then (2) noting the resistance to translation in each of these directions away from the centered position when the humeral head is pressed manually into the glenoid concavity. Absence of resistance to translation under these circumstances suggests a deficient glenoid concavity **(Fig. 8–8)**. The difference in translation between the laxity tests and the load and shift tests indicates the importance of concavity compression in centering the head in the glenoid.

## Optimizing Compression

As will be seen in the subsequent sections, the primary mechanism for centering the humeral head is compression of the humeral head in the glenoid concavity. The vector sum of all the forces acting on the humeral head is the net humeral joint reaction force. The humerus is stable in the glenoid concavity when the net humeral joint reaction force vector is within the balance stability angle of the glenoid (see next section). The body's control over the direction of the net humeral joint reaction force depends on (1) having adequate strength of the primary compressors (the supraspinatus, subscapularis, and infraspinatus), (2) having the coordination to contract these muscles so that their net vector lies within the balance stability angle, and (3) having the strength and coordination to orient the glenoid in the desired direction. If a glenoid concavity does not offer a substantial balance stability angle (for example, when the glenoid lip is excessively compliant in a case of multidirectional atraumatic glenohumeral instability), a physical training program may be quite effective by optimizing all three of the factors. Rotator strengthening exercises, scapular motor strengthening exercises, and coordination exercises often enable the patient with atraumatic instability to re-achieve the lost stability.

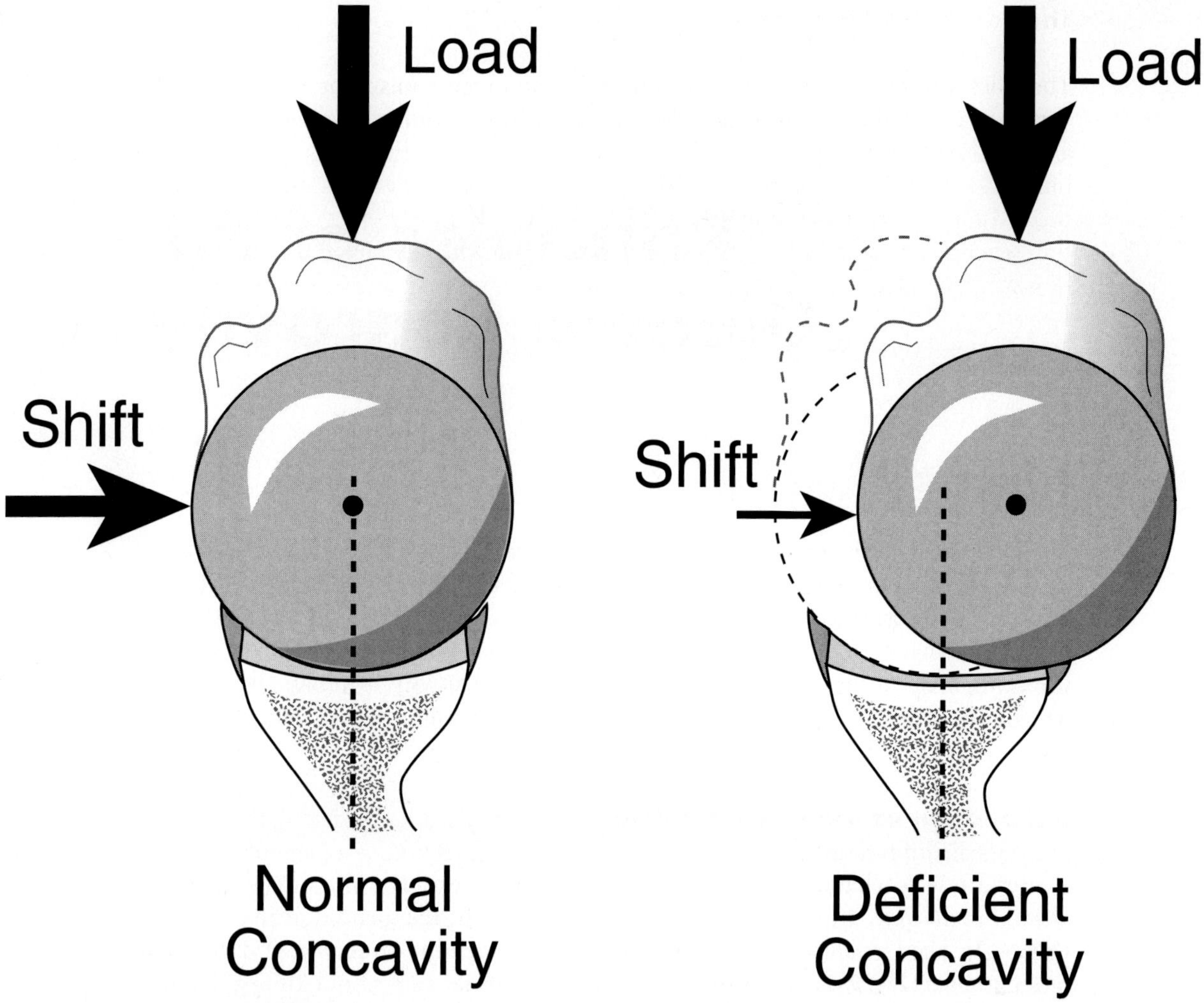


**Figure 8–8. The load and shift test**
When the normally concave glenoid is loaded in compression, a substantial force is required to shift the humeral head from its centered position (*left*). When the glenoid concavity is deficient, less force is required to shift the head from its centered position (*right*). (From Rockwood CA, Matsen FA [eds]: The Shoulder, 2nd ed. Philadelphia: WB Saunders, 1998, p. 1083.)

CHAPTER 9

# Principles of the Glenoid Concavity

## CONCEPTS

The glenoid concavity can be characterized by its orientation, shape, and size.

The glenoid concavity is formed by the sum of the contributions of the glenoid bone, glenoid cartilage, and glenoid labrum (**Fig. 9–1**). In a cadaver model system, we have found that even the simple incision of the glenoid labrum from its attachment to the glenoid compromises the ability of the glenoid concavity to center the humeral head. Loss of the cartilage of the glenoid rim further destabilizes the head.

### Orientation of the Glenoid Surface

A useful way to characterize the glenoid orientation considers the direction of the *glenoid center line*, a line perpendicular to the center of the glenoid at its midpoint (**Fig. 9–2**). The *version* of the glenoid is the angle between the center line and the *plane of the scapula* (**Fig. 9–3**). The usual center line extends laterally about 10 degrees posterior to the plane of the scapula and extends medially to exit the neck of the glenoid between the upper and lower crus of the scapula at what is called the *centering point* (**Fig. 9–4**). This centering point is a useful reference at surgery, especially when the surface anatomy is distorted (**Fig. 9–5**).

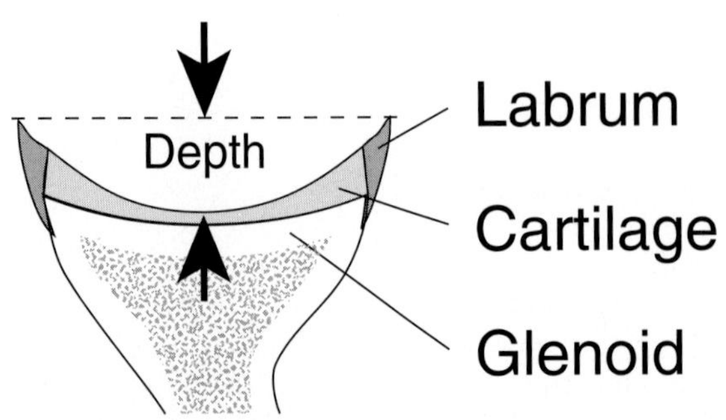


**Figure 9–1. Components of the glenoid fossa**
The glenoid fossa results from the relatively small concavity of the glenoid bone, deepened by the glenoid cartilage and by the labrum at its periphery. (Modified from Matsen FA, Lippitt SB, Sidles JA, et al [eds]: Practical Evaluation and Management of the Shoulder. Philadelphia: WB Saunders, 1994, p. 66.)

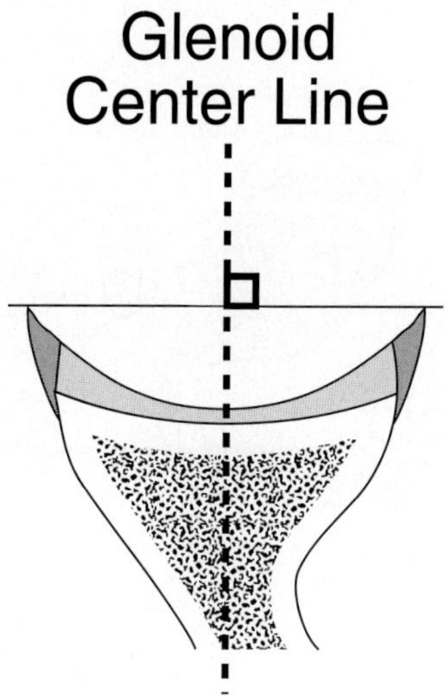


**Figure 9–2. The glenoid center line**
The glenoid center line is the line perpendicular to the surface of the glenoid at its midpoint. (Modified from Matsen FA, Lippitt SB, Sidles JA, et al [eds]: Practical Evaluation and Management of the Shoulder. Philadelphia: WB Saunders, 1994, p. 60.)

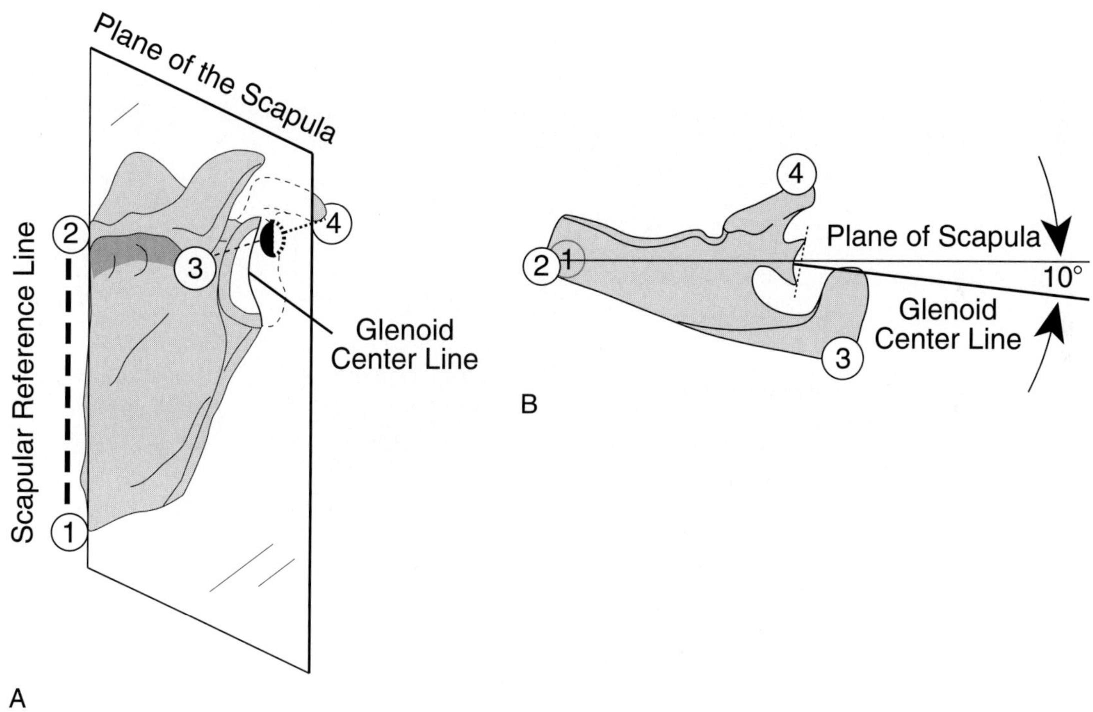


**Figure 9–3. The orientation of the glenoid center line with respect to the scapula**
The plane of the scapula is the plane passing through the inferior pole of the glenoid, through the medial extent of the spine of the scapula, and halfway between the coracoid tip and the posterior angle of the acromion. The glenoid center line lies laterally approximately 10 degrees posterior to this plane and perpendicular to the line connecting the inferior pole and the medial spine (the scapular reference line). (Modified from Matsen FA, Lippitt SB, Sidles JA, et al [eds]: Practical Evaluation and Management of the Shoulder. Philadelphia: WB Saunders, 1994, p. 30.)

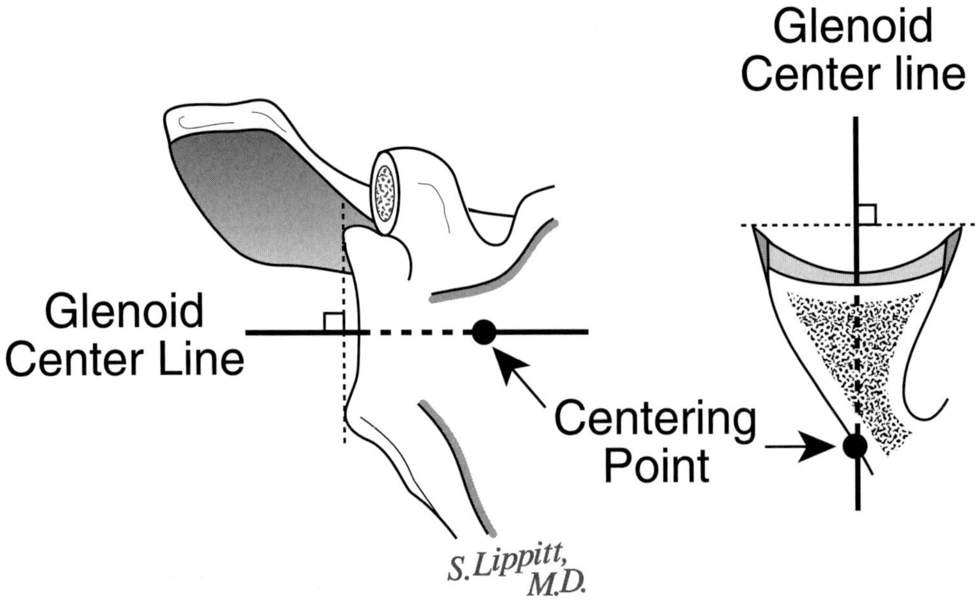


**Figure 9–4. The glenoid centering point**
The glenoid centering point is the point along the glenoid neck that is midway between the upper and lower crus of the scapula. The glenoid center line normally passes through the center of the glenoid articular surface and the centering point. (From Rockwood CA, Matsen FA [eds]: The Shoulder, 2nd ed. Philadelphia: WB Saunders, 1998, p. 850.)

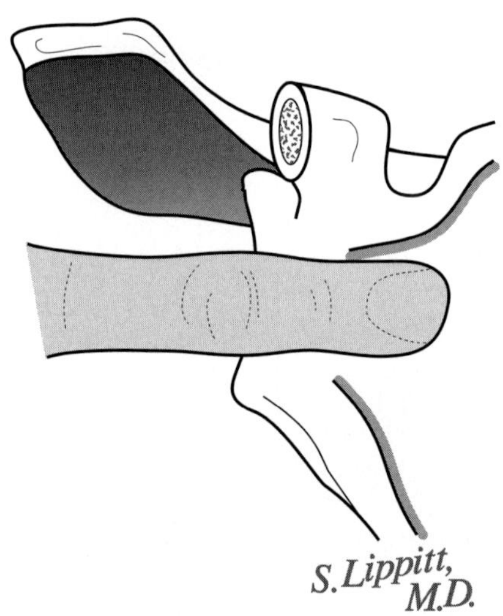


**Figure 9–5. Palpation of the glenoid centering point**
When the orientation of the glenoid surface is distorted, it is useful to orient the glenoid center line by palpating the centering point medially. This aspect of the scapula is rarely affected by arthritis or injury. (From Matsen FA, Lippitt SB, Sidles JA, et al [eds]: Practical Evaluation and Management of the Shoulder. Philadelphia: WB Saunders, 1994, p. 210.)

At rest, the scapular plane is usually directed about 30 degrees anterior to the thoracic plane (**Fig. 9–6**). In this position, the glenoid center line characteristically points 20 degrees anterior to the coronal plane, an orientation at which the glenoid can stabilize the humeral head during activities with the arm in front of the body. During shoulder activities, the scapulothoracic muscles position the scapula in a way that orients the glenoid optimally. For example, during the bench press, the pectoralis muscles can protract the scapula so that the glenoid directly supports the loaded humeral head (**Fig. 9–7**).

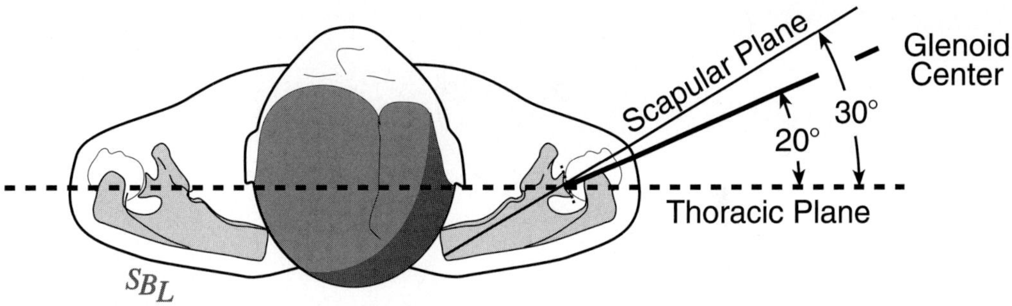


**Figure 9–6. The orientation of the glenoid center line with respect to the thorax**
While the glenoid center line passes laterally posterior to the plane of the scapula, it passes about 20° anterior to the thoracic (coronal) plane. This is because the scapular plane passes laterally about 30° anterior to the thoracic plane. This anteversion of the glenoid with respect to the body provides greater stability for the humeral head in anterior activities.

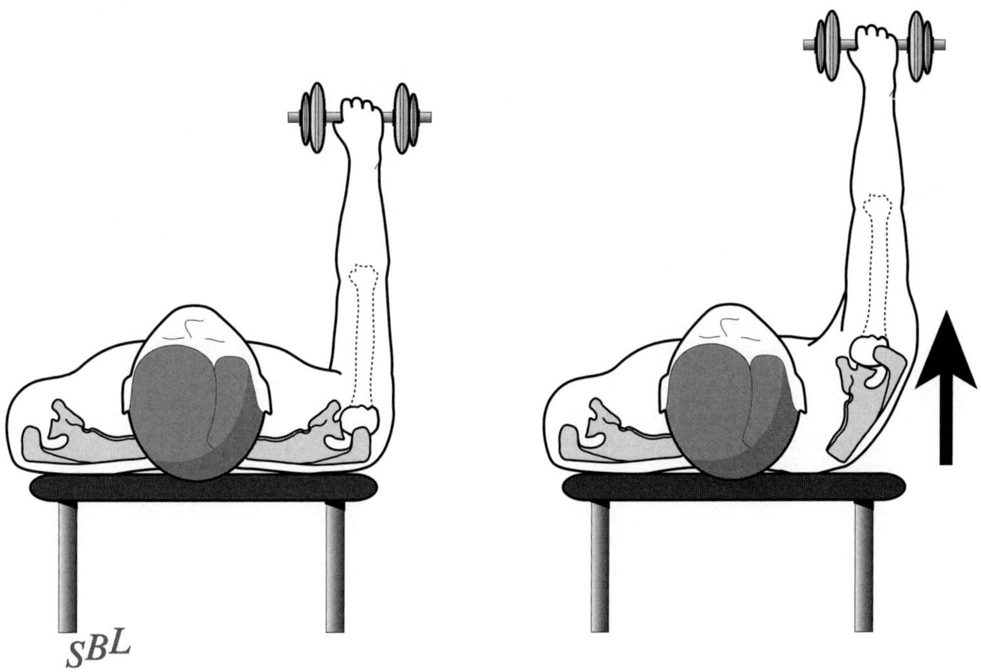


**Figure 9–7. The glenoid can be moved to support the net humeral joint reaction force**
Protraction of the scapula, for example in the bench press, places the glenoid fossa squarely beneath the force exerted on it by the loaded humerus. (From Matsen FA, Lippitt SB, Sidles JA, et al [eds]: Practical Evaluation and Management of the Shoulder. Philadelphia: WB Saunders, 1994, p. 87.)

### Net Humeral Joint Reaction Force

The net humeral joint reaction force is the vector sum of all the forces acting on the humeral head (**Fig. 9–8**).

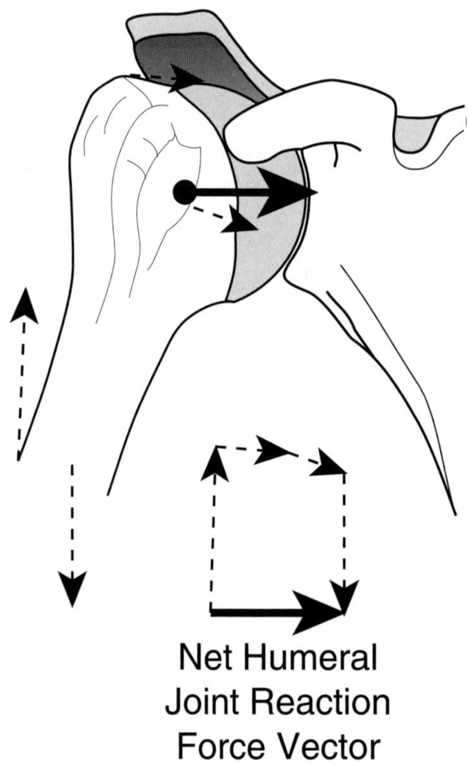


**Figure 9–8. Net humeral joint reaction force**
**A,** The vector sum of all the forces operating on the humerus is the net humeral joint reaction force. In this figure, the following forces are represented as dotted lines: the supraspinatus, the subscapularis, the deltoid, and the weight of the humerus. These sum to yield the net humeral joint reaction force (*dark arrow*).

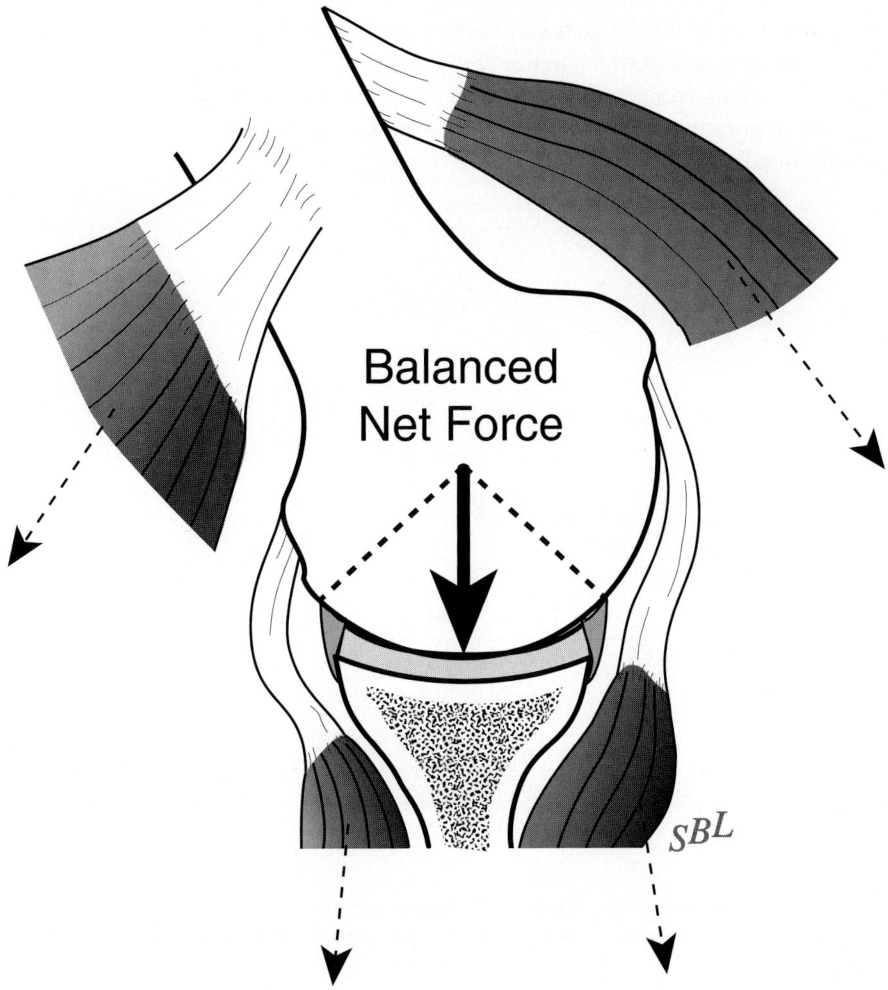


B

**Figure 9–8. Net humeral joint reaction force**—*Continued*

**B,** The shoulder is stable when the net humeral joint reaction force is contained within the glenoid. (Modified from Matsen FA, Lippitt SB, Sidles JA, et al [eds]: Practical Evaluation and Management of the Shoulder. Philadelphia: WB Saunders, 1994, pp. 60; 64.)

Each muscle force acting across on the glenohumeral head joint can be resolved into a compressive component parallel to the glenoid center line and a tangential component perpendicular to the glenoid center line. Consideration of the line of action of the cuff muscles reveals that a major component of each is parallel to the glenoid center line (i.e., they compress the humeral head into the glenoid fossa). Thus, each of the rotator cuff muscles is a major contributor to the compressive force in most glenohumeral positions (**Fig. 9–9**).

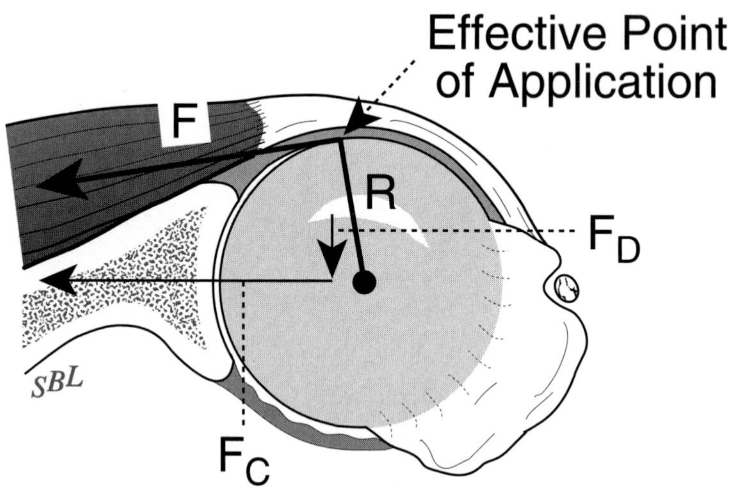


A

**Figure 9–9. The compressive component of the rotator cuff muscle action**
**A,** The subscapularis action is largely compressive. Its net force, F, consists of a compressive component, $F_C$, that is much greater than its displacing component, $F_D$.

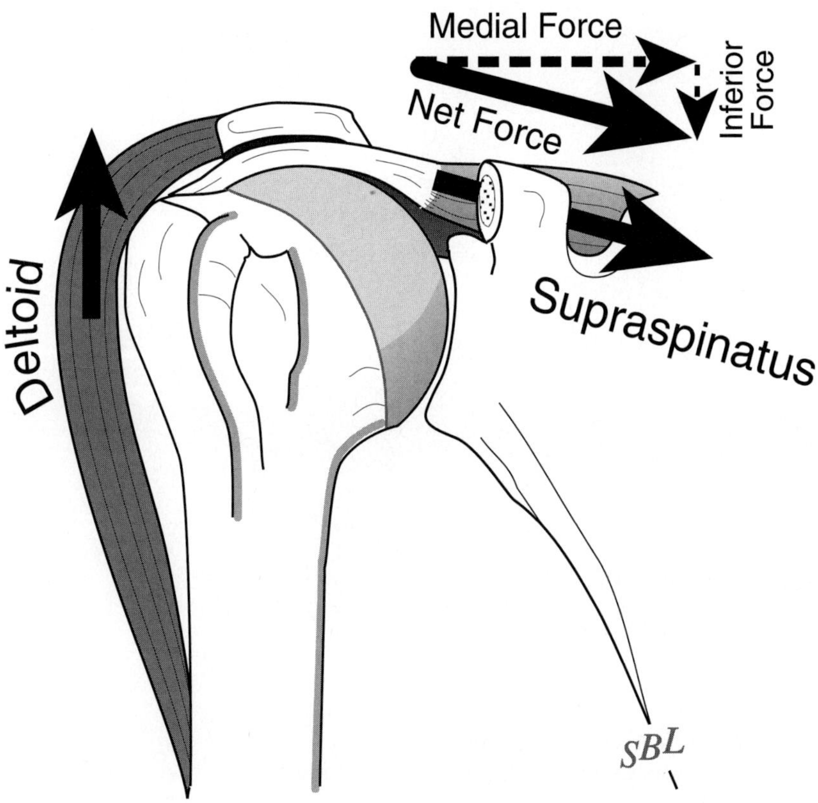


B

**Figure 9–9. The compressive component of the rotator cuff muscle action**—*Continued*

**B,** The supraspinatus action is also largely compressive. The sum of the compressive actions of the cuff muscles stabilizes the humeral head in the glenoid against the displacing component of the deltoid force. (Modified from Matsen FA, Lippitt SB, Sidles JA, et al [eds]: Practical Evaluation and Management of the Shoulder. Philadelphia: WB Saunders, 1994, pp. 70; 113.)

### Balance Stability Angle

The maximal angle that the net humeral joint reaction force can make with the glenoid center line before dislocation occurs is the *balance stability angle* **(Fig. 9–10)**. If the radius of curvature of the glenoid is R and the width of the effective glenoid concavity from the center line to the lip in a specified direction is W, the sine of the balance stability angle in that direction is W/R; thus, if we know the width and the radius, the balance stability angle is the arc sine of W/R **(Fig. 9–11)**. Because for small angles (i.e., less than 30 degrees) the sine and the tangent are about equal **(Fig. 9–12)** and because for small angles (again less than 30 degrees) the tangent is equal to the angle expressed in radians (recalling that a radian is approximately 57.3 degrees), we come up with the convenient rule of thumb that the balance stability angle in degrees is about $57.3 \times W/R$.

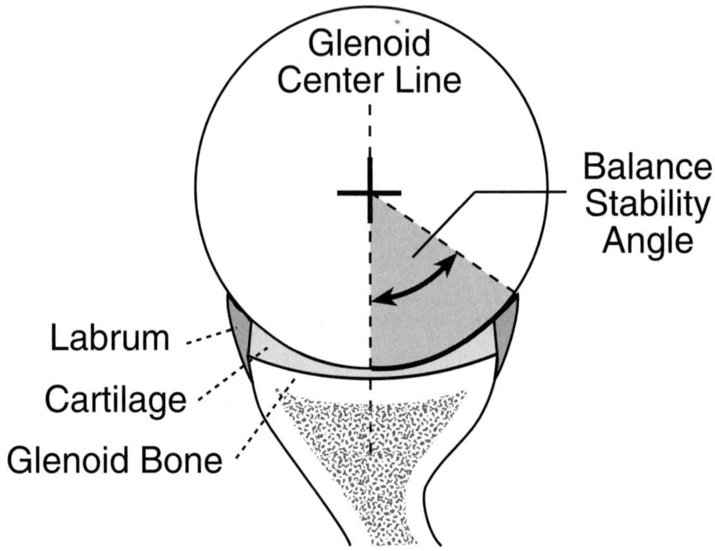


**Figure 9–10. Balance stability angle**
The balance stability angle is the maximal angle that the net humeral joint reaction force can make with the glenoid center line before dislocation occurs in a specified direction. (Modified from Matsen FA, Lippitt SB, Sidles JA, et al [eds]: Practical Evaluation and Management of the Shoulder. Philadelphia: WB Saunders, 1994, p. 62.)

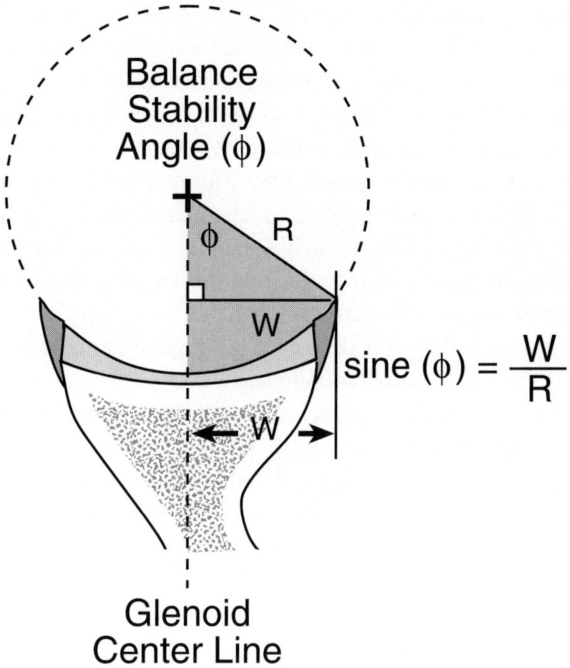


**Figure 9–11. Calculating the balance stability angle**
The balance stability angle can be predicted from the arc sine of the width of the glenoid in the direction of interest divided by the radius of curvature of the glenoid.

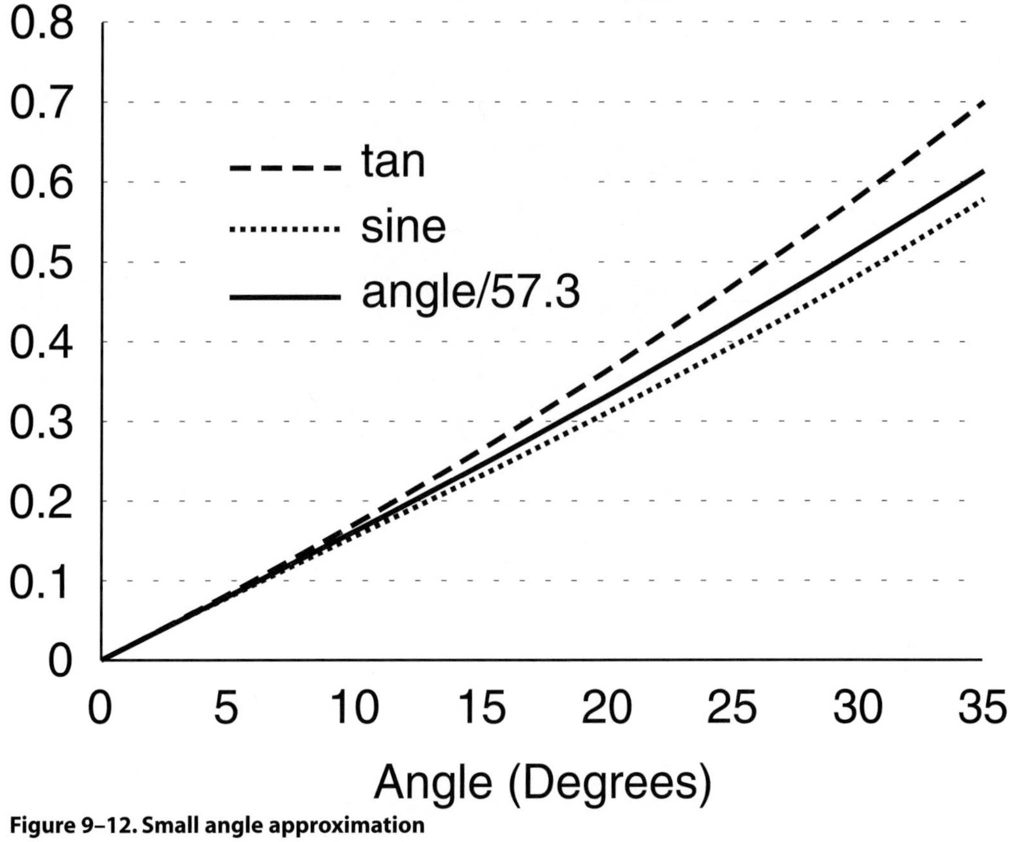


**Figure 9–12. Small angle approximation**
For small angles, the sine, the tangent, and the angle expressed in radians (degrees/57.3) are all approximately the same, making it easy to predict the balance stability angle without trigonometry calculations (BSA ~ 57.3 × W/R).

The balance stability angle can be viewed as the margin of error for the alignment of the net humeral joint reaction force with the glenoid center line. For example, if the anterior and posterior balance stability angles are each 20 degrees, it means that the glenohumeral joint will be stable if the net humeral joint reaction force is lined up ±20 degrees with the glenoid center line. If the anterior and posterior balance stability angles are only half as large, the precision of net humeral joint reaction force alignment needs to be twice as great (i.e., ±10 degrees). If the glenoid is flat (i.e., the radius is very large), the balance stability angle approaches 0, so that the net humeral joint reaction force must be precisely perpendicular to the glenoid surface; otherwise, dislocation will occur. If the posterior half of the glenoid is fractured off (**Fig. 9–13**), the width from the center line to the rim (W) will be halved and the balance stability angle in that direction (57.3 × W/R) will be substantially lessened.

It is apparent that the balance stability angle relates to the glenoid surface and the version relates the glenoid surface to the scapula. Thus, a glenoid with normal balance stability angles may not provide normal stability if its version is abnormal. To illustrate this, think how much stability a perfectly good golf tee would offer if it were set in the ground angled 30 degrees with the vertical (**Fig. 9–14**).

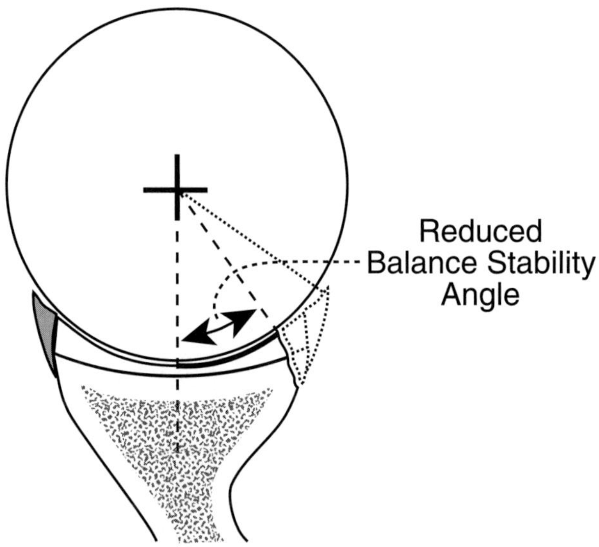


**Figure 9–13. Compromised balance stability angle**
When the glenoid width is narrowed, for example by a glenoid lip fracture, the balance stability angle is reduced. (Modified from Matsen FA, Lippitt SB, Sidles JA, et al [eds]: Practical Evaluation and Management of the Shoulder. Philadelphia: WB Saunders, 1994, p. 63.)

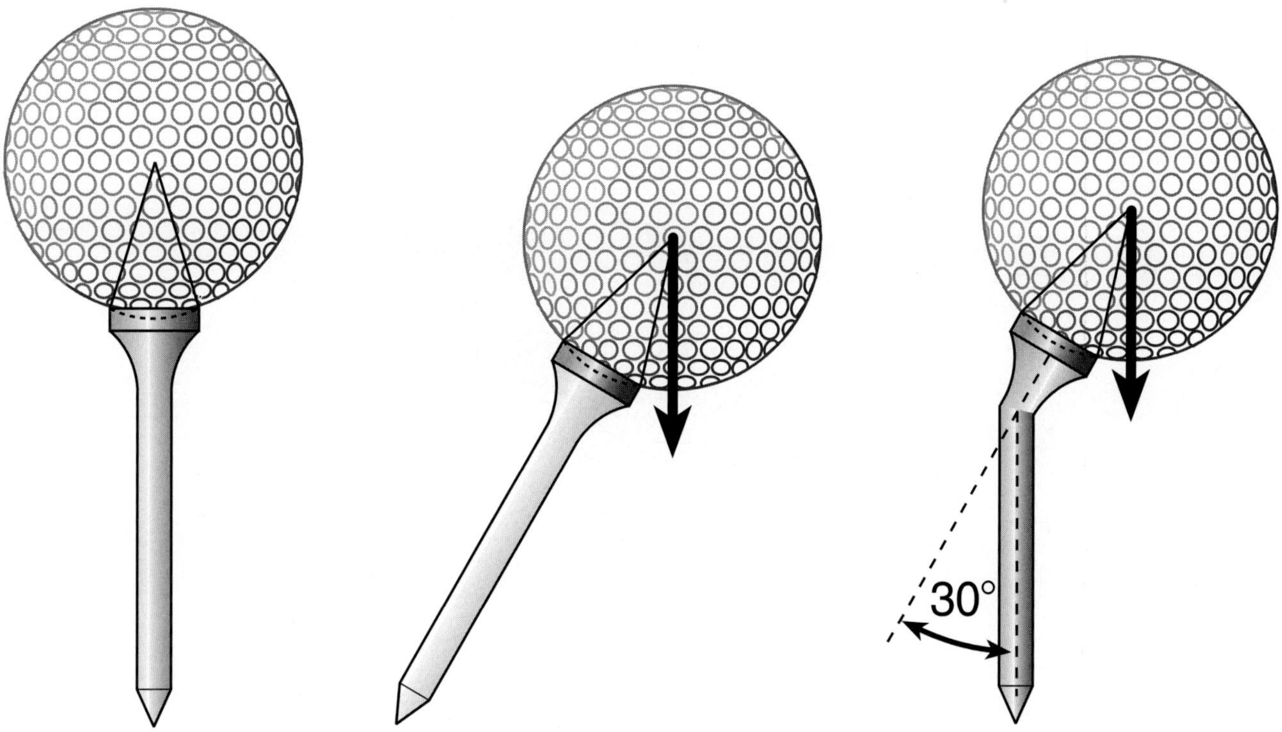


**Figure 9–14. Golf tee analogy**
A golf ball is stabilized in a golf tee when its gravitational force vector passes through the tee. When the tee is tipped substantially, the force vector passes outside the tee and the ball falls off. The ball may also dislodge if the tee is crooked.

## The Shape of the Glenoid Surface

A useful way of characterizing the functional glenoid shape is by the *glenoidogram*: the path taken by the center of the head of the humerus as it passes from the center of the glenoid over its rim in a specified direction (**Fig. 9–15**). The importance of this path lies in the fact that its vertical component represents the distance along the glenoid center line that the humeral head must be displaced against the net compressive force in order for the head to translate. Since work equals force times distance, the product of the net humeral compressive force and the height of the glenoidogram in a given direction is the work that needs to be done on the shoulder humeral head to dislocate it in that direction.

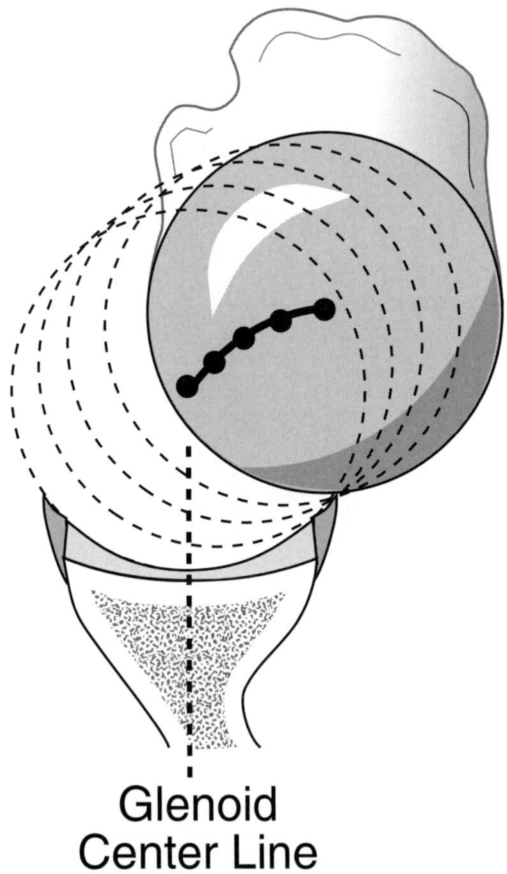


**Figure 9–15. Glenoidogram**
The glenoidogram is the path taken by the center of the humeral head as it translates across the face of the glenoid in a specified direction away from the glenoid center line. The height of the glenoidogram reflects the amount of work needed to dislocate the humeral head for a given compressive load. (Modified from Matsen FA, Lippitt SB, Sidles JA, et al [eds]: Practical Evaluation and Management of the Shoulder. Philadelphia: WB Saunders, 1994, p. 66.)

When the radius of curvature of the humeral head is equal to that of the glenoid, the glenoidogram describes a curve with a radius equal to that of the humeral head centered on the rim of the glenoid. The combination of the glenoidograms in two opposite directions yields the familiar gull-wing shape (**Fig. 9–16**). In this circumstance, the steepest part of the normal glenoidogram is when the humeral head just begins to leave the centered position. When the humeral head radius is less than that of the glenoid, there is a flatter part of the glenoidogram near the center of the glenoid

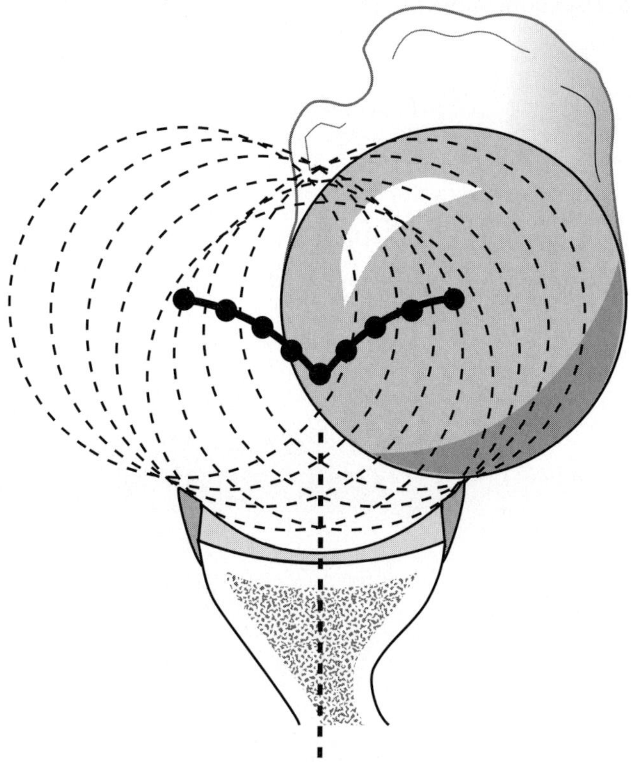

**Figure 9–16. Paired glenoidograms**
When the glenoidograms in two opposite directions are similar, they form a gull-wing shape together. The most stable position for the humeral head is that in which the two halves of the gull wing come together: at the center of the glenoid.

that extends until the head contacts the glenoid rim. This situation does not change the height of the glenoidogram and thus does not change the work necessary to dislocate the shoulder (**Fig. 9–17**). When the humeral head radius is larger than that of the glenoid, the head does not sit fully down in the glenoid; as a result, the height of the glenoidogram is less than the depth of the glenoid concavity (**Fig. 9–18**). Because the height of the glenoidogram is less, the work necessary to dislocate the shoulder is less also and, thus, the shoulder stability is reduced. While these considerations may seem esoteric, mismatches between glenoid and humeral radii of curvature exert major effects on stability in conditions such as glenoid dysplasia and osteoarthritis, as well as in surgical procedures such as prosthetic arthroplasty, glenoid osteoplasty, and the placement of glenoid bone blocks.

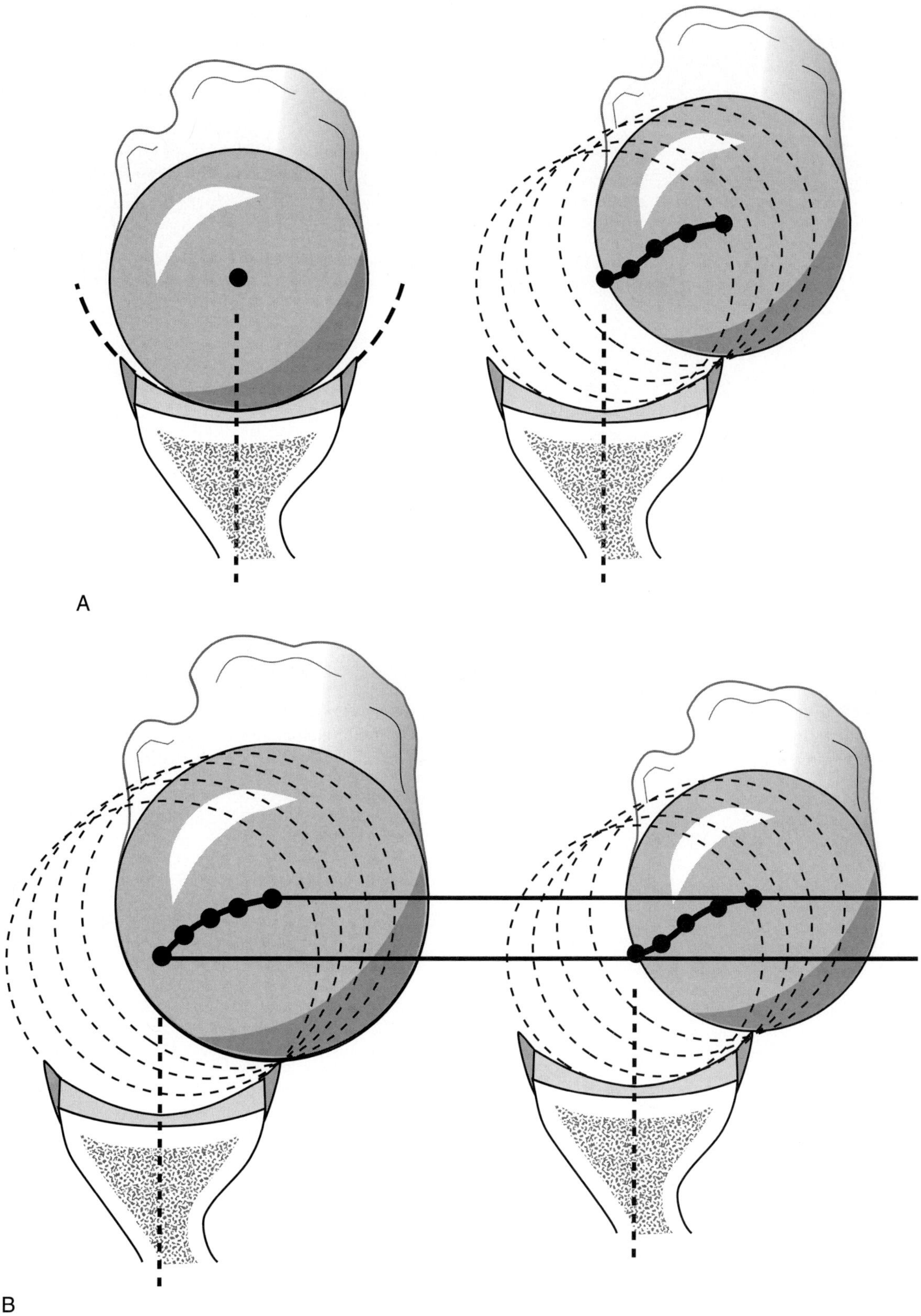

A

B

**Figure 9–17. Glenoidogram when the head has a smaller radius than the glenoid**
**A,** When the humeral radius is smaller than that of the glenoid, the glenoidogram is blunted at the center, indicating that the head will not be precisely centered. **B,** The height of the glenoidogram is not changed by a smaller head; thus, the resistance to dislocation is the same.

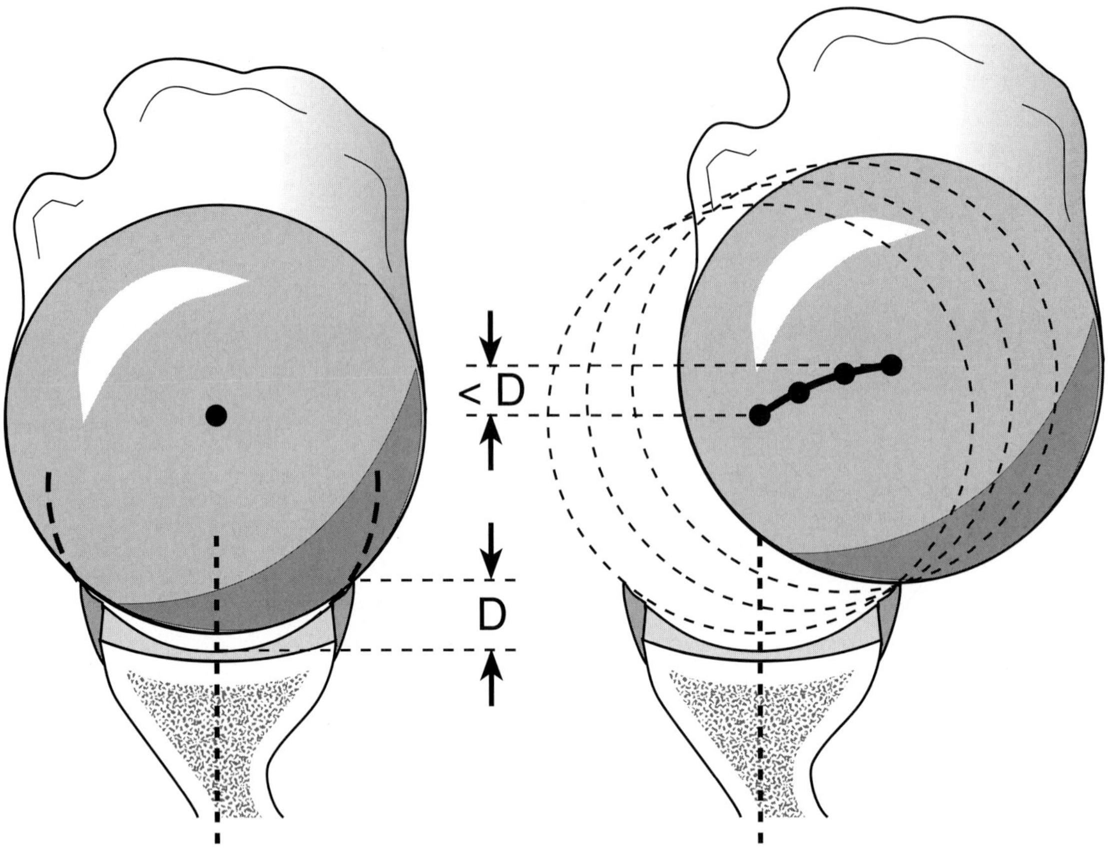


**Figure 9–18. Glenoidogram when the head has a larger radius than the glenoid**
Although the humeral head remains centered in the glenoid, the height of the glenoidogram is reduced by a larger head because the humeral head does not seat fully in the fossa; thus, the resistance to dislocation is reduced.

These considerations relate to the overall resistance to dislocation offered by different combinations of glenoid and humeral articular shapes. A bit of further analysis helps us understand how the shape of the glenoid and humeral surfaces contributes to the *centering* of the humeral head in the glenoid. The *stability ratio* is the force necessary to translate the humeral head divided by the load compressing the humeral head into the glenoid (**Fig. 9–19**). The stability ratio is not constant at every point along the surface of the glenoid. The slope of the glenoidogram at a given point is the *local stability ratio* at

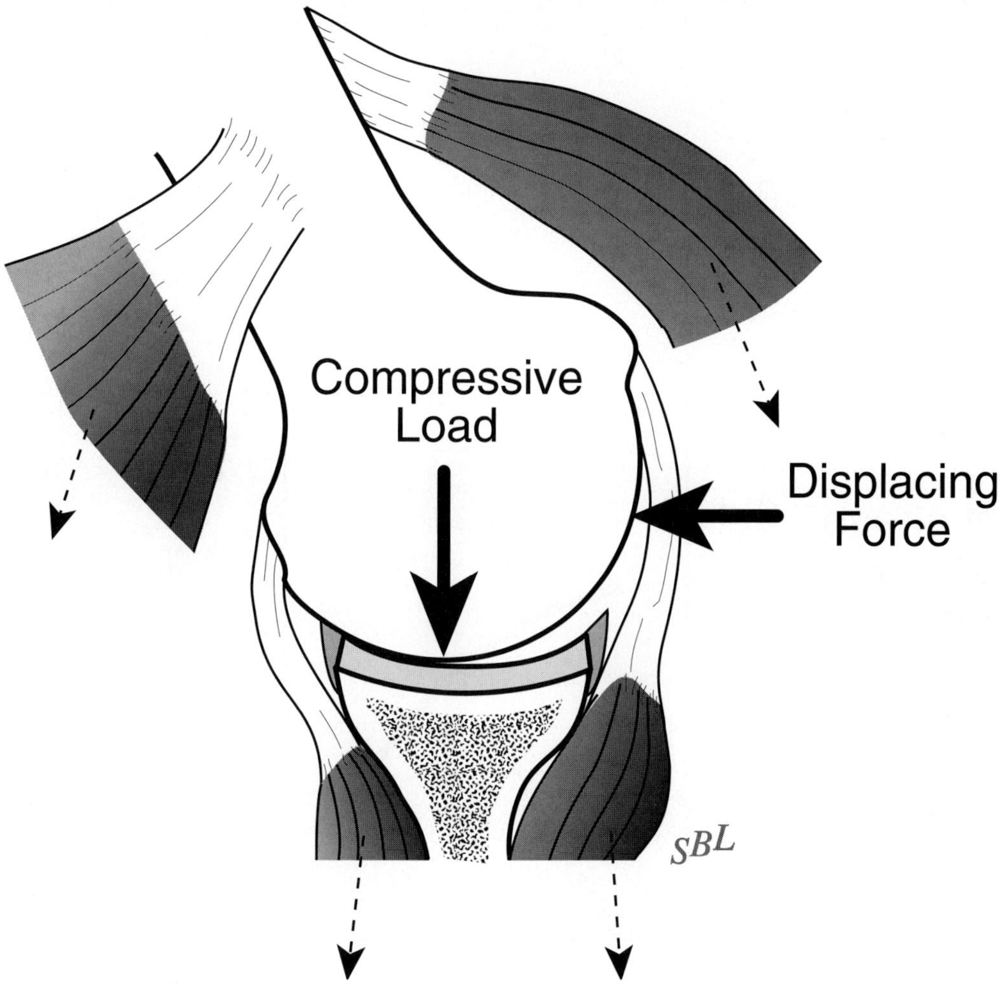


**Figure 9–19. The stability ratio**
The ratio of the force necessary to dislocate the head divided by the load compressing the humeral head into the glenoid is the stability ratio. (Modified from Matsen FA, Lippitt SB, Sidles JA, et al [eds]: Practical Evaluation and Management of the Shoulder. Philadelphia: WB Saunders, 1994, p. 64.)

that point (**Fig. 9–20**). In a joint with a humeral head and glenoid of the same radius of curvature, the plot of the local stability ratios has a peak in the center of the glenoid and drops off rapidly as the head translates toward the glenoid rim. Thus, in the normal articulation, the stability of the humeral head is greatest when it is at the center of the normal glenoid, and so it remains centered. When the humeral head has a radius greater than that of the glenoid, the maximal local stability is less than it would be if the head were of the same radius. When the humeral head is of a radius less than that of the glenoid, there are two peaks in the graph of the local stability ratio (**Fig. 9–21**). In this situation, the glenoid surface anatomy does not precisely center the humeral head but rather allows some translation at the bottom of the glenoid trough (**Fig. 9–22**).

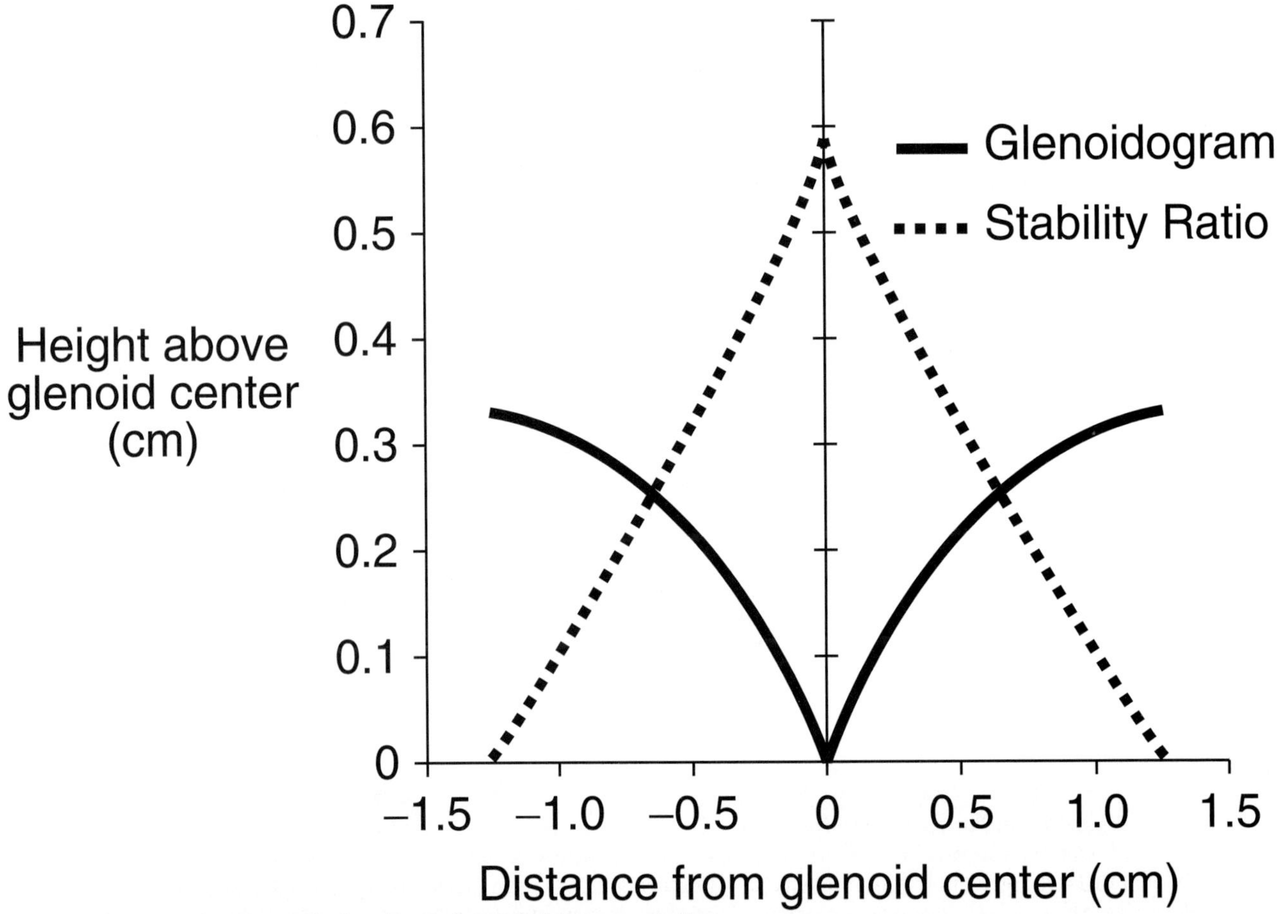


**Figure 9–20. Local stability ratio: head and glenoid of the same radius**
The stability ratio does not remain constant across the glenoid. The local stability ratio is maximal where the glenoidogram has the greatest slope. When the glenoid and humerus have the same radius, there is a peak in the local stability ratio at the center of the glenoid: the humerus is most stable in the center of the glenoid.

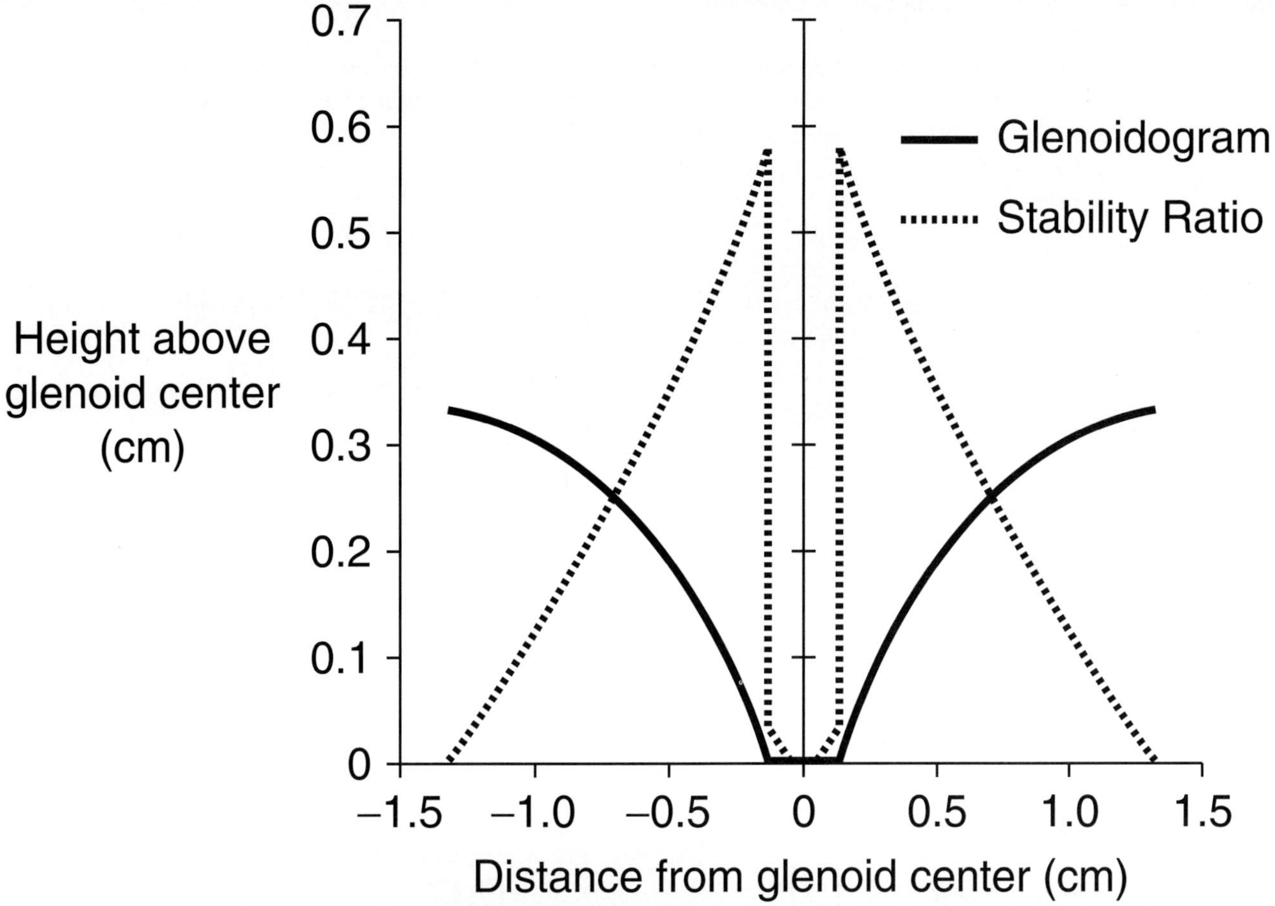


**Figure 9–21. Local stability ratio: head of smaller radius than the glenoid**
When the glenoid radius is larger than that of the humerus, the plot of the local stability ratios reveals twin peaks.

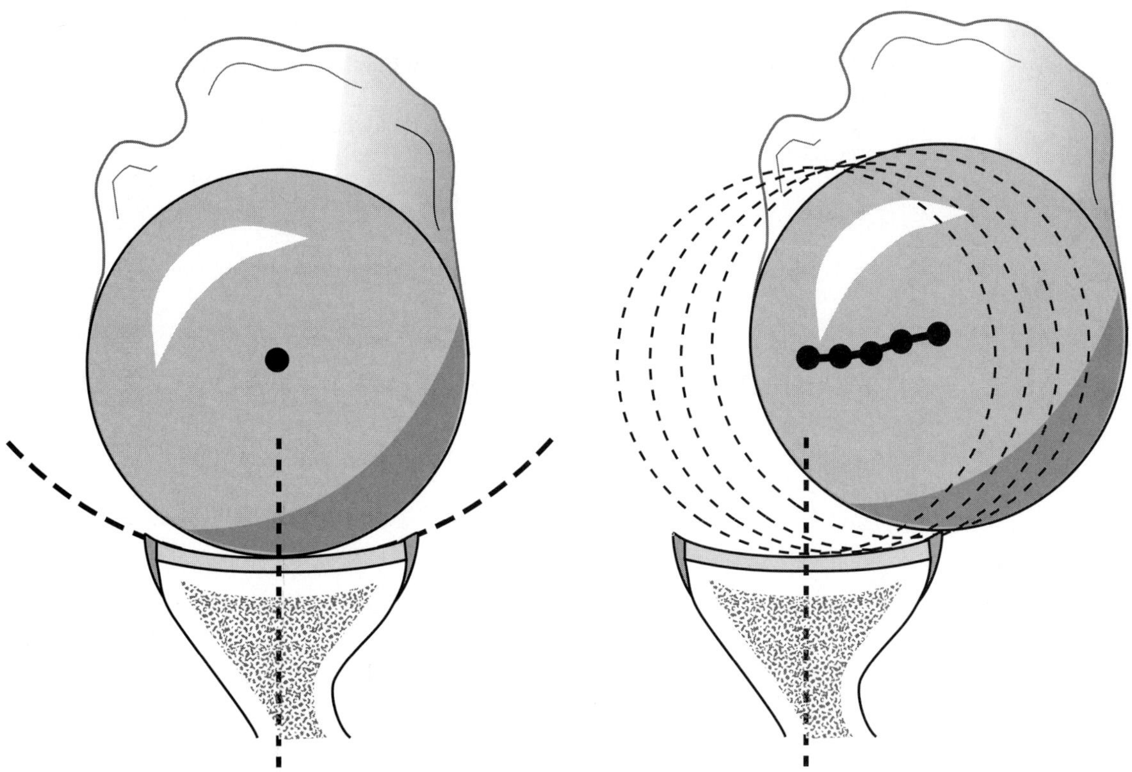

**Figure 9–22. Effect of radial mismatch on stability**
When the glenoid radius is larger than that of the humerus, the glenoid does not precisely center the head.

In the absence of frictional effects and other confounding variables, the maximal local stability ratio in a given direction is equal to the tangent of the balance stability angle in that direction (**Fig. 9–23**).

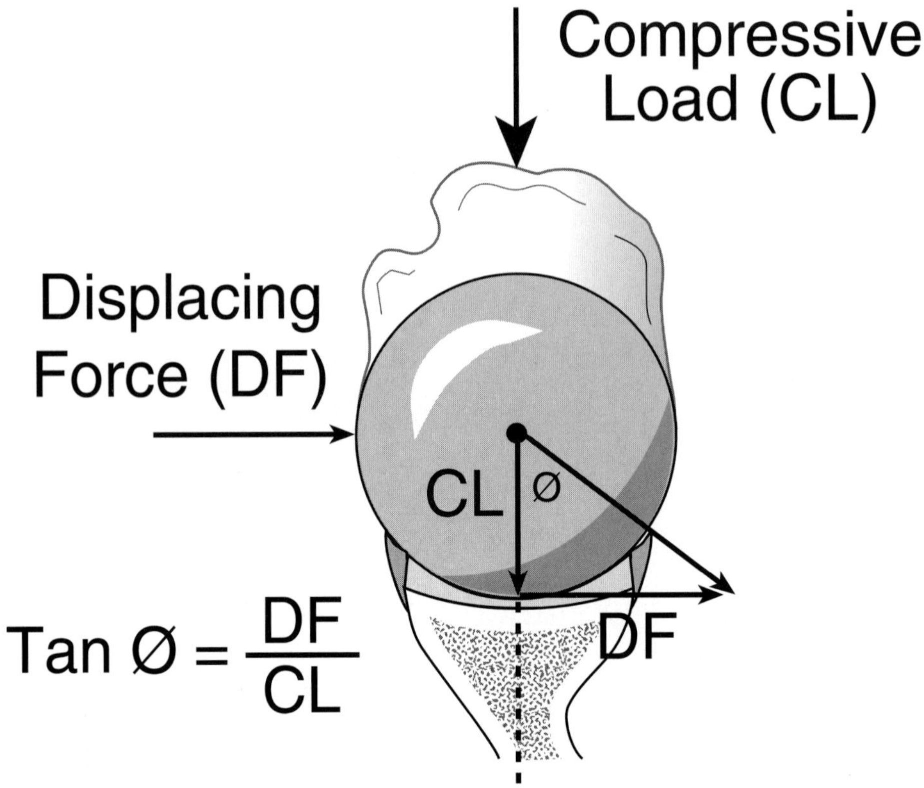


**Figure 9–23. The relationship of the maximum local stability ratio to the balance stability angle**
The tangent of the balance stability angle is equal to the ratio of the displacing force and the compressive load.

### Abnormalities of the Glenoid Concavity

The ability of the humeral head to remain centered in the glenoid can be compromised by any condition that changes the shape of the glenoid concavity.

The functional glenoid concavity may be distorted in many conditions. Some of the more common distortions include a highly compressible labrum in a case of atraumatic glenohumeral instability (**Fig. 9–24*A***), detachment of the glenoid labrum from the glenoid rim in a case of traumatic glenohumeral instability (**Fig. 9–24*B***), fracture or wear of the glenoid lip in case of traumatic glenohumeral instability (**Fig. 9–24*C***), absence of the glenoid lip in a case of glenoid hypoplasia (**Fig. 9–24*D***), and flattening of the glenoid in a case of osteoarthritis (**Fig. 9–24*E***). In each of these conditions, there is compromise of the glenoid cavity, the glenoidogram, the local stability ratio, and the ability of the

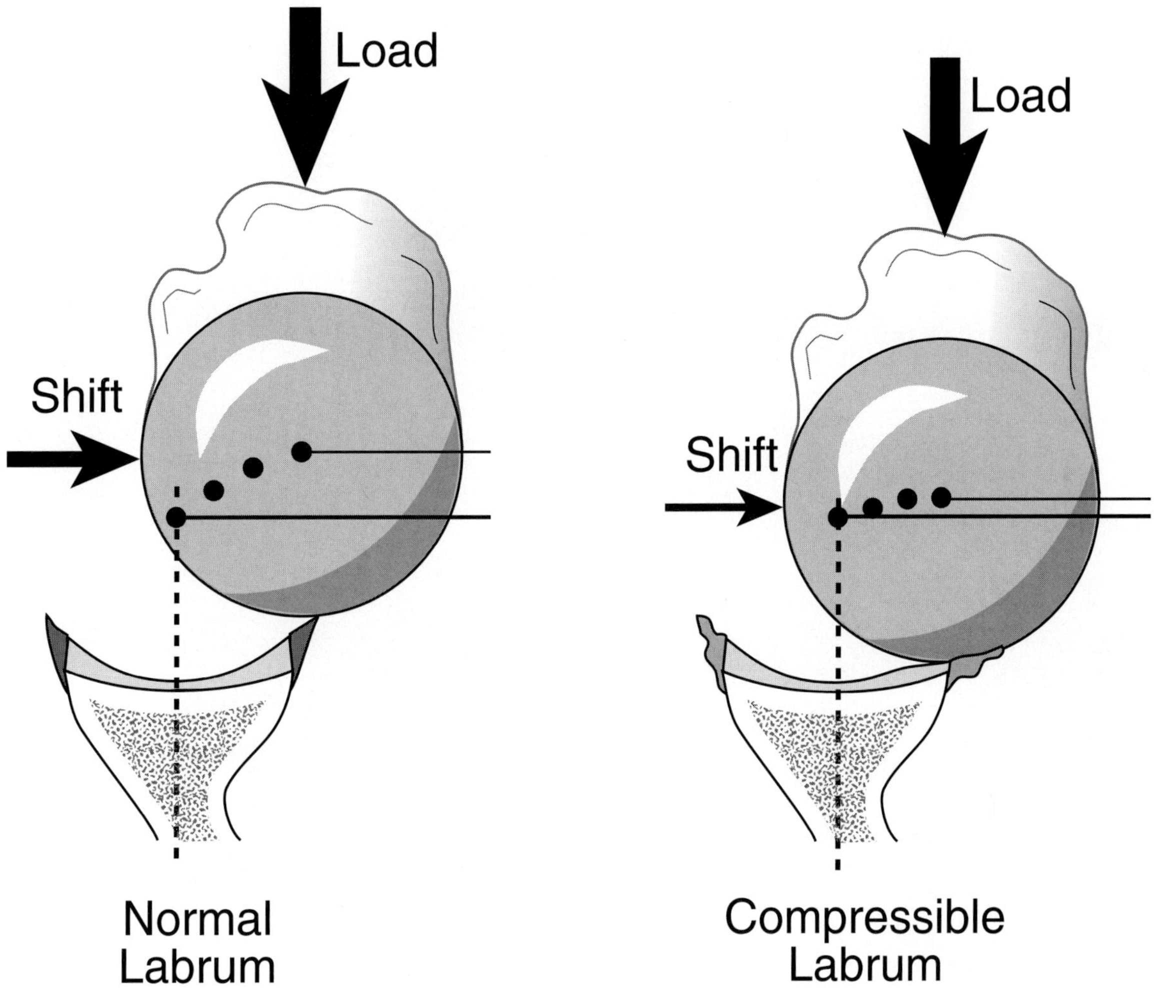


A

**Figure 9–24. Distortions of the glenoid concavity**

**A,** *Compressible labrum.* When the labrum is easily compressible, it does not contribute as much to the glenoidogram performed under loaded conditions.

*Continued*

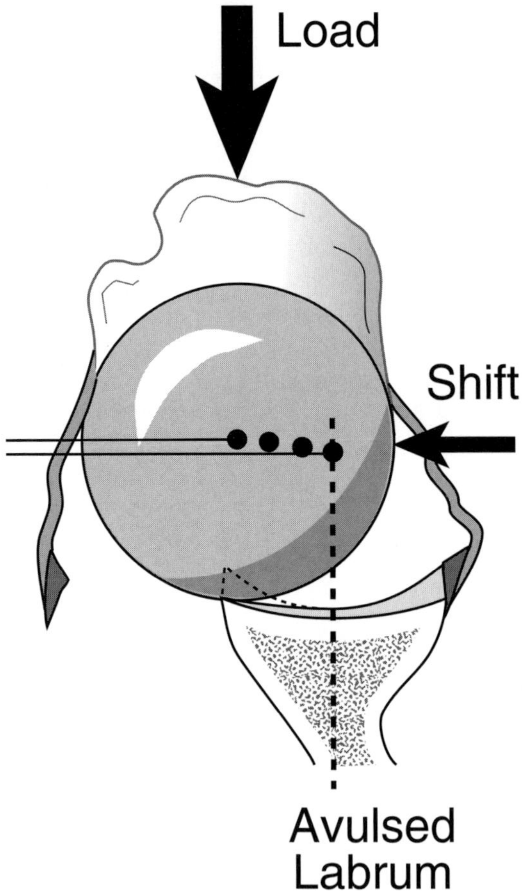


B

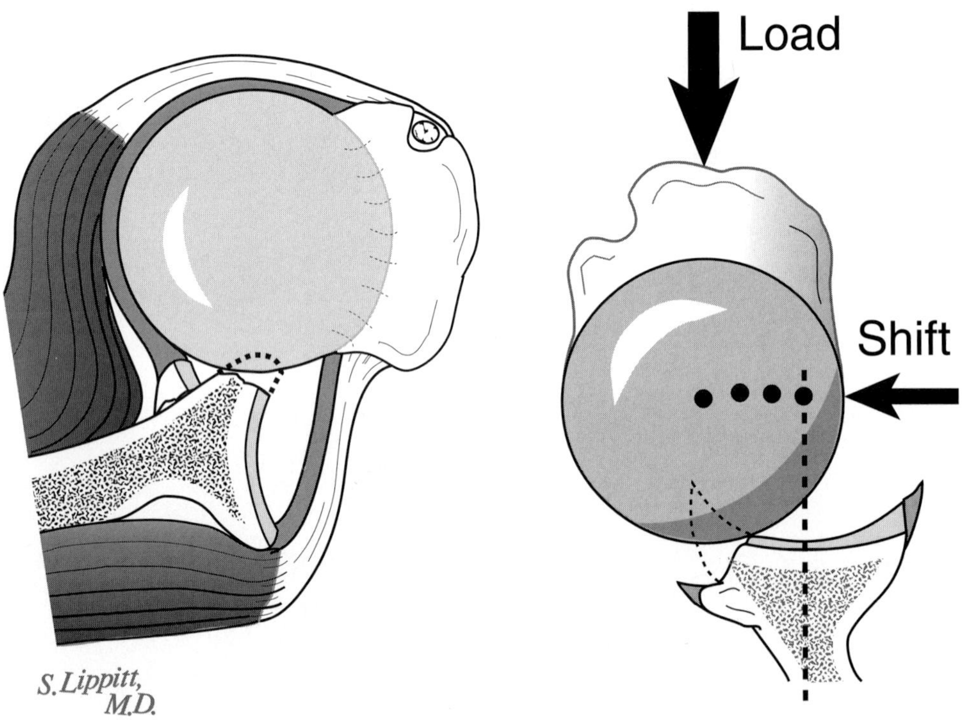


C

**Figure 9–24. Distortions of the glenoid concavity**—*Continued*
**B,** *Avulsed labrum.* When the labrum is avulsed from the glenoid, it cannot contribute to the glenoidogram. (Modified from Matsen FA, Lippitt SB, Sidles JA, et al [eds]: Practical Evaluation and Management of the Shoulder. Philadelphia: WB Saunders, 1994, p. 98.)
**C,** *Glenoid rim fracture.* When the glenoid rim is fractured, it cannot contribute to the glenoidogram. (Modified from Rockwood CA, Matsen FA [eds]: The Shoulder, 2nd ed. Philadelphia: WB Saunders, 1998, p. 615.)

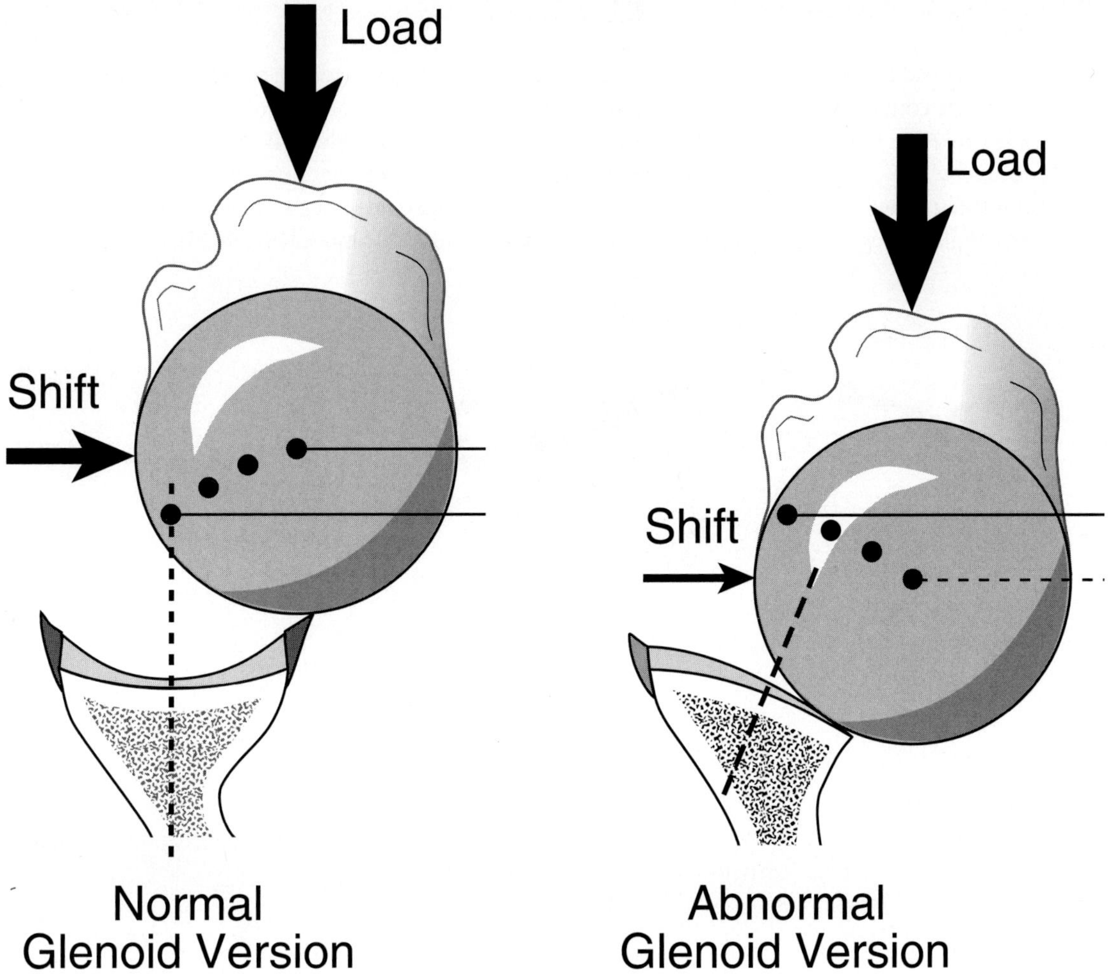


D

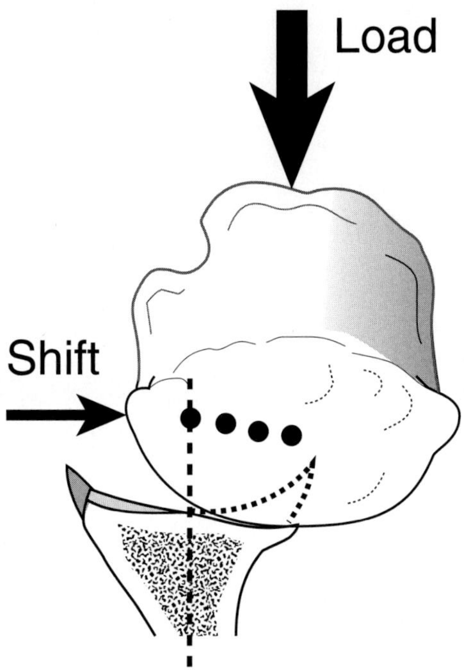


E

**Figure 9–24. Distortions of the glenoid concavity**—*Continued*
**D,** *Glenoid hypoplasia*. When the glenoid rim is hypoplastic, it cannot contribute normally to the glenoidogram. **E,** *Glenoid erosion*. When the glenoid rim is eroded, it cannot contribute normally to the glenoidogram.

humeral head to be centered. When the glenoid becomes biconcave, the stability in the pathologic concavity becomes greater than in the remaining part of the normal concavity because the pathologic concavity is deeper. Thus, resurfacing the humerus without addressing the glenoid is unlikely to recenter the humerus in the glenoid. Similarly, smoothing down the crest between the two glenoid concavities does not reestablish a normal glenoidogram, local stability ratios, or balance stability angles (**Fig. 9–25**).

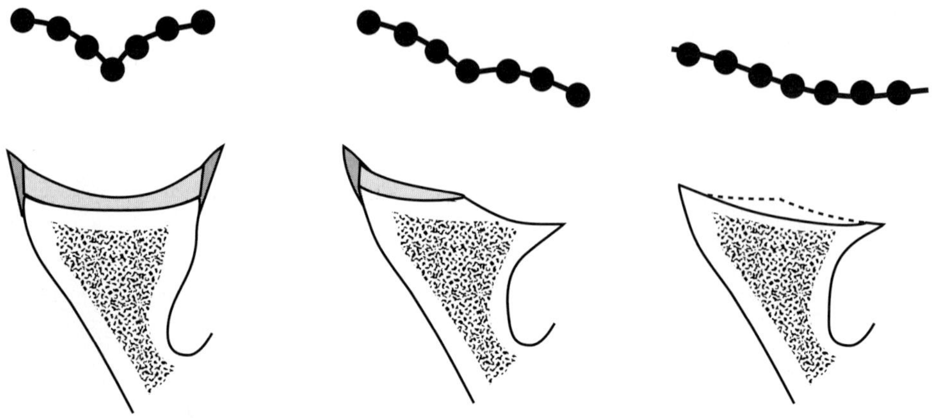

**Figure 9–25. Biconcave glenoid**
The glenoidogram associated with a biconcave glenoid, often seen in cases of osteoarthritis and capsulorrhaphy arthropathy, cannot be restored to normal by simply smoothing down the ridge between the two concavities.

## CLINICAL CONSIDERATIONS

### Clinical Tests of the Concavity

The adequacy of a patient's glenoid concavity in a defined direction is determined by the clinical analogue of the stability ratio: the *load and shift test* (**Fig. 9–26**). In this test, one hand of the examiner grasps the patient's shoulder just medial to the humeral head and the other hand grasps the patient's humeral head. While pressing the humeral head into the glenoid (load), the examiner senses the resistance to translation from the

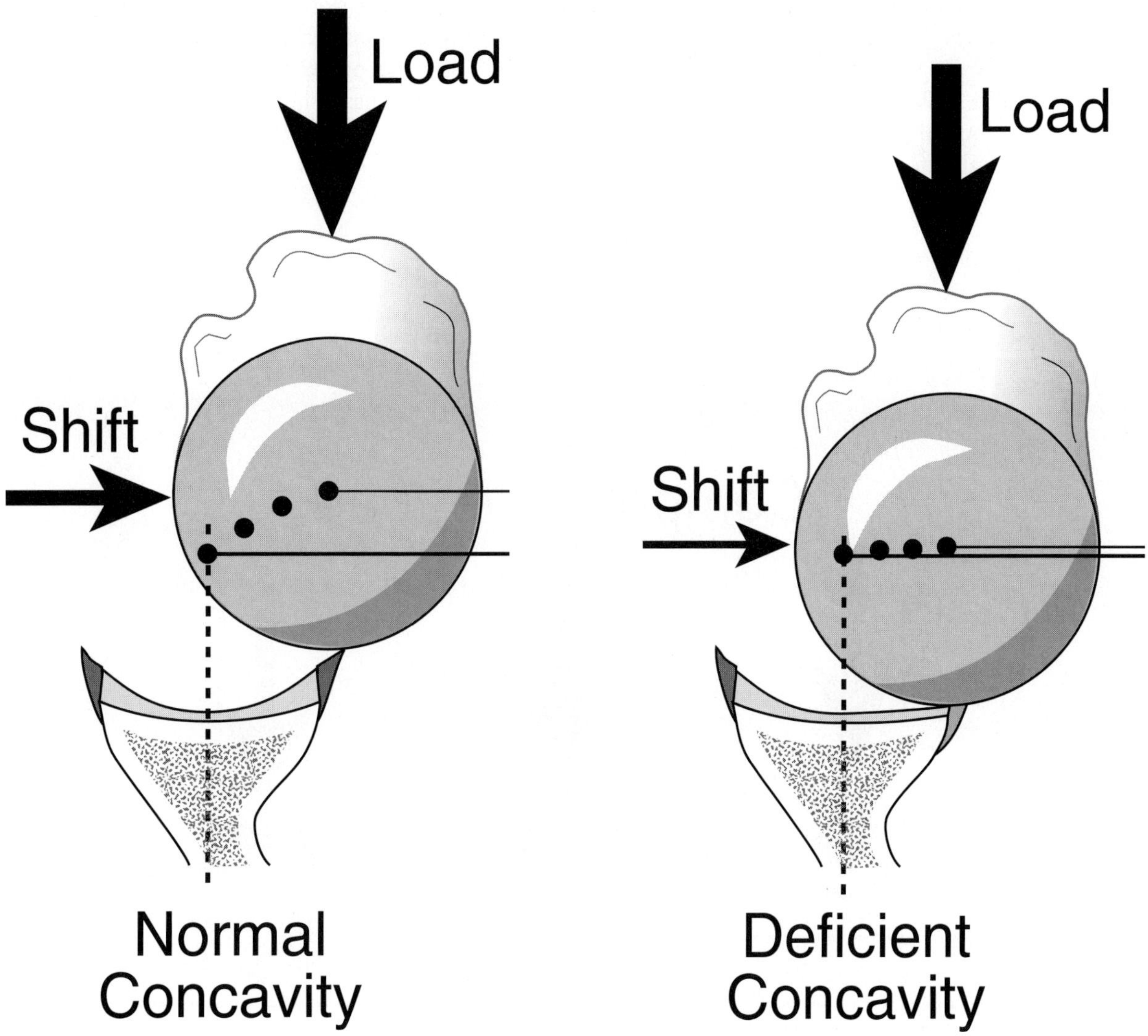


**Figure 9–26. The load and shift test**
The adequacy of the glenoid concavity in a given direction can be assessed by compressing the humeral head into the glenoid concavity and noting the amount of displacing force necessary to translate the head. The figure on the left shows a normal concavity and that on the right a diminished concavity in the direction of testing.

centered position (shift). Lack of resistance indicates a minimal glenoid concavity. For an example, compare the resistance to shift when a pool ball is pressed onto a flat table to the resistance to shift when it is pressed into a concavity (**Fig. 9–27**). The load and shift test is particularly helpful in deciding whether a socket-deepening procedure may be needed in the management of recurrent glenohumeral instability.

Another clinical relative of the stability ratio is the *active abduction test.* The examiner first performs the anterior and posterior drawer tests to assess the translational laxity with the patient's arm relaxed in slight passive abduction. Then the patient holds this same position actively while the drawer tests are repeated. In shoulders with a normal concavity, gentle active abduction creates a compressive load into the glenoid that, by virtue of the concavity compression mechanism, eliminates the examiner's ability to translate the humeral head on the drawer tests.

The *jerk test* is comparable to measuring the posterior balance stability angle. In this test, the internally rotated arm is progressively moved horizontally across the body, increasing the angle it makes with the glenoid center line while an axial load is applied to it. In the presence of posterior lip deficiency, the humeral head shoulder slips easily out of joint over the inadequate posterior glenoid lip (**Fig. 9–28**). Because of the absence of a functional lip, this translation may be unnoticed by the patient. Horizontal movement of the arm away from the body causes the humeral head to relocate in the joint with an obvious "jerk" or "clunk" as it pops back into its centered position.

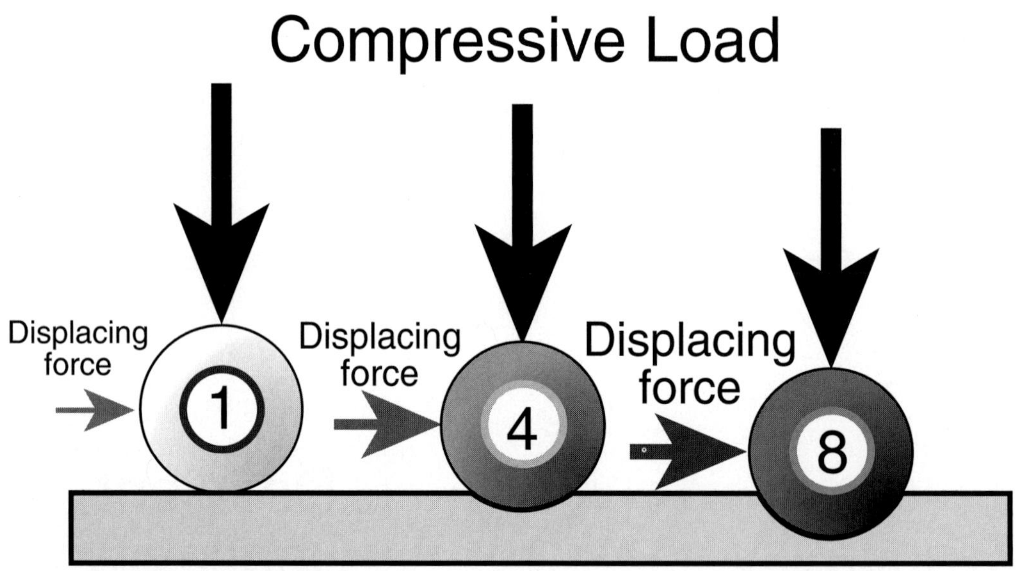


**Figure 9–27. Billiard ball analogy**
In the absence of a concavity, only a modest translational force is required to shift the sphere. As the concavity becomes deeper, a greater displacing force is required to shift the ball for a given compressive load.

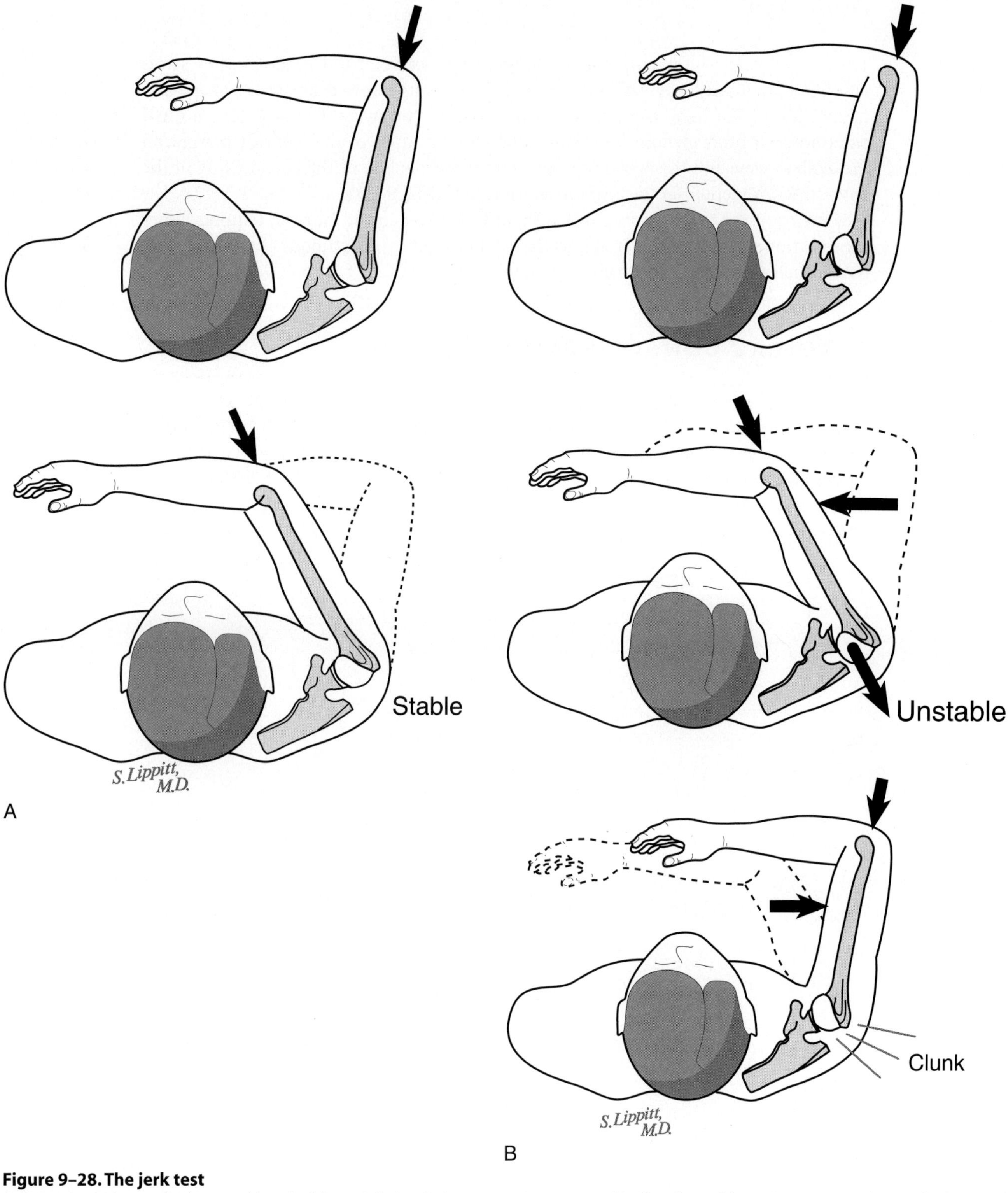


**Figure 9–28. The jerk test**

**A,** Negative jerk test: the humeral head of the axially loaded arm remains centered in the glenoid fossa. **B,** Positive jerk test: the humeral head of the axillary loaded arm slides out the back of the shoulder when the arm is adducted across the body and clunks back in when the arm position is aligned with the scapula.

## IMAGING

The most practical imaging for stability is the standardized radiographic series described previously. The axillary view enables the surgeon to evaluate the shape and orientation of the bony component of the glenoid concavity. The lack of a normal anteroinferior bony glenoid lip is suggested by truncation of the anterior margin on the axillary view and the apical oblique view as well as loss of the cortical line of the anteroinferior glenoid in the anteroposterior view (**Fig. 9–29**).

Viewing of the true glenoid surface, including cartilage and labrum, requires either the injection of contrast material into the joint or the use of techniques that image soft tissue, such as magnetic resonance imaging.

## SURGICAL CONSIDERATIONS

The intrinsic stability of the glenoid concavity can be altered by reparative and reconstructive surgery. Since the balance stability angle is approximately $57.3 \times W/R$, the balance stability angle can be increased by procedures that increase the glenoid width (W) or decrease the glenoid radius of curvature (R) to more closely match that of the humerus. For example, a posterior glenoid osteoplasty decreases R, whereas an anterior extracapsular iliac crest graft increases W. A Bankart repair does both.

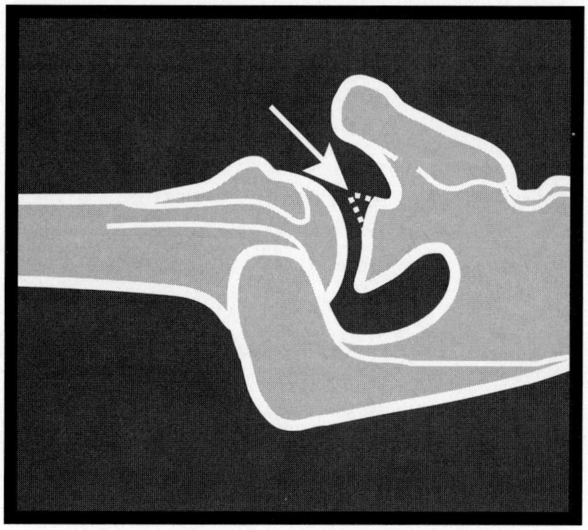

A

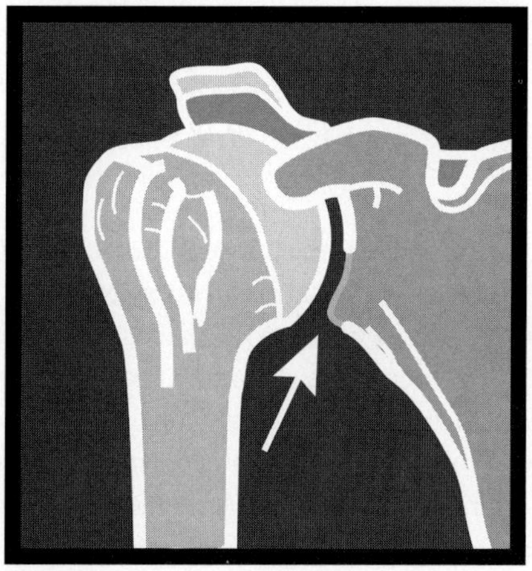

B

**Figure 9–29. Imaging for stability**

**A,** Axillary view showing anterior glenoid deficiency. This view shows a bony defect of the anterior glenoid lip. **B,** Anteroposterior view showing loss of the anteroinferior cortical line. The normally sclerotic border of the anteroinferior glenoid lip has been worn away. (Modified from Rockwood CA, Matsen FA [eds]: The Shoulder, 2nd ed. Philadelphia: WB Saunders, 1998, pp. 650; 651.)

CHAPTER 10

# Principles of the Glenohumeral Ligaments and Capsule

## CONCEPTS

The glenohumeral ligaments and capsule serve as checkreins, limiting the rotation of the humeral head. Although they limit the maximal translation of the humeral head, they are not effective in centering the head in the glenoid; this is the task of the concavity compression mechanism. They confine the baseball to the park, but they do not center it over the plate.

Laxity of movement in a specified direction is greater when the ligaments limiting that movement are slack (**Fig. 10–1**). Ligamentous stretch is a less important factor in laxity: usually ligaments are relatively noncompliant, stretching to only 110% of their resting length (**Fig. 10–2**). Ligaments are normally lax during most shoulder functions, allowing shoulder motion. If a glenohumeral joint has no laxity of its ligaments, it would not allow rotation. There is no rigorous clinical definition of "hyperlaxity" of the glenohumeral joint. Gymnasts and ballerinas provide telling examples of shoulders that are stable in the presence of substantial ligamentous laxity.

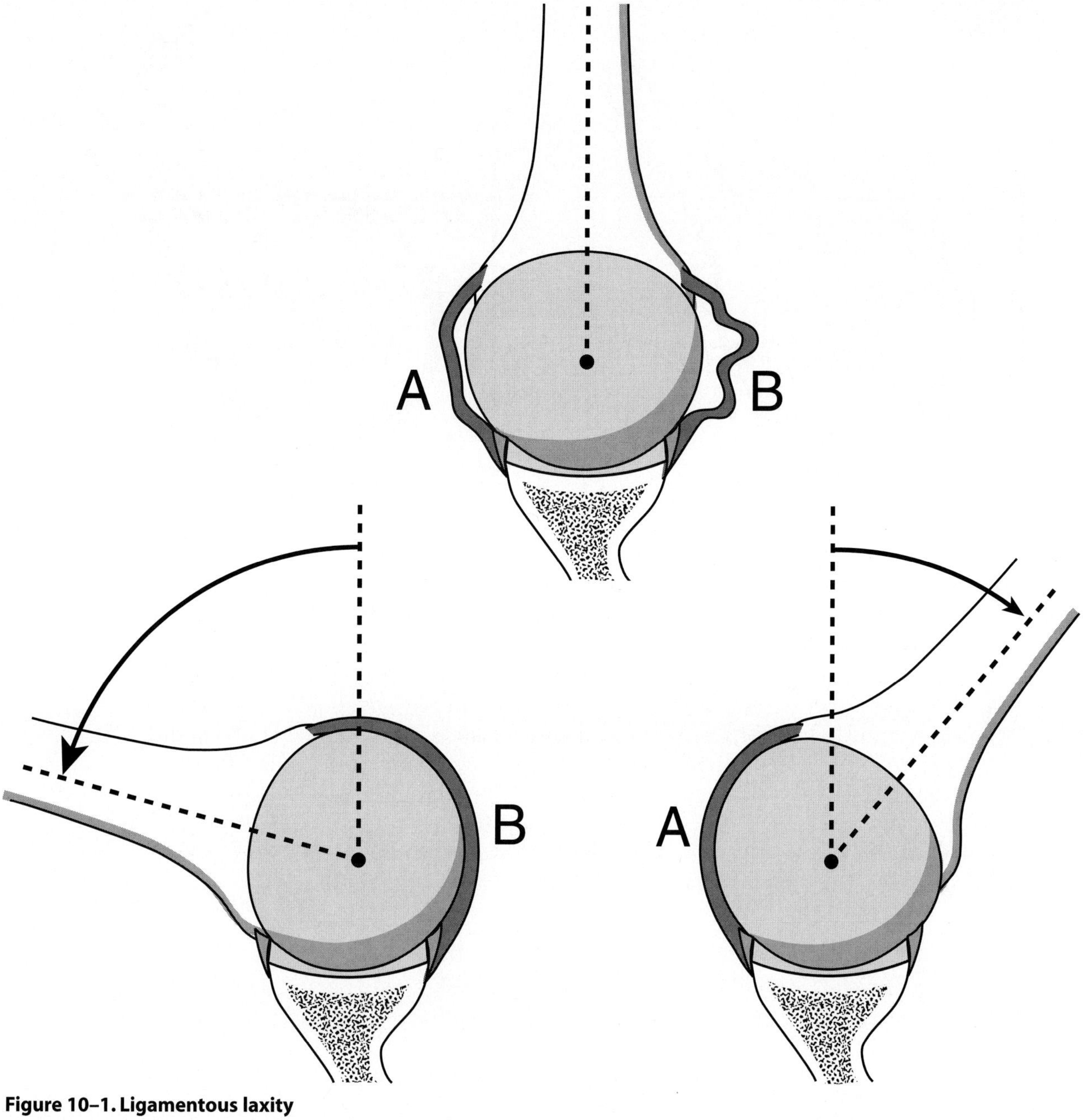


**Figure 10–1. Ligamentous laxity**
The laxity of a joint in a specified direction is determined primarily by the amount of slack (not the amount of stretch) in the ligaments, limiting that direction of movement.

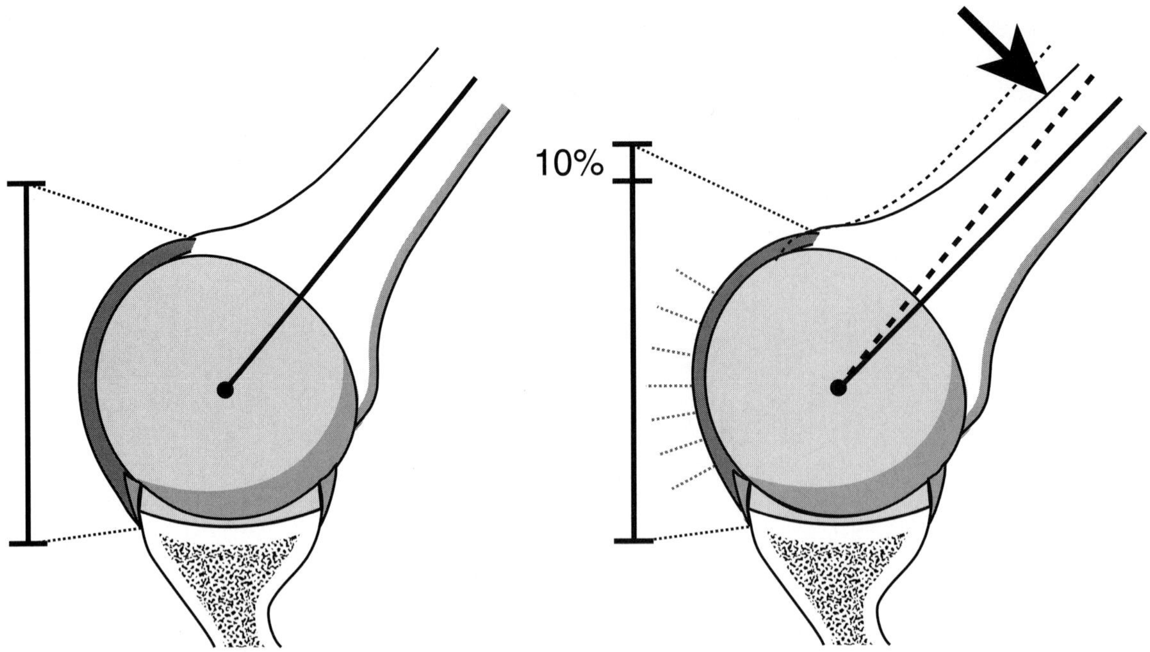


**Figure 10–2. Ligamentous compliance**
As a rule of thumb, ligaments cannot be stretched by more than 10% of their unloaded length.

## Ligamentous Disruption

Major tensile loads can avulse glenohumeral ligaments from their bony attachments **(Fig. 10–3)**. Because ligaments are normally strong and their attachments to bone secure, substantial tension is needed to disrupt them. Tensions of sufficient magnitude to disrupt ligaments are usually encountered when force is applied to the arm or hand rather than by a force applied directly to the shoulder. For example, if an anteroinferior glenohumeral ligament has a tensile strength of 500 pounds, it would require a

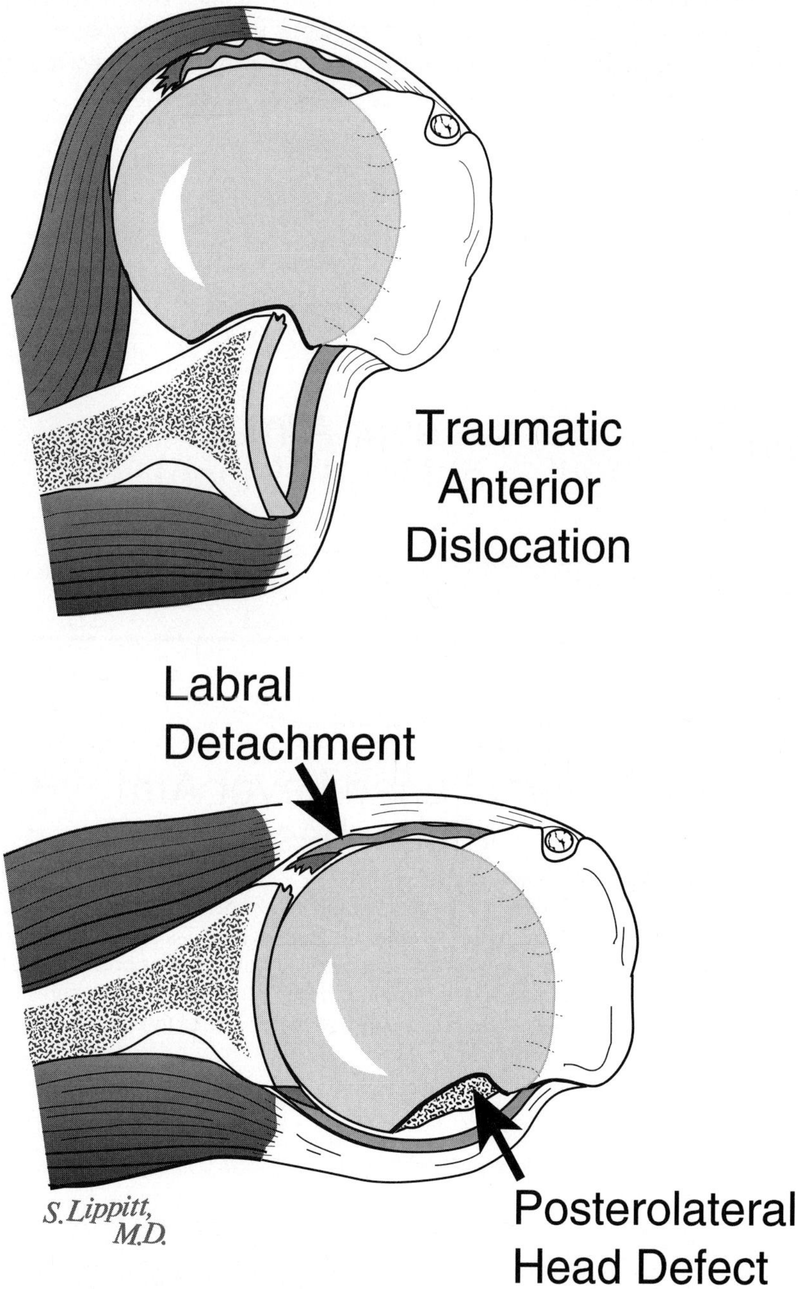


**Figure 10–3. Traumatic ligamentous disruption**
Major tensile loads on the glenohumeral ligaments can avulse their bony attachments, usually on the glenoid side. (Modified from Rockwood CA, Matsen FA [eds]: The Shoulder, 2nd ed. Philadelphia: WB Saunders, 1998, p. 613.)

force of 500 pounds to be applied to the humeral head in order to disrupt it. Such directly applied forces are not commonly encountered and, if they were, would likely produce a fracture. However, if a person falls on the arm in a way that applies a force of 20 pounds to the arm 30 inches away from the center of rotation of the humeral head and if the resulting torque is resisted by a glenohumeral ligament attached 1 inch from the center of rotation of the humeral head, the resulting load may be sufficient to disrupt the ligament. Such a load would apply 600 inch-pounds (30 in × 20 lbs) of torque to the shoulder. In that the moment arm for glenohumeral ligaments is approximately 1 inch (the radius of the humeral head), the resulting tension in the restraining ligament would be 600 pounds, sufficient to avulse the ligament **(Fig. 10–4)**.

Less compliant or stiff ligaments may be more subject to avulsion, whereas more compliant ligaments are more able to absorb the applied load without failing. Ligaments and capsules that have been weakened by previous injury, by previous surgery, or by thermal or laser treatment may be more susceptible to disruption with lower loads than the loads required to tear normal structures.

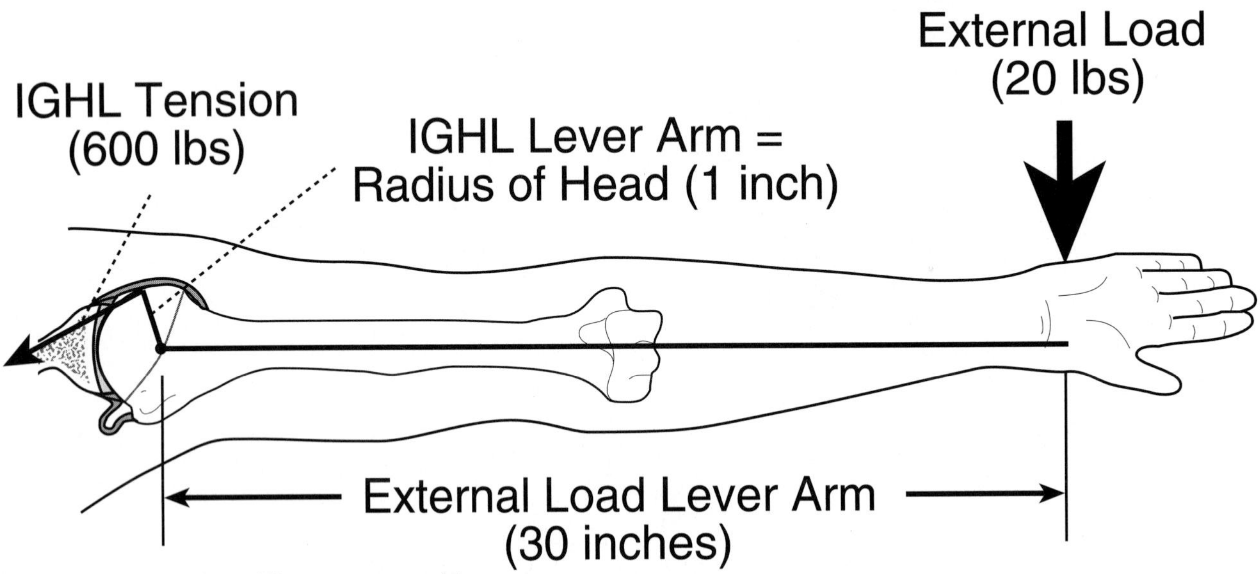


**Figure 10–4. Mechanism of ligamentous avulsion**
A load applied to the outstretched arm results in a much greater tension in the ligaments that restrain the rotation of the joint. If a load of 20 pounds applied at a distance of 30 inches from the center of the humeral head is opposed by a ligament acting 1 inch from the humeral head center, the necessary tension in the ligament would be 600 pounds, a tension sufficient to avulse the ligament attachment. If a load of 600 pounds were applied directly to the shoulder, other injuries such as fractures may well result. (Modified from Matsen FA, Lippitt SB, Sidles JA, et al [eds]: Practical Evaluation and Management of the Shoulder. Philadelphia: WB Saunders, 1994, p. 97.)

## CLINICAL CONSIDERATIONS

### Clinical Tests of the Ligaments

The laxity of a glenohumeral ligament is most easily quantified by documenting the rotation of the humerus in positions and directions in which that ligament is the primary restraint. For example, a substantial increase in the range of external rotation in comparison with the normal side suggests a tear or avulsion of the anterior capsule and ligaments (**Fig. 10–5**).

Ligamentous laxity can also be demonstrated by passive translation of the humeral head on physical examination. Examples of such translational laxity tests are the *anterior drawer*, the *posterior drawer*, and the *sulcus* tests.

It is essential to recognize that normal shoulders demonstrate rotational and translational laxity. Joint laxity of itself is not pathologic and does not require treatment. Laxity is not the same as instability.

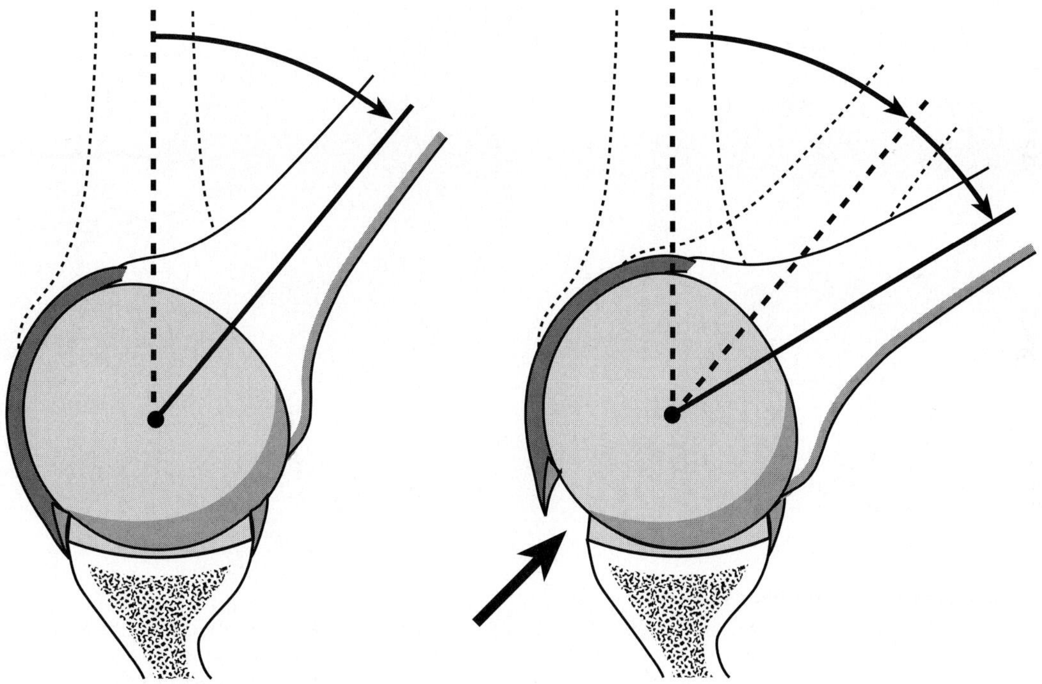

**Figure 10–5. Evidence of ligament avulsion**
When the ligament attachment is avulsed, the range of rotation may be increased in the direction usually constrained by the ligament.

## SURGICAL CONSIDERATIONS

### Procedures for the Glenohumeral Ligaments

Acute ligament tears and ligament avulsions from the glenoid lip can usually be repaired by direct suture if the tissues themselves are of sufficient quantity and quality. If the avulsion of the ligaments from the glenoid takes place lateral to the glenoid labrum, the capsule may be sutured directly to the labrum **(Fig. 10–6)**. If, as is most commonly the case, the capsule and the glenoid labrum are avulsed from the glenoid lip, a Bankart repair to freshened bone is needed (see Chapter 11) **(Fig. 10–7)**.

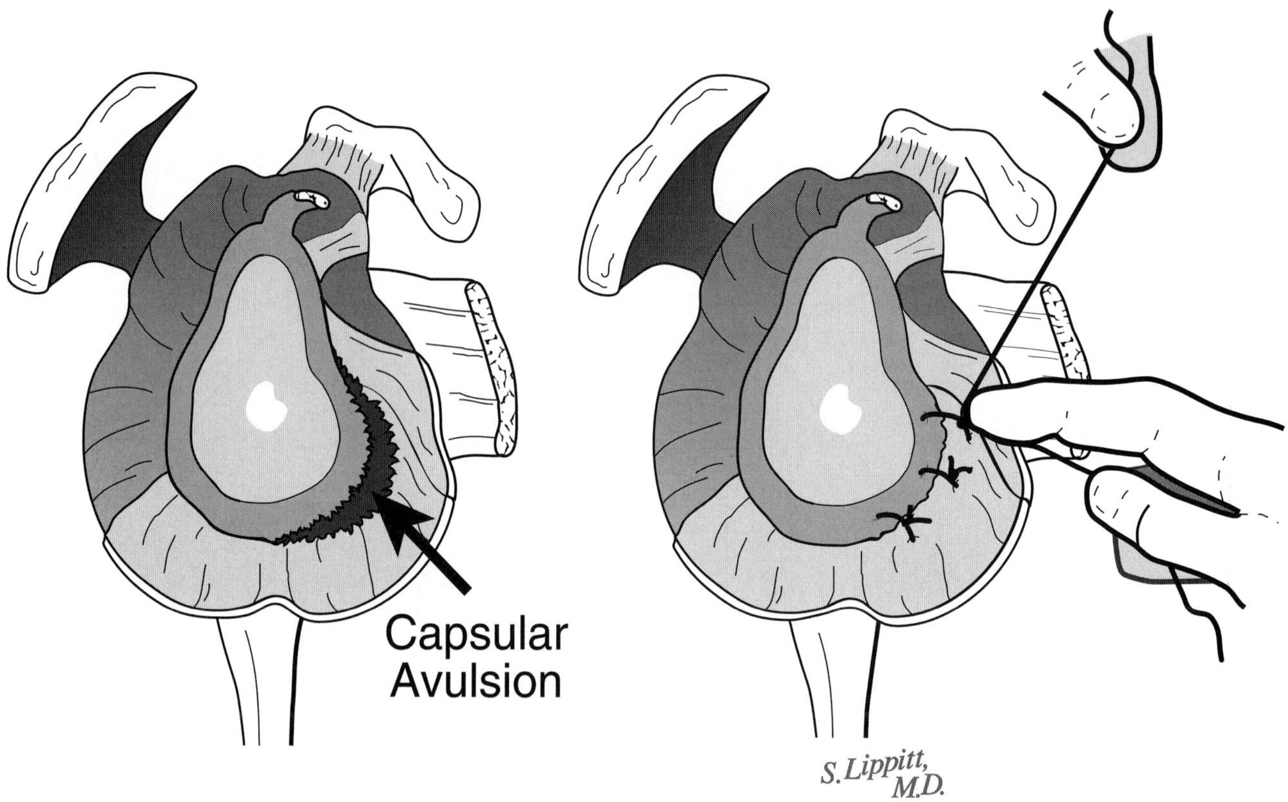


**Figure 10–6. Anatomic repair of capsular avulsion**
If the capsule is avulsed from the labrum, anatomic repair of the attachment of the ligaments to the labrum restores normal restraint of rotational laxity.

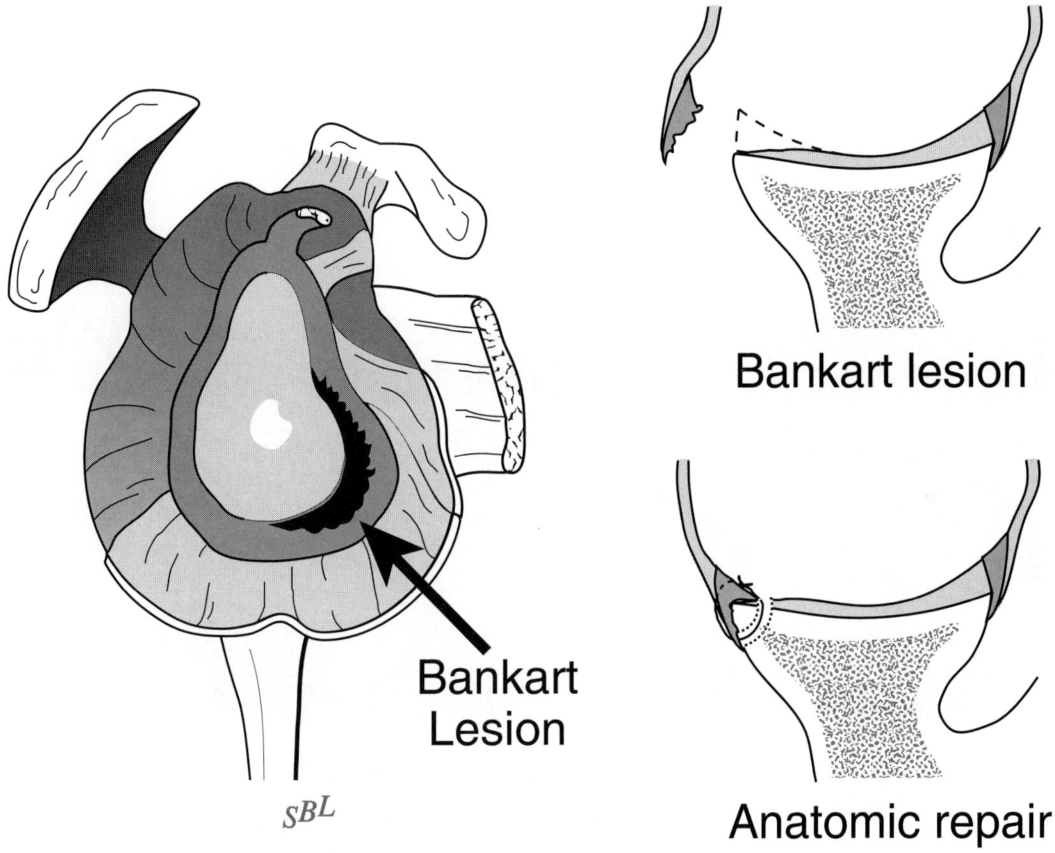


**Figure 10–7. Anatomic repair of labral avulsion**
If the labrum is avulsed from the glenoid, anatomic repair of the attachment of the labrum to the glenoid lip restores normal restraint of rotational laxity. (Modified from Matsen FA, Lippitt SB, Sidles JA, et al [eds]: Practical Evaluation and Management of the Shoulder. Philadelphia: WB Saunders, 1994, p. 103.)

If ligament deficiency leaves insufficient tissue for a robust repair, a reconstruction may be needed. In planning ligament repairs and reconstructions, it is important to determine (1) whether there is a concurrent deficiency in the glenoid labrum that also requires concurrent treatment and (2) the length of the reconstructed ligament necessary to provide the desired range of motion. We recall from the section on Principles of Glenohumeral Mobility (Chapter 6), that a loss of 10 mm of length of the capsule in an average-sized shoulder will deprive the articulation of about 20 degrees of rotation **(Fig. 10–8)**. If the capsuloligamentous tissue is of insufficient quantity or quality for a repair, for example after multiple failed repair attempts, a hamstring autograft to the capsule may be required (see Chapter 16).

Various capsular tightening and shifting procedures have been used to manage glenohumeral instability, especially when the instability is multidirectional. Because of the observation that humeral centering in the glenoid is not under ligamentous control, but rather is dependent on concavity compression, our preference is to manage multidirectional instability with physical retraining. If this program is not successful, we prefer a surgical approach that functionally deepens the glenoid fossa, as described in Chapter 14.

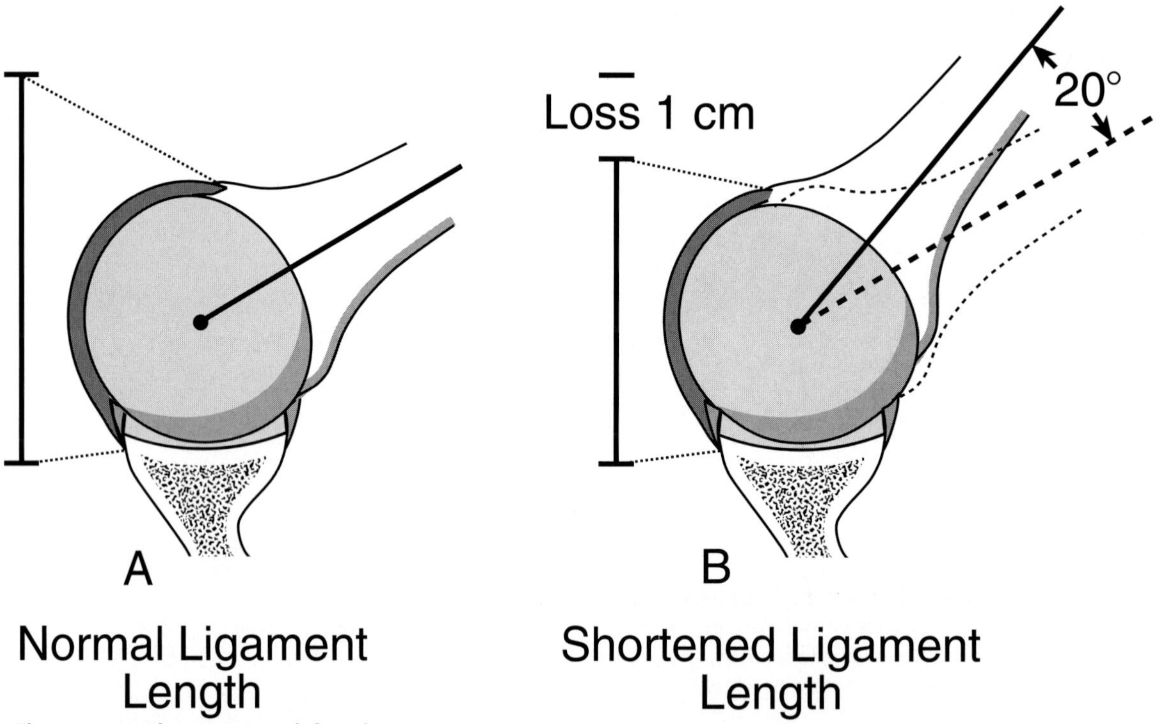


**Figure 10–8. Ligamentous tightening**
Any tightening of the ligaments will limit the range of motion in the directions that are controlled by the ligaments.

CHAPTER 11

# Procedure: Repair of the Avulsed Labrum in Traumatic Instability (Bankart Repair)

| | |
|---|---|
| ***Diagnosis*** | |
| ***Traumatic anterior instability*** | ***ICD9 CODE 718.31*** |
| ***Procedure*** | |
| ***Bankart repair*** | ***CPT CODE 23455*** |

## INDICATIONS

The patient has functionally significant recurrent anterior apprehension and instability of the shoulder from a traumatic injury forcing the arm into abduction and external rotation. The instability has been refractory to nonoperative management.

Physical examination reveals apprehension on the part of the patient when the arm is abducted and externally rotated. The shoulder demonstrates diminished resistance to the anterior load and shift test. Radiographs show a Hill-Sachs defect in the posterolateral humeral head.

Knowing the alternatives as well as the risks of infection, neurovascular injury, excessive stiffness, pain, weakness, fracture, instability, and the need for revision surgery, as well as anesthetic complications, the patient desires to proceed with the above-described procedure. The patient understands that the purpose of the procedure is to reestablish the glenoid fossa deepening effect of the glenoid labrum and to securely and anatomically reattach the anteroinferior glenohumeral capsule and ligaments with minimal reduction in the rotational laxity of the shoulder. The patient recognizes that this procedure cannot be expected to completely restore normal comfort and function to the shoulder. And, lastly, the patient understands his or her critical role in postsurgical rehabilitation.

## FINDINGS

Examination under anesthesia reveals diminished resistance to translation on the anterior load and shift test.

Surgical findings include a detachment of the labrum and capsule from the anteroinferior quadrant of the glenoid and a palpable defect in the posterolateral humeral head (**Fig. 11–1**).

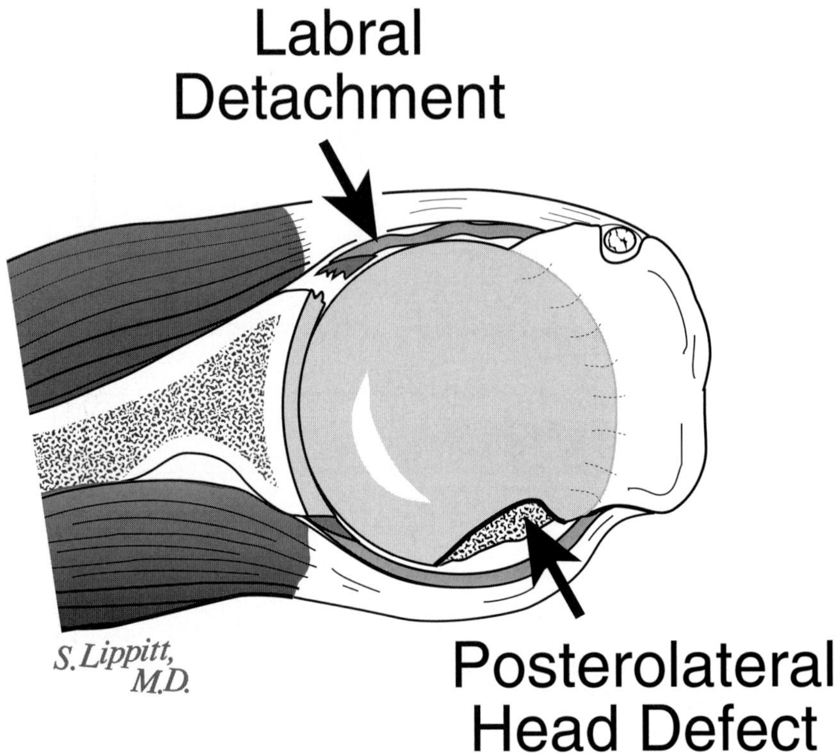


A

**Figure 11–1. Surgical findings in traumatic anterior glenohumeral instability**
**A,** The Hill-Sachs lesion is an impaction fracture of the posterior lateral humeral articular surface. The Bankart lesion is an avulsion of the glenoid labrum and capsule. (Modified from Rockwood CA, Matsen FA [eds]: The Shoulder, 2nd ed. Philadelphia: WB Saunders, 1998, p. 613.)

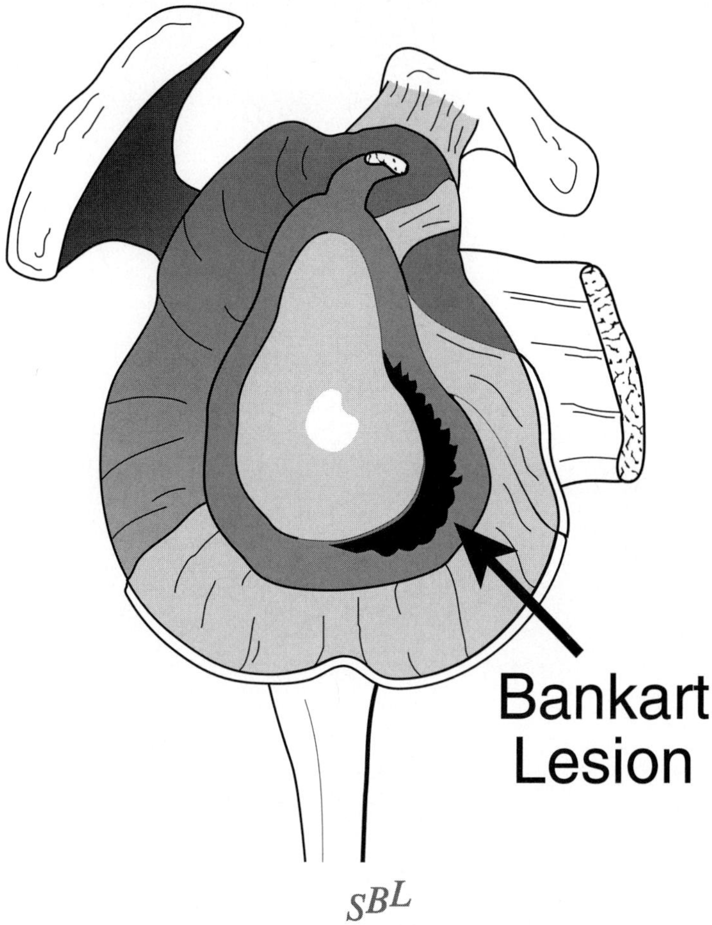


B

**Figure 11–1. Surgical findings in traumatic anterior glenohumeral instability—***Continued*

**B,** The Bankart lesion (avulsion of the glenoid labrum) usually extends from the anterior to the inferior glenoid. (Modified from Matsen FA, Lippitt SB, Sidles JA, et al [eds]: Practical Evaluation and Management of the Shoulder. Philadelphia: WB Saunders, 1994, p. 103.)

## OPERATION

Under satisfactory anesthesia, the patient is placed in a low beach chair position with the arm at the edge of the operating table. The shoulder is carefully prepped and draped. The major axillary crease is marked with a sterile pen. The shoulder is approached through a low anterior axillary incision made in this axillary crease **(Fig. 11–2)**. The skin is undermined superiorly to the level of the coracoid process **(Fig. 11–3)**. The deltopectoral interval is opened, leaving the cephalic vein on the deltoid laterally. The clavipectoral fascia is divided just lateral to the conjoined tendon and coracoid muscles, preserving the coracoacromial ligament superiorly **(Fig. 11–4)**.

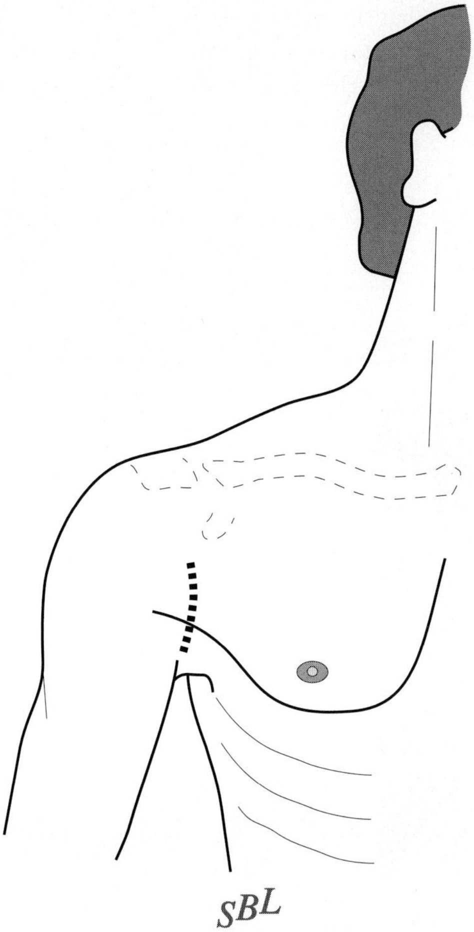

**Figure 11–2. Skin incision for Bankart repair**
If the incision is made in the major axillary crease, it usually heals with an excellent cosmetic result. (Modified from Rockwood CA, Matsen FA [eds]: The Shoulder, 2nd ed. Philadelphia: WB Saunders, 1998, p. 704.)

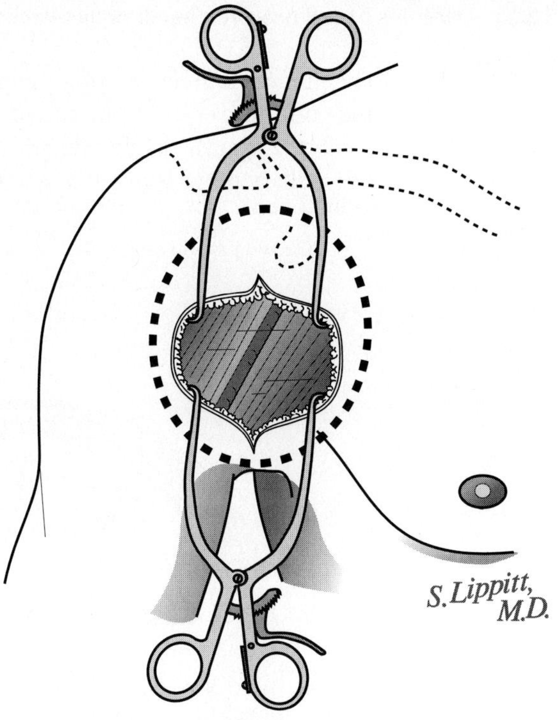

**Figure 11–3. The deltopectoral interval**
Subcutaneous dissection up to the level of the coracoid process exposes the cephalic vein in the deltopectoral groove. (Modified from Rockwood CA, Matsen FA [eds]: The Shoulder, 2nd ed. Philadelphia: WB Saunders, 1998, p. 704.)

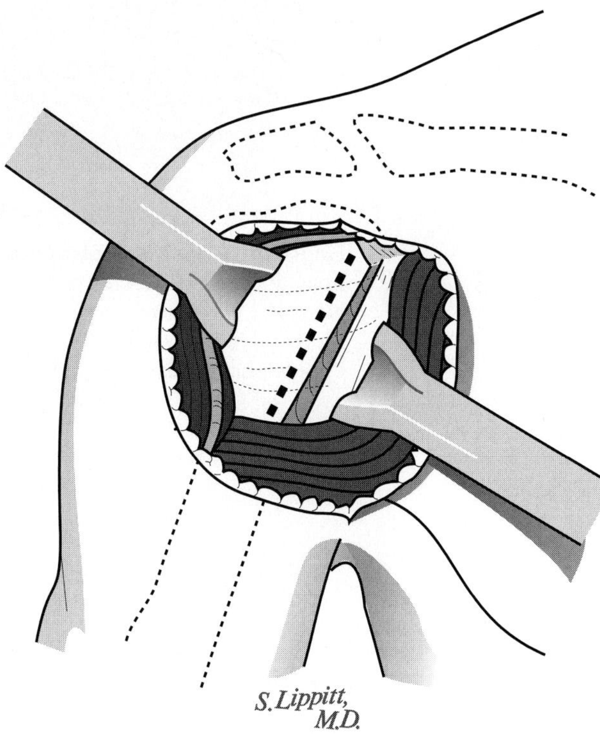

**Figure 11–4. Clavipectoral fascia**
Retraction of the deltoid and cephalic vein laterally and the pectoralis major medially exposes the clavipectoral fascia. This fascia is incised just lateral to the coracoid muscles and tendons (*dotted line*). (Modified from Rockwood CA, Matsen FA [eds]: The Shoulder, 2nd ed. Philadelphia: WB Saunders, 1998, p. 705.)

The humeroscapular motion interface is freed of adhesions so that the subscapularis and cuff muscles can be inspected **(Fig. 11–5)**. A self-retaining retractor is placed with one blade against the deltoid and the other against the coracoid muscles **(Fig. 11–6)**. The axillary nerve is palpated and protected throughout the procedure.

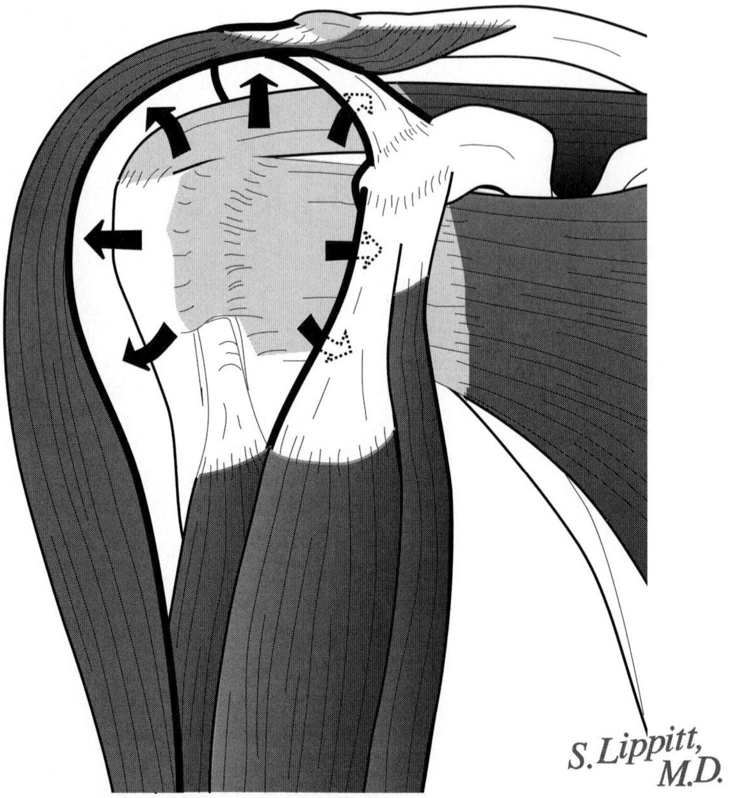


**Figure 11–5. The humeroscapular motion interface**
Any adhesions between the proximal humerus and the overlying deltoid, acromion, or coracoid are lysed. (Modified from Matsen FA, Lippitt SB, Sidles JA, et al [eds]: Practical Evaluation and Management of the Shoulder. Philadelphia: WB Saunders, 1994, p. 34.)

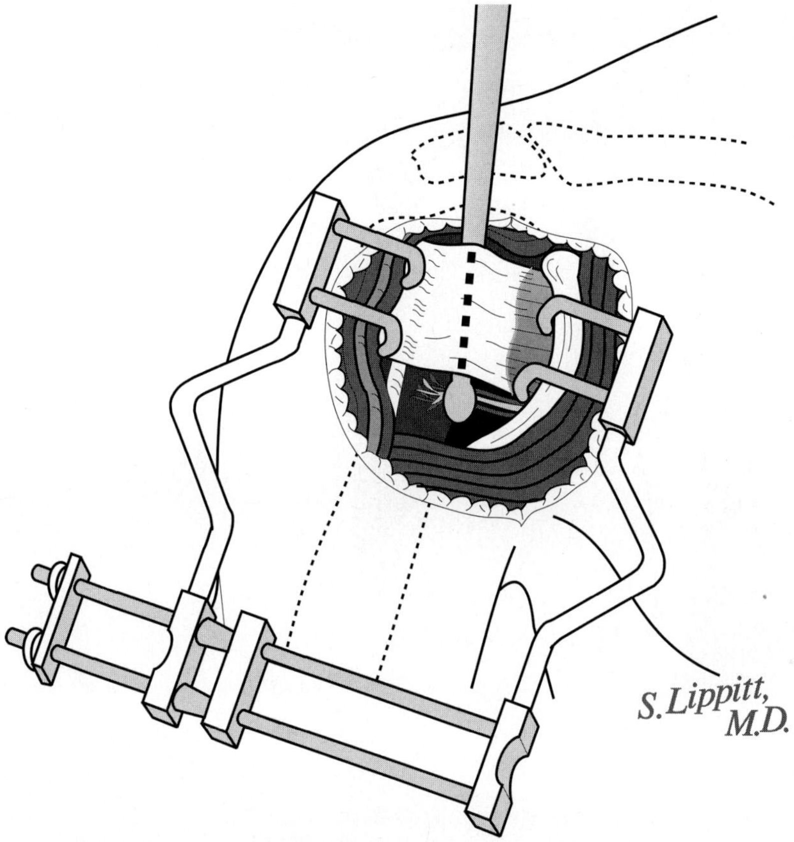


**Figure 11–6. Subscapularis incision**

The subscapularis is incised through its tendon, leaving good tissue on either side for later repair. The anterior humeral circumflex vessels are protected inferiorly. (Modified from Rockwood CA, Matsen FA [eds]: The Shoulder, 2nd ed. Philadelphia: WB Saunders, 1998, p. 705.)

The subscapularis and subjacent capsule are incised near their insertion to the lesser tuberosity, leaving sufficient tissue laterally for reattachment at the end of the procedure (**Fig. 11–7**). The tendon and capsule are not separated from each other, preserving their vascularity.

The glenohumeral joint is exposed with the above-described findings. The self-retaining retractor is removed.

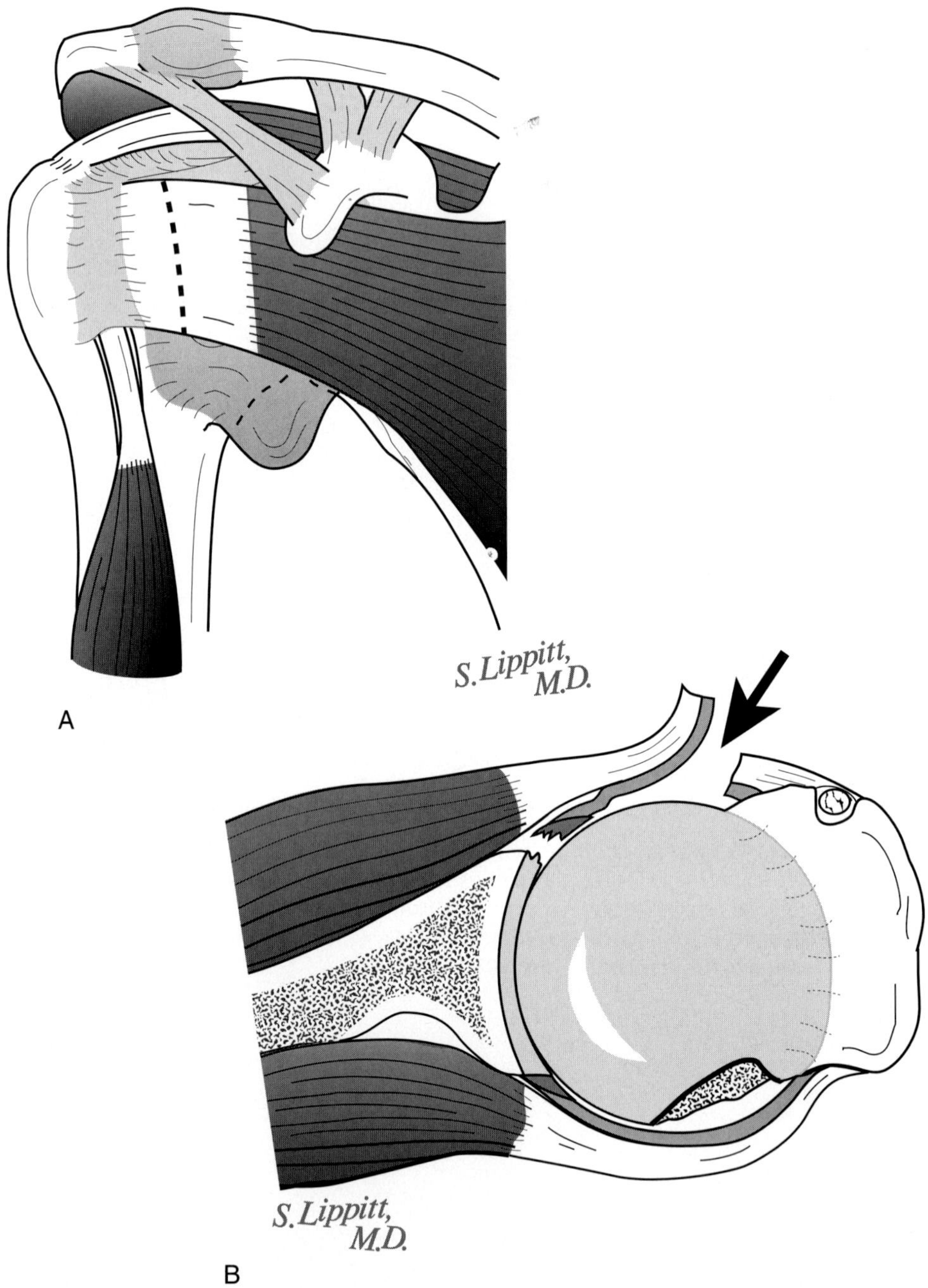


**Figure 11–7. Subscapularis and capsular incision**
**A,** The subscapularis is incised medial to the lesser tuberosity, with care taken to avoid the tendon of the long head of the biceps at the upper edge of the tendon. **B,** The subscapularis and subjacent capsule are incised so that strong tendinous tissue remains on either side of the incision. Sufficient tissue is left attached to the lesser tuberosity so that repair at the end of the case is facilitated. The subscapularis and capsule are not separated.

The glenoid is exposed using a humeral head retractor laterally and an angled retractor placed medially on the anteroinferior capsule. The area of labral detachment is identified. The insecurely attached capsule and labrum at the margins of the detachment are freed from the bony glenoid with an elevator. The angled retractor is removed and a spiked retractor is placed through the labral defect, exposing the anteroinferior glenoid lip (**Fig. 11–8**).

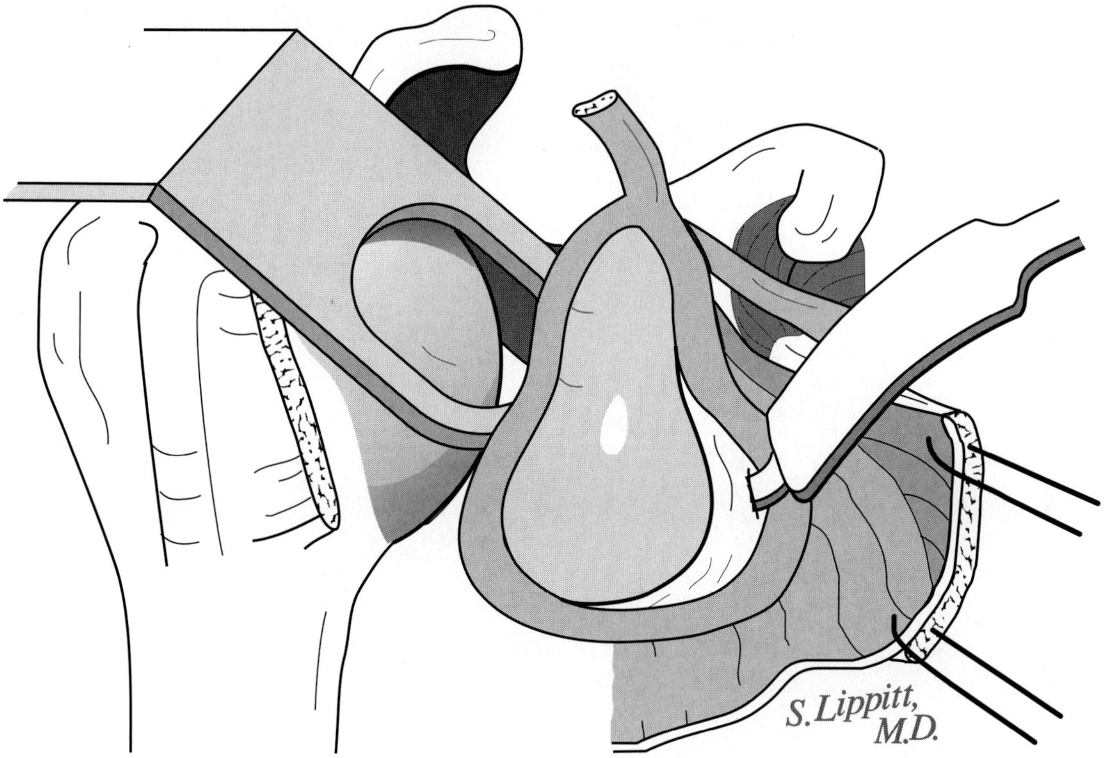


**Figure 11–8. Exposure of the anterior glenoid**
The lip of the glenoid from which the labrum has been avulsed is exposed by inserting a spiked retractor through the detachment onto the anterior glenoid neck.

The anterior nonarticular aspect of the glenoid is roughened with a pinecone burr, leaving the bone at the rim intact (**Fig. 11–9**). Along the area of the lesion, 1.8 mm holes are drilled into the glenoid articular surface 3 mm from the edge of the glenoid lip and 6 mm apart (**Fig. 11–10**). Corresponding slots are made on the anteroinferior glenoid neck opposite each drill hole, maintaining an adequate bone bridge at the

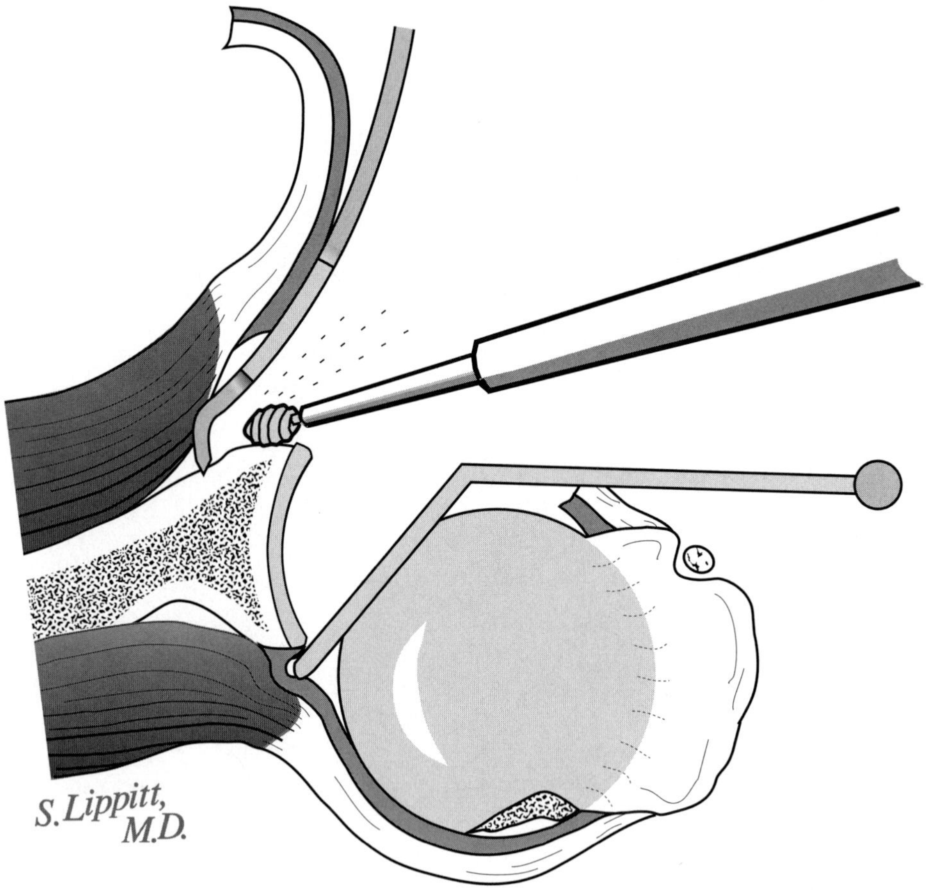


A

**Figure 11–9. Decortication of the anterior glenoid**
With the use of a pinecone burr, the cortex of the anterior, nonarticular aspect of the glenoid is roughened. (Modified from Rockwood CA, Matsen FA [eds]: The Shoulder, 2nd ed. Philadelphia: WB Saunders, 1998, p. 706.)

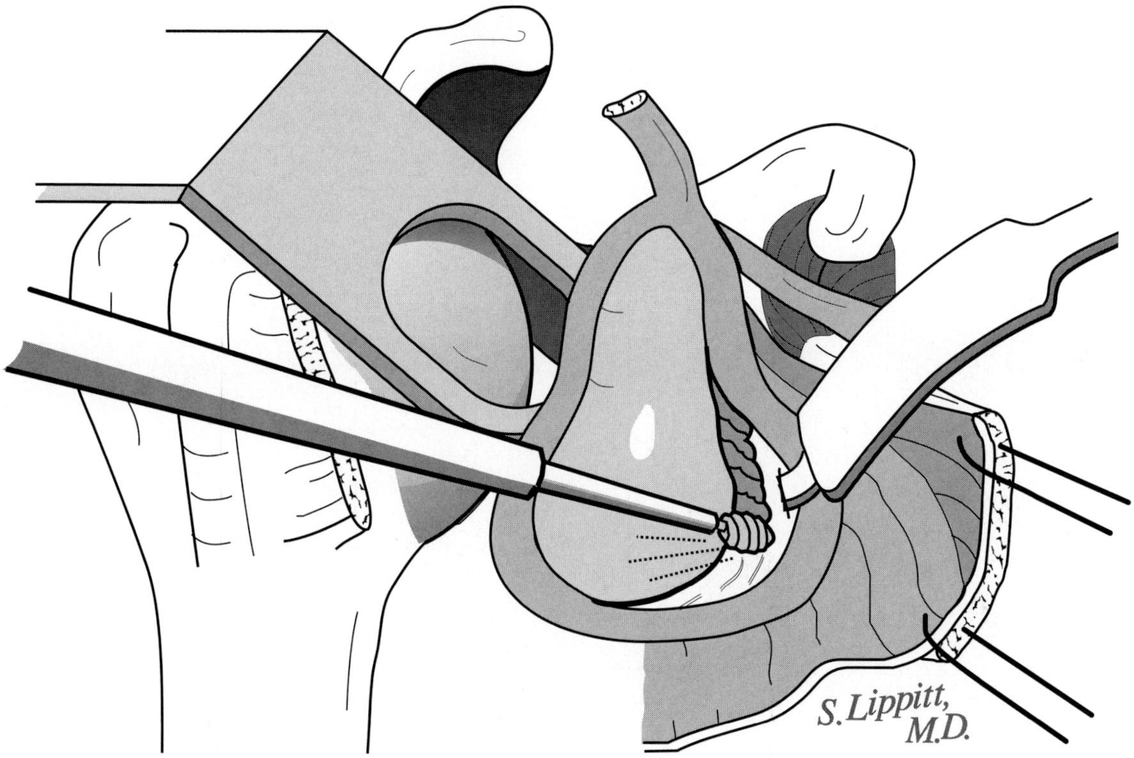


B

**Figure 11–9. Decortication of the anterior glenoid**—*Continued*
**B,** The decortication of the anterior glenoid continues for the full length of the detachment to facilitate healing of the detached labrum. (Modified from Matsen FA, Lippitt SB, Sidles JA, et al [eds]: Practical Evaluation and Management of the Shoulder. Philadelphia: WB Saunders, 1994, p. 105.)

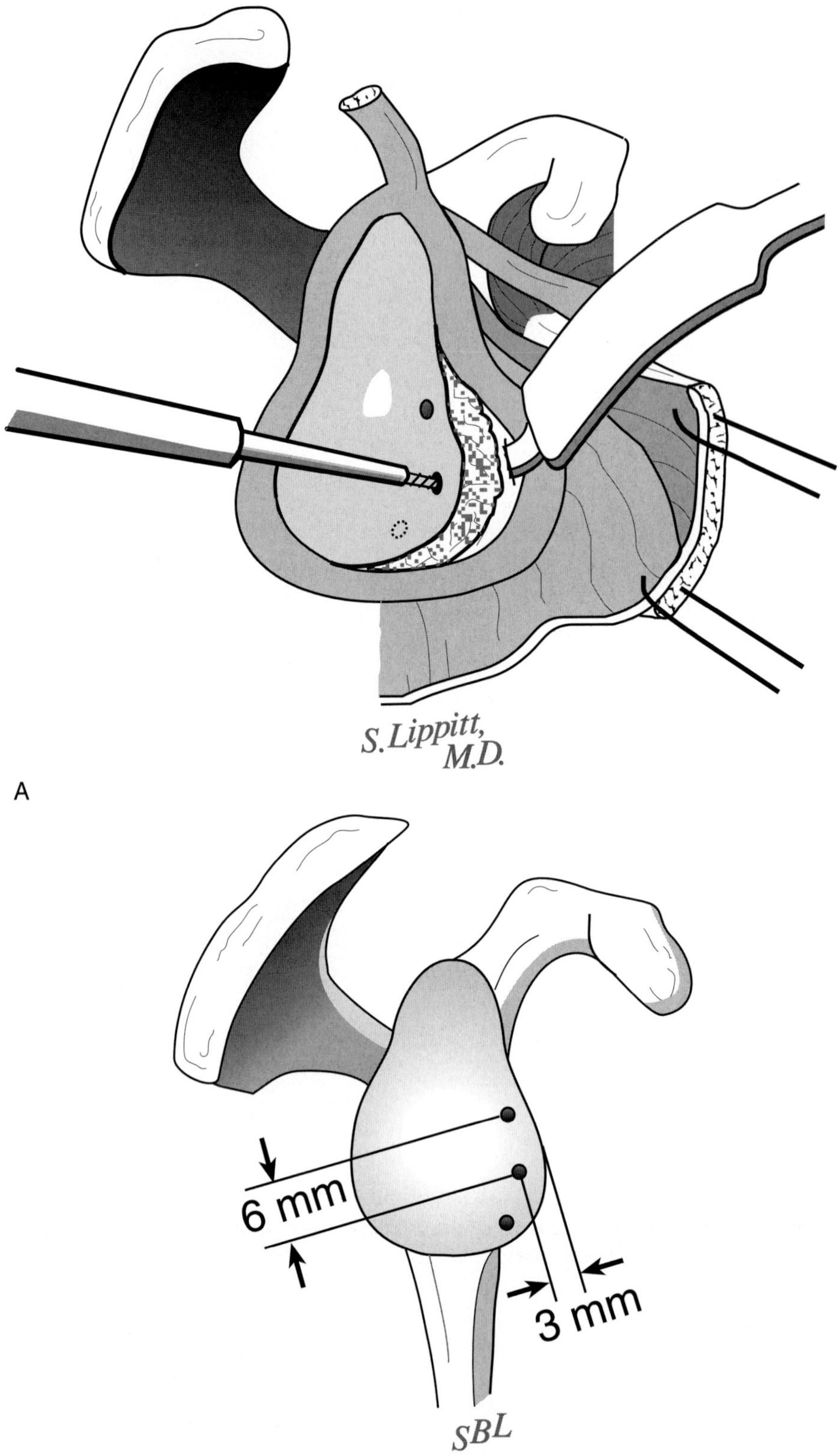


**Figure 11–10. Holes in the glenoid lip**
**A,** Holes are drilled through the cartilage and subchondral bone using a 1.8 mm drill. (Modified from Matsen FA, Lippitt SB, Sidles JA, et al [eds]: Practical Evaluation and Management of the Shoulder. Philadelphia: WB Saunders, 1994, p. 106.) **B,** The holes are placed 6 mm apart for the length of the defect and 3 mm back from the edge of the glenoid lip.

glenoid rim (**Fig. 11–11**). A 000 angled curette is used to complete the holes from the articular surface to the anterior nonarticular surface (**Fig. 11–12**). Number 2 braided nonabsorbable sutures are passed through these holes with a #5 trochar needle on an angled needle holder (**Fig. 11–13**). These sutures are then passed through the detached capsule just a bit more inferior than the corresponding drill hole so that the labrum

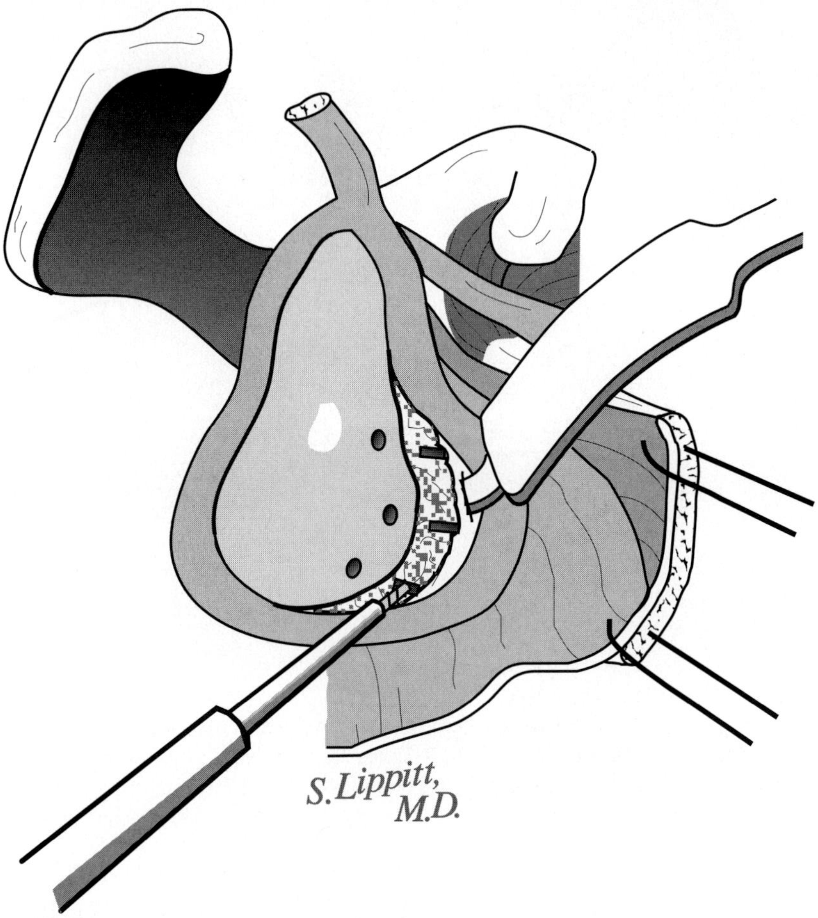


**Figure 11–11. Slots in the anterior glenoid**
If the anterior glenoid bone is dense, the 1.8 mm drill can be used to make slots to facilitate passage of the needle.

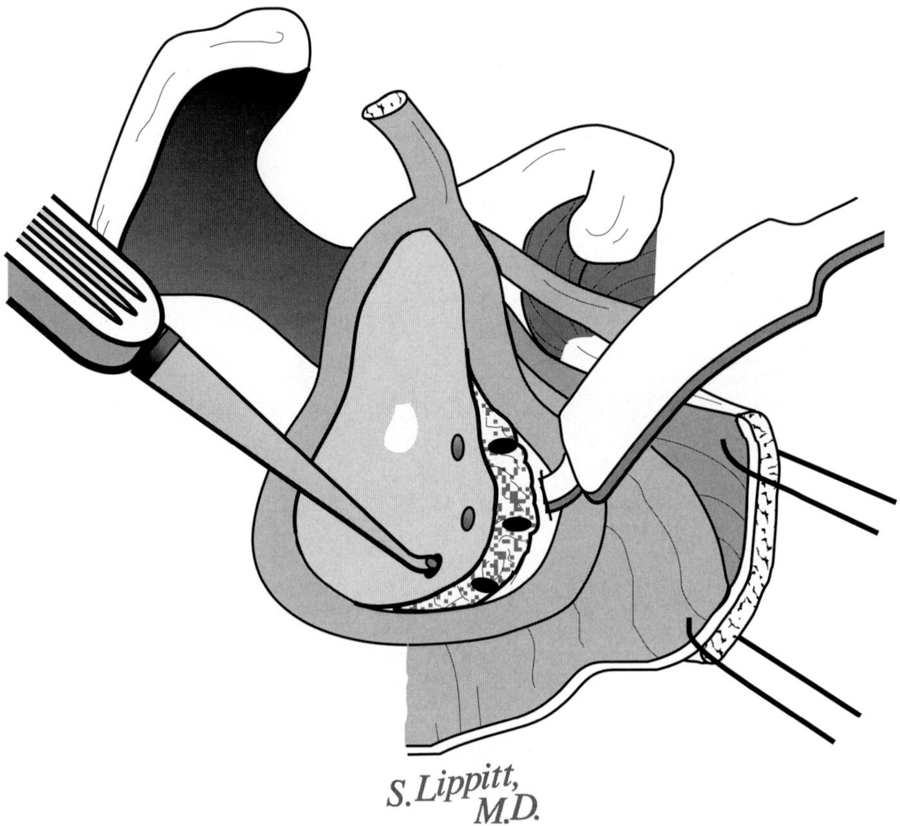


**Figure 11–12. Completing the holes**
Using a 000 angled curette, the holes are completed from the articular surface to the anterior glenoid. (Modified from Matsen FA, Lippitt SB, Sidles JA, et al [eds]: Practical Evaluation and Management of the Shoulder. Philadelphia: WB Saunders, 1994, p. 106.)

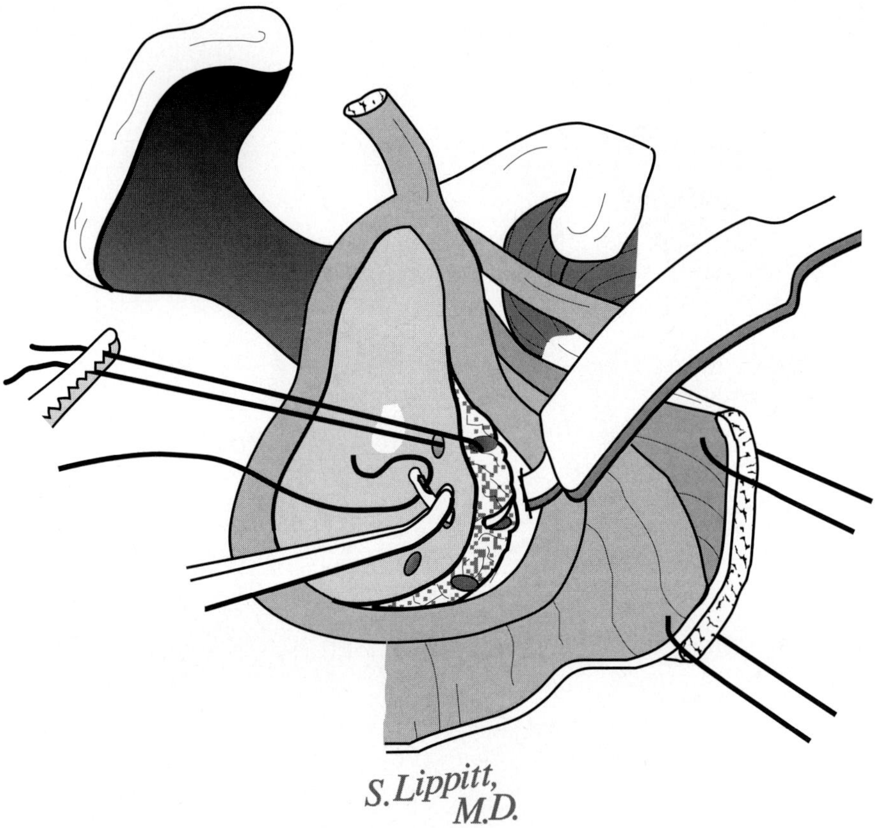


**Figure 11–13. Passing the needle**
Using an angled needle holder, a #5 trochar needle carrying #2 braided nonabsorbable suture is passed through each hole. (Modified from Matsen FA, Lippitt SB, Sidles JA, et al [eds]: Practical Evaluation and Management of the Shoulder. Philadelphia: WB Saunders, 1994, p. 106.)

will be pulled up to its normal position as the sutures are tied (**Fig. 11–14**). In that the ligaments have been torn from their glenoid attachment rather than stretched, no attempt is made to reduce the capsular laxity or to shift or tighten in this anatomic repair.

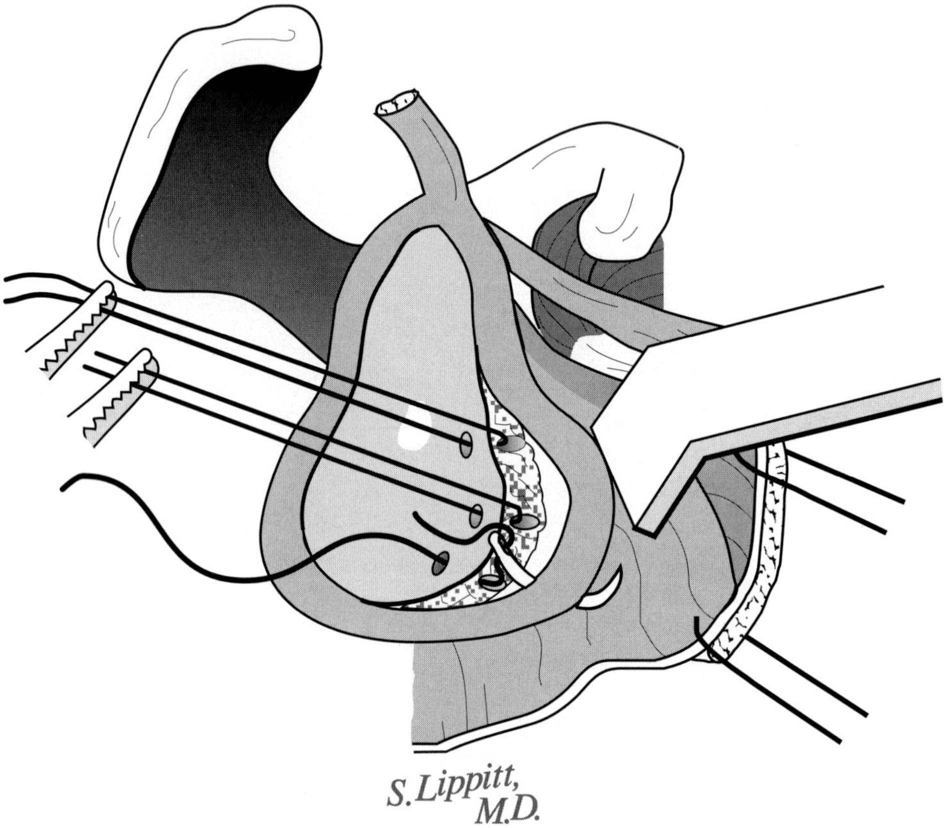


A

**Figure 11–14. Suturing the labrum and capsule**
**A,** Each suture is passed through the labrum, or if there is no residual labrum, through the trailing medial edge of the capsule. (Modified from Matsen FA, Lippitt SB, Sidles JA, et al [eds]: Practical Evaluation and Management of the Shoulder. Philadelphia: WB Saunders, 1994, p. 106.)

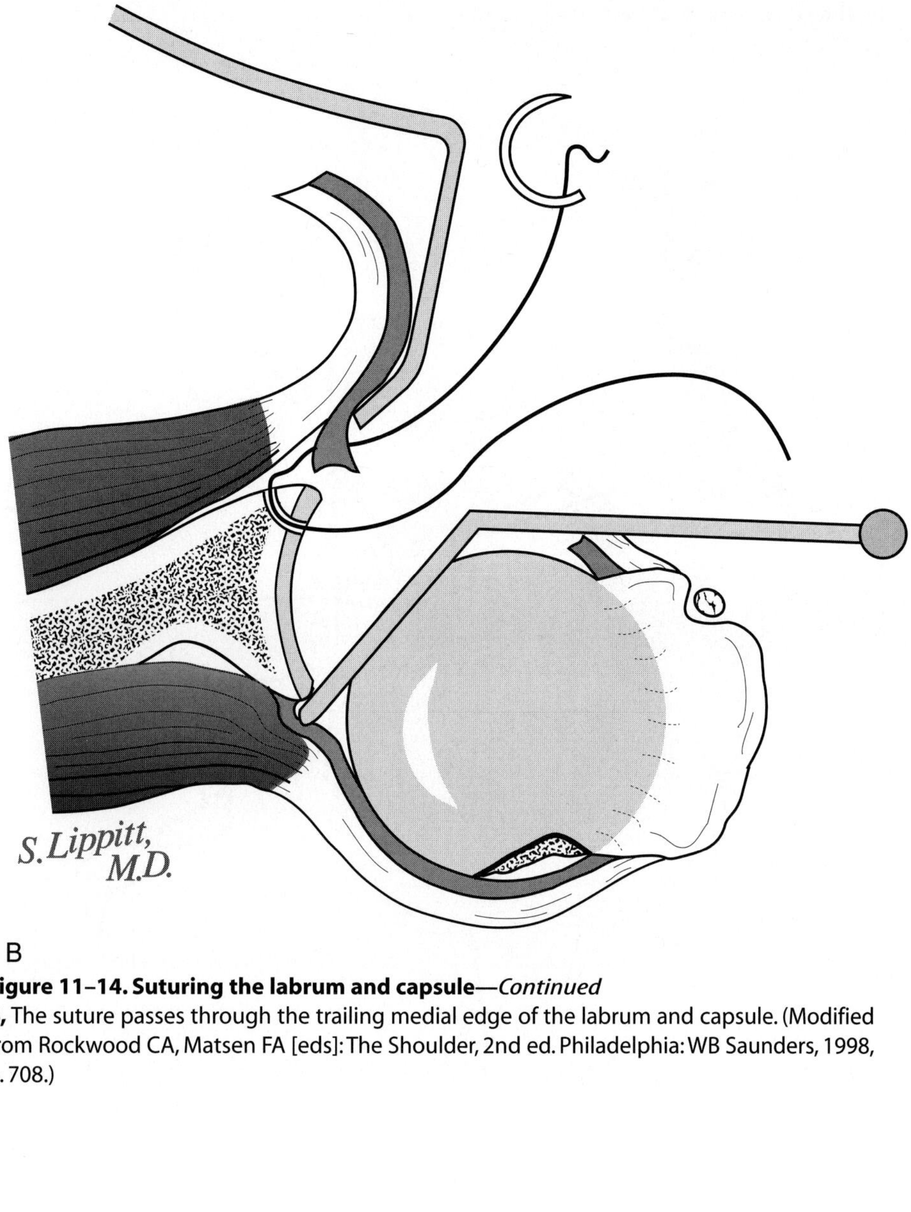


B

**Figure 11–14. Suturing the labrum and capsule**—*Continued*
**B,** The suture passes through the trailing medial edge of the labrum and capsule. (Modified from Rockwood CA, Matsen FA [eds]: The Shoulder, 2nd ed. Philadelphia: WB Saunders, 1998, p. 708.)

The sutures are tied around the limb of the suture passing through the capsule (rather than the one passing through the articular cartilage) **(Fig. 11–15)**. Tying the knots in this way pushes the capsule and labrum back up on the surface of the glenoid, restoring the fossa-deepening function of the labrum **(Fig. 11–16)**. The knots lie against the compliant capsule rather than on the articular cartilage. The security and anatomic location of the reattachment is verified. The capsule is inspected for additional lesions, which are repaired as indicated.

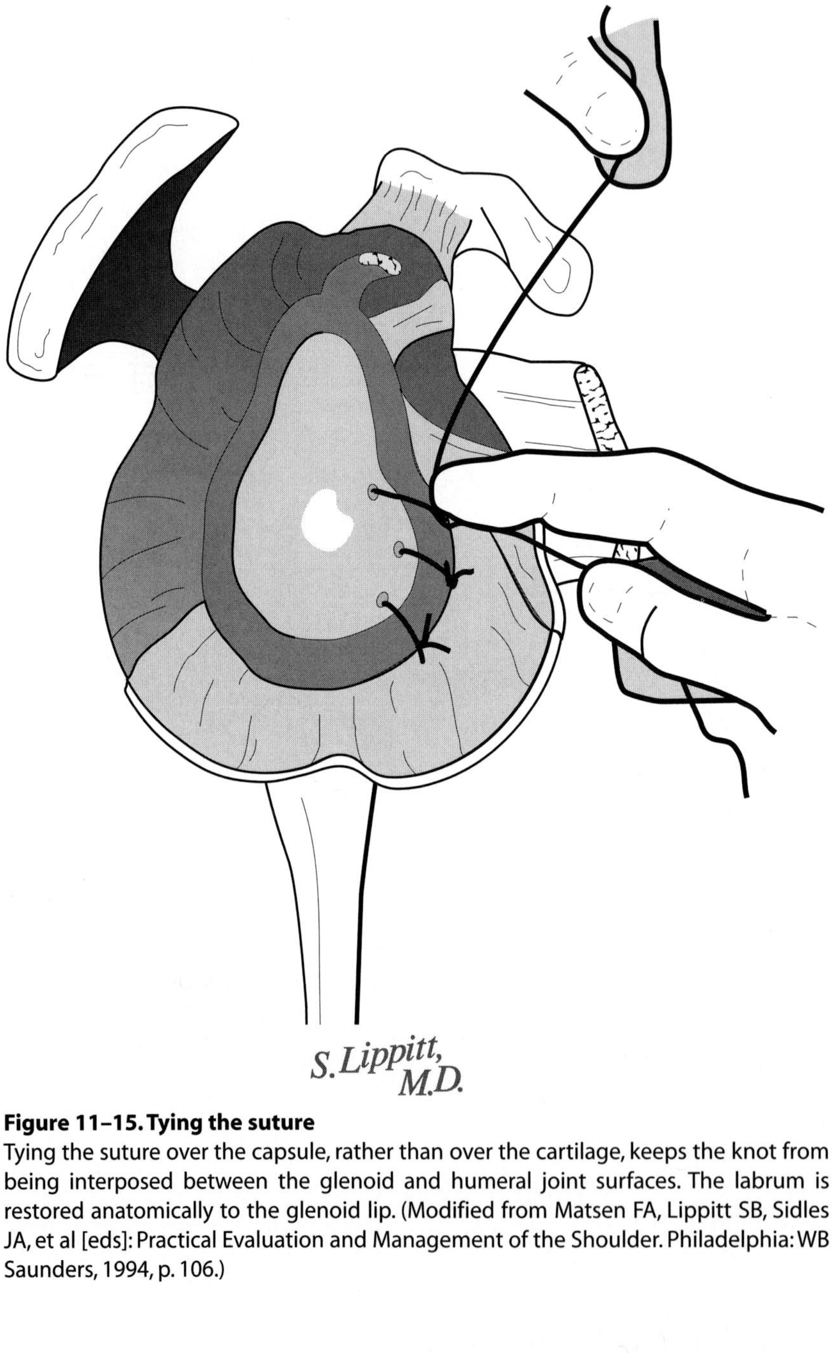


**Figure 11–15. Tying the suture**
Tying the suture over the capsule, rather than over the cartilage, keeps the knot from being interposed between the glenoid and humeral joint surfaces. The labrum is restored anatomically to the glenoid lip. (Modified from Matsen FA, Lippitt SB, Sidles JA, et al [eds]: Practical Evaluation and Management of the Shoulder. Philadelphia: WB Saunders, 1994, p. 106.)

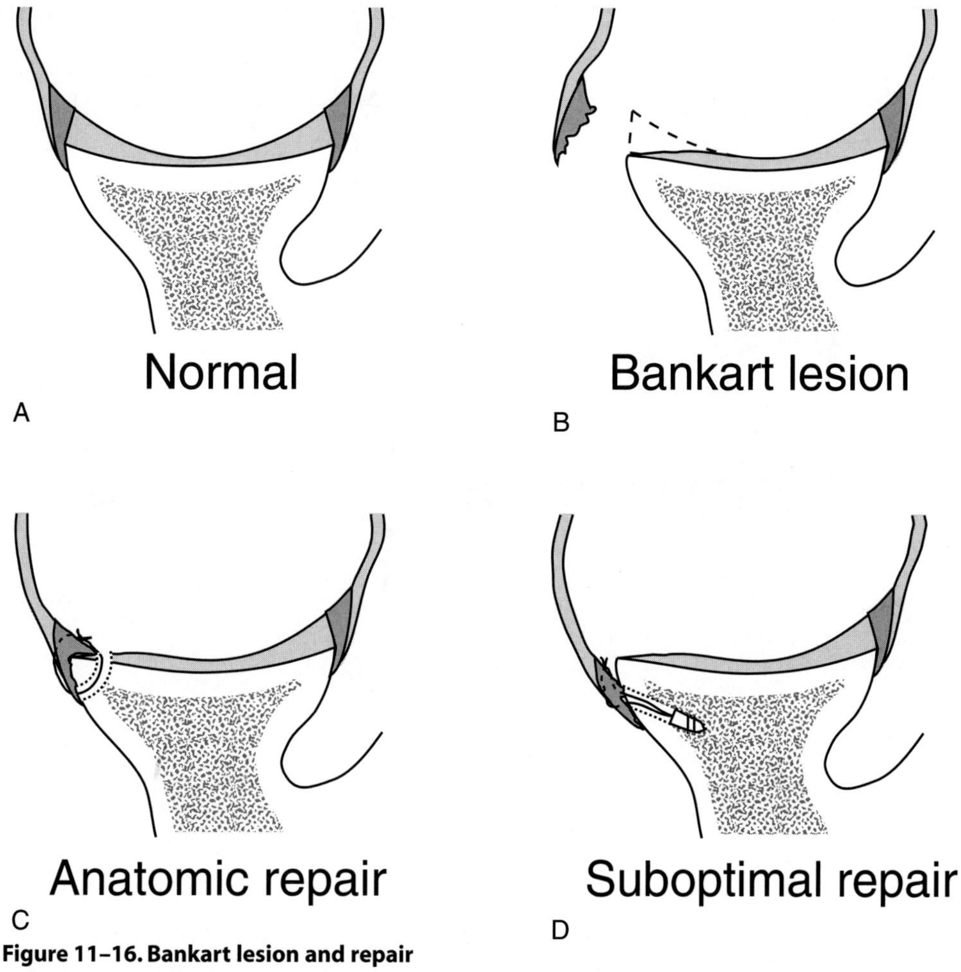


**Figure 11–16. Bankart lesion and repair**

**A,** Normally, the labrum contributes to the depth of the glenoid fossa. **B,** Detachment of this labrum compromises the glenoid concavity. **C,** Reattachment of the labrum to the lip restores the glenoid concavity. **D,** Reattachment to the neck of the glenoid does not restore the concavity. (Modified from Matsen FA, Lippitt SB, Sidles JA, et al [eds]: Practical Evaluation and Management of the Shoulder. Philadelphia: WB Saunders, 1994, p. 70.)

The wound is thoroughly irrigated. The subscapularis and lateral capsule are then closed back to the corresponding tendon and capsule at the lesser tuberosity, using six sutures of #2 nonabsorbable braided suture (**Fig. 11–17**).

The wound is closed in layers. Dry sterile dressings are applied, and the patient is returned to the recovery room with the arm in a sling.

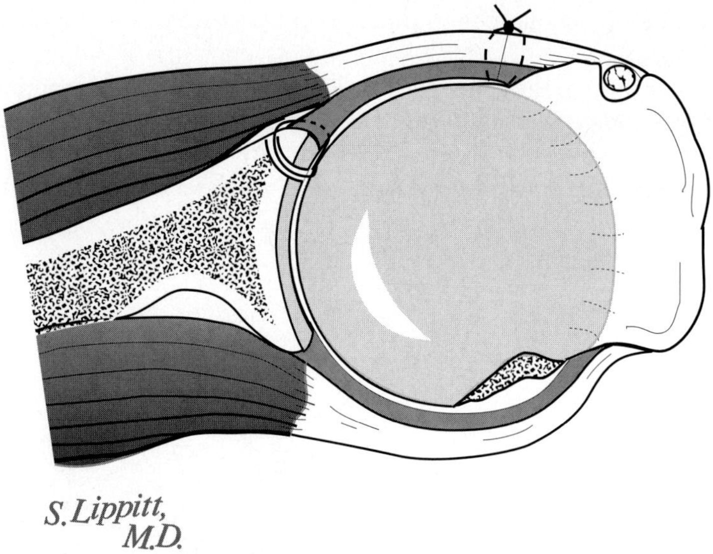


**Figure 11–17. Final repair**
Once the labrum has been reattached to the glenoid lip, the subscapularis and capsule are repaired anatomically. No capsular shift or capsular tightening is performed so that range of motion is not limited needlessly. (Modified from Rockwood CA, Matsen FA [eds]: The Shoulder, 2nd ed. Philadelphia: WB Saunders, 1998, p. 708.)

## POSTOPERATIVE PLAN

The postoperative plan includes immediate implementation of patient-conducted external rotation to 0 degrees and elevation to 90 degrees (**Fig. 11–18**). As soon as these exercises can be performed by the patient, the patient is discharged. The patient is encouraged to remove the sling and use the arm actively for gentle activities within the allowed range when functioning in a protected environment. Lifting is limited to 1 pound for 6 weeks.

At 2 weeks after surgery, the patient is instructed to begin increasing motion so that external rotation to 40 degrees and forward elevation to 140 degrees are achieved by 6 weeks. Gentle progressive strengthening exercises are started at 6 weeks. After 3 months, activities will be progressively resumed as shoulder comfort, strength, and security permit.

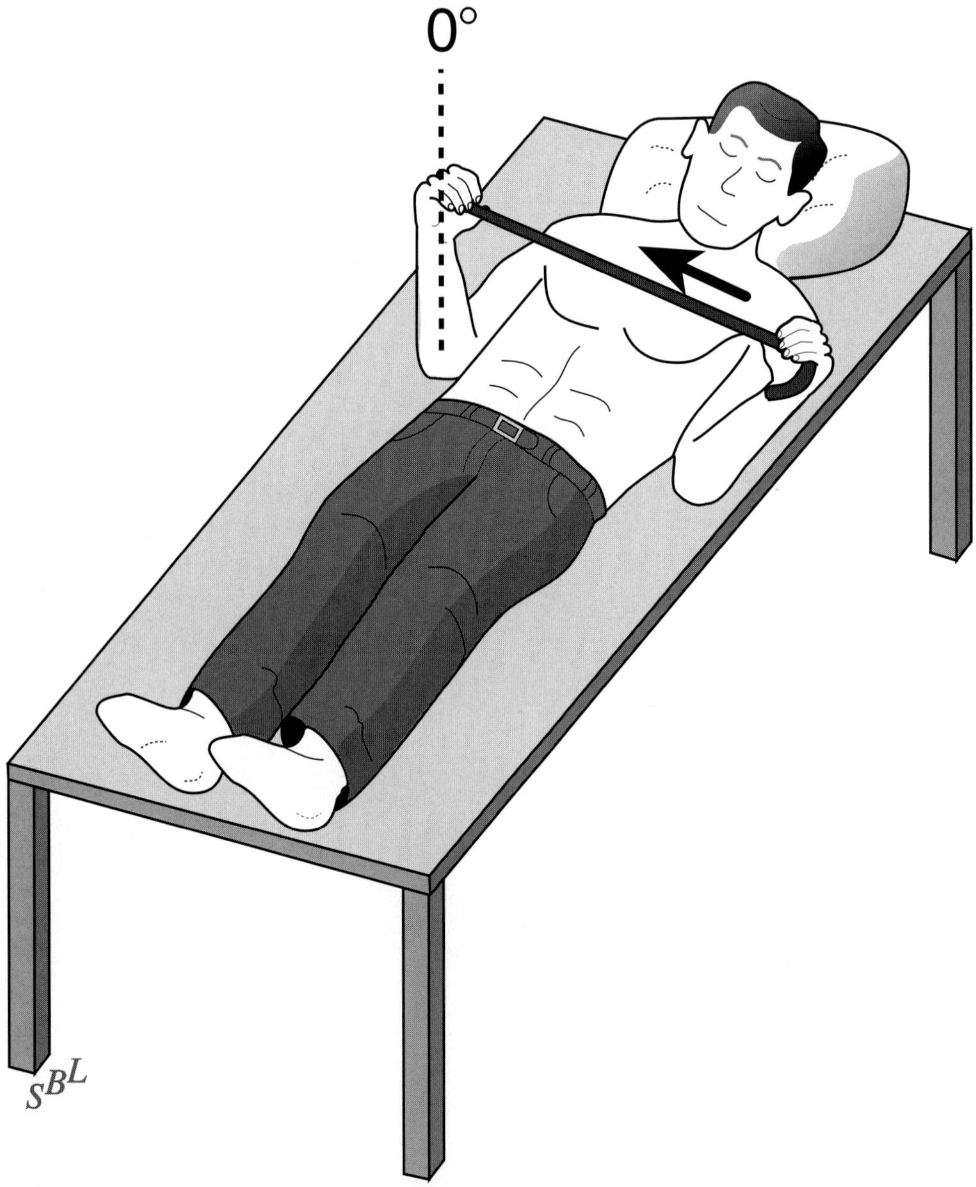


A

**Figure 11–18. Immediate postoperative rehabilitation**
**A,** Using the opposite hand and a cane or yardstick, the operated arm is passively externally rotated to 0 degrees.

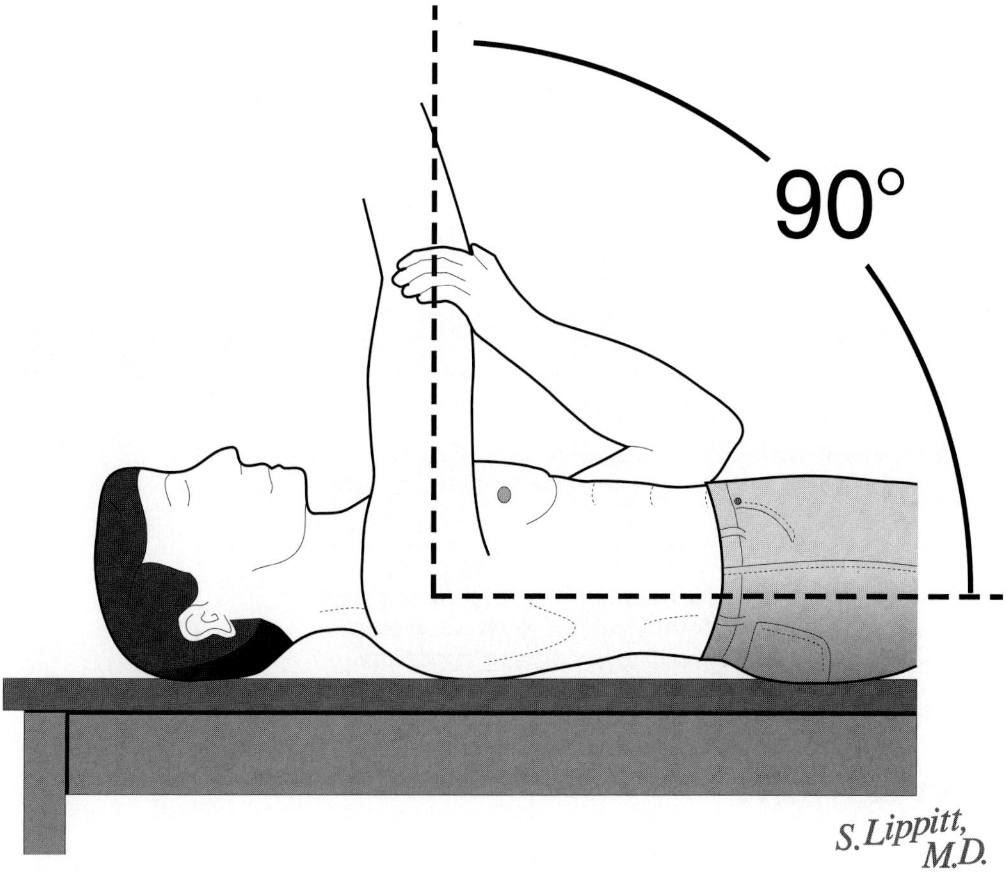


B

**Figure 11–18. Immediate postoperative rehabilitation**—*Continued*
**B,** Using the opposite hand, the operated arm is passively elevated to 90 degrees.

CHAPTER 12

# Procedure: Reconstruction of a Deficient Anterior Glenoid Lip Using an Extracapsular Anatomically Contoured Iliac Crest Graft

***Diagnosis***

***Recurrent anterior instability associated with a deficient anterior glenoid lip ICD9 CODE 718.31***

***Procedure***

***Reconstruction of anterior glenoid lip using an anatomically contoured extracapsular iliac crest autograft with screw fixation CPT CODE 23460, 20902***

## INDICATIONS

The patient has functionally significant refractory recurrent anterior glenohumeral instability, both with the arm at the side and when the arm is abducted. This instability has not responded to standard treatment, including previous surgical repairs.

Physical examination shows a lack of resistance to the anterior load and shift test (**Fig. 12–1**).

Radiographs show a bony deficiency of the anteroinferior bony glenoid, as shown by rounding of the anterior glenoid lip on the axillary radiograph and apical oblique view, as well as loss of the anteroinferior glenoid cortical line on the anteroposterior view. A moderate-sized Hill-Sachs lesion is noted on the apical oblique view.

Knowing the alternatives as well as the risks of infection, neurovascular injury, excessive stiffness, pain, weakness, fracture, instability, iliac crest donor site problems,

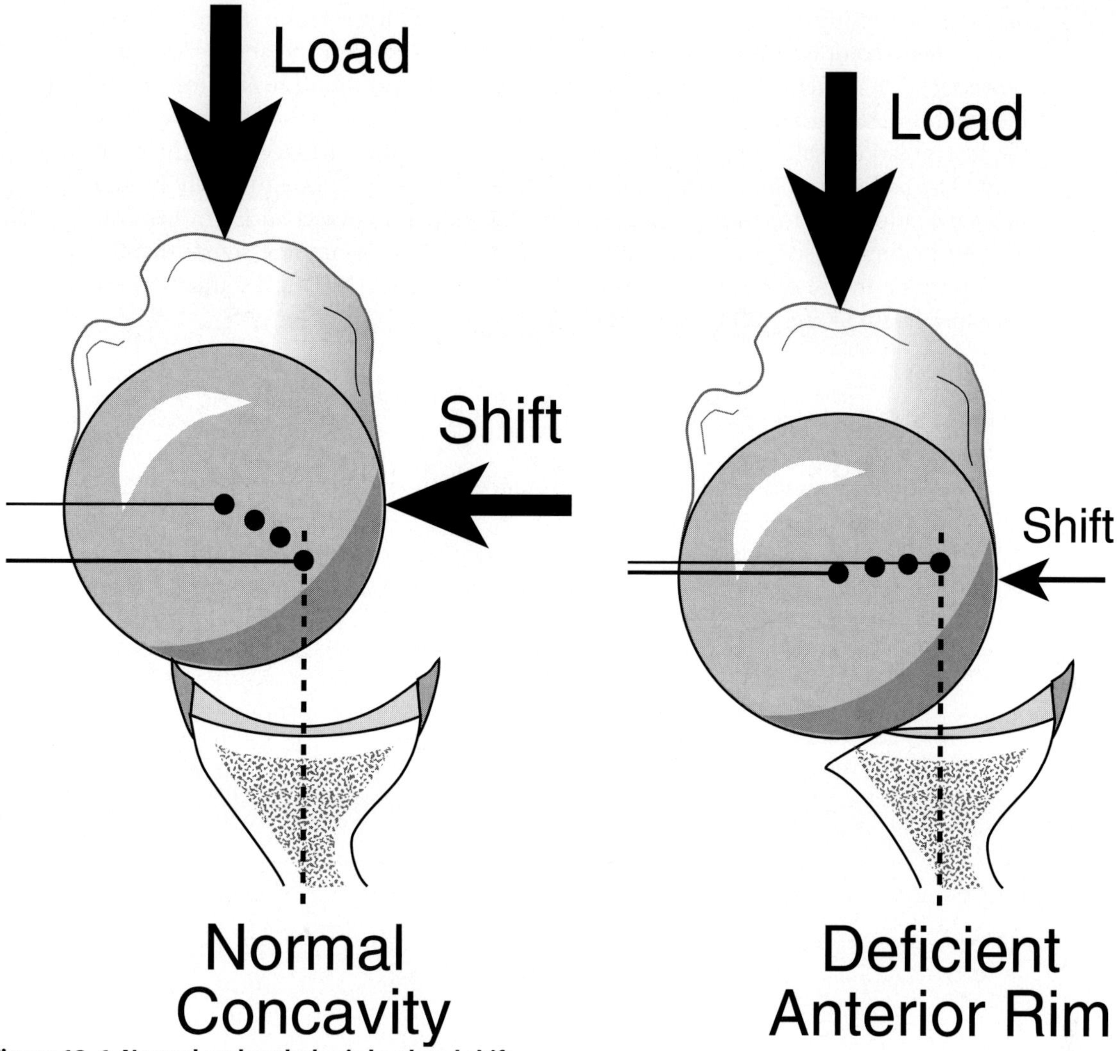


**Figure 12–1. Normal and pathologic load and shift**

In the load and shift test, the humeral head is pressed into the glenoid, and, while this loading is maintained, the examiner attempts to translate the humeral head from its position centered on the glenoid. Normally, the concavity of the glenoid provides substantial resistance to any translation. When the glenoid lip is deficient, the humeral head translates more easily from the centered position.

hardware loosening, glenohumeral arthritis, and the need for revision surgery, as well as anesthetic complications, the patient desires to proceed with the above-described procedure. The patient understands that the purpose of the procedure is to reestablish the anteroinferior glenoid width and depth with a bone graft from the iliac crest, using the interposed capsule to protect the humeral head articular cartilage from the bone graft. The patient recognizes that this procedure cannot be expected to fully restore normal comfort and function to the shoulder. The patient understands his or her critical role in the post-surgical rehabilitation. And, lastly, the patient understands that the use of a cane in the opposite hand may be necessary for several weeks after surgery because of pain in the graft harvest area.

## FINDINGS

Examination under anesthesia reveals no resistance to anterior translation on the anterior load and shift test (see **Fig. 12–1**).

Surgical findings include detachment of the anteroinferior glenoid labrum and capsule as well as loss of the anteroinferior glenoid cartilage so that there is essentially no functional anteroinferior glenoid concavity **(Fig. 12–2)**. There is a moderate-sized defect of the posterolateral humeral head (Hill-Sachs lesion).

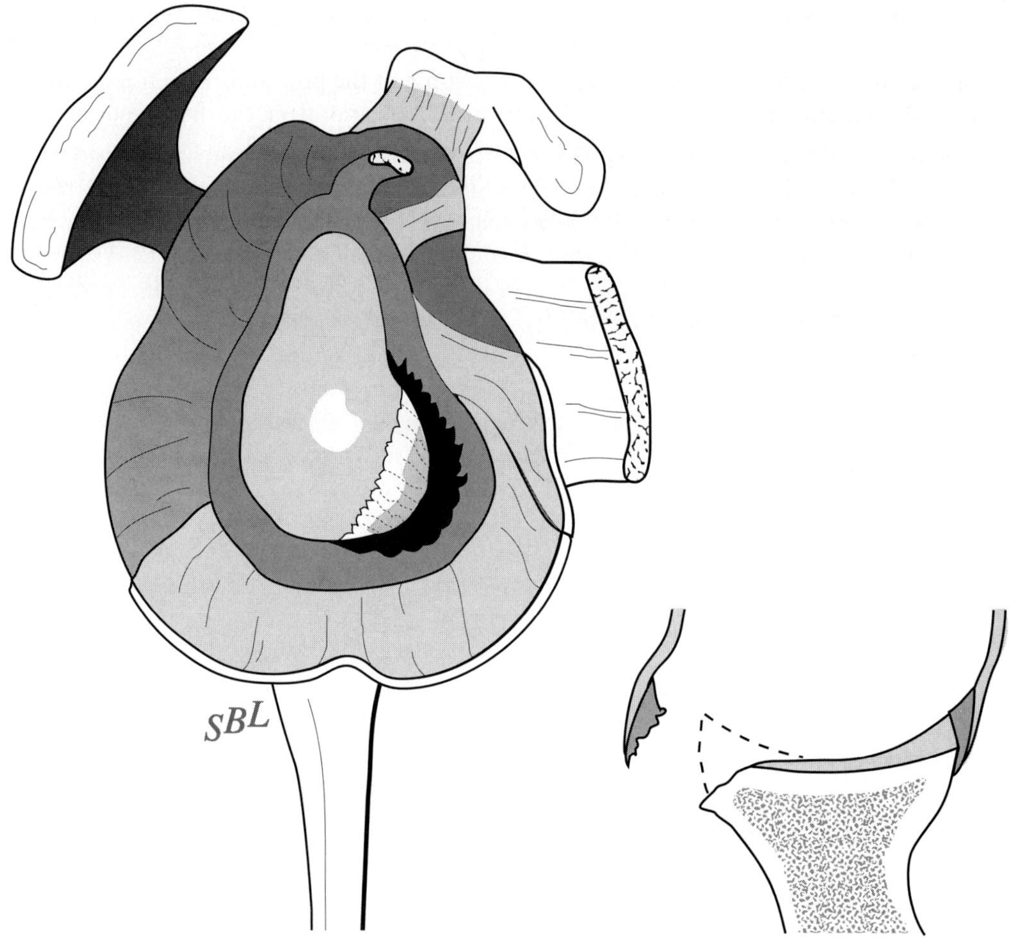


A

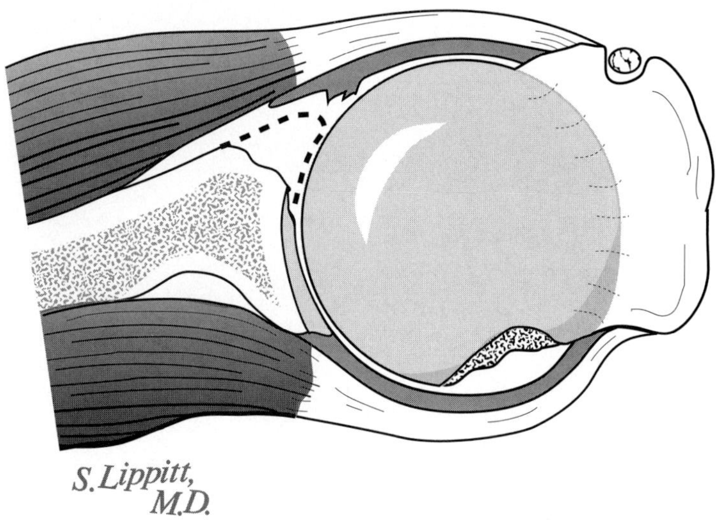


B

**Figure 12–2. Eroded anterior glenoid lip**

**A,** Deficient anterior glenoid lip. Loss of the glenoid labrum, the anterior glenoid cartilage, and the anterior glenoid bone can each contribute to diminished resistance to translation from the centered position. **B,** Loss of the anterior bony lip. Deficiency of the bony lip of the glenoid compromises the potential for reattaching the residual capsule and labrum at their physiologic length. (Modified from Rockwood CA, Matsen FA [eds]: The Shoulder, 2nd ed. Philadelphia: WB Saunders, 1998, p. 709.)

## OPERATION

Under satisfactory anesthesia, the patient is placed in a low beach chair position with the glenohumeral joint arm at the edge of the operating table. The shoulder and ipsilateral iliac crest are carefully prepped and draped. If there is a reasonable incisional scar from a previous surgery, the previous incision can be repeated. Otherwise, the major axillary crease is marked with a sterile pen and the shoulder is approached through a low anterior axillary incision made in this axillary crease (**Fig. 12–3**). The skin is undermined superiorly to the level of the coracoid process (**Fig. 12–4**). The deltopectoral interval is opened, leaving the cephalic vein on the deltoid laterally. The clavipectoral fascia is divided just lateral to the conjoined tendon, preserving the coracoacromial ligament superiorly (**Fig. 12–5**). The humeroscapular motion interface is freed of adhesions and thickened bursa from previous injury and surgery. A self-retaining retractor is placed with one blade against the deltoid and the other against the coracoid muscles. The axillary nerve is palpated and protected throughout the case.

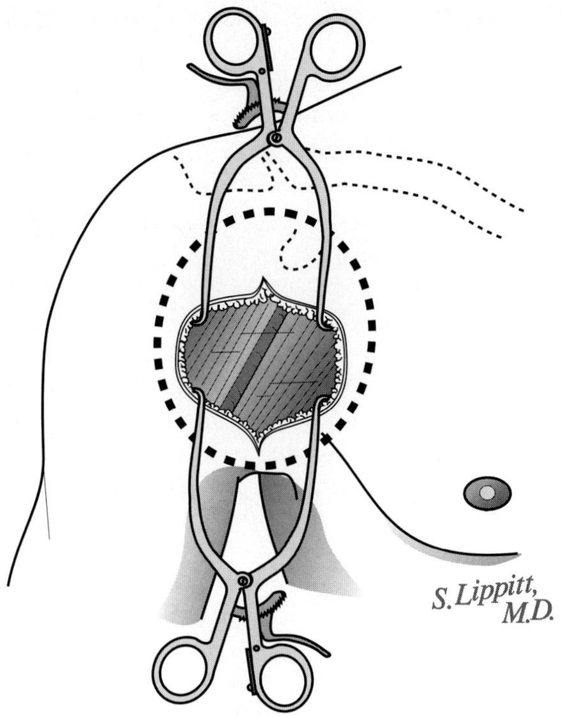


**Figure 12–4. The deltopectoral groove**
The subcutaneous tissue is mobilized to the level of the coracoid process, exposing the deltopectoral groove and the cephalic vein. (Modified from Rockwood CA, Matsen FA [eds]: The Shoulder, 2nd ed. Philadelphia: WB Saunders, 1998, p. 704.)

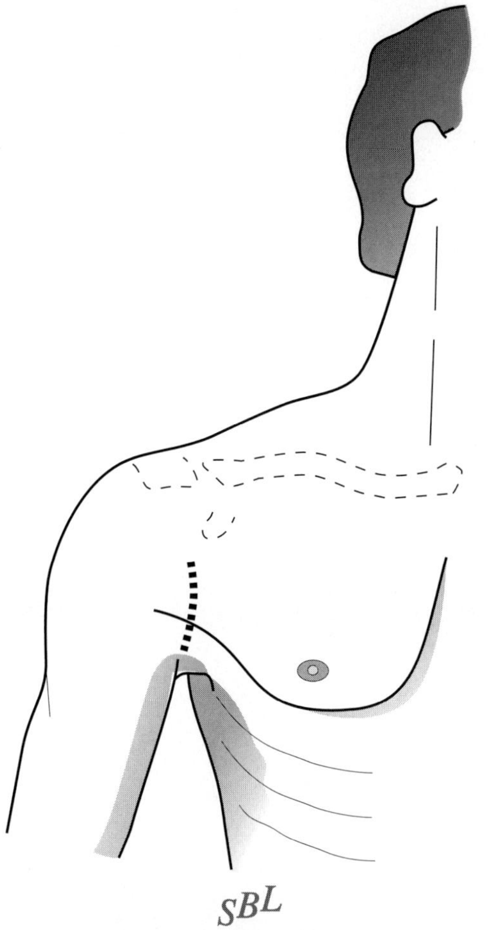


**Figure 12–3. Anteroinferior axillary incision**
The incision is made in the skin lines of the major axillary crease. (Modified from Rockwood CA, Matsen FA [eds]: The Shoulder, 2nd ed. Philadelphia: WB Saunders, 1998, p. 704.)

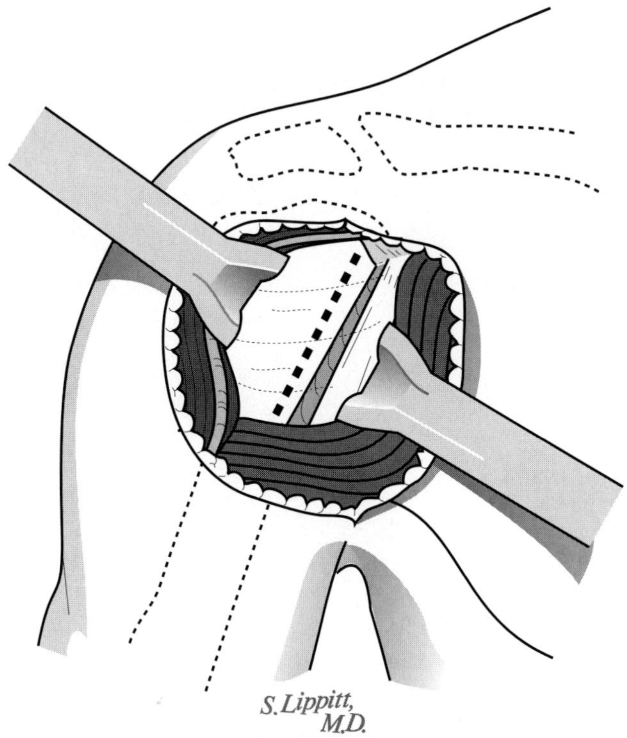


**Figure 12–5. Clavipectoral fascia**
With the deltoid and cephalic vein retracted laterally and the pectoralis major retracted medially, the clavipectoral fascia is incised just lateral to the coracoid muscles and tendons (*dotted line*). (Modified from Rockwood CA, Matsen FA [eds]: The Shoulder, 2nd ed. Philadelphia: WB Saunders, 1998, p. 705.)

The subscapularis tendon and subjacent capsule are incised near their insertion to the lesser tuberosity, leaving sufficient tissue laterally for reattachment at the end of the procedure (**Fig. 12–6**).

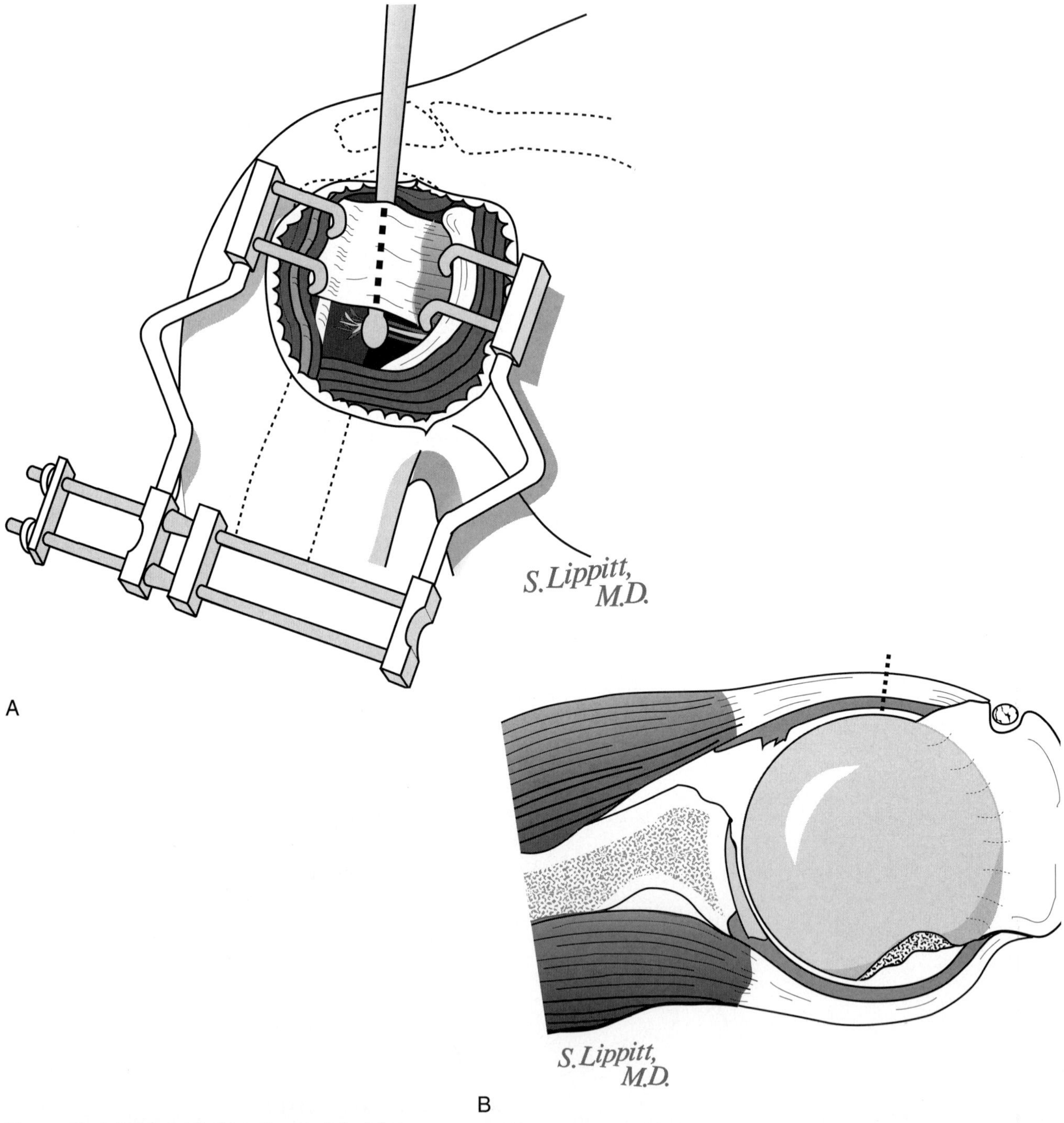


**Figure 12–6. Subscapularis and capsule incision**

**A,** The subscapularis is incised through its tendon. The anterior humeral circumflex vessels are protected inferiorly. (Modified from Rockwood CA, Matsen FA [eds]: The Shoulder, 2nd ed. Philadelphia: WB Saunders, 1998, p. 705.) **B,** The incision is positioned to leave good tissue on either side for later repair. (Modified from Rockwood CA, Matsen FA [eds]: The Shoulder, 2nd ed. Philadelphia: WB Saunders, 1998, p. 709.)

The glenohumeral joint is exposed with the above-described findings.

Tag sutures are placed in the superior and inferior corners of the capsule and of the subscapularis tendon. With the use of a sharp knife, the capsule and subscapularis are dissected free of each other. The plane of dissection is carried down to the anterior glenoid neck (**Fig. 12–7**).

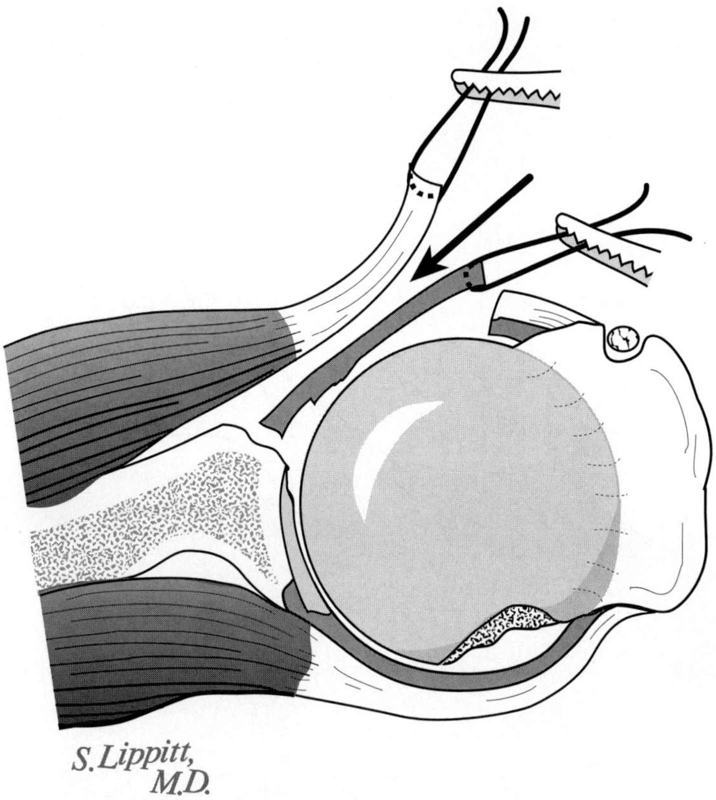


**Figure 12–7. Splitting of the capsule from the subscapularis**
The capsule is dissected sharply from the subscapularis. (Modified from Churchill RS, Moskal MJ, Lippitt SB, Matsen FA: Extracapsular anatomically countoured anterior glenoid bone grafting for complex glenohumeral instability. Techn Shoulder Elbow Surg 2:214, 2001.)

The self-retaining retractor is removed and a humeral head retractor is used to expose the glenoid. A spiked retractor is placed on the medial glenoid neck. With the axillary nerve protected, a second spiked retractor is placed under the inferior glenoid neck.

The anterior glenoid neck is identified by palpation (**Fig. 12–8**). A 25 × 25 mm flat area on the inferior aspect of the anterior of the glenoid neck is identified as the

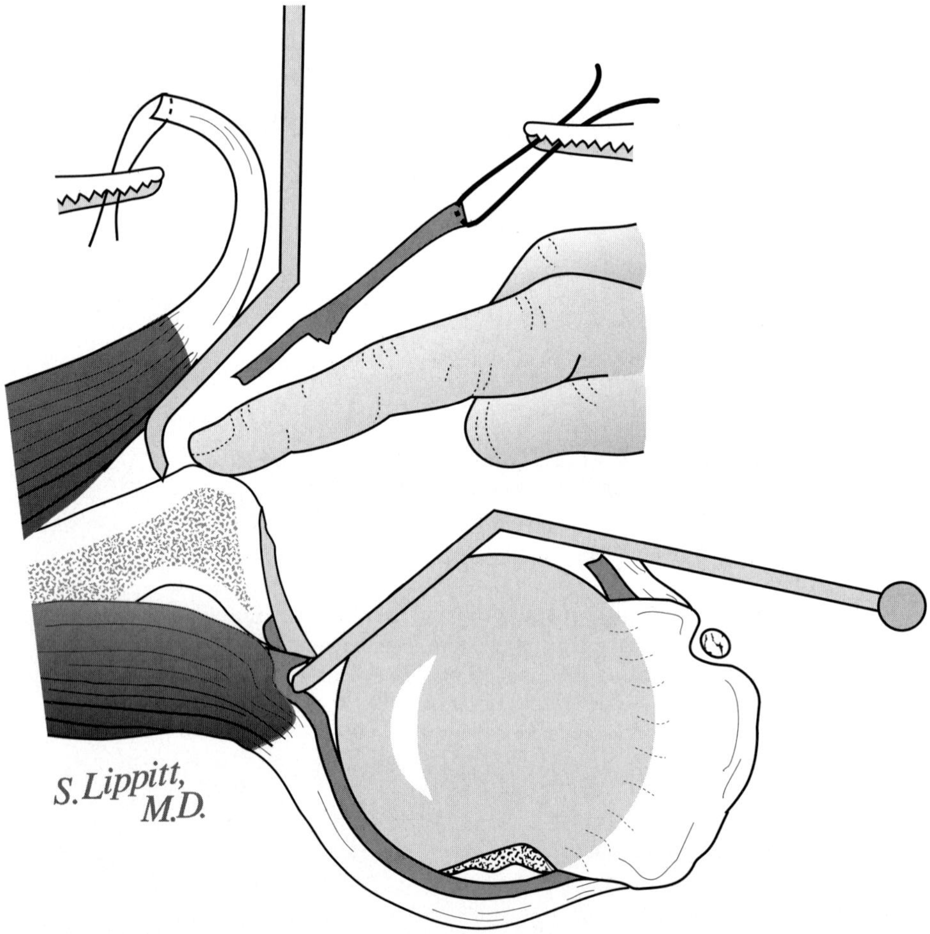


**Figure 12–8. Palpating the host site**
The anterior glenoid is palpated to identify the optimal site to receive the graft.

"docking area" for the graft, and the area is curetted free of soft tissue. A straight 25 mm osteotome is used to ensure its flatness and that the bone is freshened for healing of the graft (**Fig. 12–9**). The docking area is checked to be sure that the straight osteotome lies flat on it.

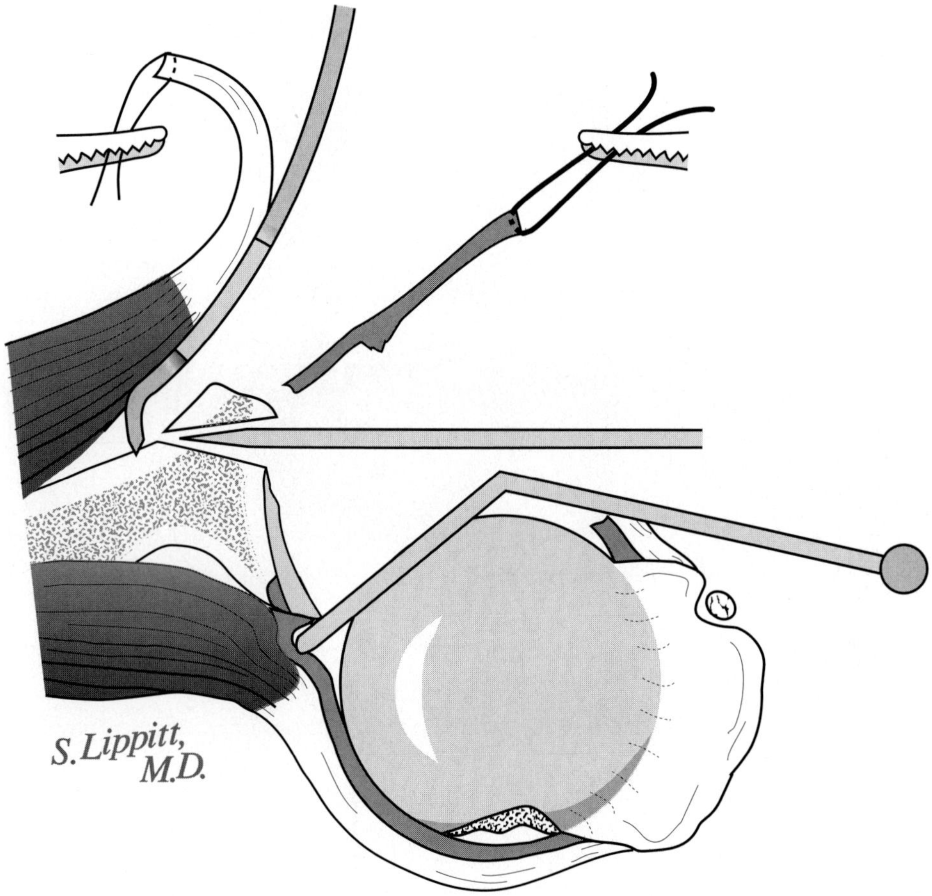


**Figure 12–9. Flattening the host site**
The selected host site is flattened with an osteotome, preserving the intact portion of the glenoid concavity. Ideally, the host site should measure 25 × 25 mm.

Drill holes are then made on the edge of the remaining glenoid articular surface with a 1.8 mm drill (**Fig. 12–10**). Sutures of #2 nonabsorbable suture material are passed through these holes for later repair of the capsule to the remaining cartilaginous rim (**Fig. 12–11**). These sutures are placed 6 mm apart and 3 mm from the glenoid edge of the remaining articular surface and roughened slightly with a pinecone burr to encourage healing of the graft.

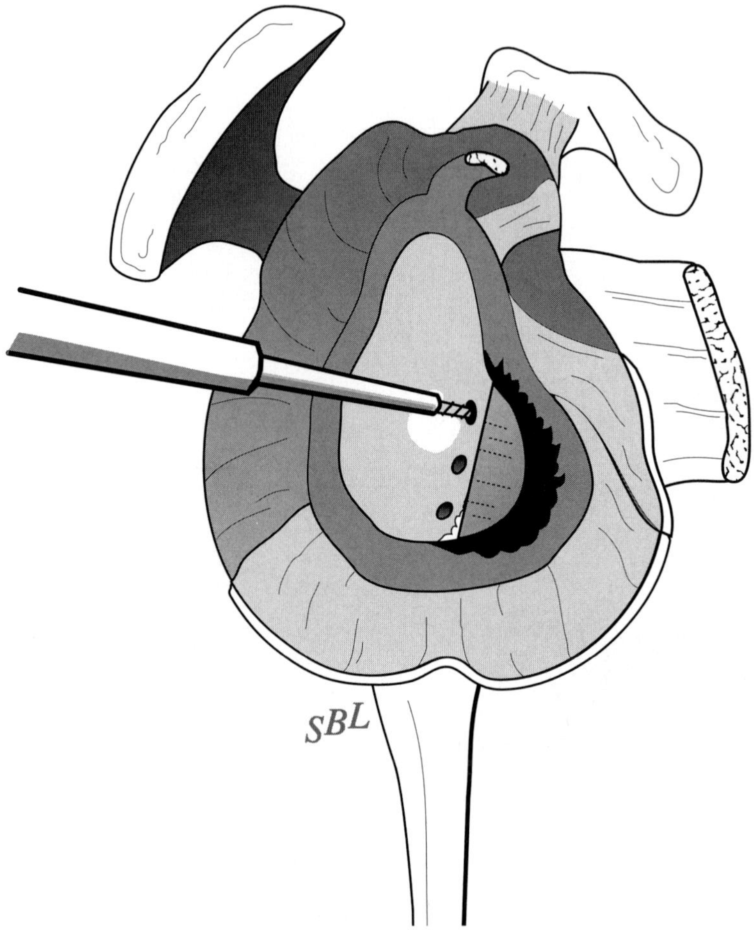


**Figure 12–10. Capsular fixation holes**
Drill holes are made at the margin of the intact glenoid for attachment of the capsule.

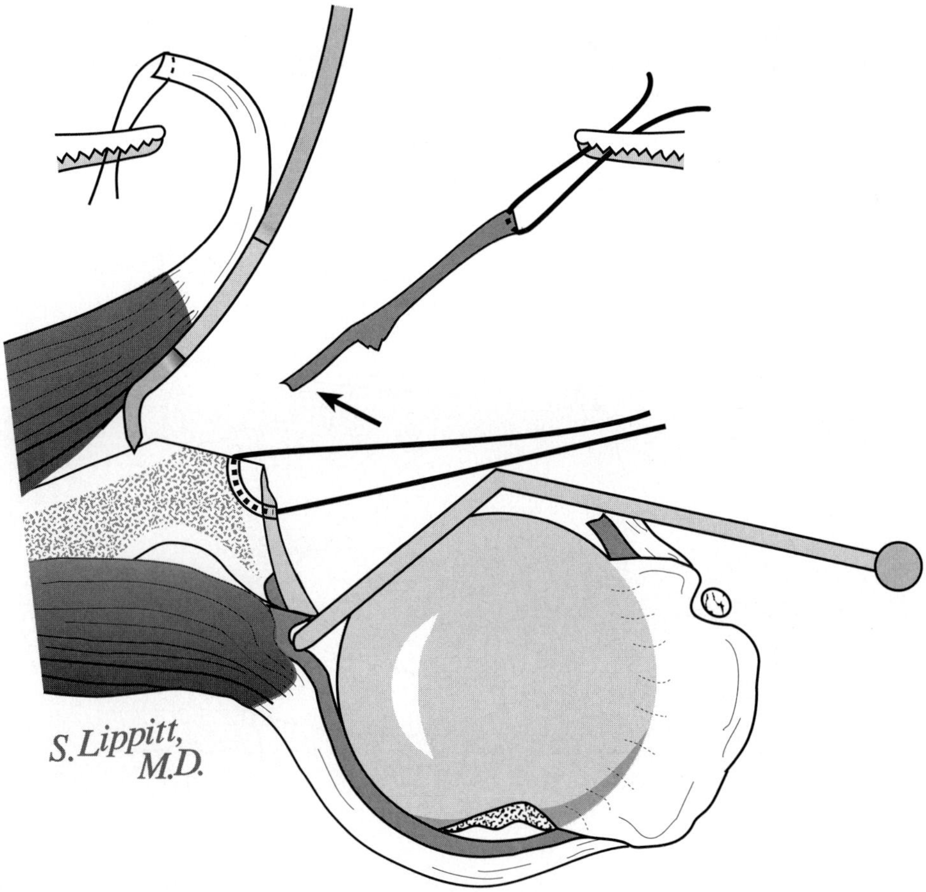


**Figure 12–11. Suture passage**
Strands of #2 braided nonabsorbable suture are passed through each hole in the glenoid lip.

Attention is then directed to the ipsilateral iliac crest where a skin incision is made below the crest line, just behind the anterior iliac spine (**Fig. 12–12**). The muscles are sharply dissected from the superolateral crest. Using straight sharp osteotomes, a 25 × 25 × 10 mm bicortical lateral graft is harvested, taking care to avoid violating the inner table of the pelvis and to avoid fracturing the graft (**Fig. 12–13**). Several cubic centimeters of cortical graft are also harvested. The muscles are then reattached securely to the iliac crest and the wound is closed.

The flat cancellous surface of the graft is placed on the flat docking area so that it can be slid medially and laterally as necessary (**Fig. 12–14**). It is important that the flat aspect of the graft sit flat on the docking area without interposed tissue. The spiked retractor beneath the glenoid neck helps ensure that the graft is not placed too inferiorly.

The humeral head retractor is removed and the humeral head is reduced in the glenoid by application of a gentle compressive load on the proximal humerus directed toward the glenoid center.

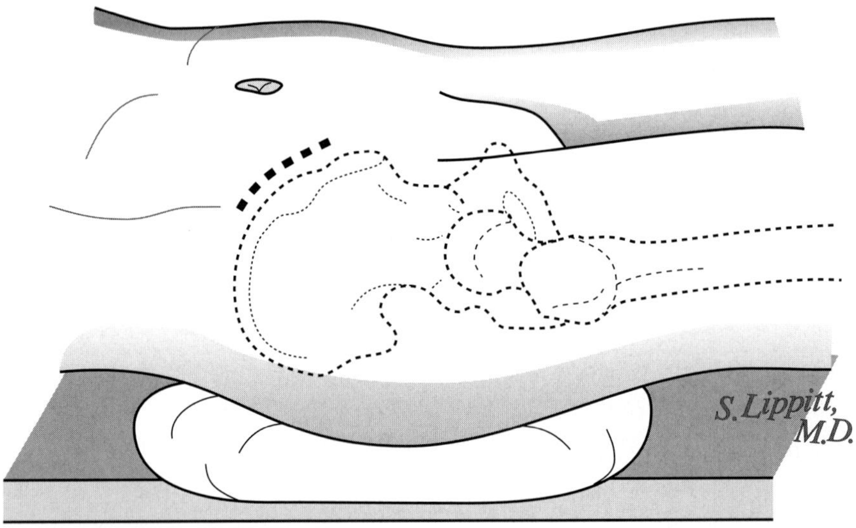


**Figure 12–12. Graft incision**
A skin incision is made over the anterior iliac crest.

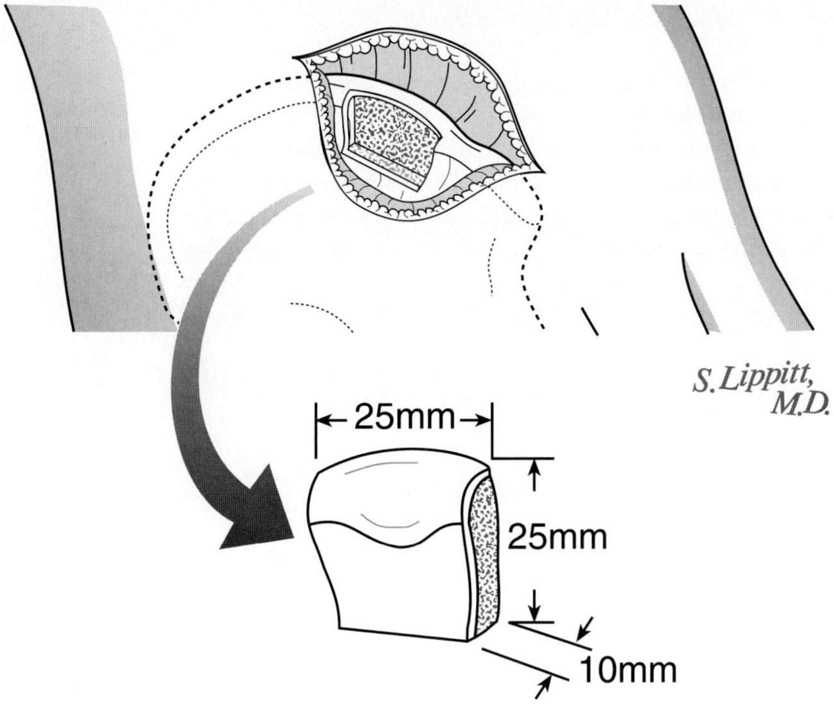


**Figure 12–13. The graft**
A 25 × 25 × 10 mm graft is harvested from the superolateral iliac crest. (Modified from Churchill RS, Moskal MJ, Lippitt SB, Matsen FA: Extracapsular anatomically contoured anterior glenoid bone grafting for complex glenohumeral instability. Techn Shoulder Elbow Surg 2:215, 2001.)

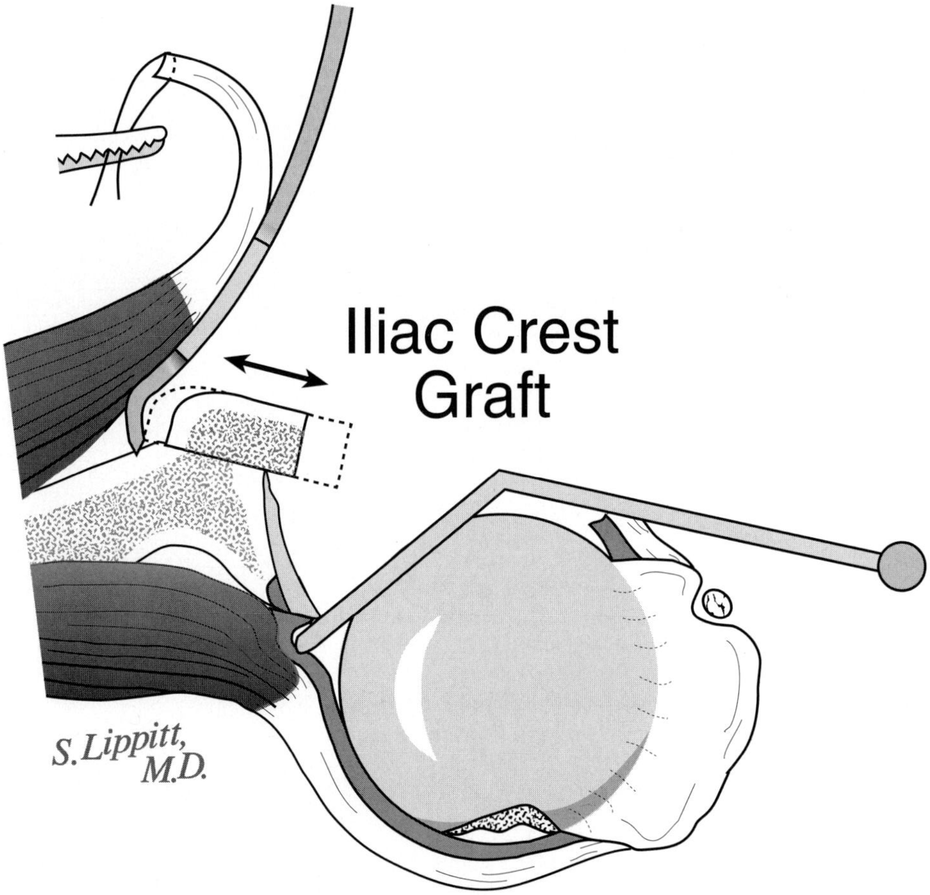


**Figure 12–14. Docking the graft**
The flat surface of the graft is placed on the flat surface of the host site. The graft is positioned so that it extends a few millimeters more laterally than the joint surface.

The graft is then slid laterally until it presses gently against the reduced humeral head. The desired position of the graft has it extending 8 mm beyond the glenoid lip (see **Fig. 12–14**). The graft is temporarily fixed into position using two 2 mm Kirschner wires placed so that they do not enter the joint and so that they do not interfere with the subsequent placement of the three fixation screws (**Fig. 12–15**). The fit of the graft on the anterior neck and the gentle contact of the graft with the humeral head are verified.

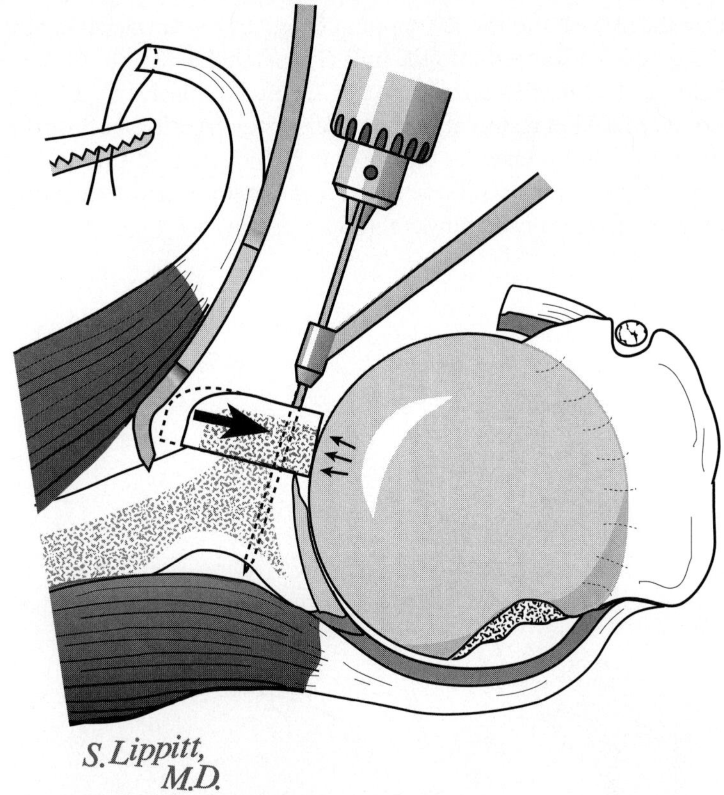


**Figure 12–15. Pinning the graft**
Once the desired position of the graft is identified, it is temporarily fixed in position using two Kirschner wires.

The drill hole for the first screw is placed as far medially as the graft will allow so that the screw will hold the graft flat on the docking area glenoid neck (**Fig. 12–16**). The depth of the drill is carefully controlled so that the nerve to the infraspinatus is not jeopardized in the spinoglenoid notch. The direction of the drill hole is aimed below the midequator of the glenoid (**Fig. 12–17**). The depth of the hole is measured. A 3.5 mm self-tapping cortical screw is selected with a length 2 mm longer than the hole (to accommodate the washer and the self-tapping flutes). A metal washer is placed on this screw and the screw is advanced into the hole. The washer is used to minimize the risk of splitting the graft. Once this screw has been secured in place, two additional screws with washers are placed in a similar manner nearer the lateral aspect of the graft, fixing it into position. Care is taken to ensure that each screw is of proper length, enters the bone of the glenoid neck, and does not enter the joint, and that the screw heads and washers are well clear of the humeral head.

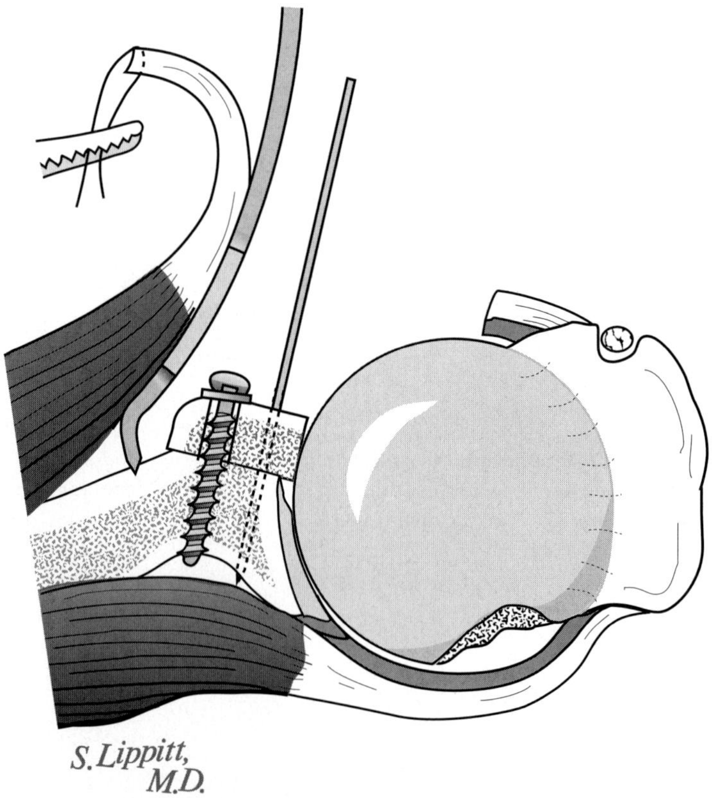


**Figure 12–16. The first screw**

A 3.5 mm self-tapping cortical screw with a washer is placed as far medially as the graft will allow.

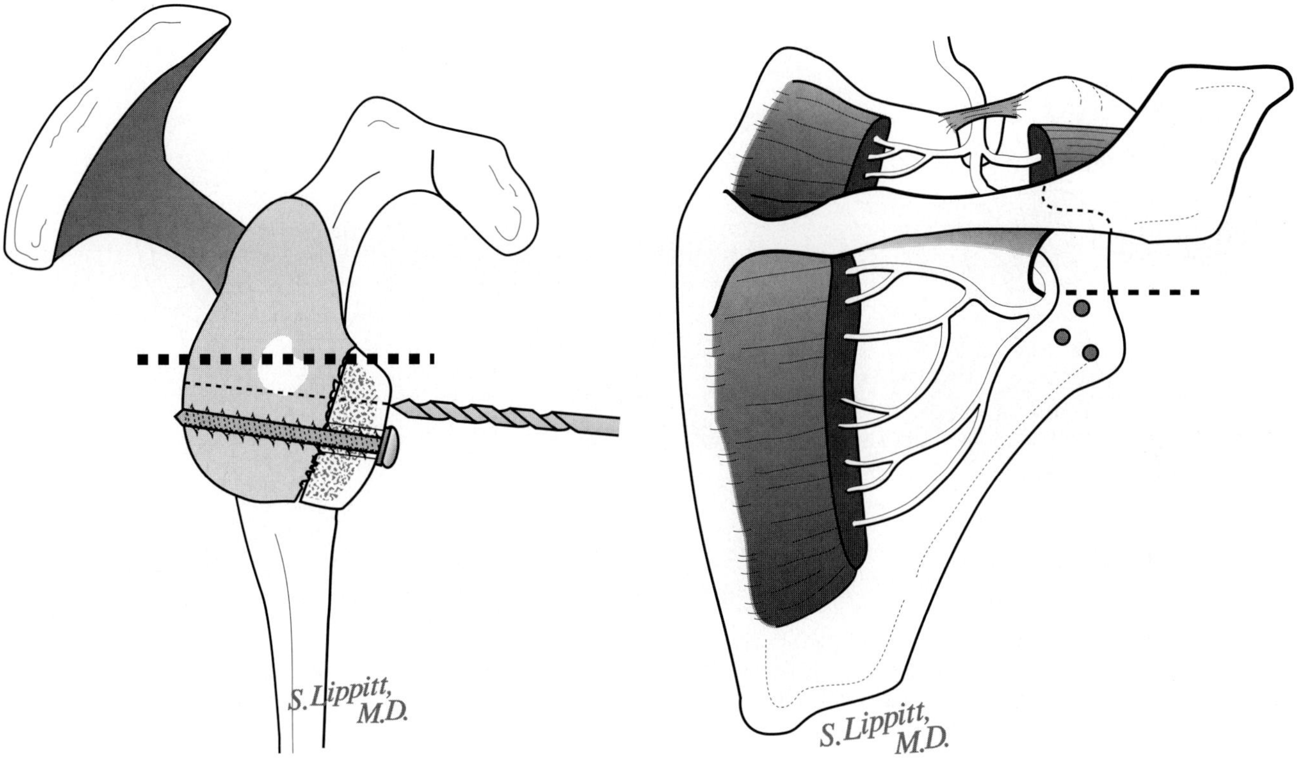


A B

**Figure 12–17. Second and third screws**

**A,** Two additional self-tapping cortical screws are placed further laterally in the graft. These screws are directed below the mid-glenoid and clear of the joint surface. **B,** Placing the screws below the mid-glenoid reduces the risk to the nerve to the infraspinatus posteriorly. (Modified from Churchill RS, Moskal MJ, Lippitt SB, Matsen FA: Extracapsular anatomically contoured anterior glenoid bone grafting for complex glenohumeral instability. Techn Shoulder Elbow Surg 2:215, 2001.)

Once the three screws are in position, the Kirschner wires are removed (**Fig. 12–18**).

Now that the graft is in its final position, a pinecone burr is used to contour the graft so that there is a small (2 mm) clearance between the graft and the reduced humeral head and also that the surface presented by the graft to the humeral head is smooth (**Fig. 12–19**). The desired clearance is verified by the ability to pass a thin dissector between the head and the graft (**Fig. 12–20**). This step ensures that the graft is not pressing the humeral head posteriorly out of the joint.

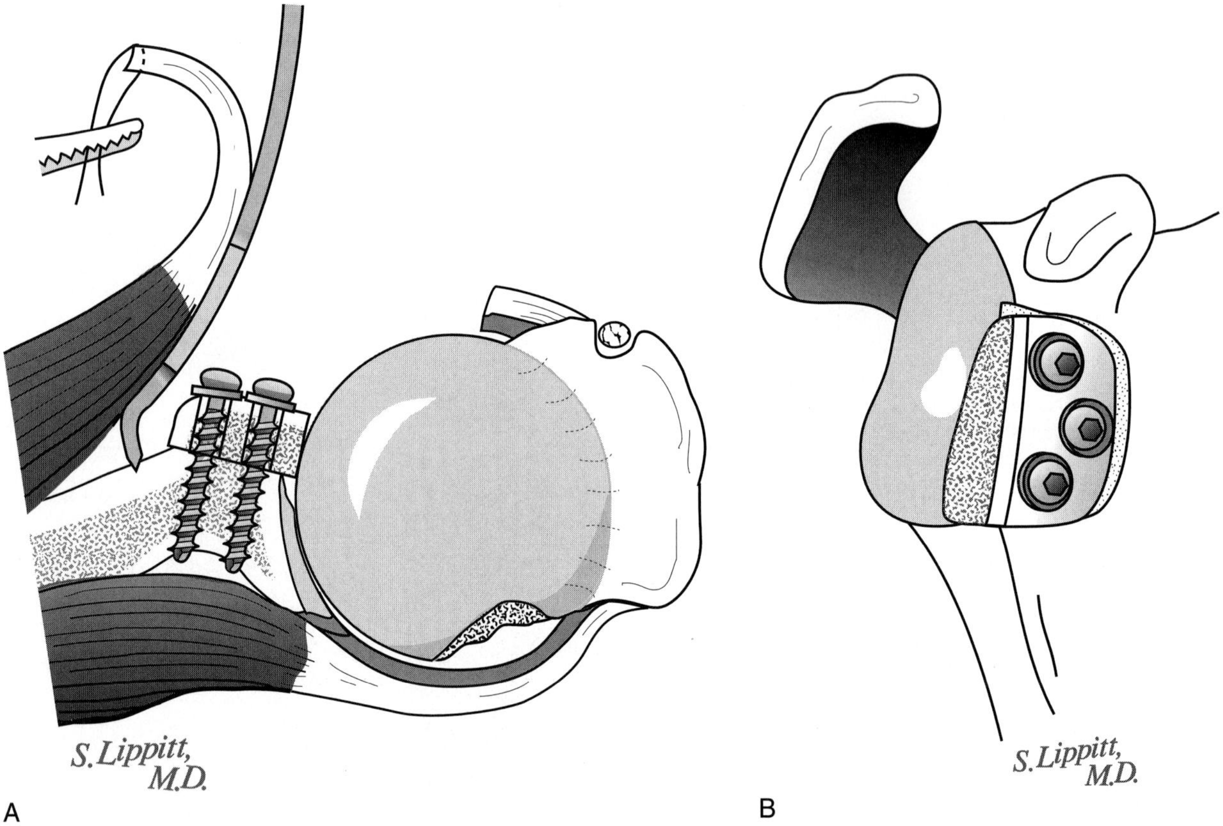


**Figure 12–18. Screw fixation**
**A,** The graft is now securely fixed with its flat side against the flat side of the host site. **B,** Arrangement of the three screws in a triangular configuration minimizes the risk of loosening.

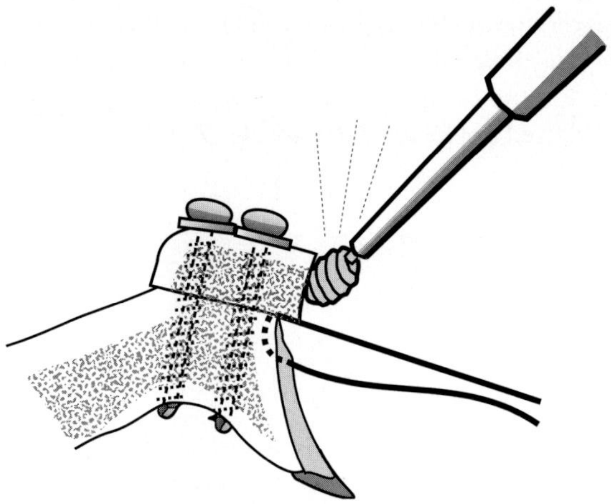

**Figure 12–19. Graft contouring**
The graft is contoured in situ using a pinecone burr. (Modified from Churchill RS, Moskal MJ, Lippitt SB, Matsen FA: Extracapsular anatomically contoured anterior glenoid bone grafting for complex glenohumeral instability. Techn Shoulder Elbow Surg 2:215, 2001.)

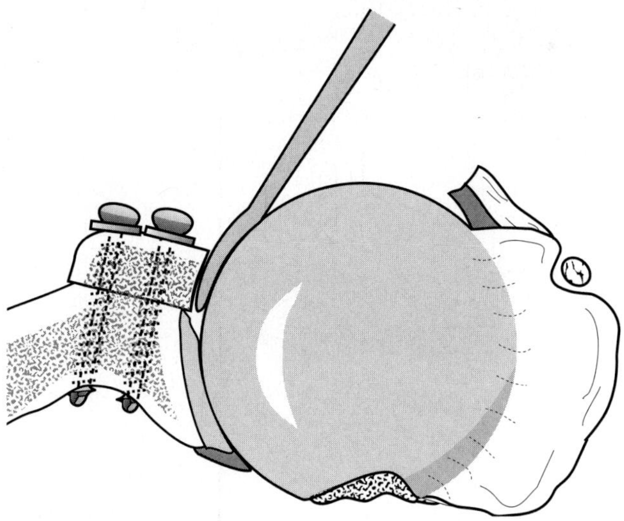

**Figure 12–20. Fine-tuning**
Shaping of the graft is continued until a thin elevator just passes between the graft and the humeral head centered in the glenoid. It is important that the graft not press the humeral head posteriorly.

The #2 braided nonabsorbable sutures passed through the glenoid holes, exiting at the graft-glenoid junction, are then placed in the detached edge of the capsule. Tying these sutures brings the capsule down to the graft-glenoid junction, rendering the graft extra-articular (**Fig. 12–21**).

The surgeon places a finger on the articular side of the capsule to palpate the aspect of the graft adjacent to the humeral articular surface. Sharp corners on the graft are smoothed with a pinecone burr. The joint is carefully inspected to ensure that the graft does not press the head posteriorly on the glenoid. Fine bits of cancellous bone graft are then inserted between the graft and the capsule to allow for a contoured bone surface to develop in support of the repaired anteroinferior capsule (**Fig. 12–22**).

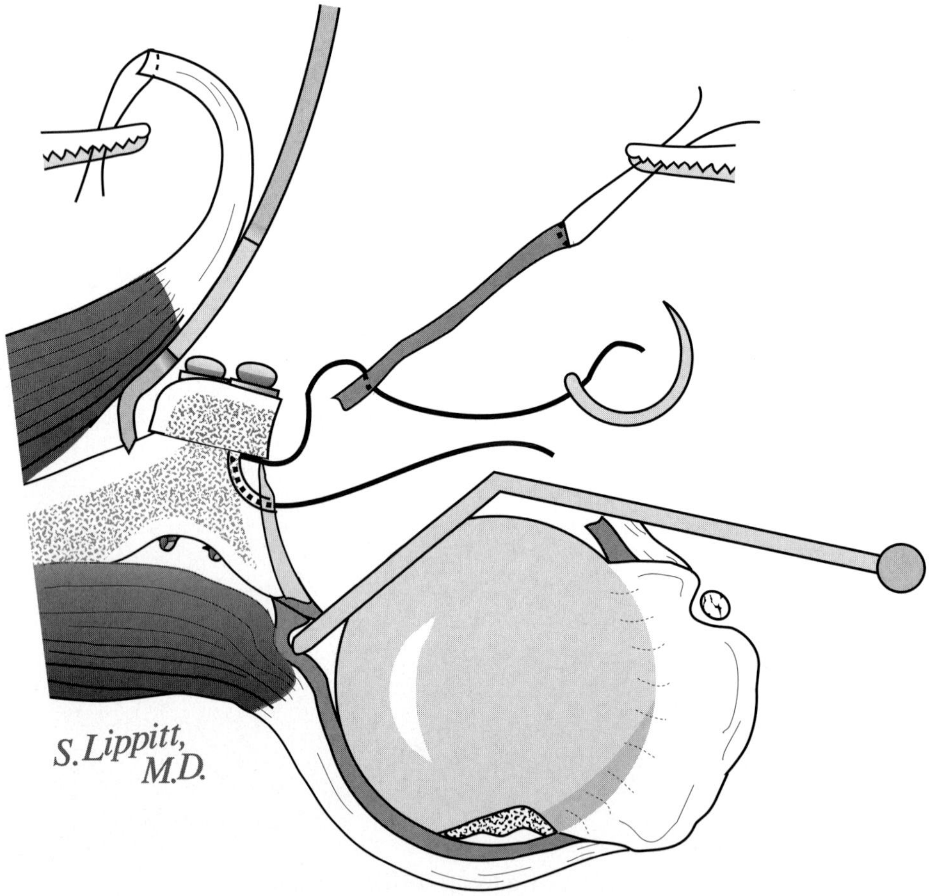


**Figure 12–21. Capsule suturing**
The capsule is closed to the margin of the glenoid using the previously placed sutures.

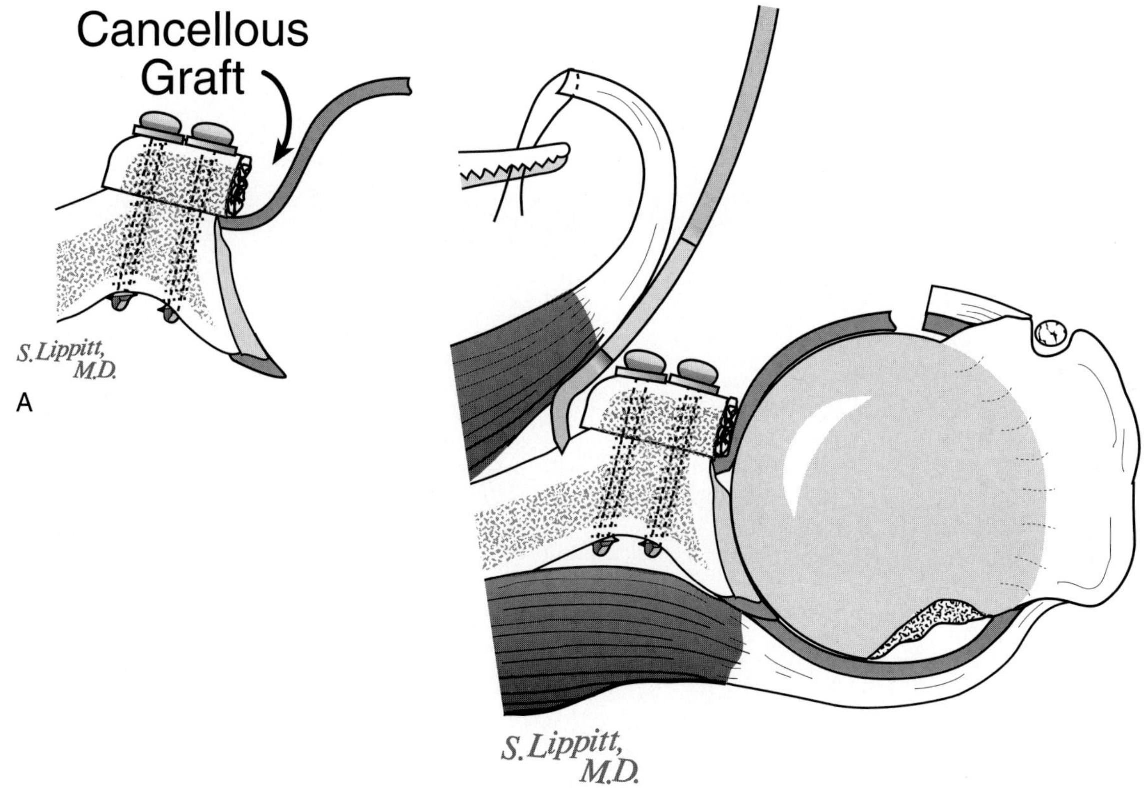


**Figure 12–22. Cancellous grafting**
**A,** Cancellous bone graft is added between the fixed graft and the capsule. **B,** The cancellous graft on top of the fixed graft provides moldable extracapsular support for the anterior capsule.

The security of the graft fixation and the capsular interposition are verified. The load and shift test is performed to ensure that the graft provides the desired stability (**Fig. 12–23**). The humerus is rotated to ensure that the articulation is smooth. The glenoid is inspected once more to ensure that no screws penetrate the articular surface and that the capsule is interposed between the graft and humeral head.

Anteroposterior and axillary x-rays are obtained to document the position of the graft and the screws.

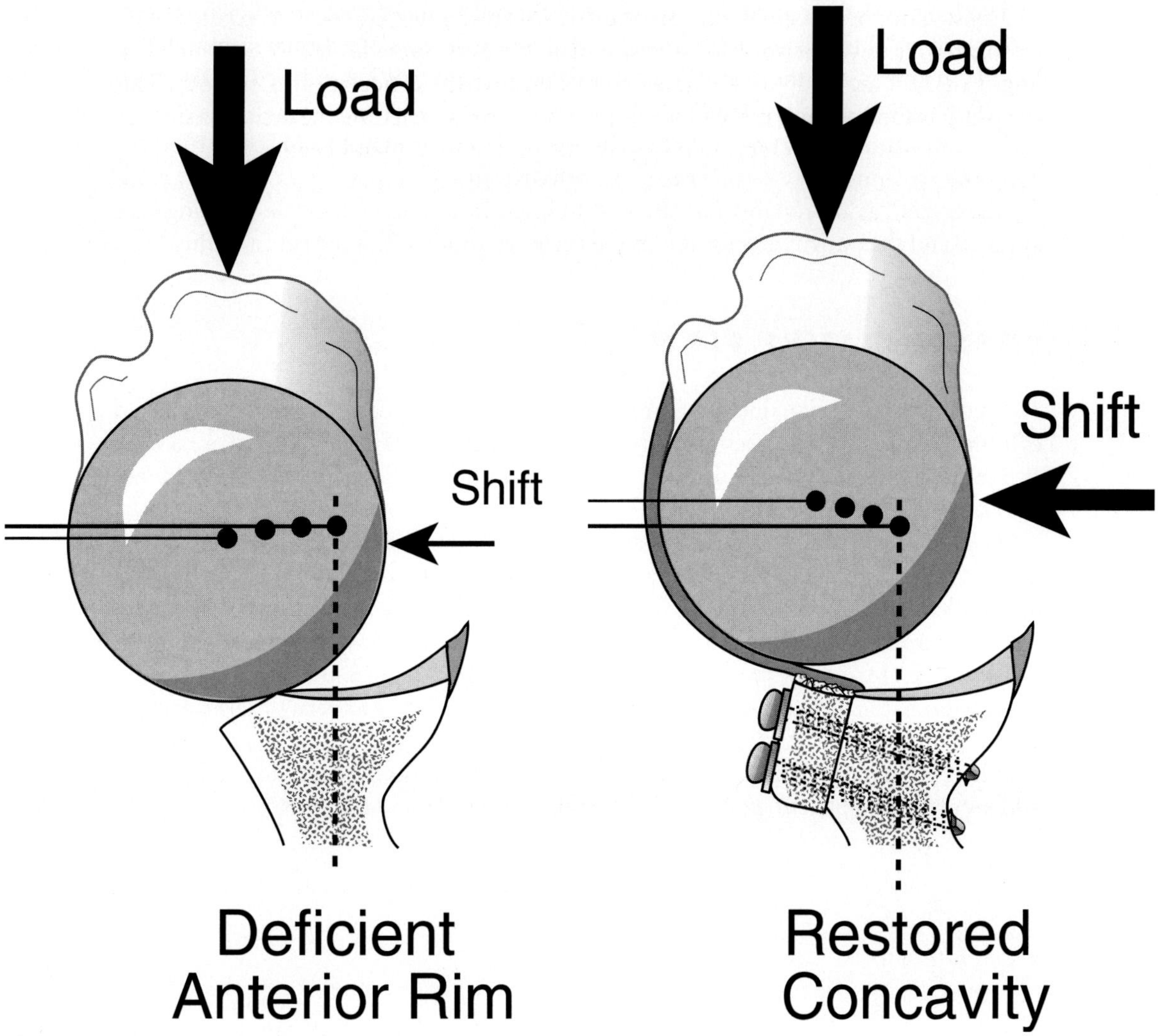


**Figure 12–23. Restored concavity**
After the reconstruction, the load and shift test confirms the restoration of centering of the humeral head and restoration of stability.

The length of the remaining capsule is evaluated to determine whether its lateral extent will reach to the lesser tuberosity and allow 20 degrees of external rotation (**Fig. 12–24**). If this is not the case, the lateral edge of the capsule is sutured to the deep aspect of the subscapularis tendon.

The subscapularis and capsule are then repaired to their mates at the lesser tuberosity, using six sutures of #2 nonabsorbable braided suture.

The wound is thoroughly irrigated and closed in layers. Dry sterile dressings are applied, and the patient is returned to the recovery room with the arm in a sling.

## POSTOPERATIVE PLAN

The postoperative plan includes immediate implementation of patient-conducted external rotation to 0 degrees and elevation to 90 degrees. The patient is given a cane to use in the hand opposite the side of surgery until the iliac crest site is no longer bothersome with ambulation.

As soon as the patient can ambulate and perform the shoulder exercises, he or she is discharged. The patient is encouraged to remove the sling and use the arm actively for gentle activities within the allowed range of motion when functioning in a protected environment. Lifting is limited to 1 pound for 6 weeks. After 6 weeks, range of motion is increased by the patient gently toward 140 degrees of elevation and 40 degrees of external rotation. After 3 months, x-rays are taken to verify the security of the fixation and stability of the screw position. Rigorous activities may be progressively resumed as soon as the shoulder is comfortable, has the desired range, and feels strong and secure to the patient, and the graft appears healed on radiographs.

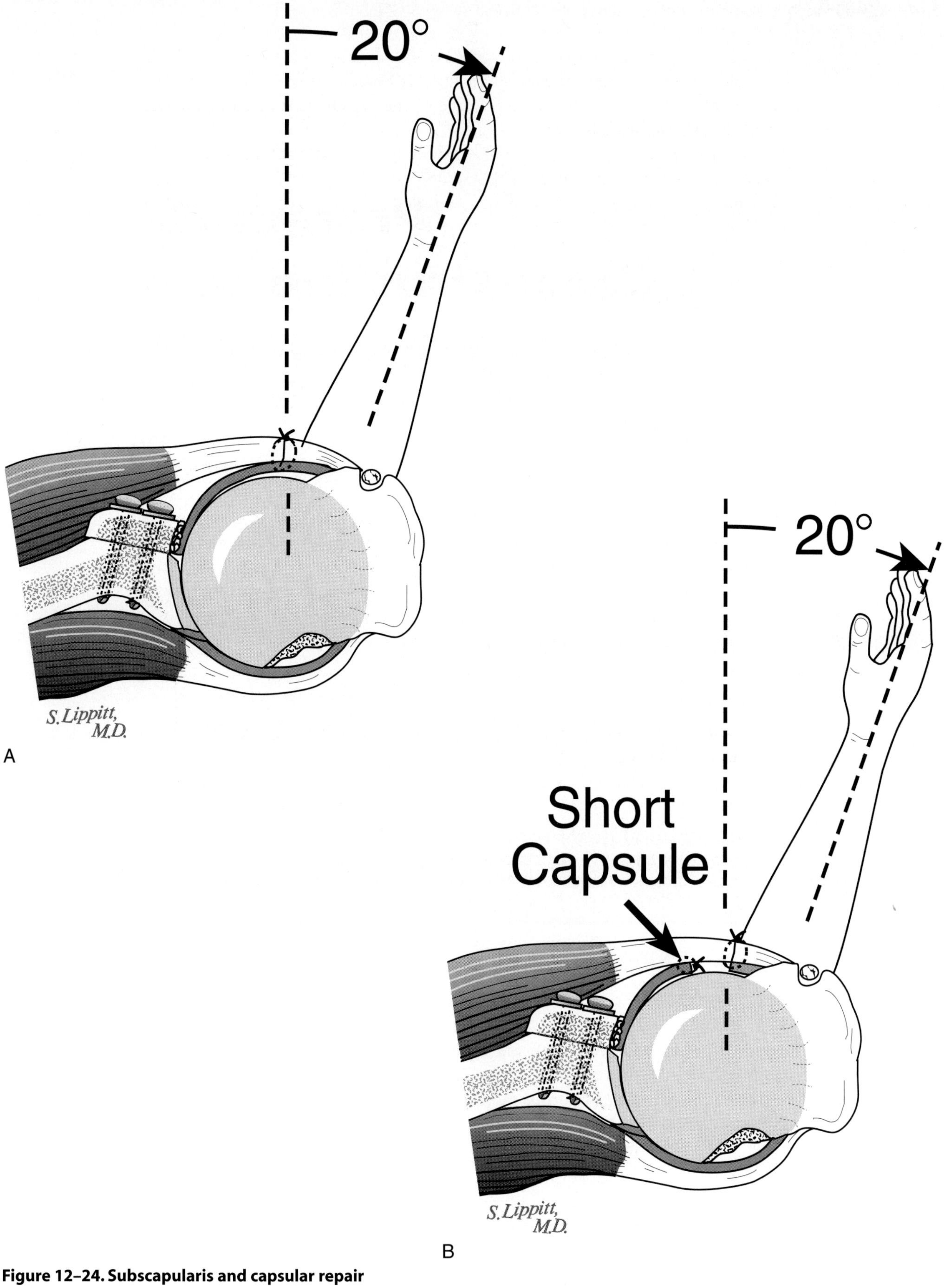


**Figure 12–24. Subscapularis and capsular repair**

**A,** If the capsule is of sufficient length, it is repaired back to its counterpart at the lesser tuberosity along with the subscapularis. **B,** If the capsule is too short to repair itself, the lateral edge of the capsular flap is sewn to the deep surface of the subscapularis tendon that is then repaired to the tendon remaining at the lesser tuberosity.

CHAPTER 13

# Procedure: Reconstruction of a Deficient Posterior Glenoid Lip Using an Extracapsular Anatomically Contoured Iliac Crest Graft

***Diagnosis***

***Recurrent posterior instability associated with a deficient posterior glenoid lip ICD9 CODE 718.31***

***Procedure***

***Reconstruction of posterior glenoid lip through an "infraspinatus on" approach using an anatomically contoured, extracapsular iliac crest autograft with screw fixation CPT CODE 23465, 20902***

## INDICATIONS

The patient has functionally significant refractory recurrent posterior glenohumeral instability, especially when the arm is flexed. This instability has not responded to standard treatment, including a rigorous exercise program.

Physical examination reveals diminished resistance to the posterior load and shift test (**Fig. 13–1**) and a positive "jerk" test (**Fig. 13–2**).

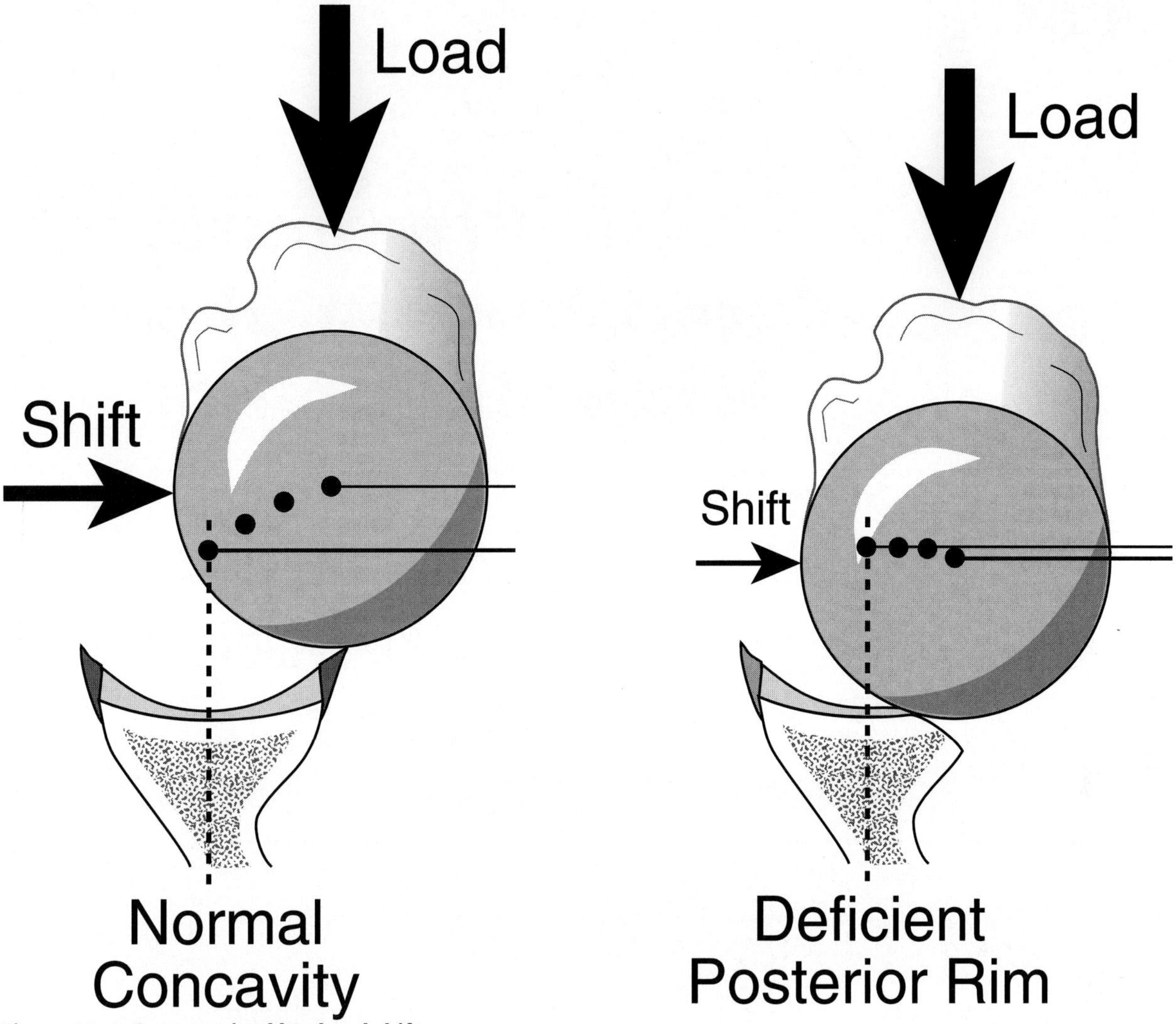


**Figure 13–1. Compromised load and shift**
A compromised posterior glenoid lip is indicated by diminished resistance to translation of the loaded humeral head away from the glenoid center.

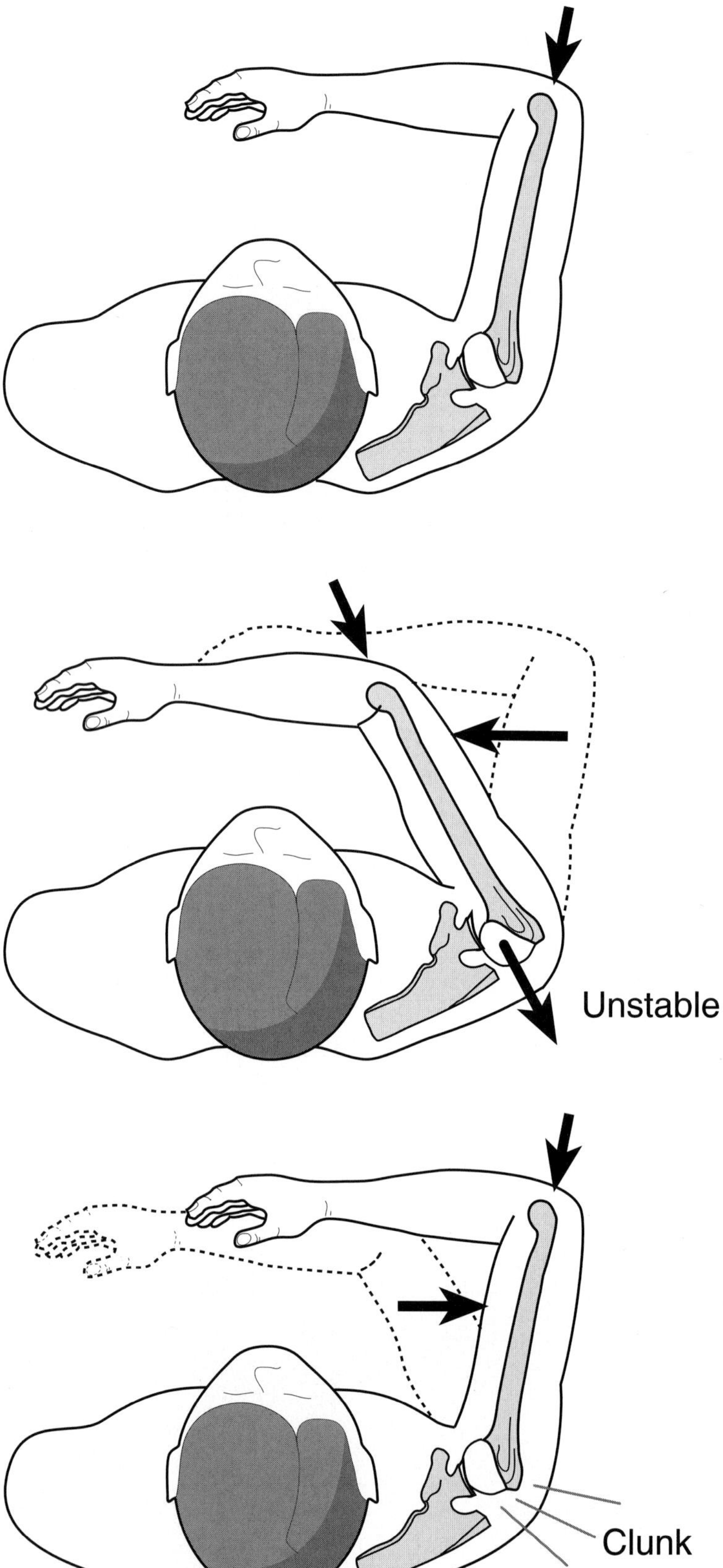


**Figure 13–2. The jerk test**
The humeral head is reduced when the arm is in the plane of the scapula. In the posteriorly unstable shoulder, adducting the arm across the body can cause the humeral head to slide over the posterior glenoid rim. Abduction of the arm back to the plane of the scapula reduces the humeral head, often with a pronounced "clunk."

Axillary radiographs demonstrate a deficiency of the posterior glenoid such that a posterior glenoid osteoplasty would be unlikely to restore the posterior glenoid lip **(Fig. 13–3)**.

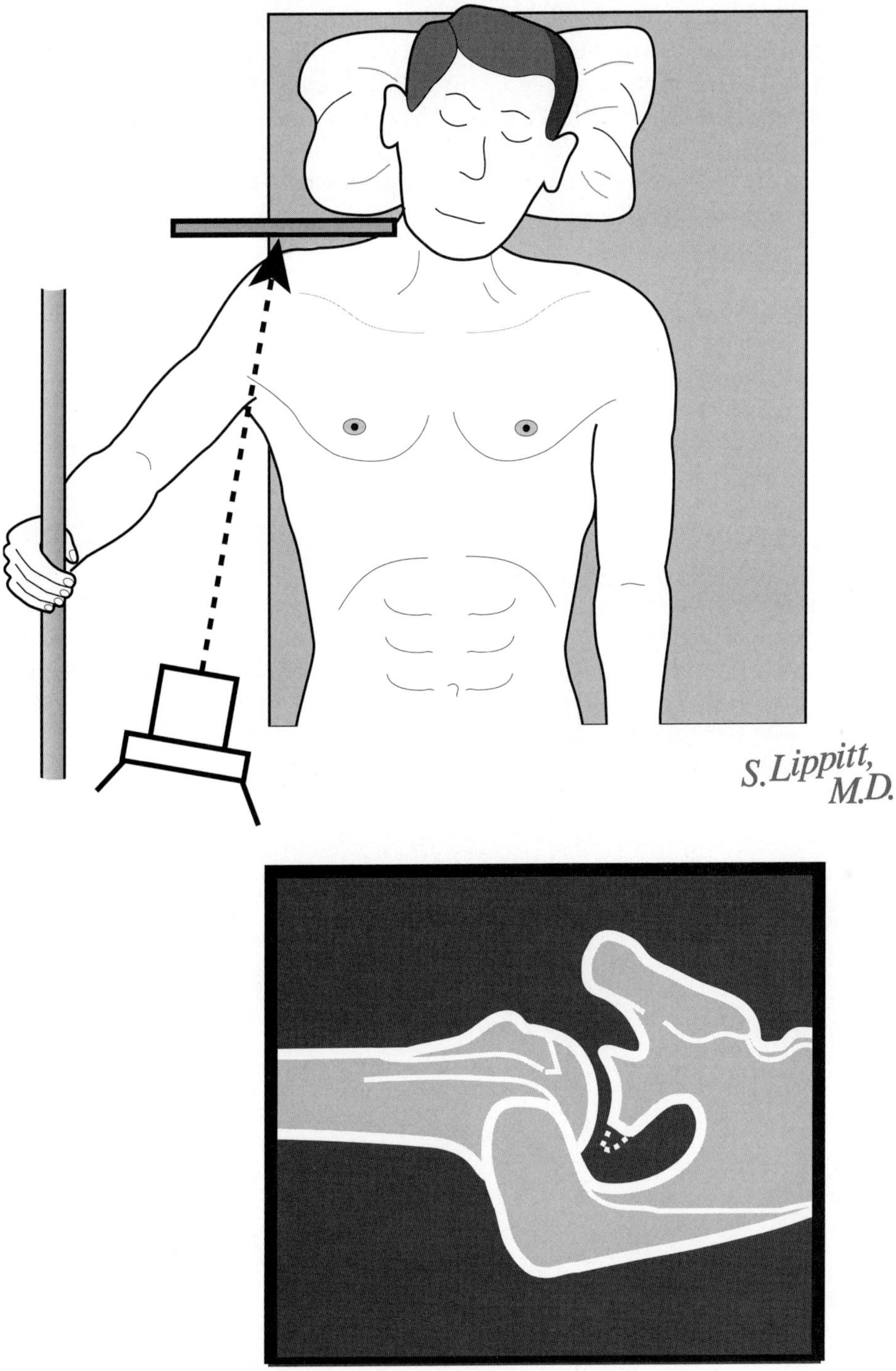


**Figure 13–3. Axillary x-ray**
An axillary x-ray may reveal a deficiency of the bony posterior glenoid lip.

Knowing the alternatives as well as the risks of infection, neurovascular injury, excessive stiffness, pain, weakness, fracture, instability, iliac crest donor site problems, hardware loosening, glenohumeral arthritis, and the need for revision surgery, as well as anesthetic complications, the patient desires to proceed with the above-described procedure. The patient understands that the purpose of the procedure is to reestablish the posteroinferior glenoid depth with a bone graft from the iliac crest, using interposed capsule to protect the humeral head articular cartilage from the bone graft. The patient recognizes that this procedure cannot be expected to completely restore normal comfort and function to the shoulder. The patient understands his or her critical role in the post-surgical rehabilitation. And lastly, the patient understands that the use of a cane in the opposite hand may be necessary for several weeks after surgery because of pain in the graft harvest area.

## FINDINGS

Examination under anesthesia in the supine position reveals diminished resistance to translation on the posterior load and shift test and a positive jerk test.

Surgical findings include thinning of the posterior glenohumeral joint capsule.

## OPERATION

Under satisfactory anesthesia, the patient is positioned prone on the operating table with appropriate attention to padding, arm position, and airway. The shoulder is prepped and draped to the posterior midline with the arm free. The ipsilateral posterior iliac crest is prepped and draped. A 6 cm incision based on the major posterior axillary crease is marked with a sterile pen (**Fig. 13–4**).

The deltoid is split between its posterior one third and anterior two thirds beginning at the posterior corner of the acromion (**Fig. 13–5**).

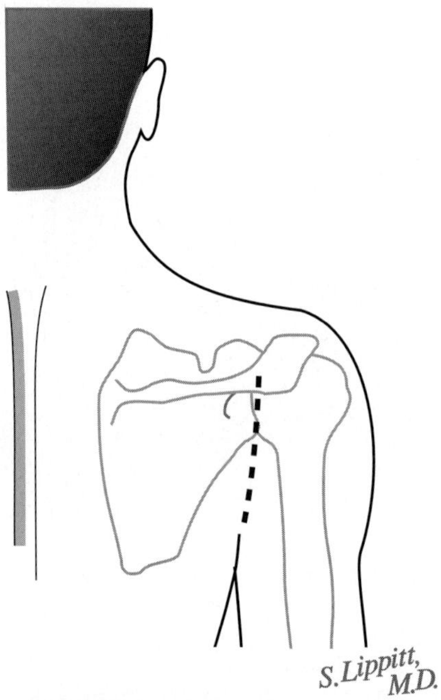


**Figure 13–4. Skin incision**
The posterior skin incision is made in the posterior axillary crease.

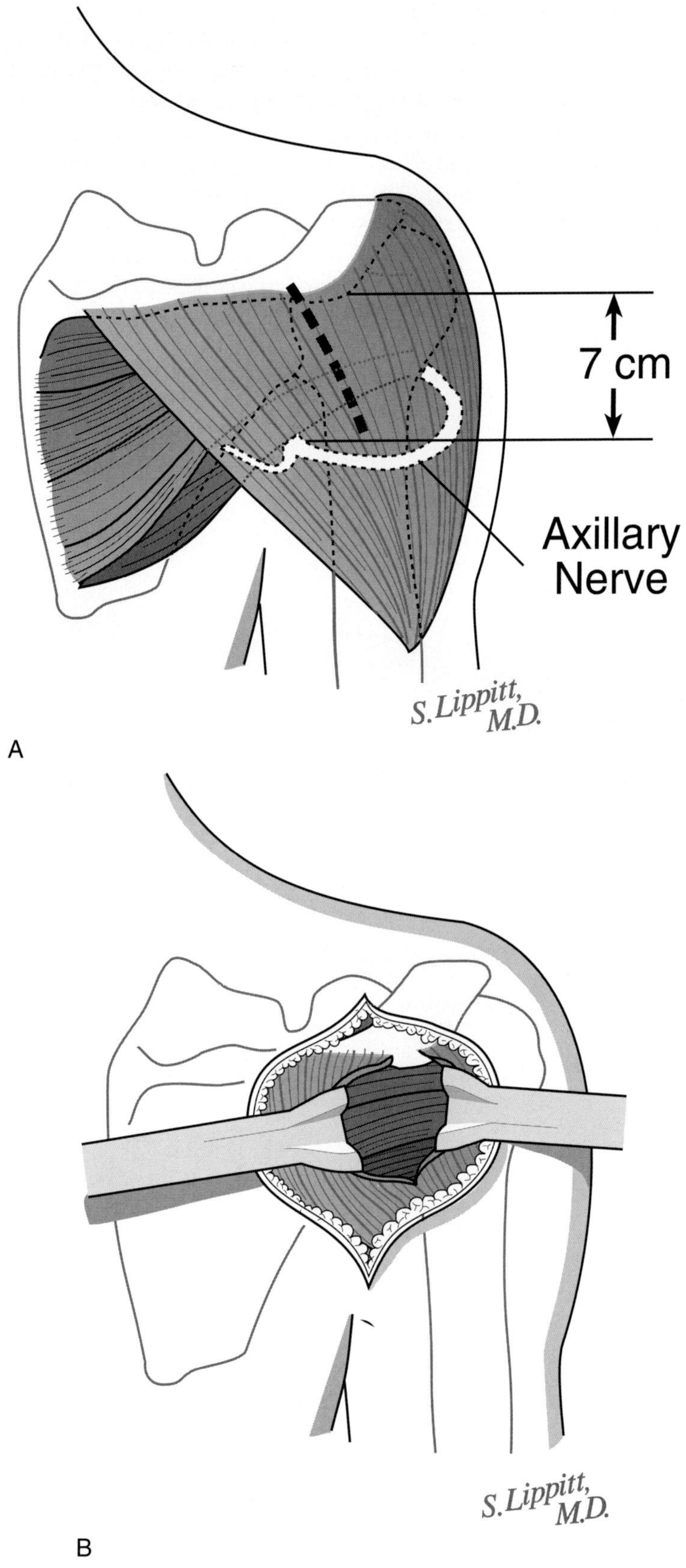


**Figure 13–5. Posterior deltoid split**

**A,** The deltoid is split between the anterior two thirds and the posterior one third of the muscle, mindful of the axillary nerve inferiorly. **B,** Retracting the deltoid reveals the infraspinatus muscle.

The bursa is incised to expose the infraspinatus.

The interval between the infraspinatus and teres minor is opened horizontally, leaving the teres minor protecting the axillary nerve (**Fig. 13–6*A***). These muscles are relaxed by passive external rotation (**Fig. 13–6*B***). The axillary nerve is identified by palpation as it exits the quadrilateral space and is protected throughout the case (**Fig. 13–6*C***). A spiked retractor is placed beneath the glenoid neck, reflecting the teres minor and axillary nerve inferiorly and to serve as a guide to the level of the inferior aspect of the glenoid.

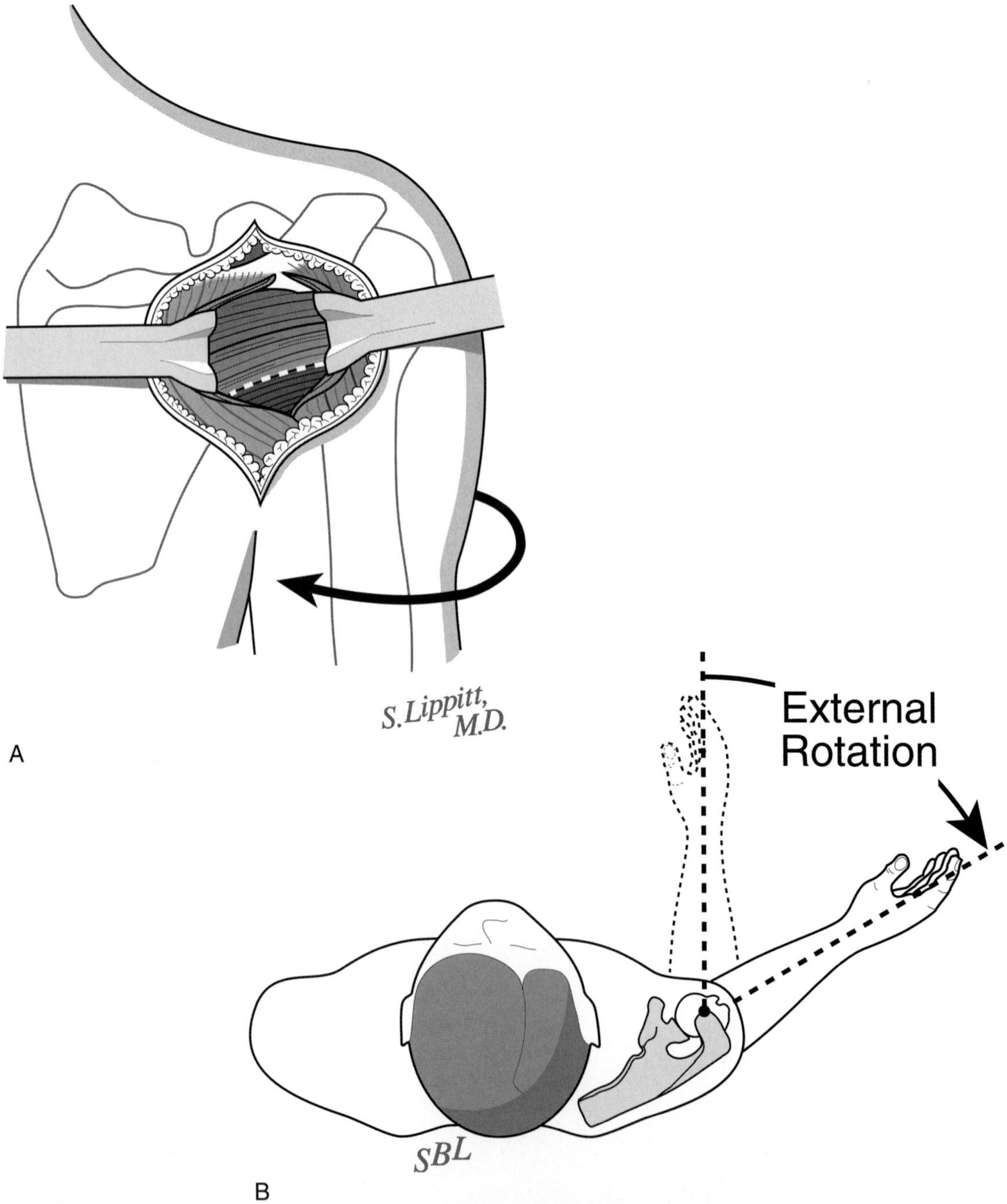


A

B

**Figure 13–6. Splitting the external rotators**

**A,** The external rotators are split between the infraspinatus and the teres minor. **B,** These muscles are relaxed by external rotation of the humerus.

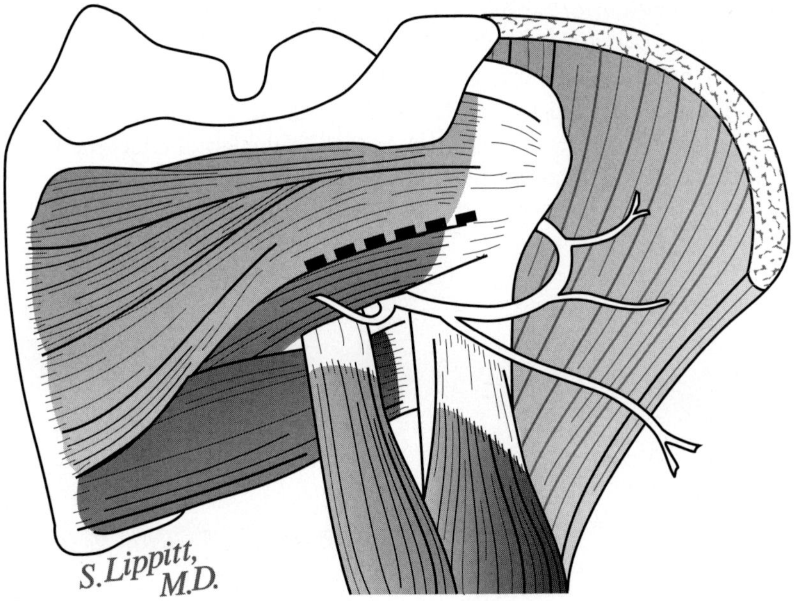


C

**Figure 13–6. Splitting the external rotators—***Continued*

**C,** Splitting the external rotators above the teres minor leaves it in a position to protect the axillary nerve.

The lateral infraspinatus muscle and tendon are bluntly dissected from the posterior glenoid neck and capsule.

The periosteum of the glenoid neck is elevated with a periosteal elevator.

A spiked retractor is placed beneath the glenoid neck, reflecting the teres minor and axillary nerve inferiorly (**Fig. 13–7**).

A second spiked retractor is placed in the body of the scapula to hold the infraspinatus superiorly (see Fig. 13–7).

The posterior glenohumeral capsule is exposed and inspected. Often a defect or very thin portion of the capsule is identified.

A horizontal posterior capsulotomy is created through the thinnest part of the capsule; the edges of the capsulotomy are tagged with #2 braided sutures (**Fig. 13–8**). The attachment of the posterior capsule to the glenoid is carefully preserved.

The integrity of the posterior labrum is verified by palpation with a blunt elevator. If a posterior labral detachment is identified, it is repaired to bone.

The plane of the glenoid articular surface is determined, using a blunt elevator.

A 25 × 25 mm area of the glenoid neck medial to the labral attachment is curetted free of soft tissue and flattened with a pinecone burr for flat seating of the graft and to encourage graft healing to the posterior glenoid neck (**Fig. 13–9**).

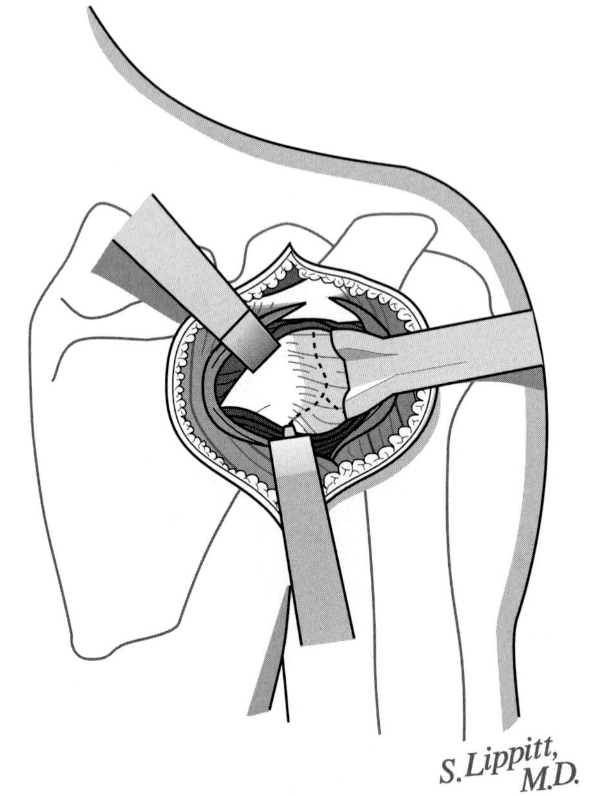


**Figure 13–7. Exposure of the inferior glenoid neck**
With the teres minor and axillary nerve retracted inferiorly, a spiked retractor is placed below the glenoid neck. The infraspinatus is retracted superiorly (toward its nerve supply) with a second spiked retractor.

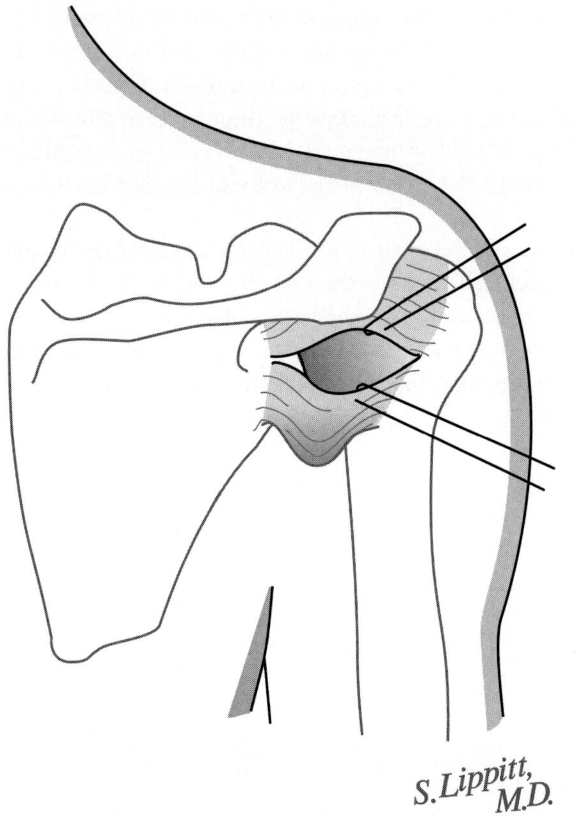


**Figure 13–8. Capsulotomy**
The posterior capsule is opened horizontally, with the incision made through the weakest part of the capsule.

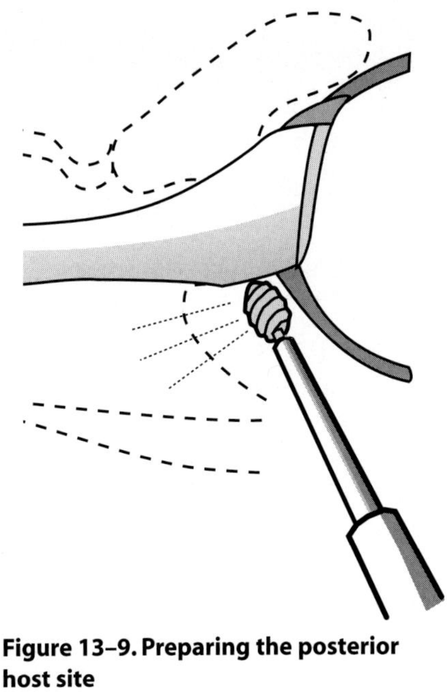

**Figure 13–9. Preparing the posterior host site**
The area of posterior glenoid just outside the capsule is flattened with a pinecone burr.

Attention is then directed to the ipsilateral posterior iliac crest, where a skin incision is made below the crest line (**Fig. 13–10**). The muscles are sharply dissected from the superolateral crest. The surgeon harvests a 25 × 25 × 10 mm unicortical graft using straight sharp osteotomes, taking care to avoid violating the inner table of the pelvis and to avoid fracturing the graft (**Fig. 13–11**). A few cubic centimeters of cancellous graft is also harvested. The muscles are then reattached securely to the iliac crest and the wound is closed.

The flatness of the cancellous surface of the graft is verified so that it will fit on the flat prepared surface of the glenoid neck. The graft is then inserted between the infraspinatus and the capsule so that its flat surface lies on the flattened posteroinferior glenoid neck. The desired position of the graft has it extending a few millimeters beyond the glenoid lip so that it supports the humeral head through the posterior capsule.

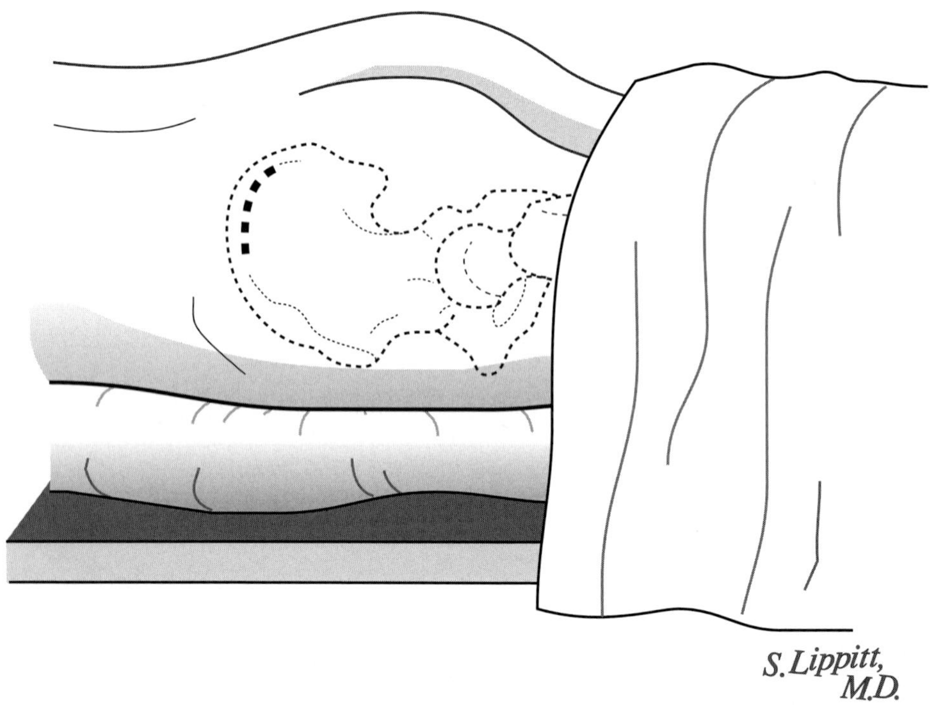


**Figure 13–10. Graft harvest incision**
The skin incision is made over the posterior iliac crest.

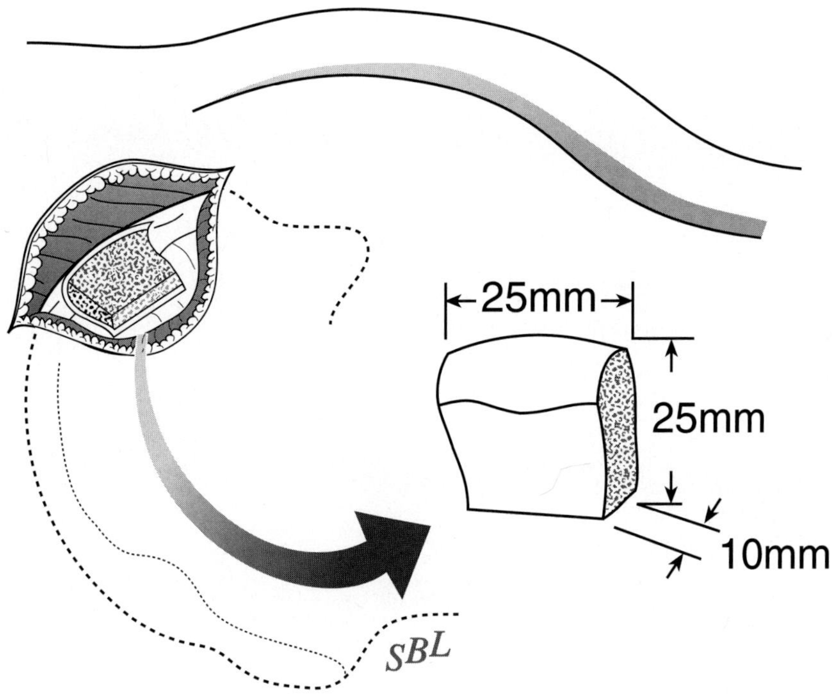


**Figure 13–11. Iliac crest harvest**
A 25 × 25 × 10 mm graft is harvested from the posterior iliac crest.

The humeral head is reduced. The graft is inspected to ensure that there is no soft tissue interposed between it and the glenoid neck and that it does not extend below the inferior glenoid neck.

The graft is positioned so that there is a slight gap between it and the reduced humeral head. The graft is fixed into position using two 2 mm Kirschner wires placed so that they do not enter the joint and do not interfere with the placement of the screws (**Fig. 13–12**). When the graft is verified to be in the desired position, three 3.5 mm self-tapping cortical screws are then used to fix the graft to the glenoid, with care taken that they enter the bone of the glenoid neck but not the joint and that the screw heads and washers will be well clear of the humeral head. The length of the screws is measured carefully so that they extend only 2 mm beyond the anterior aspect of the glenoid bone. A washer is applied to each screw before insertion to minimize the risk of splitting the graft (**Fig. 13–13**). The security of graft fixation is verified and the Kirschner wires are removed.

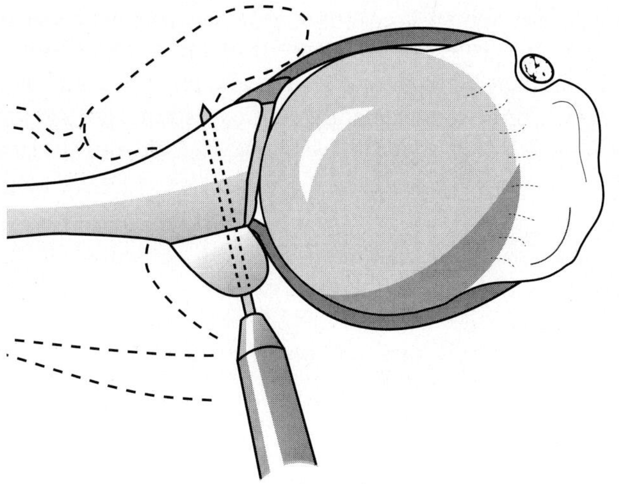

**Figure 13–12. Graft pinning**
The posterior iliac crest graft is pinned with Kirschner wires so that its flat side lies flat on the prepared site on the posterior glenoid neck adjacent to the capsule.

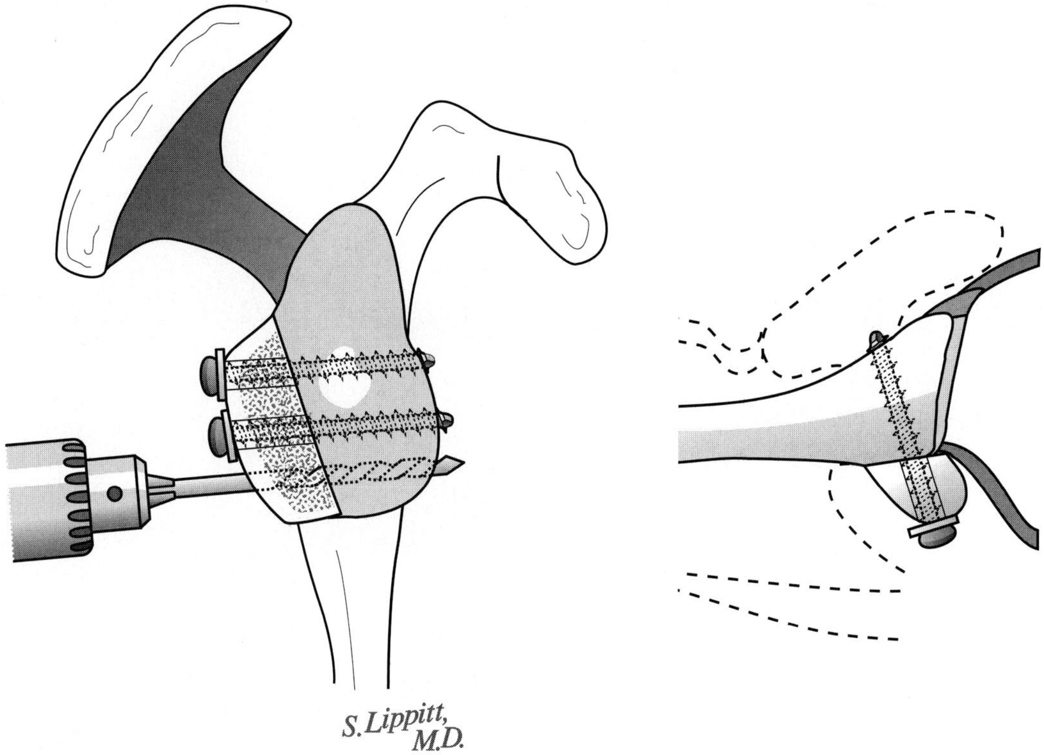


**Figure 13–13. Screw fixation**
Three 3.5 mm self-tapping cortical screws are used to fix the graft to the host site. The arthrotomy is inspected to ensure that the screws are extra-articular.

A finger is placed on the articular side of the capsule to palpate the aspect of the graft adjacent to the humeral articular surface. The contour of the graft is modified with a pinecone burr so that it conforms to the humeral head and to remove any sharp edges, leaving a 2 mm gap (which can be conveniently verified with a thin elevator) (**Fig. 13–14*A***). Bits of cancellous graft are added between the capsule and the graft (**Fig. 13–14*B***).

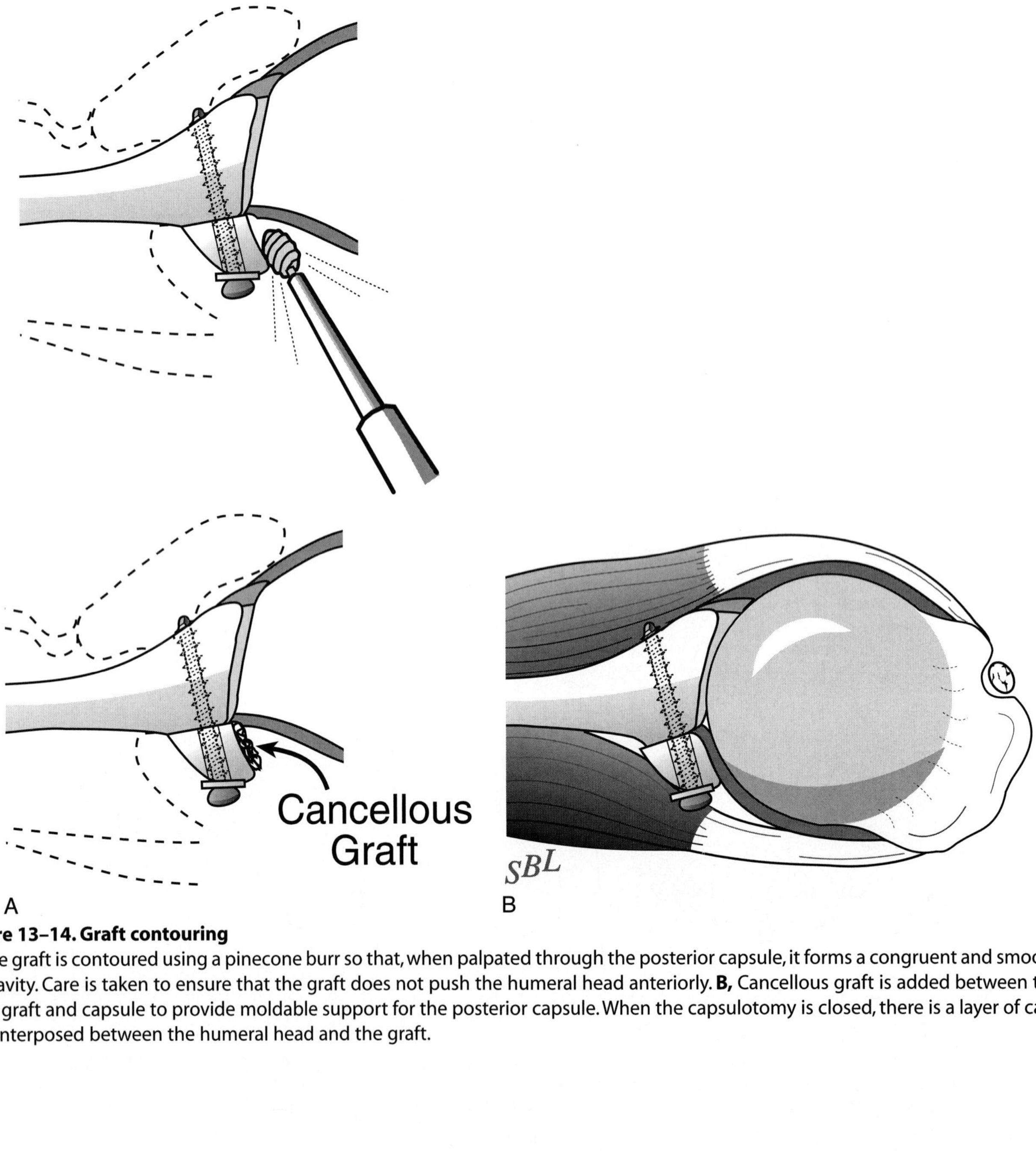


**Figure 13–14. Graft contouring**
**A,** The graft is contoured using a pinecone burr so that, when palpated through the posterior capsule, it forms a congruent and smooth concavity. Care is taken to ensure that the graft does not push the humeral head anteriorly. **B,** Cancellous graft is added between the fixed graft and capsule to provide moldable support for the posterior capsule. When the capsulotomy is closed, there is a layer of capsule interposed between the humeral head and the graft.

The humerus is rotated to ensure that the articulation is smooth. The glenoid is inspected once more to ensure that no screws penetrate the articular surface. The load and shift test is performed to ensure that the graft provides the desired stability **(Fig. 13–15)**. Anteroposterior and axillary x-rays are obtained to document the position of the graft and screws.

The relationship of the graft to the axillary nerve is examined; any rough edges or encroachment can be resolved by trimming of the graft.

The infraspinatus is allowed to fall back into position. The humerus is once again rotated to ensure that there is no crepitance from rubbing of the infraspinatus over the posterior graft.

The wound is thoroughly irrigated and closed in layers. Dry sterile dressings are applied, and the patient is returned to the recovery room with the arm in a sling.

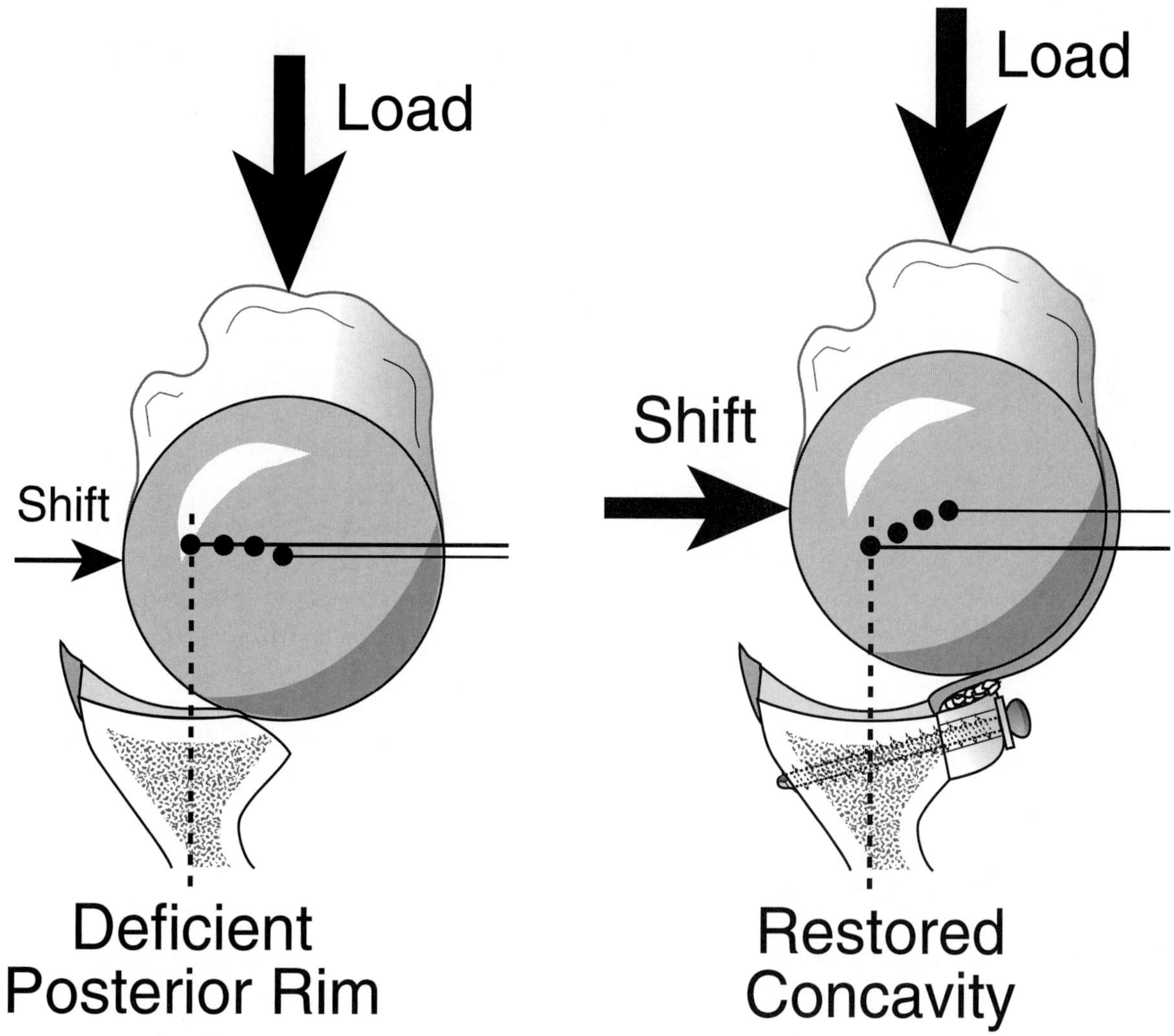


**Figure 13–15. Restored concavity**
After the reconstruction, the load and shift test demonstrates restored centering of the humeral head on the glenoid.

## POSTOPERATIVE PLAN

On the first postoperative day, the patient begins active assisted internal and external rotation exercises, keeping the elbow at the side, using the 0 degrees flexion, 40 degrees internal rotation, and 40 degrees external rotation program (**Fig. 13–16**). The patient is given a cane to use in the hand opposite the side of surgery until the iliac crest site is no longer bothersome with ambulation.

As soon as the patient can ambulate and perform the shoulder exercises, the patient is discharged.

For 6 weeks, the patient avoids moving the elbow from the side and develops progressive strength of internal and external rotation.

At 6 weeks, the patient begins abduction in the plane of the body. Only when the arm can be lifted comfortably and strongly in abduction is elevation started in more anterior planes.

At 3 months after surgery, x-rays are taken to verify the security of the fixation and stability of the screw position and graft. At this point, the patient is allowed to progressively increase the use of the arm.

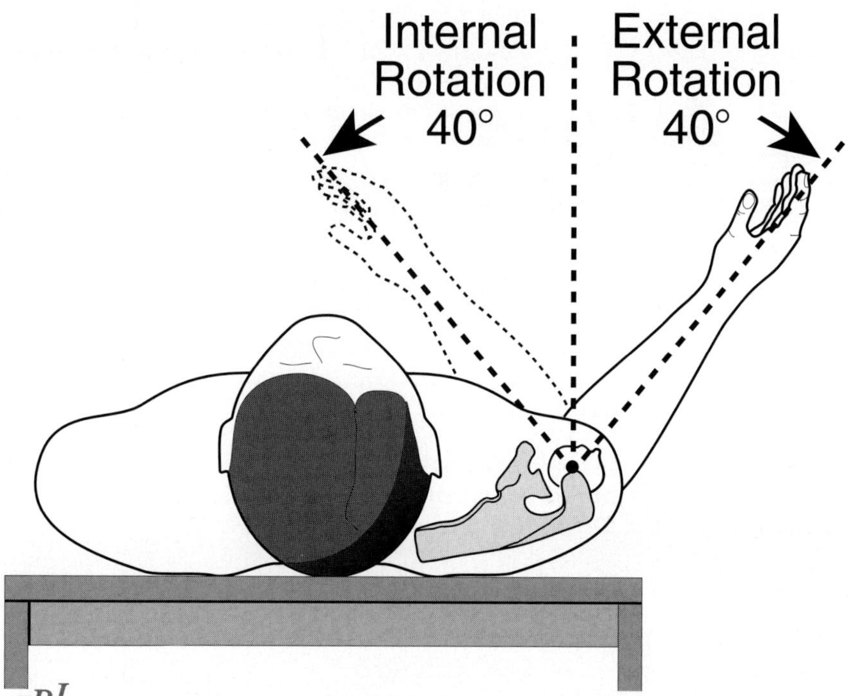


**Figure 13–16. Postsurgical rehabilitation**
Immediately after surgery, the patient begins passive and active internal and external rotation range of motion exercise, keeping the elbow at the side.

CHAPTER 14

# Procedure: Augmentation of an Excessively Compliant Glenoid Labrum

***Diagnosis***

***Recurrent atraumatic glenohumeral instability associated with an excessively compliant glenoid labrum ICD9 CODE 718.31***

***Procedure***

***Reconstruction and augmentation of a deficient glenoid labrum CPT CODE 23466***

## INDICATIONS

The patient has functionally significant recurrent atraumatic instability of the glenohumeral joint in multiple directions. This instability has been refractory to nonoperative management with rotator cuff strengthening and stability training.

Physical examination shows diminished resistance to the load and shift test in multiple directions (**Fig. 14–1**). There is no clinical evidence of traumatic injury to the supporting structures of the glenohumeral joint.

Radiographs show no bony abnormalities of the glenohumeral joint.

Knowing the alternatives as well as the risks of infection, neurovascular injury, excessive stiffness, pain, weakness, instability, and the need for revision surgery, as well as anesthetic complications, the patient desires to proceed with the above-described procedure. The patient recognizes that the purpose of the procedure is to increase the functional depth of the glenoid by augmenting the size and reducing the compliance of the glenoid labrum. The patient recognizes that this procedure cannot be expected to completely restore normal comfort and function to the shoulder. And, lastly, the patient understands his or her critical role in post-surgical rehabilitation.

## FINDINGS

Examination under anesthesia reveals diminished resistance to translation on the load and shift test in multiple directions.

Surgical findings include diminished functional height of the glenoid lip.

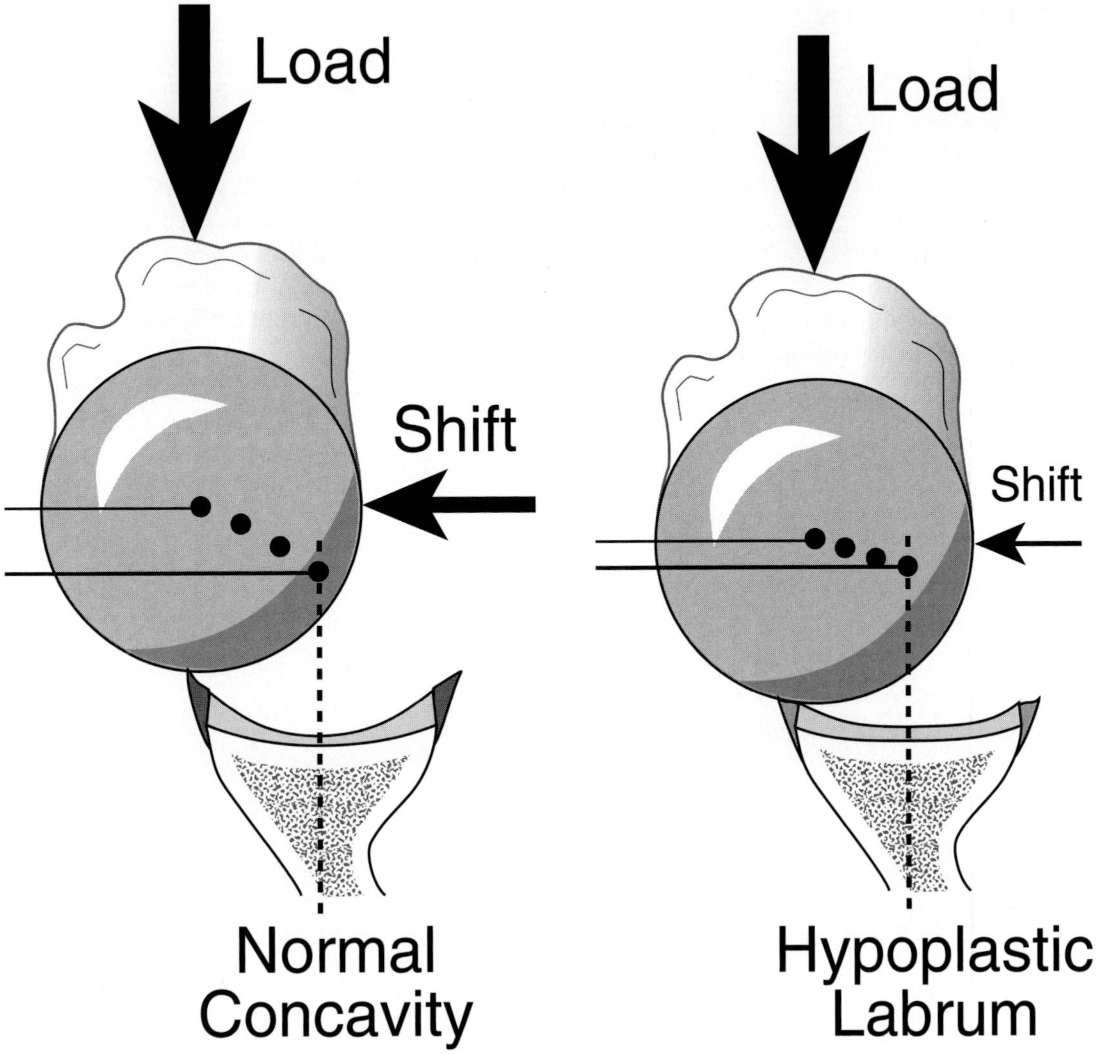


**Figure 14–1. Compromised humeral head centering**
When the labrum is excessively compliant, there is diminished resistance to the load and shift test.

## OPERATION

Under satisfactory anesthesia, the patient is placed in a low beach chair position with the arm at the edge of the operating table. The shoulder is carefully prepped and draped. The major axillary crease is marked with a sterile pen. The shoulder is approached through a low anterior axillary incision made in this axillary crease (**Fig. 14–2**). The deltopectoral interval is opened, leaving the cephalic vein on the deltoid laterally (**Fig. 14–3**). The humeroscapular motion interface is freed of adhesions. A self-retaining retractor is placed with one blade against the deltoid and the other against the coracoid muscles (**Fig. 14–4**). The subscapularis tendon is incised along with the subjacent capsule (**Fig. 14–5**).

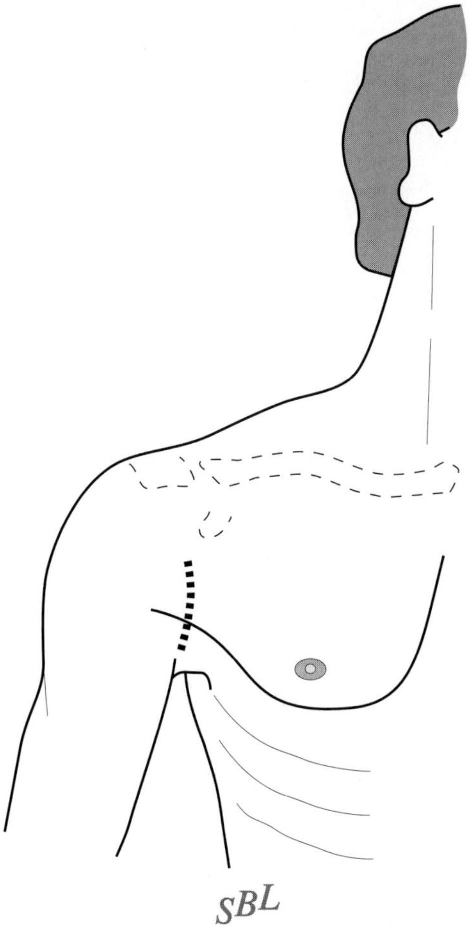


**Figure 14–2. Skin incision for glenoid augmentation**
If the incision is made in the major axillary crease, it usually heals with an excellent cosmetic result. (Modified from Rockwood CA, Matsen FA [eds]: The Shoulder, 2nd ed. Philadelphia: WB Saunders, 1998, p. 704.)

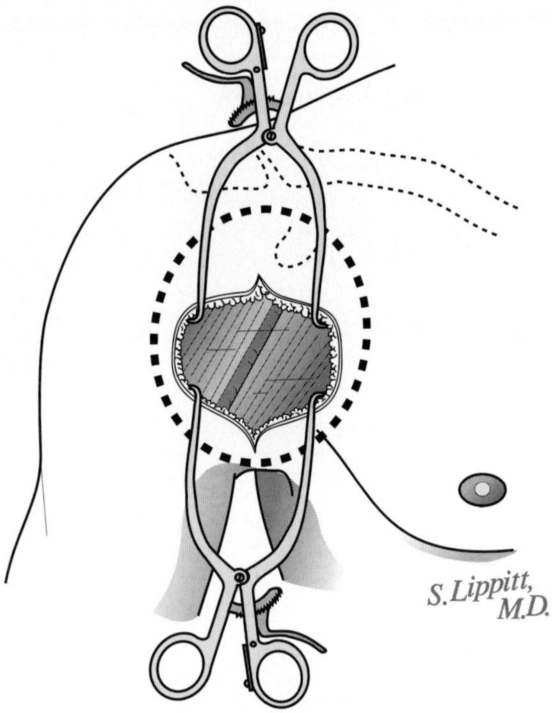


**Figure 14–3. Opening of the deltopectoral interval**
Subcutaneous dissection up to the level of the coracoid process exposes the cephalic vein in the deltopectoral groove. (Modified from Rockwood CA, Matsen FA [eds]: The Shoulder, 2nd ed. Philadelphia: WB Saunders, 1998, p. 704.)

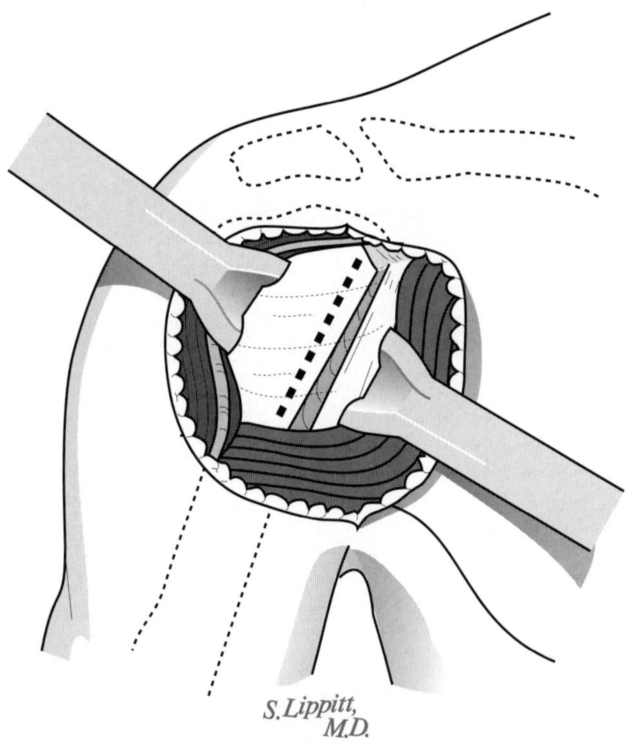


**Figure 14–4. Placement of self-retaining retractors**
Retraction of the deltoid and cephalic vein laterally and the pectoralis major medially exposes the clavipectoral fascia. This fascia is incised just lateral to the coracoid muscles and tendons (*dotted line*). (Modified from Rockwood CA, Matsen FA [eds]: The Shoulder, 2nd ed. Philadelphia: WB Saunders, 1998, p. 705.)

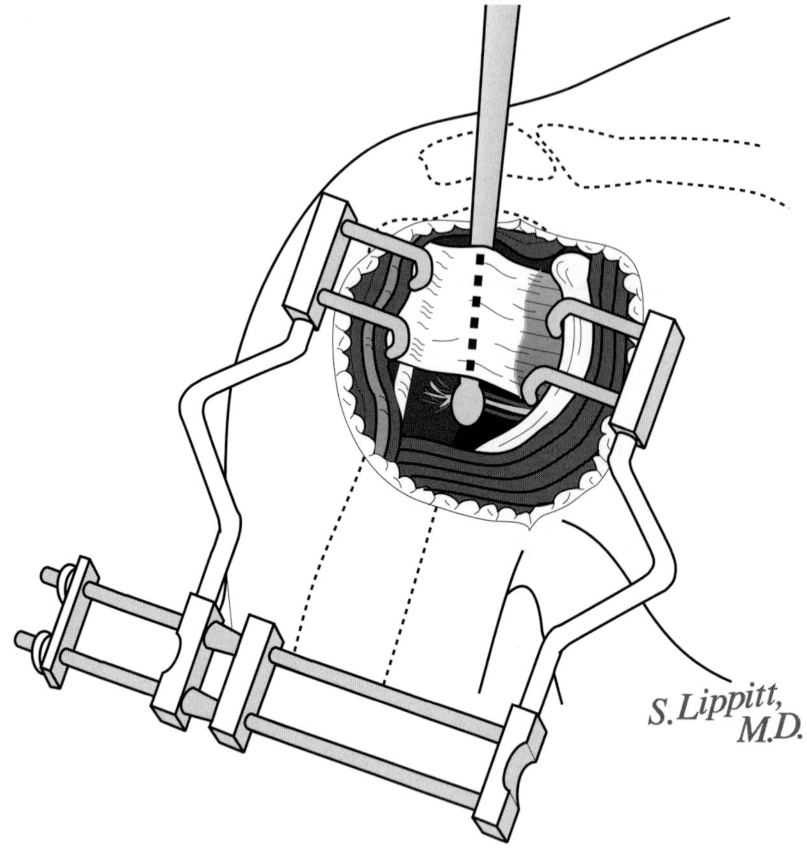


**Figure 14–5. Subscapularis incision**
The subscapularis is incised through its tendon, leaving good tissue on either side for later repair. The anterior humeral circumflex vessels are protected inferiorly. (Modified from Rockwood CA, Matsen FA [eds]: The Shoulder, 2nd ed. Philadelphia: WB Saunders, 1998, p. 705.)

The subscapularis and subjacent capsule are incised so that there is sufficient tissue laterally for reattachment at the end of the procedure (**Fig. 14–6**).

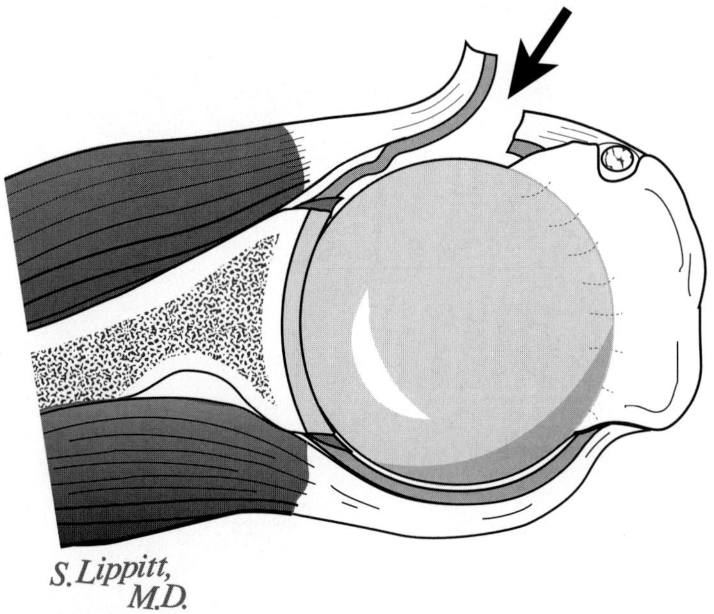


**Figure 14–6. Subscapularis and capsular incision**
The subscapularis and subjacent capsule are incised so that strong tendinous tissue remains on either side of the incision. Sufficient tissue is left attached to the lesser tuberosity so that repair at the end of the case is facilitated. The subscapularis and capsule are not separated.

The glenohumeral joint is exposed with the above-described findings. A humeral head retractor is inserted. Placing the shoulder in its mid-range position relaxes the capsule and ligaments. Twisting the humeral head retractor exposes the inferior half of the posterior labrum (**Fig. 14–7**). A needle carrying #0 absorbable suture is passed through the junction of the labrum and the glenoid articular cartilage, around the labrum, and through the capsule so that when this suture is tied, an imbrication of 1 cm of capsule is accomplished (**Fig. 14–8**). One such suture is placed every 6 mm around the perimeter of the inferior half of the glenoid from posterior mid-glenoid to anterior mid-glenoid (**Fig. 14–9**).

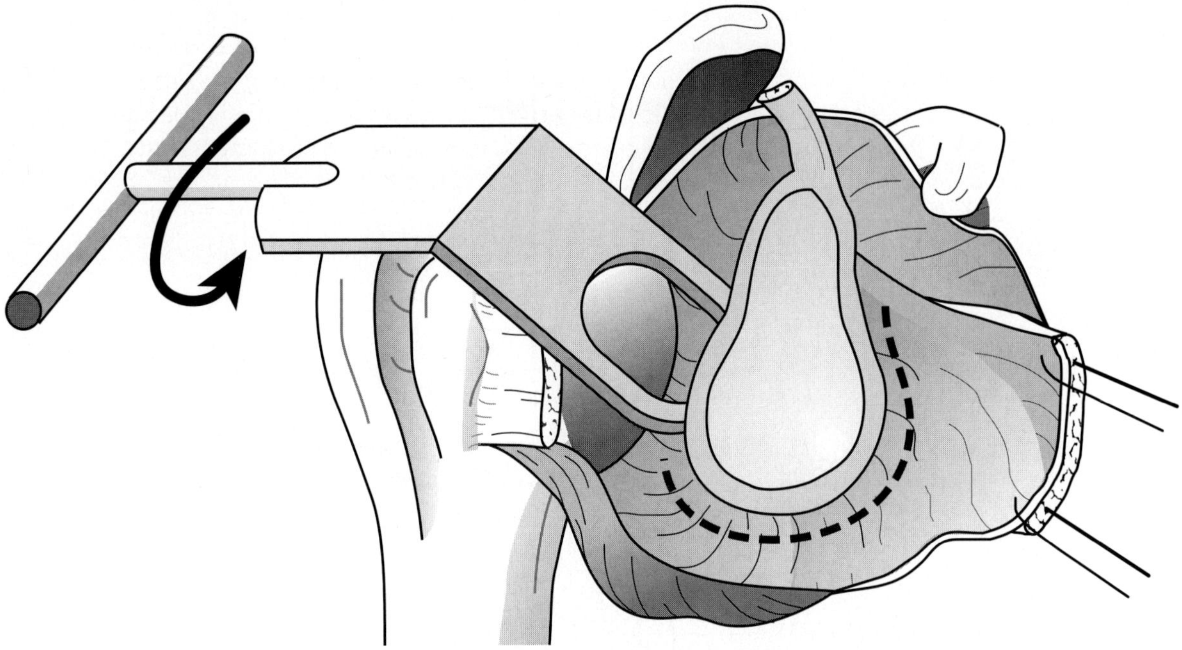

**Figure 14–7. Capsular exposure**
Twisting the inferior part of the humeral head retractor away from the glenoid exposes the inferior capsule.

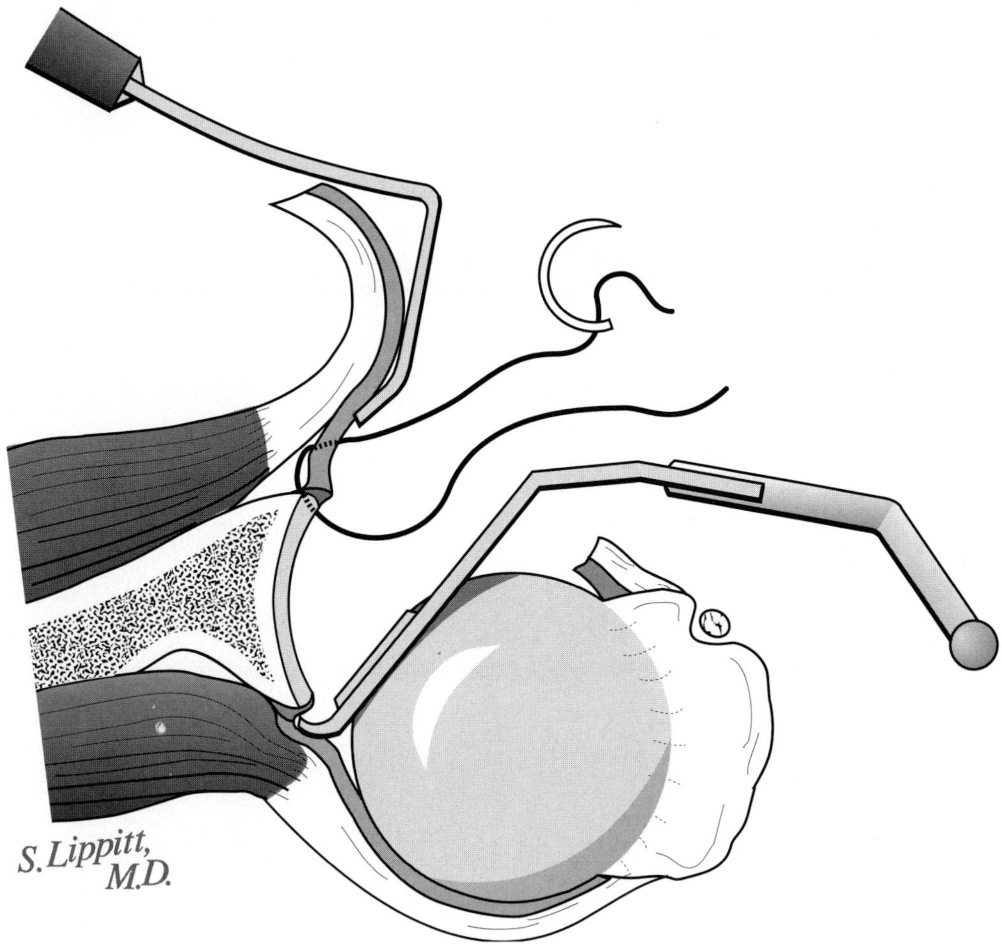


**Figure 14–8. Suture passage**
The suture is passed through the margin of the articular cartilage, around the labrum, and around 1 cm of capsule.

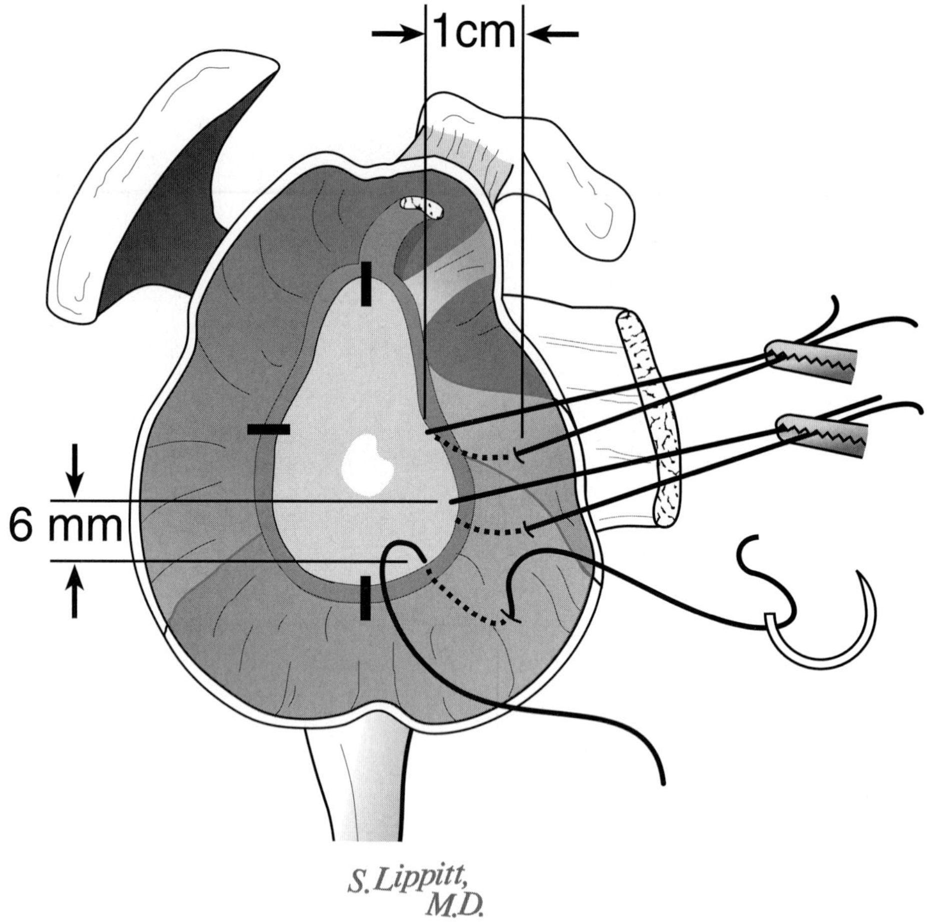


A

**Figure 14–9. Suture placement and tying**

**A,** Sutures are placed around the perimeter of the glenoid from three o'clock to nine o'clock.

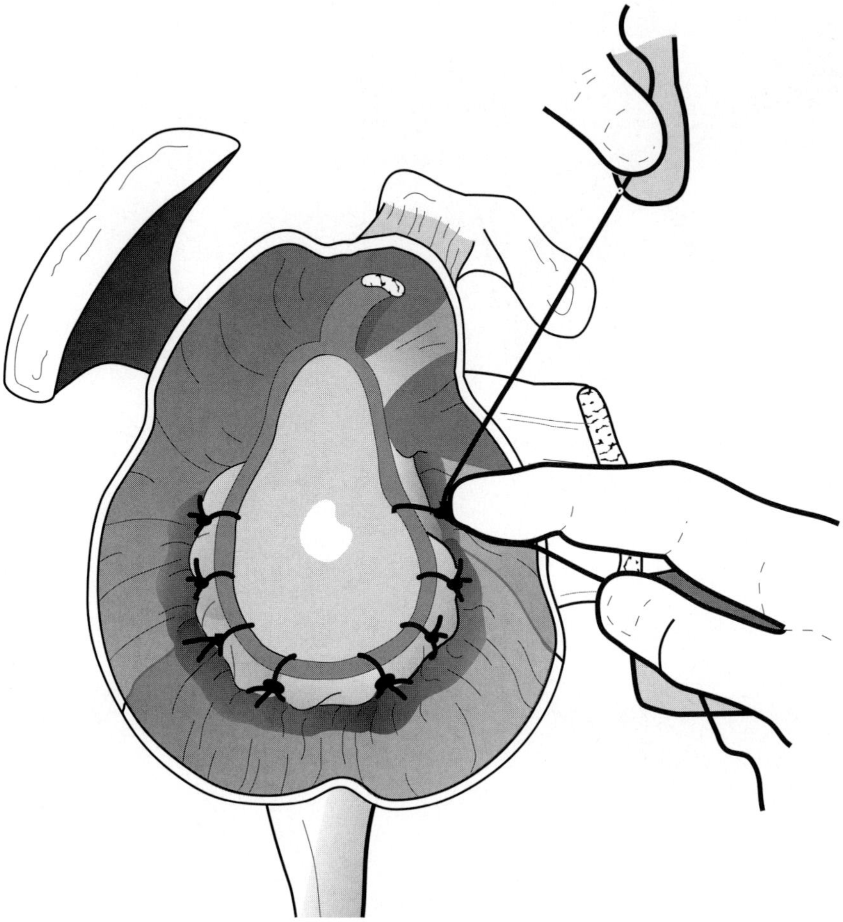


B

**Figure 14–9. Suture placement and tying**—*Continued*
**B,** These sutures are tied so that the knots overlie the capsule.

*Continued*

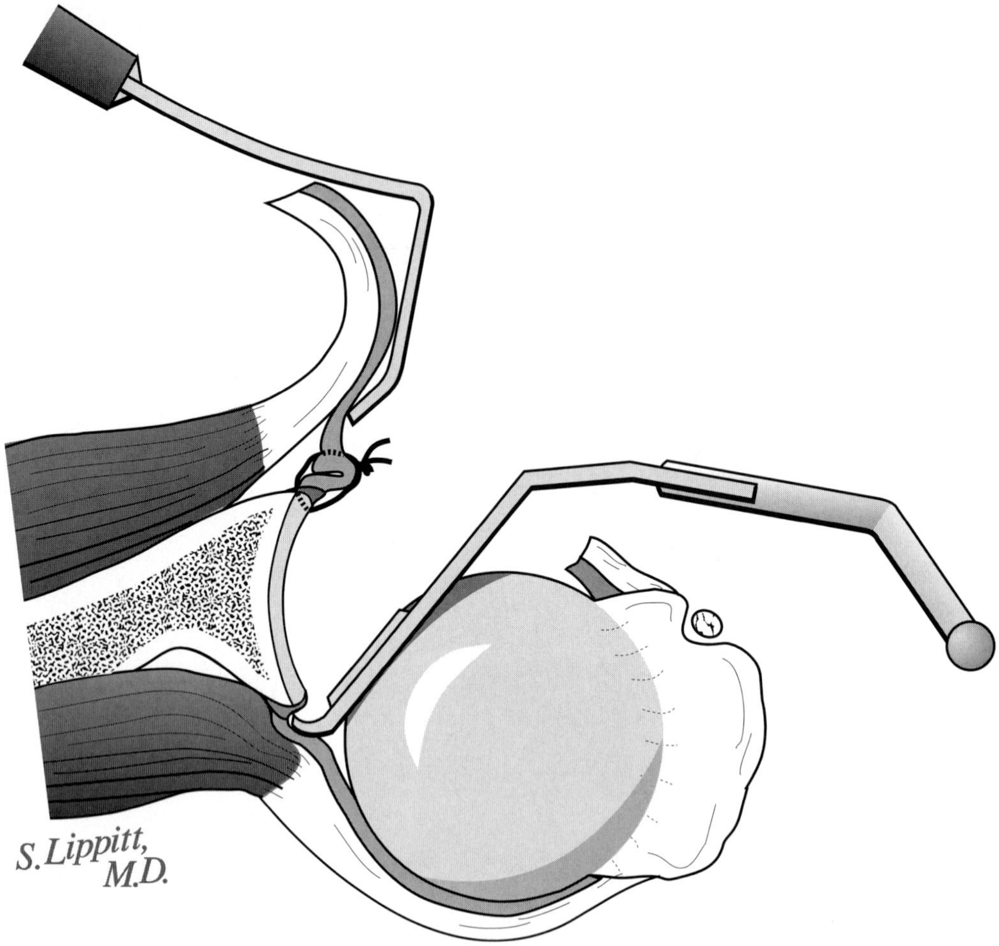


C

**Figure 14–9. Suture placement and tying**—*Continued*
**C,** Tying these sutures creates a substantial "bumper," augmenting the glenoid concavity.

Twenty milliliters of blood is drawn from the antecubital fossa of the ipsilateral elbow (**Fig. 14–10**). Using a flat beveled needle, blood is injected into the imbricated labrum and capsule between the sutures, with care taken to avoid cutting them. Injection of the blood swells the rolled-up tissue and provides additional stem cells for

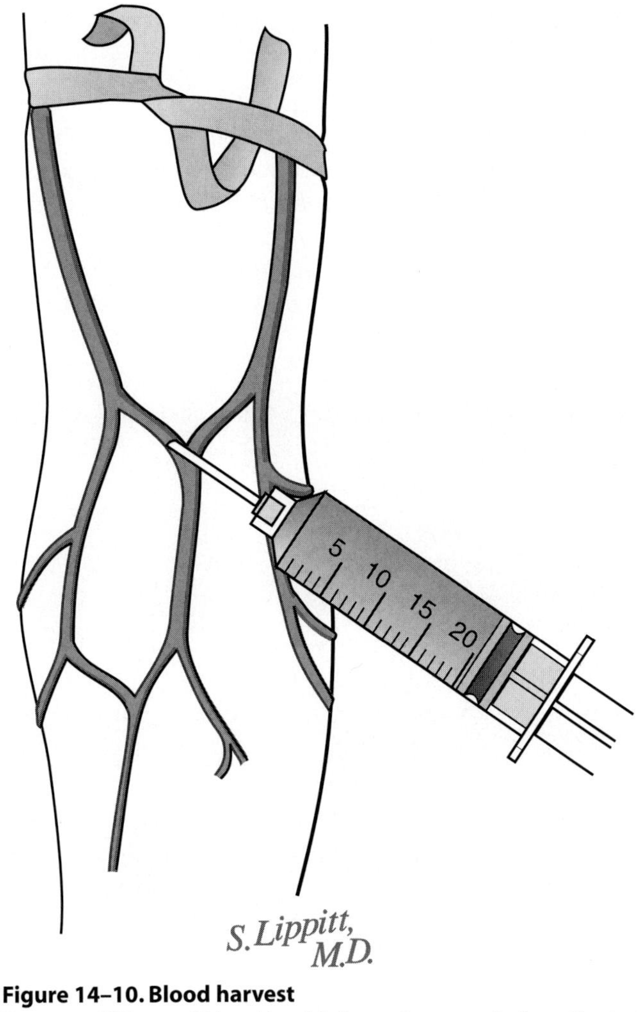


**Figure 14–10. Blood harvest**
Twenty milliliters of blood is withdrawn from a vein from the ipsilateral antecubital fossa.

a substantial healing response (**Fig. 14–11**). Injection is repeated until the reconstructed labrum is maximally inflated.

The labral augmentation functionally deepens the glenoid concavity (**Fig. 14–12**). Post-repair findings reveal improved load and shift test results (**Fig. 14–13**).

The subscapularis and capsule are then repaired to their mates at the lesser tuberosity using six sutures of #2 nonabsorbable braided suture.

The wound is thoroughly irrigated and closed in layers. Dry sterile dressings are applied, and the patient is returned to the recovery room with the arm in a sling.

## POSTOPERATIVE PLAN

The postoperative plan calls for early implementation of gentle isometric deltoid and rotator cuff maintenance exercises, with the patient avoiding elevating the arm away from the side but allowing up to 40 degrees each of internal and external rotation. For 2 months, the patient confines the use of the arm to activities in the mid-range of shoulder motion and does not lift more than 1 pound.

After 2 months, additional emphasis is placed on strengthening of the cuff and gentle progression of activities. Stretching exercises are not performed.

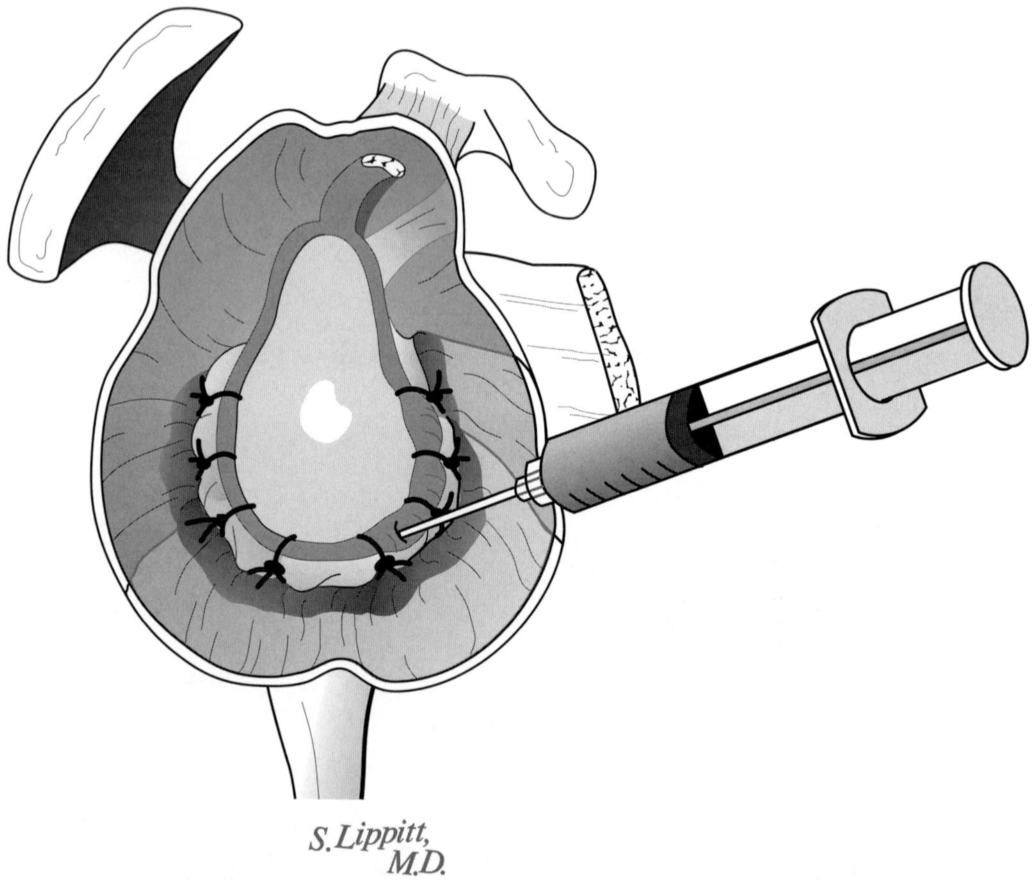


**Figure 14–11. Labral inflation**
The harvested blood is immediately injected into the rolled-up capsule and labrum before clotting takes place. A flat beveled needle is helpful here.

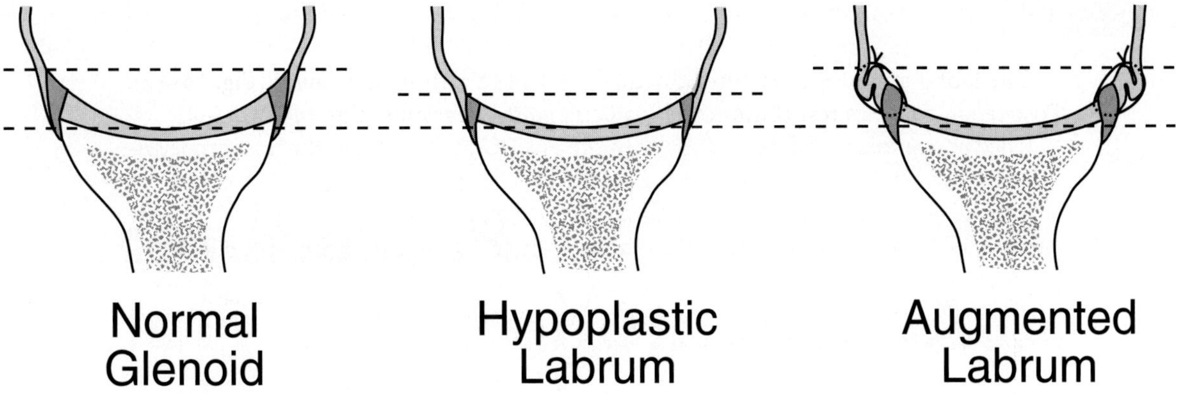


**Figure 14–12. Augmented glenoid depth**
The functional depth of the glenoid is increased by this labral augmentation.

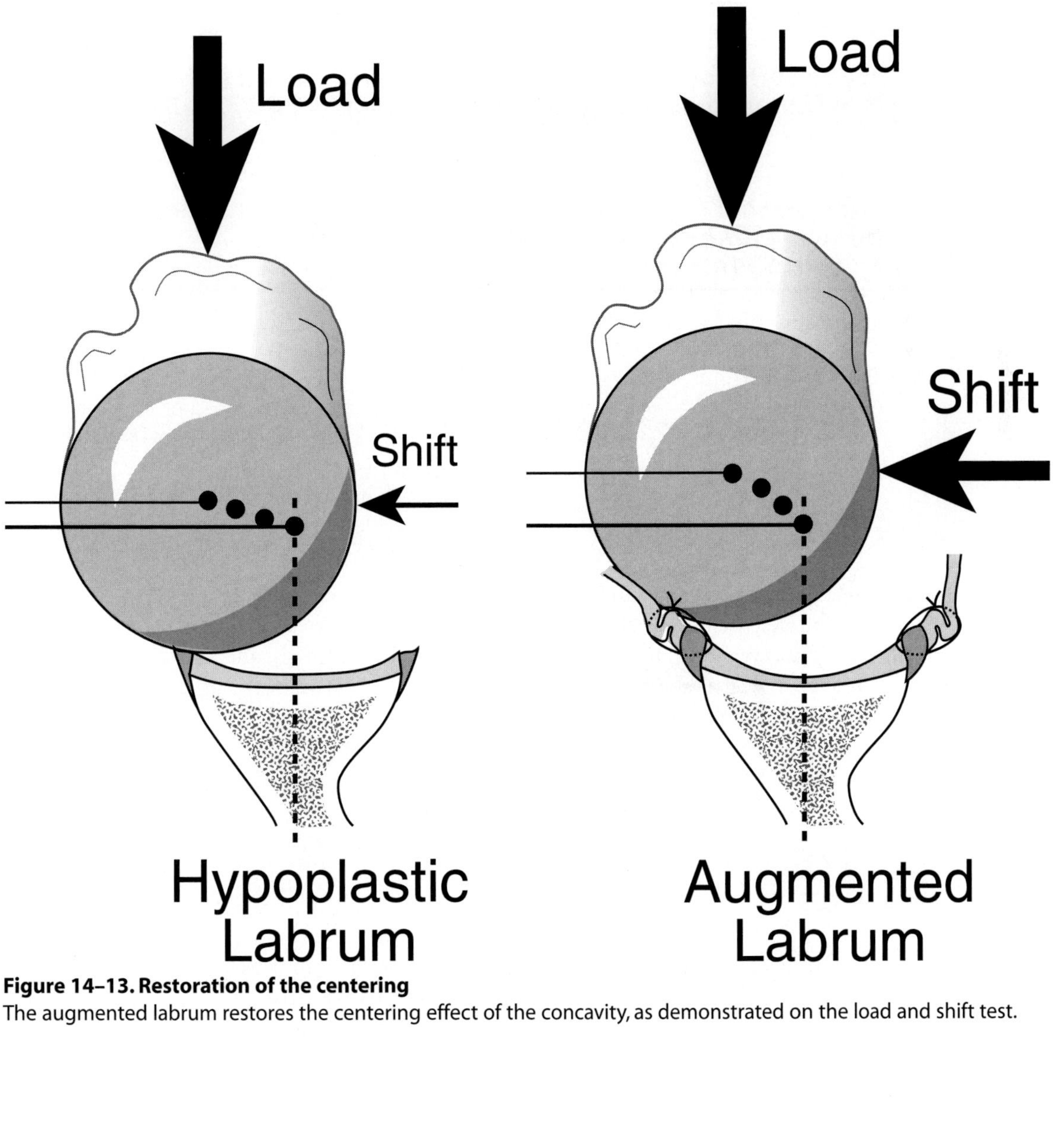


**Figure 14–13. Restoration of the centering**
The augmented labrum restores the centering effect of the concavity, as demonstrated on the load and shift test.

CHAPTER 15

# Procedure: Augmentation of a Flat Glenoid Lip by Posterior Glenoid Osteoplasty

***Diagnosis***

***Recurrent posterior instability of the shoulder associated with a flattened posterior glenoid lip ICD9 CODE 718.31***

***Procedure***

***Posterior glenoid osteoplasty through an "infraspinatus-on" approach with harvest of scapular bone graft CPT CODE 23465***

## INDICATIONS

The patient has functionally significant recurrent posterior apprehension and instability of the shoulder that has been refractory to nonoperative management.

Physical examination reveals diminished resistance to the posterior load and shift test (**Fig. 15–1**).

The axillary radiograph shows normal glenoid width, sufficient for osteoplasty, and a suggestion of increased posterior inclination of the glenoid joint surface.

Knowing the alternatives as well as the risks of infection, neurovascular injury, excessive stiffness, pain, weakness, fracture, continued instability, arthritis, and the need for revision surgery, as well as anesthetic complications, the patient desires to proceed with the above-described procedure. The patient understands that the purpose of the procedure is to increase the posteroinferior glenoid concavity with an osteotomy and graft from the scapula. The patient recognizes that this procedure cannot be expected to completely restore normal comfort and function to the shoulder. And lastly, the patient understands his or her critical role in the post-surgical rehabilitation.

## FINDINGS

Examination under anesthesia in the supine position reveals diminished resistance to translation on the posterior load and shift test and a positive jerk test.

Surgical findings include thinning of the posterior glenohumeral joint capsule.

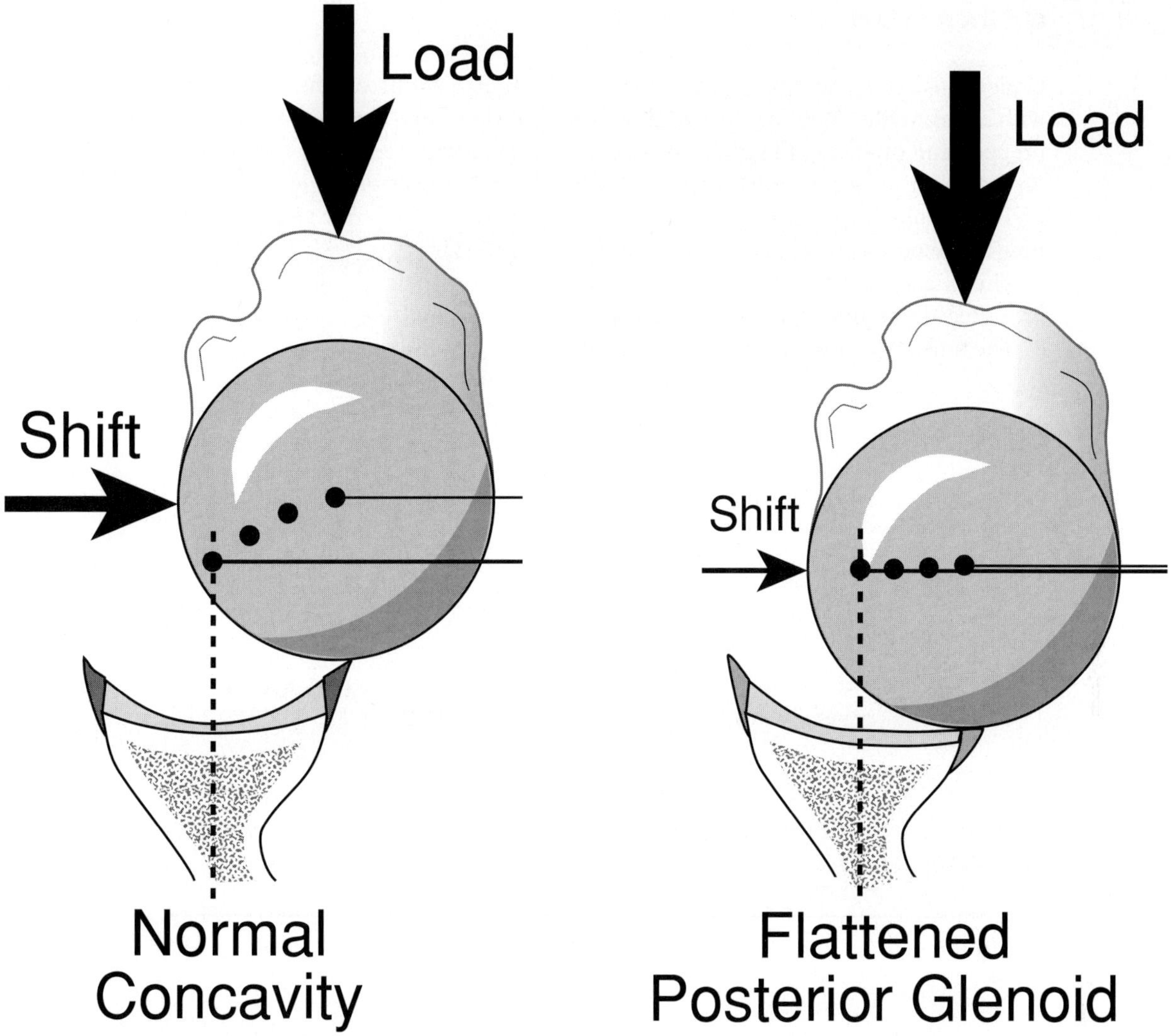


**Figure 15–1. Diminished resistance to load and shift**
A flat posterior glenoid diminishes the centering of the humeral head as reflected by the load and shift test.

## OPERATION

Under satisfactory anesthesia, the patient is positioned prone on the operating table with appropriate attention to padding, arm position, and airway. The shoulder is prepped and draped to the posterior midline with the arm free. A 6 cm incision based on the major posterior axillary crease is marked with a sterile pen **(Fig. 15–2)**.

The deltoid is split between its posterior one third and anterior two thirds beginning at the posterior corner of the acromion **(Fig. 15–3)**.

The axillary nerve is identified by palpation as it exits the quadrilateral space and is protected throughout the case **(Fig. 15–4)**.

The bursa is incised to expose the infraspinatus.

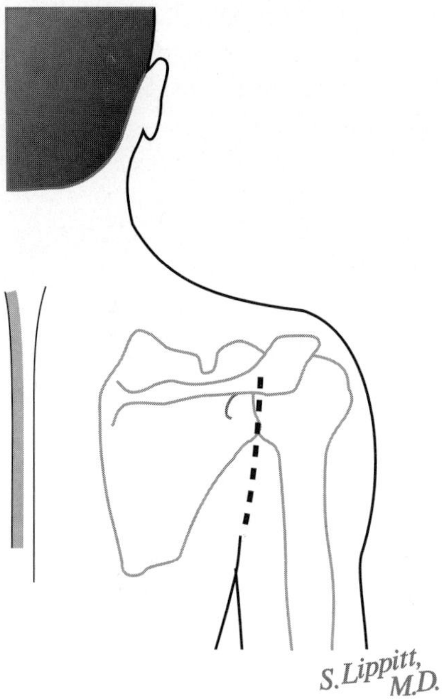


**Figure 15–2. Skin incision**
The posterior skin incision is made in the posterior axillary crease.

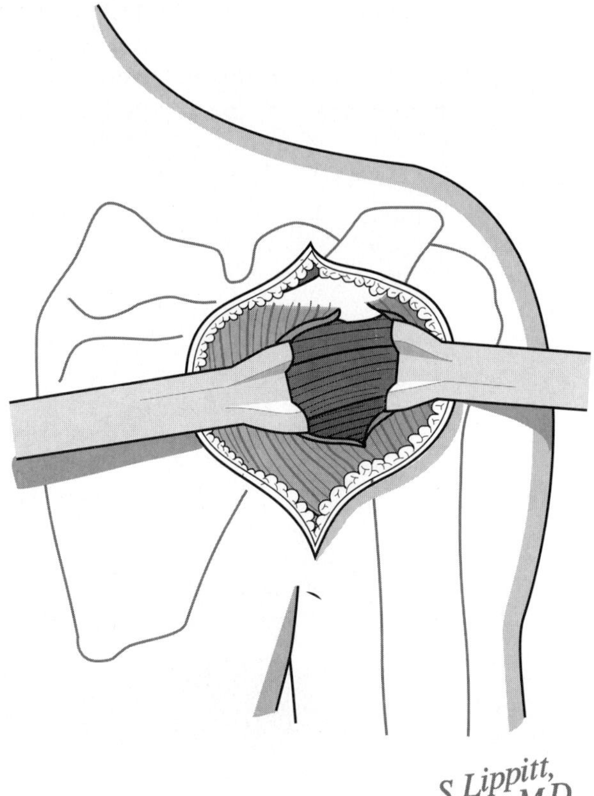


**Figure 15–3. Opening the deltoid**
Retracting the deltoid reveals the infraspinatus muscle.

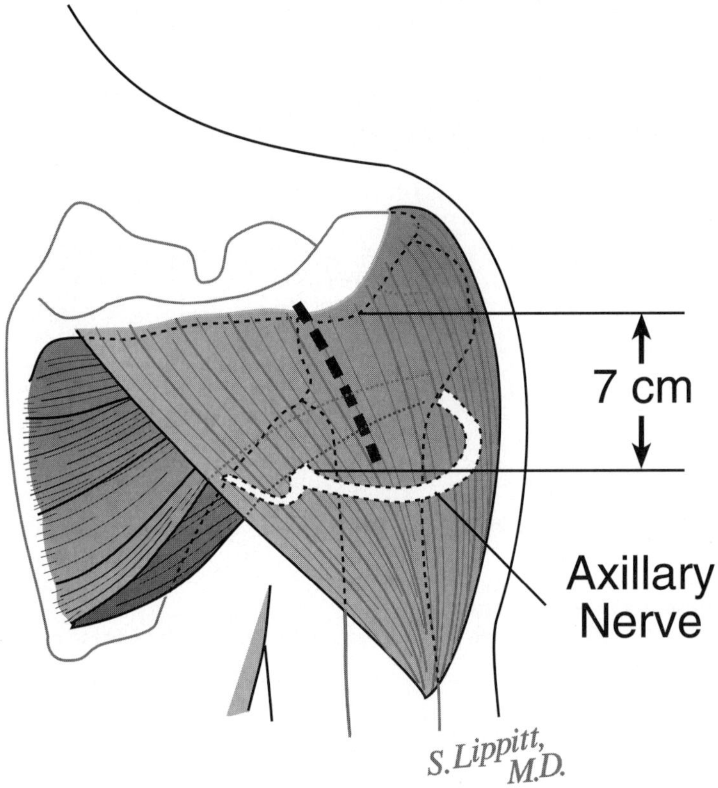


**Figure 15–4. Posterior deltoid split**
The deltoid is split between the anterior two thirds and the posterior one third of the muscle, being mindful of the axillary nerve inferiorly.

The interval between the infraspinatus and teres minor is opened horizontally, leaving the teres minor protecting the axillary nerve (**Fig. 15–5**). Passive external rotation relaxes the infraspinatus and teres minor. A spiked retractor is placed beneath the glenoid neck, reflecting the teres minor and axillary nerve inferiorly.

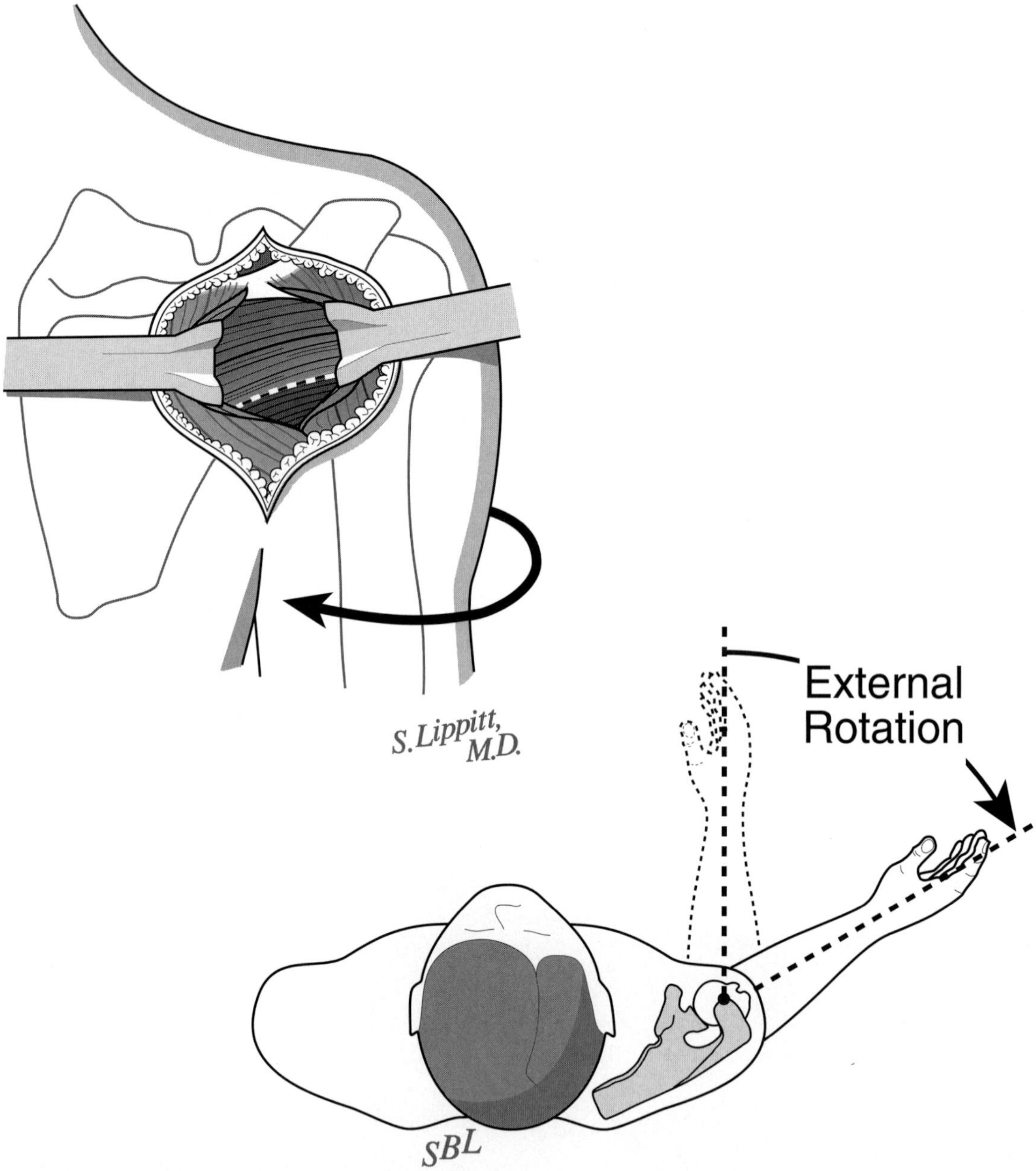


**Figure 15–5. Splitting the external rotators**
The external rotators are split between the infraspinatus and the teres minor. These muscles are relaxed by external rotation of the humerus.

The lateral infraspinatus muscle and tendon are bluntly dissected from the posterior glenoid neck and capsule. A second spiked retractor is placed in the body of the scapula to hold the lateral infraspinatus superiorly **(Fig. 15–6)**.

The periosteum of the glenoid neck is elevated with a periosteal elevator. The posterior glenohumeral capsule is exposed and inspected. Often a defect or very thin portion of the capsule is identified.

A horizontal posterior capsulotomy is created through the thinnest part of the capsule; the edges of the capsulotomy are tagged with sutures of #2 braided suture **(Fig. 15–7)**.

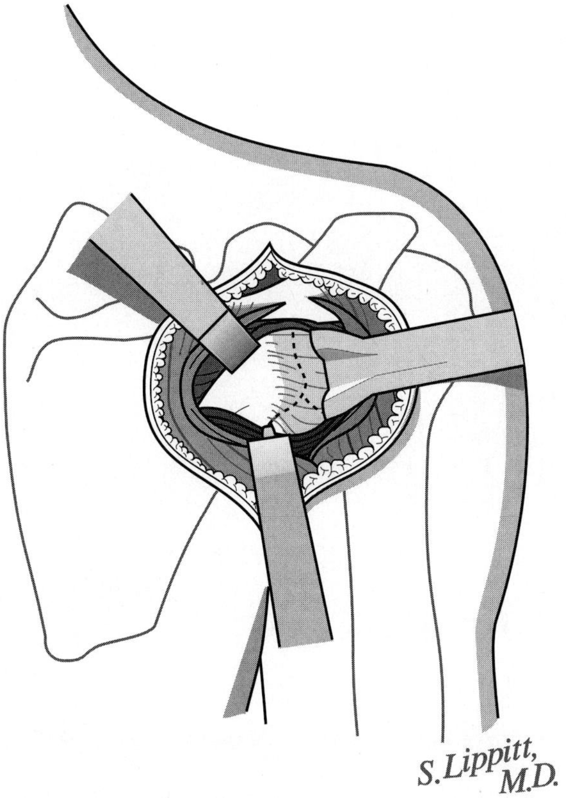


**Figure 15–6. Exposure of the inferior glenoid neck**
With the teres minor and axillary nerve retracted inferiorly, a spiked retractor is placed below the glenoid neck. The infraspinatus is retracted superiorly (toward its nerve supply) with a second spiked retractor. This provides an excellent exposure of the capsule.

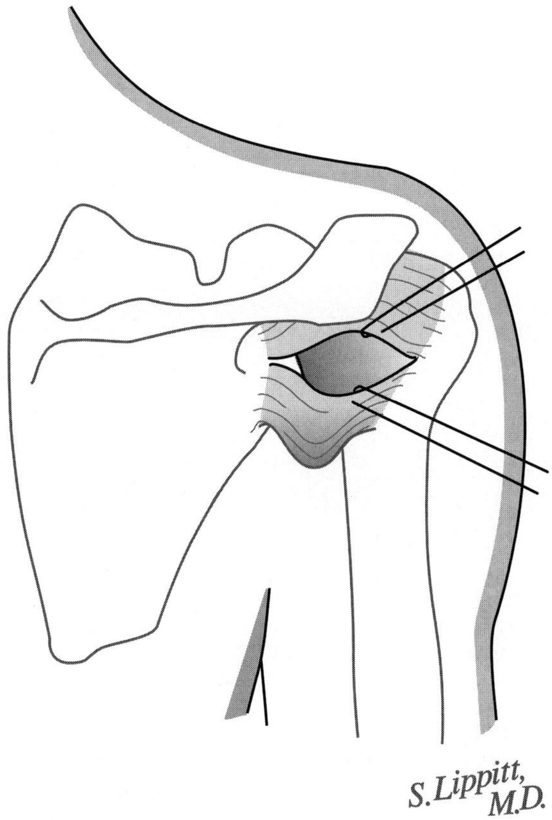


**Figure 15–7. Capsulotomy**
The posterior capsule is opened horizontally, making the incision through the weakest part of the capsule.

The integrity of the posterior labrum is verified by palpation with a blunt elevator. If a posterior labral detachment is identified, it is repaired to bone.

The plane of the glenoid articular surface is determined using a blunt elevator.

The plane of the osteotomy is 1 cm medial to and parallel to the plane of the joint surface. A small drill hole is made in the plane of the osteotomy at the superoinferior midpoint of the glenoid (**Fig. 15–8**). The depth of this drill hole is measured with a depth gauge (**Fig. 15–9**).

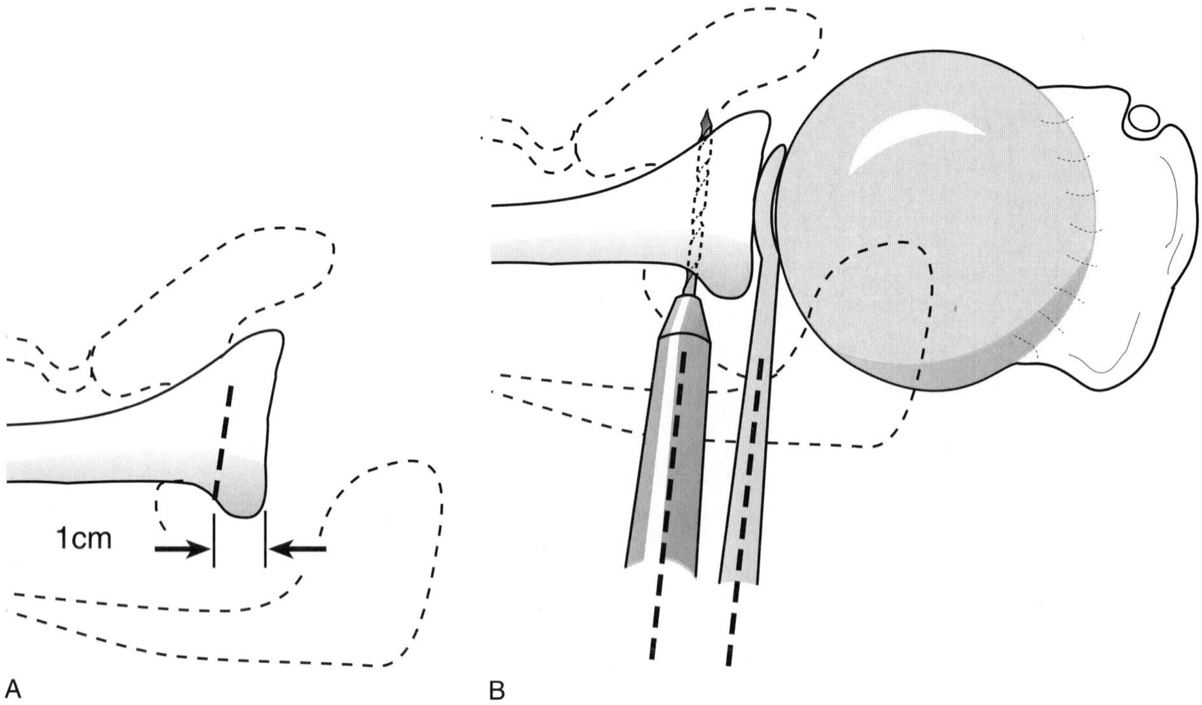


**Figure 15–8. Osteotomy**
**A,** The intended osteotomy is marked 1 cm medial to the joint surface. **B,** With a smooth elevator on the joint surface, a 2 mm hole is drilled parallel to the joint in the plane of the osteotomy.

A 3/4 inch flat and strong osteotome is marked with sterile tape at a length equal to three quarters of the anteroposterior dimension of the glenoid as indicated by the depth gauge (see Fig. 15–9).

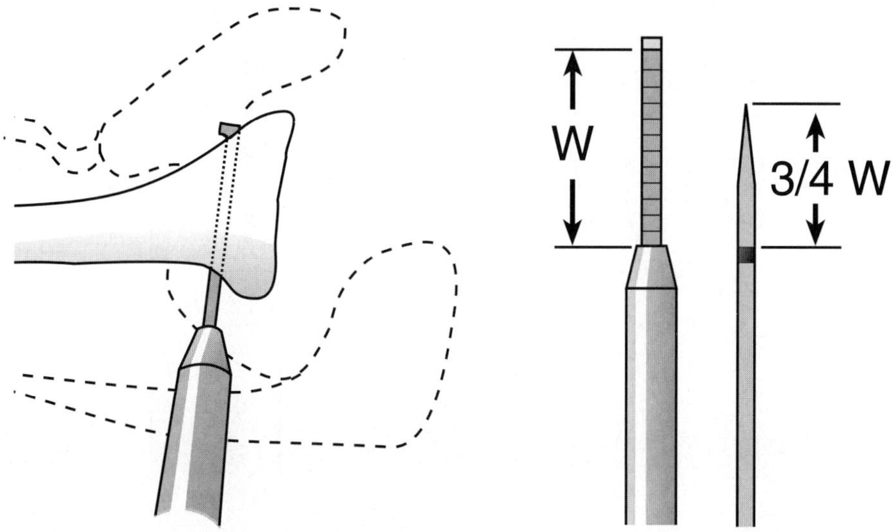


**Figure 15–9. The depth of the osteotomy**
The depth of the drill hole is measured with a depth gauge. A sterile paper tape is placed on the osteotomy at a distance from the tip equal to three quarters of the depth of the hole.

A posteroinferior opening wedge osteoplasty is created 1 cm medial and parallel to the plane of the glenoid, with the recognition that making the cut closer to the joint may endanger the articular surface and that making it farther away may make it difficult to open the osteoplasty (**Fig. 15–10**). The depth of the osteotome is controlled by paying attention to the sterile tape mark.

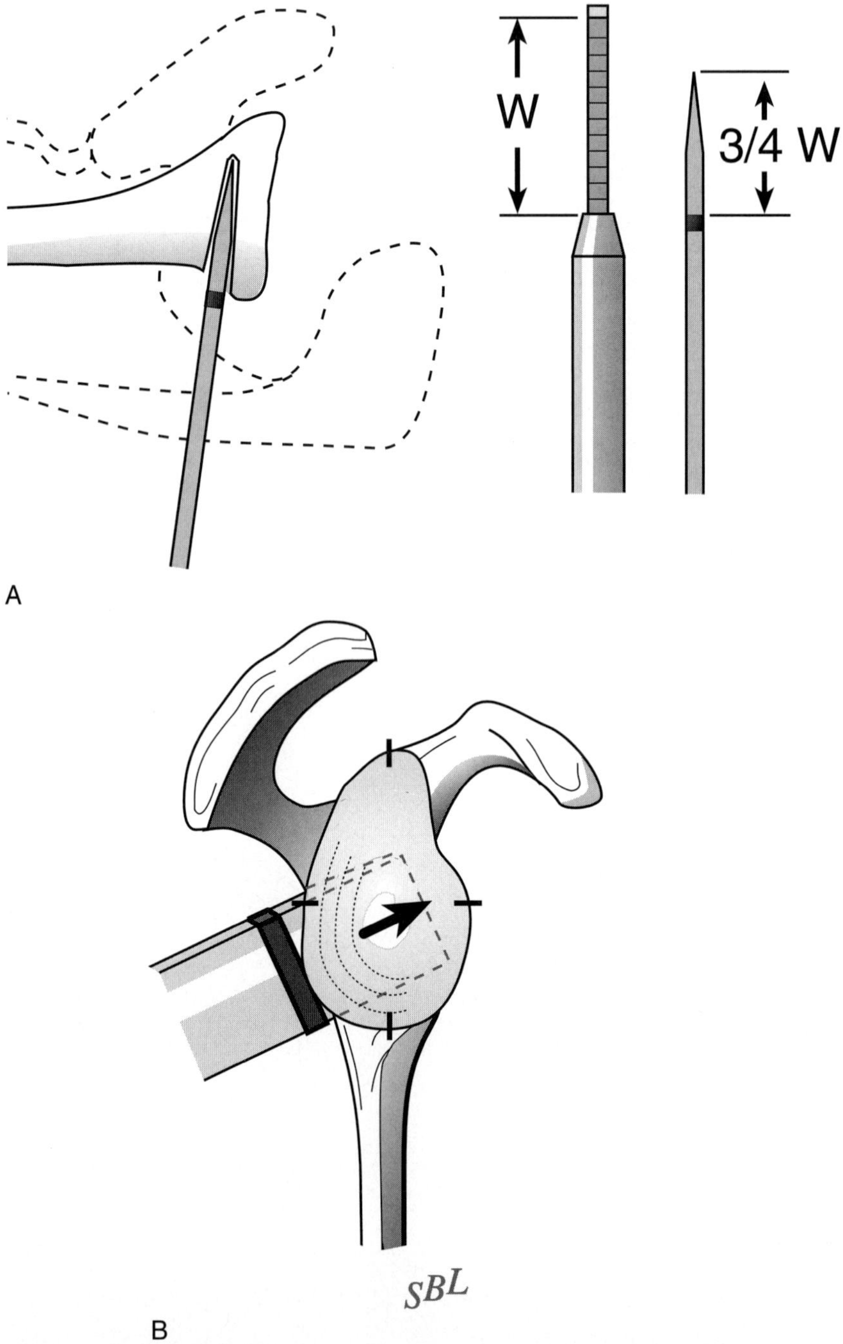


**Figure 15–10. The cut**
**A,** The osteotome is inserted parallel to the joint surface to the depth marked with the sterile tape. This should be three quarters of the anteroposterior thickness of the glenoid at the site of the osteotomy. **B,** The osteotome is inserted from posteroinferior to anterosuperior.

This osteoplasty is opened with successive levering steps to "bend" the bone, rather than breaking it. The glenoid surface is observed as the cut is deepened to prevent penetration of the joint surface (**Fig. 15–11**).

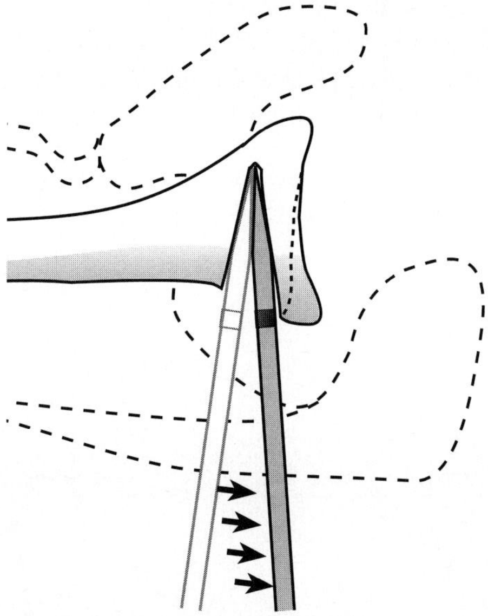

**Figure 15–11. Opening the osteotomy**
One opens the osteotomy with progressive gentle levering motions, attempting to bend, rather than fracture, the glenoid.

Through the same skin incision, a bicortical bone graft is harvested from the posterior scapular spine. A 25 mm wide segment of the posterior spine is exposed by incising the fibers of deltoid origin, keeping these fibers with the deltoid muscle. A graft 25 × 5 × 10 mm is harvested using a thin oscillating saw. The inferior aspect of the scapular spine is left intact (**Fig. 15–12**). At the end of the case, the deltoid will be repaired to itself, and, as necessary, to drill holes in the remaining scapular spine.

The graft is fashioned into a sharp wedge (**Fig. 15–13**).

The glenoid osteoplasty is pried open using a narrow osteotome, and the graft is placed in the defect with its thickest aspect inferiorly (**Fig. 15–14**). The bone graft is driven into position using a bone tamp. When fully inserted, the cortex of the graft is slightly deeper than the medial and lateral posterior cortex of the osteotomized glenoid (**Fig. 15–15**). No internal fixation is needed.

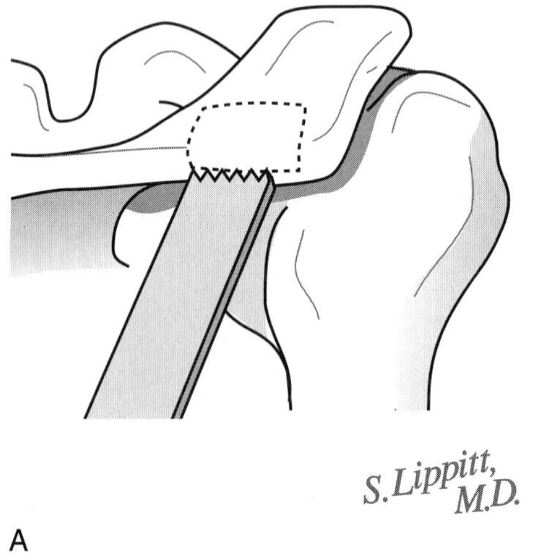


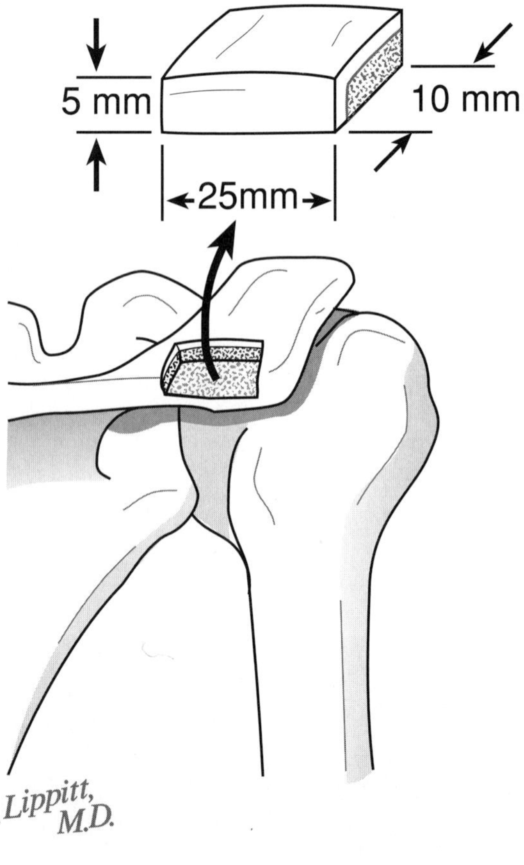


**Figure 15–12. Graft harvest**
**A,** The bone graft is harvested from the posterosuperior scapular spine. **B,** The graft should be approximately 25 mm wide, 5 mm thick, and 10 mm deep.

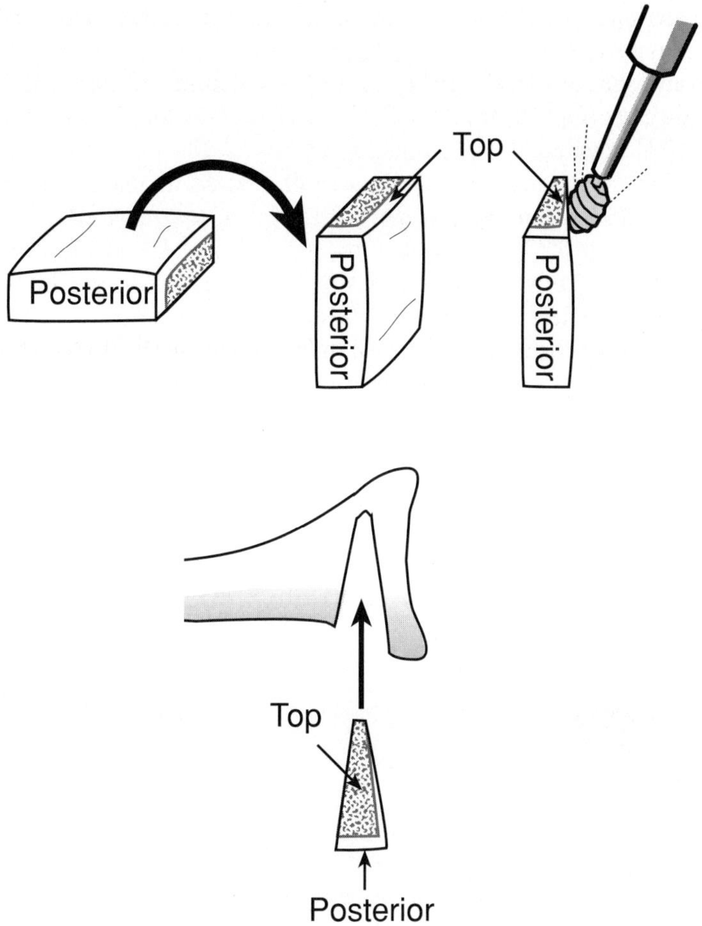


**Figure 15–13. Shaping the graft**
The graft is shaped to form a wedge with a base of 5 mm.

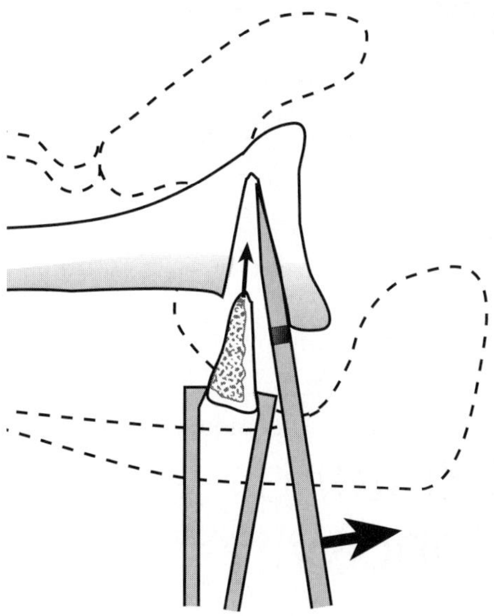

**Figure 15–14. Inserting the graft**
As the osteotomy is pried open, the graft is inserted with its cortical side toward the articular surface.

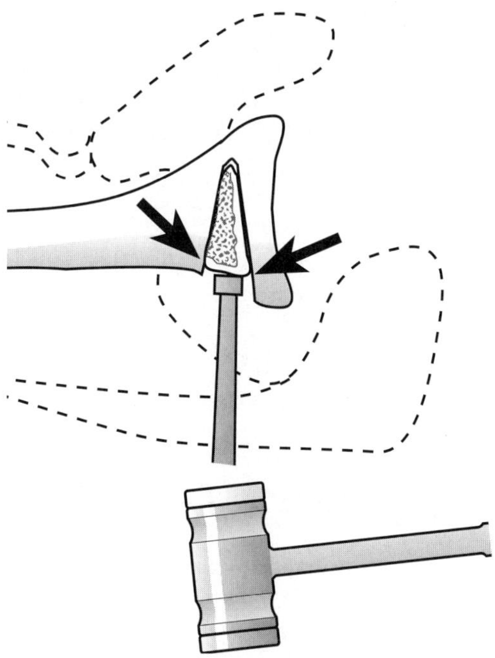

**Figure 15–15. Recessing the graft**
The graft is impacted until its base is within the cortex of the posterior glenoid.

Anteroposterior and axillary x-rays are obtained to document the position of the osteotomy and graft.

The load and shift test is repeated to confirm the stability of the joint as well as the security of the graft (**Fig. 15–16**).

The wound is irrigated.

The posterior capsulotomy is closed using #2 nonabsorbable suture. The deltoid is repaired to itself, and, as necessary, to drill holes in the remaining scapular spine (**Fig. 15–17**).

The retractors are removed, allowing the infraspinatus to fall back into position.

The security of the deltoid closure is verified.

The wound is again irrigated and closed in layers. Dry sterile dressings are applied, and the patient is returned to the recovery room in satisfactory condition with the arm in a sling.

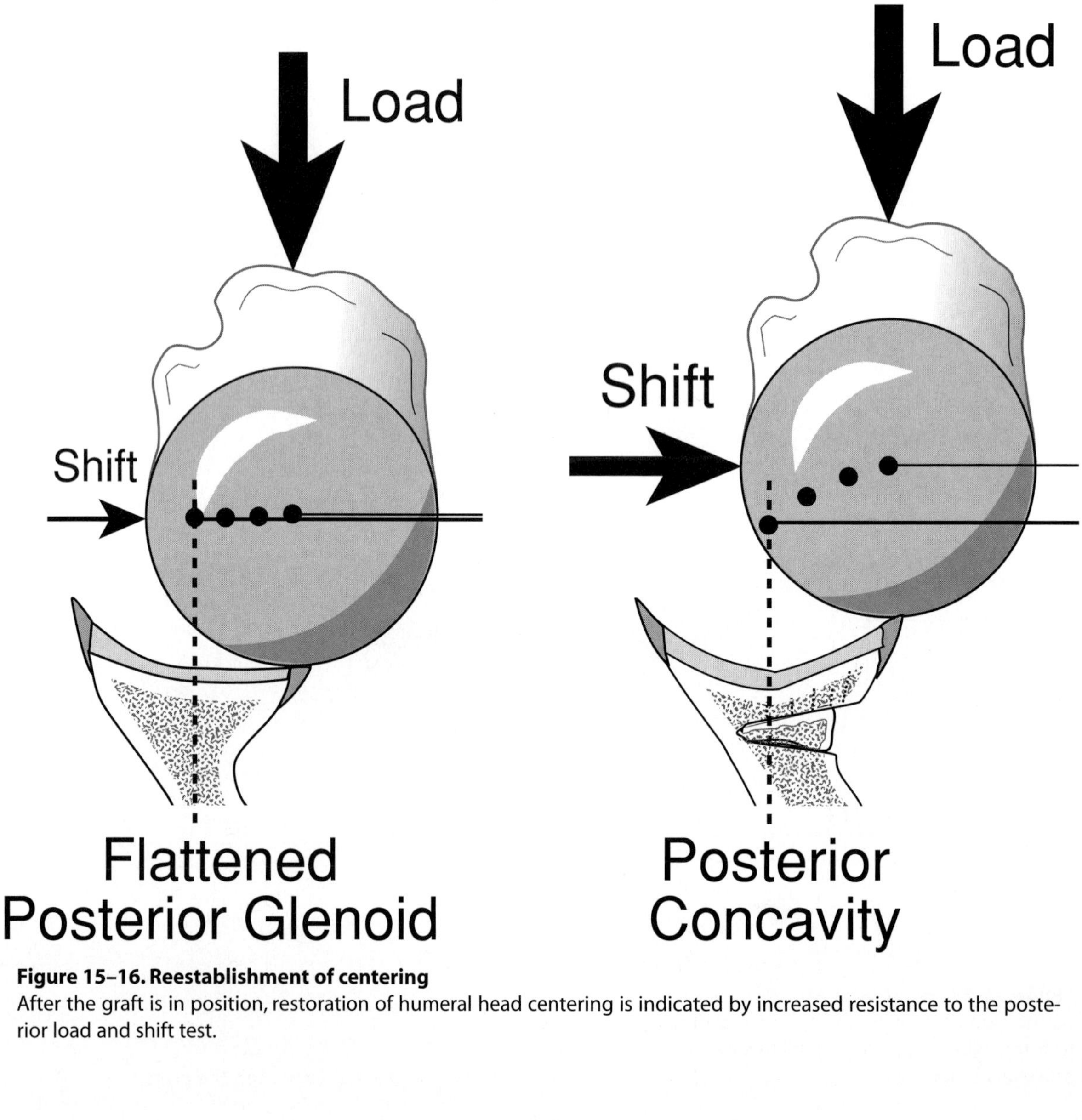


**Figure 15–16. Reestablishment of centering**
After the graft is in position, restoration of humeral head centering is indicated by increased resistance to the posterior load and shift test.

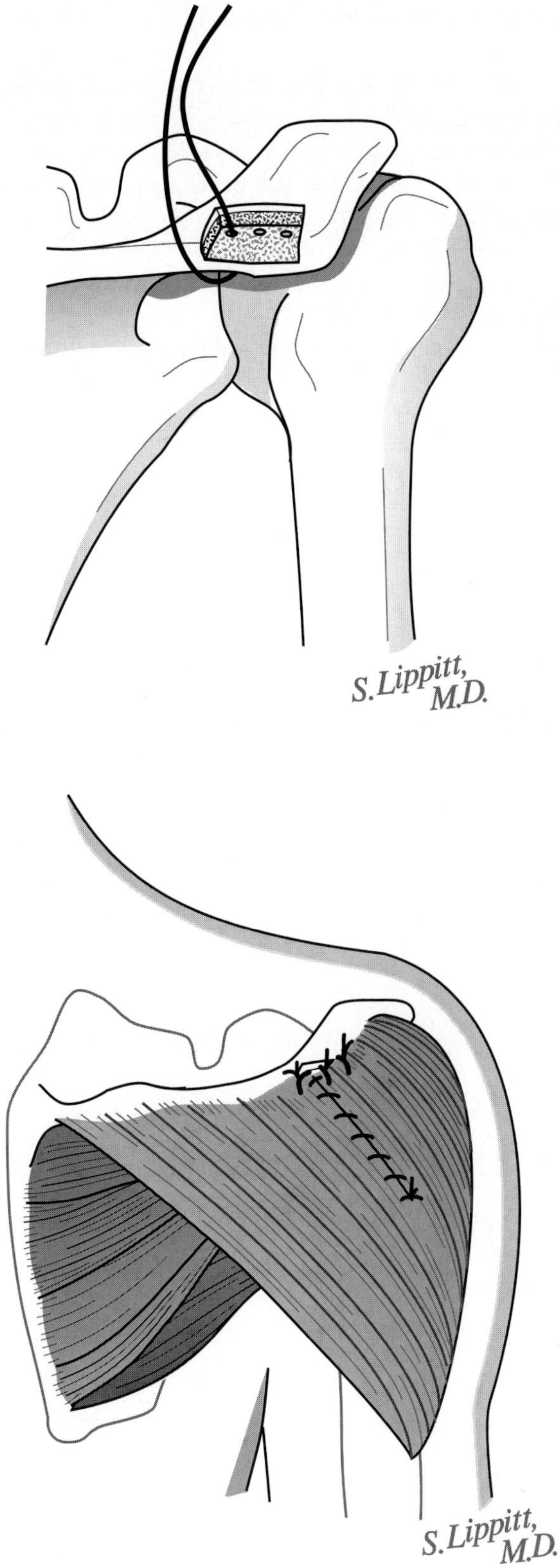


**Figure 15–17. Deltoid repair**
The deltoid is repaired to drill holes at the osteotomy harvest site. The deltoid is then closed side-to-side.

## POSTOPERATIVE PLAN

On the first postoperative day, the patient begins active assisted internal and external rotation exercises, keeping the elbow at the side, using the 0 degrees of elevation, 40 degrees internal and external rotation program (**Fig. 15–18**). For 6 weeks, the patient avoids moving the elbow from the side and develops progressive strength of internal and external rotation.

At 6 weeks, the patient begins abduction in the plane of the body. Only when the arm can be lifted comfortably and strongly in abduction is elevation started in more anterior planes.

By 3 months after surgery, the patient should be able to return to progressive use of the arm.

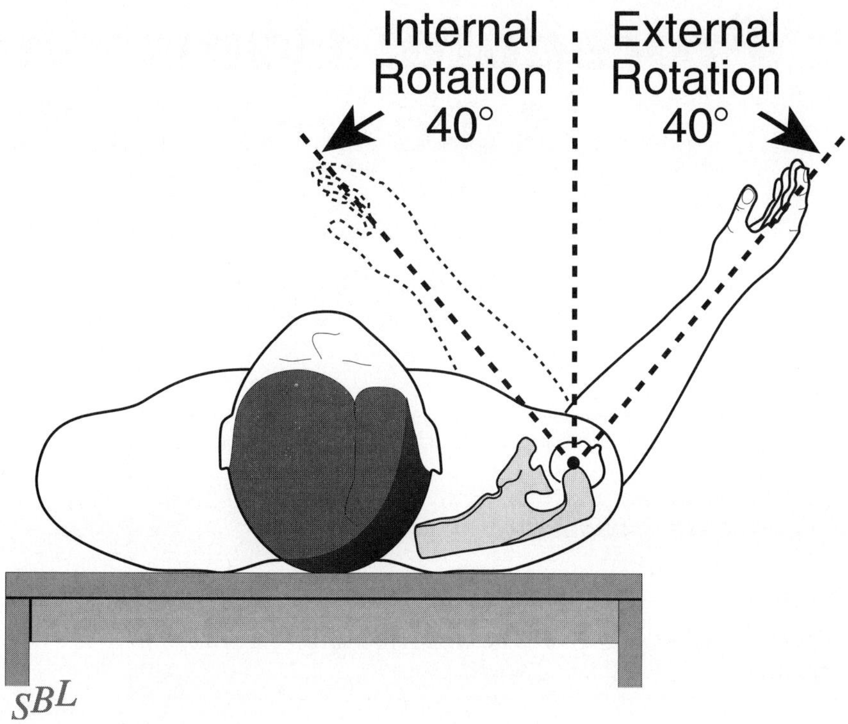


**Figure 15–18. Rehabilitation**
Immediately after surgery, the patient begins active and passive rotation with the elbow at the side.

CHAPTER 16

# Procedure: Hamstring Autograft to the Anterior Glenohumeral Joint Capsule

**Diagnosis**

***Traumatic anterior instability ICD9 CODE 718.31***
***Failed anterior stabilization procedure***

**Procedure**

***Hamstring autograft to the anterior glenohumeral capsule CPT CODE 23460***

## INDICATIONS

The patient has functionally significant anterior apprehension and instability after failed previous anterior repairs, especially when the arm is in external rotation and abduction.

Physical examination demonstrates increased range of external rotation and thinning of the tissues anterior to the humeral head by palpation through the intact skin (**Fig. 16–1**). The load and shift test result is normal, indicating an intact labral concavity.

Radiographs of the shoulder show minimal bony deficiencies.

The patient understands that there is a suspicion of insufficient quantity and quality of the anterior capsular tissue and the potential need for autogenous tissue from the hamstrings. Knowing the alternatives as well as the risks of infection, neurovascular injury, excessive stiffness, pain, weakness, fracture, instability, symptoms at the donor site at the knee, and the need for revision surgery, as well as anesthetic complications, the patient desires to proceed with the above-described procedure. The patient understands that the graft is to be harvested from the same side as the shoulder and that a cane may be needed in the hand opposite the leg graft donor site to assist with walking until the leg allows for comfortable ambulation. The patient has not been smoking for at least 3 months prior to the procedure and will not resume smoking following the procedure. The patient understands that the purpose of this procedure is to reestablish the capsuloligamentous checkrein anteriorly to limit excess external rotation. The patient recognizes that this procedure cannot be expected to completely restore normal comfort and function to the shoulder. And, lastly, the patient understands his or her critical role in the post-surgical rehabilitation.

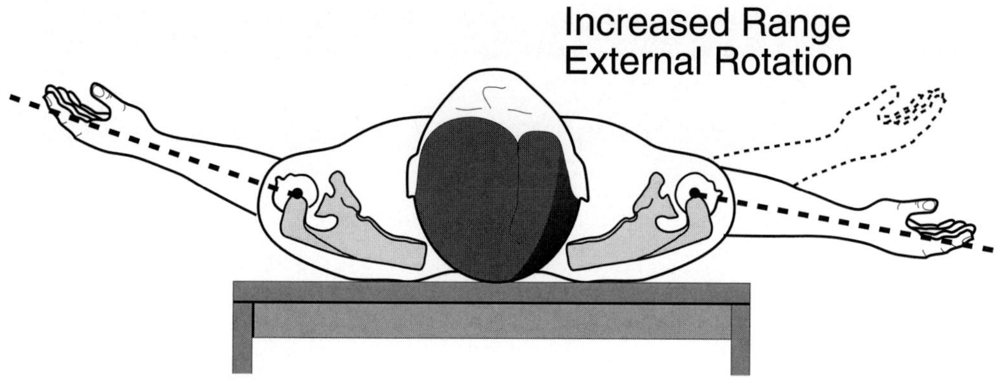


**Figure 16–1. Loss of checkrein**
When the anterior capsule is disrupted, the glenohumeral joint lacks its normal limitation of external rotation.

## FINDINGS

Examination with the patient under anesthesia reveals increased external rotation in comparison with the normal shoulder (see Fig. 16–1) and a palpable thinning of the anterior capsule.

Surgical findings include a defect in the subscapularis tendon and anterior capsule. There is insufficient quantity and quality of the anterior capsuloligamentous tissue to allow for a robust anterior repair (**Fig. 16–2**).

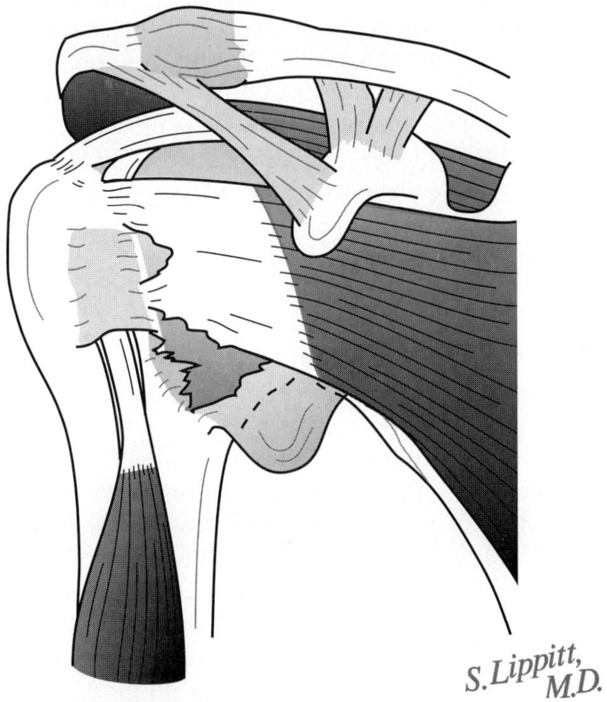


**Figure 16–2. Compromised tissue quality**
The quality of the subscapularis tendon and anterior capsule is insufficient for repair.

## OPERATION

Under satisfactory anesthesia, the patient is placed in a low beach chair position with the glenohumeral joint at the edge of the operating table. The shoulder and ipsilateral lower extremity are carefully prepped and draped. The shoulder is approached through the previous incisional scar. The deltopectoral interval is opened, leaving the cephalic vein on the deltoid laterally. The humeroscapular motion interface is freed of adhesions, especially the scarring around the subscapularis and axillary nerve. A self-retaining retractor is placed with one blade against the deltoid and the other against the coracoid muscles. The axillary nerve is palpated and protected throughout the case.

The quality and quantity of the subscapularis tendon are found to be deficient, as is the capsule in the area of the previous repair. The subscapularis incision is made through the weakest part of the subscapularis tendon, leaving the strongest parts intact for inclusion in the repair at the conclusion of the case.

The subjacent capsular defect is identified. It is apparent that a robust repair cannot be achieved at the desired length without additional tissue of quality. The residual tissues at the lesser tuberosity and at the glenoid are left intact.

At this time, the integrity of the glenoid labrum is verified. If there is a deficiency of the labrum, it is repaired at this time.

The glenoid insertion site for the graft is selected immediately medial to the glenoid lip at distances 25% and 50% superior from the inferior aspect of the glenoid. At each of these insertion sites, sufficient bone is exposed to allow the creation of a 5 mm diameter hole (**Fig. 16–3**). The surgeon connects the two holes below the cortical bridge between them by removing the intervening cancellous bone with an angled curette. A suture is passed in one of the holes and out the other. Similarly, two 5 mm diameter holes are made 25% and 50% up the base of the lesser tuberosity where the capsule normally attaches. The cancellous bone beneath the cortical bridge between the two holes is removed as on the glenoid side (**Fig. 16–4**). A suture is passed in one of these two holes and out the other.

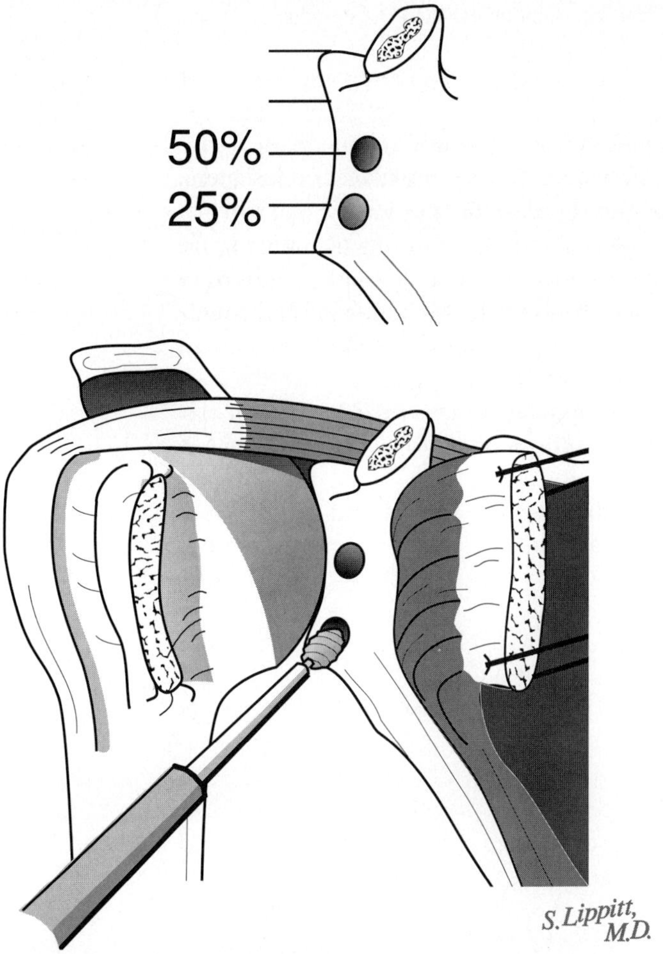


**Figure 16–3. Glenoid drill holes**
Using a pinecone burr, drill holes are placed in the middle and inferior aspects of the anterior glenoid, near the lip.

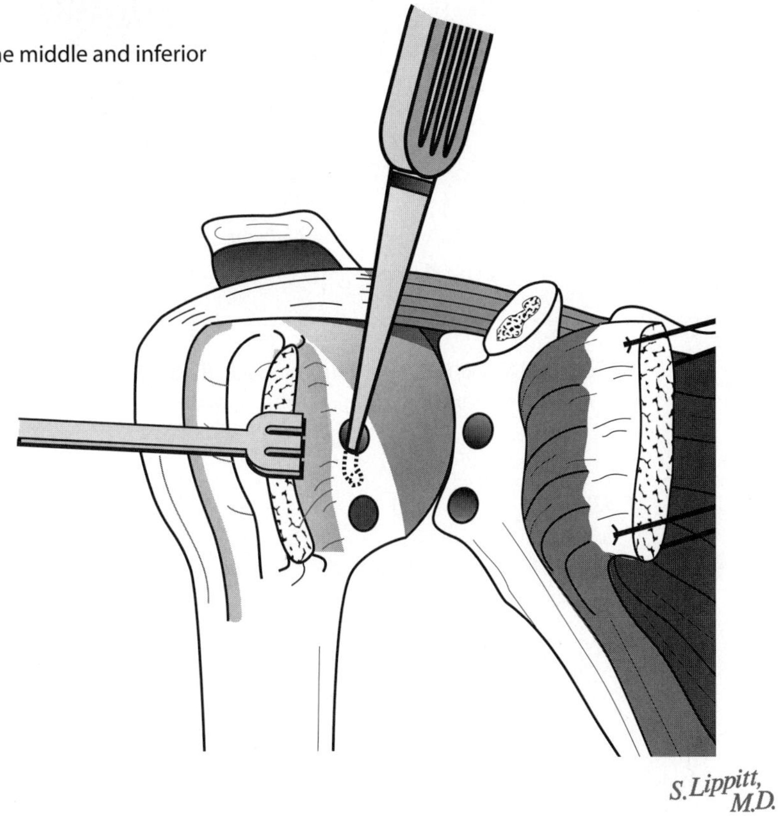


**Figure 16–4. Humeral drill holes**
Similarly, holes connected with a curette are made in the middle and inferior aspects of the proximal humerus, near the articular surface.

The semitendinosus tendon is harvested in a sterile fashion from the ipsilateral knee. At least 15 cm of robust graft is desired. It is cleaned of muscle, and a suture is woven in each end. One end of the graft is passed from the lower to the upper glenoid hole **(Fig. 16–5)**. The other end of the graft is passed from the lower to the upper humeral hole **(Fig. 16–6)**. The length of the graft between the two lower holes is set to allow 20 degrees of external rotation. The two ends of the graft exiting the upper holes are sewn to each other with #2 nonabsorbable braided suture so that, again, the length is set to become tight at 20 degrees of external rotation **(Fig. 16–7)**. Medial and lateral soft tissues are sewn to the graft to reinforce it. The additional length of graft tissue available is used to reinforce the reconstruction **(Fig. 16–8)**.

The wound is thoroughly irrigated. The subscapularis is then closed back to the tissue left attached to the lesser tuberosity with six sutures of #2 nonabsorbable braided suture.

The wounds are closed in layers. Dry sterile dressings are applied, and the patient is returned to the recovery room with the arm in a sling.

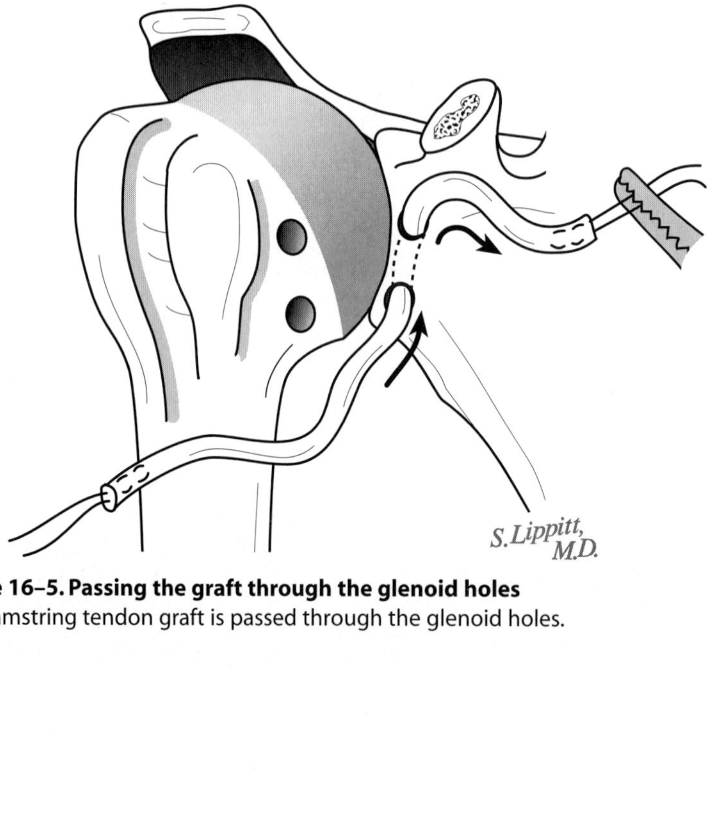


**Figure 16–5. Passing the graft through the glenoid holes**
The hamstring tendon graft is passed through the glenoid holes.

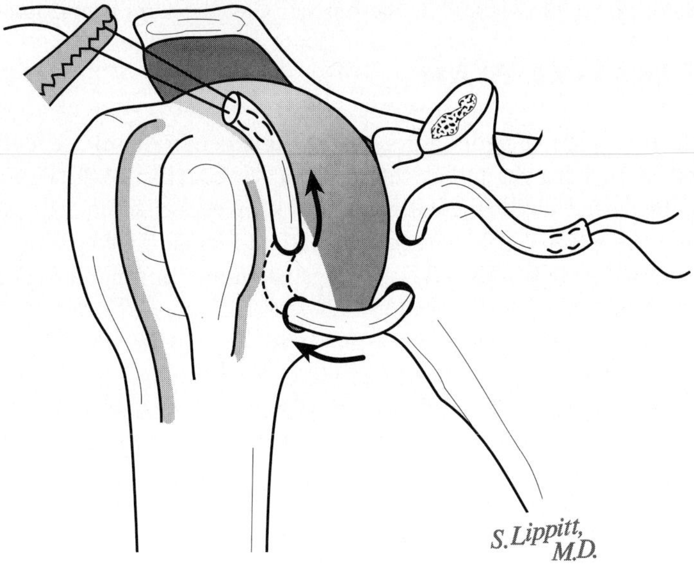


**Figure 16–6. Passing the graft through the humeral holes**
The hamstring tendon graft is then passed through the humeral holes.

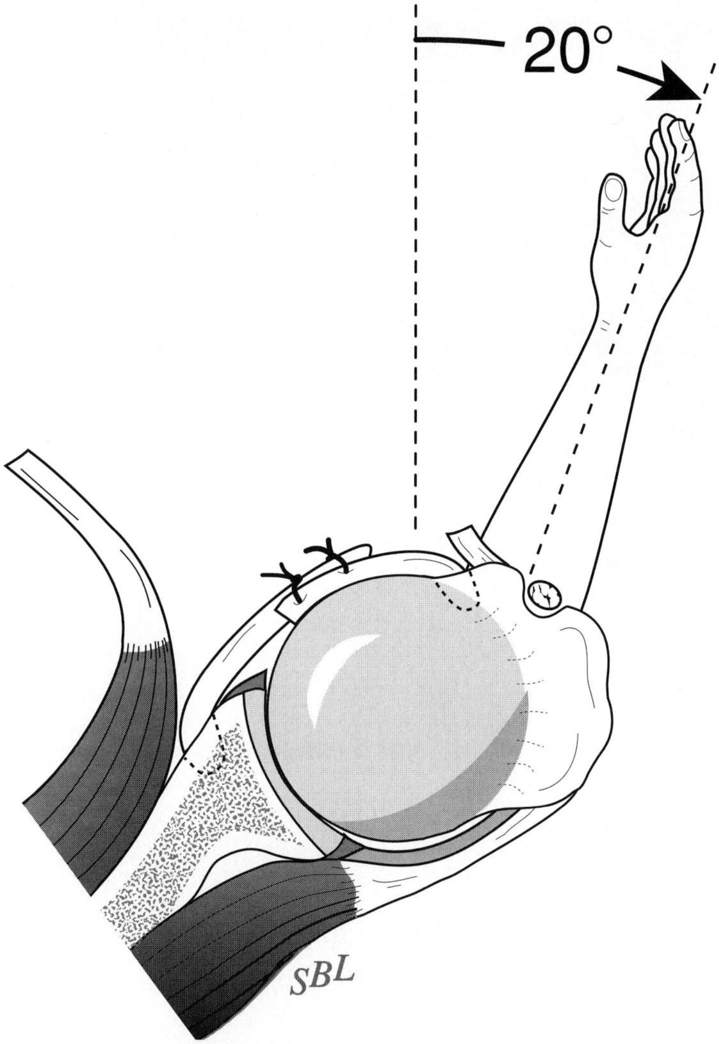


**Figure 16–7. Tying the graft**
The graft is tied so that external rotation is checked at 20 degrees.

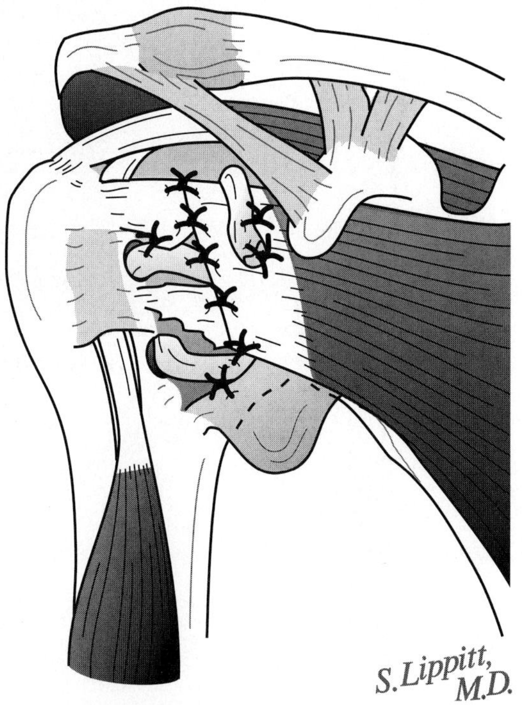


**Figure 16–8. Reinforcing the graft**
Any available capsular or tendon tissue is anchored to the graft.

## POSTOPERATIVE PLAN

The postoperative plan includes immediate implementation of patient-conducted external rotation to 0 degrees and elevation to 90 degrees (**Fig. 16–9**). As soon as these exercises can be performed by the patient and as soon as the patient can walk well and independently, the patient is discharged. The patient is encouraged to remove the sling and move the arm actively in the allowed range when functioning in a protected environment. Lifting is limited to 1 pound for 12 weeks.

At 2 weeks after surgery, the patient is instructed to increase external rotation to 20 degrees and forward elevation to 120 degrees, maintaining external rotation at 0 degrees. Gentle progressive strengthening exercises may be started at 12 weeks. The shoulder is not used for forceful activities until at least 6 months after the surgery. Smoking is prohibited following the surgery.

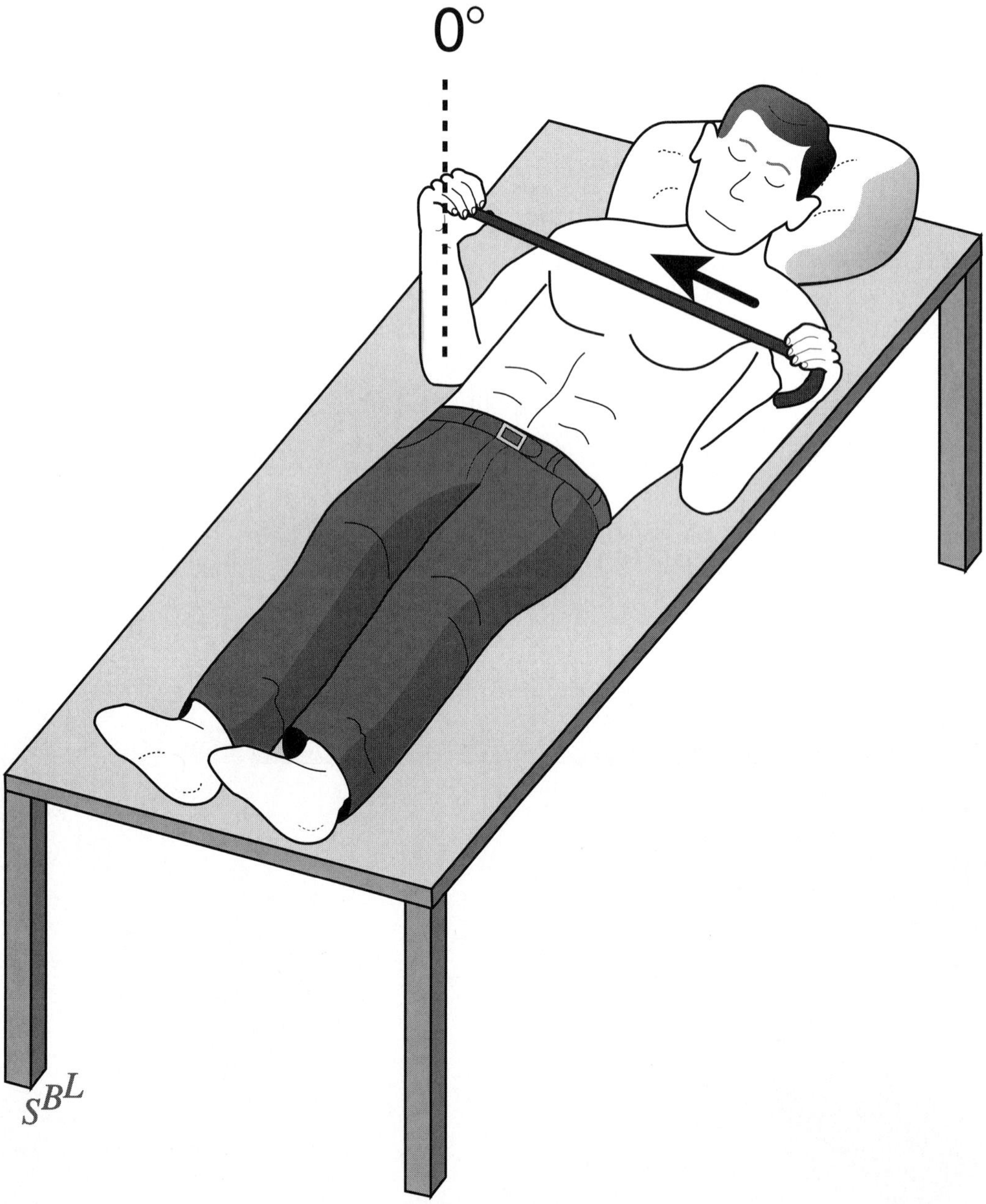


A

**Figure 16–9. Postoperative exercises**

**A,** External rotation. Passive and active external rotation are initiated to 0 degrees.

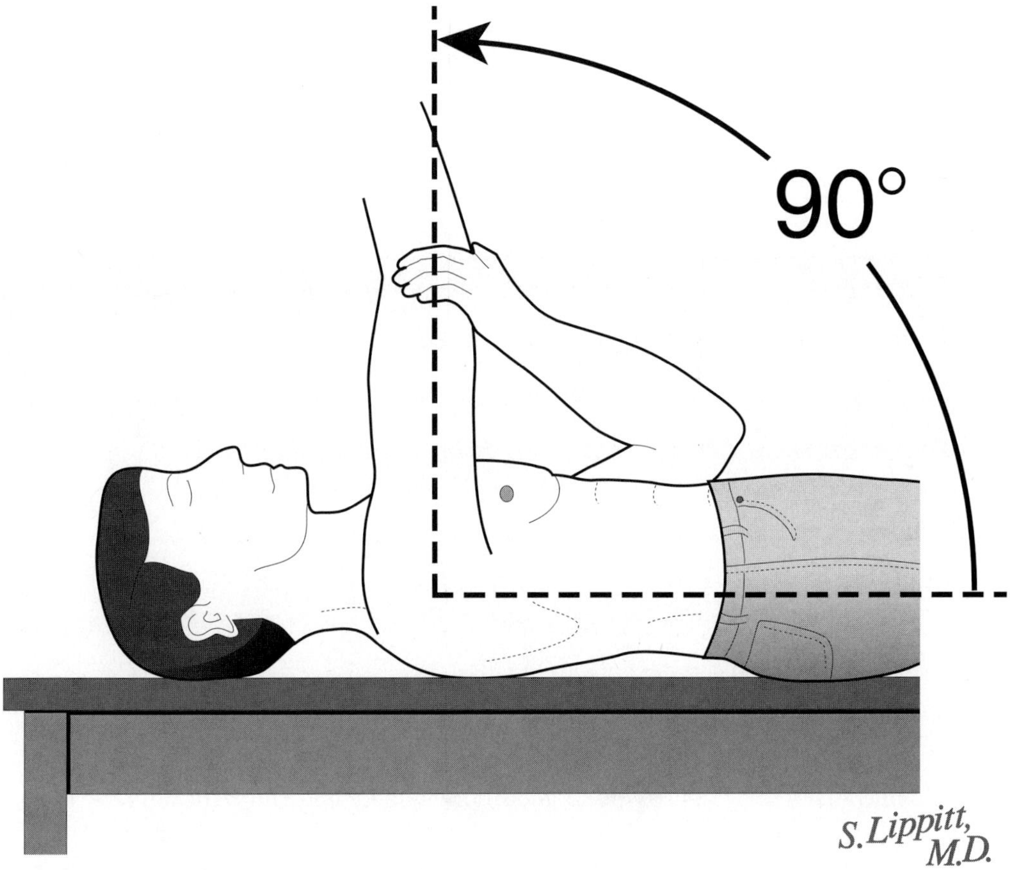


B

**Figure 16–9. Postoperative exercises—***Continued*
**B,** Forward elevation. Forward elevation is initiated to 90 degrees.

CHAPTER 17

# Procedure: Glenohumeral Arthrodesis Using Autogenous Iliac Crest Graft

***Diagnosis***

***Uncorrectable instability ICD9 CODE 718.31***

***Procedure***

***Glenohumeral arthrodesis with internal fixation and autogenous iliac crest graft CPT CODE 23802***

## INDICATIONS

The patient has severe glenohumeral instability, that cannot be managed by ordinary approaches.

Preoperative radiographs indicate good bone quality and sufficient humeral and glenoid bone stock to achieve arthrodesis without the use of a scapulohumeral plate.

The patient desires to proceed with the fusion, knowing in detail the alternatives as well as the substantial and permanent restriction of shoulder motion expected from a glenohumeral arthrodesis along with the risks of infection, fracture, neurovascular injury, pain, scapulothoracic discomfort, weakness, nonunion, hardware problems, the need for revision surgery, complications of iliac crest autograft harvest as well as anesthetic complications.

The patient recognizes that a shoulder fusion is disabling, that the range of humerothoracic motions will be severely limited, and that new demands will be placed on the scapulothoracic muscles and the scapulothoracic articulation, which may become painful. The patient understands that this procedure will not restore normal comfort and function to the shoulder. The patient understands the need for graft from the iliac crest and the possible need for a cane in the opposite hand after surgery. And, lastly, the patient understands his or her critical role in the postsurgical rehabilitation and that this rehabilitation period make take up to 1 year. The patient has not been smoking for one month prior to the procedure and will not smoke afterward.

## FINDINGS

The examination under anesthesia and surgical findings supports the diagnosis of major glenohumeral instability.

## DESCRIPTION OF PROCEDURE

The goal of the procedure is to achieve a solid arthrodesis by maximizing the contact between the humeral head and the glenoid and retaining the maximal nerve, muscle, and tendon integrity around the shoulder.

Under satisfactory anesthesia, the patient is placed in a low beach chair position. The entire forequarter is carefully prepped and draped in the usual sterile fashion with the arm free to be moved. The ipsilateral anterior iliac crest is also prepared and draped for the bone graft harvest.

The shoulder is approached through a low anterior deltopectoral incision in the axillary skin crease. The humeroscapular motion interface is cleared of hypertrophic bursa and scar. The subscapularis and subjacent capsule are incised near their insertion to the lesser tuberosity. The glenohumeral joint is exposed by gentle external rotation. The articular cartilage is removed from the entire humeral head and glenoid, preserving the convexity and concavity of the subchondral bone, respectively (**Figs. 17–1** and **17–2**). The center of the glenoid is curetted a bit more than its periphery to optimize the convex–concave fit of the humeral head to the glenoid.

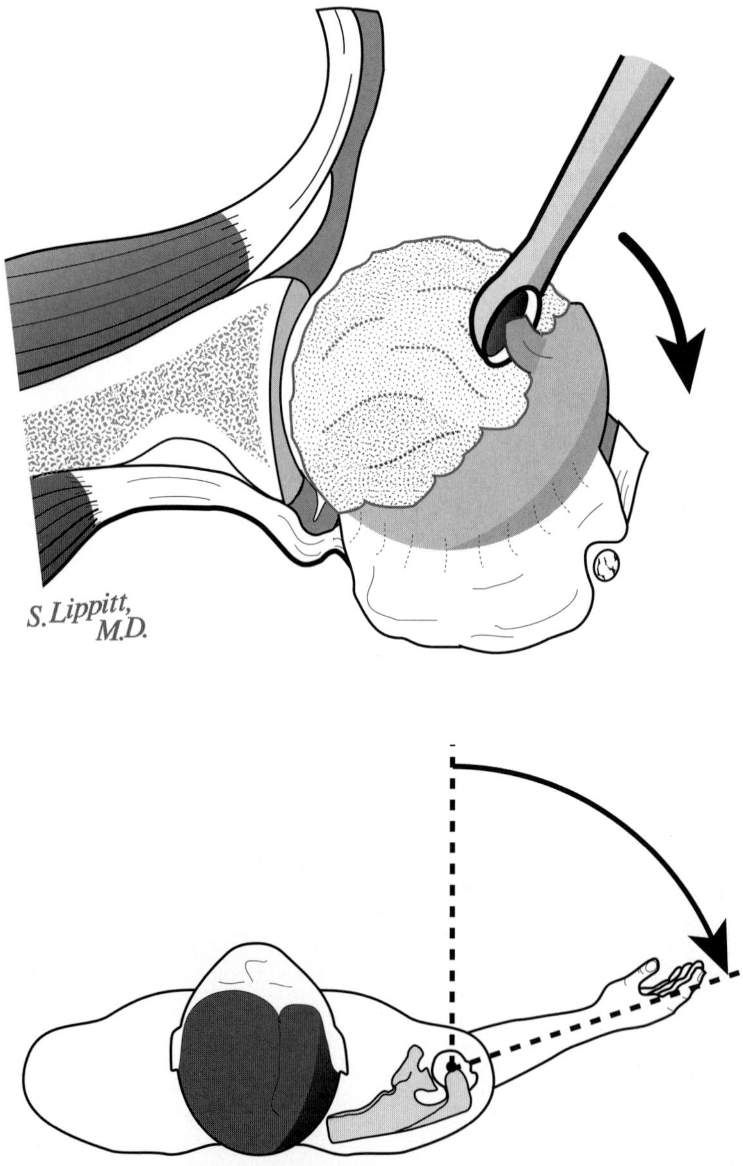


**Figure 17–1. Humeral head curettage**
The articular cartilage is removed from the head of the humerus without sacrificing subchondral bone. Access to the joint surface is achieved by external rotation.

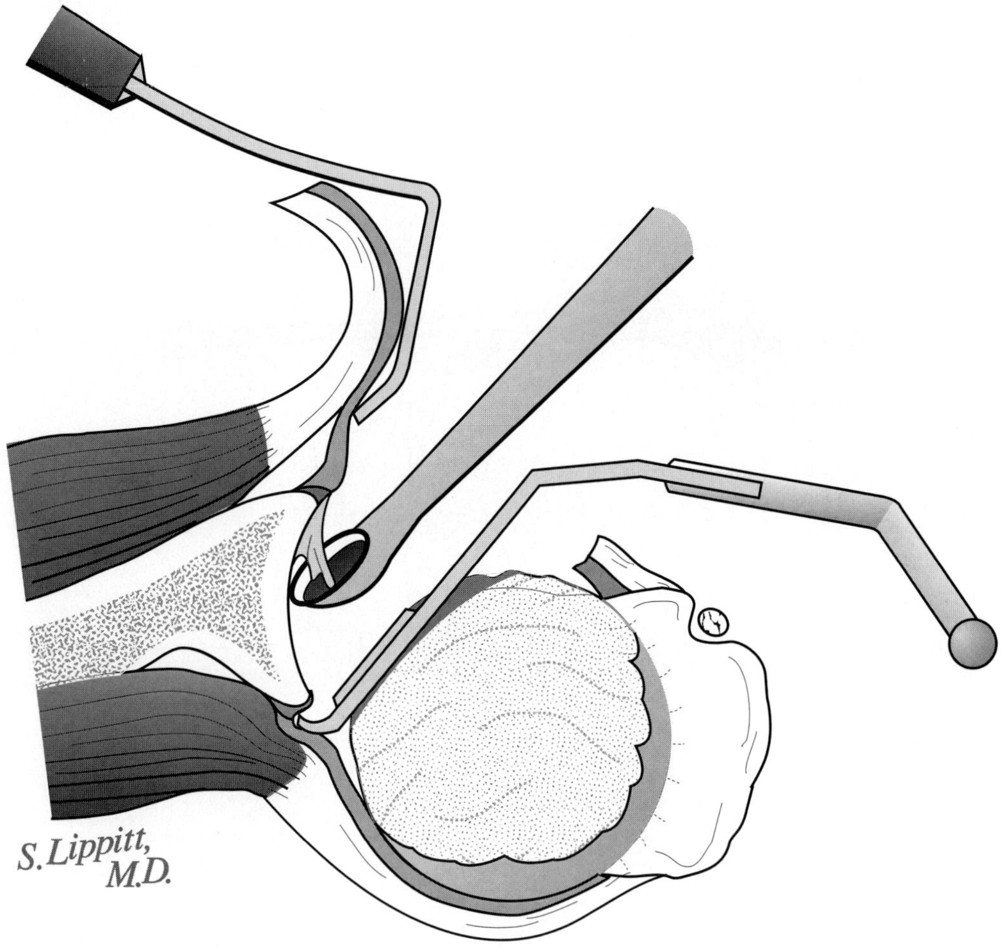


**Figure 17–2. Glenoid curettage**
The articular cartilage of the glenoid is removed with a curette without compromising its subchondral bone.

The undersurface of the acromion is dissected free of soft tissues and curetted down to raw bone **(Fig. 17–3)**.

The labrum and anterior capsule are dissected from the anterior aspect of the glenoid. An index finger is passed down the front of the glenoid neck to palpate the target for the humeroscapular screws **(Fig. 17–4)**.

The position of arthrodesis is selected as 0, 0, 60 (0 degrees of flexion and abduction and 60 degrees of internal rotation) **(Fig. 17–5)**. A folded towel is placed in the axilla to ensure that there will be "breathing space" between the medial humerus and the lateral chest wall. With the arm in this position, the hand should reach both the mouth and the anterior perineum. The supraspinatus tendon lying between the humeral head and the acromion is resected, leaving the remaining rotator cuff intact.

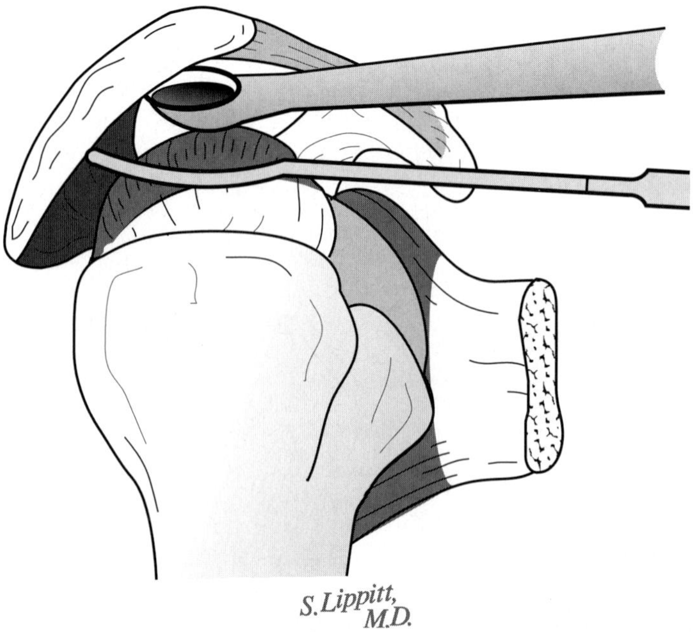


**Figure 17–3. Acromion curettage**
The periosteum of the undersurface of the acromion is curetted without compromising the cortical bone.

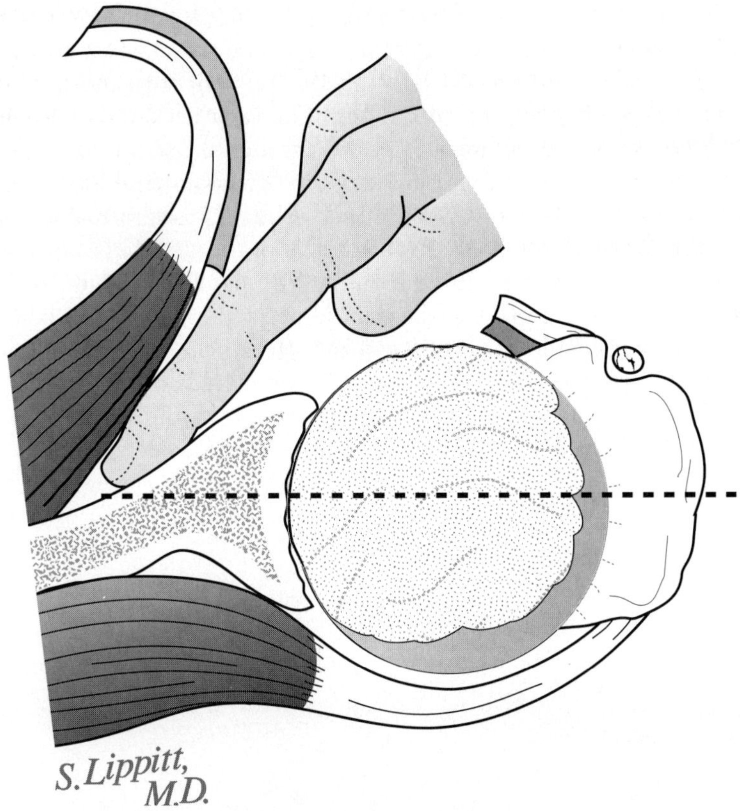


**Figure 17–4. Identifying the subscapularis fossa**
The anterior aspect of the glenoid neck is palpated. This area will be the target for the compression screws.

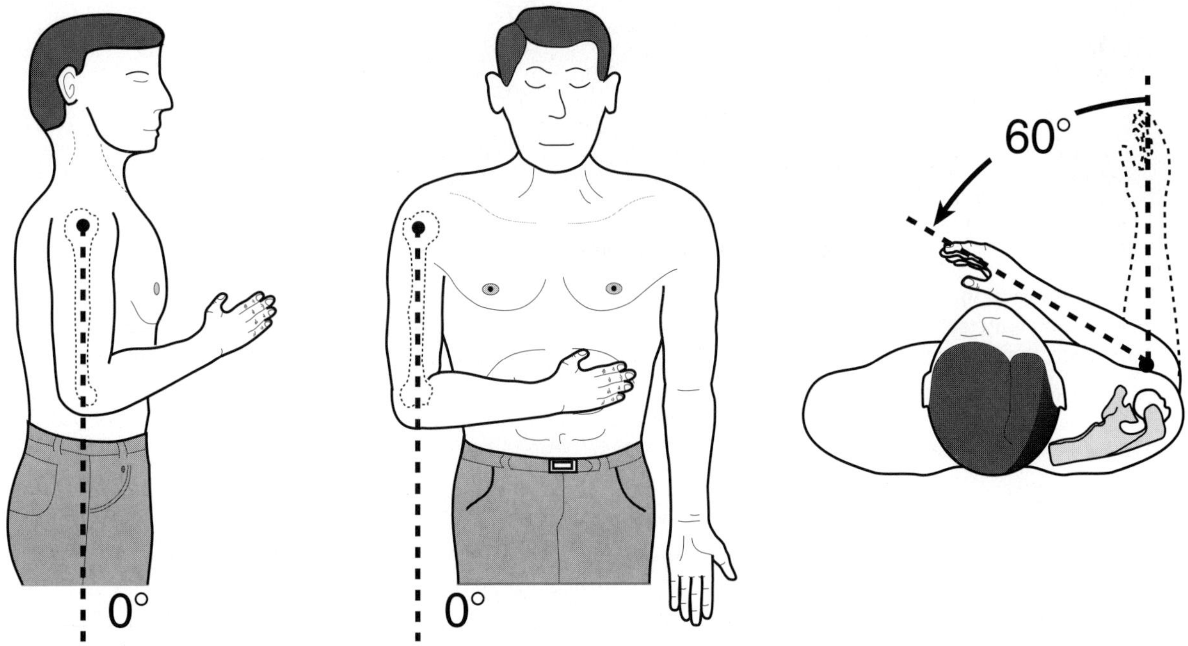


**Figure 17–5. Position of fusion**
For many patients, the most comfortable position of fusion is that of 0 degrees of flexion, 0 degrees of abduction, and 60 degrees of internal rotation. This position allows the scapula to sit in its normal position on the chest wall when the arm is at the side. (Modified from Matsen FA, Lippitt SB, Sidles JA, et al [eds]: Practical Evaluation and Management of the Shoulder. Philadelphia: WB Saunders, 1994, p. 149.)

The surgeon uses four 3.2 mm drills, ensuring before their use that they are all the same length. A stab incision is made over the mid-lateral aspect of the greater tuberosity. With the humeral head pressed into the glenoid concavity and the arm in the desired position, a guiding finger is placed on the anterior neck of the glenoid to indicate the drill target. One 3.2 mm drill is passed through the stab wound, through the deltoid, through the proximal humerus, across the glenohumeral joint, and into the glenoid so that it exits the anterior glenoid neck at least 25 mm medial to the anterior glenoid lip (**Fig. 17–6**). If this drill exits the middle of the glenoid neck, a second drill is passed parallel and 1 cm superior to it and a third parallel and 1 cm inferior to it. Each drill is left in place and all exit the glenoid neck anteriorly. If the first drill exits near the top of the glenoid, the second two are placed below it. If the first drill exits near the bottom of the glenoid, the second two are placed above it (**Fig. 17–7**). The position of the arm is again verified as being the desired position of fusion. The length of each of the first three drills in the humerus and glenoid is determined by subtraction using a fourth drill. Three fully threaded 6.5 mm cancellous screws (or, if the bone

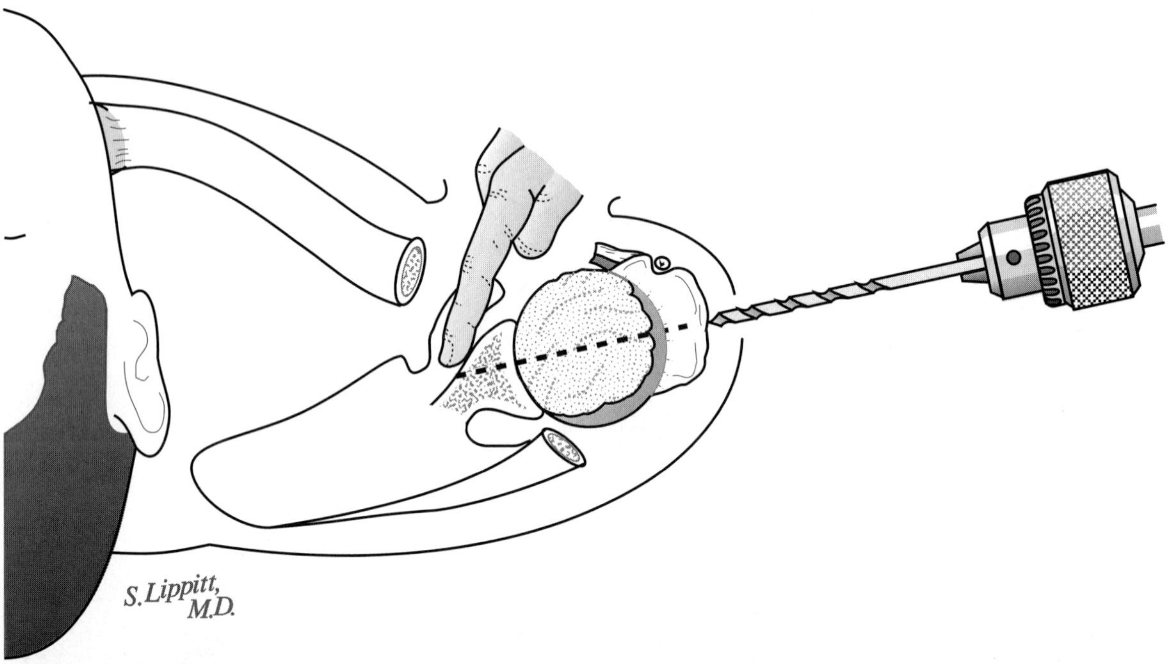


**Figure 17–6. Drilling**
While the humeral head is held reduced in the glenoid fossa and in the proper position, a drill bit is passed through a stab incision, through the deltoid, through the proximal humerus, through the glenoid, and out the neck anteriorly.

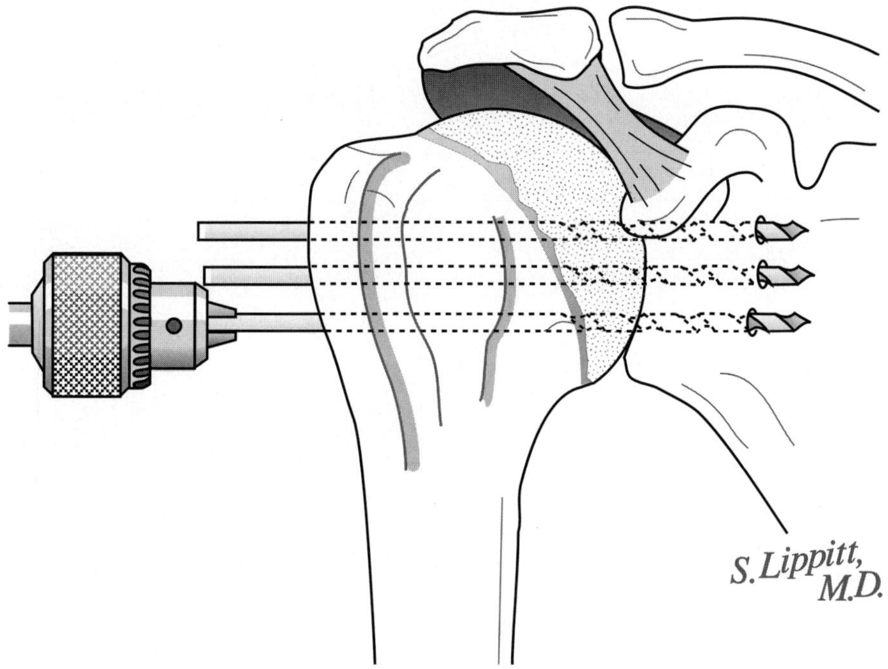


**Figure 17–7. Subsequent drill placement**
Two additional drills are placed parallel to the first, equally spaced across the glenohumeral joint. The position and orientation of the humerus in relation to the glenoid is again checked.

is of particularly good quality, 4.5 mm cortical screws) are selected of lengths 2 mm longer than the intraosseous lengths of the drills. Washers are placed on each of these screws. One by one, the drills are removed and replaced by the screw of the corresponding length (**Fig. 17–8**). Each screw is tightened, compressing the humeral head into the glenoid concavity. A finger along the anterior neck of the glenoid is used to ensure that the screw takes the correct path and is of the optimal length (**Fig. 17–9**). The screws function as lag screws (even though the hole in the humerus is not over-drilled) because the humeral bone is less dense than that of the glenoid.

The shape and size of the space between the upper aspect of the denuded humeral head and the denuded undersurface of the acromion is measured (**Fig. 17–10**).

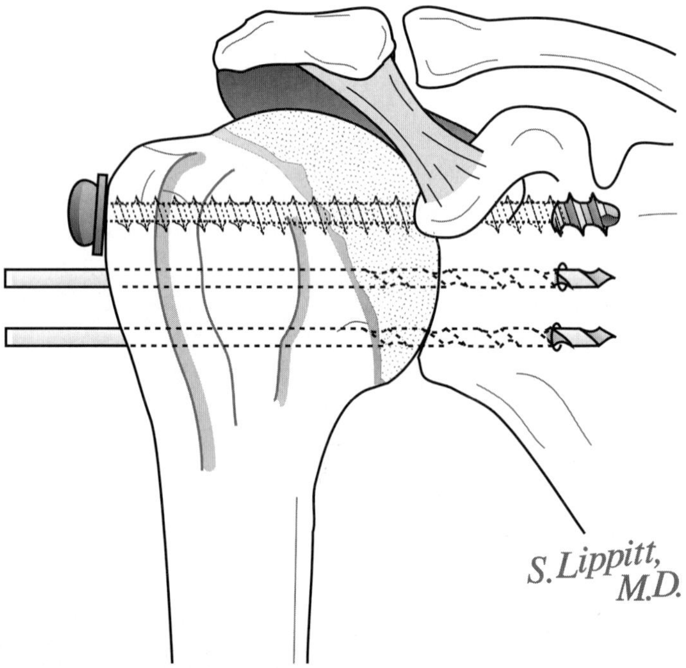


**Figure 17–8. Screw placement**
The drills are sequentially replaced with 6.0 mm fully threaded cancellous screws with washers.

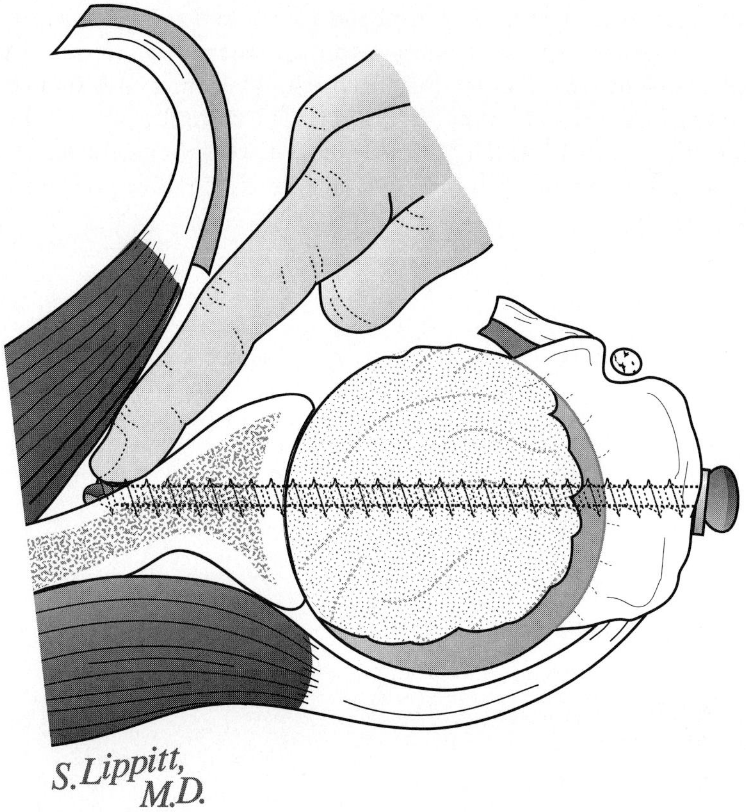


**Figure 17–9. Screw length**
Each screw should just penetrate the subscapularis fossa at the base of the glenoid neck.

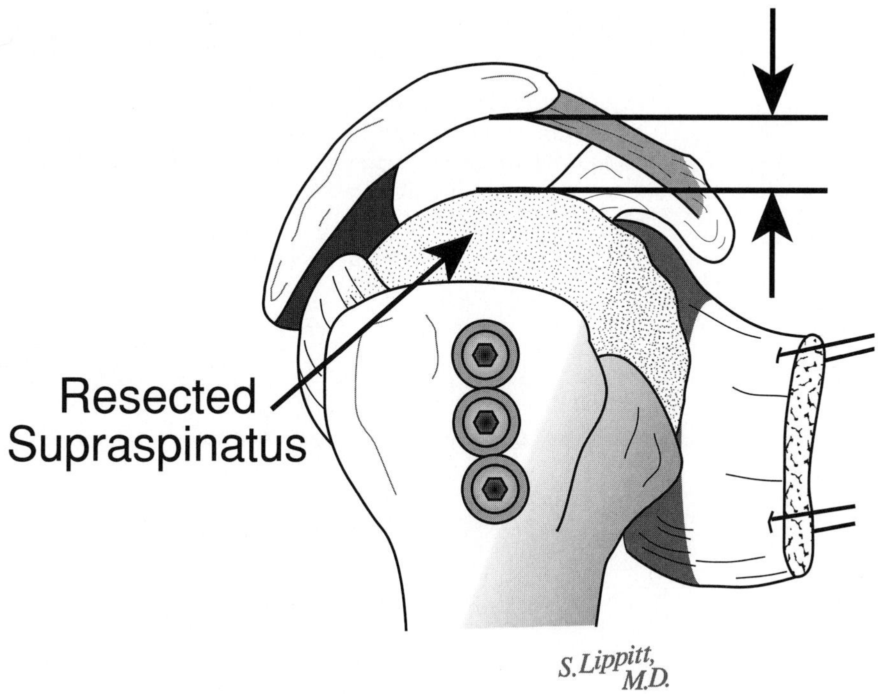


**Figure 17–10. Acromiohumeral distance**
After the supraspinatus tendon has been resected, the distance between the humeral head and the acromion is measured.

A structural graft is harvested from the iliac crest and shaped so that opposing cancellous surfaces fit precisely between the acromion and the humeral head in the area previously occupied by the supraspinatus tendon. This graft usually measures about 8 mm in thickness and is 2 cm wide and deep **(Fig. 17–11)**. The cortical surface of the graft is positioned anteriorly **(Fig. 17–12)**. A 3.2 mm drill is passed through a stab incision over the posterior acromion, through the graft, anterior to the three previously

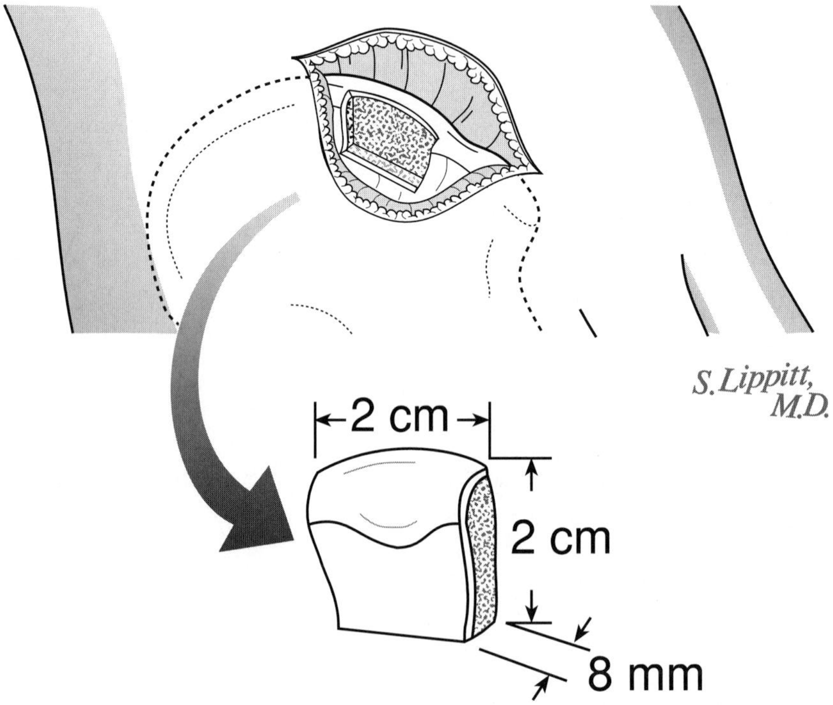


**Figure 17–11. Graft harvest**
A segment of graft measuring 20 × 20 × 8 mm is harvested from the iliac crest. (Churchill RS, Moskal MJ, Lippitt SB, Matsen FA: Extracapsular anatomically contoured anterior glenoid bone grafting for complex glenohumeral instability. Techn Shoulder Elbow Surg 2:215, 2001.)

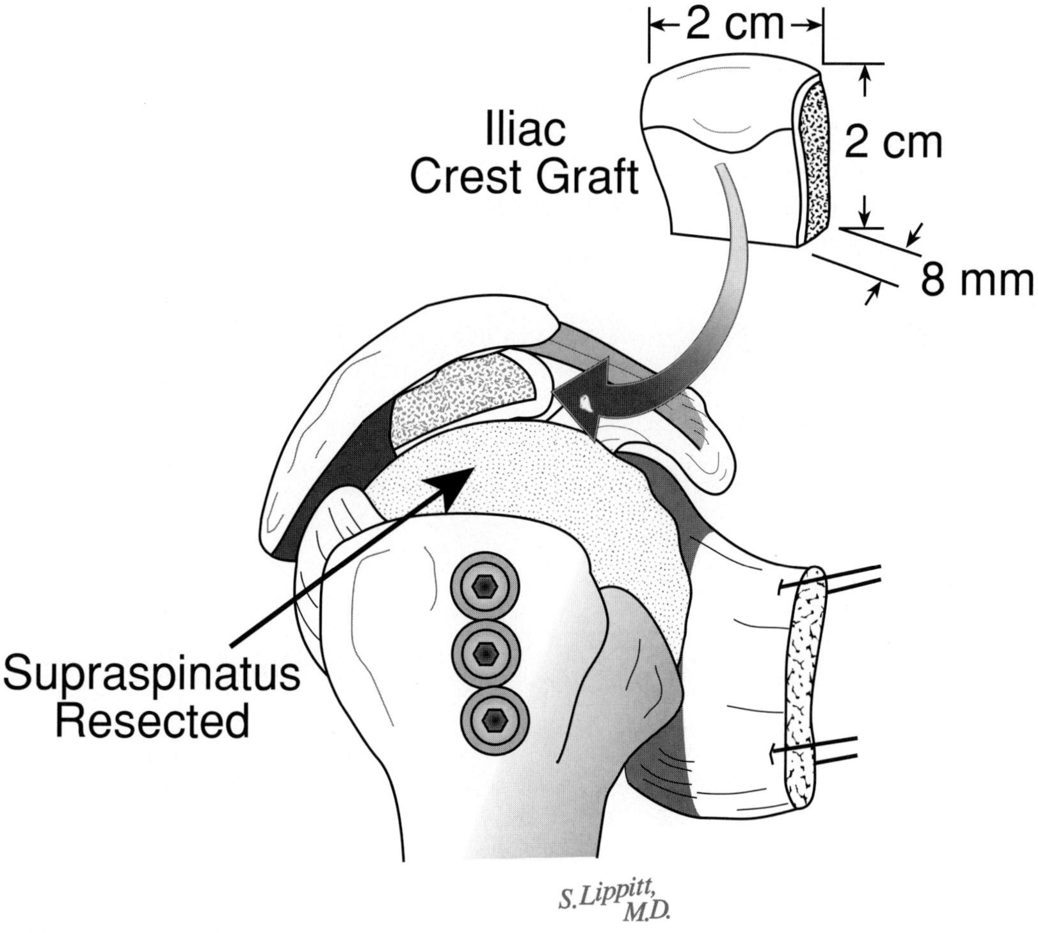


**Figure 17–12. Graft placement**
The graft is placed between the humeral head and the acromion in the area normally occupied by the supraspinatus tendon. This graft increases the quality of the fixation while helping to maintain the position of the humeral head in the glenoid concavity.

placed screws, and out the front of the humeral neck, where it can be palpated as it penetrates the bone. A fourth 6.5 mm fully threaded cancellous screw (or 4.5 mm cortical screw) is selected with a length just longer than the intraosseous aspect of this drill **(Fig. 17–13)**. The screw is passed through the stab incision, through the acromion, and out the anterior humerus where it can be easily palpated.

At this point, the heads and points of all four screws are in known positions. The position of the humerus on the scapula is secure.

The ability of the hand to be positioned at the mouth and at the anterior perineum is verified.

Radiographs are obtained of the anteroposterior scapular and axillary projections to verify the position and apposition of the humeral head and glenoid.

Additional cancellous iliac crest graft is morcelized and packed into the joint space so that it bridges the glenoid and the humerus **(Fig. 17–14)**.

The subscapularis is repaired to the tissues at the lesser tuberosity.

The wound is irrigated and closed in layers.

An abdominal pad is placed in the axilla to avoid maceration.

Dry sterile dressings are applied to both incisions.

The arm is placed in a sling, and the patient is returned to the recovery room in satisfactory condition.

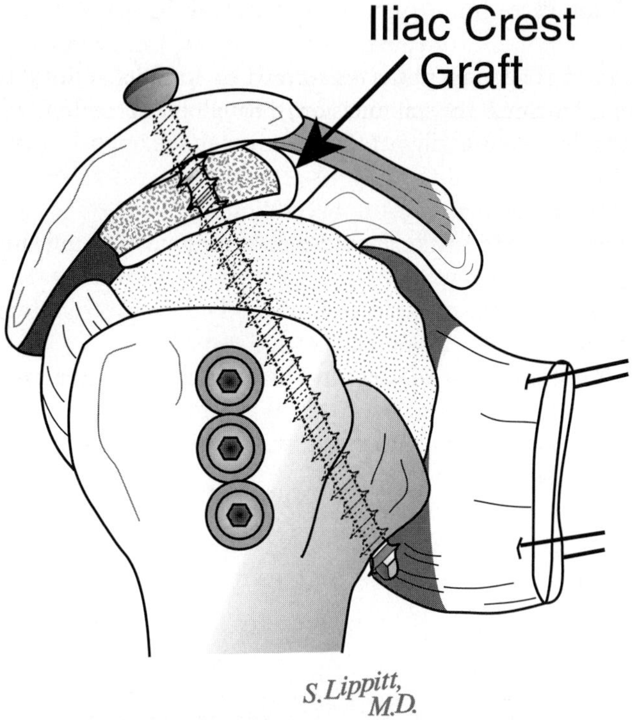


**Figure 17–13. Graft fixation**
A fourth screw is passed through the acromion, through the graft, and out the firm bone at the humeral neck.

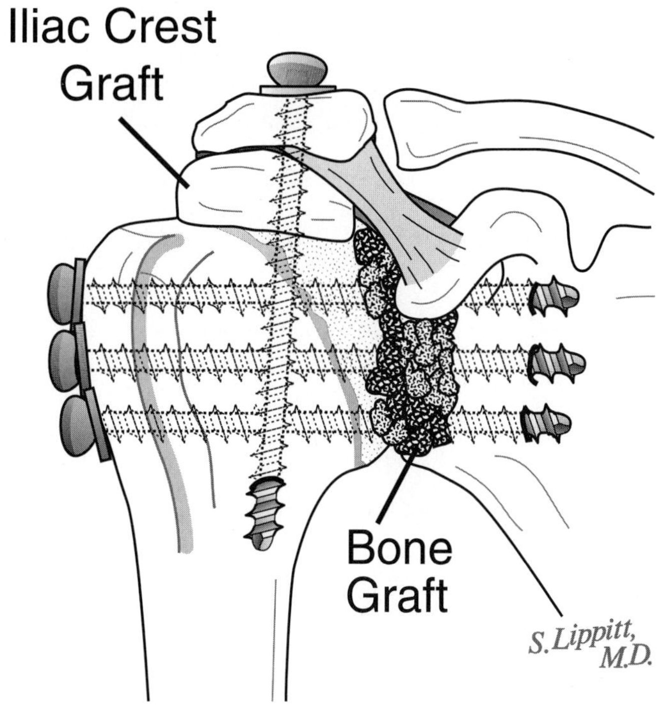


**Figure 17–14. Cancellous grafting**
Cancellous bone graft is added across the area of glenohumeral arthrodesis.

## POSTOPERATIVE PLAN

The patient will keep the arm in a sling for 6 weeks, using the arm for hand-to-mouth activities only, avoiding lifting anything greater than 1 pound. Rotation of the arm away from the body will be avoided. A cane will be offered for use in the opposite hand during ambulation as needed.

An axillary pad will be kept in place to avoid skin maceration.

Radiographs are repeated at 2 months. If the shoulder appears solid clinically and radiographically at this time, additional gentle activities involving flexion and extension of the elbow, but no shoulder rotation, are added slowly and progressively as long as they are comfortable.

Radiographs are repeated at 4 months. If the shoulder is solid clinically and radiographically at this time, other activities are added slowly as comfort permits. Gentle scapulothoracic mobility and strengthening exercises are started at this point. Activities are added progressively as tolerated.

# PART IV

# STRENGTH

CHAPTER 18

# Principles of Glenohumeral Strength

## CONCEPTS

When a muscle contracts, it approximates its effective origin and insertion with a force limited by its physiologic cross-sectional area. Muscles that have large cross-sections, such as the deltoid, can provide a larger maximal force than a muscle with a small cross-section, such as the subclavius. The contractile elements within a muscle are connected to tendon fibers that connect to the bony origin and insertion. The tendon insertion is structured so that there is a smooth mechanical transition from flexible tendon to stiff bone (**Fig. 18–1**). This smooth transition enables the insertion to manage the repeated bending loads to which it is subject (**Fig. 18–2**). When the tissues providing this smooth transition degenerate, they become stiff and weak, so that the tendon insertion becomes increasingly vulnerable to failure (**Fig. 18–3**).

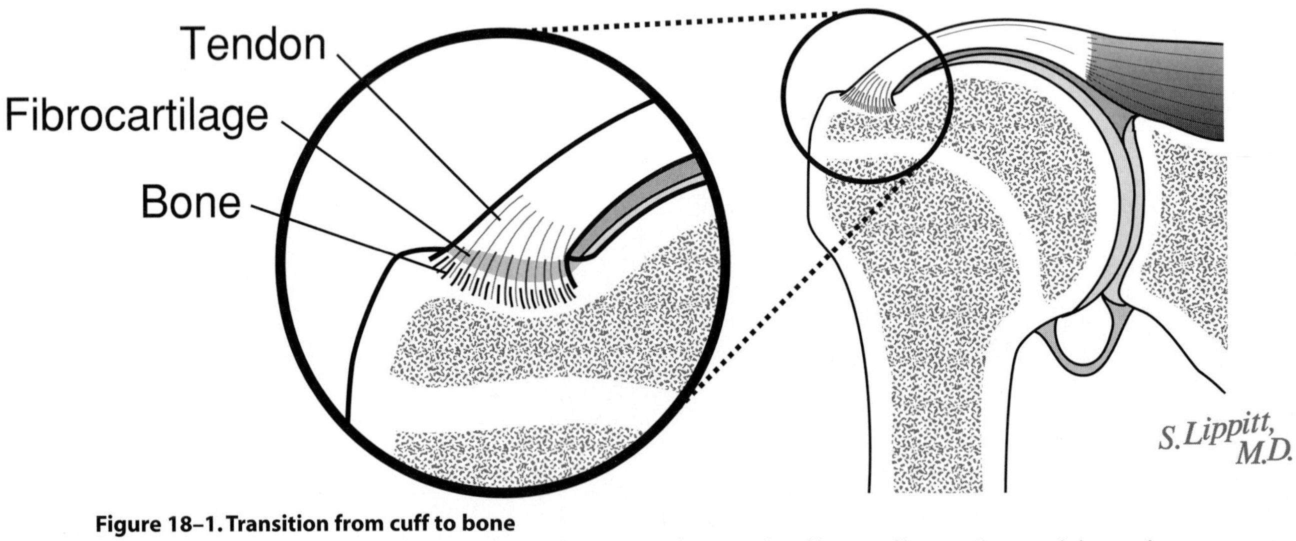


**Figure 18–1. Transition from cuff to bone**
The normal tendon insertion to bone is a smooth transition from tendon fibers to fibrocartilage and then to bone.

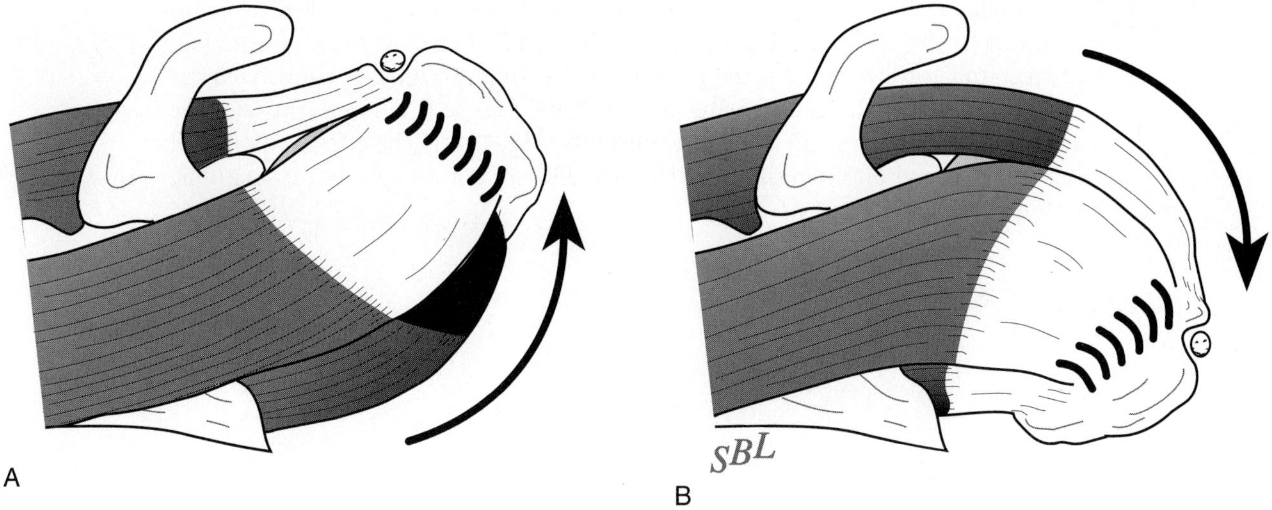


**Figure 18–2. Bending loads**
The cuff insertion is subjected to continuous bending loads that, if it were not supple, would fatigue it as a paper clip fatigues when it is bent back and forth. (Modified from Matsen FA, Lippitt SB, Sidles JA, et al [eds]: Practical Evaluation and Management of the Shoulder. Philadelphia: WB Saunders, 1994, p. 116.)

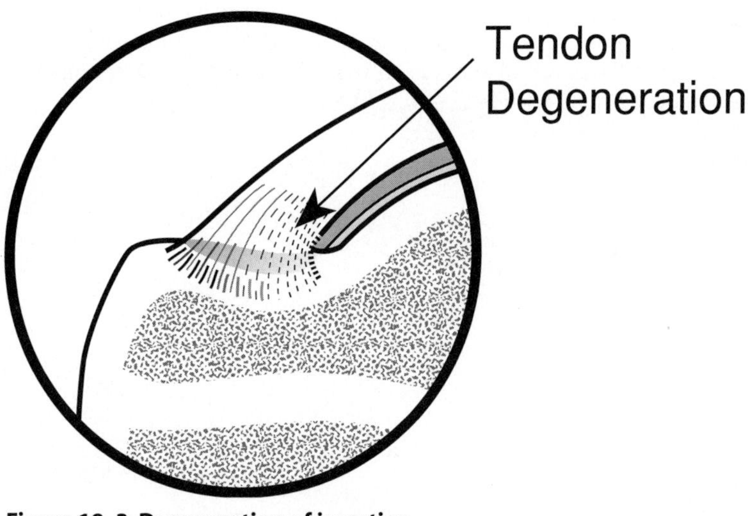


**Figure 18–3. Degeneration of insertion**
Degeneration of the cuff insertion results in its becoming stiff, weak, and subject to progressive failure. This process usually begins on the deep surface of the tendon insertion to bone.

The strength of a muscle is noted in terms of the torque it can generate. We recall that torque results when a force is exerted at a distance from a fixed center of rotation. The magnitude of the torque is the product of the length of the line connecting the center of rotation to the effective attachment of the muscle (the lever arm) and the magnitude of the force perpendicular to this line **(Fig. 18–4)**. The effective points of attachment depend on the position of the arm and are not necessarily the anatomic insertions **(Fig. 18–5)**.

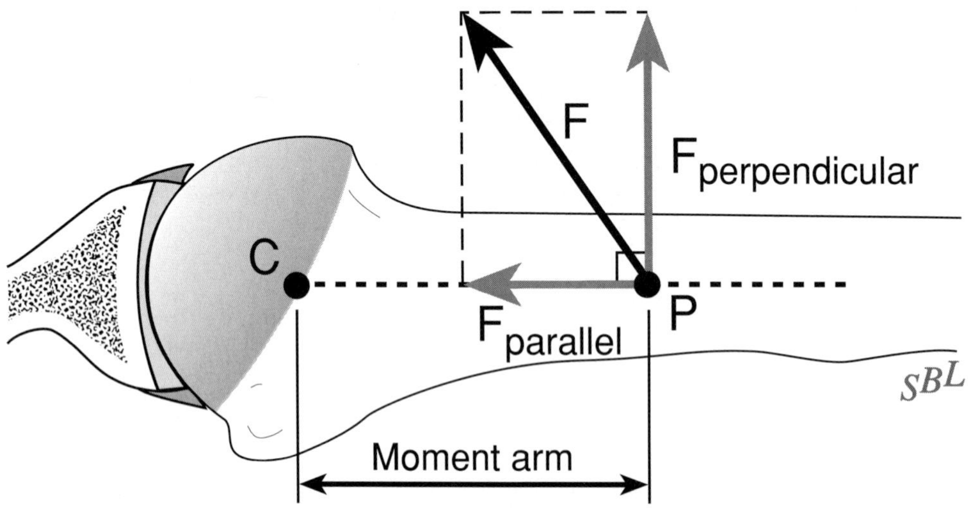


**Figure 18–4. Torque**
The magnitude of the torque resulting from a muscle force is the product of the moment or lever arm (the length of the line connecting the center of rotation to the effective attachment of the muscle, C to P) and the magnitude of the force perpendicular to this line (F perpendicular). (Modified from Matsen FA, Lippitt SB, Sidles JA, et al [eds]: Practical Evaluation and Management of the Shoulder. Philadelphia: WB Saunders, 1994, p. 112.)

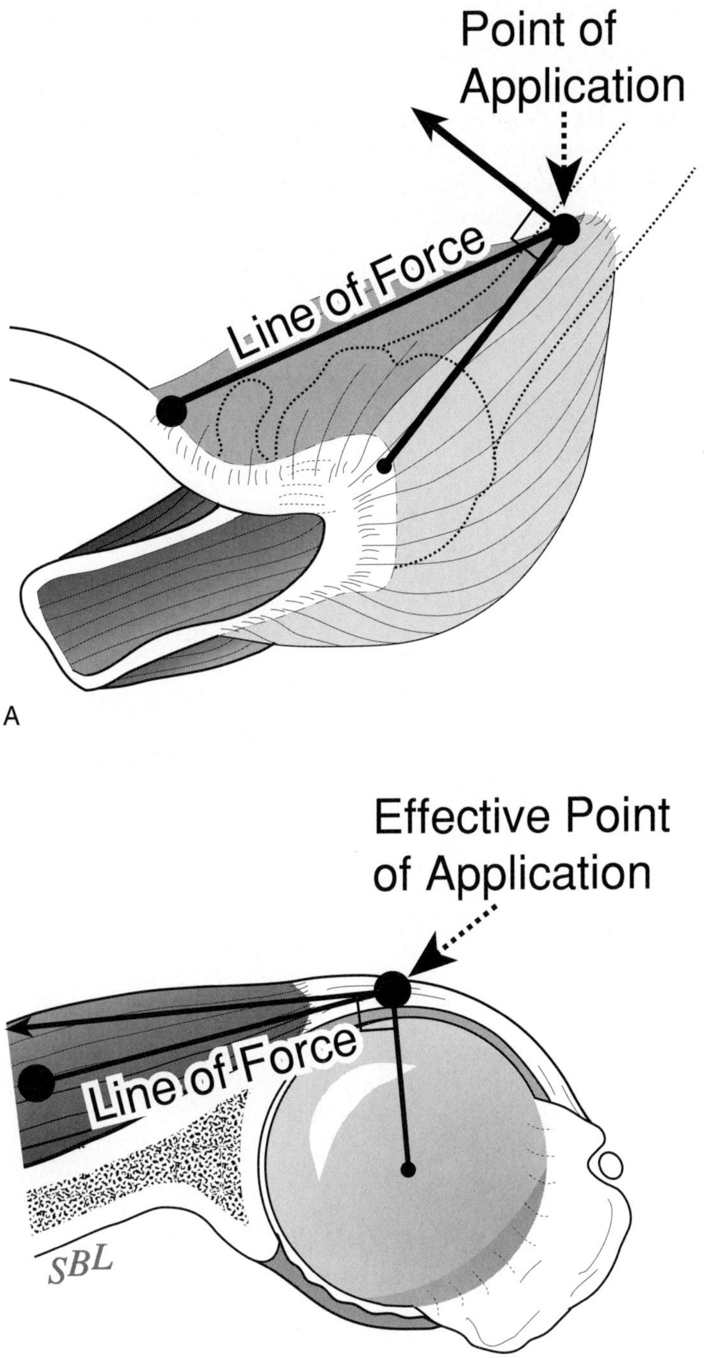


A

B

**Figure 18–5. Effective point of application of muscle force**

The torque the muscle exerts is the product of the length of the line from the center of rotation to the effective point of application of the force multiplied by the component of the muscle force vector perpendicular to this line. As shown for the deltoid muscle (**A**), the part of the muscle force vector contributing to adduction torque is only the component of the vector perpendicular to the moment arm.

The effective point of application of a muscle force is not necessarily its anatomic insertion (**B**). (Modified from Matsen FA, Lippitt SB, Sidles JA, et al [eds]: Practical Evaluation and Management of the Shoulder. Philadelphia: WB Saunders, 1994, p. 113.)

The weight of a dumbbell that can be held with the arm out to the side is determined by the net upward torque divided by the lever arm of the weight to be lifted **(Fig. 18–6)**.

Throughout this discussion, the lever arms have been described as the distance between the point of action of the muscle force and the center of rotation. For torques to be realized, the humerus must rotate around a stable center. This is why we have placed such emphasis on the mechanisms for centering of the head in the section on Stability (Part III). Without this precise centering, the effectiveness of the muscle contractions would be lost.

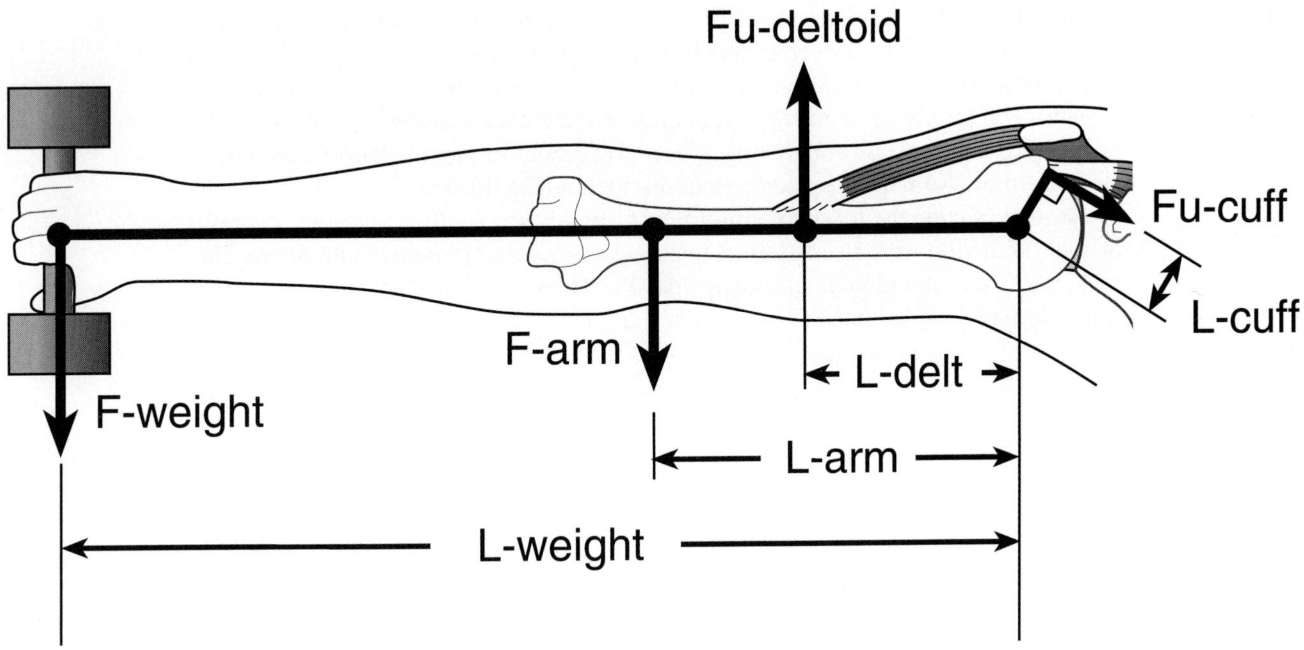


**Figure 18–6. Torque diagram**
The weight that can be lifted by the extended arm can be determined from the forces and lever arms in a free-body diagram. In this example, it is equal to (a) the product of the length of the cuff lever arm (L-cuff = the distance from the effective cuff insertion to the center of rotation of the head) and the maximal upward rotating force that can be exerted by the rotator cuff perpendicular to this lever arm (Fu-cuff) plus (b) the product of the length of the deltoid lever arm (L-deltoid = the distance from the effective deltoid insertion to the center of rotation of the head) and the maximal upward rotating force that can be exerted by the deltoid perpendicular to this lever arm (Fu-deltoid) minus (c) the product of the distance from the center of rotation of the head to the center of arm mass (L-arm) and the downward rotating gravitational force on the arm perpendicular to this lever arm (F-arm), all divided by the lever arm of the weight (L-weight = the distance from the weight to the center of rotation of the head).

$$\text{Weight that can be lifted (F-weight)} = (\text{Fu-cuff} \times \text{L-cuff} + \text{Fu-deltoid} \times \text{L-deltoid} - \text{F-arm} \times \text{L-arm})/\text{L-weight}.$$

Muscles are also characterized by their excursion: the change in length over which they can provide force. To be effective throughout a range of motion, the centimeters of excursion of a muscle must match the product of the muscle's lever arm in centimeters and the range of motion in degrees divided by the number of degrees in a radian (**Fig. 18–7**). So, although longer lever arms result in more torque per unit muscle force, they also require greater muscle excursion (**Fig. 18–8**).

Muscles provide the maximal amount of force when operating close to the middle of their excursion with a drop-off in maximal force as the muscle length approaches maximal extension or maximal contraction (**Fig. 18–9**). Muscles that have been chronically detached, as in long-standing cuff tears, tend to lose their excursion. Even if they are reattached, the length over which they can exert an effective force is often diminished.

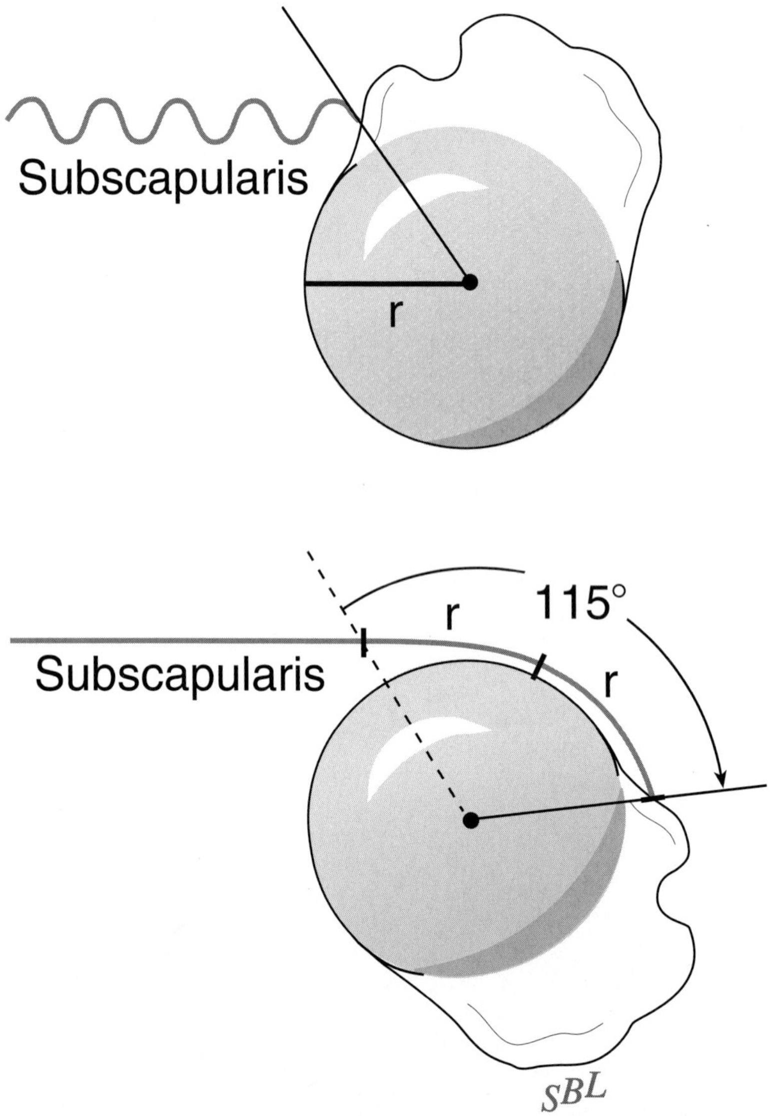


**Figure 18–7. Subscapularis excursion**
To power the shoulder through a range of motion, the excursion of a muscle must equal the product of the effective lever arm (in the case of the subscapularis, the radius of the humeral head, r) times the rotational range of motion in the direction of action of the muscle divided by the number of degrees in a radian (57.3). Thus, if we wish the subscapularis to power the shoulder through a 115-degree arc of rotation acting through a lever arm equal to the radius of the humeral head (say 25 mm), its excursion would need to be 25 mm × 115 degrees/57.3 degrees, or 50 mm.

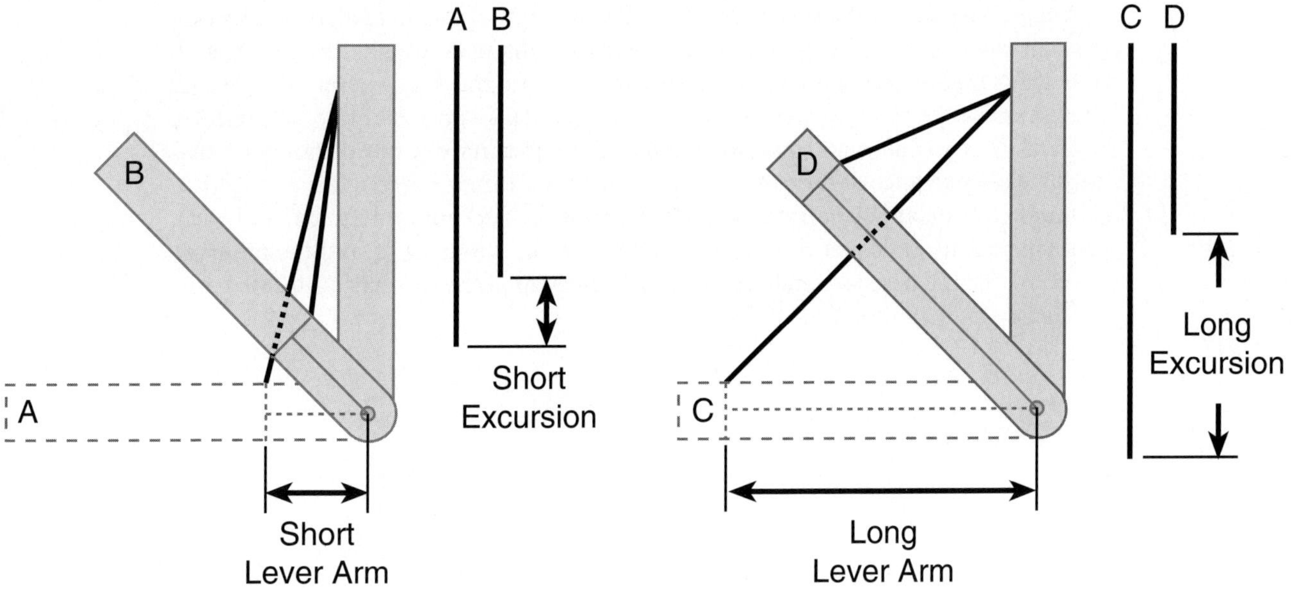


**Figure 18–8. Lever arm and excursion**
Muscles acting through longer lever arms (right figure) generate more torque per unit force (torque = force × lever arm), but require greater excursion for a given arc of motion (see difference between dark lines representing muscle length in extension and flexion) than muscles acting through shorter lever arms, which require less excursion but which result in less torque (left figure).

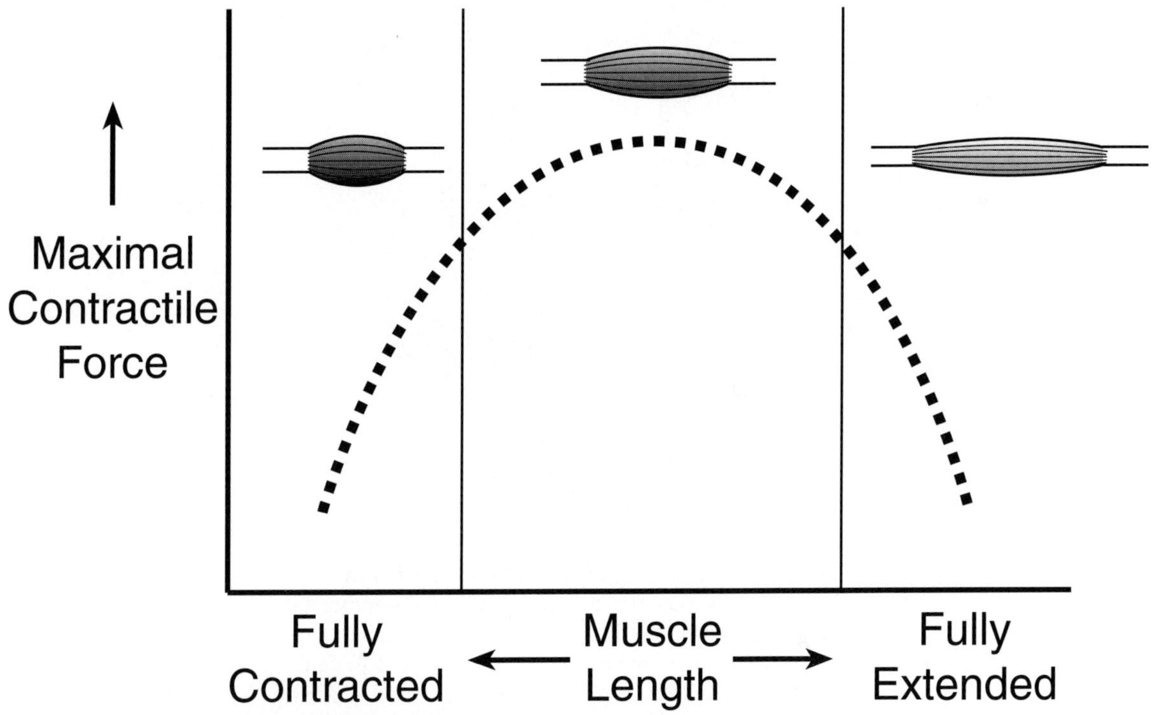


**Figure 18–9. Muscle length and force**
A typical relationship between a muscle's length and the maximal force that it can produce. Note that the maximal force is less at the extremes of the range of motion.

A special feature of the shoulder is that the powerful thoracoscapular muscles can position the entire glenohumeral joint along with the deltoid and the rotator cuff through a range of approximately 40 degrees of adduction/abduction (**Fig. 18–10**) and 40 degrees of protraction/retraction (**Fig. 18–11**). This "portability" of the glenohumeral joint enables the scapulohumeral muscles to carry out most shoulder functions in the mid-range of their excursion, where they are the strongest. It is of note that the humeroscapular position is essentially the same for the knockout punch, the bench press, the point of racquet contact with the ball in the tennis serve, and the moment of release for the baseball pitch, even though the scapulothoracic positions are quite different.

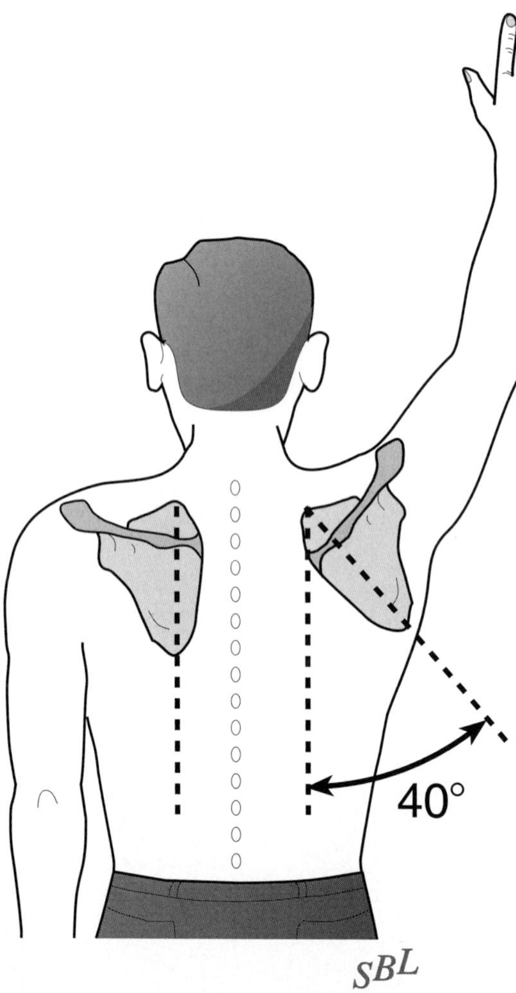


**Figure 18–10. Scapular adduction and abduction**
The range of motion through which the scapulohumeral muscles (i.e., the deltoid and the rotator cuff) can exert their power is enhanced by the fact that the scapula can be moved on the chest wall by powerful thoracoscapular muscles. The 40 degrees of scapular abduction enables the scapulohumeral muscles of the elevated arm to function near the middle of their excursions, where they are most powerful.

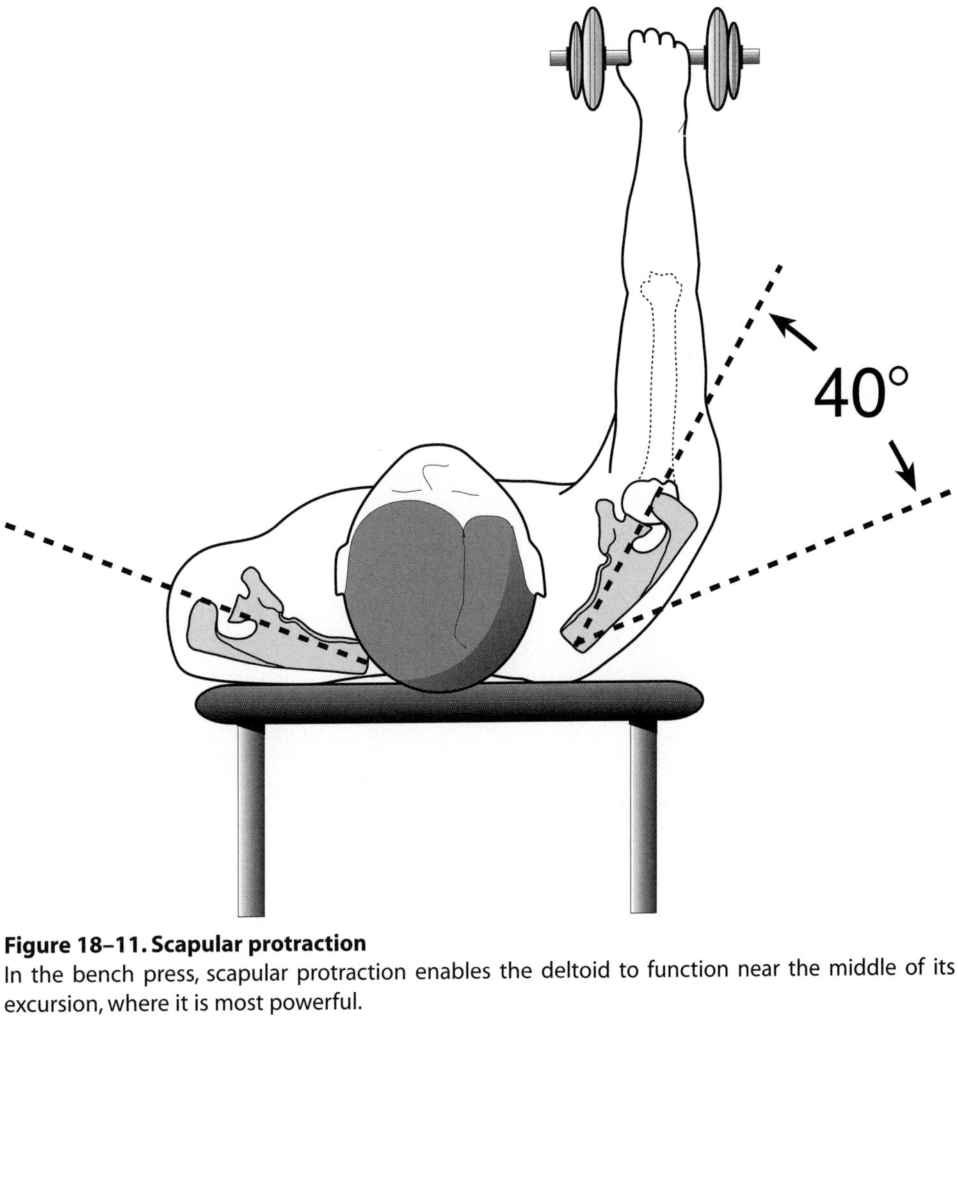


**Figure 18–11. Scapular protraction**
In the bench press, scapular protraction enables the deltoid to function near the middle of its excursion, where it is most powerful.

One of the relatively unexplored facets of active shoulder strength is the requirement for muscular balance. In the knee, the muscles generate torques about a relatively fixed axis: that of flexion-extension. If the quadriceps pull is a bit off-center, the knee still extends. In the shoulder, no such fixed axis exists. In a specified position, each muscle creates a unique set of rotational moments. Imagine a rope attached to a sphere. The motion resulting from pulling on the rope depends on the orientation of the sphere as well as the direction of pull on the rope. If some of the resulting motion were undesired, it would need to be cancelled out by attaching another rope and pulling on it to resist the unwanted motion. So, for example, the anterior deltoid exerts moments in forward elevation, internal rotation, and cross-body movement (**Fig. 18–12**). If elevation without cross-body movement is desired, the posterior deltoid must negate the cross-body moment of the anterior deltoid (**Fig. 18–13**). Similarly, if elevation without rotation is desired, the cross-body and internal rotation moments of this muscle must be resisted by other muscles (such as the posterior deltoid and infraspinatus). These balancing activities take place at an additional energy cost.

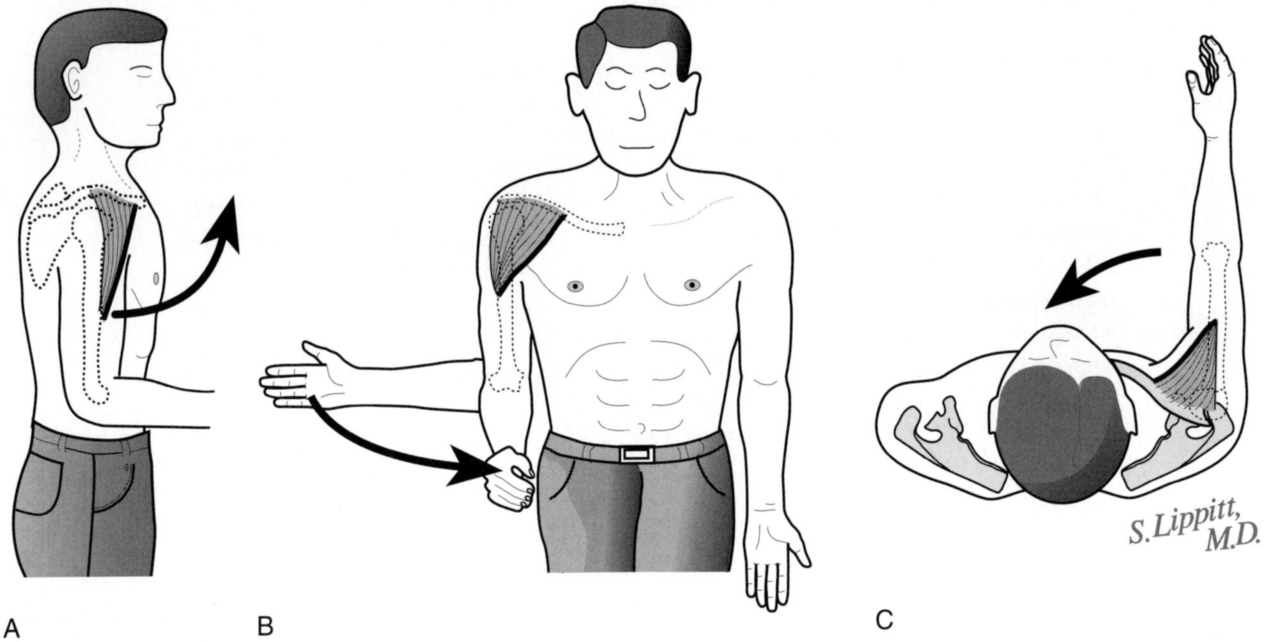


**Figure 18–12. Deltoid moment**
The anterior deltoid generates moments in forward elevation (**A**), internal rotation (**B**), and cross-body movement (**C**). (Modified from Matsen FA, Lippitt SB, Sidles JA, et al [eds]: Practical Evaluation and Management of the Shoulder. Philadelphia: WB Saunders, 1994, p. 115.)

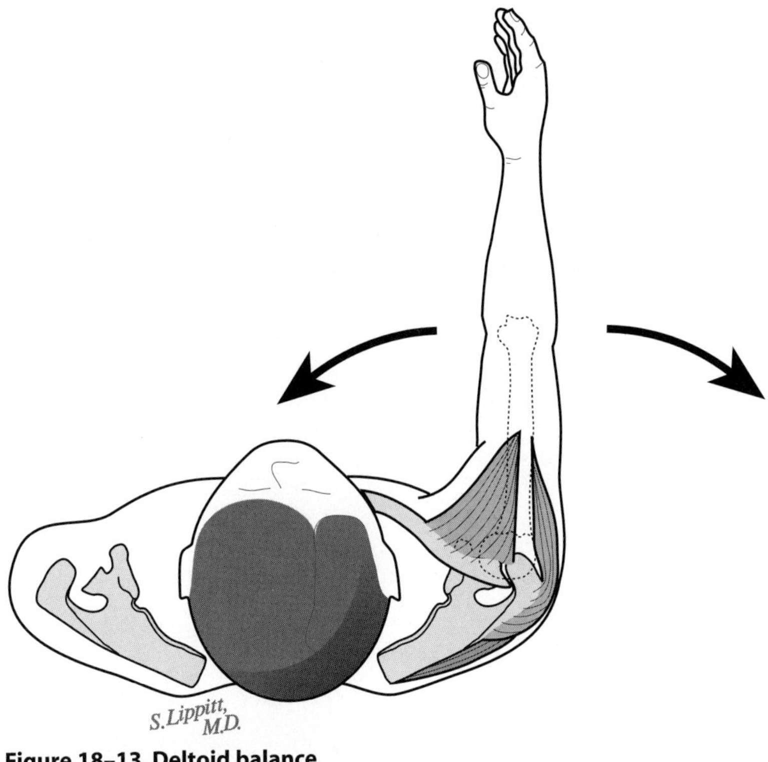


**Figure 18–13. Deltoid balance**
Pure elevation requires that the internal rotation and cross-body moments of the anterior deltoid be opposed by other muscle action. For example, even though it is an antagonist to the anterior deltoid, the posterior deltoid must contract during elevation to resist the cross-body moment of the anterior deltoid. (From Matsen FA, Lippitt SB, Sidles JA, et al [eds]: Practical Evaluation and Management of the Shoulder. Philadelphia: WB Saunders, 1994, p. 115.)

# CLINICAL CONSIDERATIONS

## Clinical Conditions Relating to Shoulder Strength

### *Neurogenic and Muscular Causes*

The most devastating injury to a muscle is the loss of its nerve supply. Losses of the innervation of the deltoid, supraspinatus, and infraspinatus can be congenital (Erb's palsy), inflammatory (brachial neuritis), degenerative (cervical radiculopathy), traumatic (penetrating or stretch), compressive (a ganglion in the spinoglenoid notch), or iatrogenic (dissection or screw placement). These conditions, along with myopathies such as facioscapular muscular dystrophy, must be considered when the shoulder is weak.

The day this paragraph was written, we saw a patient sent in for a cuff repair. He had been in a water-skiing accident and landed on the water in a way that pressed his head to the left and his right shoulder down. At the moment of impact, he experienced a shock down his right arm and noted severe weakness of his right shoulder. His physician sent him for a magnetic resonance imaging (MRI) scan that showed a partial tear of his supraspinatus. On examination in our office, he had, 6 weeks after injury, atrophy and weakness of his spinati, deltoid, and biceps—a classic Erb's type injury.

Electromyography, nerve conduction velocities, and muscle biopsies may be needed to sort out these diagnoses.

### *Loss of the Humeral Fulcrum*

If the humeral head does not remain centered during muscle contraction, the forces intended to cause rotation will cause translation. An example is the shoulder with posterior instability: when forward elevation is attempted, the humeral head slips out the back. In this situation, valuable muscle excursion is consumed by displacement of the head, and the strength of elevation is lost. The effects of loss of centering are also seen with the cuff- and superior labral–deficient shoulder in which contraction of the deltoid produces ascension of the humeral head rather than abduction **(Fig. 18–14)**. However, if the glenoid concavity remains intact (**Fig. 18–15**), the humeral head may remain stabilized in the glenoid in spite of superior cuff deficiency.

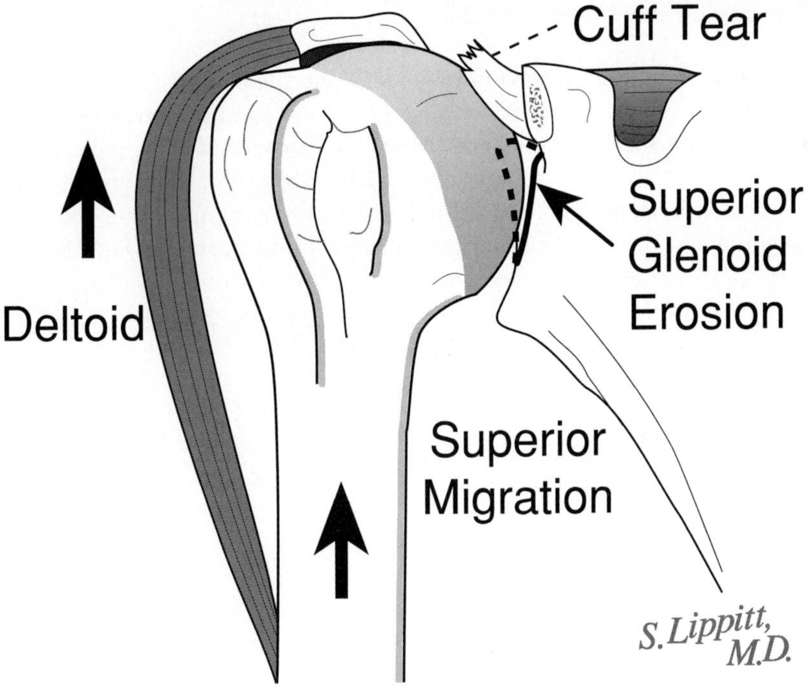


**Figure 18–14. Loss of centering**
The combination of loss of the rotator cuff and loss of the superior glenoid concavity allows the destabilized humeral head to move upward, rather than to abduct on contraction of the deltoid. (Modified from Matsen FA, Lippitt SB, Sidles JA, et al [eds]: Practical Evaluation and Management of the Shoulder. Philadelphia: WB Saunders, 1994, p. 71.)

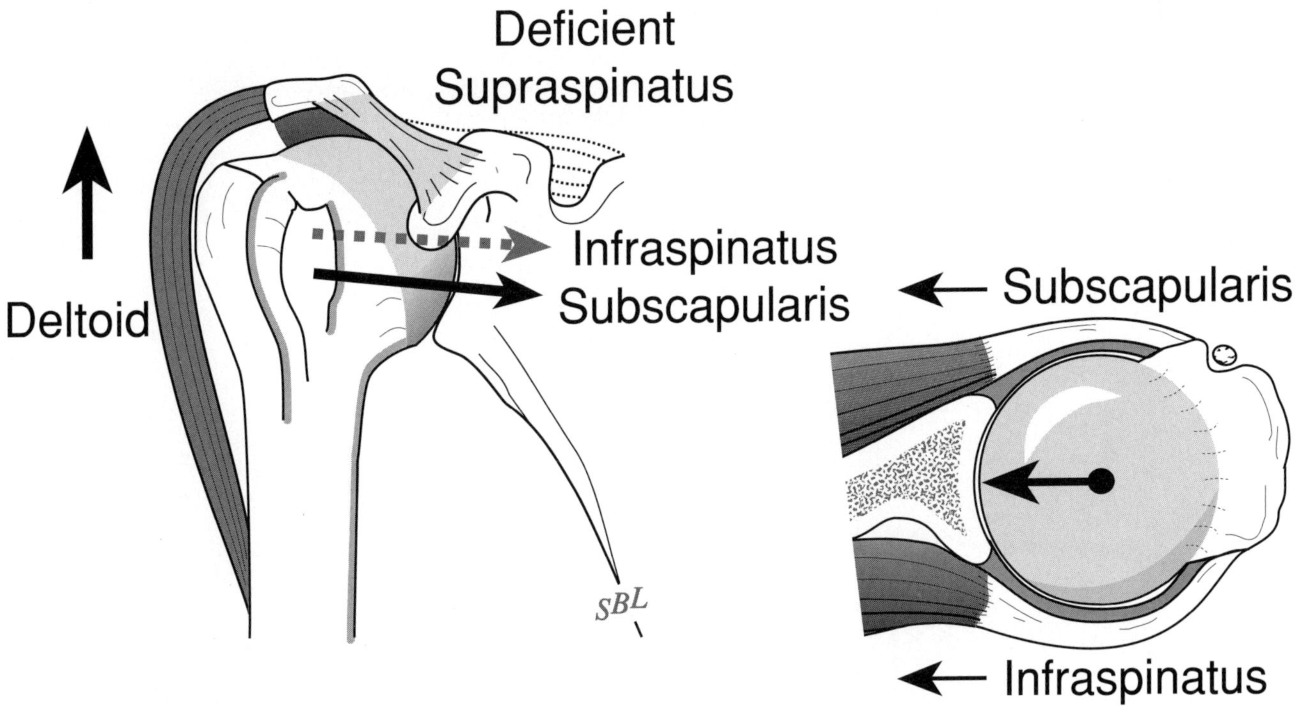


**Figure 18–15. Intact glenoid cavity**
If the glenoid concavity is intact, the compressive action of the subscapularis and infraspinatus may stabilize the humeral head in the center of the glenoid socket against the upward pull of the deltoid. (Modified from Matsen FA, Lippitt SB, Sidles JA, et al [eds]: Practical Evaluation and Management of the Shoulder. Philadelphia: WB Saunders, 1994, p. 71.)

If the coracoacromial arch remains intact, the humeral head of the cuff-deficient shoulder may be secondarily stabilized in a new position, superiorly displaced against the arch (**Fig. 18–16**). Thus, in the presence of cuff deficiency, it is vitally important to protect and maintain the coracoacromial arch. Without it, the humeral head will escape anterosuperiorly when the deltoid contracts—a complication that can result from acromioplasty and resection of the coracoacromial ligament (**Fig. 18–17**).

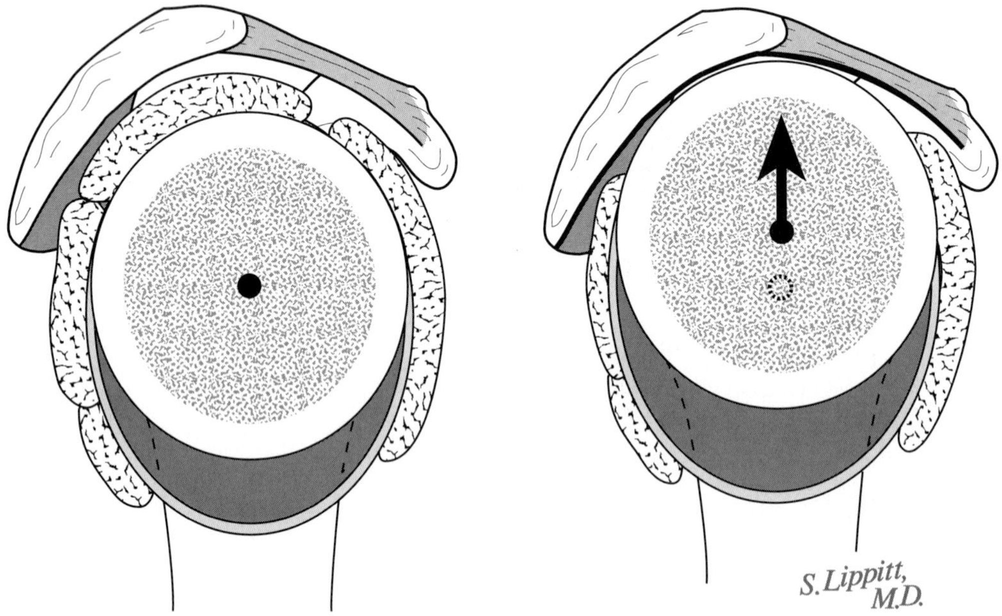


A B

**Figure 18–16. Intact coracoacromial arch**

If the coracoacromial arch remains intact (i.e., not damaged by acromioplasty or coracoacromial arch section), the humeral head may be secondarily stabilized by the arch against the upward pull of the deltoid.

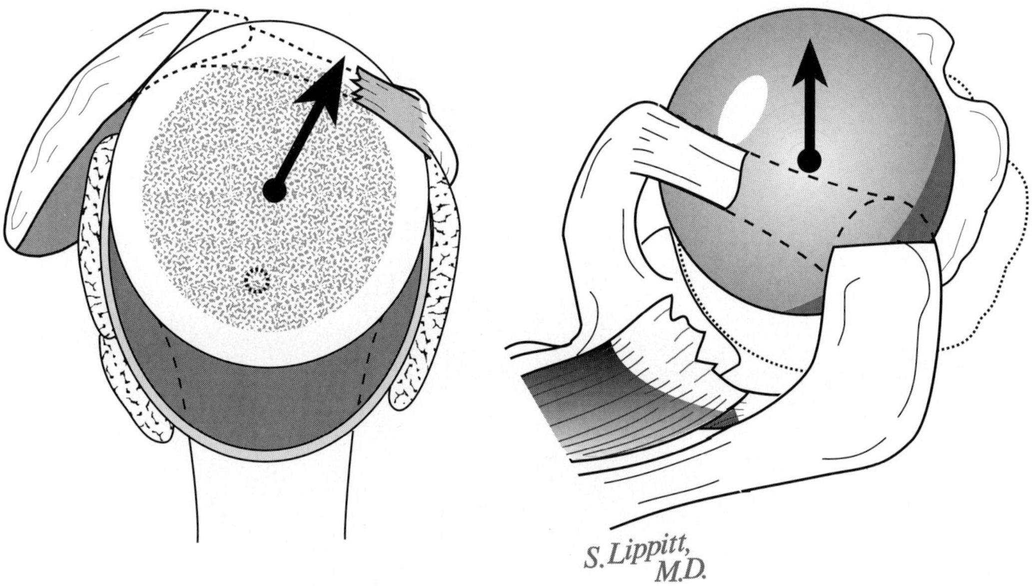


**Figure 18–17. Escape of the humeral head**
Resection of the coracoacromial ligament and anterior acromioplasty may allow the humeral head of the cuff-deficient shoulder to escape anterosuperiorly.

### *Loss of Muscle Attachment to Bone*

The bony connections of the deltoid muscle are rarely damaged, except by surgery. However, the fact that the deltoid muscle originates directly from the clavicle and acromion without much of a tendon makes this muscle attachment difficult to restore once it has been compromised. Resection of the anterior undersurface of the acromion removes part of the bony origin of the deltoid (**Fig. 18–18**). Taking down the anterior deltoid for surgical exposure risks failure of the surgical reinsertion because there is no tendon to suture back to the bone. For these reasons, we advocate the "deltoid-on" approach to the rotator cuff (**Fig. 18–19**).

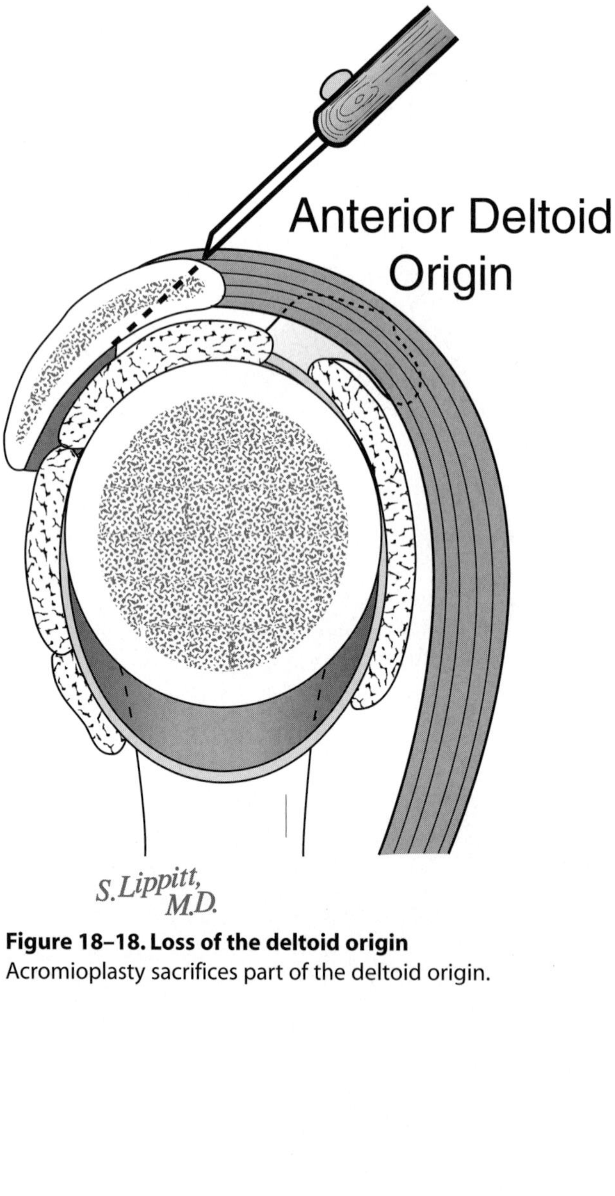


**Figure 18–18. Loss of the deltoid origin**
Acromioplasty sacrifices part of the deltoid origin.

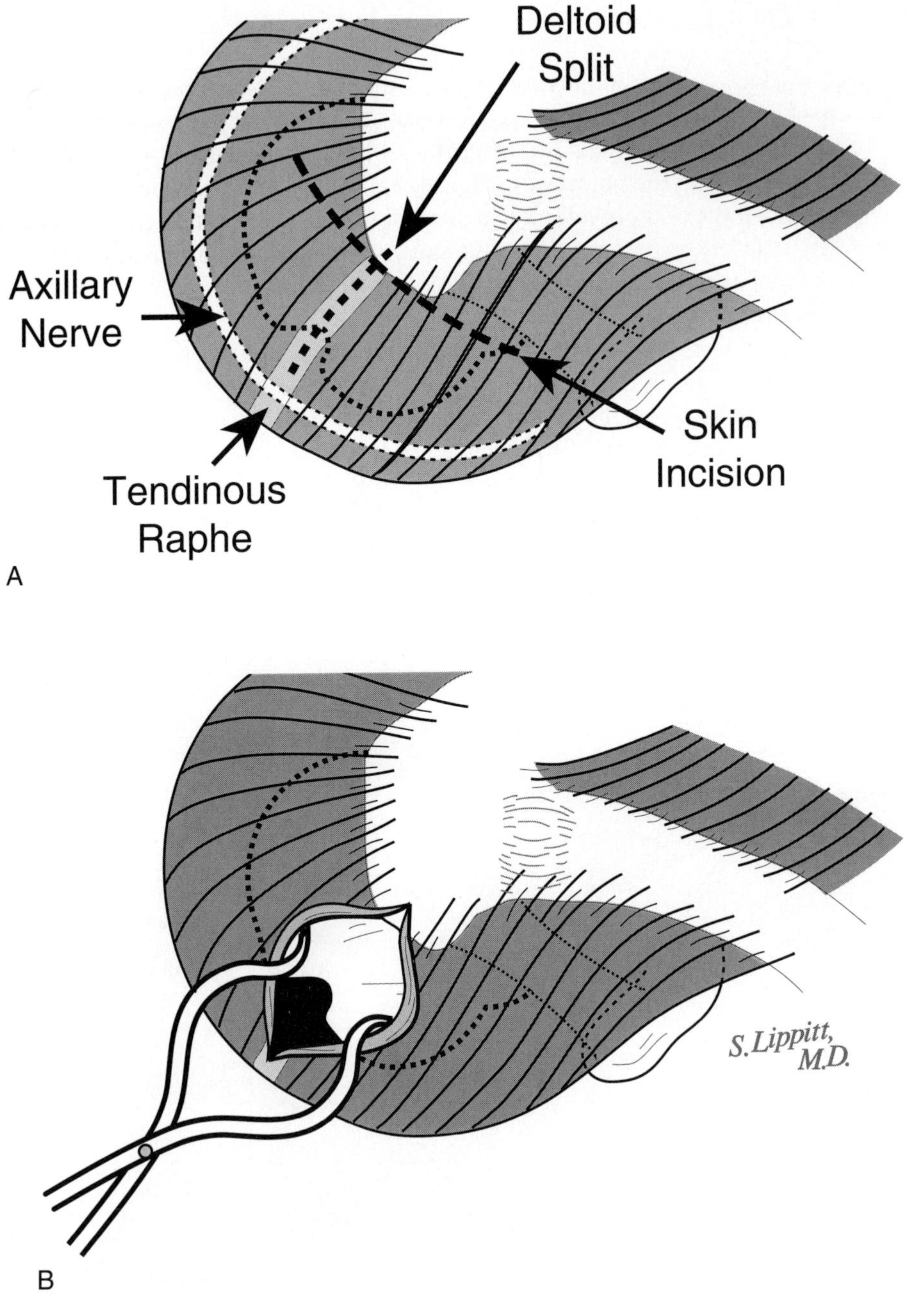


**Figure 18–19. Deltoid split**
The deltoid-on approach to the rotator cuff includes a cosmetic skin incision in Langer's lines and a deltoid split in the tendinous raphe between the anterior and lateral thirds of the deltoid. This approach preserves all the deltoid origin, avoiding the risk of failure of a repair. (Modified from Matsen FA, Lippitt SB, Sidles JA, et al [eds]: Practical Evaluation and Management of the Shoulder. Philadelphia: WB Saunders, 1994, p. 135.)

### *Patterns of Tearing*

In partial-thickness cuff tears, loss of some of the tendon fibers reduces the ability of the attached muscle fibers to deliver force to the bone. This disruption typically starts on the deep surface of the cuff (**Fig. 18–20**) but may also occur within the tendon (**Fig. 18–21**) or on the bursal side (**Fig. 18–22**). Partial tears may be accompanied by avulsion of a piece of the greater tuberosity (**Fig. 18–23**). A thinned tendon contains fewer fibers than one of normal thickness; thus, a muscle with a thinned tendon has lost the optimal attachment of its contractile elements, and increasing load is placed on the remaining fibers (**Fig. 18–24**).

Partial tendon tears can also prevent effective use of the muscle by producing pain on muscle contraction. In this respect, a partial-thickness cuff tear resembles a tennis elbow, a condition in which the extensor carpi radialis brevis is partially torn from the latter epicondyle. Contraction of the muscle produces pain at the tendon attachment to bone. This condition is also similar to partial thickness tears at the insertion of the Achilles and patellar tendons. While these conditions are often thought to be inflammatory ("tendonitis"), the problem is actually mechanical.

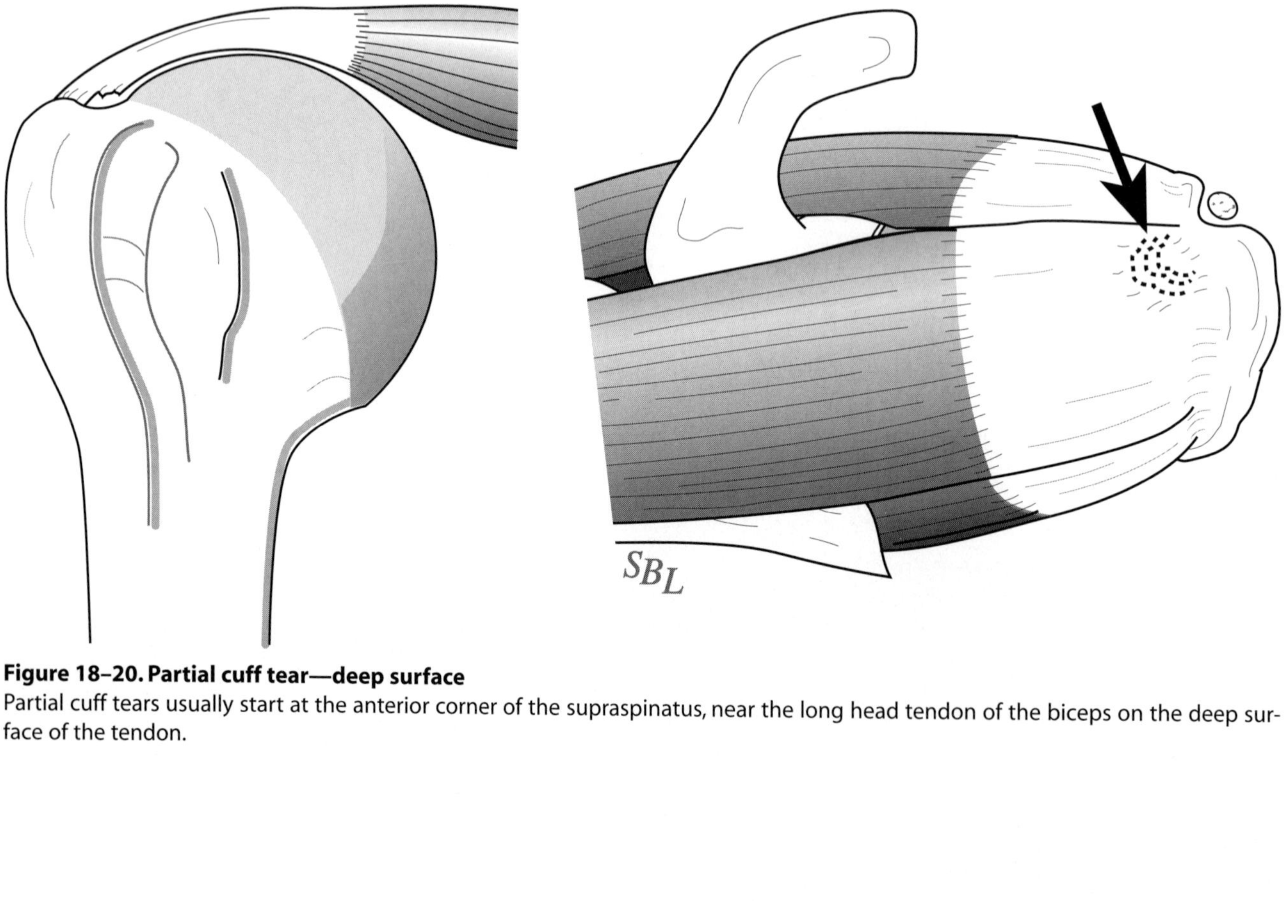


**Figure 18–20. Partial cuff tear—deep surface**
Partial cuff tears usually start at the anterior corner of the supraspinatus, near the long head tendon of the biceps on the deep surface of the tendon.

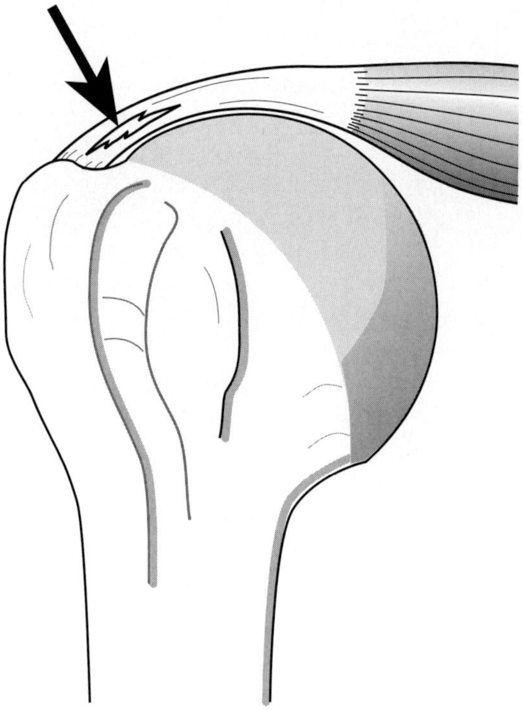

**Figure 18–21. Partial-thickness tear—intratendinous**
An intrasubstance partial-thickness cuff tear.

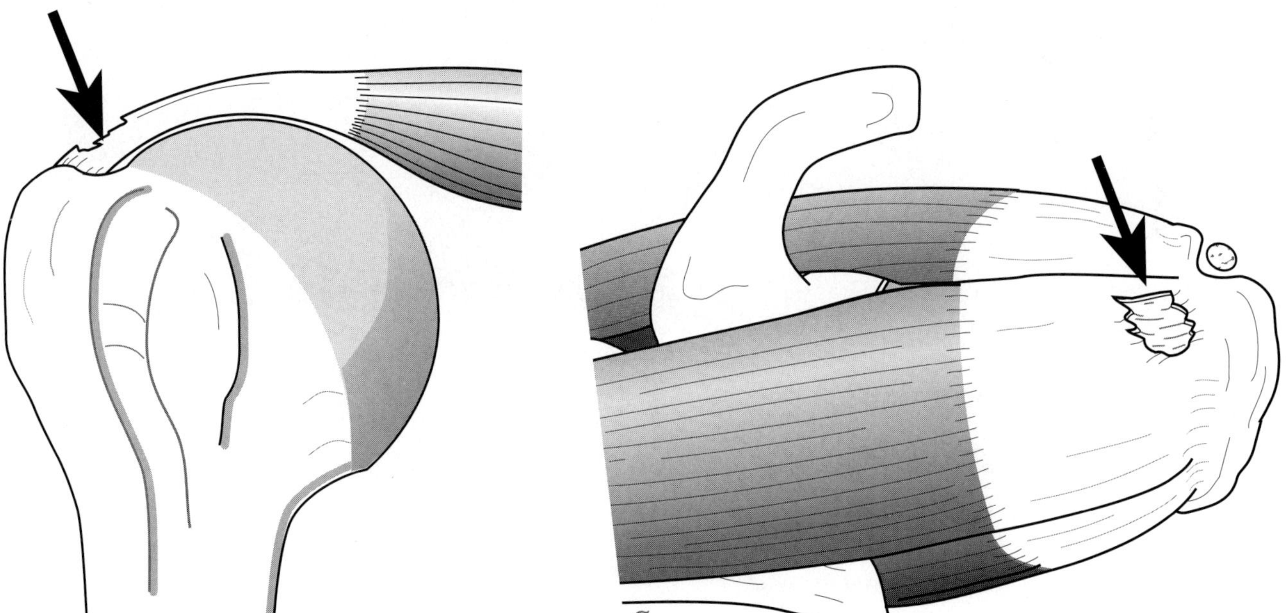


**Figure 18–22. Partial-thickness tear—bursal side**
A bursal side partial-thickness cuff tear.

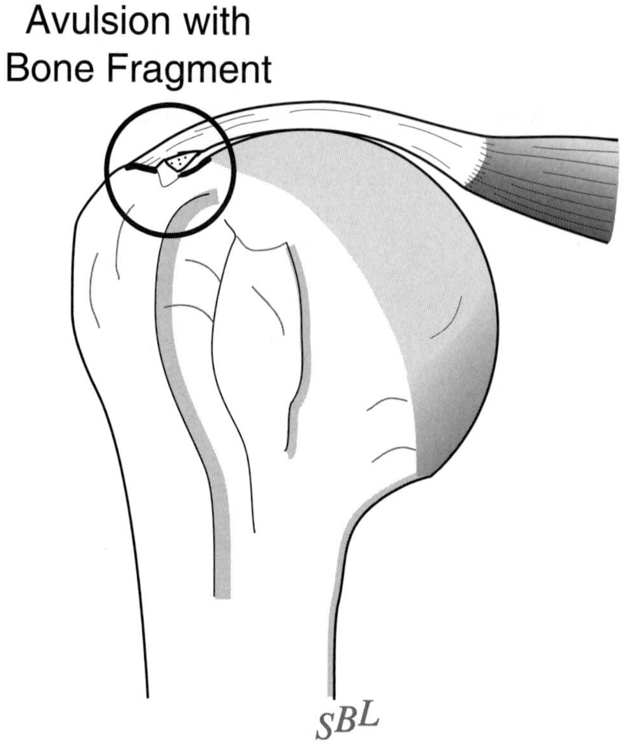


**Figure 18–23. Bone avulsion**
Especially in younger individuals, the cuff insertion may fail by avulsion of the bony attachment of the deep cuff fibers. This bony fragment should not be confused with calcific tendonitis. (Modified from Matsen FA, Lippitt SB, Sidles JA, et al [eds]: Practical Evaluation and Management of the Shoulder. Philadelphia: WB Saunders, 1994, p. 119.)

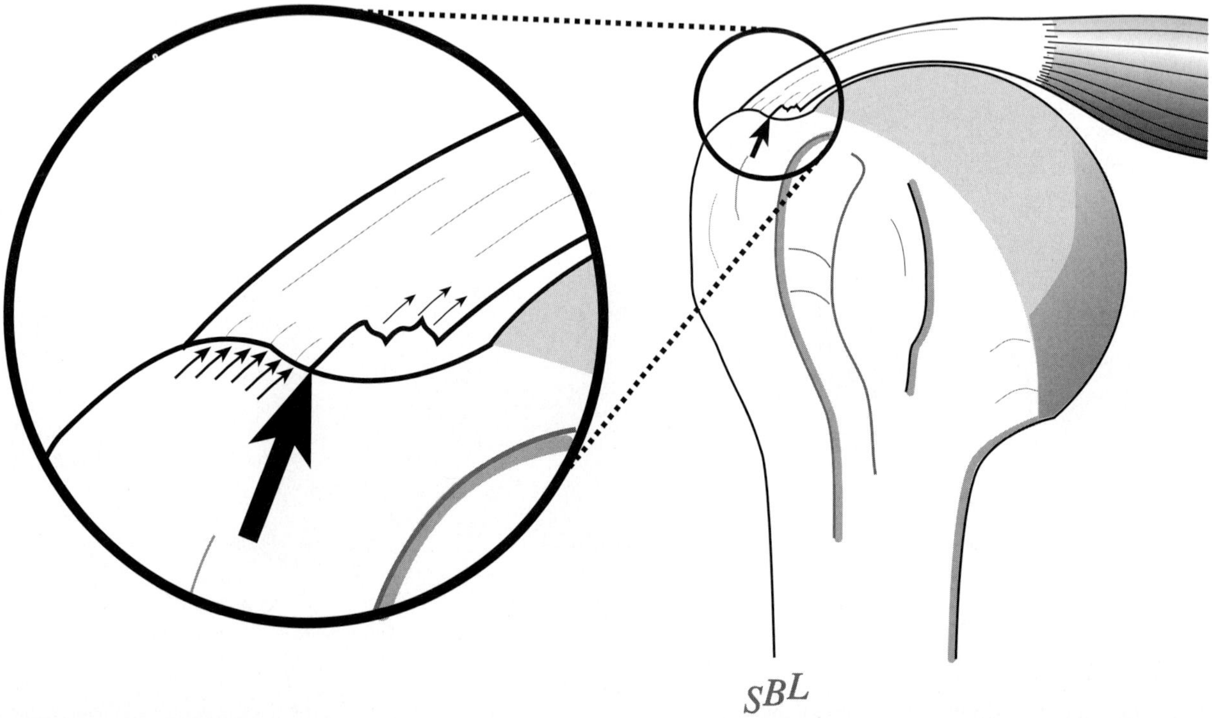


**Figure 18–24. Load concentration**
In partial-thickness tears, the disruption of fibers on the deep surface places excess load on the remaining superficial fibers, especially those at the edge of the defect.

When a tendon is partially torn, there is disproportionate load on the fibers at the edge of the tear, like when a zipper is pulled open, like a nylon stocking developing a run in it, or like a piece of paper that is partially torn: the load is on the connection adjacent to the tear. This force concentration is sometimes referred to as the "notch" phenomenon—a mechanism by which partial tears can propagate progressively (**Fig. 18–25**). In this progressive tendon tearing, each step in the progression may be interpreted as an episode of "tendonitis" until it is established that the problem is a cuff tear (**Fig. 18–26**).

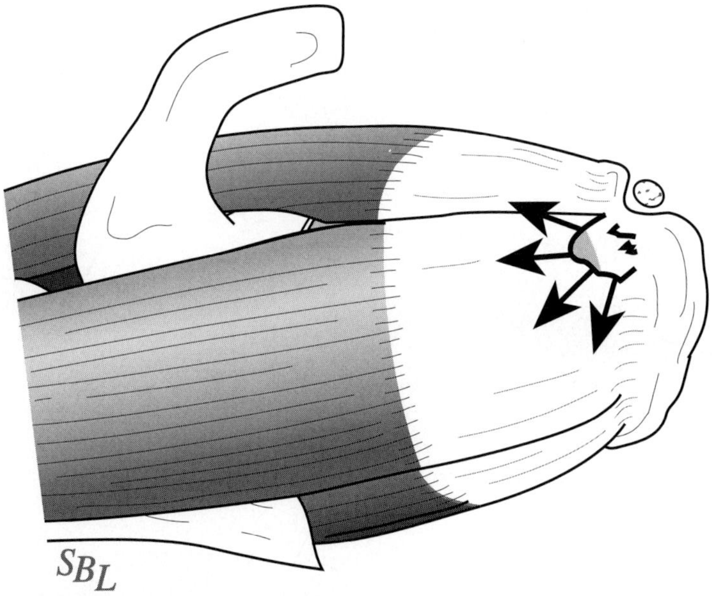


**Figure 18–25. Notch phenomenon**
In a partial cuff tear, the force of the muscle contraction is concentrated at the margin of the tear, facilitating extension of the defect. (Modified from Matsen FA, Lippitt SB, Sidles JA, et al [eds]: Practical Evaluation and Management of the Shoulder. Philadelphia: WB Saunders, 1994, p. 121.)

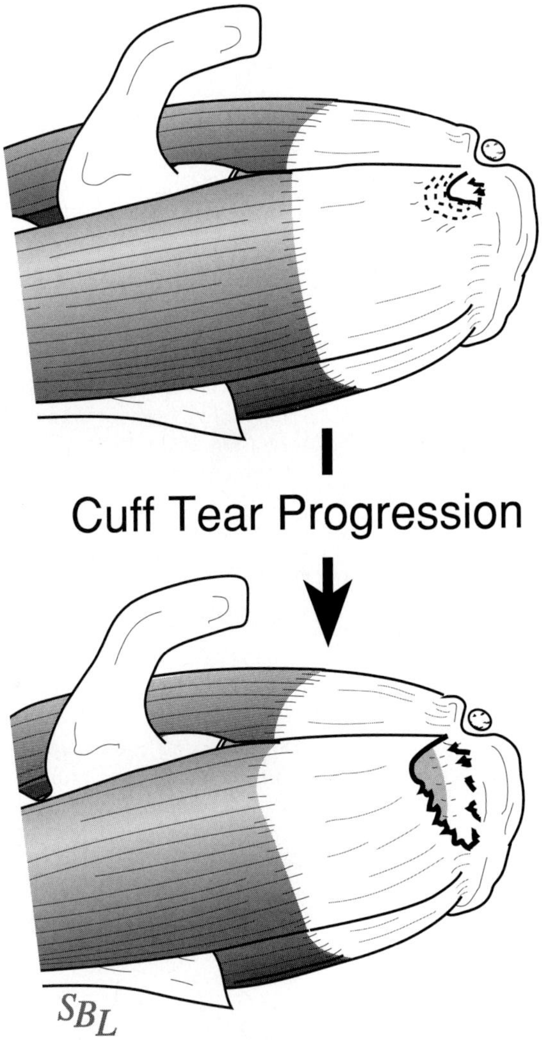


**Figure 18–26. Progression of a cuff tear**
The extension of the cuff tear may continue, stopping only when the tendon attachments at the margin of the tear are able to manage the forces applied to them. (Modified from Matsen FA, Lippitt SB, Sidles JA, et al [eds]: Practical Evaluation and Management of the Shoulder. Philadelphia: WB Saunders, 1994, p. 119.)

*Initiation of Cuff Failure*

Cuff fiber failure commonly results from the sudden application of eccentric loads **(Fig. 18–27)** while the cuff insertion seems to be better able to tolerate concentric loads **(Fig. 18–28)**.

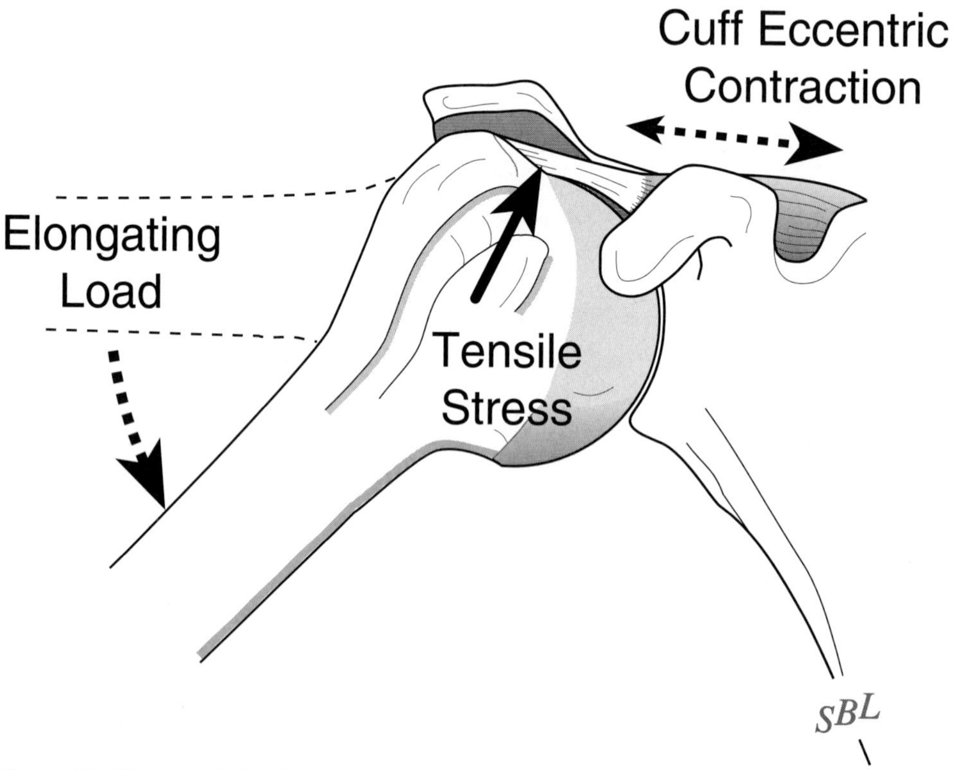


**Figure 18–27. Eccentric loading**
Cuff tendon fibers are susceptible to eccentric loading, for example when attempting to actively resist a sudden downward force on the arm. (Modified from Matsen FA, Lippitt SB, Sidles JA, et al [eds]: Practical Evaluation and Management of the Shoulder. Philadelphia: WB Saunders, 1994, p. 116.)

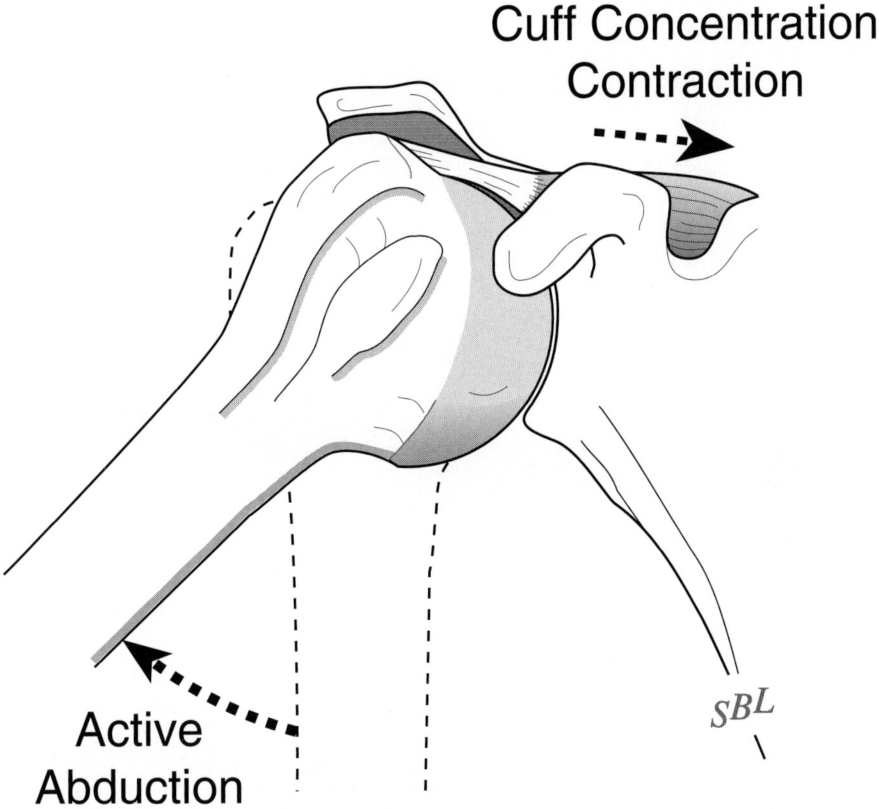


**Figure 18–28. Concentric loading**

Loads from concentric contractions are better tolerated by the cuff insertion, for example, when the arm abducts against resistance. Note that the cuff insertion clears the acromion at low angles of elevation, protecting it from impingement by the coracoacromial arch. (Modified from Matsen FA, Lippitt SB, Sidles JA, et al [eds]: Practical Evaluation and Management of the Shoulder. Philadelphia: WB Saunders, 1994, p. 116.)

An anatomic factor predisposing to deep surface failure of the cuff insertion is internal abutment, in which the corner of the glenoid contacts the deep aspect of the cuff at its tuberosity insertion (**Fig. 18–29**). This is most likely to be a problem for throwers who have stretched out their anterior capsule, allowing increased external rotation.

It is apparent that the most common form of cuff fiber failure, that which occurs on the articular surface of the cuff tendon, cannot be attributed to scuffing of the bursal surface by the acromion: so-called subacromial "impingement." In fact, the cuff insertion is well under the acromion at relatively small angles of elevation where it is protected from contact with the coracoacromial arch (see Fig. 18–28).

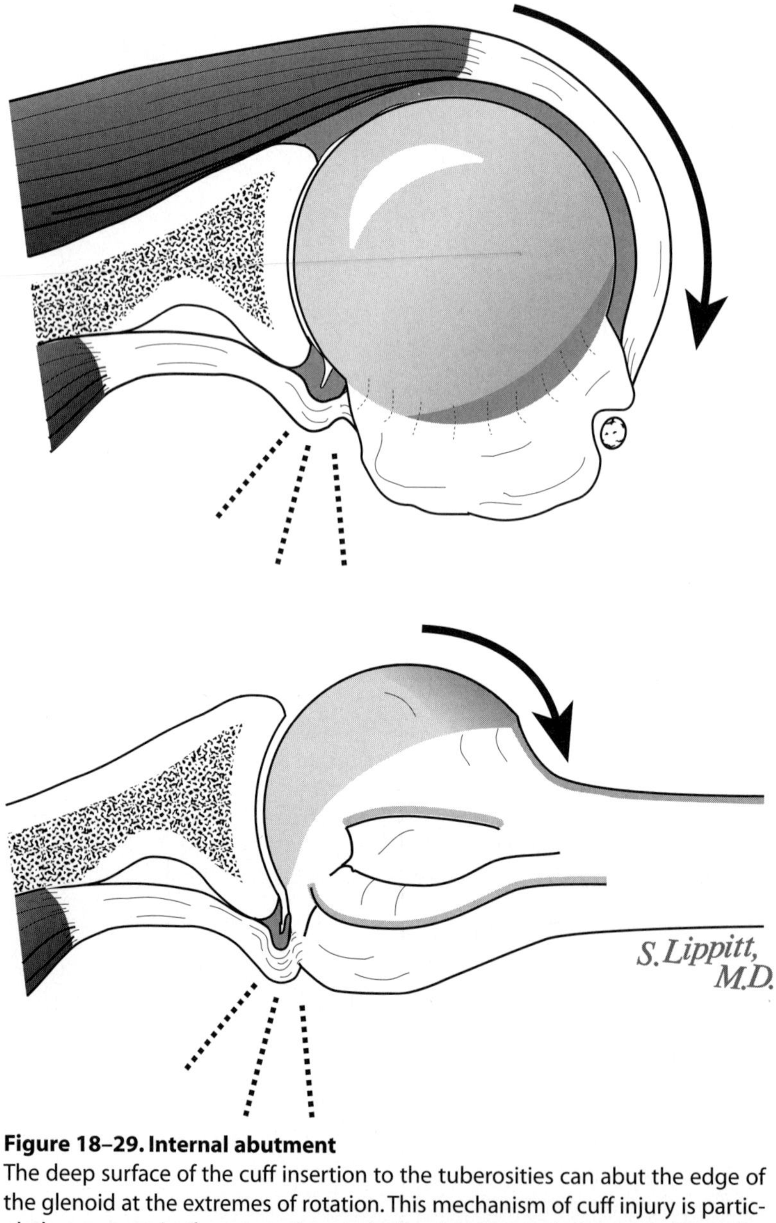


**Figure 18–29. Internal abutment**
The deep surface of the cuff insertion to the tuberosities can abut the edge of the glenoid at the extremes of rotation. This mechanism of cuff injury is particularly common in throwers who gradually stretch out their anterior capsular restraints, allowing very large ranges of external rotation. (Modified from Matsen FA, Lippitt SB, Sidles JA, et al [eds]: Practical Evaluation and Management of the Shoulder. Philadelphia: WB Saunders, 1994, p. 117.)

### *Factors Compromising Tendon Healing*

Deep surface rotator cuff fiber failure exposes the defect to joint fluid. This joint fluid prevents the formation of a fibrin clot and, thus, healing is contravened **(Fig. 18–30)**. Furthermore, tension at the edge of the cuff tear compromises the circulation to the margin of the tendon **(Fig. 18–31)**. For these reasons, left to their own devices, cuff defects tend to progress rather than heal. An optimal cuff repair surgery will bring healthy tendon into contact with vascularized bone and exclude joint fluid from the repair site (see Chapter 21).

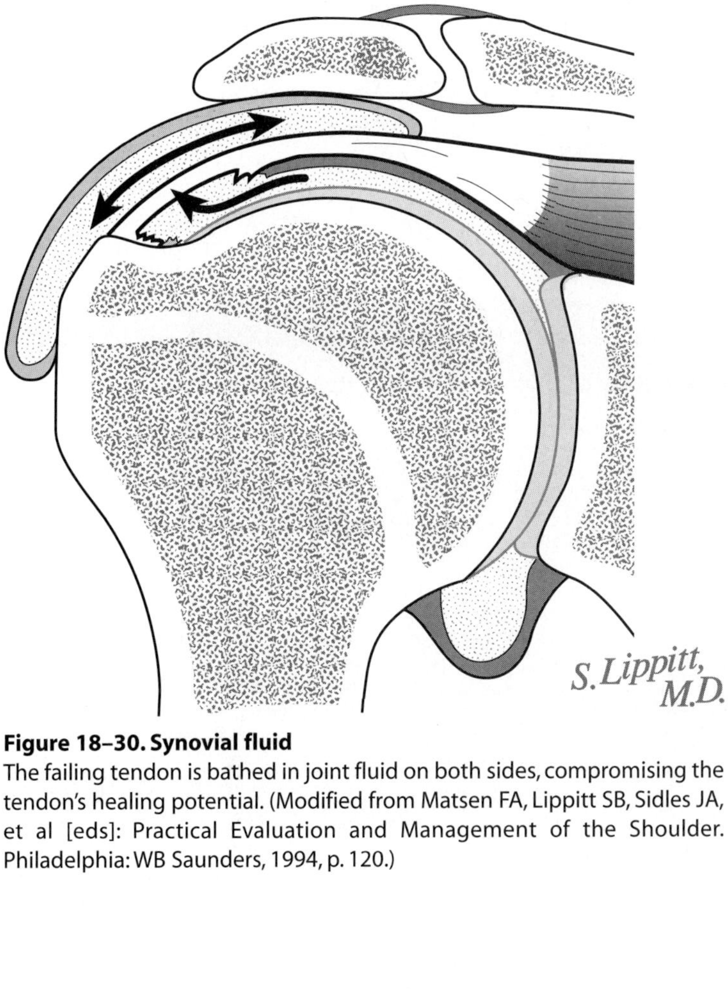


**Figure 18–30. Synovial fluid**
The failing tendon is bathed in joint fluid on both sides, compromising the tendon's healing potential. (Modified from Matsen FA, Lippitt SB, Sidles JA, et al [eds]: Practical Evaluation and Management of the Shoulder. Philadelphia: WB Saunders, 1994, p. 120.)

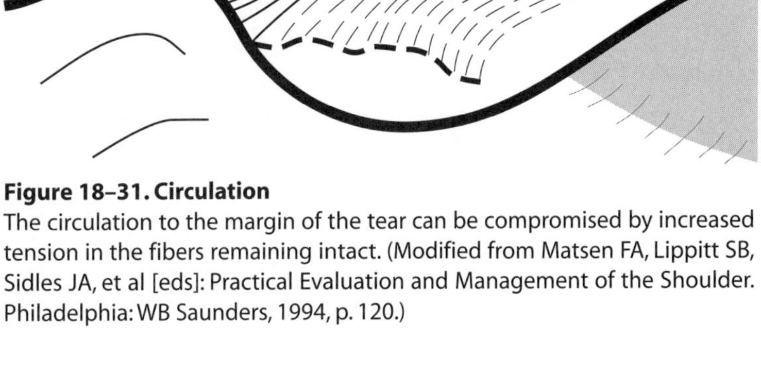

**Figure 18–31. Circulation**
The circulation to the margin of the tear can be compromised by increased tension in the fibers remaining intact. (Modified from Matsen FA, Lippitt SB, Sidles JA, et al [eds]: Practical Evaluation and Management of the Shoulder. Philadelphia: WB Saunders, 1994, p. 120.)

### *Factors Affecting Reparability*

In considering the potential for surgically restoring a durable tendon insertion to bone, the surgeon needs to consider the quality of the tissue to be used in the repair. The ability of the cuff tendon tissue to withstand tensile loads is compromised by age, disuse, steroid injections, smoking, and poor general health (**Table 18–1**). These factors can predispose the cuff tendons to fail with minimal force—essentially an atraumatic fiber failure. Cuff fibers that fail atraumatically may be so constitutionally weak that they cannot hold up even if repaired back to the bone. Thus, in chronic atraumatic cuff tears, there is reason to consider a nonoperative approach to improving shoulder function by rehabilitating the muscle-tendon units that remain intact.

Acute cuff detachments that result from major force application are likely to be repairable (**Fig. 18–32**). If acute traumatic cuff tears are not repaired promptly, the muscle may undergo intramuscular contracture, atrophy, and fatty degeneration (**Fig. 18–33**), and the tendon may become progressively reabsorbed. These degenerative changes compromise the opportunity for surgical repair. Thus, as with any other tendon avulsion from bone, time is of importance in the repair of acute tears of the rotator cuff.

**Table 18–1**

**Encouraging and Discouraging Prospects for a Durably Reparable Cuff Tear**

| Encouraging | Discouraging |
|---|---|
| ***History*** | |
| Age younger than 55 years | Age older than 65 years |
| Acute traumatic onset | Insidious, atraumatic onset |
| No relation to work | Attribution of tear to work |
| Short duration of weakness | Weakness over 6 months |
| No history of smoking | Many smoking pack-years |
| No steroid injections | Repeated steroid injections |
| No major medications | Systemic steroids or antimetabolites |
| No concurrent disease | Inflammatory joint disease, other chronic illnesses |
| No infections | History of previous shoulder infection |
| No previous shoulder surgery | Previous cuff surgery |
| Benign surgical history | History of failed soft tissue repairs (e.g., dehiscence, infections complicating herniorrhaphy) |
| ***Physical Examination*** | |
| Good nutrition | Poor nutrition |
| Mild to moderate weakness | Severe weakness |
| No spinatus atrophy | Severe spinatus atrophy |
| Stable shoulder | Anterior superior instability |
| Intact acromion | Previous acromioplasty |
| No stiffness | Stiffness |
| ***Radiographs*** | |
| Normal radiographs | Upward displacement of head against coracoacromial arch<br>Cuff tear arthropathy |

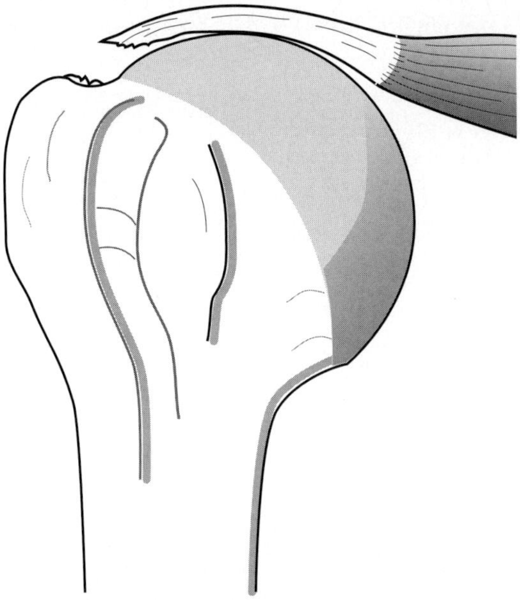

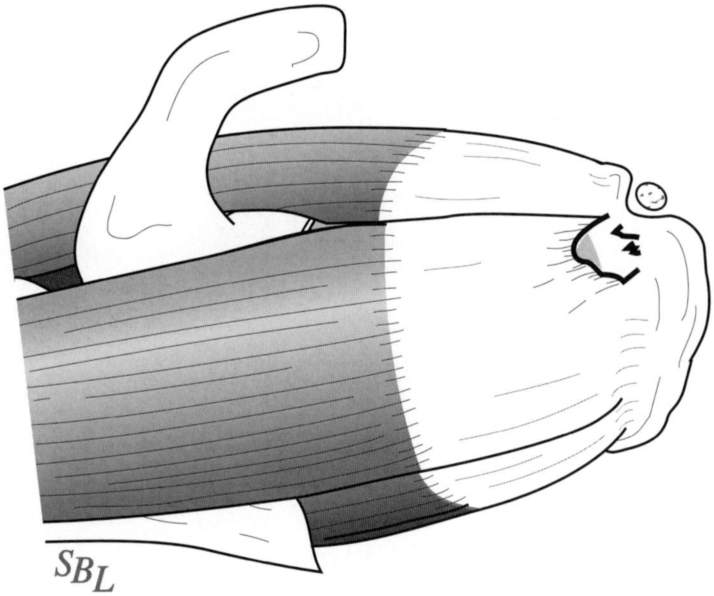


**Figure 18–32. Acute cuff tear**
An acute traumatic cuff tear through strong tendon presents the optimal opportunity for surgical repair.

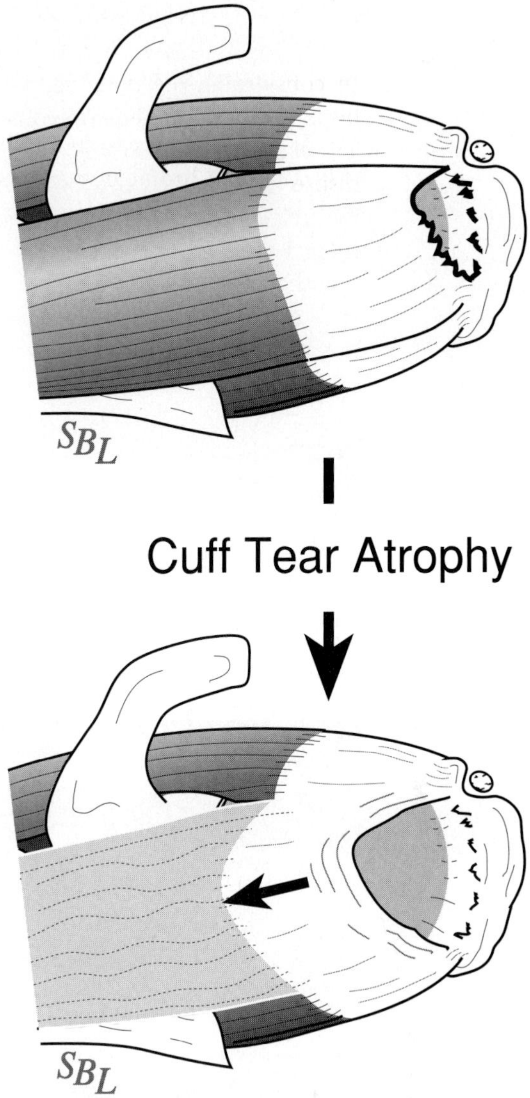


**Figure 18–33. Atrophy**
In chronic tears, the muscle becomes atrophic and infiltrated with fat, and the tendon edge becomes weaker and less able to hold the suture of a surgical repair.

Loss of the rotator cuff subjects the superior glenoid to increased loads that can contribute to its erosion (**Fig. 18–34**). Progressive upward displacement of the humeral head produces secondary changes in the coracoacromial arch (**Fig. 18–35**). Once the humeral head has ascended so that its equator is above the residual cuff, contraction of the cuff muscles lock the humeral head in the superiorly displaced position (**Fig. 18–36**). Chronic upward displacement of the humeral head from cuff deficiency and superior glenoid erosion are elements of cuff tear arthropathy (**Fig. 18–37**).

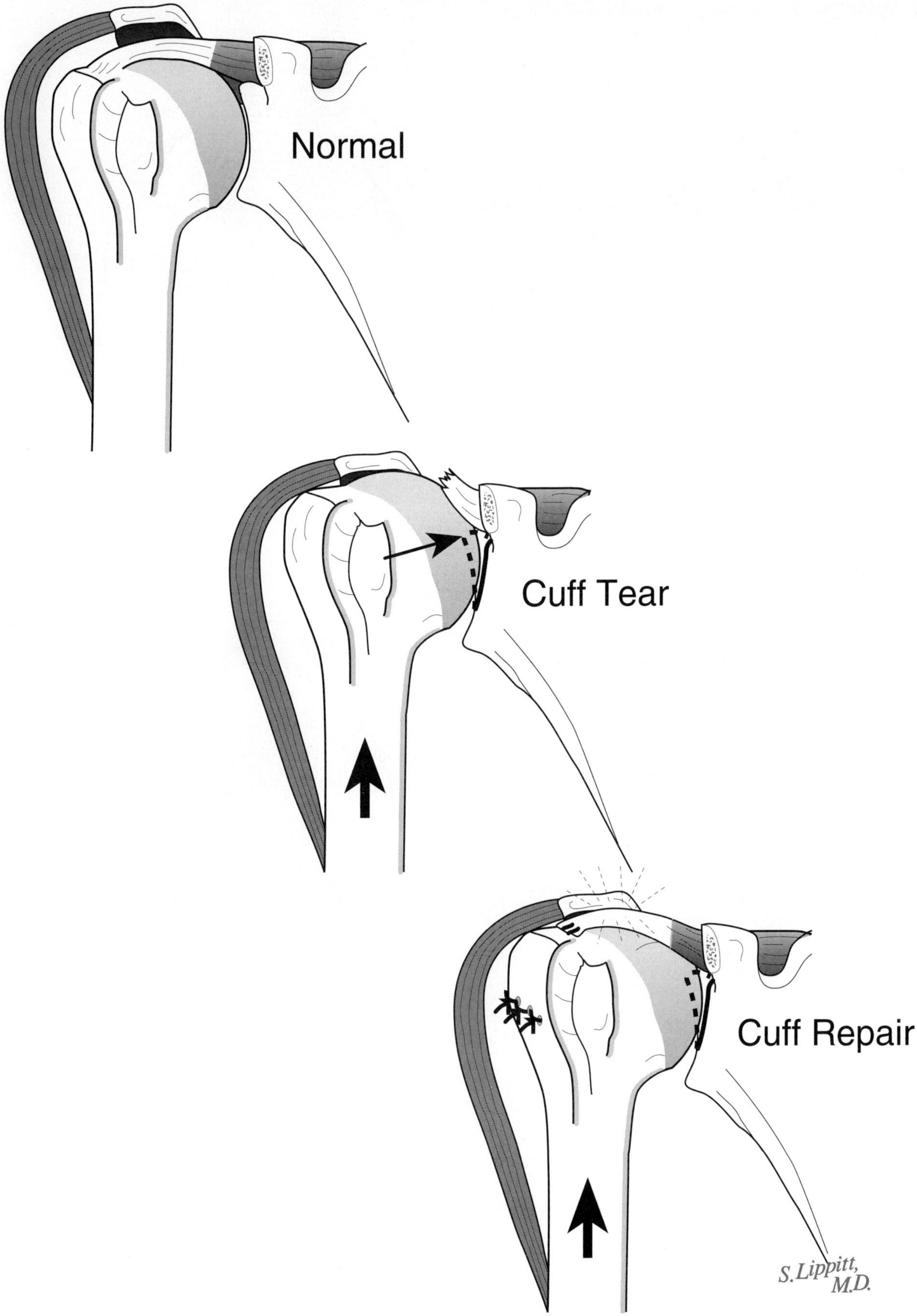


**Figure 18–34. Loss of the superior rim**

Chronic cuff tears can allow the humeral head to migrate superiorly and to wear progressively the superior glenoid concavity. Loss of the superior glenoid lip leaves the shoulder with a permanent tendency to superior subluxation that cannot be reversed by cuff repair surgery. (Modified from Rockwood CA, Matsen FA [eds]: The Shoulder, 2nd ed. Philadelphia: WB Saunders, 1998, p. 778.)

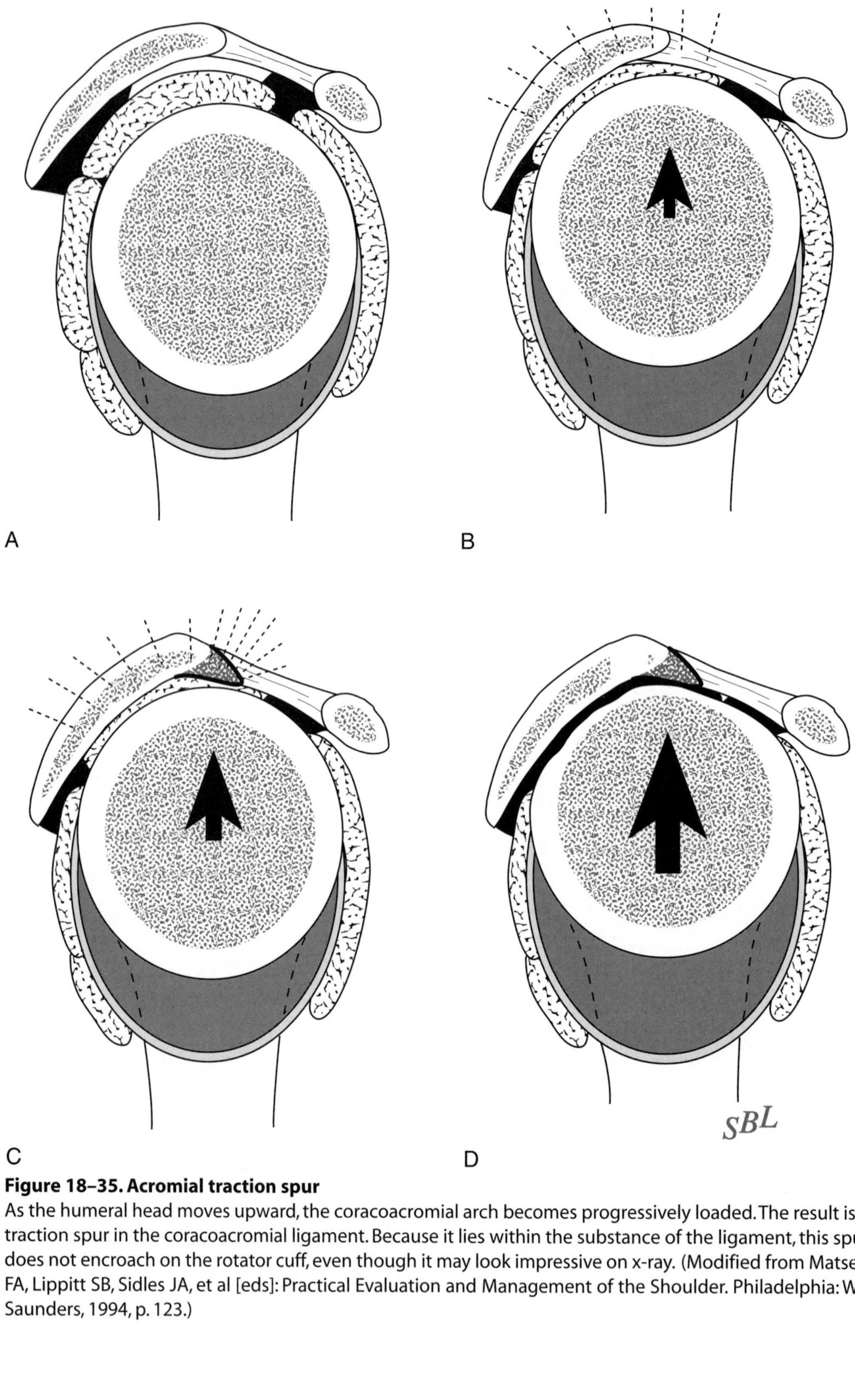


**Figure 18–35. Acromial traction spur**
As the humeral head moves upward, the coracoacromial arch becomes progressively loaded. The result is a traction spur in the coracoacromial ligament. Because it lies within the substance of the ligament, this spur does not encroach on the rotator cuff, even though it may look impressive on x-ray. (Modified from Matsen FA, Lippitt SB, Sidles JA, et al [eds]: Practical Evaluation and Management of the Shoulder. Philadelphia: WB Saunders, 1994, p. 123.)

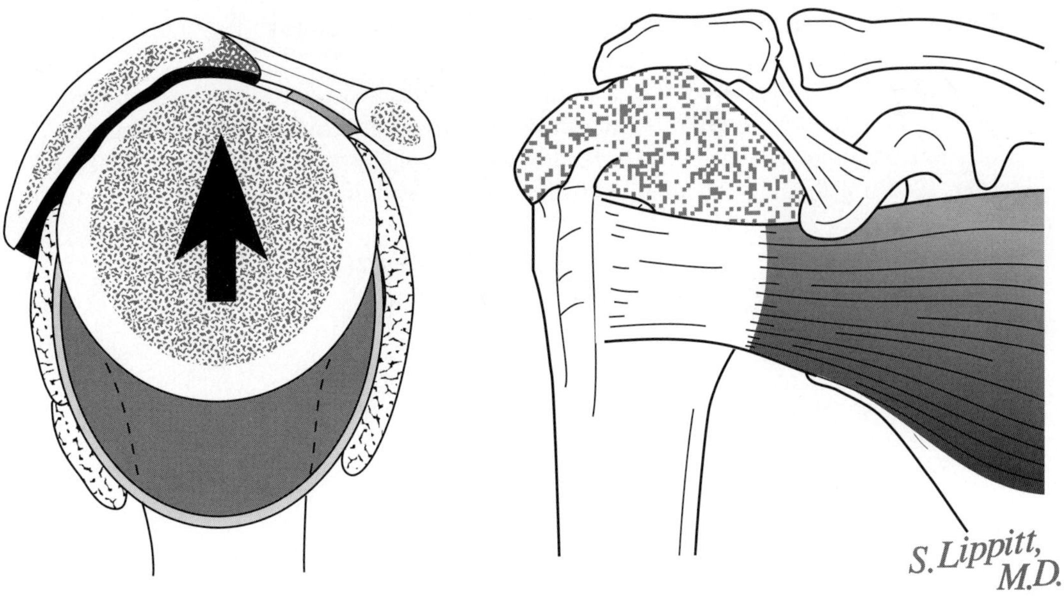


**Figure 18–36. Boutonnière deformity**
The boutonnière deformity is present when the upper edges of the residual infraspinatus and subscapularis slide below the equator of the humeral head. Contraction and contracture of these muscles contributes to locking the humeral head in its superiorly displaced position. (Modified from Matsen FA, Lippitt SB, Sidles JA, et al [eds]: Practical Evaluation and Management of the Shoulder. Philadelphia: WB Saunders, 1994, p. 123.)

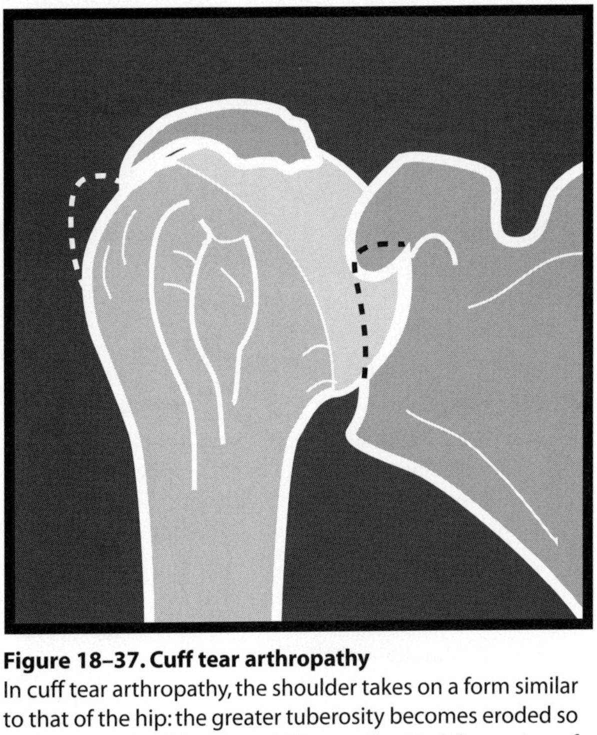

**Figure 18–37. Cuff tear arthropathy**
In cuff tear arthropathy, the shoulder takes on a form similar to that of the hip: the greater tuberosity becomes eroded so that the proximal humerus is "femoralized" while erosion of the coracoacromial arch and upper glenoid results in their "acetabularization." (Modified from Matsen FA, Lippitt SB, Sidles JA, et al [eds]: Practical Evaluation and Management of the Shoulder. Philadelphia: WB Saunders, 1994, p. 128.)

## Clinical Examination Related to Shoulder Weakness

Inspection can reveal atrophy as well as incisions and scars indicating previous surgery. The physical examination may reveal subacromial roughness from hypertrophic bursa or from the superior edges of torn tendon rubbing against the coracoacromial arch (**Fig. 18–38**). Palpation can reveal gaps in the cuff tendon (**Figs. 18–39, 18–40,** and **18–41**).

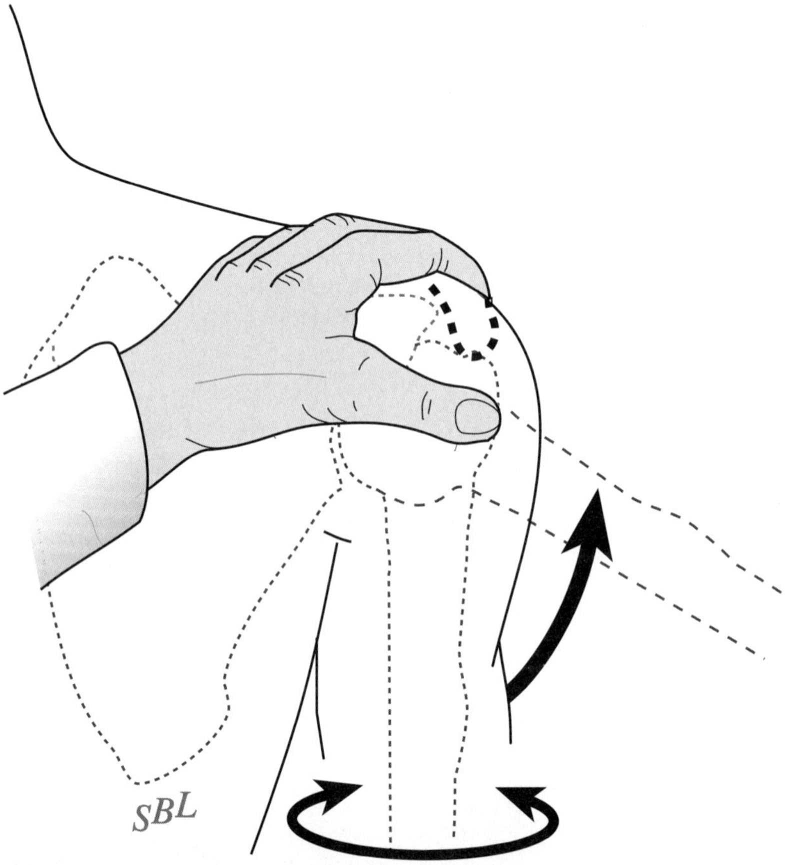


**Figure 18–38. Palpation for crepitance**
The examiner can palpate the rotator cuff for crepitance by placing one hand on the scapula with the index finder just anterior to the acromion while the arm is moved through its full range of motion.

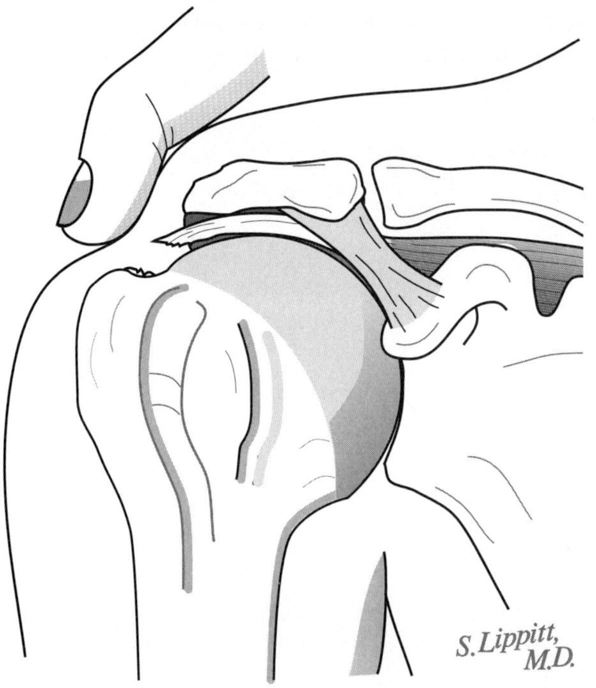


**Figure 18–39. Palpation of defect cuff**
Defects in the tendinous cuff can often be palpated through the overlying skin and deltoid.

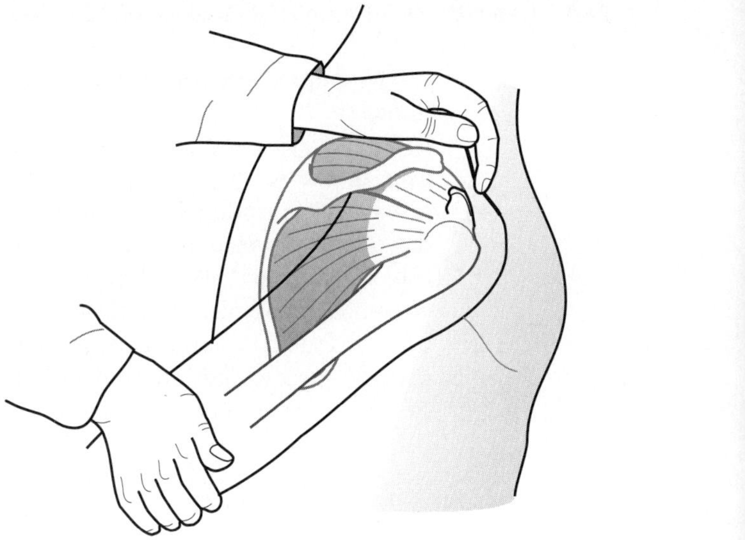

**Figure 18–40. Palpation of supraspinatus defect**
The accessibility of the supraspinatus tendon for palpation can be enhanced by extending the arm.

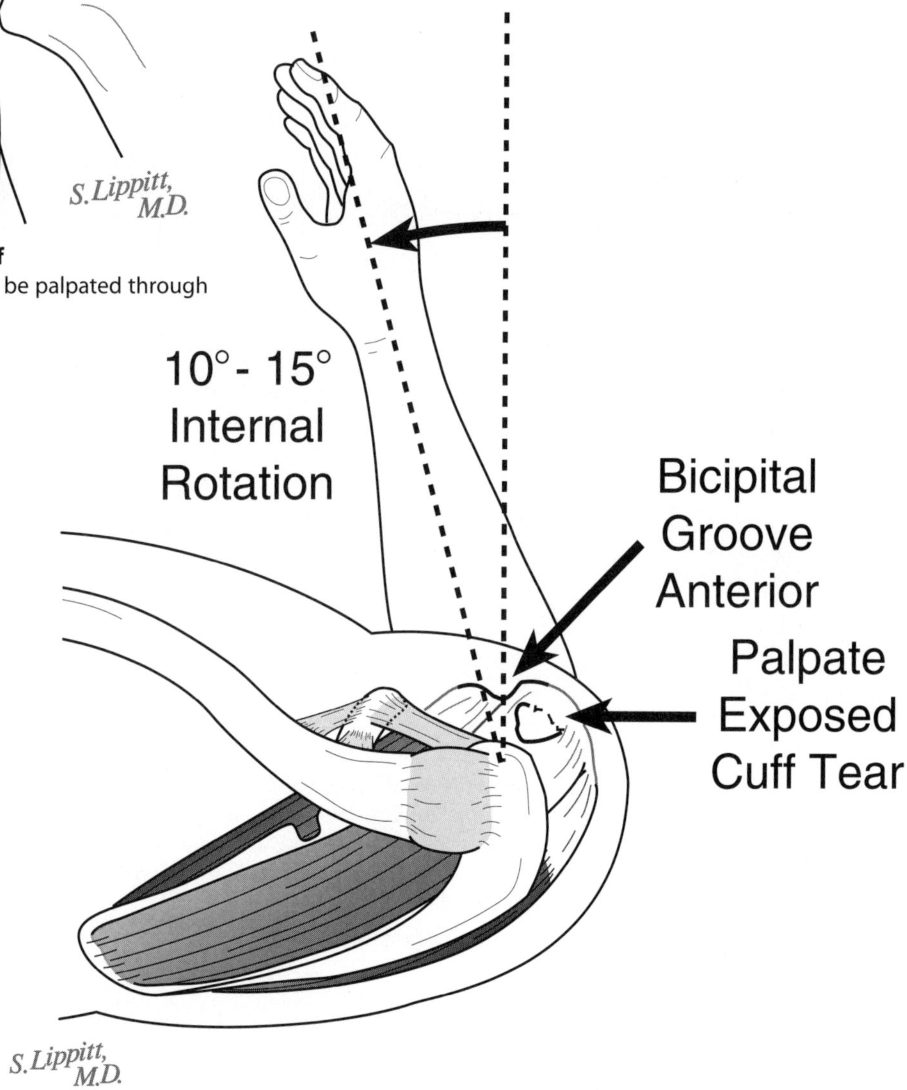


**Figure 18–41. Reference to bicipital groove**
The bicipital groove is normally straight anterior when the arm (with flexed elbow) is in 10 to 15 degrees internal rotation. Reference to these anatomical landmarks can help locate the tear.

The range of motion examination can reveal restrictions due to contracture surrounding the area of injury or scarring in the humeroscapular motion interface. Limited range of motion is particularly common in the presence of partial-thickness tears of the rotator cuff. The most common partial-thickness tear is that of the supraspinatus tendon. In this situation, it is characteristic to have loss of the motions that place this tendon under tension: internal rotation with the arm at the side (**Fig. 18–42**), internal rotation of the arm in 90 degrees of abduction (**Fig. 18–43**), and cross-body movement (**Fig. 18–44**). Although in the past, pain on these maneuvers has been attributed to "impingement," it is now recognized as being due to the pull on the partially torn tendon attachment, which is analogous to the pain experienced on stretching the origin of the extensor carpi radialis brevis in tennis elbow.

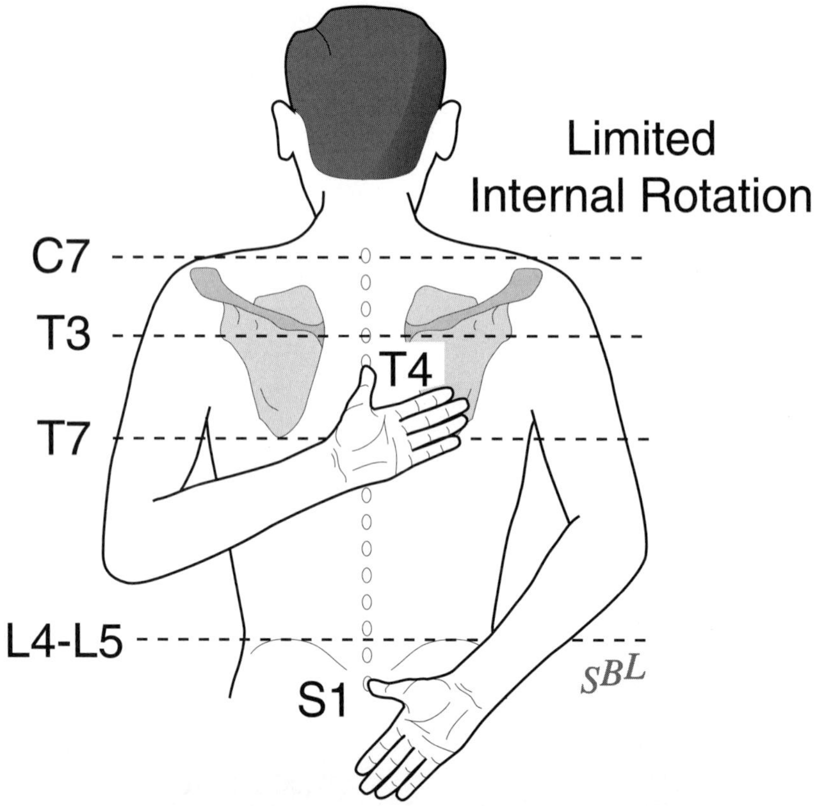


**Figure 18–42. Internal rotation in adduction**
Examination of internal rotation with the arm at the side. The motion is recorded as the segment of the posterior midline anatomy that can be reached with the thumb. (Modified from Rockwood CA, Matsen FA [eds]: The Shoulder, 2nd ed. Philadelphia: WB Saunders, 1998, p. 1083.)

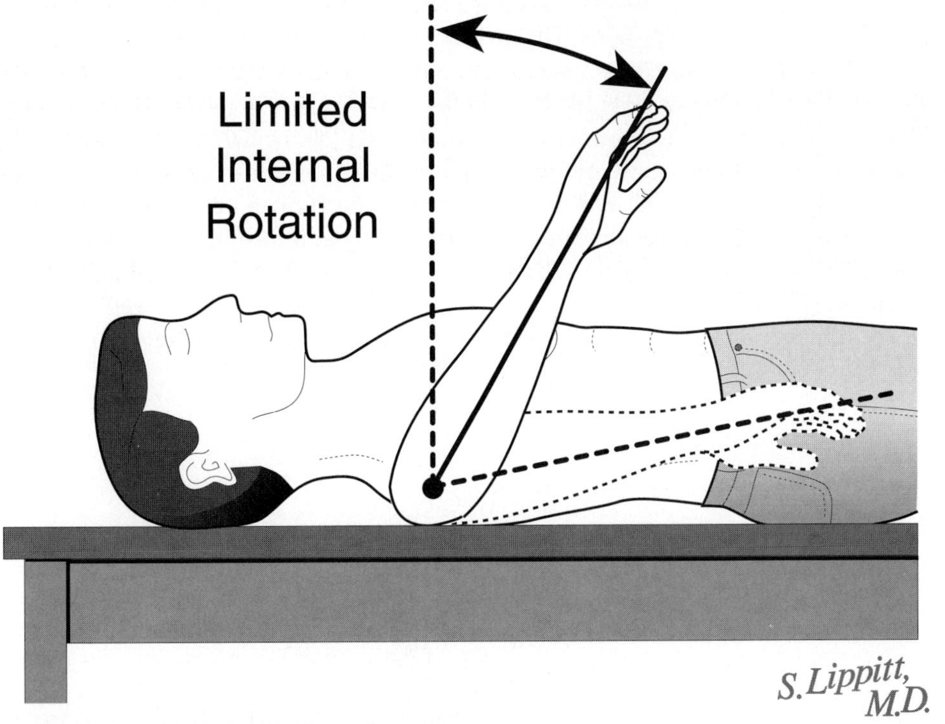


**Figure 18–43. Internal rotation in abduction**
Examination of internal rotation with the arm in 90 degrees of abduction. The motion is recorded as the number of degrees the arm can be rotated from the position where the forearm points straight ahead. (Modified from Rockwood CA, Matsen FA [eds]: The Shoulder, 2nd ed. Philadelphia: WB Saunders, 1998, p. 1083.)

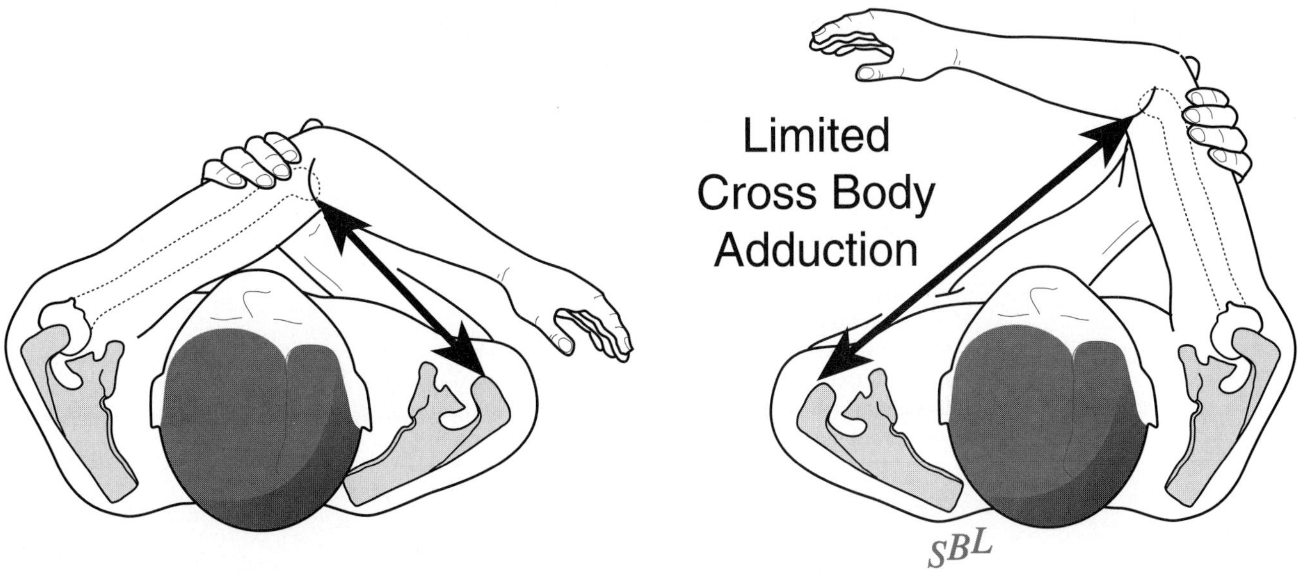


**Figure 18–44. Cross-body movement**
Examination of cross-body movement. The motion is recorded as distance between the antecubital fossa and the contralateral acromion. (Modified from Rockwood CA, Matsen FA [eds]: The Shoulder, 2nd ed. Philadelphia: WB Saunders, 1998, p. 1083.)

Cuff strength is conveniently examined using manual tests of isometric torque. Isometric testing removes potential interference from pain on motion, from crepitance, or from stiffness. These tests examine the integrity of the supraspinatus (**Fig. 18–45**), the infraspinatus (**Fig. 18–46**), and the subscapularis (**Figs. 18–47** and **18–48**). Pain or weakness on these maneuvers constitutes an abnormal tendon sign for the specified tendon-muscle unit. These tests are relatively specific to each muscle but are not specific to the cause of weakness; for example, a suprascapular nerve lesion or a cuff tear may each produce abnormal supraspinatus and infraspinatus tendon signs.

Clinical assessment can yield substantial information on the potential reparability of the rotator cuff. Table 18–1 is a summary of the findings that have been shown to be encouraging and discouraging about the prospect of finding a durably reparable cuff tear.

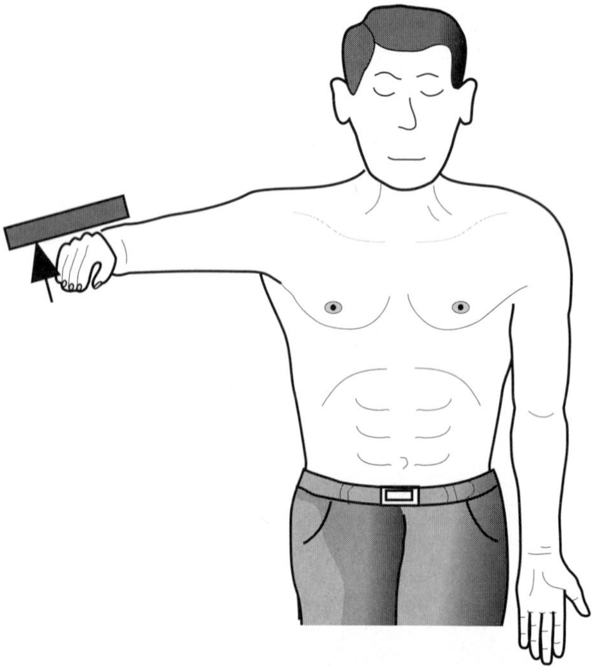

**Figure 18–45. Supraspinatus test**
The supraspinatus is tested by positioning the arm in 90 degrees of abduction in the plane of the scapula and in slight internal rotation—this puts the supraspinatus tendon on top of the humeral head. The patient is asked to hold this position while the examiner attempts to adduct the arm. (Modified from Matsen FA, Lippitt SB, Sidles JA, et al [eds]: Practical Evaluation and Management of the Shoulder. Philadelphia: WB Saunders, 1994, p. 127.)

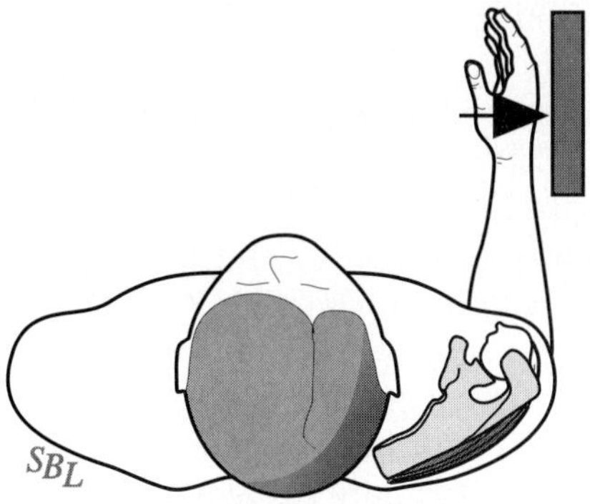

**Figure 18–46. Infraspinatus test**
The infraspinatus is tested by positioning the humerus with the elbow at the side and the forearm pointing straight ahead. The patient is asked to hold this position while the examiner attempts to push the arm into internal rotation. (Modified from Matsen FA, Lippitt SB, Sidles JA, et al [eds]: Practical Evaluation and Management of the Shoulder. Philadelphia: WB Saunders, 1994, p. 127.)

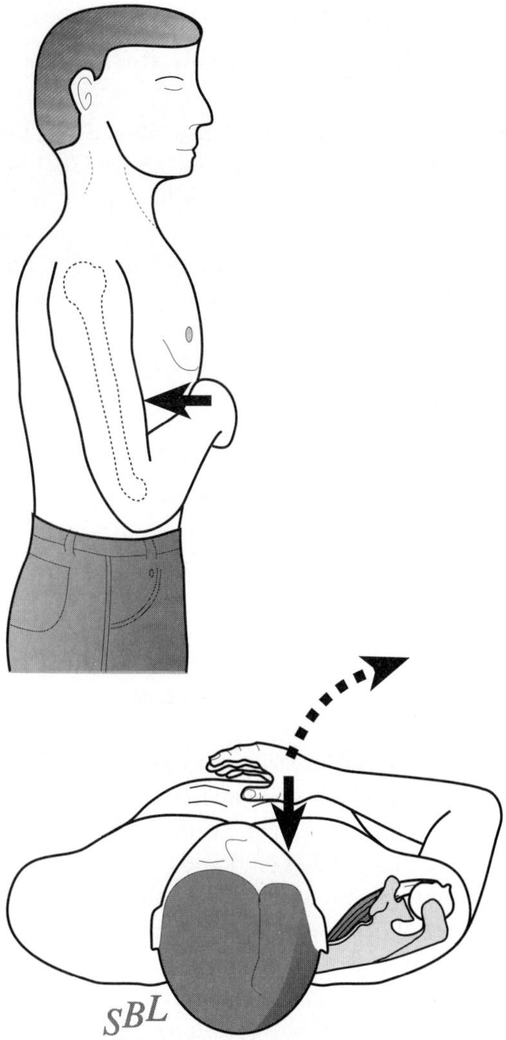

**Figure 18–47. Subscapularis test**
The subscapularis is tested by having the patient press the hand in toward the stomach.

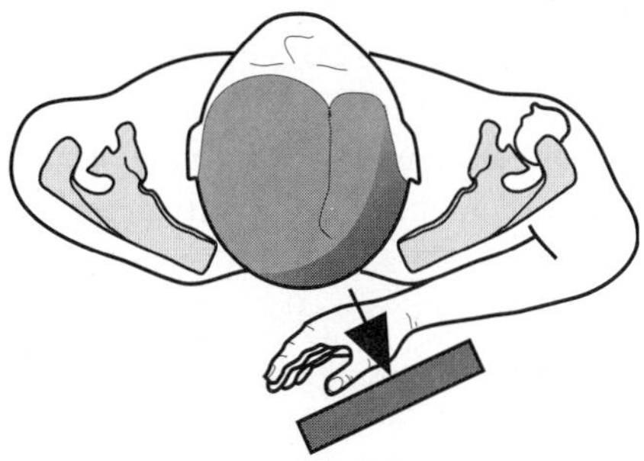

**Figure 18–48. Lift-off test**
The subscapularis can also be tested by having the patient push the hand away from the lumbar area posteriorly against resistance. (Modified from Matsen FA, Lippitt SB, Sidles JA, et al [eds]: Practical Evaluation and Management of the Shoulder. Philadelphia: WB Saunders, 1994, p. 127.)

# IMAGING

## Imaging the Rotator Cuff

Plain radiographs can provide indirect information regarding the integrity of the rotator cuff. On the anteroposterior (AP) view in the plane of the scapula, an acromiohumeral interval of less than 6 mm indicates thinning of the supraspinatus tendon. This is because the thickness of the normal supraspinatus tendon between the humeral head and the acromion is 6 mm (**Fig. 18–49**). Acromiohumeral contact indicates that the superior cuff tendon cannot be intact (**Fig. 18–50**).

Imaging of the rotator cuff tendons can be used to confirm the diagnosis of cuff tear, to establish the extent of the tear, and to evaluate the degree of tendon retraction.

In many cases, these determinations can be made from the clinical history and the examination. MRI or expert dynamic sonography are now the gold standards for cuff tear imaging, replacing arthrography. Recently, the advent of surgeon-performed in-office sonography has provided a real-time opportunity for integration of cuff imaging with the physical examination as well as the opportunity to demonstrate the pathologic lesion to the patient.

# MANAGEMENT

## Partial-Thickness Tears

Partial-thickness rotator cuff tears produce symptoms because the muscle is pulling on an unstable tendon attachment to bone, resulting in uneven distribution of force. As in the case of the conditions known as tennis elbow (lateral epicondylitis), biceps tendonitis, Achilles tendonitis, and patellar tendonitis, the primary pathologic condition is not inflammation, as the suffix "-itis" might imply, but rather a partial tendon detachment from bone. In these situations, a disproportionate share of the load is borne by the fibers at the edge of the tear; as when a zipper is pulled apart, the load is on the last intact link. When load is applied to the affected tendon, the area of the partial tear becomes painful—a positive tendon sign. If the detachment were complete, as in a complete rupture of the biceps or Achilles tendons, pull on the tendon would be painless. Often these conditions are associated with stiffness of the joint in the direction that stretches the tendon: lack of extension of the elbow in tennis elbow, lack of ankle dorsiflexion in Achilles tendonitis, or lack of internal rotation in partial-thickness cuff tears.

For each of these conditions, treatment may include (1) stretching the tendon until the stiffness is resolved and the load at the tendon attachment is distributed evenly among the fibers remaining intact, (2) release of insecurely attached fibers so that the load is borne only by those fibers that robustly connect the tendon to bone (as in a tennis elbow release), or (3) reattachment of the partially detached fibers. The difficulty with the last approach lies in reconstructing the isometry of the tendon attachment. Taking the Achilles tendon with a lateral one-third tear as an example, reattachment of the torn portion of tendon is likely to result in its being disproportionately tight, so that when the attached muscle contracts, the repaired part of the tendon takes the preponderance of the load and risks re-tear. For the same reason, repairs of tennis elbow are less successful in relieving symptoms than are selective releases.

## Full-Thickness Tears

Acute full-thickness tears merit consideration for early repair before tendon resorption and muscle atrophy can occur. Chronic tears merit consideration for repair if there is evidence of good residual muscle and tendon. Symptoms from irreparable tears may respond to smoothing of the humeroscapular motion interface.

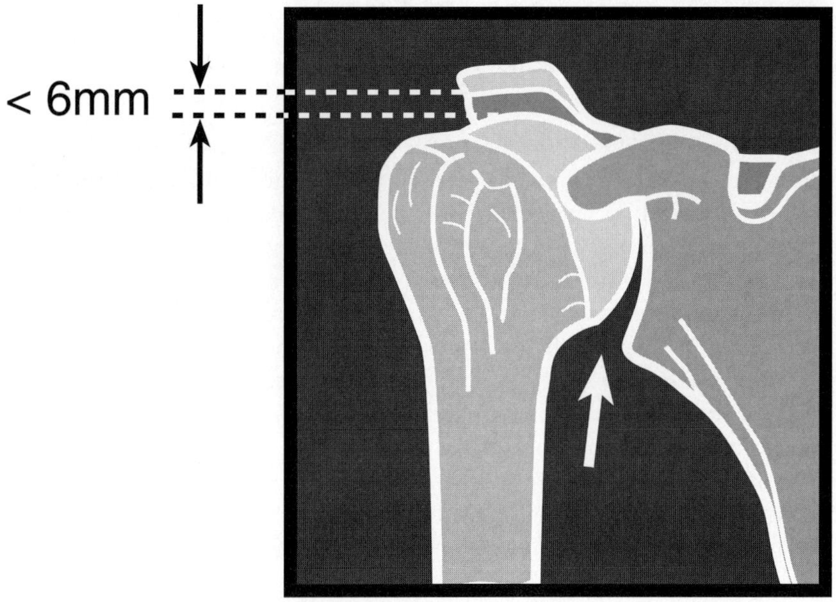


**Figure 18–49. Narrowed acromiohumeral interval**
With thinning of the cuff and ascension of the humeral head, the acromiohumeral interval narrows. This narrowing can be seen on an anteroposterior x-ray of the shoulder. Because the normal cuff is about 6 mm thick, an acromiohumeral interval of less than 6 mm suggests cuff tendon thinning or failure.

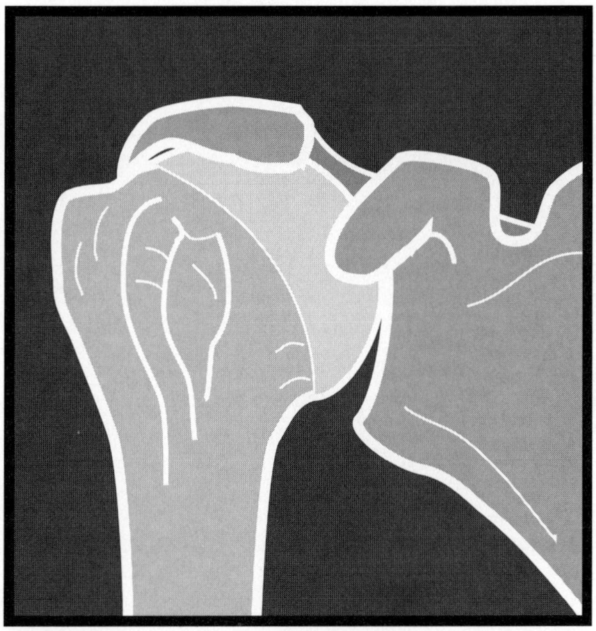

**Figure 18–50. Acromiohumeral contact**
If radiographs indicate contact between the humeral head and the acromion, the superior rotator cuff must be deficient.

# SURGICAL CONSIDERATIONS

## Principles of Rotator Cuff Surgery

The priorities in treating disorders of the rotator cuff are as follows:

1. Preserve the deltoid. Thus, surgical approaches are conducted through either the superior deltoid-on approach (for subacromial smoothing, cuff curettage or cuff repair; see Chapters 19–22) or the deltopectoral approach (for humeral hemiarthroplasty for cuff tear arthropathy; see Chapter 23).
2. Ensure smoothness of the humeroscapular motion interface. Thus, the upper aspect of the humerus and cuff must present a smooth convexity to articulate with the concave undersurface of the coracoacromial arch. All hypertrophic bursa and excrescences of the tuberosities are removed, leaving a smooth proximal humeral convexity (**Fig. 18–51**). Sutures are placed so that the knots do not lie on the superior aspect of the cuff or tuberosity.
3. Maintain the normal mobility of the glenohumeral joint. Thus, limiting scar must be resolved and the cuff tendons must be released from the glenoid and coracoid before reattachment.
4. Ensure an even distribution of tension on the cuff insertion. Thus, differential tightness at the area of cuff repair is avoided.
5. Ensure that if cuff tendon reattachment is performed, it is sufficiently robust to heal and to allow early motion after surgery. Thus, multiple sutures securing the tendon edge into a bony trough are preferred. The trough excludes joint fluid from the repair site and allows for some slip of the tendon while maintaining tendon-to-bone contact (**Fig. 18–52**).

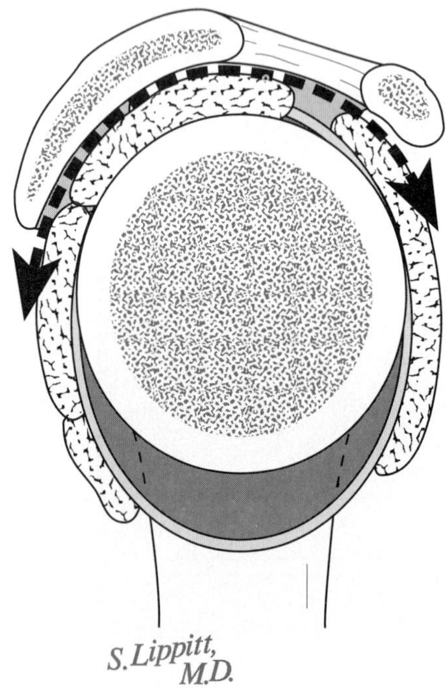


**Figure 18–51. Humeroscapular interface**
Smoothness of the humeroscapular motion interface is a critical goal of rotator cuff surgery. Most potential causes of roughness are on the humeral side of the interface: hypertrophic bursa, prominences of the tuberosities, rough cuff edges, sutures placed on the top of the tendon, and prominent suture anchors. The ideal repair technique leaves this interface smooth. (Modified from Rockwood CA, Matsen FA [eds]: The Shoulder, 2nd ed. Philadelphia: WB Saunders, 1998, p. 758.)

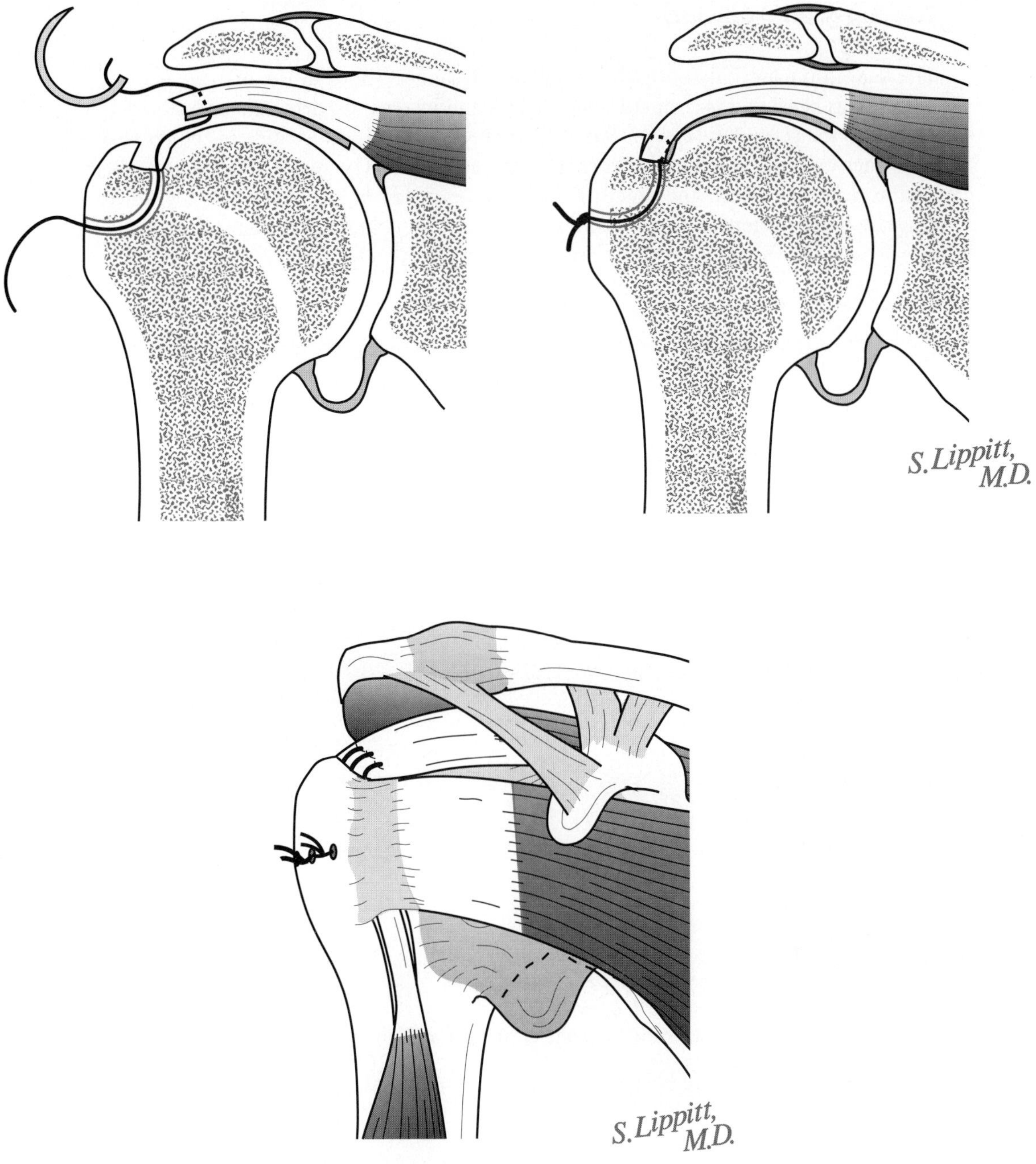


**Figure 18–52. Suturing to the trough for a smooth upper surface**
The cuff tendon is repaired into a trough in the tuberosity, tongue-in-groove style. This technique excludes joint fluid from the repair site and also allows the potential for some slip of the tendon without losing contact with the bone. Note the low placement of the knots on the lateral tuberosity so that they do not cause roughness in the humeroscapular motion interface.

## The Surgical Approach

The deltoid-on surgical approach has offered a major advance in the management of cuff lesions because it is cosmetic and efficient and involves no detachment of the deltoid from the acromion (**Fig. 18–53**). A 6 cm long skin incision is made in the normal skin lines over the anterolateral corner of the acromion. The major tendinous raphe of the deltoid between the anterior and middle thirds of the deltoid is identified (**Fig. 18–54**). This tendon is split, with half of it left on either side of the split to facili-

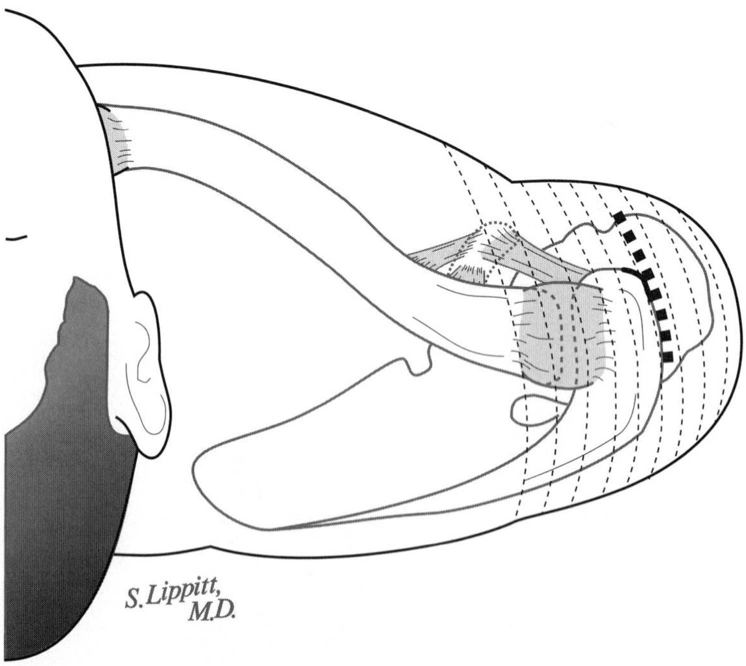


**Figure 18–53. Langer's line incision**
The skin incision is made in Langer's lines for an optimal cosmetic result after wound closure.

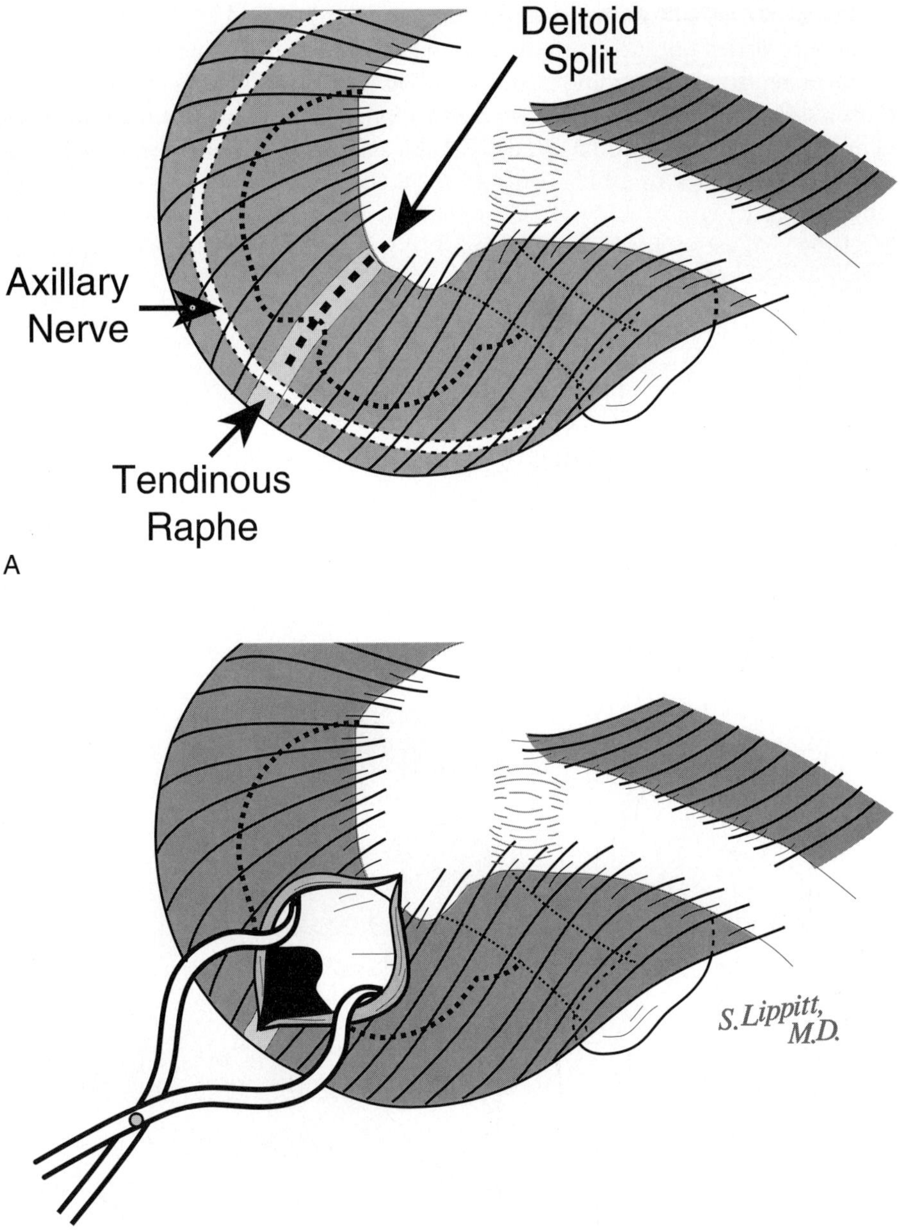


B

**Figure 18–54. Deltoid split**
The deltoid is split along the raphe between the anterior and middle thirds of the muscle without detaching any fibers from the acromion. (Modified from Matsen FA, Lippitt SB, Sidles JA, et al [eds]: Practical Evaluation and Management of the Shoulder. Philadelphia: WB Saunders, 1994, p. 135.)

tate the repair. The split is carried down through the bursa and to the cuff, where the procedure is carried out. Access to different parts of the cuff is achieved by rotation of the arm, rather than by extending the incision (**Fig. 18–55**). At the conclusion of the procedure, a side-to-side repair of the deltoid and a subcuticular closure of the skin are carried out, leaving an uncompromised deltoid and a cosmetic skin incision (**Fig. 18–56**).

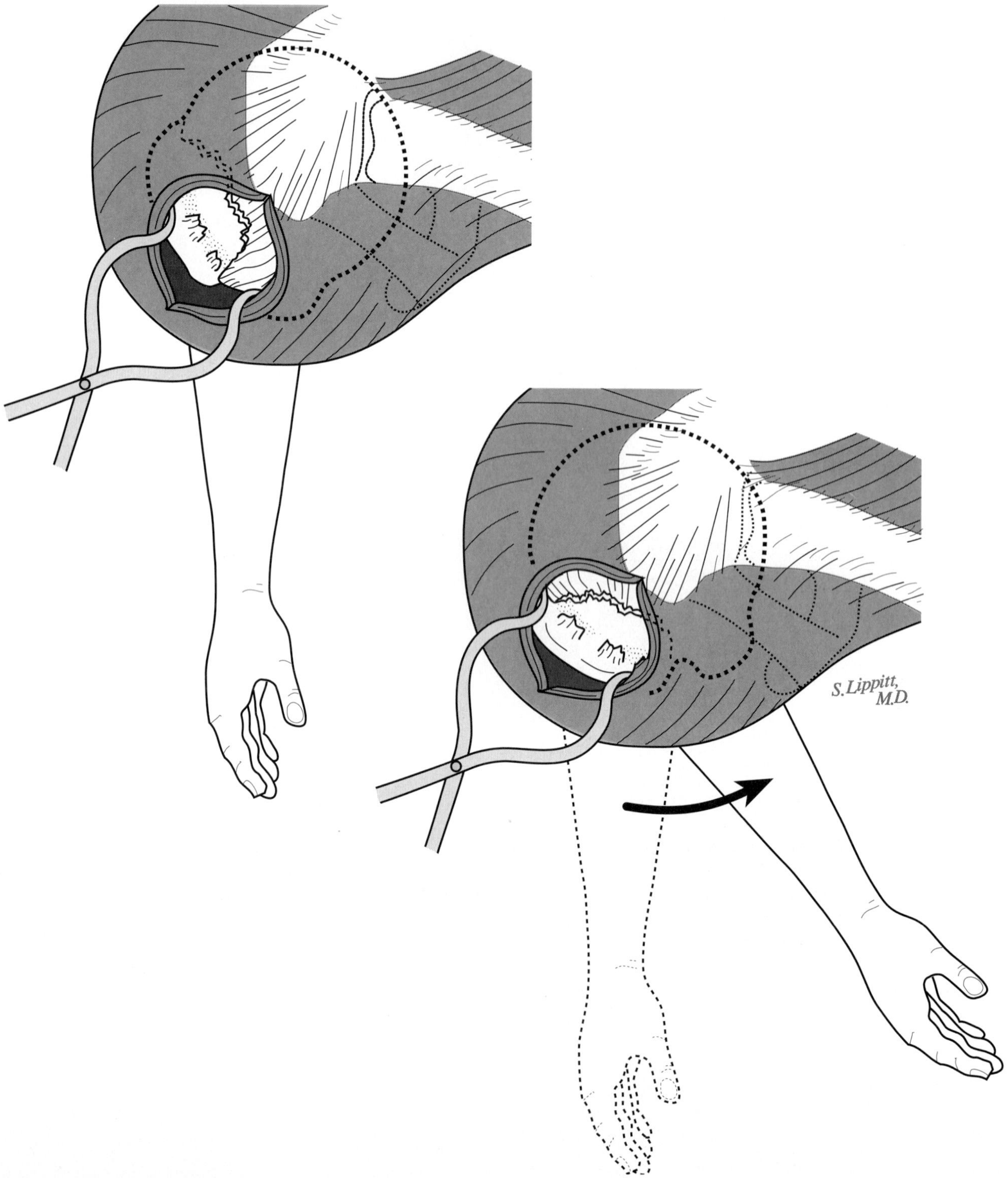


**Figure 18–55. View of cuff tear**
By rotating the arm, the different elements of the cuff can be brought to this split, rather than making a bigger exposure by detaching the deltoid origin.

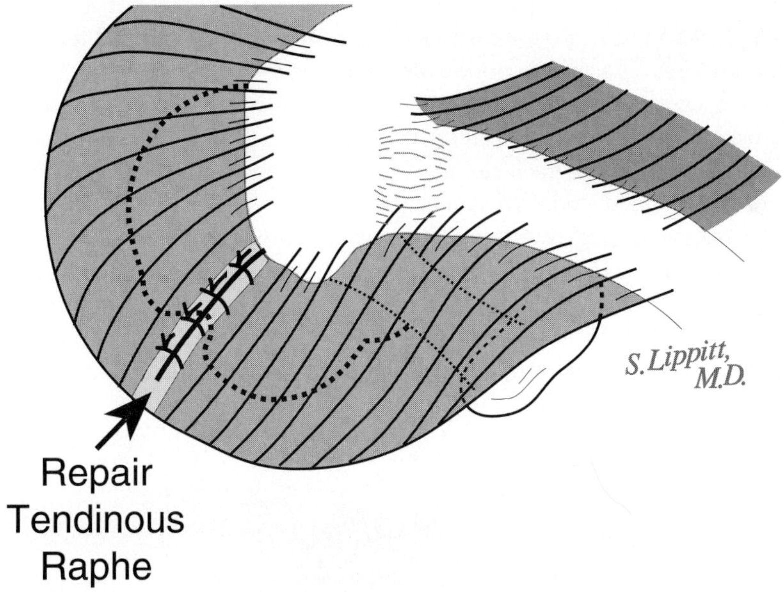


**Figure 18–56. Deltoid split repair**
The tendinous raphe of the deltoid split is repaired, ensuring that the knots are out of the humeroscapular motion interface and that they are not prominent subcutaneously. (Modified from Matsen FA, Lippitt SB, Sidles JA, et al [eds]: Practical Evaluation and Management of the Shoulder. Philadelphia: WB Saunders, 1994, p. 135.)

## Management of Partial-Thickness Tears

In the management of partial-thickness cuff tears, the first line of treatment is stretching the shoulder to eliminate any tightness of internal rotation with the arm at the side (**Fig. 18–57**), internal rotation of the arm in 90 degrees of abduction (**Fig. 18–58**), and cross-body adduction (**Fig. 18–59**). Often, as is the case with tennis elbow, progressive stretching exercises will eliminate the tightness and even out the distribution of force so that comfort and function are restored in the presence of a thinned tendon.

If symptoms are refractory to nonoperative management, consideration can be given to a surgical release of the insecurely attached fibers at the margin of the tear, a procedure we refer to as cuff curettage (see Chapter 19). This can be accomplished through a small deltoid split through which the location of the partial detachment can be confirmed by palpation of the thinned tendon. A small curette is inserted in the area of the detachment and used to release the weakly attached fibers around the periphery of the defect, leaving only the securely attached fibers to transmit the force of the muscle to bone. Since there is no deltoid detachment and no cuff repair, stretching and active use can be started immediately after surgery using the same exercises that were learned by the patient as a part of the nonoperative program described in the previous paragraph.

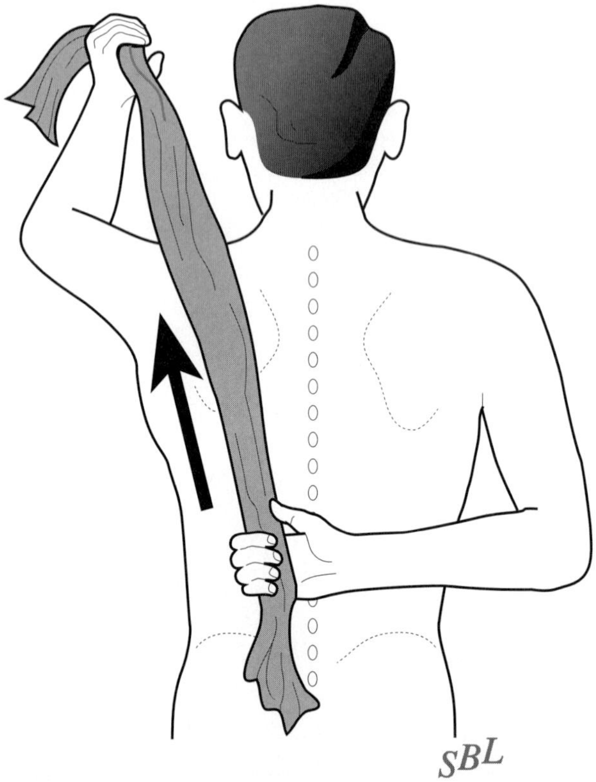


**Figure 18–57. Stretching the shoulder in internal rotation in abduction**
Internal rotation with the arm at the side can be stretched using a towel held in the hand of the sound arm to pull the hand of the involved arm up the back. (Modified from Matsen FA, Lippitt SB, Sidles JA, et al [eds]: Practical Evaluation and Management of the Shoulder. Philadelphia: WB Saunders, 1994, p. 48.)

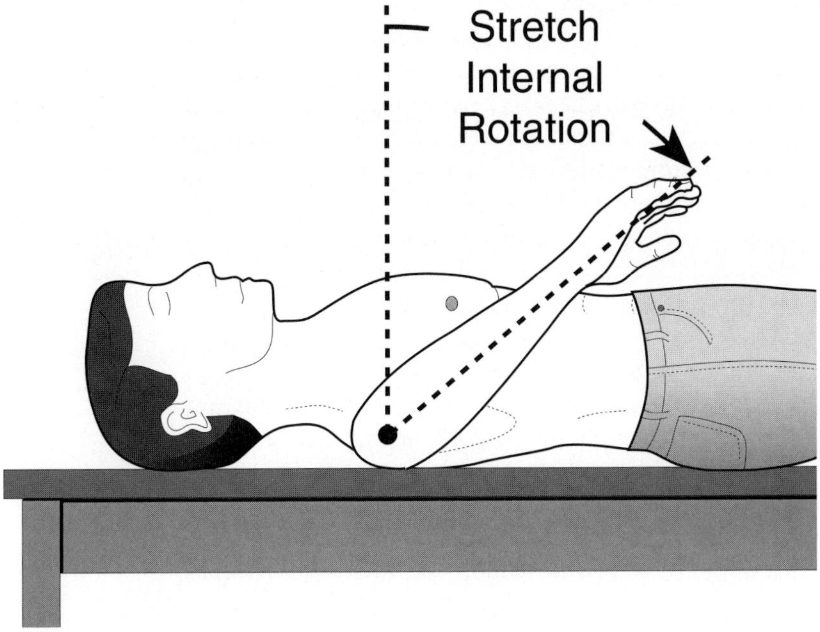


**Figure 18–58. Stretching the shoulder in internal rotation in abduction**
Internal rotation with the arm in abduction can be stretched while the patient lies supine with the arm supported in 90 degrees of abduction; the internal rotation force is gently applied by the patient using the other hand or by a friend. (Modified from Rockwood CA, Matsen FA [eds]: The Shoulder, 2nd ed. Philadelphia: WB Saunders, 1998, p. 1083.)

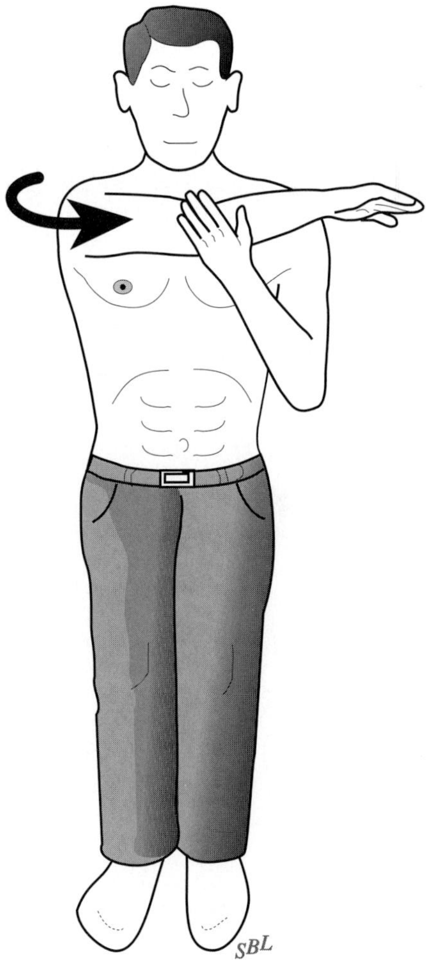


**Figure 18–59. Stretching the shoulder in cross-body movement**
Cross-body adduction can be stretched by drawing the involved arm across the chest using the sound arm. (Modified from Matsen FA, Lippitt SB, Sidles JA, et al [eds]: Practical Evaluation and Management of the Shoulder. Philadelphia: WB Saunders, 1994, p. 49.)

In all cuff surgery, an important goal is to ensure the smooth passage of the rotator cuff beneath the coracoacromial arch. Roughness can be detected at surgery by placing the fingers of one hand on the acromion while the arm is passively rotated throughout its range of motion with the other (**Fig. 18–60**). The positions productive of crepitance are noted and, before wound closure, relief of this crepitance is verified. The source of subacromial crepitance is usually some combination of bursal hypertrophy, roughness on the upper surface of the cuff, and roughness around the humeral tuberosities. While it is our surgical routine to palpate the undersurface of the coracoacromial arch for sources of roughness, the acromion and the coracoacromial ligament are almost always smooth. The presence of "spurs" may be suggested on preoperative radiographs, but these are usually only calcifications in the coracoacromial ligament and, as such, do not encroach on the free movement of the cuff beneath it (see Fig. 18–35).

Smoothness of the humeroscapular motion interface is assured by resecting any abnormal bursa or scar in this interface from the axillary nerve inferomedially, between the subscapularis and the coracoid muscles, under the acromion, and down to the axillary nerve posteroinferiorly: a complete nerve-to-nerve release (**Fig. 18–61**). Complete release of the external surface of the supraspinatus and infraspinatus can be verified by passing a smooth elevator between each tendon and the coracoacromial arch (**Fig. 18–62**).

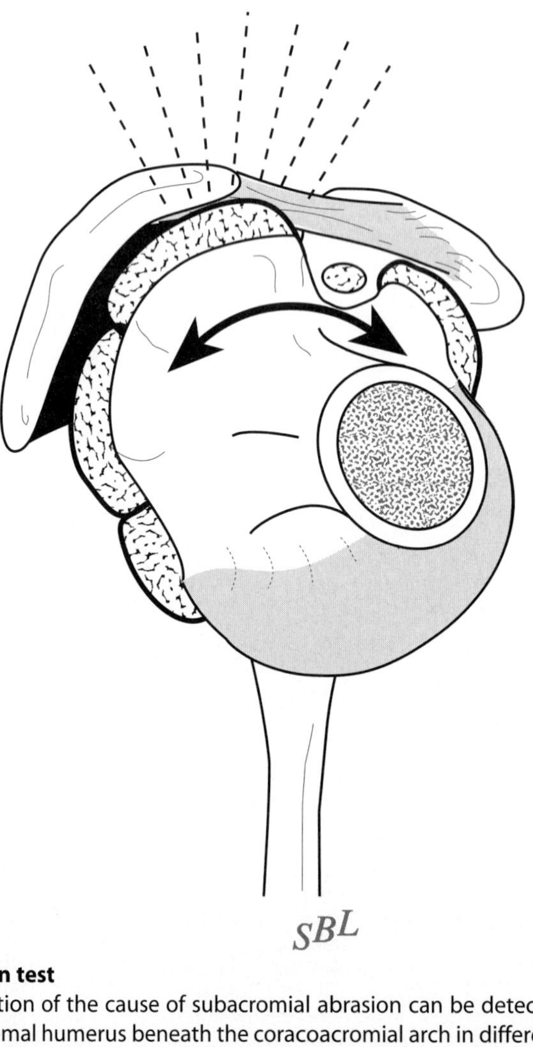


**Figure 18–60. Abrasion test**
The existence and location of the cause of subacromial abrasion can be detected at surgery by passively rotating the proximal humerus beneath the coracoacromial arch in different positions of flexion and abduction. The cause of the roughness is almost universally on the proximal humeral convexity rather than on the coracoacromial concavity. (Modified from Matsen FA, Lippitt SB, Sidles JA, et al [eds]: Practical Evaluation and Management of the Shoulder. Philadelphia: WB Saunders, 1994, p. 126.)

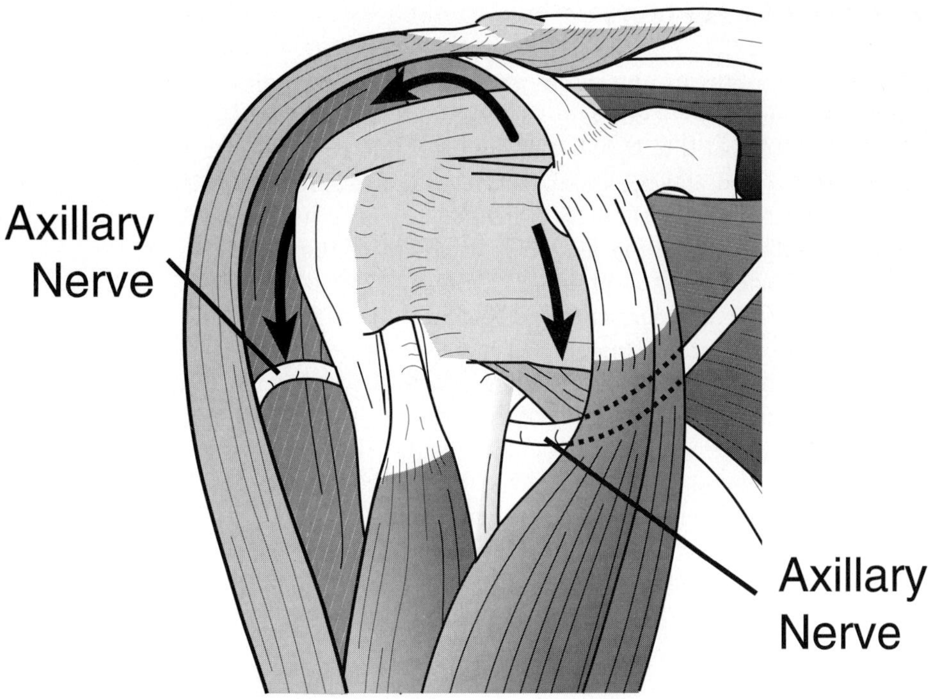


**Figure 18–61. Nerve-to-nerve release**
All scar tissue in the humeroscapular motion interface is released from the axillary nerve medially as it crosses the subscapularis, then under the coracoid, then under the coracoacromial ligament, then under the acromion, and then finally under the deltoid to the axillary nerve posteriorly as it exits the quadrilateral space: the nerve-to-nerve release.

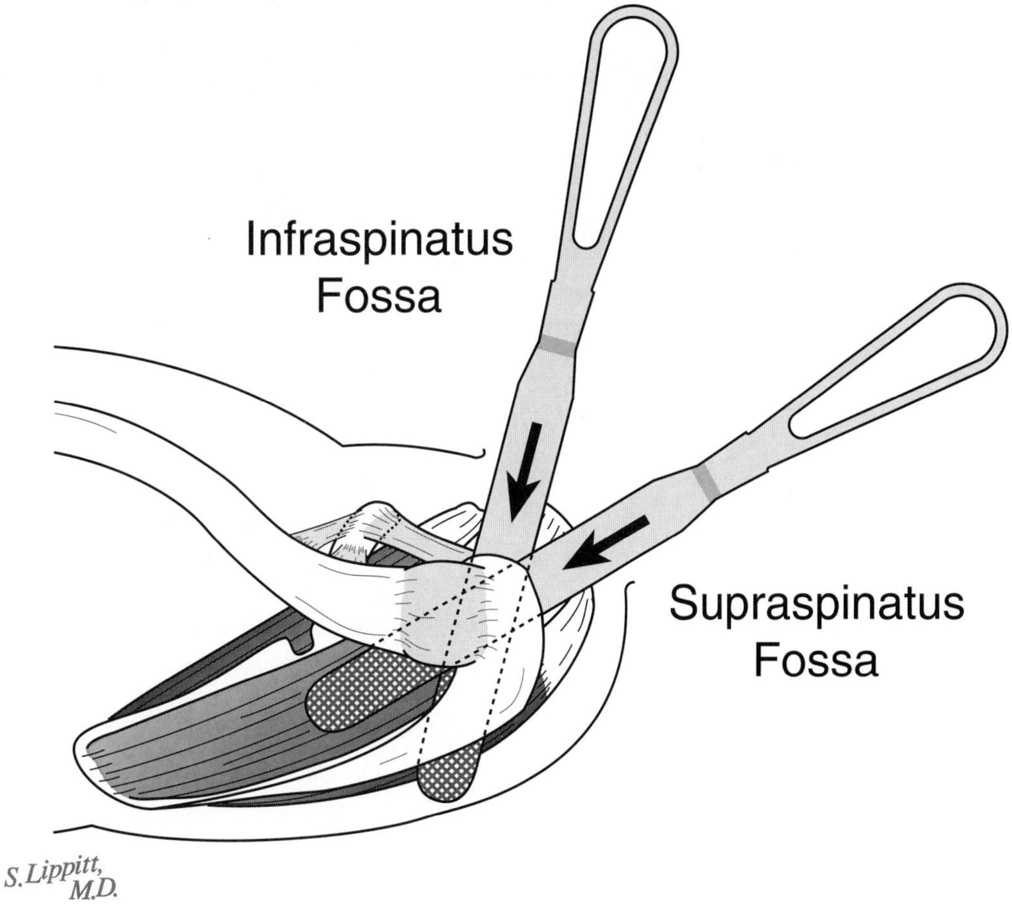


**Figure 18–62. Verifying complete release**
A smooth elevator is passed superficially to the supraspinatus and infraspinatus to ensure their freedom from the overlying coracoacromial arch.

## Management of Full-Thickness Tears

Full-thickness rotator cuff tears are treated by secure reattachment to bone, provided there is sufficient quantity and quality of tendon for a robust attachment with the arm at the side (see Chapter 21). The goal is to have a smooth distribution of load that is continuous across both the repaired and the intact tendon so that disproportionate force concentration on the repair is avoided. Because there is often a loss of tendon substance, repair to bone relatively shortens the tendon. The ability of the muscle to be extended laterally to compensate for this shortening is limited by (1) the attachment of the capsule to the tendon on one hand and to the glenoid labrum on the other and (2) the attachment of the coracohumeral ligament to the tendon of the supraspinatus and subscapularis laterally and the coracoid medially. Thus, unless the tear is acute, it is usually necessary to release the coracohumeral ligament from the coracoid **(Fig. 18–63)** and to release the capsule from its attachment to the glenoid labrum **(Fig. 18–64)** so that the muscle and tendon can be drawn out further laterally to the insertion. Without such releases, the repair may be under undue tension and at risk for failure. After the releases have been performed and after any scar has been dissected from the humeroscapular motion interface, traction sutures are placed in the tendon edge. If good-quality tendon can be brought close to its normal insertion site with the arm in adduction, a robust repair can be carried out.

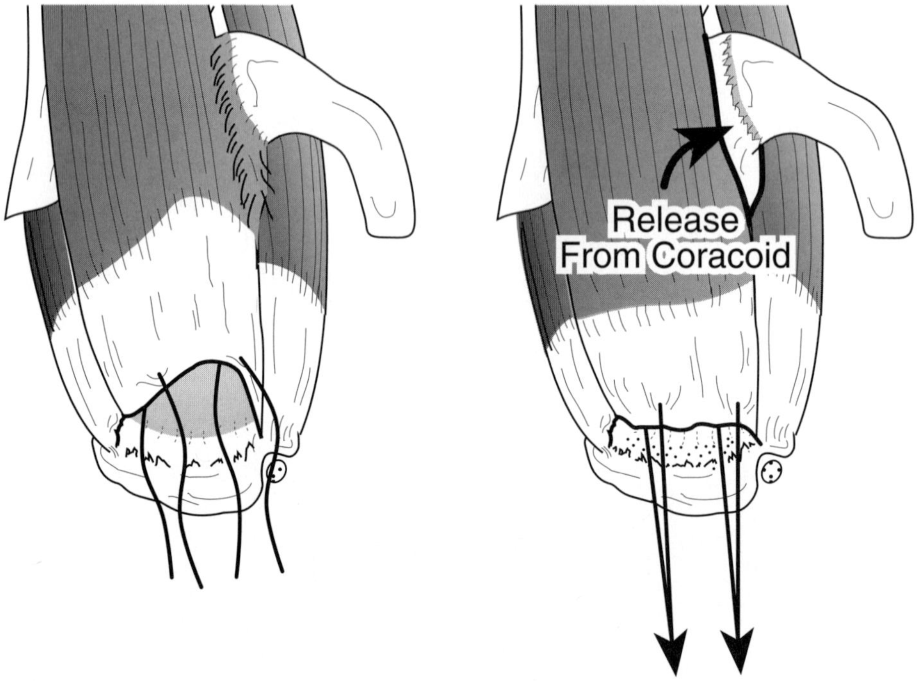


**Figure 18–63. Release from coracoid**
Release of the cuff tendon from the coracoid allows lateral advancement of the tendon edge toward the desired insertion site. (Modified from Matsen FA, Lippitt SB, Sidles JA, et al [eds]: Practical Evaluation and Management of the Shoulder. Philadelphia: WB Saunders, 1994, p. 138.)

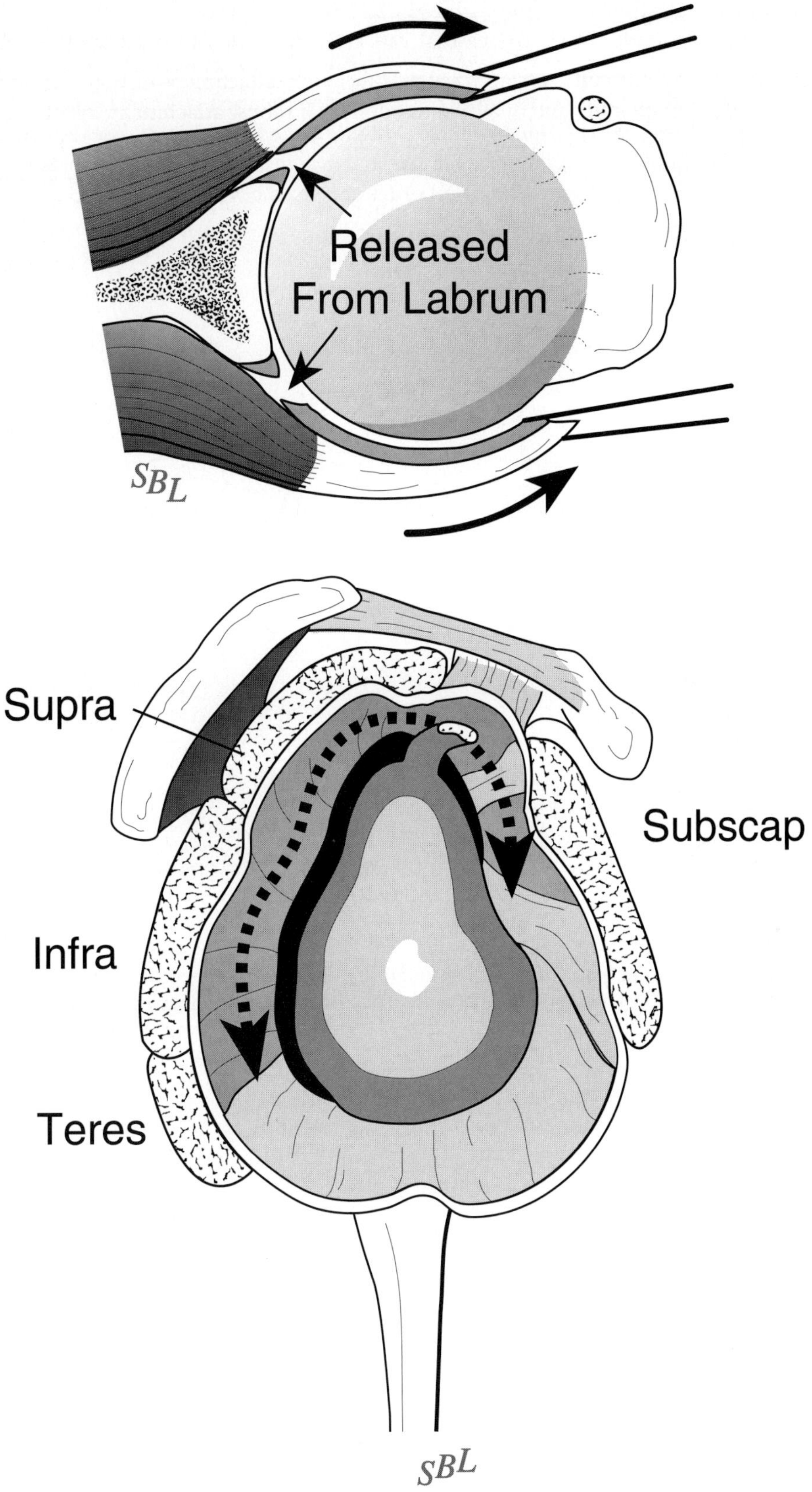


**Figure 18–64. Release from labrum**

Release of the capsule from the labrum allows further lateral advancement of the tendon edge. (Modified from Matsen FA, Lippitt SB, Sidles JA, et al [eds]: Practical Evaluation and Management of the Shoulder. Philadelphia: WB Saunders, 1994, p. 138.)

The ideal reattachment technique has the following properties:

1. It yields a smooth upper surface that can articulate congruously with the intact undersurface of the coracoacromial arch (**Fig. 18–65,** and see Fig. 18–52) and avoids knots or tendon edges on the upper aspect of the repaired cuff, where they could rub under the coracoacromial arch (**Fig. 18–66**).
2. It excludes joint fluid from the repair site and accommodates some slippage in the sutures and knots without separation of tendon from bone (see Fig. 18–52).

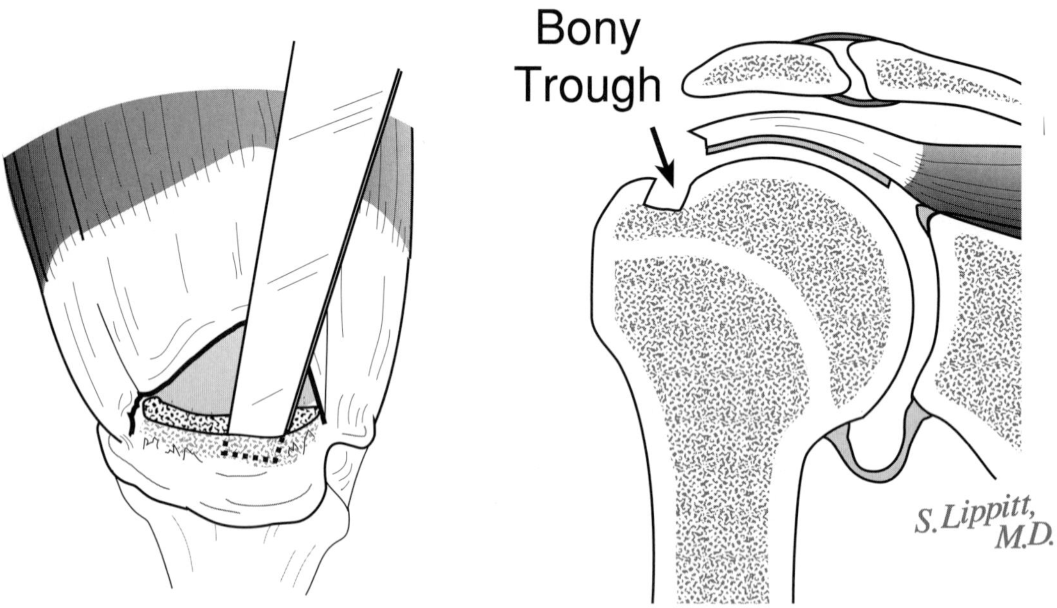


**Figure 18–65. Bony trough**

A bony trough is made at the base of the greater tuberosity, just lateral to the articular surface. The trough extends the full length of the tendon detachment. (Modified from Matsen FA, Lippitt SB, Sidles JA, et al [eds]: Practical Evaluation and Management of the Shoulder. Philadelphia: WB Saunders, 1994, p. 139.)

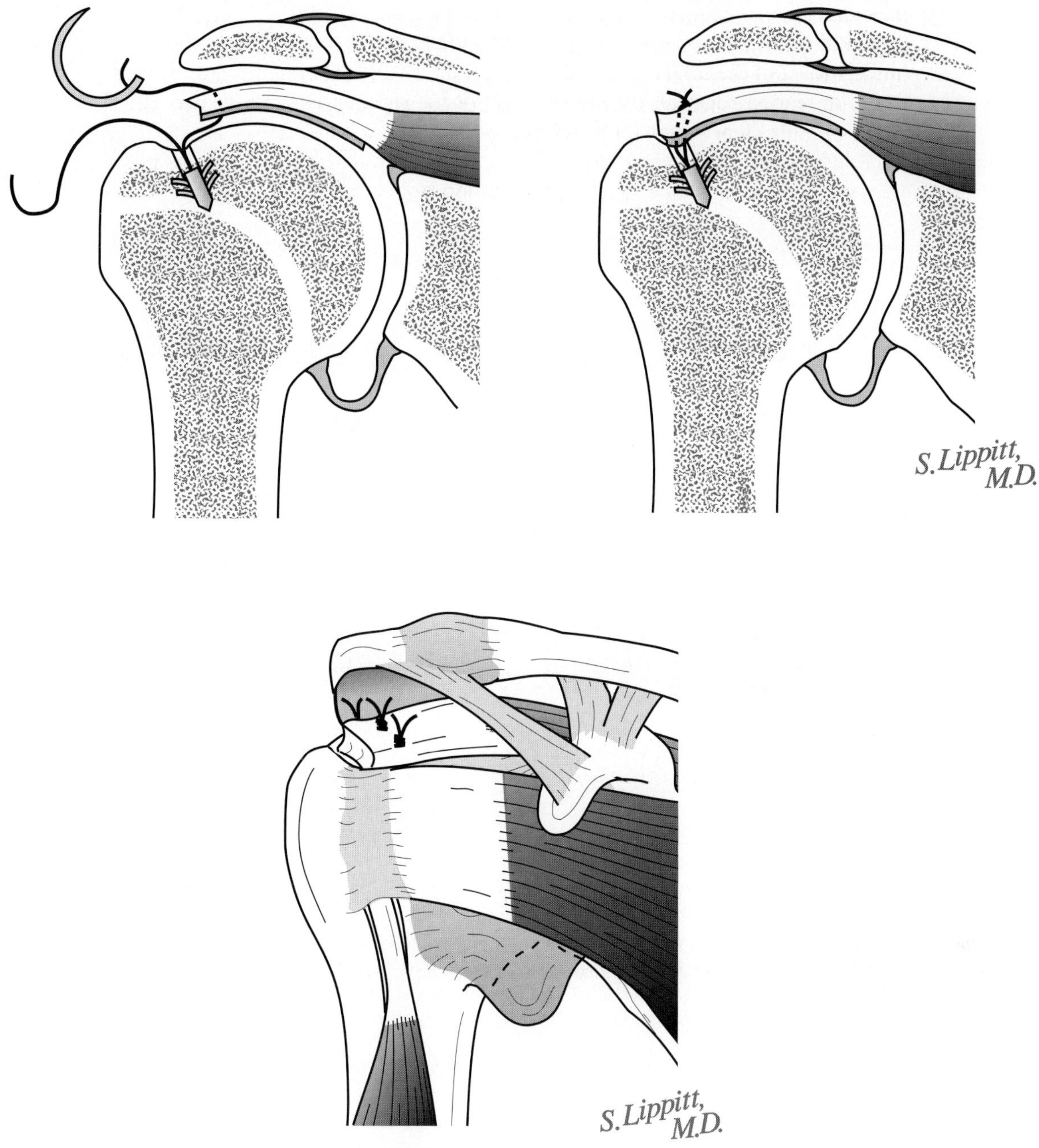


**Figure 18–66. Repairs with a rough upper surface**
Surgical techniques that attach the tendon on to (rather than in to) the humerus leave a tendon edge that can catch on the coracoacromial arch. Techniques that leave suture knots on the upper surface of the tendon position these knots so that they can catch on the coracoacromial arch.

3. It creates a secure isometric junction between the tendon and bone, spreading the load among numerous sutures (**Figs. 18–67** and **18–68**).
4. It can accommodate weakened bone at the greater tuberosity (**Fig. 18–69**).
5. It can be accomplished without sacrificing acromion, the acromioclavicular joint, or the deltoid origin (see Fig. 18–19).

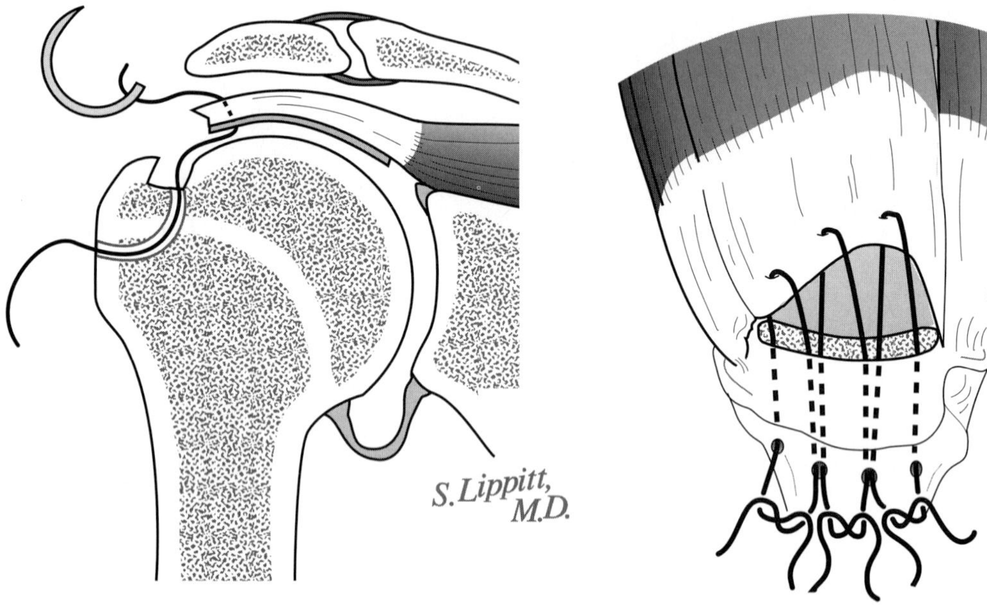


**Figure 18–67. Placement of sutures**
Multiple, closely placed sutures distribute the load of reattachment broadly across the tendon and bone. Three such sutures are shown in this figure; twice this number would be used to repair a cuff defect this size. The sutures are placed far enough medially so that they gain purchase in solid tissue. These sutures incorporate the full thickness of the tendon along with the capsule on its deep surface. As each suture is placed, the security of its "bite" in the tendon is verified. (Modified from Matsen FA, Lippitt SB, Sidles JA, et al [eds]: Practical Evaluation and Management of the Shoulder. Philadelphia: WB Saunders, 1994, p. 139.)

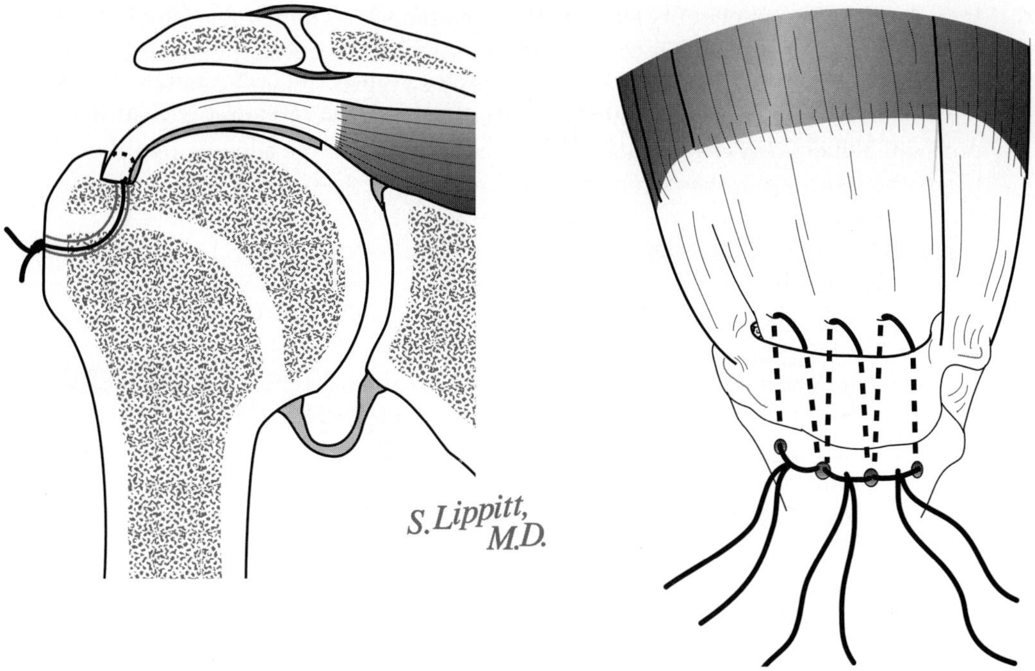


**Figure 18–68. Tying the sutures**

Tying these sutures reapproximates the tendon into the bone with good load distribution and a smooth upper surface to articulate with the coracoacromial arch. Only three sutures are shown in this figure, although twice this number would be used for a tear of this size. (Modified from Matsen FA, Lippitt SB, Sidles JA, et al [eds]: Practical Evaluation and Management of the Shoulder. Philadelphia: WB Saunders, 1994, p. 138.)

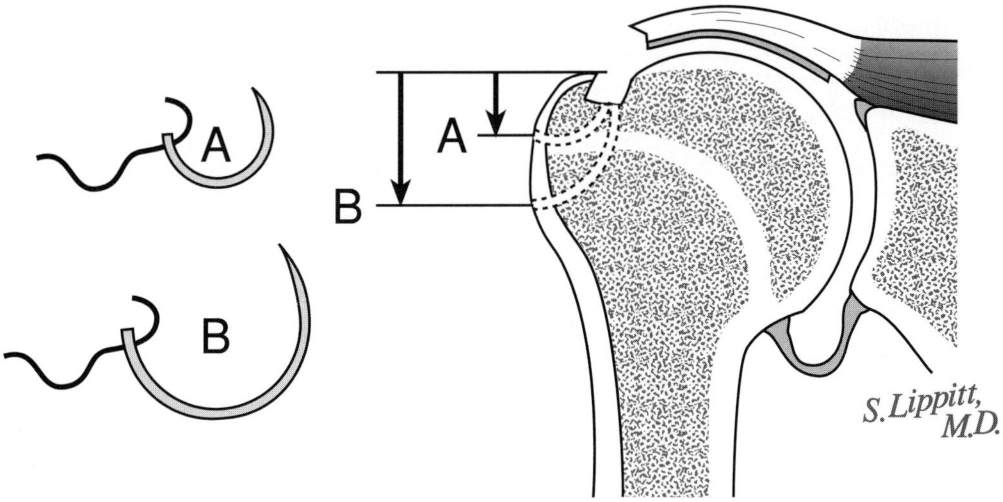


**Figure 18–69. Suturing to adequate bone**

If the bone near the edge of the trough is weak, sutures can be passed more distally through denser cortical bone.

If there is insufficient quantity and quality of tendon to reach the tuberosity with the arm at the side, consideration can be given to moving the insertion site up to 1 cm medially on the humeral articular surface. If a robust repair cannot be performed, the priority shifts from repair to achieving the smoothest possible upper aspect of the proximal humerus for articulating with the undersurface of the coracoacromial arch. Often the head is translated superiorly because of the loss of the spacer effect of the superior cuff tendon and secondary erosion of the superior glenoid lip (see Fig. 18–34). This situation may call for smoothing of the upper aspect of the residual cuff as well as recession of the tuberosities if they are prominent, so that the surface presented by the proximal humerus to the coracoacromial arch is smooth. We refer to this as a "smooth and move," the goal of which is to convert the upper aspect of the proximal humerus into a smooth convexity that articulates congruously with the concave undersurface of the coracoacromial arch (see Chapters 20 and 22). Because the procedure is performed through a deltoid-on approach, no postoperative restrictions are placed so that the patient can move the joint actively immediately after surgery. We have found that when the cuff will not reach to a reasonable insertion site, abducting the shoulder so that repair can be achieved (**Fig. 18–70**) and then "protecting" the arm in an abduction pillow (**Fig. 18–71**) tends to lead to cuff insertion failure once the arm is returned to the patient's side.

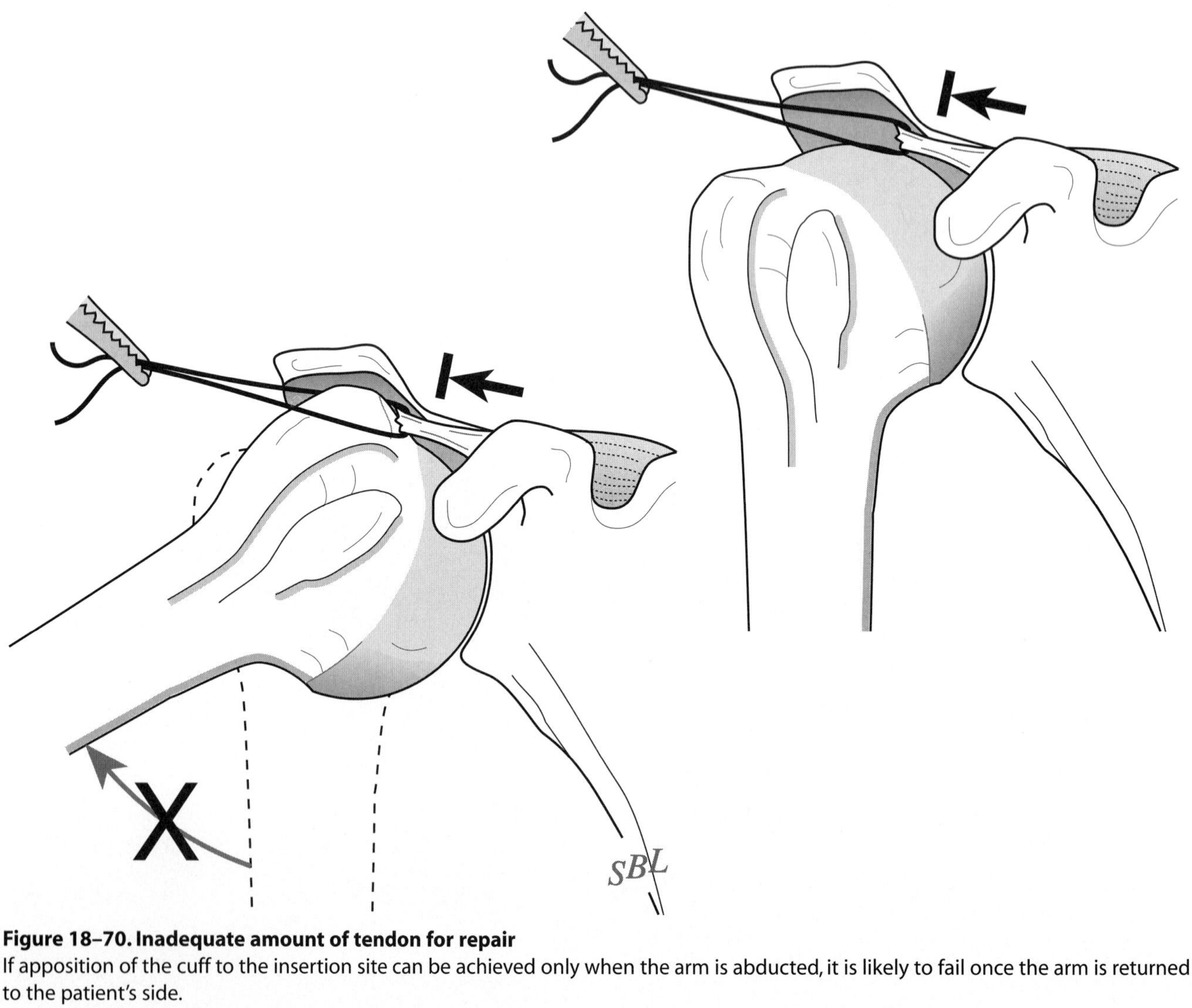


**Figure 18–70. Inadequate amount of tendon for repair**
If apposition of the cuff to the insertion site can be achieved only when the arm is abducted, it is likely to fail once the arm is returned to the patient's side.

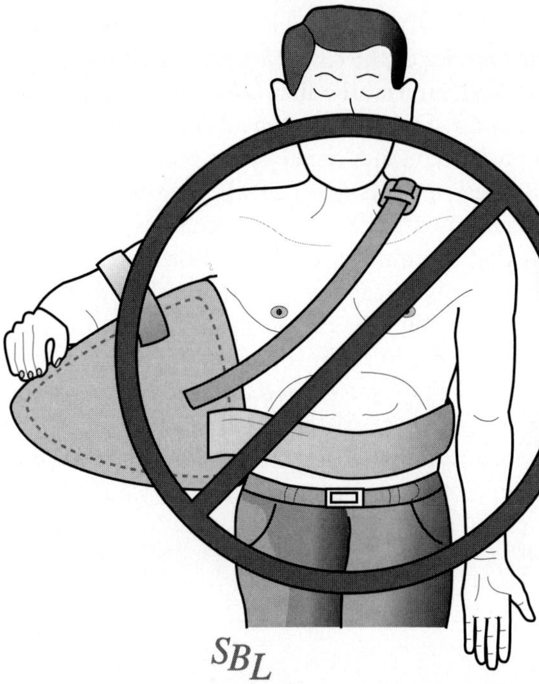

**Figure 18–71. Abduction pillow—potential problems**
An abduction pillow cannot prevent tension in the cuff repair. In fact, some patients actively abduct their shoulder to move the pillow around. Once the pillow is removed, the tendon is placed under tension, which may rupture the repair.

In cuff tear arthropathy, there is an irreparable cuff lesion and substantial roughness of the humeral articular surface (see Fig. 18–37). In this circumstance, a prosthetic hemiarthroplasty can be considered. In this procedure, an anatomically restored humeral articular surface articulates with the undersurface of the coracoacromial arch and the eroded upper glenoid (**Fig. 18–72**). This procedure is described in the section on glenohumeral smoothness (see Chapter 27).

In that smoothness of the articulation between the upper aspect of the proximal humerus and the undersurface of the coracoacromial arch is essential for a good clinical result after rotator cuff surgery, the final surgical step prior to closure is to once more check that there is no crepitance on movement of the upper humerus beneath the coracoacromial arch. If crepitance remains, it is pursued until smooth subacromial motion is ensured. Because the repair process begins immediately after surgery, we wish to give the repairing tissues the desired mechanical signals as soon as possible after the surgery. By using continuous passive motion starting in the recovery room, we inform the cells in the humeroscapular motion interface that smoothness is desired throughout this articulation (**Fig. 18–73**). By ensuring that the motion is limited to passive flexion and external rotation after rotator cuff repair, we avoid undue stress on the cuff attachment, informing the repairing cells that a robust reconnection is desired. Patients understand that stem cells are stimulated in a healing environment and easily comprehend that the correct mechanical signals will enable some stem cells to become "sliders" (i.e., in the humeroscapular motion interface) while others differentiate into "stickers" (i.e., at the site of cuff repair).

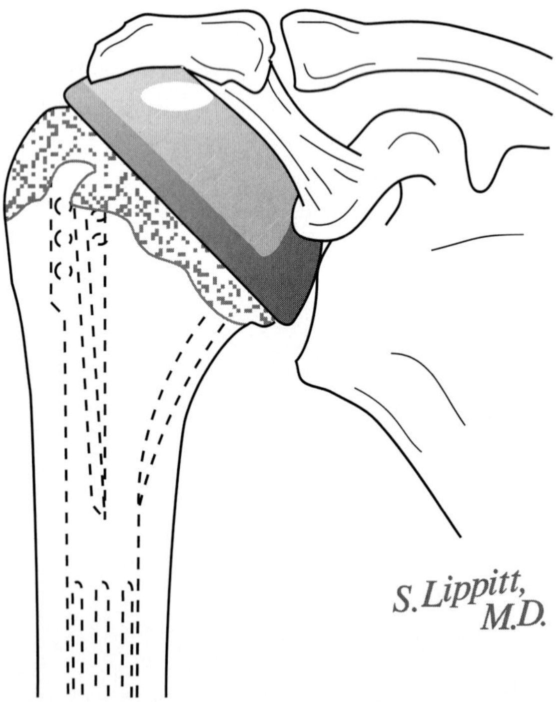


**Figure 18–72. Humeral hemiarthroplasty for cuff tear arthropathy**
In cuff tear arthropathy, provided the coracoacromial arch is intact, the humeroscapular articulation can be resurfaced with a humeral hemiarthroplasty that articulates with the concavity formed by the erosion of the coracoacromial arch and upper glenoid.

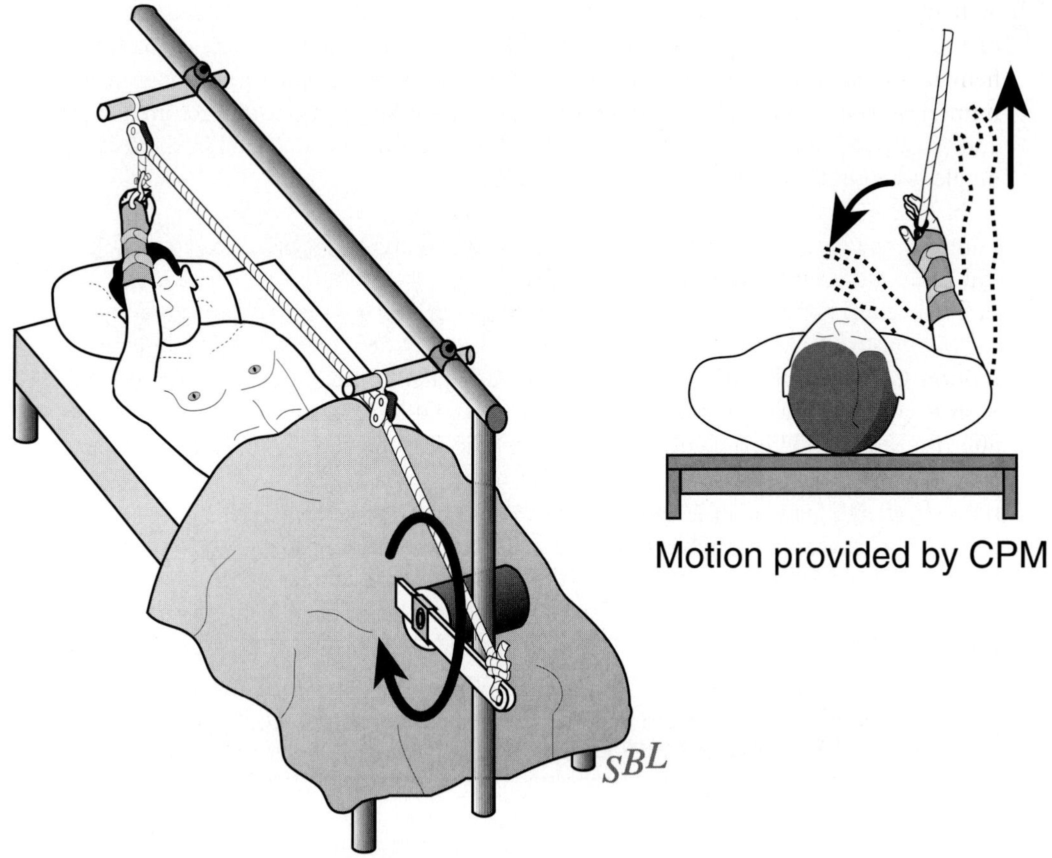


**Figure 18–73. Continuous passive motion**

Continuous passive motion used for the first 36 hours after rotator cuff surgery helps ensure that the healing in the humeroscapular motion interface proceeds in a way that yields smooth articulating surfaces rather than adhesions that can develop rapidly if the shoulder is immobilized during the early healing response after surgery. Continuous passive motion provides mechanical signals to the healing cells, differentiating those that are to heal the tendon to the bone from those that are to facilitate sliding of the cuff surface on the undersurface of the coracoacromial arch. (Modified from Matsen FA, Lippitt SB, Sidles JA, et al [eds]: Practical Evaluation and Management of the Shoulder. Philadelphia: WB Saunders, 1994, p. 50.)

CHAPTER 19

# Procedure: Cuff Curettage

***Diagnosis***

***Partial-thickness cuff tear involving the deep surface of the anterior supraspinatus near the tuberosity and the bicipital groove  ICD9 CODE 726.1***

***Procedure***

***Rotator cuff exploration, lysis of adhesions, resection of bursal tissue, curettage of partial-thickness cuff tear  CPT CODE 23405 or 23130***

## INDICATIONS

The patient has functionally significant pain on elevation of the shoulder. The symptoms have not responded to a program of stretching exercises even though the range of motion is now full. The shoulder continues to manifest a positive supraspinatus tendon sign, that is, pain on active isometric elevation in the plane of the scapula at 90 degrees of elevation while the arm is in slight internal rotation. There is minimal atrophy of the supraspinatus and a slight local depression in the tendon near its insertion.

Cuff imaging tests reveal thinning of the supraspinatus tendon due to a partial-thickness deep surface tear near its anterior insertion without retraction of the tendon.

Knowing the alternatives as well as the risks of infection, neurovascular injury, excessive stiffness, pain, weakness, irreparability, re-rupture, and the need for revision surgery, as well as complications related to anesthesia, the patient desires to proceed with rotator cuff surgery. The patient understands that this surgery will probably consist of curetting the cuff lesion so that its tenuous attachments are released, but could also possibly include a rotator cuff repair if the tear is essentially full thickness and if the cuff tendons are of sufficient quantity and quality, and possibly include a smooth-and-move procedure without repair if a large irreparable cuff lesion is encountered. The patient recognizes that the goal of this procedure is to release weakly attached tendon fibers and understands that it cannot be expected to completely restore normal comfort and function to the shoulder. And, lastly, the patient understands his or her critical role in the postsurgical rehabilitation.

## FINDINGS

Examination under anesthesia reveals a slightly diminished range of motion and a slight palpable thinning of the cuff near the supraspinatus insertion to the greater tuberosity.

Surgical findings include mild scarring in the humeroscapular motion interface as well as bursal thickening. There is a partial-thickness, deep surface defect involving the anterior supraspinatus tendon. The other aspects of the cuff tendons are of good quality and the long head of the biceps and the subscapularis are intact. The undersurface of the coracoacromial arch is smooth.

## OPERATION

Under satisfactory anesthesia, the patient is placed in a low beach chair position. The entire forequarter is carefully prepped and draped in the usual sterile fashion with the arm free to be moved (**Fig. 19–1**).

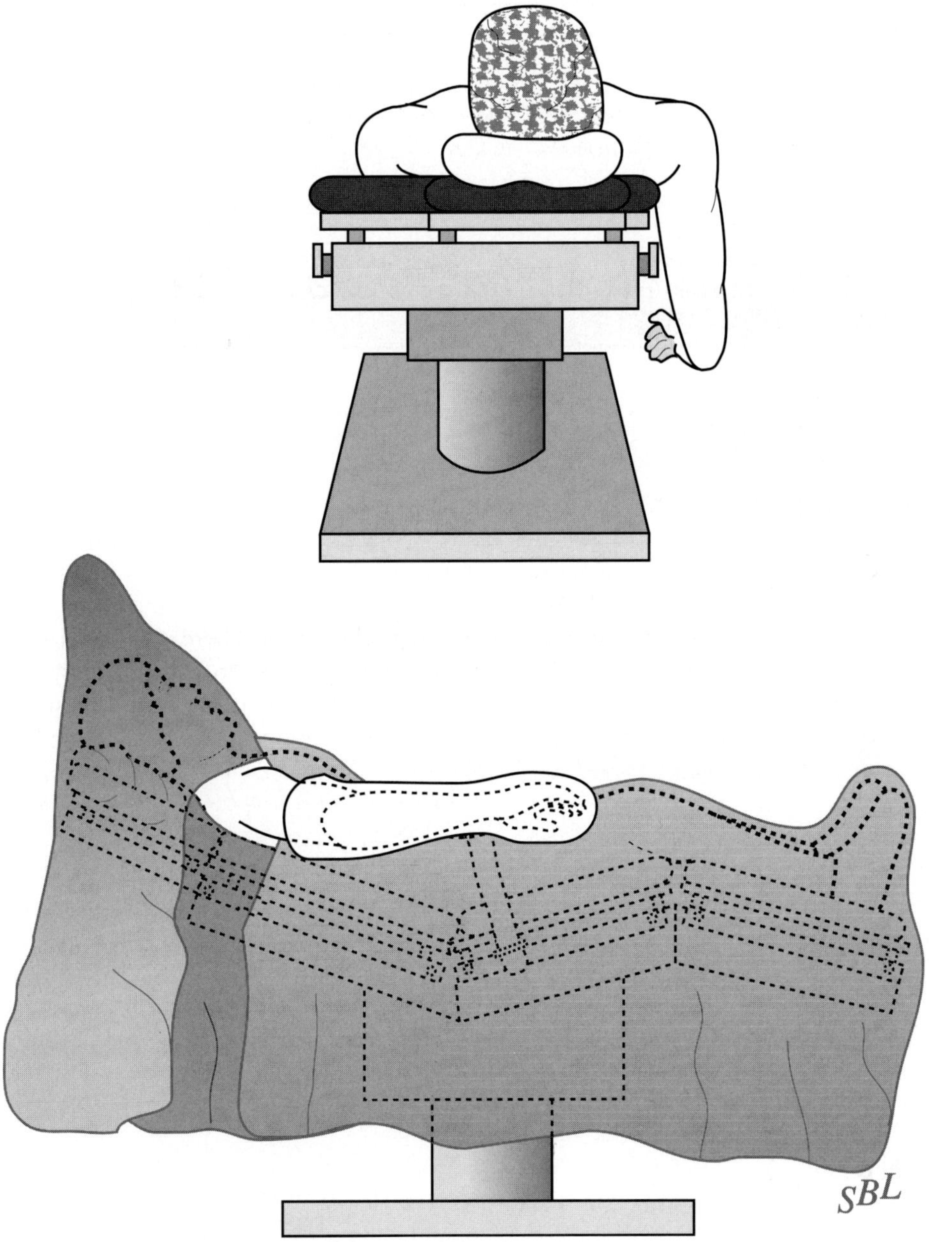


**Figure 19–1. Positioning and draping the shoulder**
The patient is placed in beach chair position with the arm draped free. Note that the patient is positioned with the glenohumeral joint at the edge of the table so that the arm can be moved through a full range of motion.

The shoulder is approached through a superior incision in the skin line crossing the anterior corner of the acromion (**Fig. 19–2**). The deltoid-on approach is used (**Fig. 19–3**). The deltoid tendon of origin running between the anterior and lateral thirds of the deltoid is identified and split longitudinally, leaving half of the tendon on either side of the split; no deltoid is detached from the acromion. This split is carried down to the subdeltoid bursa, which is divided in line with the deltoid split (**Fig. 19–4**). The total length of the deltoid split is limited to 4 cm from the acromion.

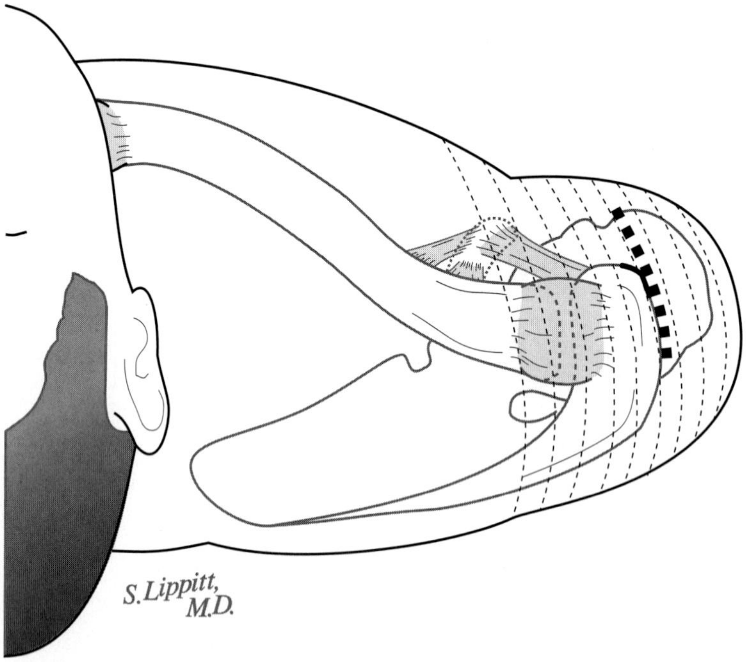


**Figure 19–2. Deltoid-on approach**
The deltoid-on approach, showing the skin incision in Langer's lines.

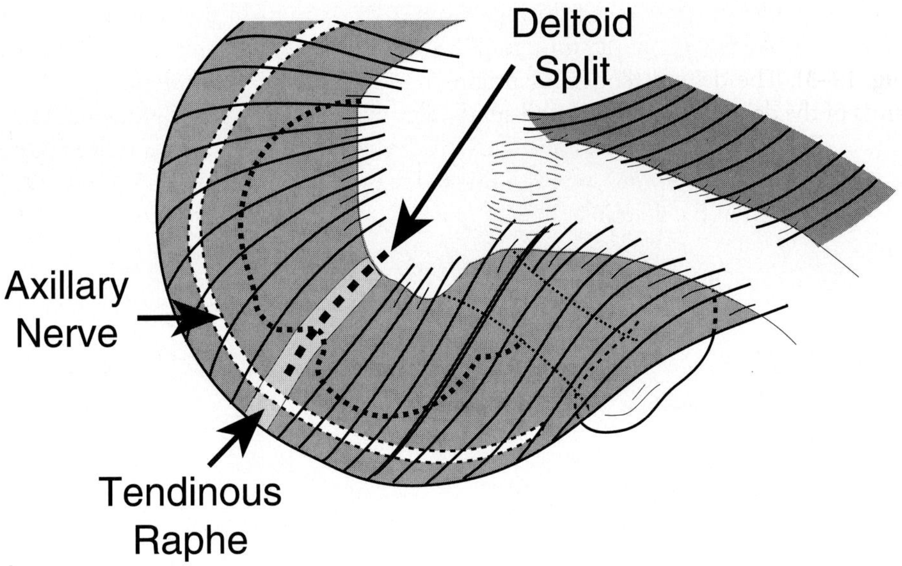


A

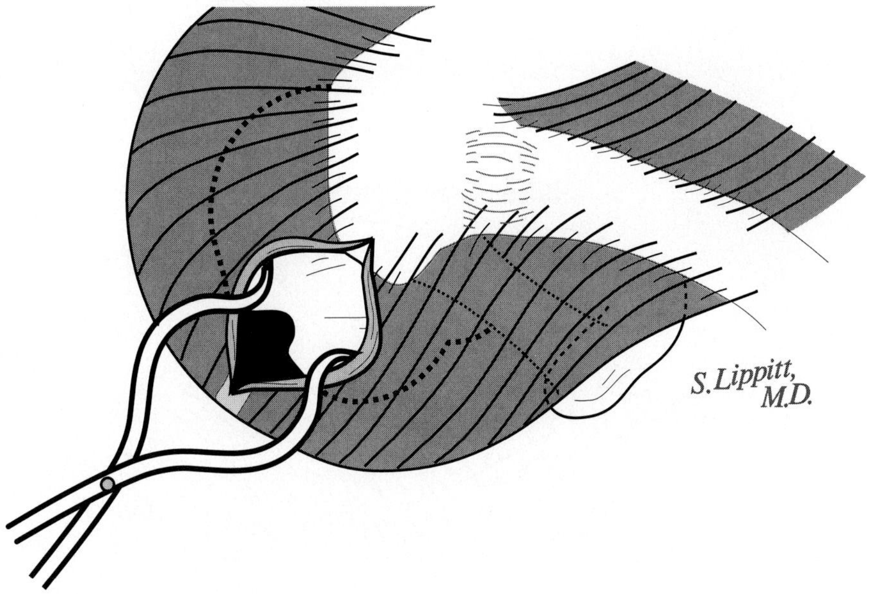


B

**Figure 19–3. Deltoid split**

The deltoid is split along the raphe between the anterior and lateral thirds of the muscle without detaching any of it from the acromion. (Modified from Matsen FA, Lippitt SB, Sidles JA, et al [eds]: Practical Evaluation and Management of the Shoulder. Philadelphia: WB Saunders, 1994, p. 135.)

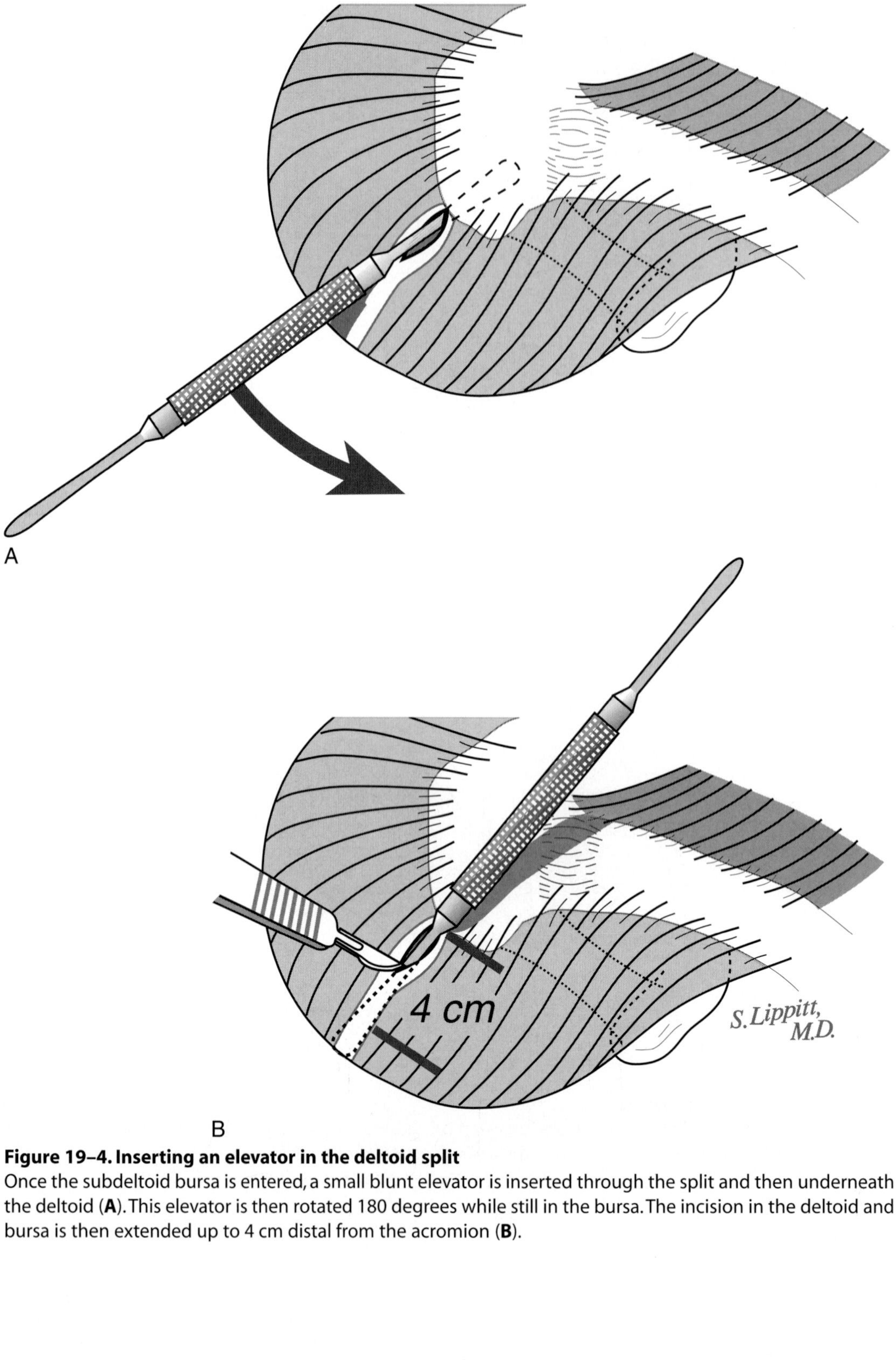


**Figure 19–4. Inserting an elevator in the deltoid split**
Once the subdeltoid bursa is entered, a small blunt elevator is inserted through the split and then underneath the deltoid (**A**). This elevator is then rotated 180 degrees while still in the bursa. The incision in the deltoid and bursa is then extended up to 4 cm distal from the acromion (**B**).

The humeroscapular motion interface is mobilized by blunt finger dissection. A small, self-retaining retractor is inserted into the split. The hypertrophic bursa is dissected from the surface of the rotator cuff. The humeroscapular motion interface is mobilized beneath the coracoid muscles until the axillary nerve can be palpated medially on the front of the subscapularis. The interface is dissected laterally until the axillary nerve can be palpated laterally as it exits the quadrilateral space (**Fig. 19–5**).

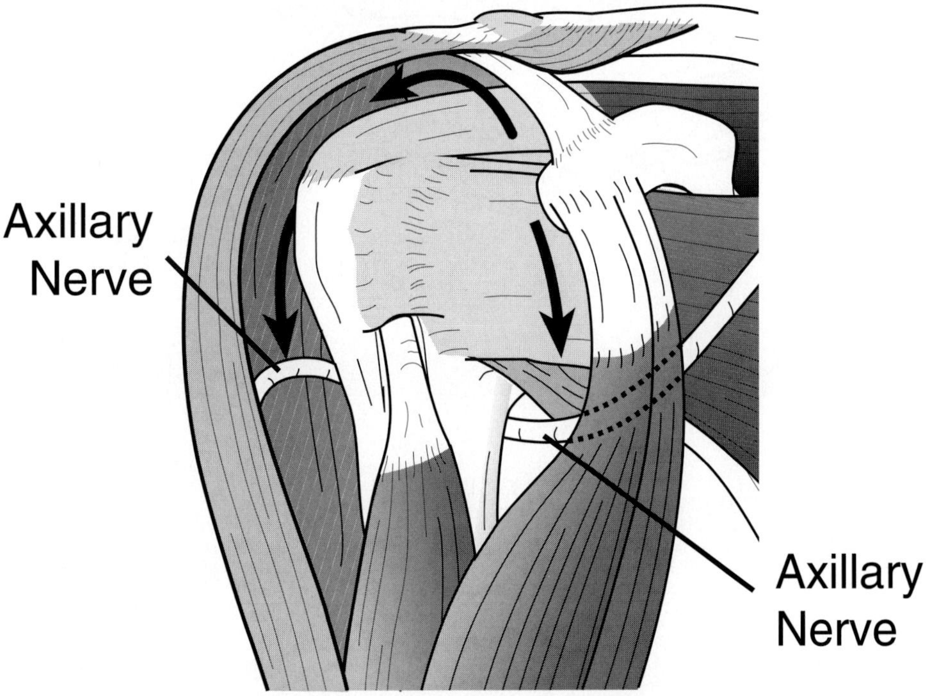


**Figure 19–5. Nerve-to-nerve release**
All scar tissue in the humeroscapular motion interface is released from the axillary nerve medially as it crosses the subscapularis, then under the coracoid, then under the coracoacromial ligament, then under the acromion, and then finally under the deltoid to the axillary nerve posteriorly as it exits the quadrilateral space: the nerve-to-nerve release.

The thickened subacromial/subdeltoid bursa is excised (**Fig. 19–6**). This dissection provides excellent exposure of the rotator cuff. The thinned area of the cuff can be identified by palpation, even though the bursal side of the tendon is intact (**Fig. 19–7**).

A small 000 curette is inserted through the thinnest part of the cuff without making a cuff incision (**Fig. 19–8**). The curette is felt to scrape against the uncovered bone from where cuff has been torn. This area is curetted from the anterior to the posterior

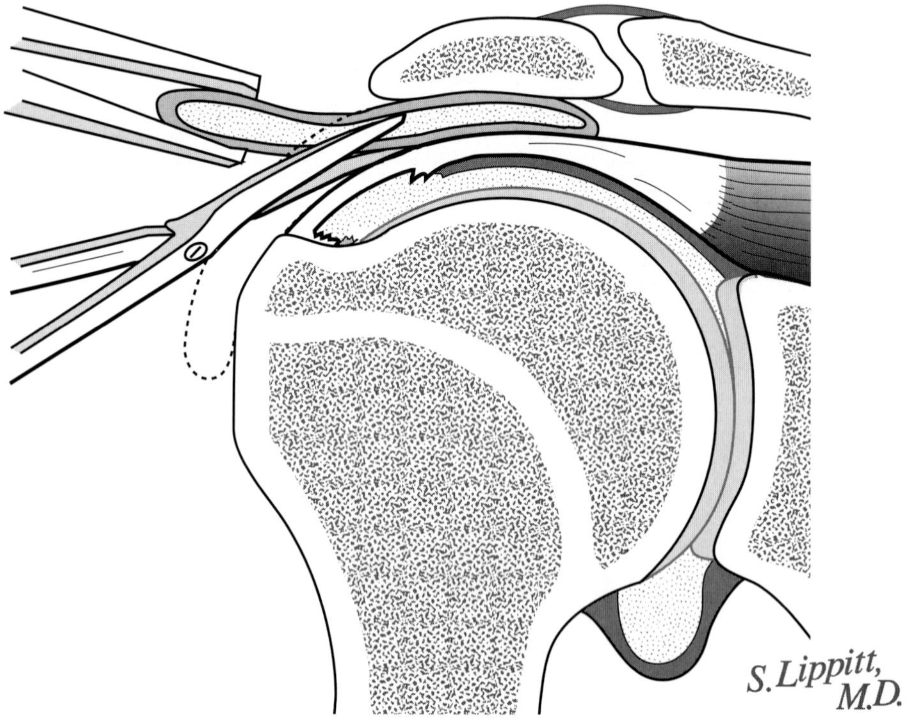


**Figure 19–6. Removing the bursa**
The hypertrophic bursa is removed by sharp dissection.

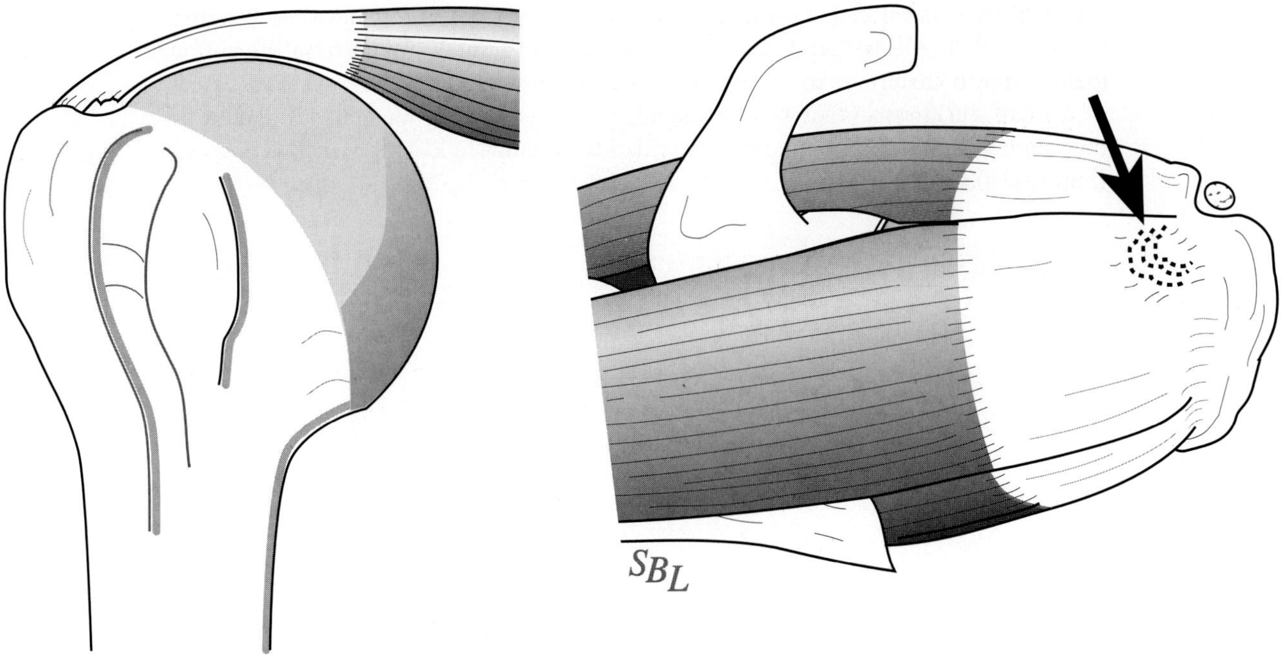


**Figure 19–7. Locating the defect**
The defect is usually palpable just behind the long head of the biceps and just medial to the greater tuberosity.

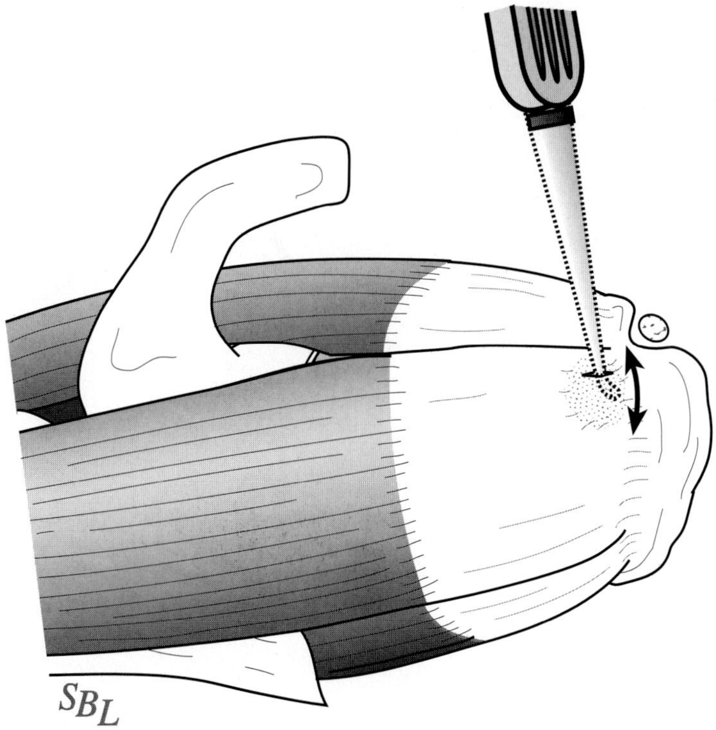


**Figure 19–8. Inserting the curette**
A 000 angled curette is inserted through the thinnest part of the supraspinatus tendon near its insertion to the greater tuberosity.

extent of the tendon detachment until secure cuff insertion is encountered at either end **(Fig. 19–9)**. On withdrawing of the curette, only a small puncture in the cuff is present, so no closure of this defect is needed. If the defect had been through most of the cuff thickness so that the tendon insertion was severely weakened, the detachment would have been completed and a formal repair would have been carried out **(Fig. 19–10)**.

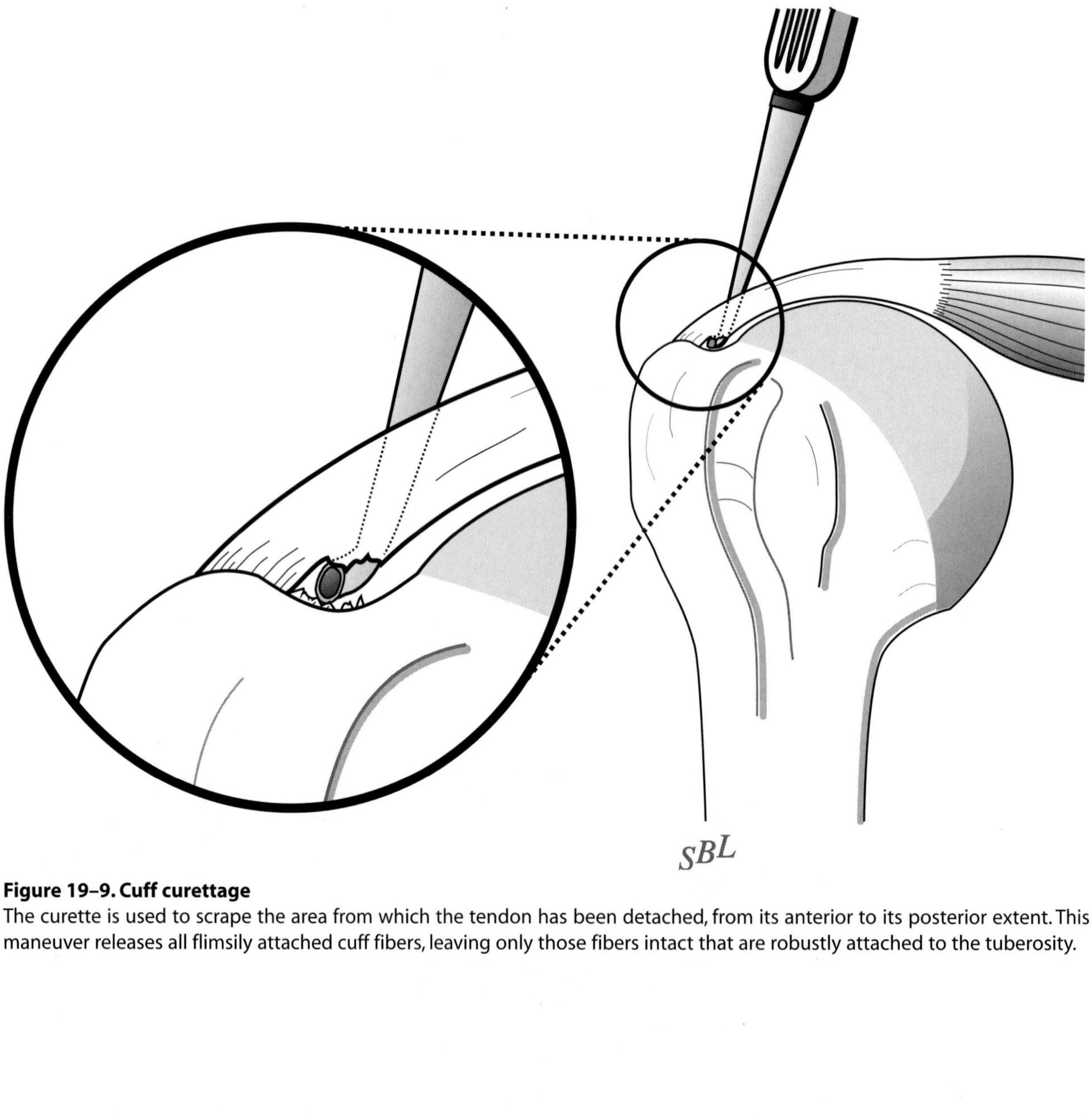


**Figure 19–9. Cuff curettage**
The curette is used to scrape the area from which the tendon has been detached, from its anterior to its posterior extent. This maneuver releases all flimsily attached cuff fibers, leaving only those fibers intact that are robustly attached to the tuberosity.

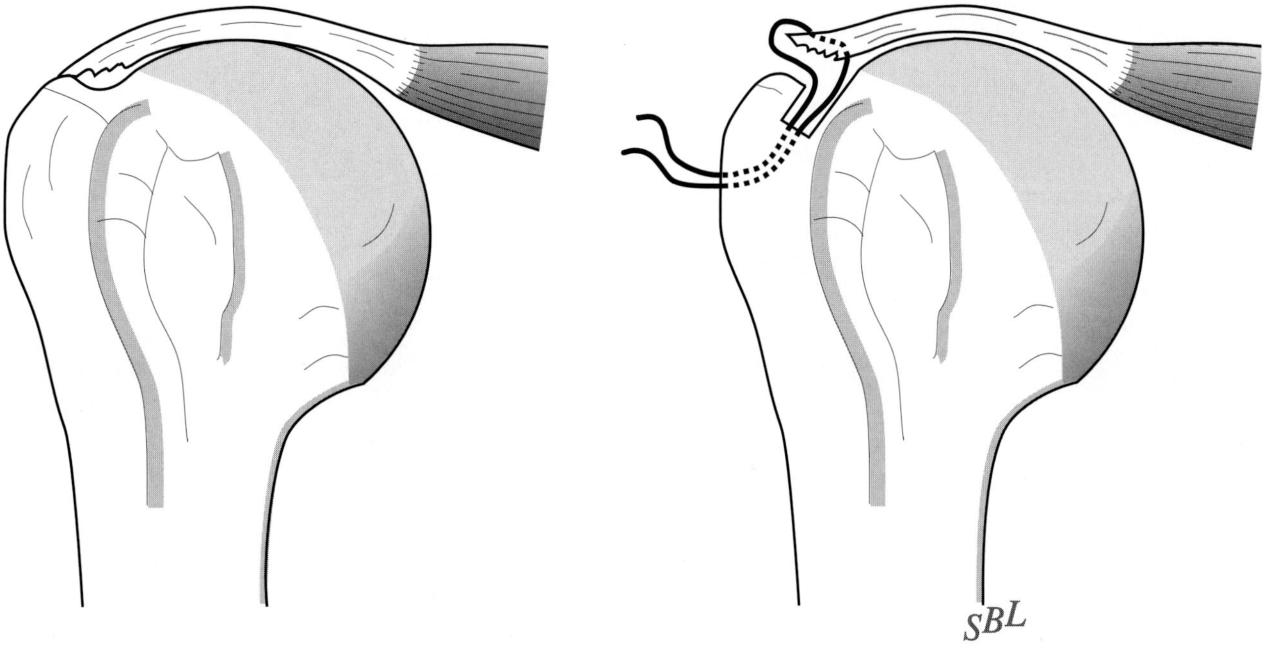


**Figure 19–10. Completing the detachment and repair**
When the majority of the thickness of the tendon is torn, the few remaining fibers are incised and the tendon is formally repaired to a groove in bone. (Modified from Matsen FA, Lippitt SB, Sidles JA, et al [eds]: Practical Evaluation and Management of the Shoulder. Philadelphia: WB Saunders, 1994, p. 142.)

Full motion of the glenohumeral joint is ensured by gentle manipulation. The acromion is palpated while the shoulder is put through a complete range of motion to verify the absence of any crepitance. The undersurface of the coracoacromial arch is palpated to ensure its smoothness. If there is a prominence that encroaches on the cuff, it is smoothed with a pinecone burr (**Fig. 19–11**). Routine acromioplasty is avoided to preserve the coracoacromial concavity as well as to minimize the risk of adhesions and weakening of the deltoid origin (**Fig. 19–12**).

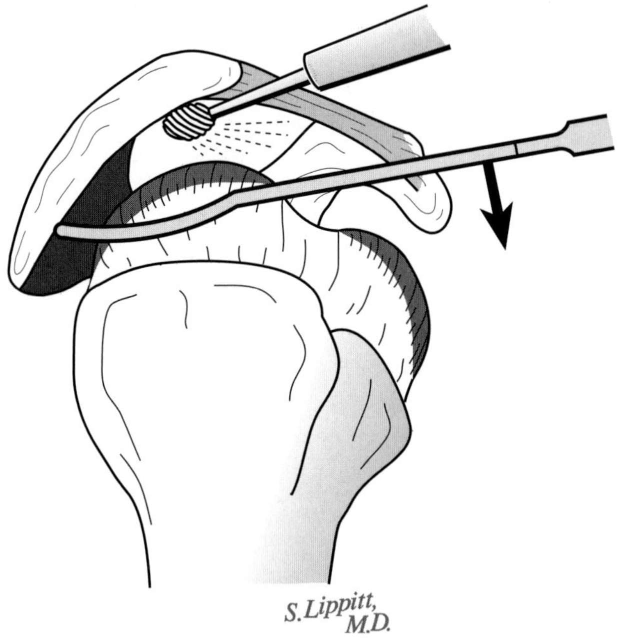


**Figure 19–11. Smoothing the coracoacromial arch**
If, as is rarely the case, there is roughness on the underside of the coracoacromial arch, it can be smoothed with a pinecone burr, leaving the arch intact. (Modified from Matsen FA, Lippitt SB, Sidles JA, et al [eds]: Practical Evaluation and Management of the Shoulder. Philadelphia: WB Saunders, 1994, p. 136.)

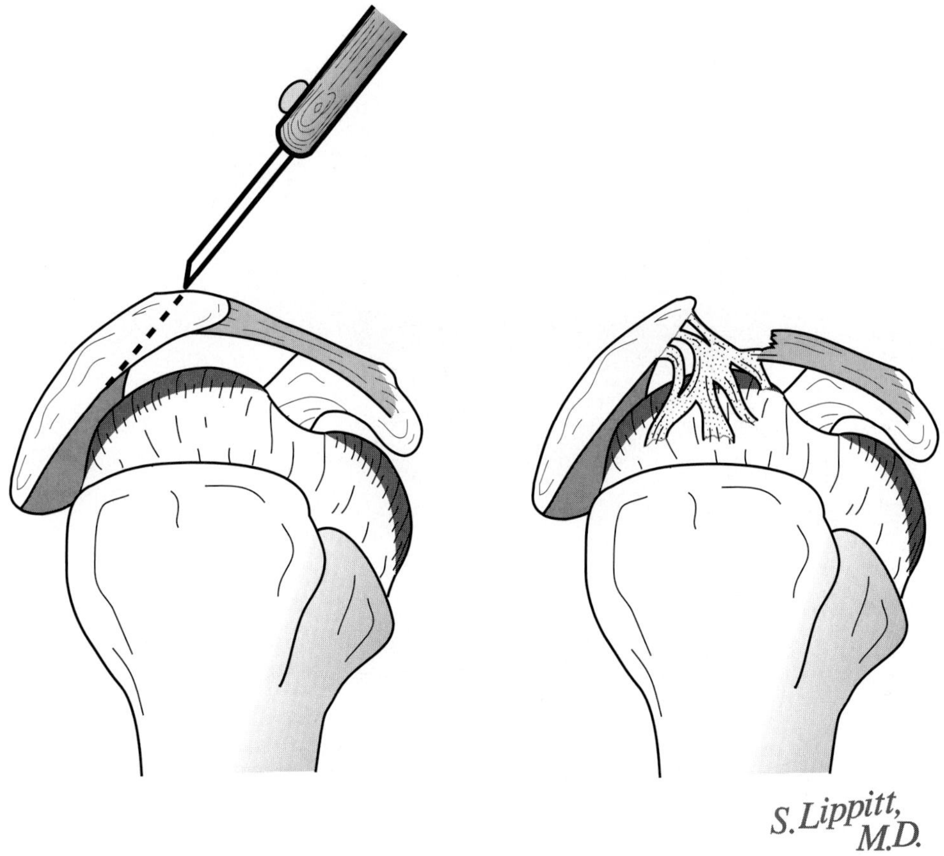


**Figure 19–12. Disadvantages of acromioplasty**
Acromioplasty is avoided because it sacrifices the stability provided by the coracoacromial arch, it compromises the deltoid origin, and it risks adhesion to the underlying cuff.

Hemostasis is seen to be excellent. The wound is thoroughly irrigated. The deltoid origin is intact at the conclusion of the case. The deltoid split is closed side-to-side-to-side with absorbable sutures (**Fig. 19–13**). A standard subcutaneous and subcuticular skin incision is carried out, followed by the application of sterile tape closures and sterile dressings.

The patient is returned to the recovery room in satisfactory condition, with the arm in continuous passive motion (**Fig. 19–14**).

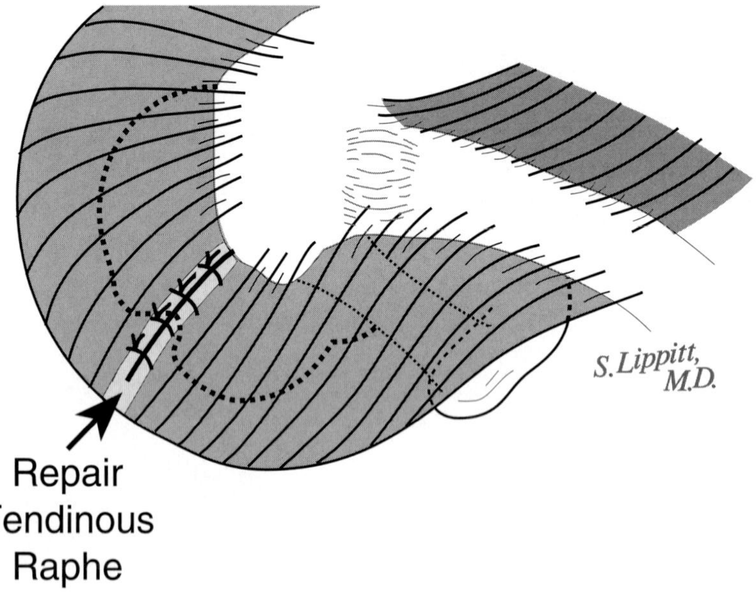


**Figure 19–13. Deltoid split repair**
The tendinous raphe of the deltoid split is repaired, with care taken to ensure that the knots are out of the humeroscapular motion interface and that they are not prominent subcutaneously.

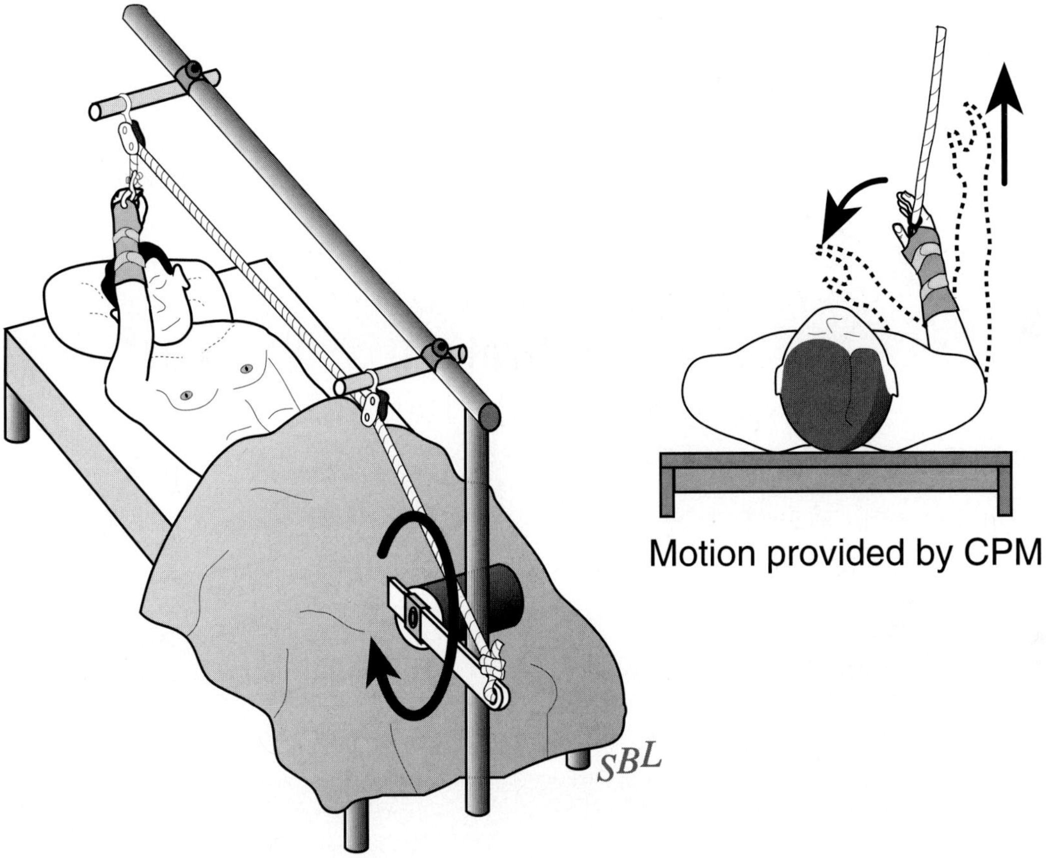


**Figure 19–14. Continuous passive motion**
Continuous passive motion is started immediately in the recovery room and continued while the patient is in the hospital during the times the patient is in bed. It moves the shoulder from adduction and internal rotation to 90 degrees of elevation in neutral rotation using a slow adjustable cam rotating at four cycles per minute. (Modified from Matsen FA, Lippitt SB, Sidles JA, et al [eds]: Practical Evaluation and Management of the Shoulder. Philadelphia: WB Saunders, 1994, p. 50.)

## POSTOPERATIVE PLAN

Our postoperative plan is for the 140 degrees of flexion, 40 degrees of external rotation, full motion active program, including stretches in forward flexion (**Fig. 19–15**), external rotation (**Fig. 19–16**), up the back (**Fig. 19–17**), and cross-body (**Fig. 19–18**) as well as internal rotation in abduction (**Fig. 19–19**). There is no need for protection in that there has been no cuff repair and the deltoid has only been split along its fibers. Forward elevation can also be assisted using a pulley (**Fig. 19–20**). The ranges of motion are charted on a wall chart twice daily; the patient is discharged when the assisted range of motion goals are achieved (**Fig. 19–21**).

Strengthening exercises are started at 6 weeks after surgery when the shoulder is completely comfortable.

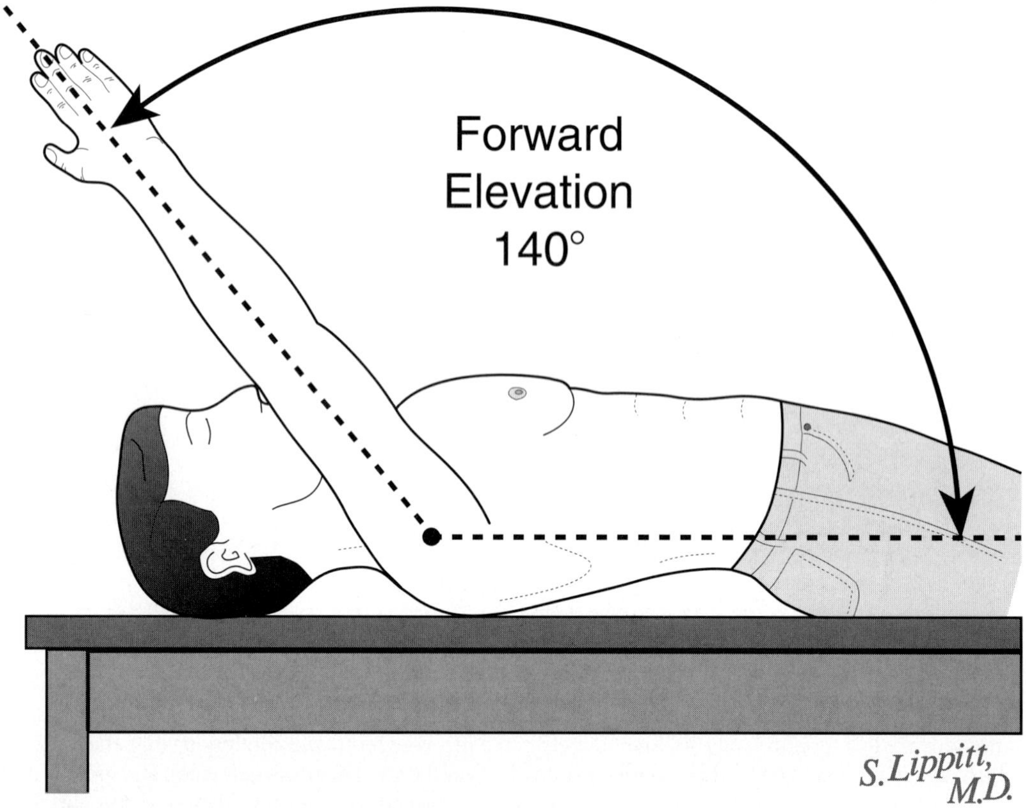


**Figure 19–15. Active assisted forward elevation**
With assistance of the other hand as necessary, the arm is elevated to 140 degrees.

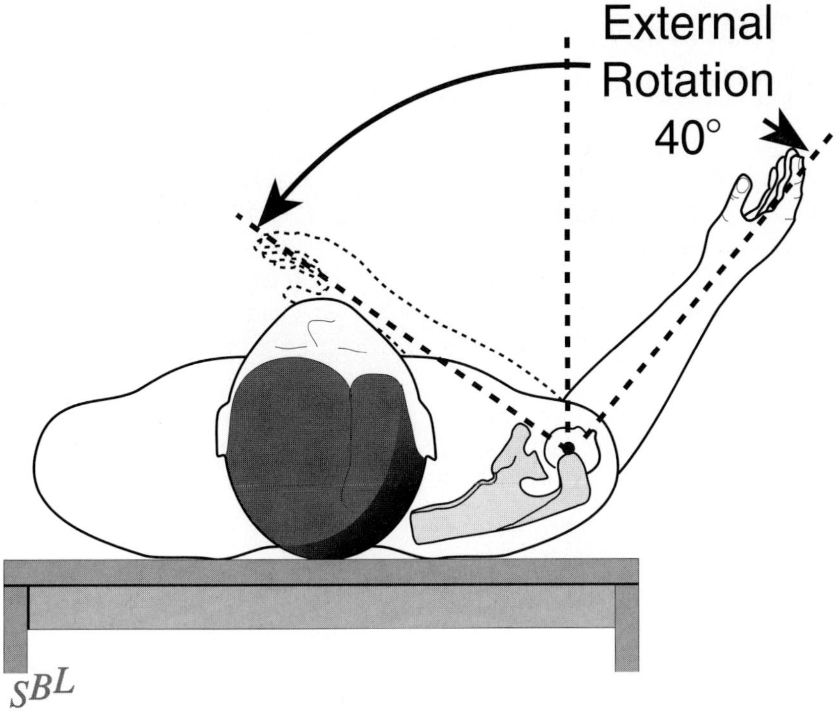


**Figure 19–16. Active assisted external rotation**
With assistance of the other hand as necessary, the arm is externally rotated to 40 degrees.

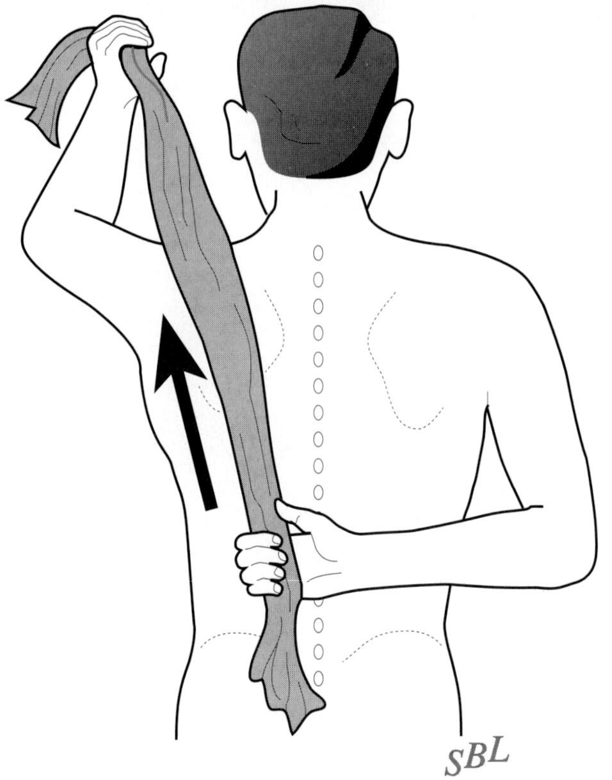

**Figure 19–17. Internal rotation in adduction**
With the assistance of the other hand as necessary, the hand of the involved arm is brought up the back. (Modified from Matsen FA, Lippitt SB, Sidles JA, et al [eds]: Practical Evaluation and Management of the Shoulder. Philadelphia: WB Saunders, 1994, p. 48.)

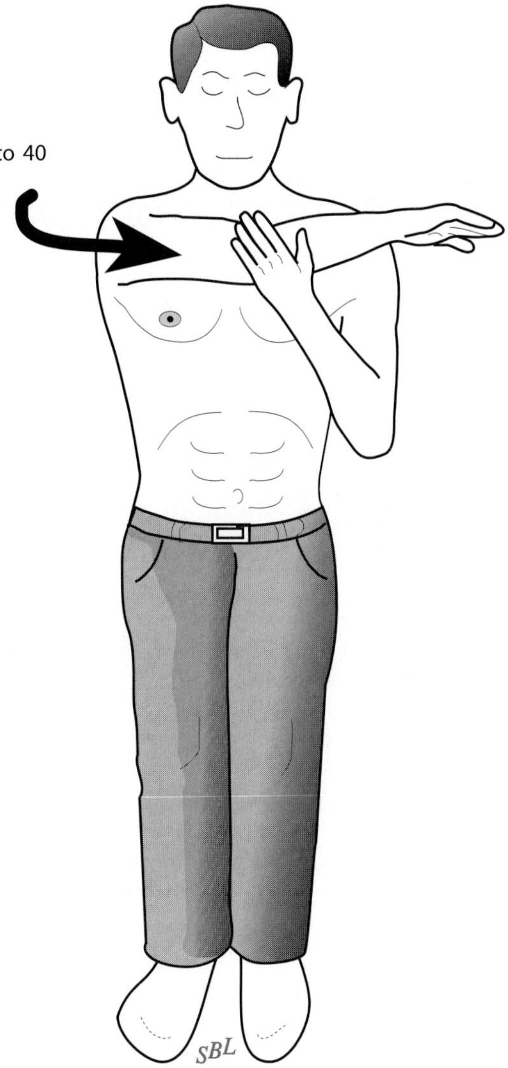

**Figure 19–18. Cross-body adduction**
With the assistance of the other hand as necessary, the involved arm is brought across the body toward the opposite shoulder. (Modified from Matsen FA, Lippitt SB, Sidles JA, et al [eds]: Practical Evaluation and Management of the Shoulder. Philadelphia: WB Saunders, 1994, p. 49.)

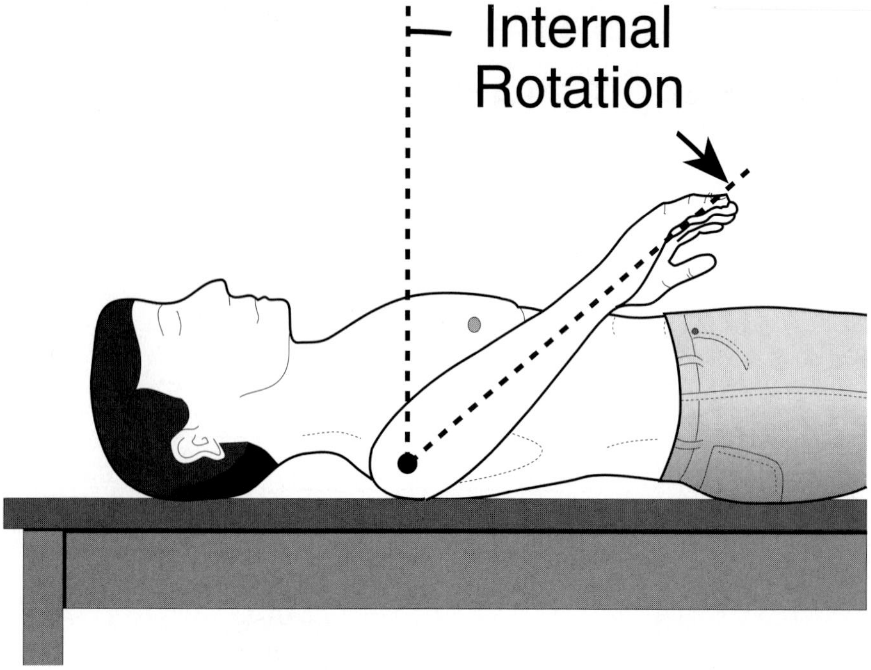


**Figure 19–19. Internal rotation in abduction**
With the arm abducted to 90 degrees, the involved arm is internally rotated using the opposite arm or with the help of a friend. (Modified from Rockwood CA, Matsen FA [eds]: The Shoulder, 2nd ed. Philadelphia: WB Saunders, 1998, p. 1083.)

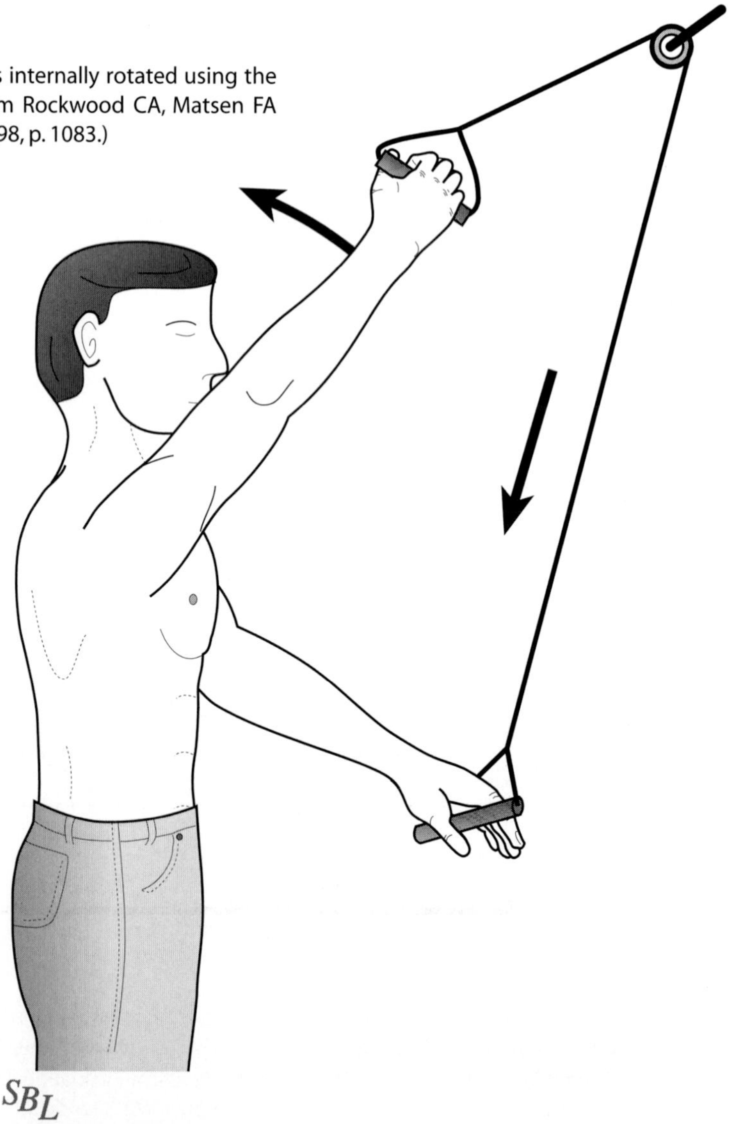

**Figure 19–20. Door pulley**
A pulley mounted on the door can be helpful in achieving elevation, especially when the opposite shoulder is involved.

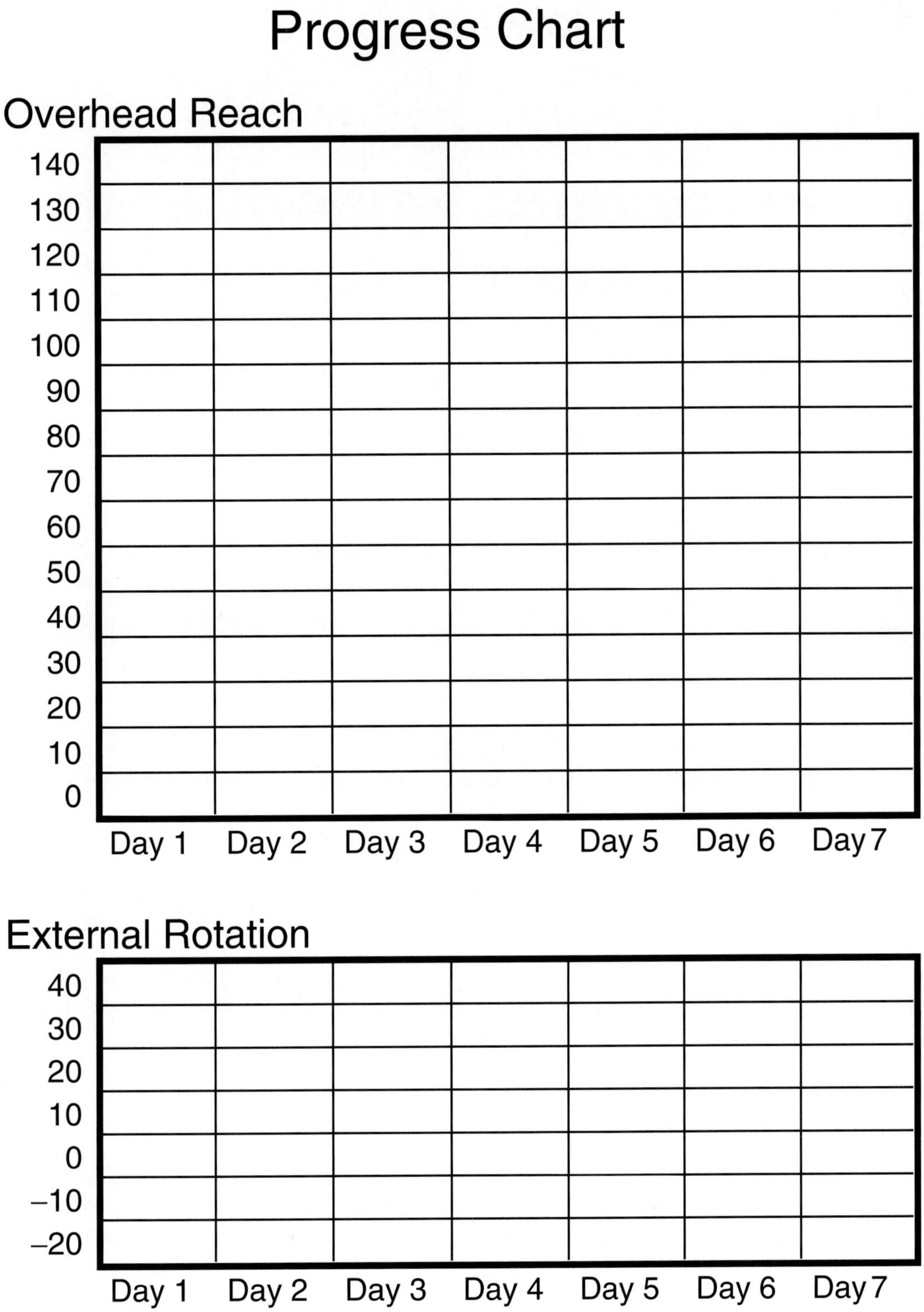


**Figure 19–21. Wall chart**
Daily progress is recorded on a wall chart so that positive feedback is provided to patients as they increase their range of motion. (Modified from Matsen FA, Lippitt SB, Sidles JA, et al [eds]: Practical Evaluation and Management of the Shoulder. Philadelphia: WB Saunders, 1994, p. 56.)

CHAPTER 20

# Procedure: Smooth and Move—Cuff Intact

***Diagnosis***

***Humeroscapular/subacromial roughness ICD9 CODE 726.10***

***Procedure***

***Smoothing of humeroscapular motion interface through a deltoid-on approach CPT CODE 23415***

## INDICATIONS

The patient has crepitance, catching, and popping in the subacromial/subdeltoid area that limits the comfort and function of the shoulder and has proven refractory to a sustained program of flexibility exercises.

Physical examination and rotator cuff imaging indicate that the rotator cuff is intact.

Knowing the alternatives as well as the risks of infection, neurovascular injury, excessive stiffness, pain, weakness, fracture, instability, and the need for revision surgery as well as anesthetic complications, the patient desires to proceed with the above-described procedure. The patient understands that the goal of this procedure is to smooth the area around the humerus and rotator cuff. The patient recognizes that this procedure cannot be expected to completely restore normal comfort and function to the shoulder. The patient understands his or her critical role in the post-surgical rehabilitation.

## FINDINGS

Examination under anesthesia reveals crepitance palpated anterior to the acromion on humeral rotation. Shoulder motion is restricted approximately 20% in all directions.

Surgical findings include thickened bursal tissue and adhesions across the humeroscapular motion interface restricting humeroscapular motion. These adhesions are particularly prevalent between the coracoid muscles and the subscapularis tendon. The rotator cuff is intact.

## OPERATION

Under satisfactory anesthesia, the patient is placed in a low beach chair position with the glenohumeral joint at the edge of the operating table (**Fig. 20–1**). The entire

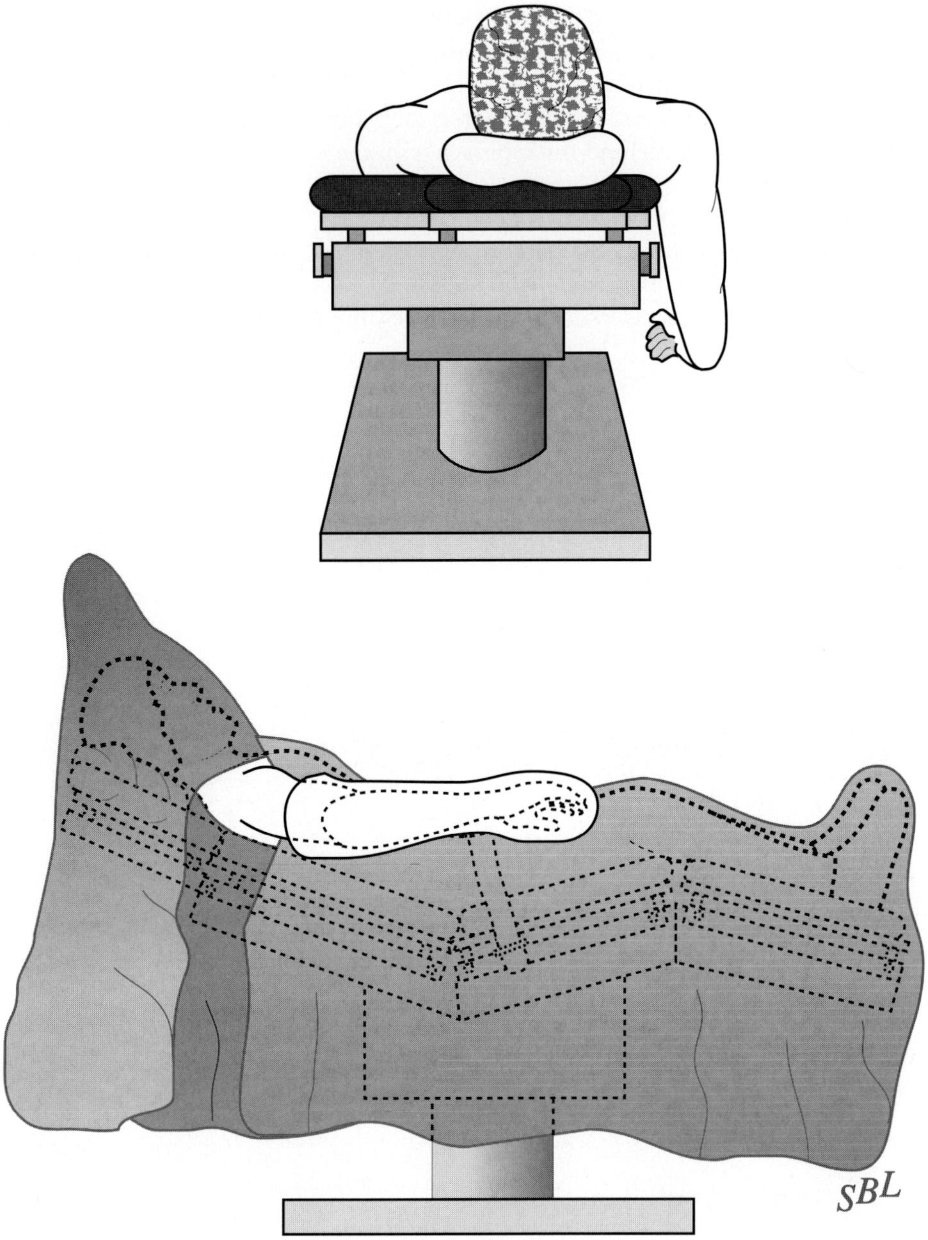


**Figure 20–1. Positioning and draping the shoulder**
The patient is placed in beach chair position with arm draped free. Note that the patient is positioned with the glenohumeral joint at the edge of the table so that the arm can be moved through a full range of motion.

forequarter is carefully prepped and draped in the usual sterile fashion with the arm free to be moved. The shoulder is examined during passive motion to identify the positions that are associated with crepitance.

The anterolateral corner of the acromion is identified by palpation. The shoulder is approached through the deltoid-on approach with the incision in the skin line crossing the anterior corner of the acromion and perpendicular to the anterolateral fibers of the deltoid (**Fig. 20–2**).

The major raphe between the anterior and lateral thirds of the deltoid is identified and split sharply so that some white tendon remains on either side of the split (**Fig. 20–3**). No deltoid is taken down from the acromion. Care is taken not to cut the

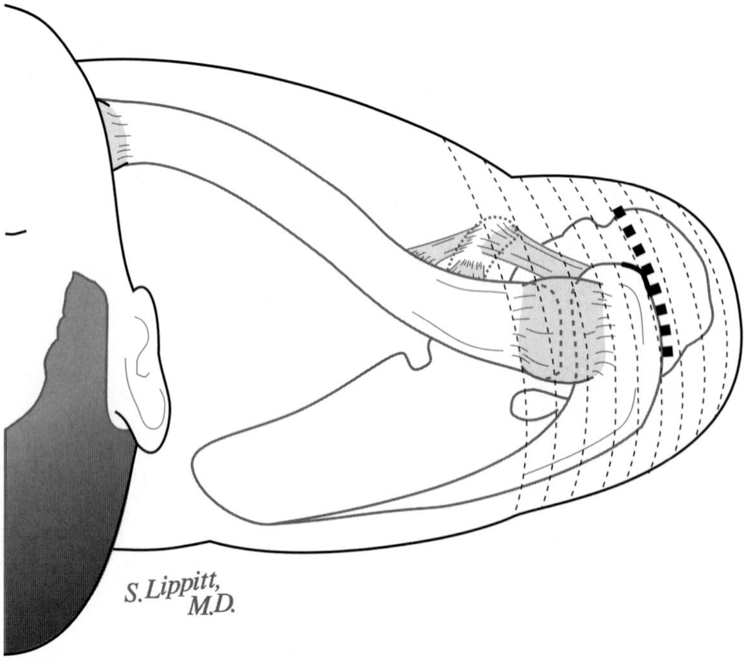


**Figure 20–2. Deltoid-on approach**
The deltoid-on approach, showing the skin incision in Langer's lines.

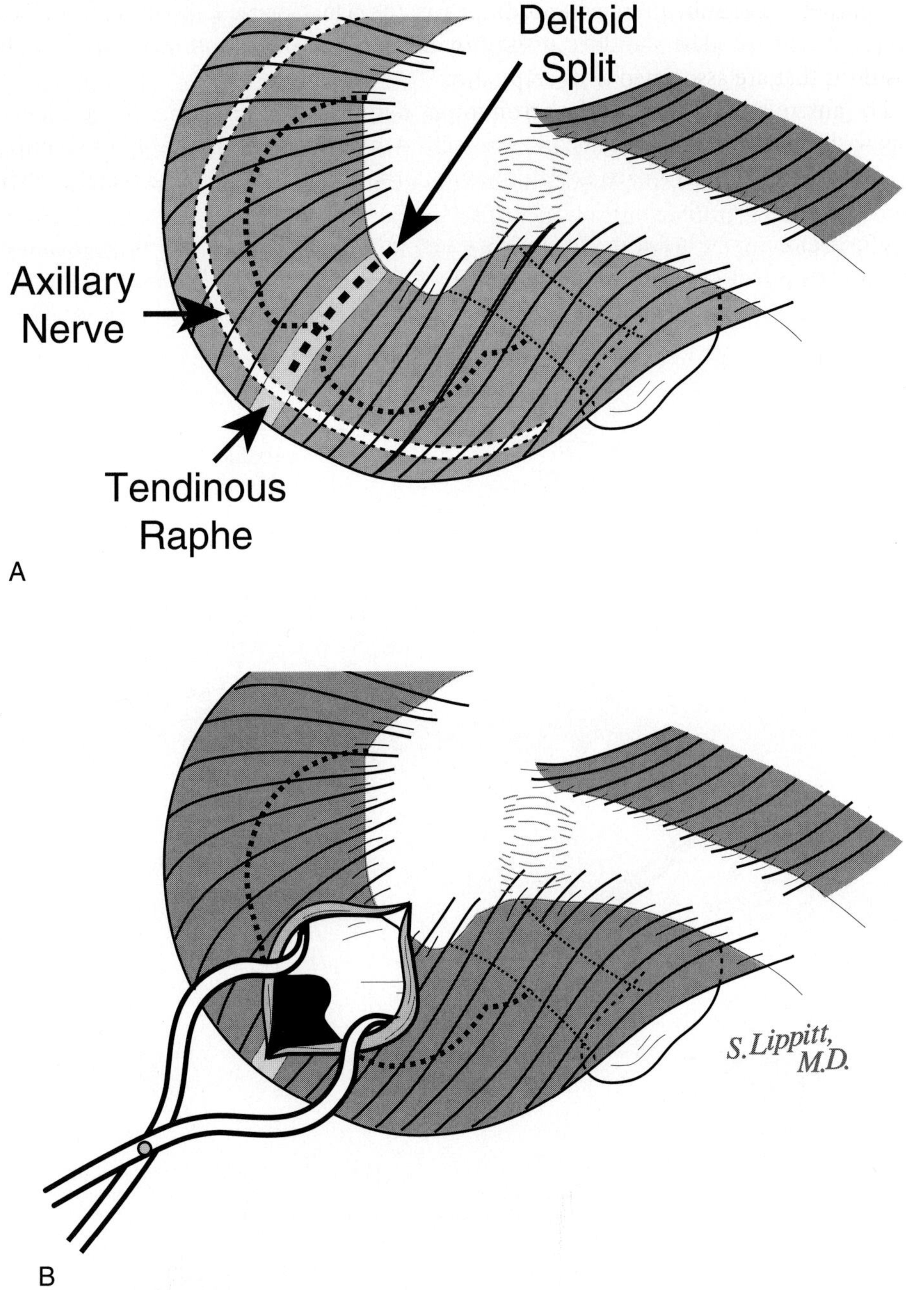


**Figure 20–3. Deltoid split**
The deltoid is split along the raphe between the anterior and lateral thirds of the muscle without any of it being detached from the acromion. (Modified from Matsen FA, Lippitt SB, Sidles JA, et al [eds]: Practical Evaluation and Management of the Shoulder. Philadelphia: WB Saunders, 1994, p. 135.)

cuff deep to this incision. Once the deltoid raphe has been split, a small smooth elevator is passed beneath the acromion (**Fig. 20–4**). Rotating this elevator so that it points distally allows safe incision of the bursa attached to its deep surface. The total length of the deltoid split is limited to 4 cm from the acromion.

Small, self-retaining retractors are placed in the deltoid split to hold it open. Bursal scar is noted creating "spot welds" across the humeroscapular motion interface (**Fig. 20–5**). The hypertrophic bursa is identified by the "roll, no-roll test"; that is, the bursa can be differentiated from the underlying cuff by the fact that it does not move with the humerus as the arm is rotated. All of the bursa is resected, along with any scar in the humeroscapular motion interface (**Fig. 20–6**). A nerve-to-nerve release is carried

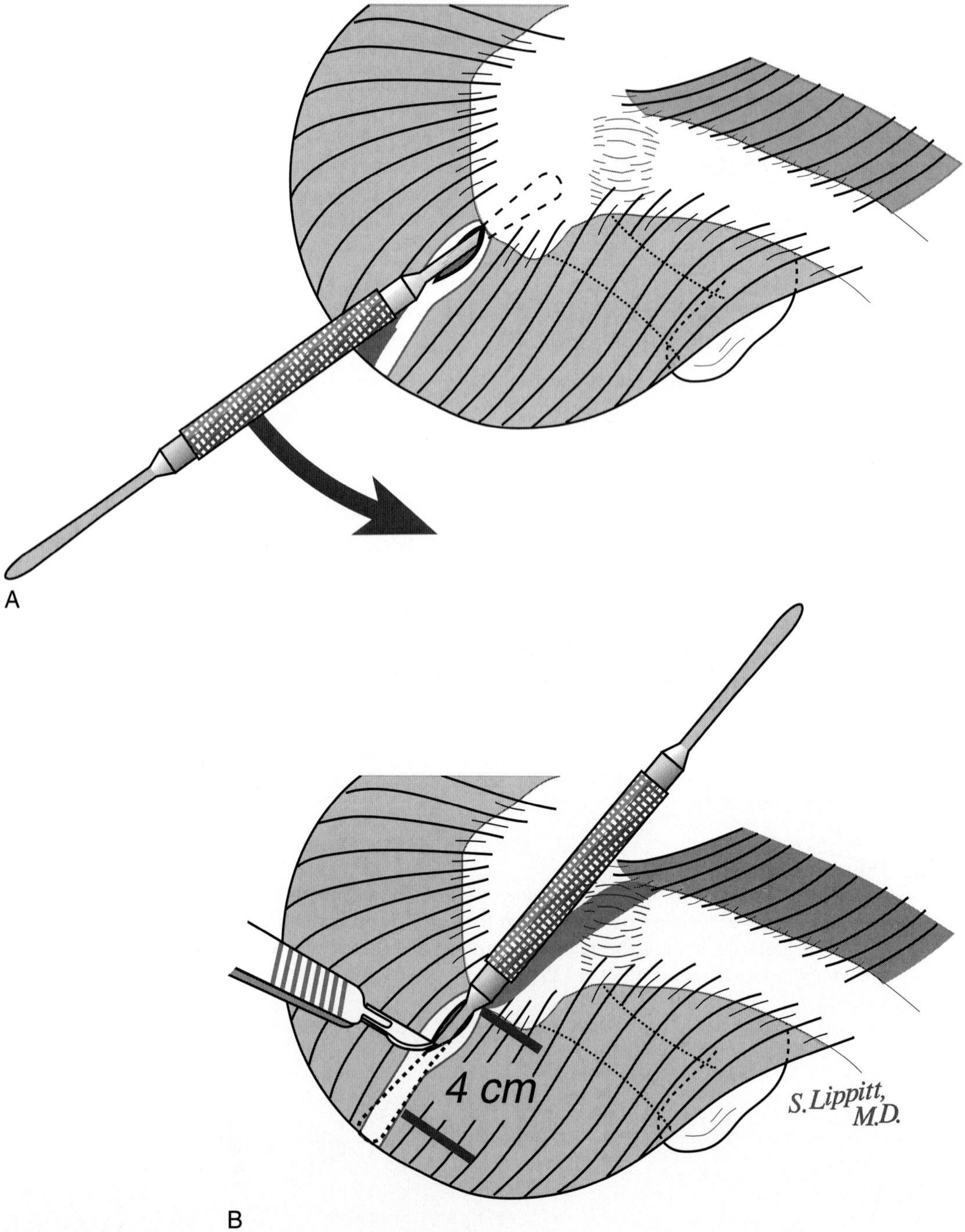


**Figure 20–4. Inserting an elevator in the deltoid split**
Once the subdeltoid bursa is entered, a small blunt elevator is inserted through the split and then underneath the deltoid (**A**). This elevator is then rotated 180 degrees while still in the bursa. The incision in the deltoid and bursa is then extended up to 4 cm distal from the acromion (**B**).

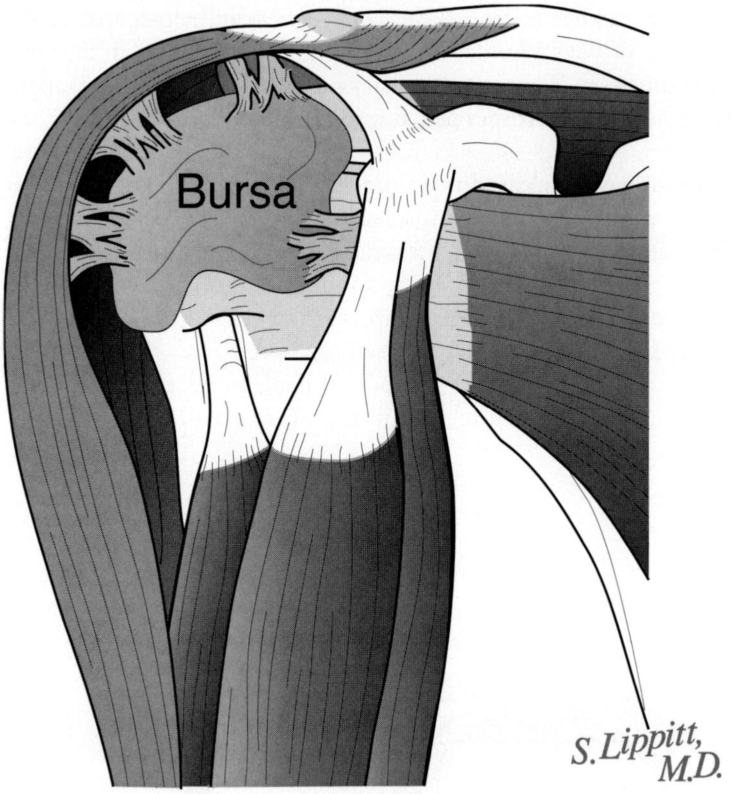


**Figure 20–5. Adhesions in the motion interface**
Scar tissue across the humeroscapular motion interface limits motion and smoothness.

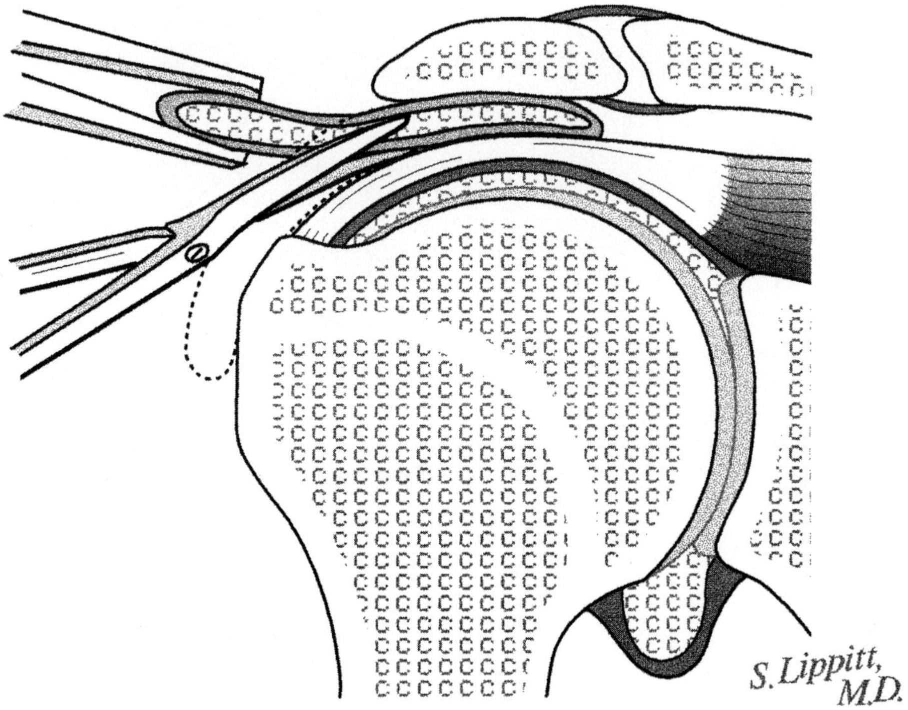


**Figure 20–6. Removal of bursa**
The hypertrophic bursa is removed by sharp dissection.

out so that at the conclusion of the release, the axillary nerve can be palpated in the axilla as it runs across the subscapularis and lateral to the humerus as it traverses around it just below the tuberosities. Since the axillary nerve lies in the humeroscapular motion interface, the fact that it becomes palpable indicates the completeness of the release (**Fig. 20–7**).

The coracohumeral ligament is released from the coracoid process (**Fig. 20–8**). At this point, the shoulder is gently manipulated to ensure a full range of flexion, abduction, and cross-body adduction rotation at the side and rotation at 90 degrees of abduction. The obligate anterior and posterior translations that occur at, respectively, the extremes of internal and external rotation are observed to ensure that this translation occurs only at the end of the physiologic range of rotation.

The purpose of the procedure is to restore a smooth articulation between the coracoacromial concavity and the proximal humeral convexity (**Fig. 20–9**). This is accomplished in two steps.

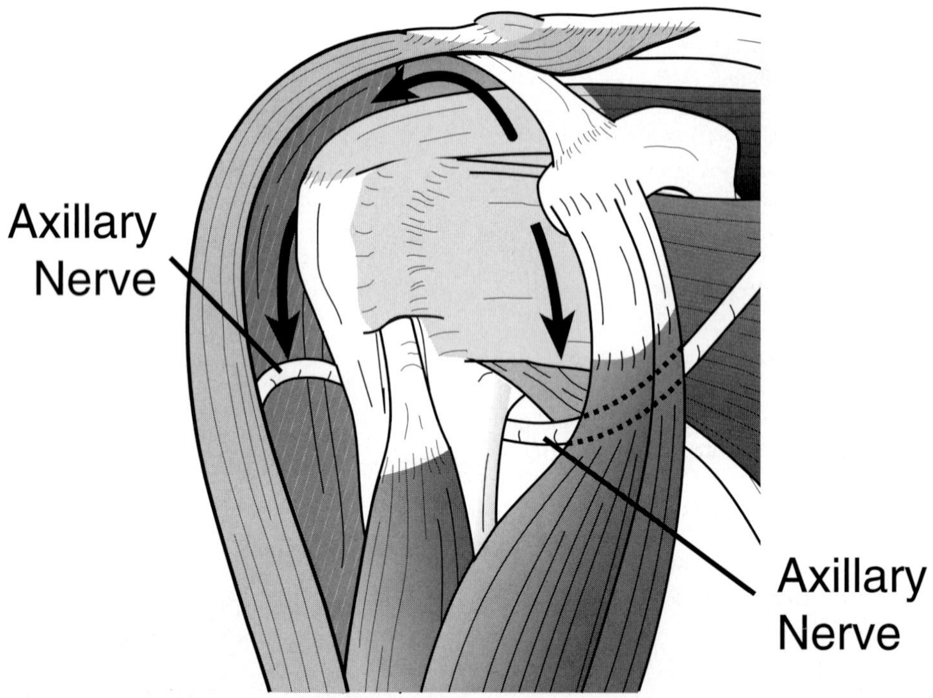


**Figure 20–7. Nerve-to-nerve release**
All scar tissue in the humeroscapular motion interface is released from the axillary nerve medially as it crosses the subscapularis, then under the coracoid, then under the coracoacromial ligament, then under the acromion, and then finally under the deltoid to the axillary nerve posteriorly as it exits the quadrilateral space: the nerve-to-nerve release.

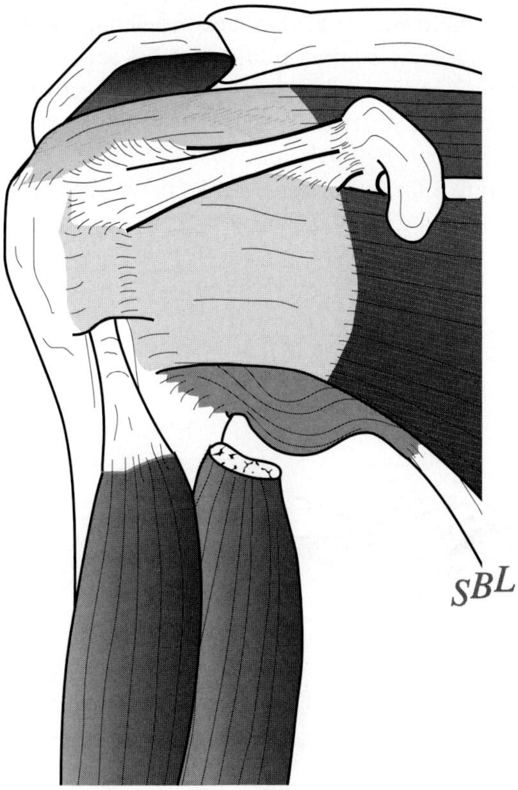


**Figure 20–8. Coracohumeral ligament**
The coracohumeral ligament runs from the base of the coracoid to the transverse humeral ligament. It can restrict external rotation and internal rotation when the arm is in adduction. It is most easily released at the base of the coracoid process. (Modified from Matsen FA, Lippitt SB, Sidles JA, et al [eds]: Practical Evaluation and Management of the Shoulder. Philadelphia: WB Saunders, 1994, p. 37.)

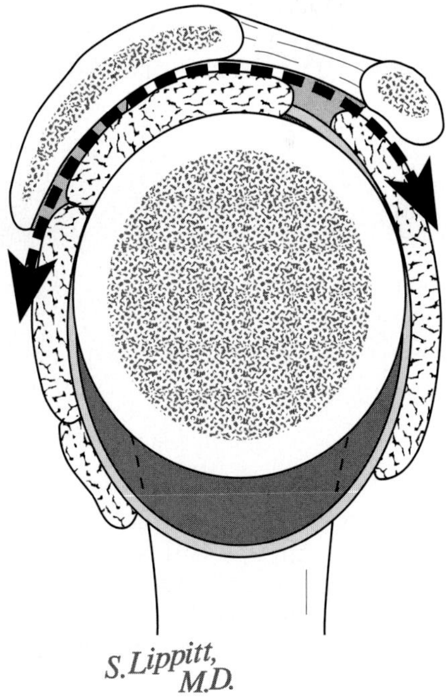


**Figure 20–9. Humeroscapular motion interface**
Normal shoulder function requires a smooth articulation between the proximal humeral convexity and the coracoacromial concavity via the humeroscapular motion interface. (Modified from Rockwood CA, Matsen FA [eds]: The Shoulder, 2nd ed. Philadelphia: WB Saunders, 1998, p. 618.)

First, the surface of the proximal humerus and cuff is palpated to be sure of its smoothness. Any prominence of cuff or tuberosity is smoothed so that the convex proximal humeral convexity surface is smoothly spherical (**Fig. 20–10**). Next, the concave undersurface of the coracoacromial arch is palpated to be sure of its smoothness. If there is a prominence that encroaches on the cuff, it is smoothed with a pinecone burr (**Fig. 20–11**). Conventional acromioplasty is avoided to preserve the coracoacromial concavity and as well as to minimize the risk of adhesions and weakening of the deltoid origin (**Fig. 20–12**).

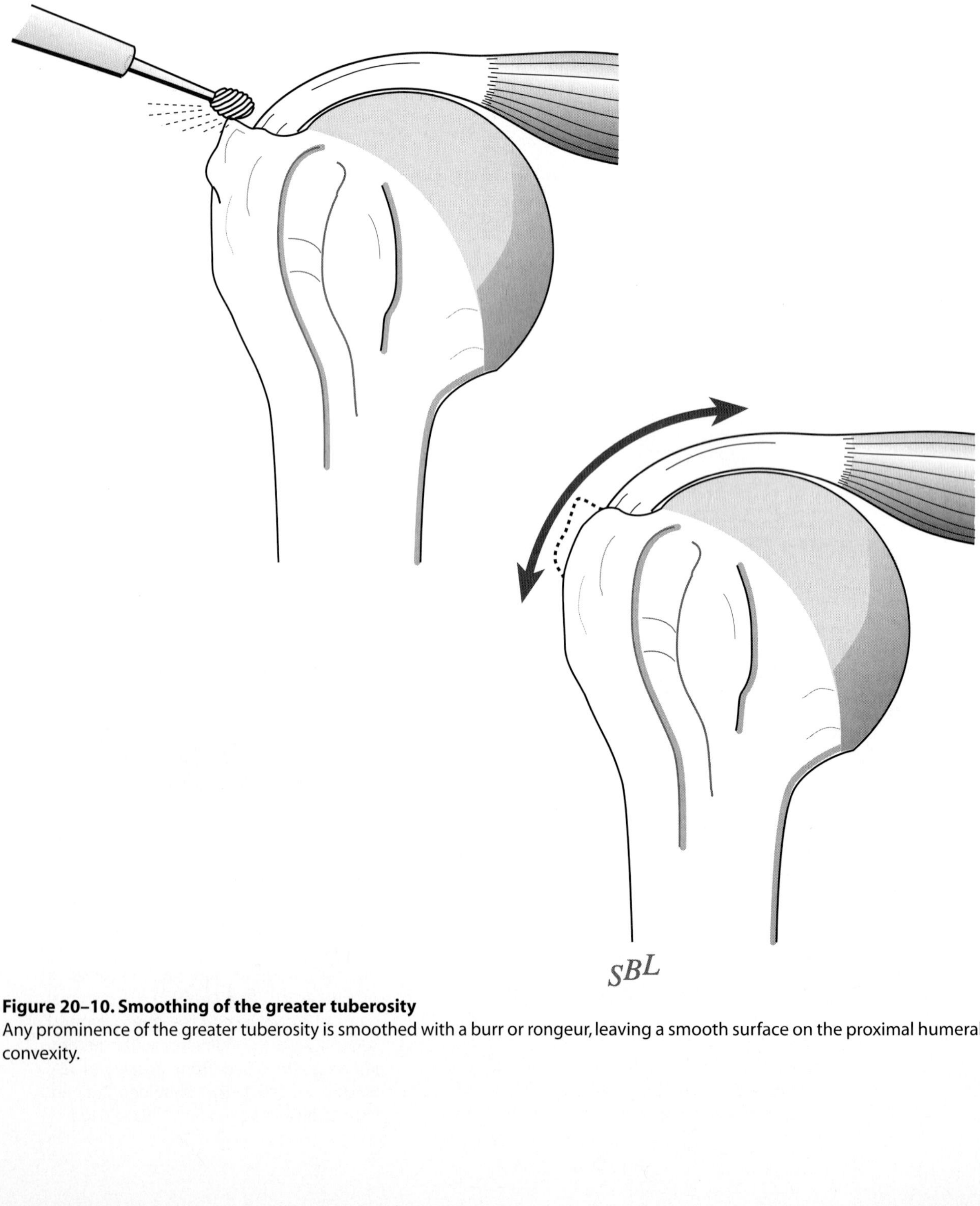

**Figure 20–10. Smoothing of the greater tuberosity**
Any prominence of the greater tuberosity is smoothed with a burr or rongeur, leaving a smooth surface on the proximal humeral convexity.

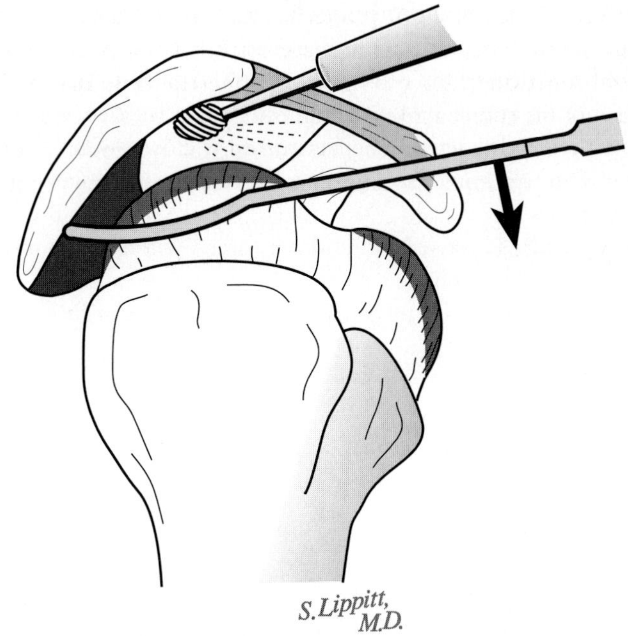


**Figure 20–11. Smoothing of the coracoacromial arch**
If, as is rarely the case, there is roughness on the underside of the coracoacromial arch, it can be smoothed with a pinecone burr, leaving the arch intact.

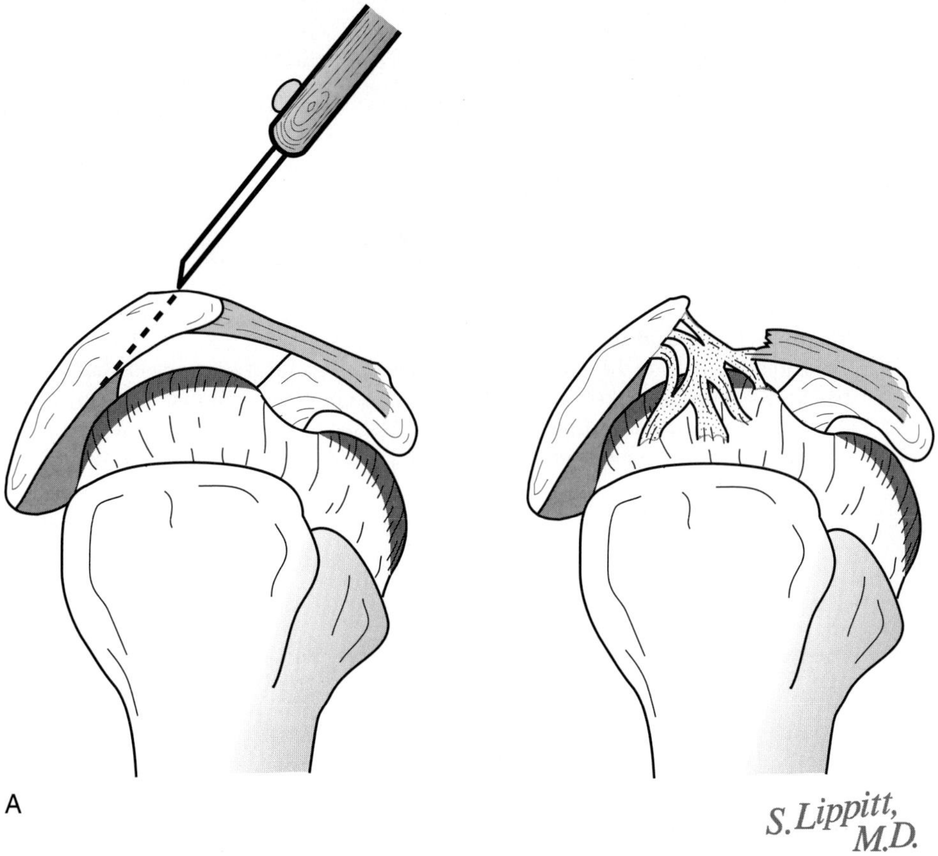


**Figure 20–12. Acromioplasty—potential hazards**
Acromioplasty is avoided because it sacrifices the stability provided by the coracoacromial arch, it compromises the deltoid origin, and it risks adhesion to the underlying cuff.

At the conclusion of the smoothing, the shoulder is put through a range of motion while the area anterior to the acromion is palpated. Any residual crepitance is managed by smoothing of the aspect of the proximal humeral convexity that is responsible.

The range of motion and lack of crepitance are again verified.

The wound is thoroughly irrigated. The deltoid is closed with absorbable sutures, with care taken that all knots are out of the humeroscapular motion interface (**Fig. 20–13**).

A subcuticular closure is carried out and reinforced with sterile tapes.

Dry sterile dressings are applied.

The patient is returned to the recovery room with the arm in continuous passive motion (**Fig. 20–14**).

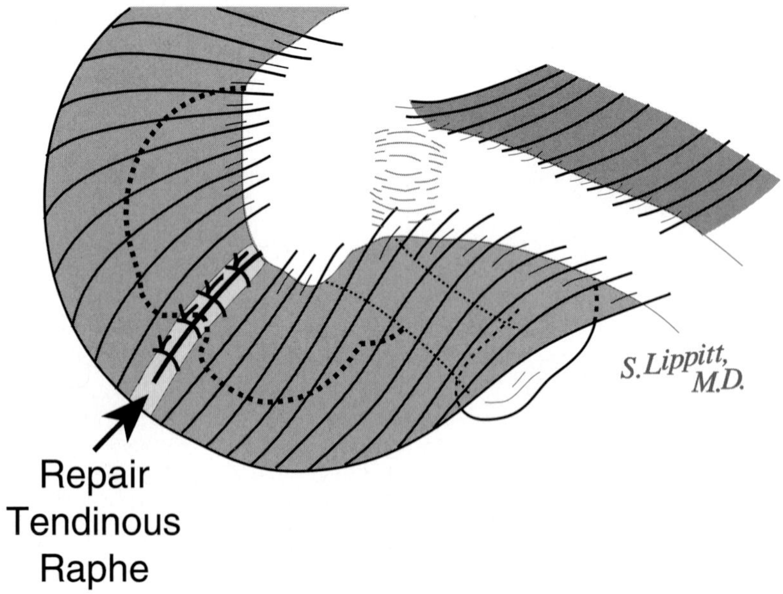


**Figure 20–13. Deltoid split repair**
The tendinous raphe of the deltoid split is repaired, with care taken to ensure that the knots lie outside of the humeroscapular motion interface and that they are not prominent subcutaneously. (Modified from Matsen FA, Lippitt SB, Sidles JA, et al [eds]: Practical Evaluation and Management of the Shoulder. Philadelphia: WB Saunders, 1994, p. 136.)

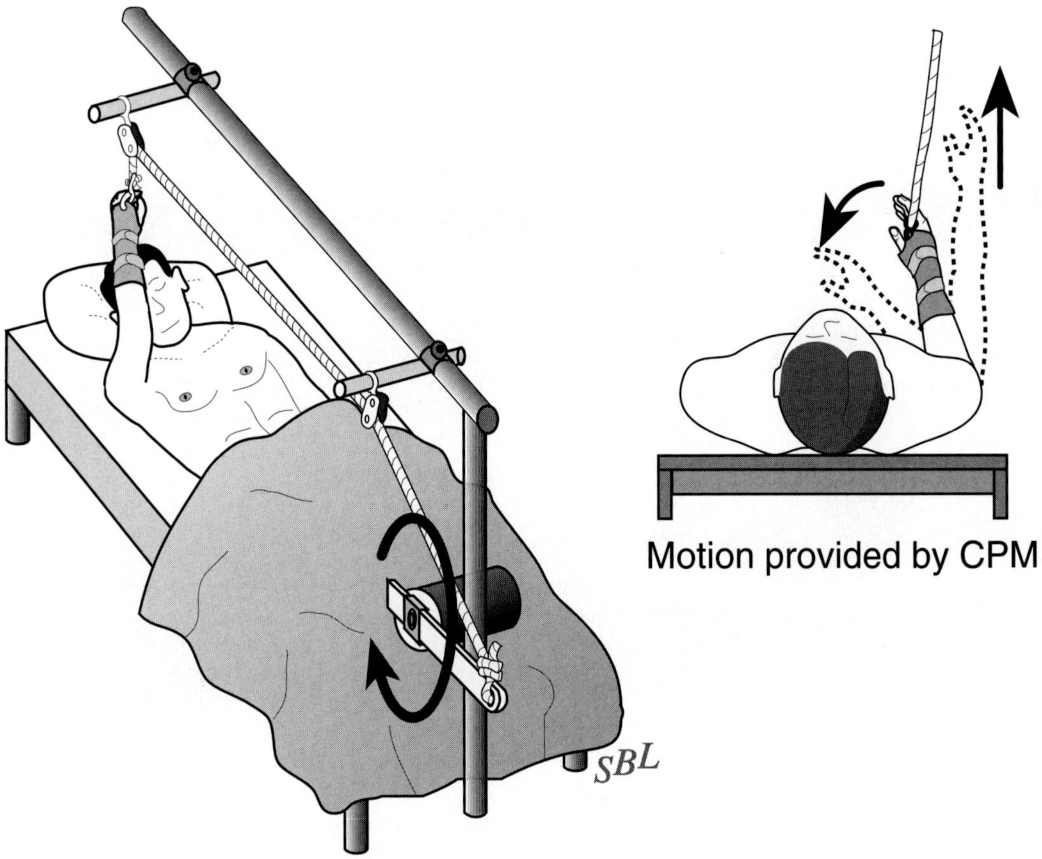


**Figure 20–14. Continuous passive motion**

Continuous passive motion is started immediately in the recovery room and continued while the patient is in the hospital during the times the patient is in bed. It moves the shoulder from adduction and internal rotation to 90 degrees of elevation in neutral rotation using a slow adjustable cam rotating at four cycles per minute. (Modified from Matsen FA, Lippitt SB, Sidles JA, et al [eds]: Practical Evaluation and Management of the Shoulder. Philadelphia: WB Saunders, 1994, p. 50.)

## POSTOPERATIVE PLAN

Continuous passive motion is provided for the first 36 hours whenever the patient is in bed and not doing assisted exercises.

The patient is instructed in a full motion program including assisted flexion (**Fig. 20–15**), external rotation at the side (**Fig. 20–16**), internal rotation up the back (**Fig. 20–17**), cross-body adduction (**Fig. 20–18**), and internal rotation in abduction (**Fig. 20–19**). If the contralateral shoulder is involved, a pulley is used to achieve the range of motion (**Fig. 20–20**). The range of flexion, external rotation, and cross-body adduction are charted on a wall chart twice daily.

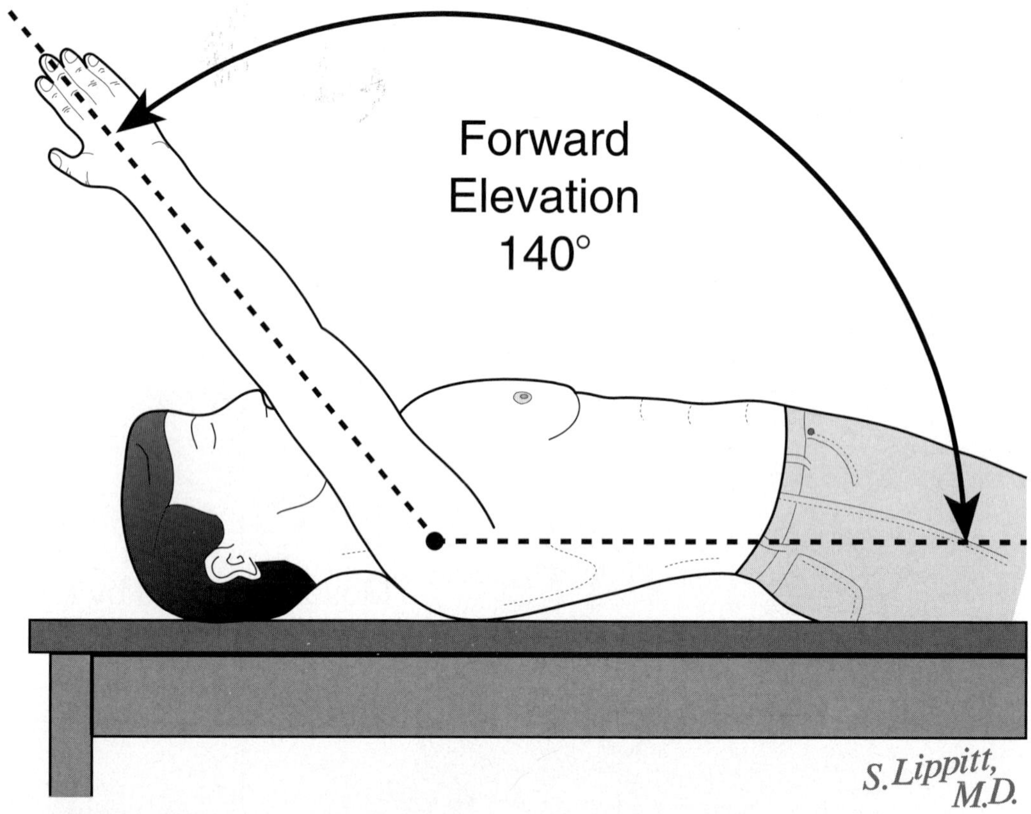


**Figure 20–15. Active assisted forward elevation**
With the assistance of the other hand as necessary, the arm is elevated to 140 degrees.

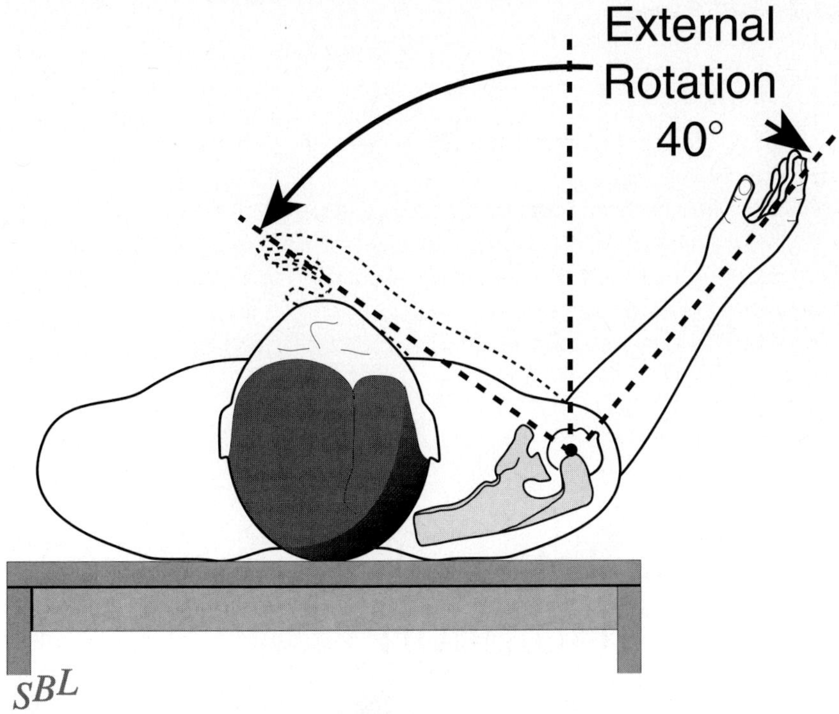


**Figure 20–16. Active assisted external rotation**
With the assistance of the other hand as necessary, the arm is externally rotated to 40 degrees.

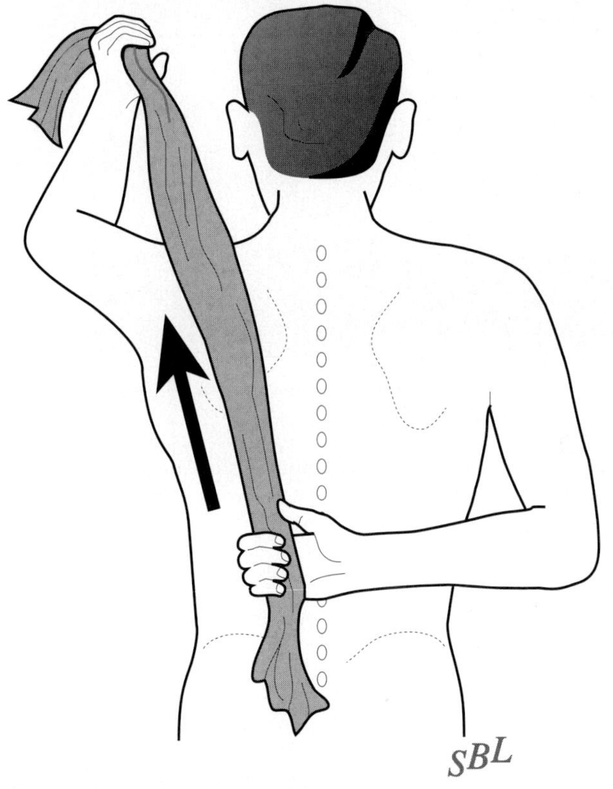


**Figure 20–17. Internal rotation in adduction**
With the assistance of the other hand as necessary, the hand of the involved arm is brought up the back. (Modified from Matsen FA, Lippitt SB, Sidles JA, et al [eds]: Practical Evaluation and Management of the Shoulder. Philadelphia: WB Saunders, 1994, p. 48.)

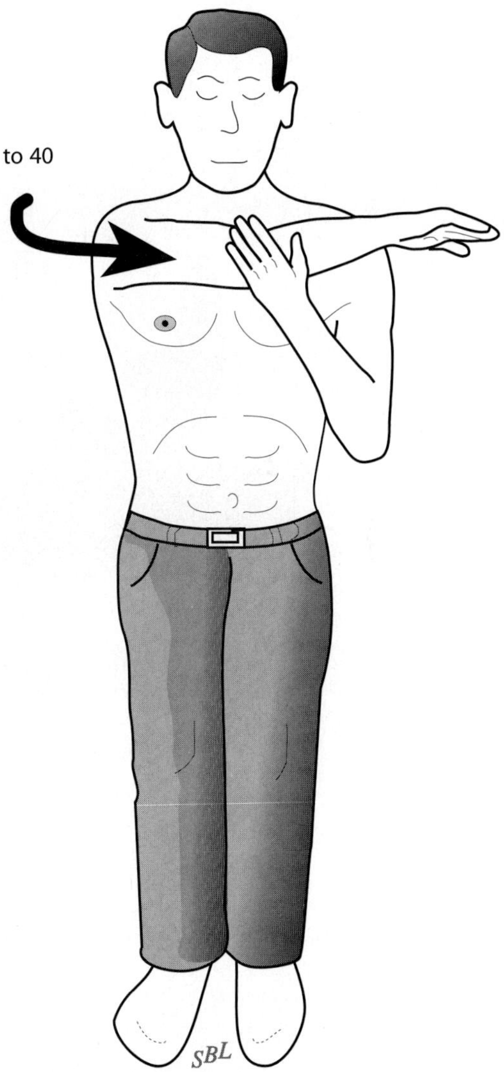


**Figure 20–18. Cross-body adduction**
With the assistance of the other hand as necessary, the involved arm is brought across the body toward the opposite shoulder. (Modified from Matsen FA, Lippitt SB, Sidles JA, et al [eds]: Practical Evaluation and Management of the Shoulder. Philadelphia: WB Saunders, 1994, p. 49.)

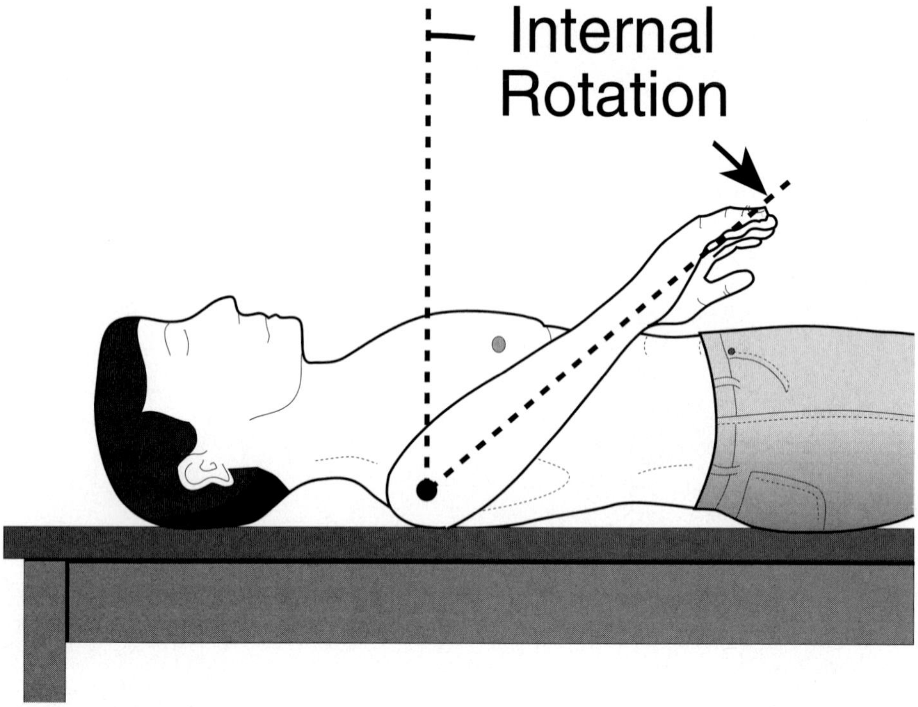


**Figure 20–19. Internal rotation in abduction**
With the arm abducted to 90 degrees, the involved arm is internally rotated using the opposite arm or with the help of a friend. (Modified from Rockwood CA, Matsen FA [eds]: The Shoulder, 2nd ed. Philadelphia: WB Saunders, 1998, p. 1083.)

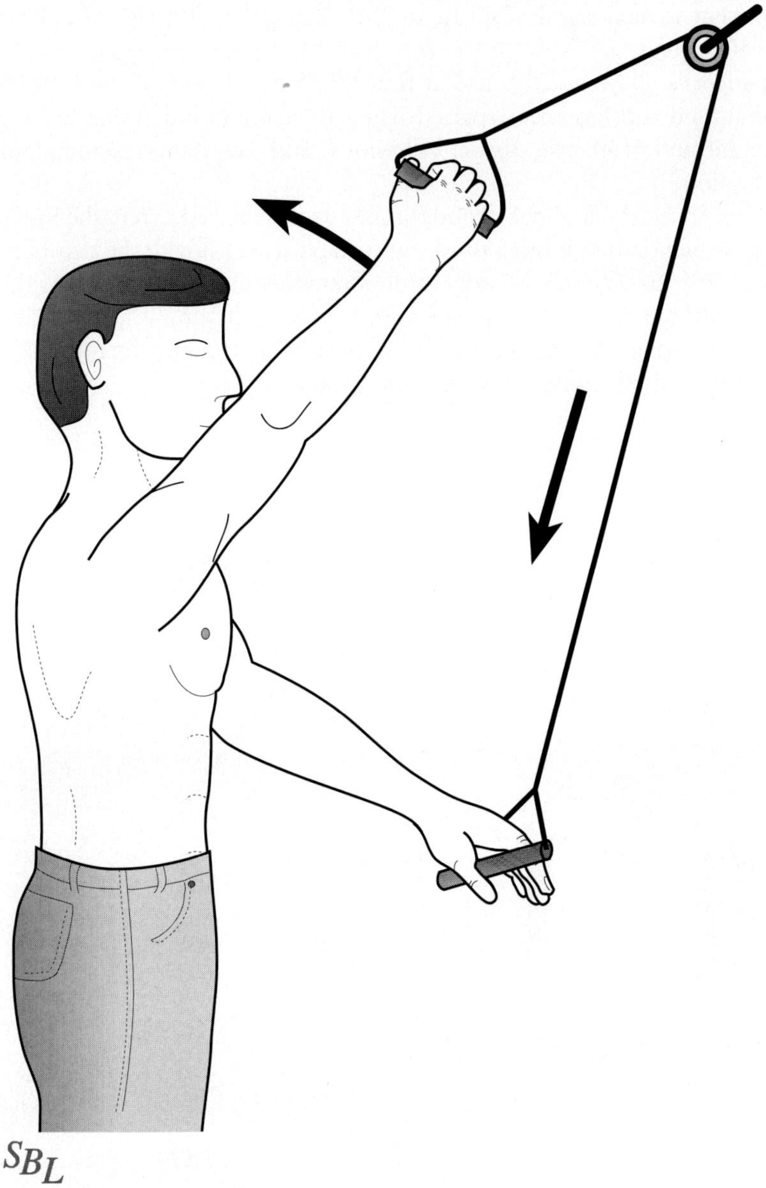

**Figure 20–20. Door pulley**
A pulley mounted on the door can be helpful in achieving elevation, especially when the opposite shoulder is involved.

The patient is discharged when he or she can flex to 140 degrees and externally rotate to 40 degrees.

The patient is allowed active use of the shoulder as tolerated, since no deltoid is detached and no cuff has been repaired. The patient is reminded that the key to preventing reformation of scar tissue, adhesions, and crepitance is maintaining full assisted motion.

After full, comfortable range of motion has been achieved, strengthening exercises are started sequentially. It is often most comfortable to begin with the two-hand supine press series (**Fig. 20–21**) and shoulder girdle strengthening (**Fig. 20–22**). As the patient advances in the supine press, scapula protractor strengthening is added (**Fig. 20–23**). Finally, internal (**Fig. 20–24**) and then external rotator strengthening (**Fig. 20–25**) are added as long as these exercises remain comfortable.

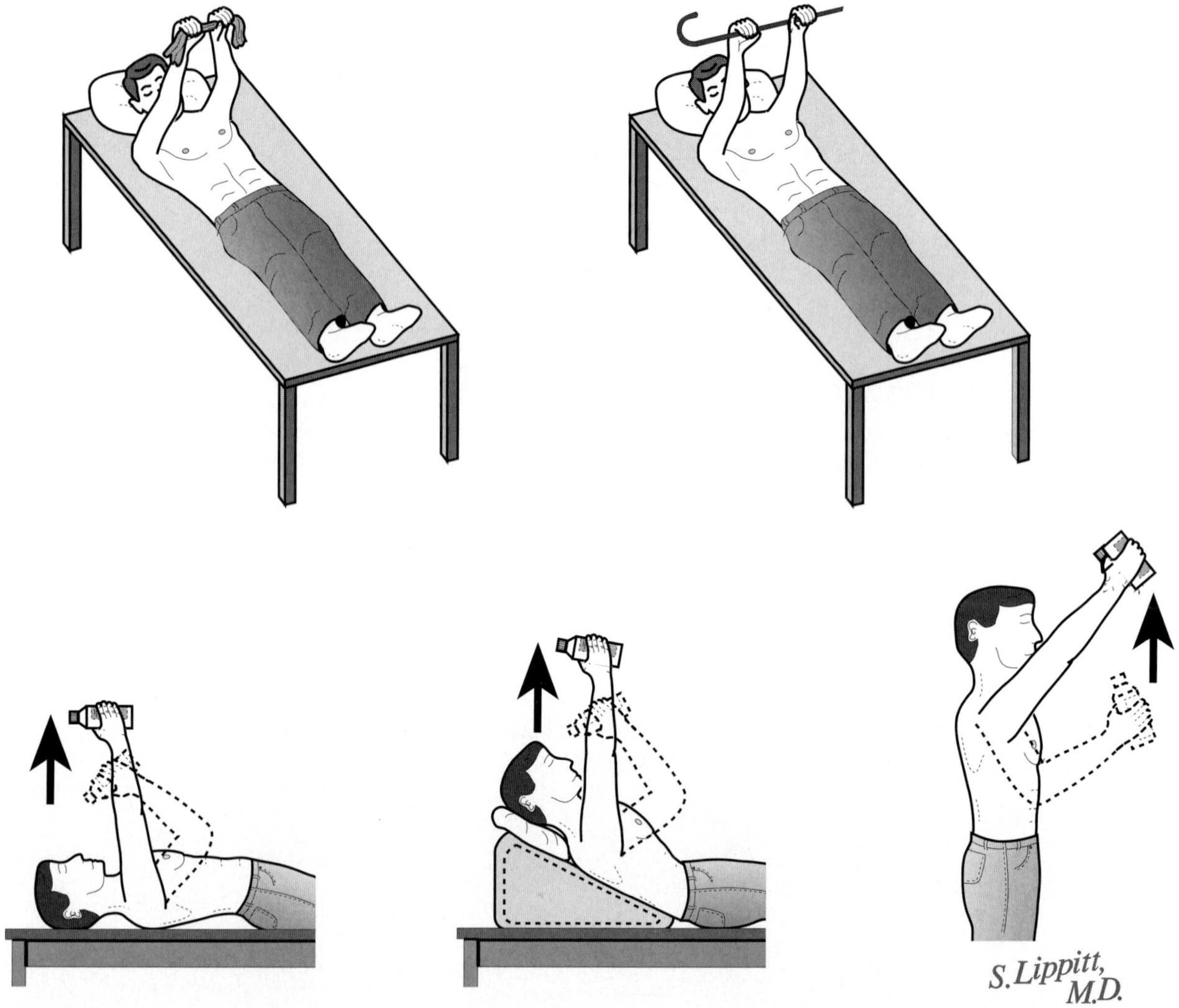


**Figure 20–21. Incremental press**

Integrated forward elevation is developed by a series of exercises that can be progressed in small increments. First, two hands are placed close to each other on a light stick or towel and both hands are pressed upward toward the ceiling while the patient is in the supine position. Next, the same exercise is repeated with the arms progressively farther apart. Next, the arm does the supine press unassisted. Next, small amounts of weight are added to the hand until 2 pounds can be pressed upward 20 times. Then the patient's back is elevated slightly while the weight is pressed vertically upward. The amount of elevation is increased when 2 pounds can be pressed upward 20 times. The progression is continued until the exercise can be performed with the back in a vertical position. (Modified from Matsen FA, Lippitt SB, Sidles JA, et al [eds]: Practical Evaluation and Management of the Shoulder. Philadelphia: WB Saunders, 1994, p. 131.)

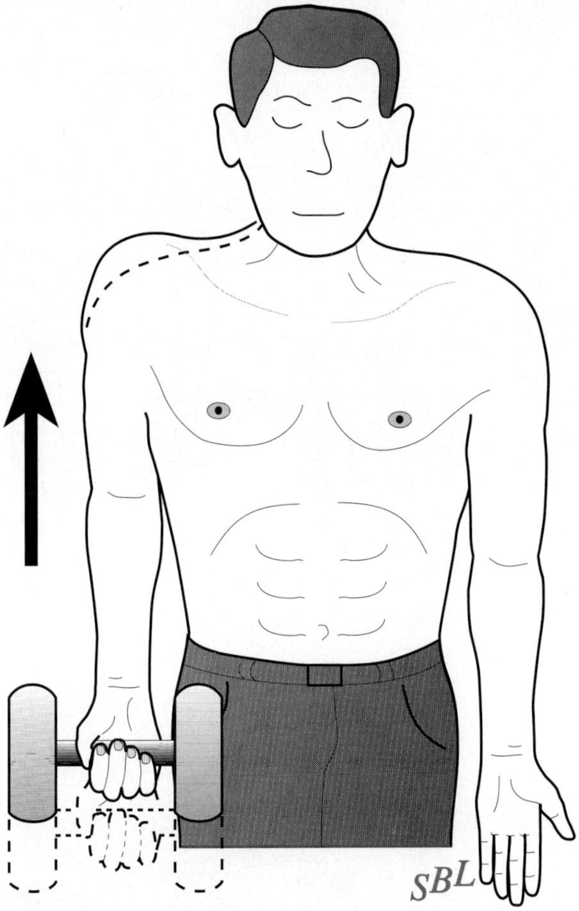


**Figure 20–22. Trapezius shrug**
The trapezius is strengthened by the patient's shrugging the shoulder upward while holding a weight in the hand. (Modified from Matsen FA, Lippitt SB, Sidles JA, et al [eds]: Practical Evaluation and Management of the Shoulder. Philadelphia: WB Saunders, 1994, p. 87.)

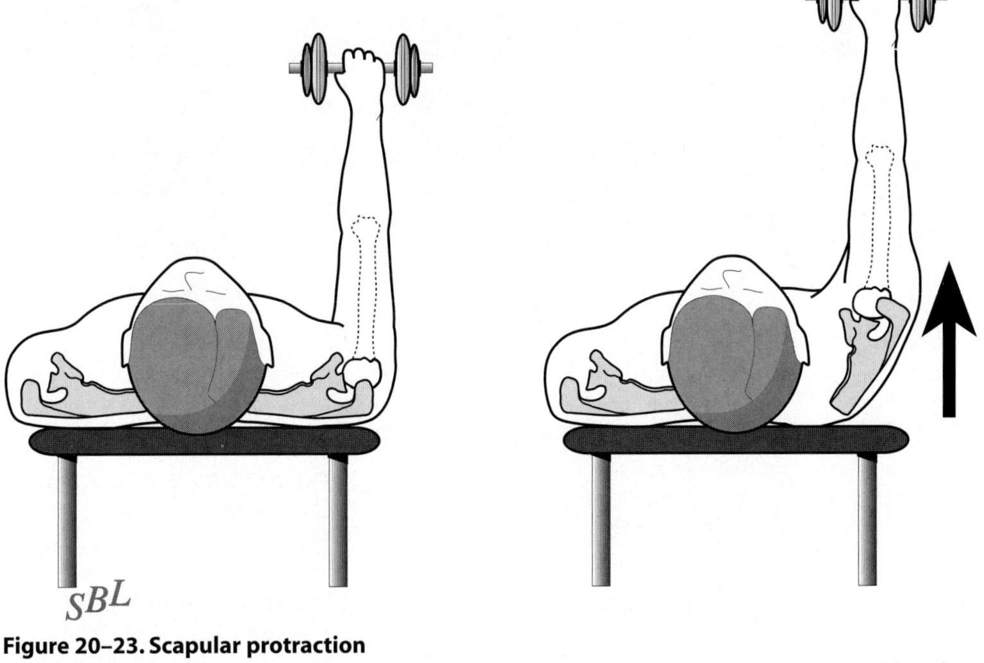


**Figure 20–23. Scapular protraction**
The hand is pressed upward. The press is completed by protracting the scapula. (Modified from Matsen FA, Lippitt SB, Sidles JA, et al [eds]: Practical Evaluation and Management of the Shoulder. Philadelphia: WB Saunders, 1994, p. 87.)

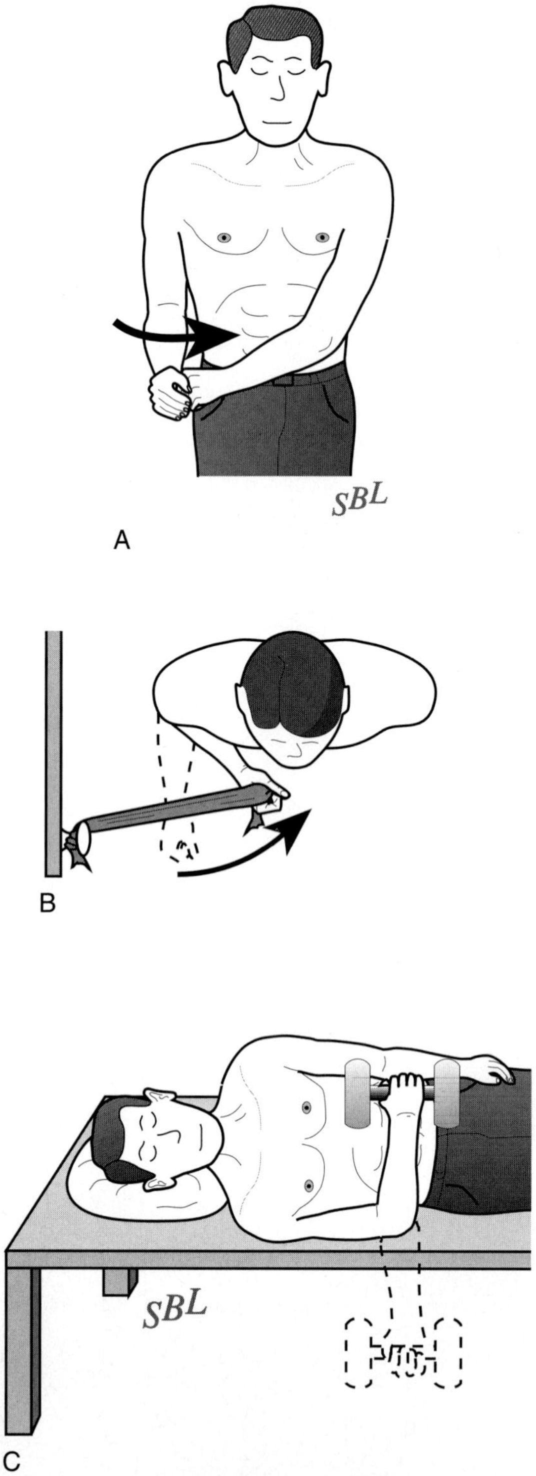


**Figure 20–24. Internal rotation strengthening**
The muscles of internal rotation are strengthened by exercising them against isometric resistance, against elastic tubing, and against weights. (Modified from Matsen FA, Lippitt SB, Sidles JA, et al [eds]: Practical Evaluation and Management of the Shoulder. Philadelphia: WB Saunders, 1994, p. 86.)

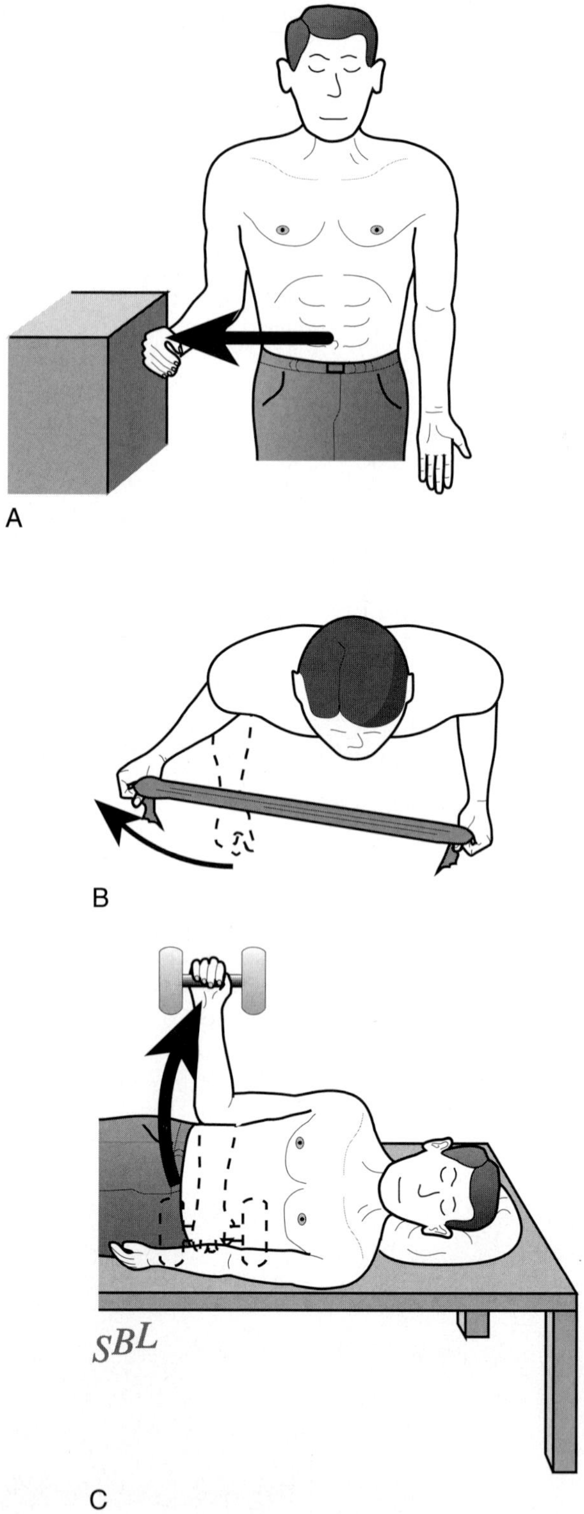


**Figure 20–25. External rotation strengthening**
The muscles of external rotation are strengthened by exercising them against isometric resistance, against elastic tubing, and against weights. (Modified from Matsen FA, Lippitt SB, Sidles JA, et al [eds]: Practical Evaluation and Management of the Shoulder. Philadelphia: WB Saunders, 1994, p. 86.)

CHAPTER 21

# Procedure: Rotator Cuff Repair

***Diagnosis***

***Full-thickness rotator cuff tear involving the supraspinatus tendon ICD9 CODE 840.6***

***Surgical Procedure***

***Rotator cuff repair CPT CODE 23412 or 23410***

## INDICATIONS

The patient has persistent and functionally significant weakness of the shoulder after a definite injury. The shoulder is weak on supraspinatus testing. A defect in the cuff near the supraspinatus insertion to the greater tuberosity is noted by palpation. The supraspinatus muscle is mildly atrophic.

A rotator cuff tear involving the supraspinatus is demonstrated on rotator cuff tendon imaging. The symptoms have not responded to nonoperative management.

Knowing in detail the alternatives as well as the risks of infection, neurovascular injury, excessive stiffness, pain and weakness, irreparability, re-rupture, and the need for revision surgery, as well as the risks of anesthesia, the patient desires to proceed with rotator cuff surgery—including rotator cuff repair if the cuff tendons are of sufficient quantity and quality. The patient recognizes that this procedure cannot be expected to completely restore normal comfort and function to the shoulder. And lastly, the patient understands his or her critical role in post-surgical rehabilitation.

## FINDINGS

Examination under anesthesia indicates subacromial crepitance on passive motion and a palpable defect at the supraspinatus insertion to the greater tuberosity.

Surgical findings include scarring in the humeroscapular motion interface as well as bursal thickening. There is a full-thickness defect involving the entire supraspinatus tendon. The quality of the residual tendon is excellent. The tendon edge comes to within 15 mm of the anatomical insertion site. The long head of the biceps is intact. The undersurface of the coracoacromial arch is smooth.

## OPERATION

Under satisfactory anesthesia, the patient is placed in a low beach chair position with the glenohumeral joint at the edge of the operating table (**Fig. 21–1**). The entire forequarter is carefully prepped and draped in the usual sterile fashion with the arm free to be moved.

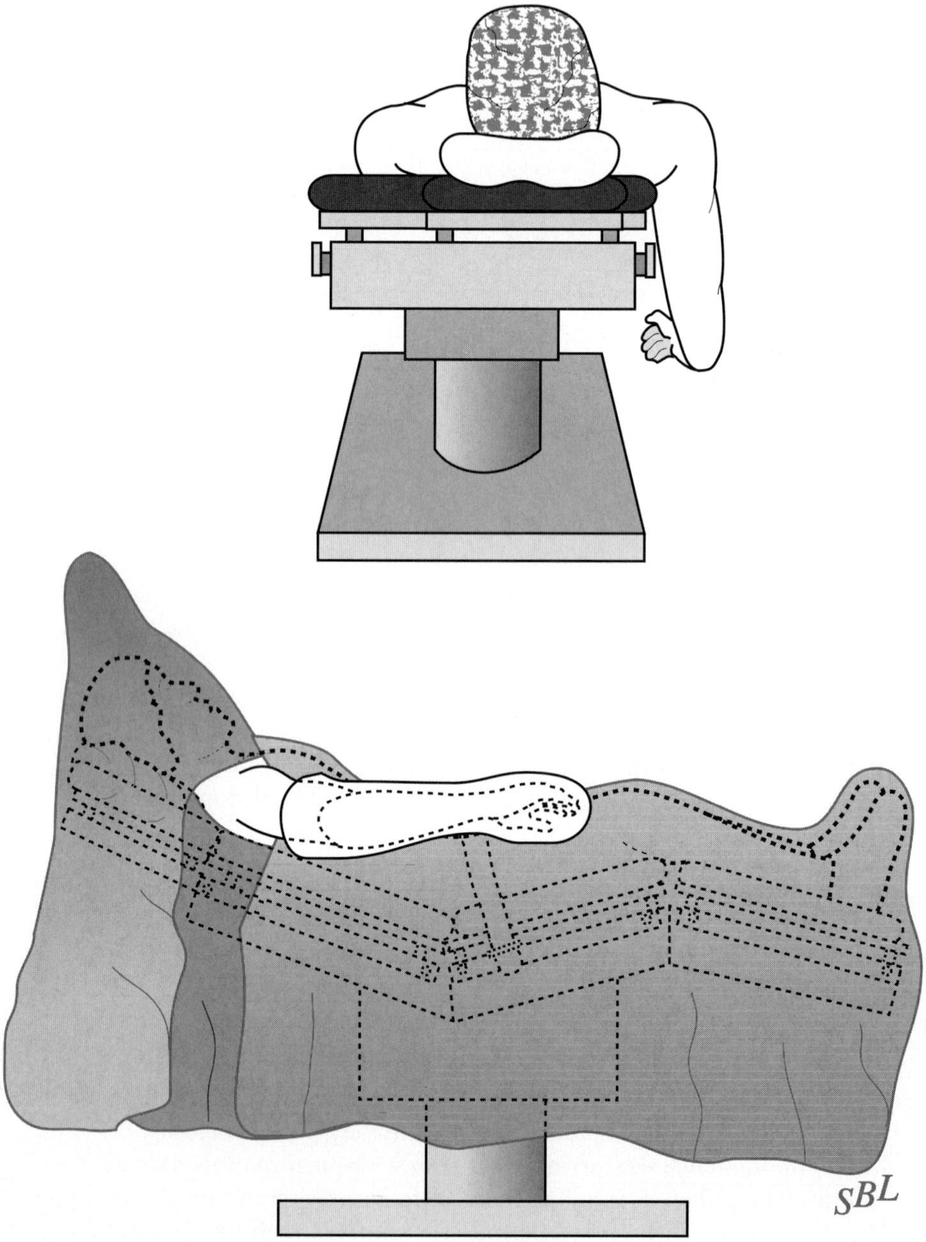


**Figure 21–1. Draping the shoulder**
The patient is placed in beach chair position with arm draped free. Note that the patient is positioned with the glenohumeral joint at the edge of the table so that the arm can be moved through a full range of motion.

The shoulder is approached through a superior incision in the skin line crossing the anterior corner of the acromion (**Fig. 21–2**). The deltoid-on approach is used (**Fig. 21–3**). The deltoid tendon of origin running between the anterior and lateral thirds of the deltoid is identified and split longitudinally, leaving half of the tendon on either side of the split; no deltoid is detached from the acromion. This split is carried down to the subdeltoid bursa that is divided in line with the deltoid split (**Fig. 21–4**).

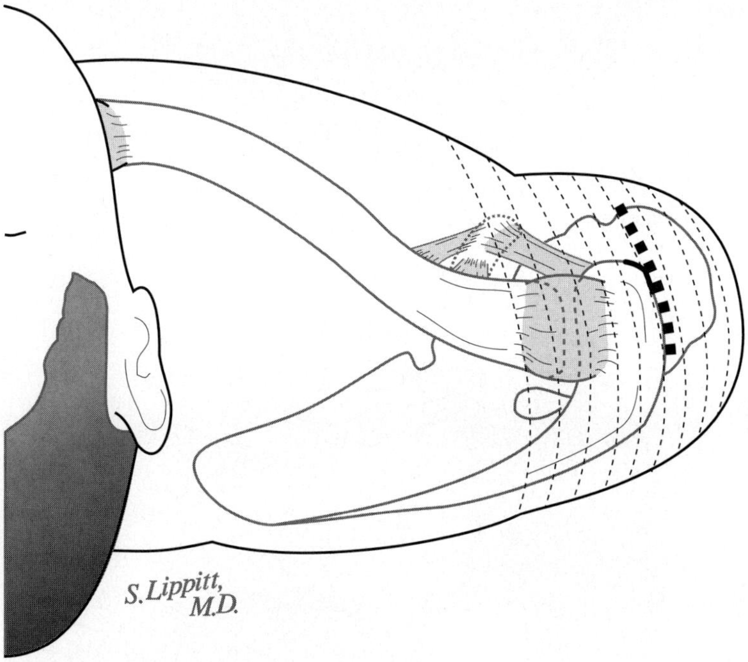


**Figure 21–2. Deltoid-on approach**
The deltoid-on approach, showing the skin incision in Langer's lines.

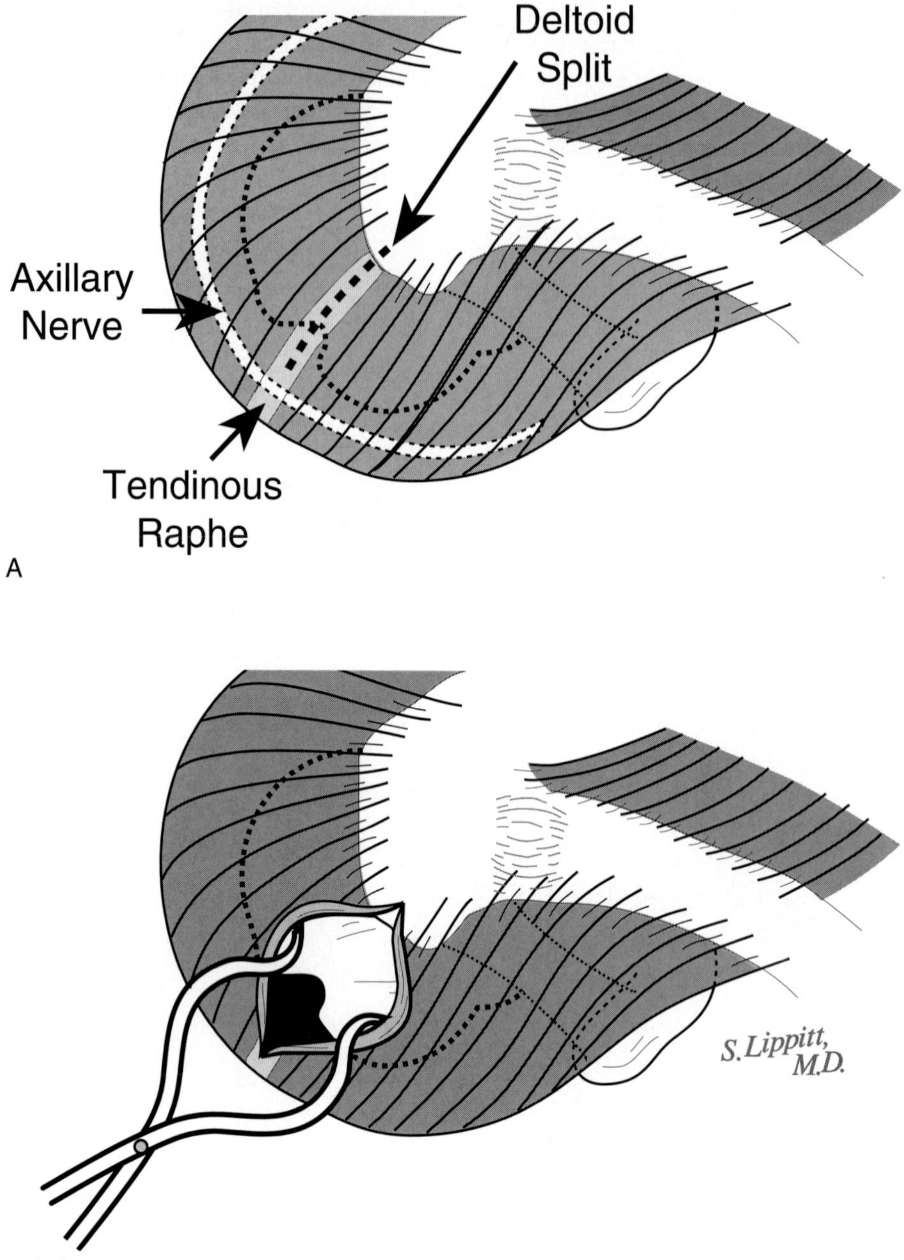


**Figure 21–3. Deltoid split**
The deltoid is split along the raphe between the anterior and lateral thirds of the muscle without any of it being detached from the acromion. (Modified from Matsen FA, Lippitt SB, Sidles JA, et al [eds]: Practical Evaluation and Management of the Shoulder. Philadelphia: WB Saunders, 1994, p. 135.)

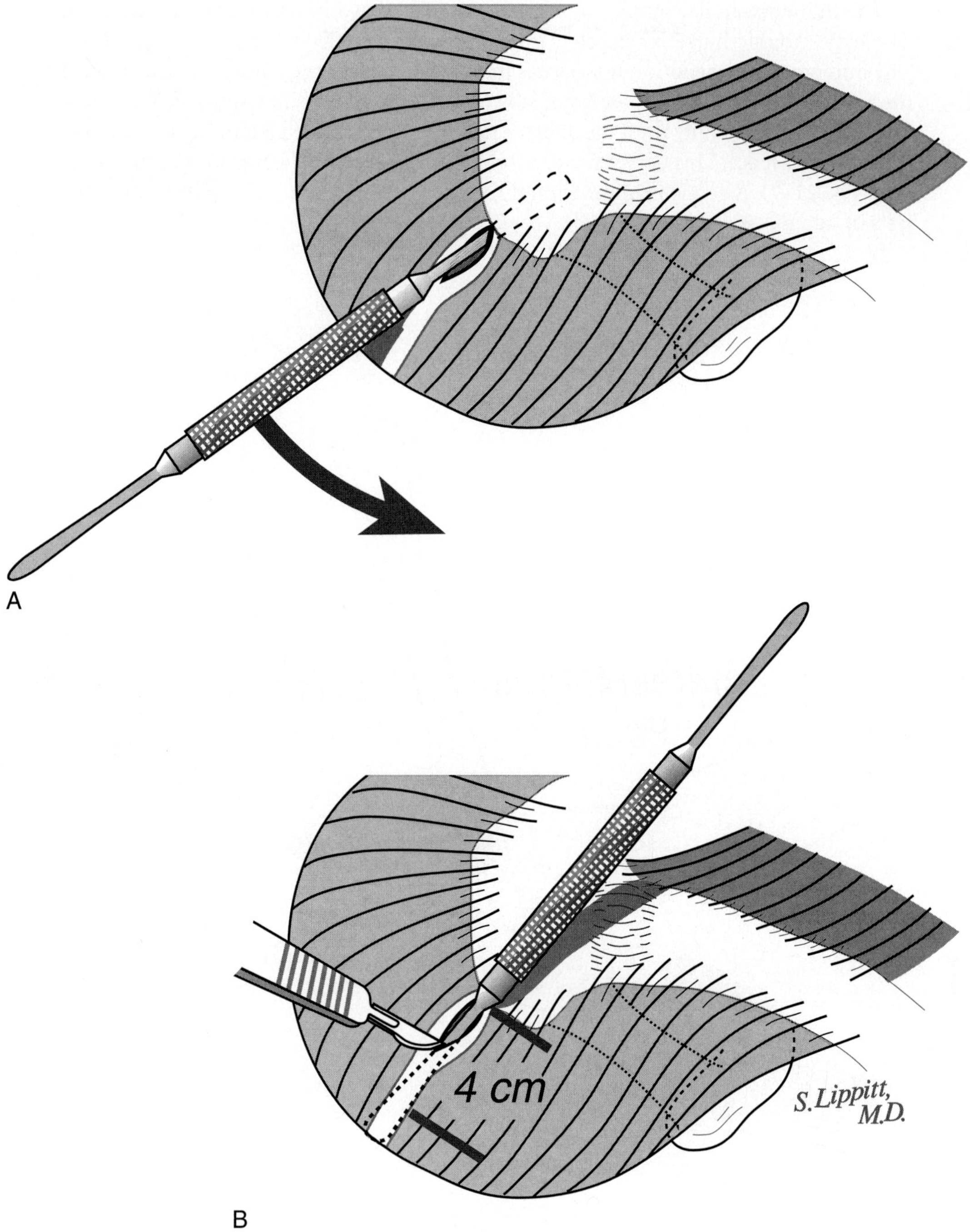


**Figure 21–4. Inserting an elevator in the deltoid split**
Once the subdeltoid bursa is entered, a small blunt elevator is inserted through the split and then underneath the deltoid (**A**). This elevator is then rotated 180 degrees while still in the bursa. The incision in the deltoid and bursa is then extended 4 cm distal from the acromion (**B**).

The humeroscapular motion interface is mobilized by blunt dissection (**Fig. 21–5**). The hypertrophic bursa is dissected from the surface of the rotator cuff (**Fig. 21–6**). The humeroscapular motion interface is mobilized beneath the coracoid muscles until the axillary nerve can be palpated medially on the front of the subscapularis. The interface is dissected laterally until the axillary nerve can be palpated laterally as it exits the quadrilateral space. This nerve-to-nerve release ensures complete freedom of the interface (**Fig. 21–7**). A gentle manipulation through a full range of motion ensures that the lysis of adhesions is complete.

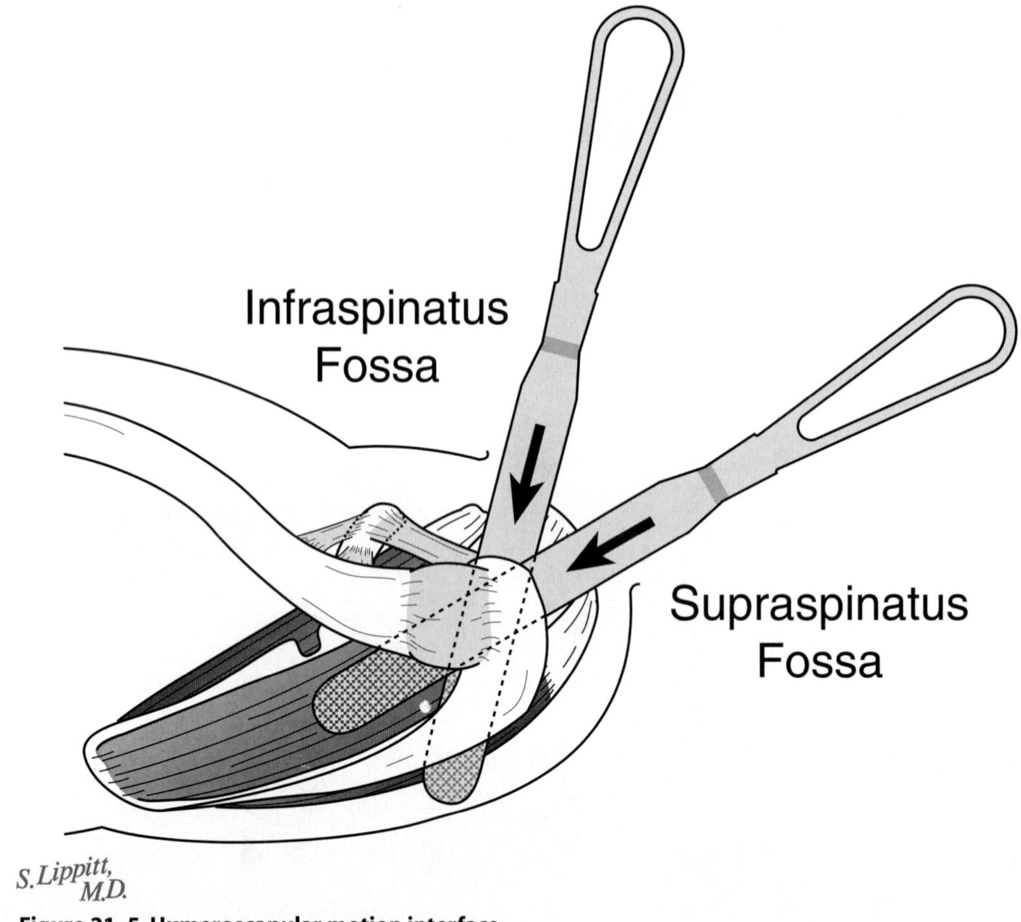


**Figure 21–5. Humeroscapular motion interface**
A smooth elevator is passed superficially to the supraspinatus and infraspinatus to ensure their freedom from the overlying coracoacromial arch.

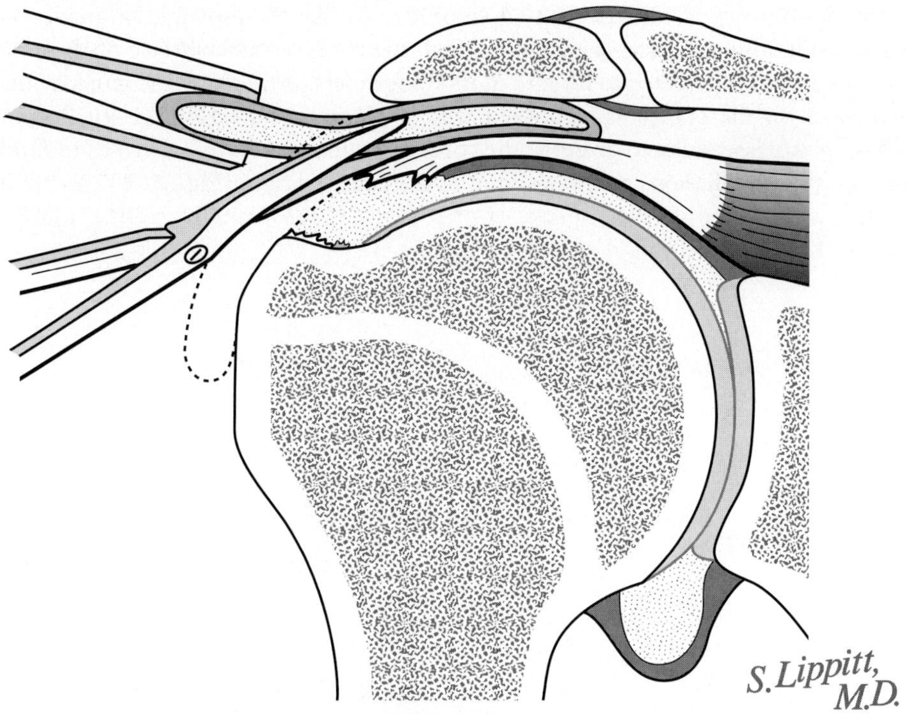


**Figure 21–6. Removal of the bursa**
The hypertrophic bursa is removed by sharp dissection.

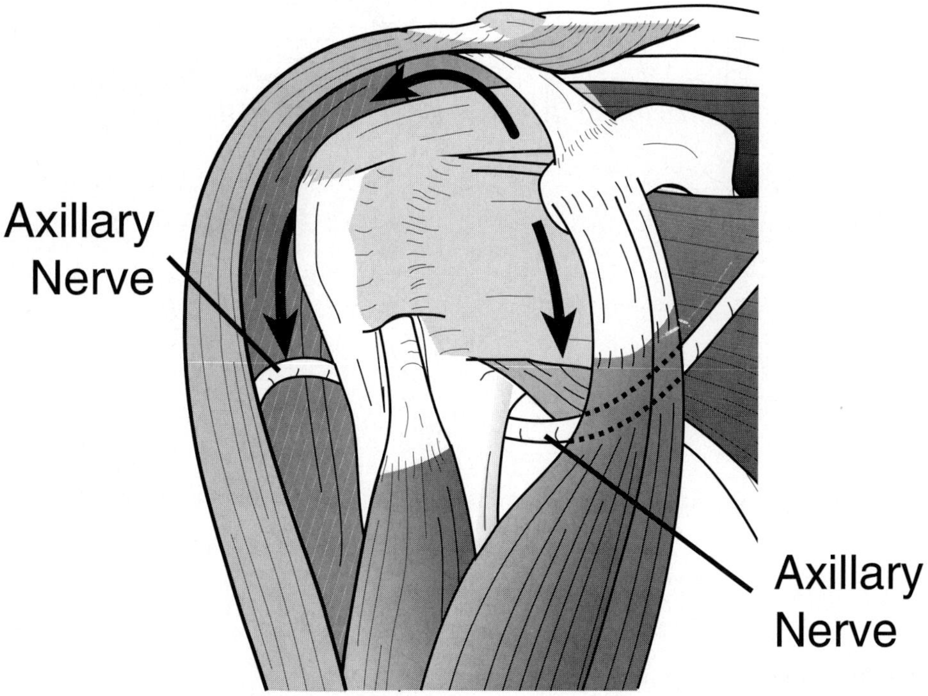


**Figure 21–7. Nerve-to-nerve release**
All scar tissue in the humeroscapular motion interface is released from the axillary nerve medially as it crosses the subscapularis, then under the coracoid, then under the coracoacromial ligament, then under the acromion, and then finally under the deltoid to the axillary nerve posteriorly as it exits the quadrilateral space: the nerve-to-nerve release.

Any prominence of the tuberosity is smoothed so that the proximal humeral convexity is smoothly spherical (**Fig. 21–8**). Next, the concave undersurface of the coracoacromial arch is palpated to be sure of its smoothness. If there is a prominence that encroaches on the cuff, it is smoothed with a pinecone burr (**Fig. 21–9**). Routine acromioplasty is avoided to preserve the coracoacromial concavity as well as to minimize the risk of adhesions and weakening of the deltoid origin (**Fig. 21–10**). By rotating the arm, the different aspects of the tear can be brought to the incision (**Fig. 21–11**).

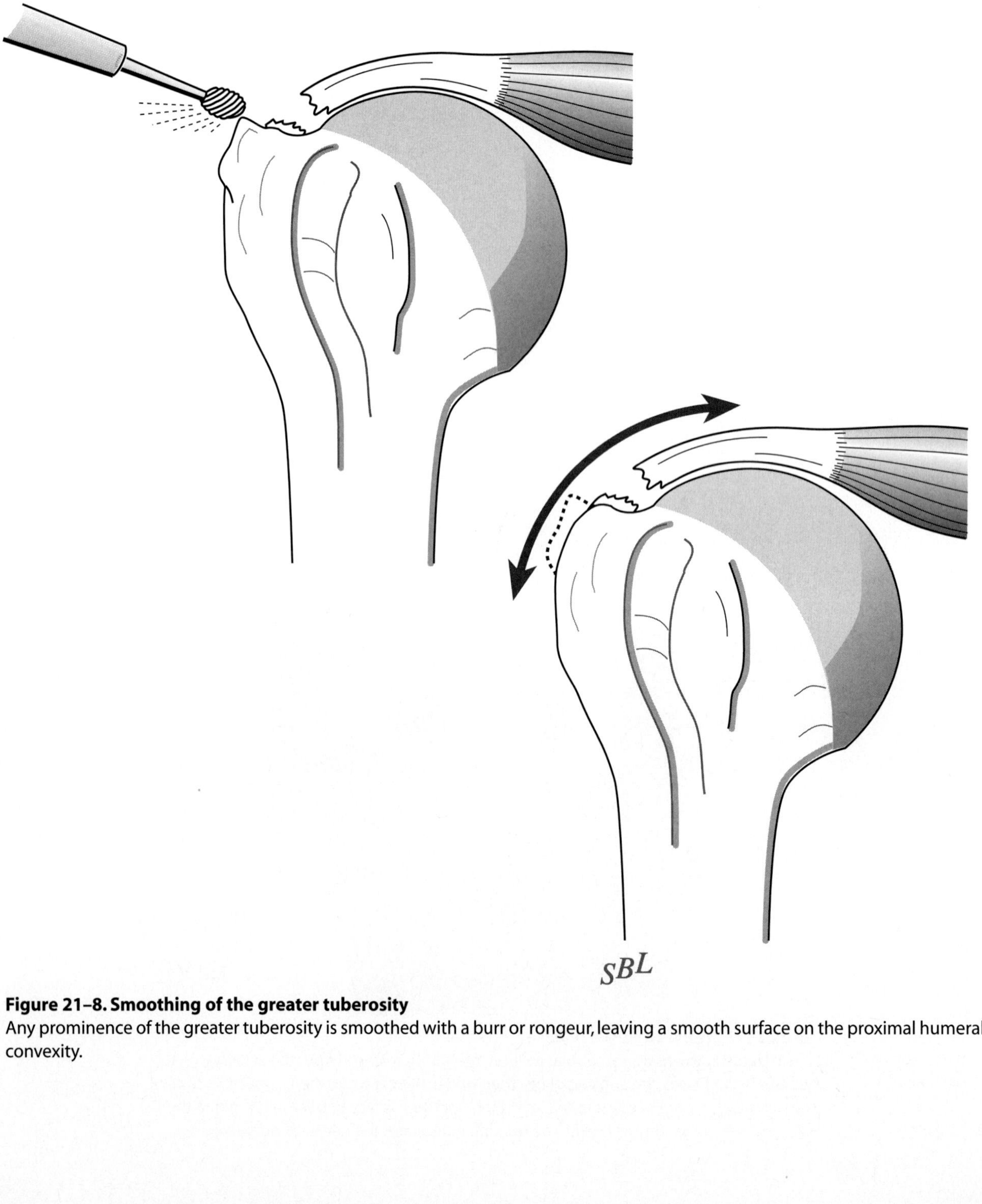


**Figure 21–8. Smoothing of the greater tuberosity**
Any prominence of the greater tuberosity is smoothed with a burr or rongeur, leaving a smooth surface on the proximal humeral convexity.

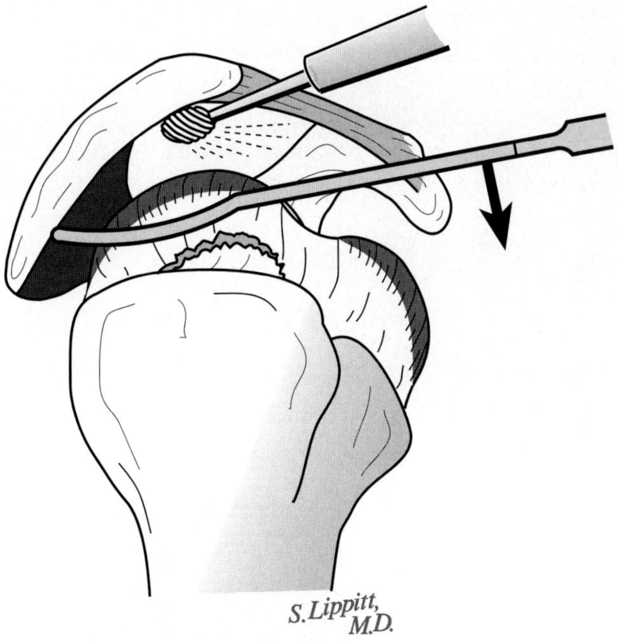


**Figure 21–9. Smoothing of the coracoacromial arch**
If, as is rarely the case, there is roughness on the underside of the coracoacromial arch, it can be smoothed with a pinecone burr, leaving the arch intact.

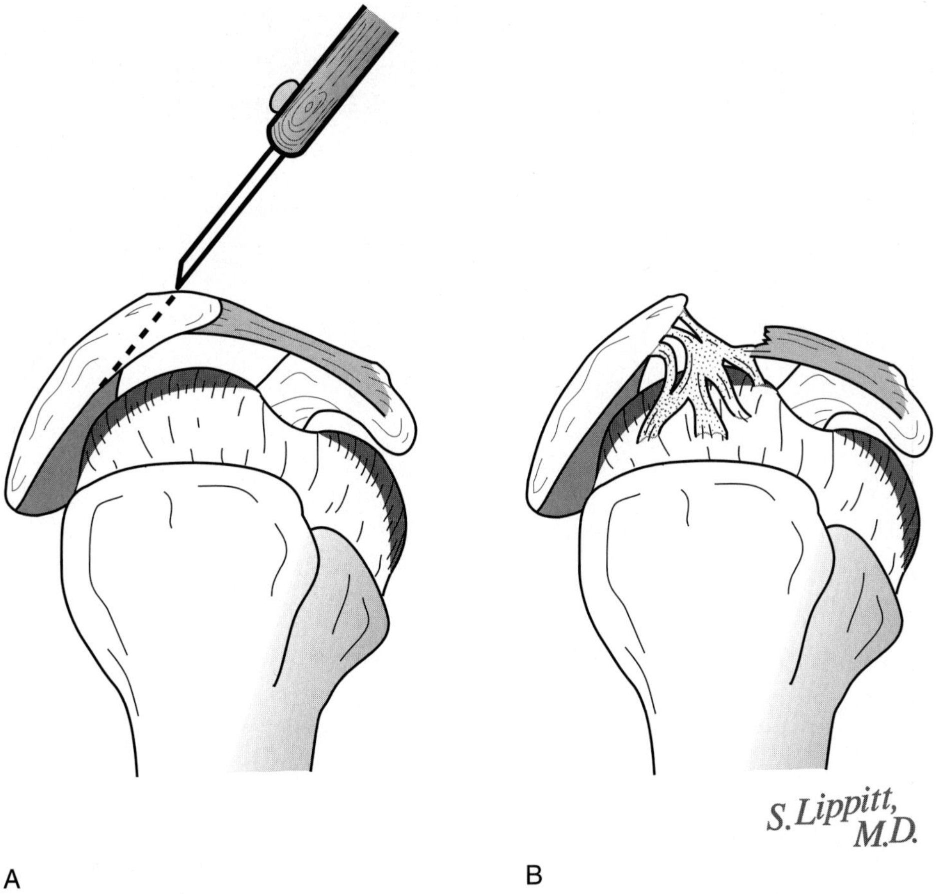


**Figure 21–10. Acromioplasty hazards**
Acromioplasty is avoided because it sacrifices the stability provided by the coracoacromial arch, it compromises the deltoid origin, and it risks adhesion to the underlying cuff.

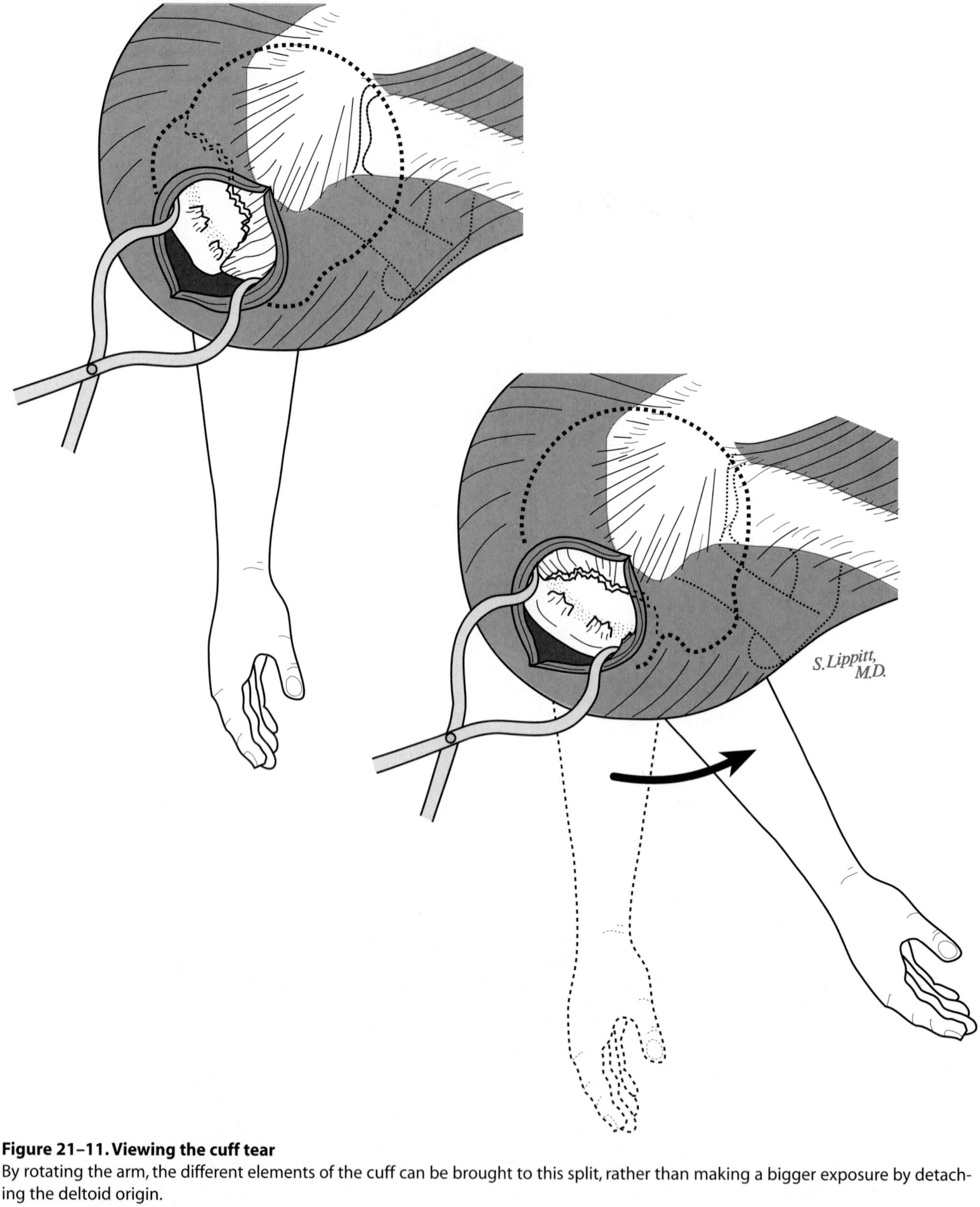


**Figure 21–11. Viewing the cuff tear**
By rotating the arm, the different elements of the cuff can be brought to this split, rather than making a bigger exposure by detaching the deltoid origin.

This dissection provides excellent exposure of the torn edge of the supraspinatus tendon as well as a split between the supraspinatus and the infraspinatus. Traction sutures are placed in the tendon edge (**Fig. 21–12**). Traction on these sutures indicates that the tendon is robust. If the cuff is retracted so that it will not reach the desired insertion site with the arm in adduction, the tendons are released

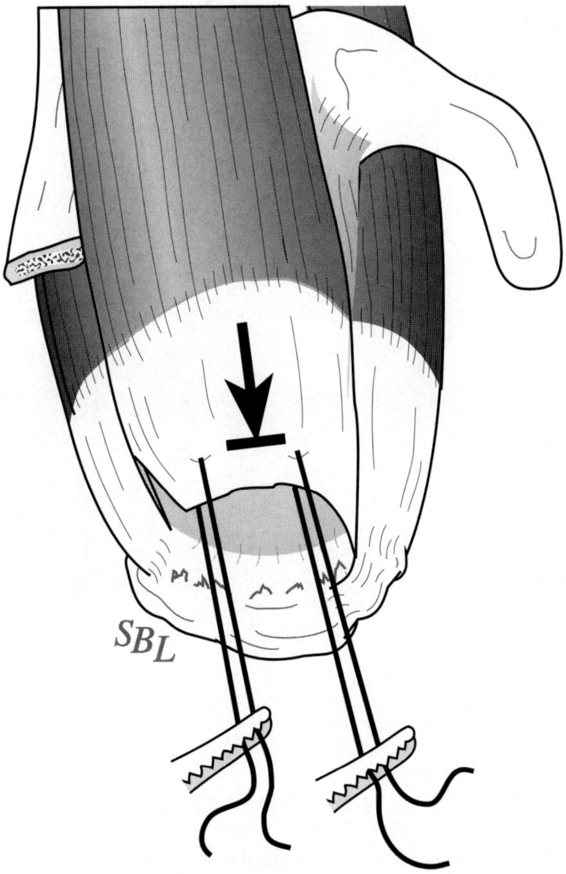


**Figure 21–12. Traction sutures**
Traction sutures are placed in the cuff tendon. These sutures should be able to withstand a strong pull without pulling through the tendon.

from the coracoid process (**Fig. 21–13**). If the cuff tendon edge still does not reach to the insertion site with the arm in adduction, an extralabral release is performed by passing a sharp periosteal elevator deep to the supraspinatus tendon, releasing the capsule from the glenoid labrum (**Fig. 21–14**). This release enables the tendon to be pulled laterally so that with physiologic tension, its lateral edge easily reaches the tuberosity of the adducted arm. The glenoid labrum remains intact to the glenoid.

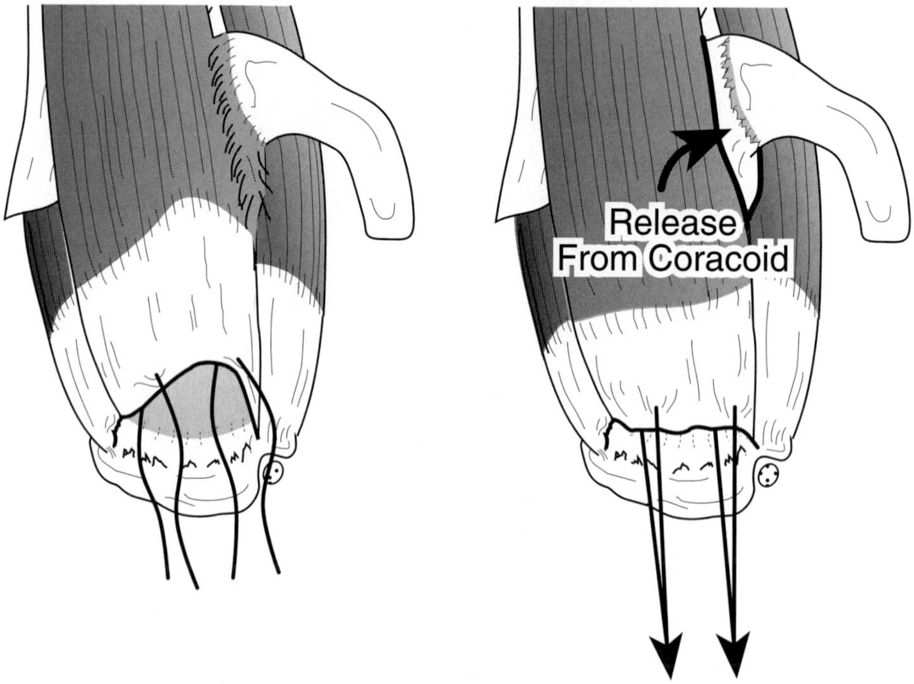


**Figure 21–13. Cuff release from coracoid**
Release of the cuff tendon from the coracoid allows lateral advancement of the tendon edge toward the desired insertion site. (Modified from Matsen FA, Lippitt SB, Sidles JA, et al [eds]: Practical Evaluation and Management of the Shoulder. Philadelphia: WB Saunders, 1994, p. 138.)

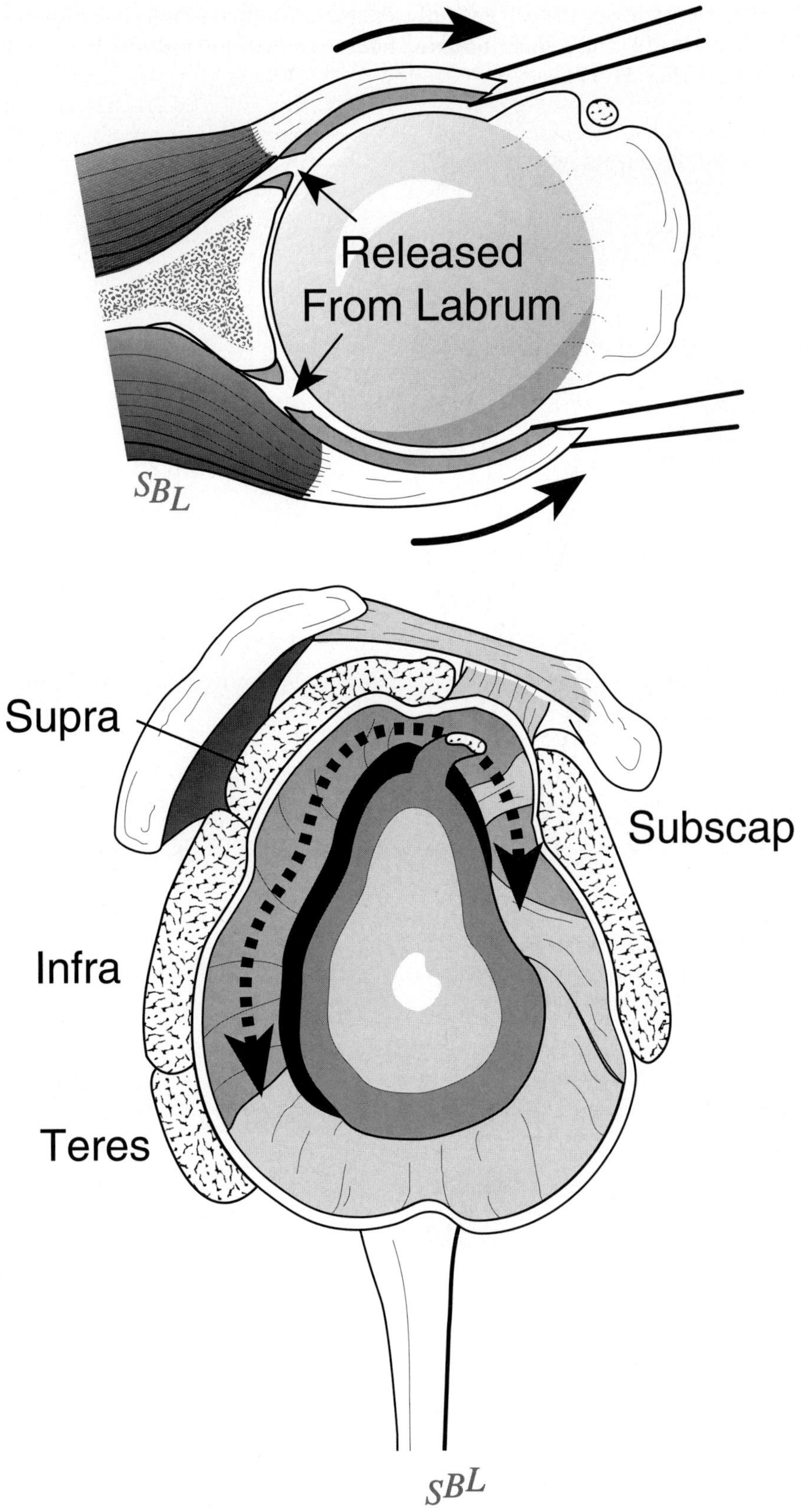


**Figure 21–14. Cuff release from labrum**
Release of the capsule from the labrum allows further lateral advancement of the tendon edge. (Modified from Matsen FA, Lippitt SB, Sidles JA, et al [eds]: Practical Evaluation and Management of the Shoulder. Philadelphia: WB Saunders, 1994, p. 138.)

After these releases, the cuff has sufficient excursion to reach the insertion site (**Figs. 21–15** and **21–16**) and a good "bounce," indicating that the tendon is free of restricted movement (**Fig. 21–17**).

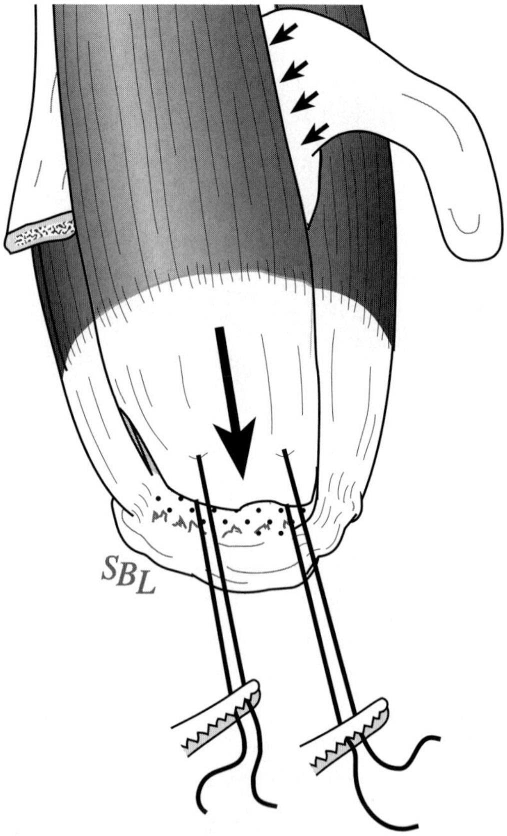


**Figure 21–15. After the release**
The lateral edge of the supraspinatus can now reach the base of the greater tuberosity.

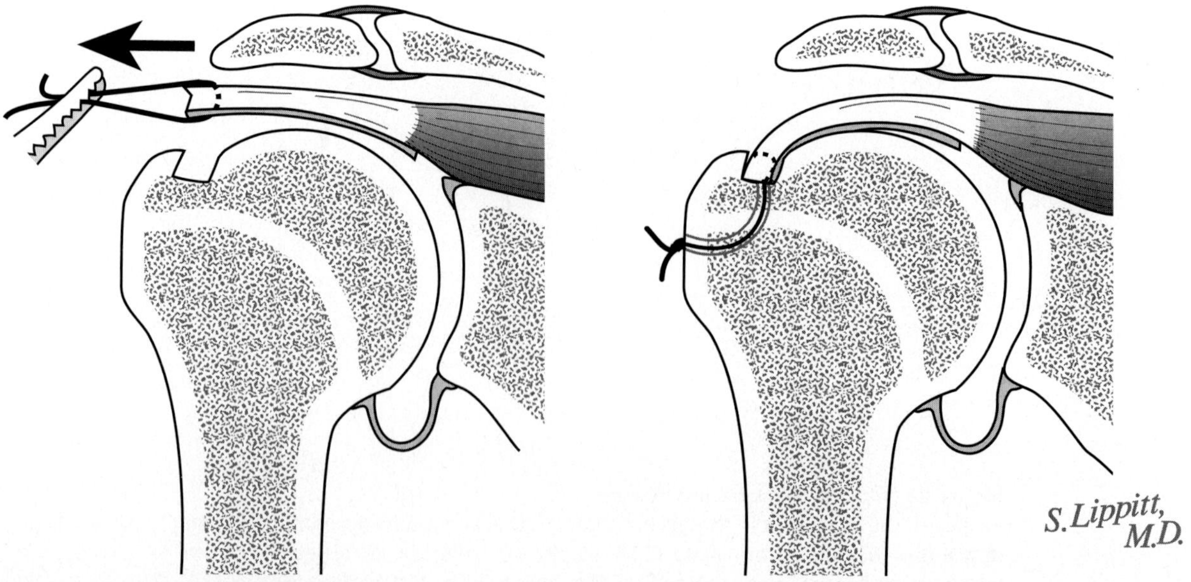


**Figure 21–16. Adequate excursion**
If a durable repair is to be carried out, the tendon margin should reach the insertion site with the arm in adduction without the application of excess tension.

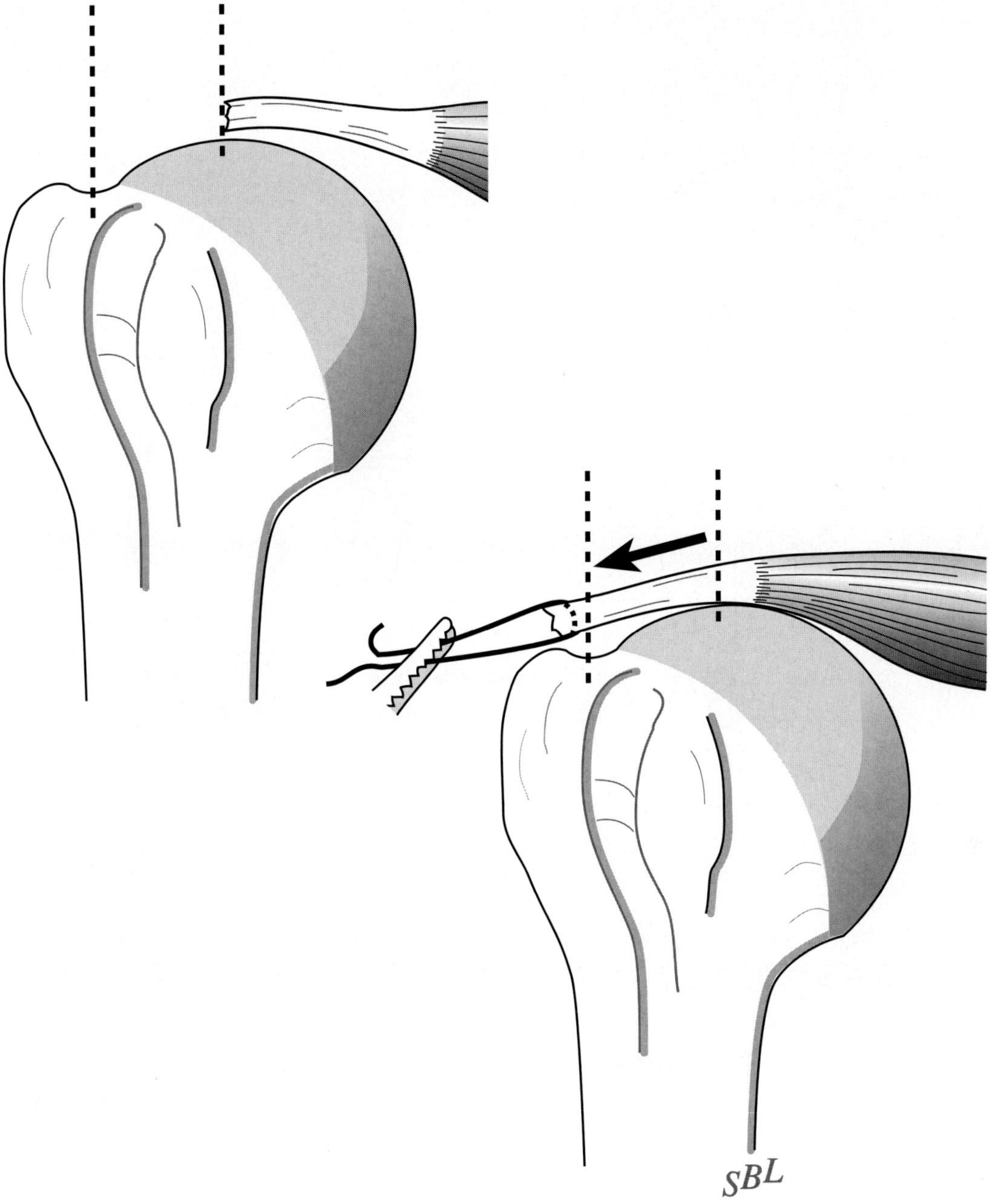


**Figure 21–17. Cuff bounce**
Once the tendon is freed of adhesions, the muscle should have a springy feel when traction is applied and released.

The tear pattern may resemble a three-corner tear (**Fig. 21–18**). Any split between the supraspinatus and the infraspinatus (**Fig. 21–19**) is closed with side-to-side sutures of #2 nonabsorbable braided suture using a buried knot technique so that the upper surface of the repaired cuff is smooth and free of knots (**Fig. 21–20**).

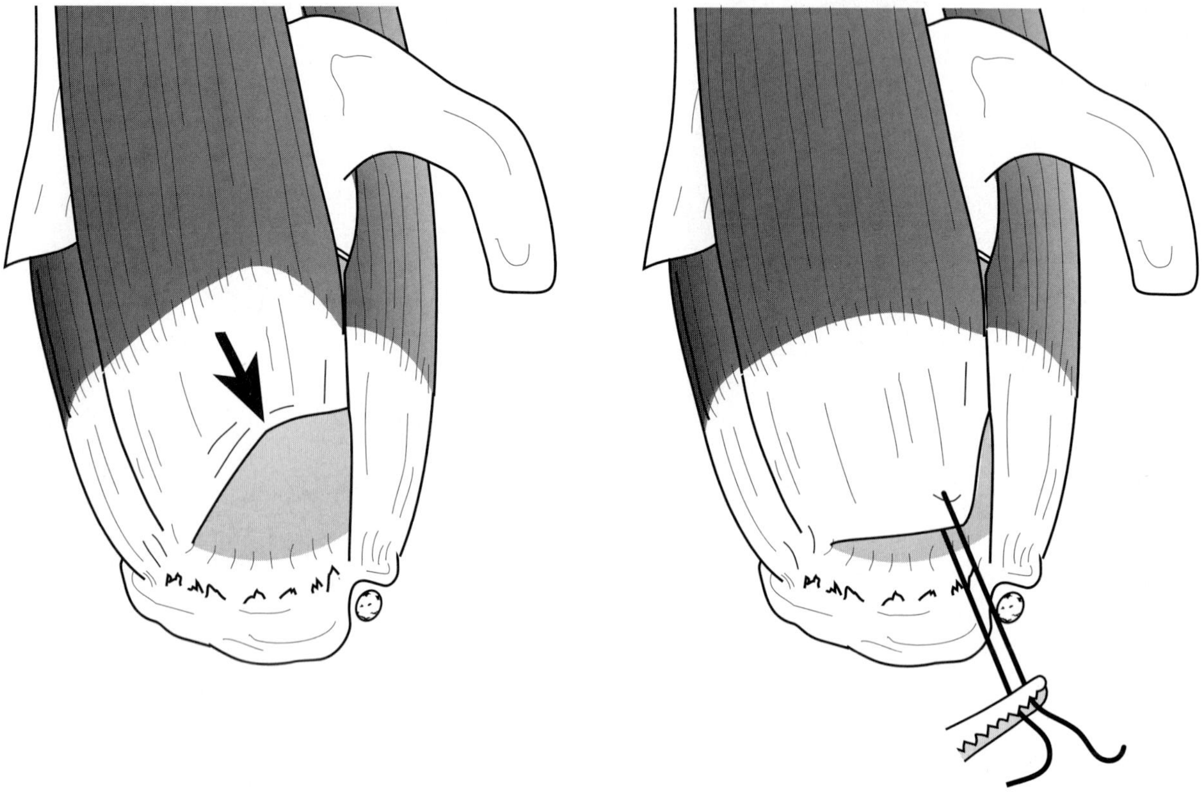

**Figure 21–18. Three-corner tear**
A tendon defect that begins at the anterior corner of the supraspinatus may propagate posteriorly toward the infraspinatus and medially between the supraspinatus and subscapularis, resulting in a three-corner tear.

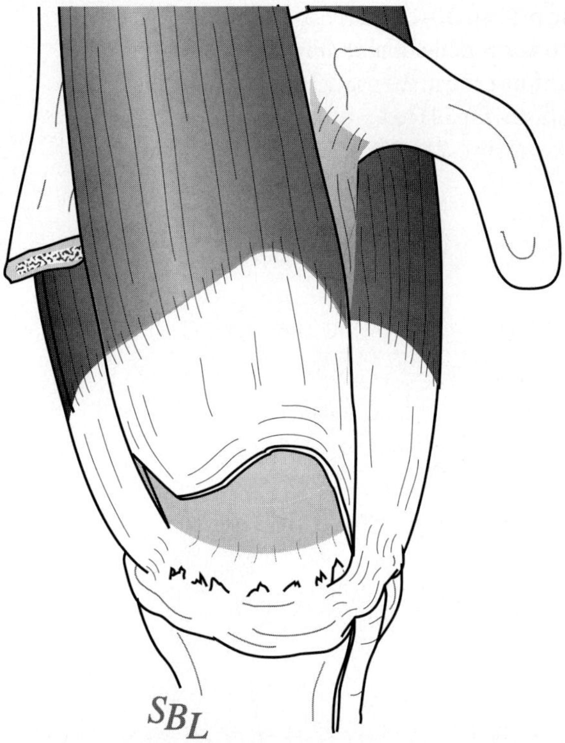

**Figure 21–19. Secondary split**
Not infrequently, there is a secondary split between the supraspinatus and the infraspinatus.

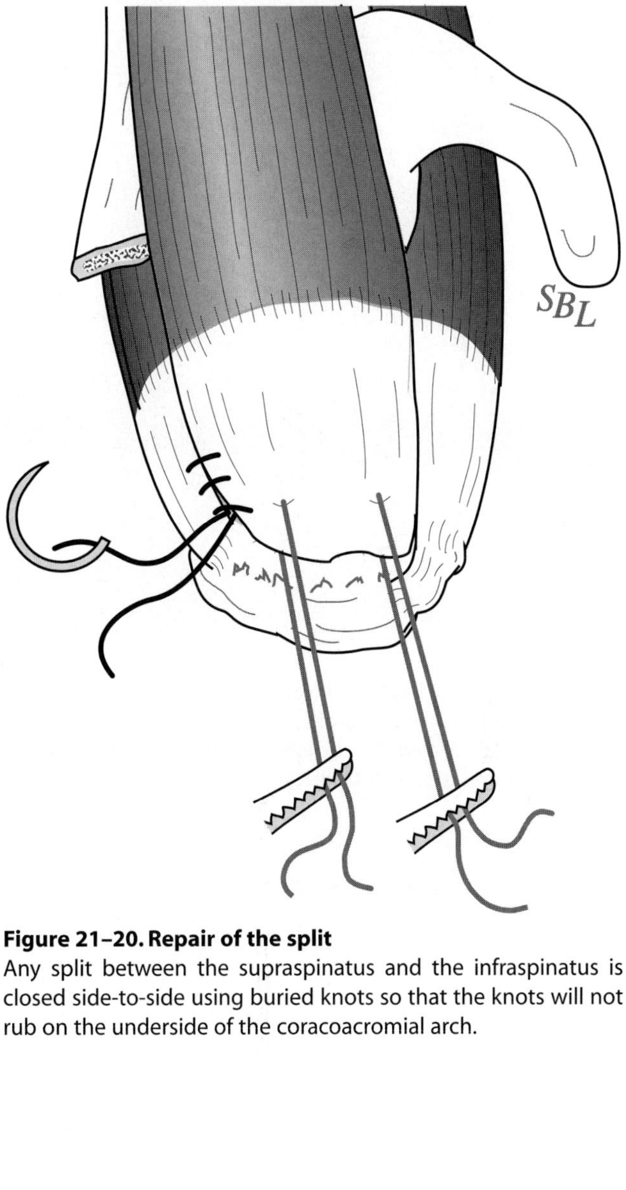

**Figure 21–20. Repair of the split**
Any split between the supraspinatus and the infraspinatus is closed side-to-side using buried knots so that the knots will not rub on the underside of the coracoacromial arch.

A 7 mm wide trough is created at the margin of the articular surface at the base of the greater tuberosity extending the length of the tendon detachment (**Fig. 21–21**). If good-quality tendon could not reach the normal cuff insertion, the trough would have been made more medially (**Fig. 21–22**). Staggered holes are placed 5 mm apart in the lateral aspect of the tuberosity where the bone is robust (**Fig. 21–23**). If the bone of the

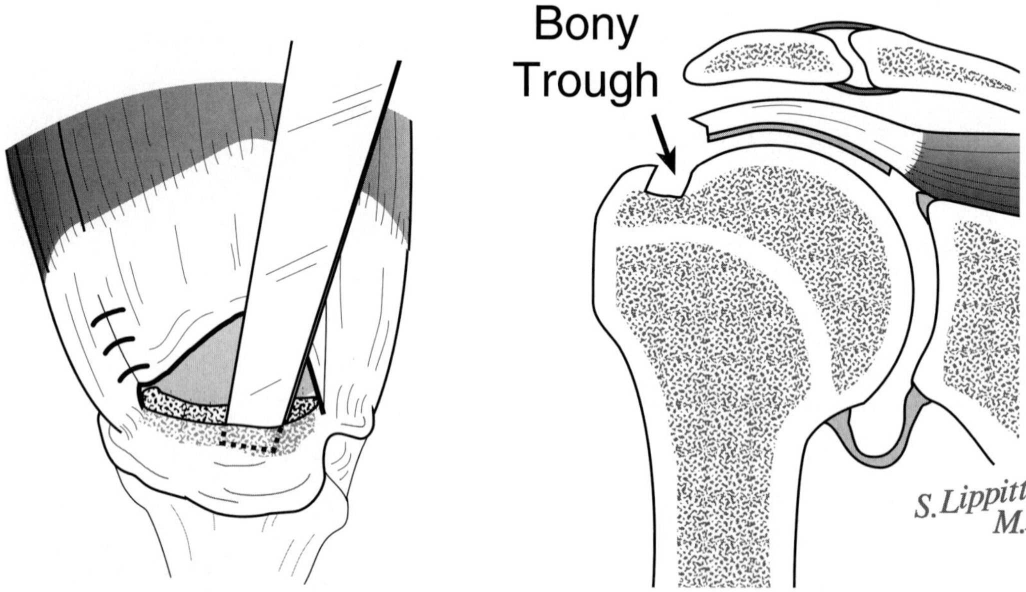


**Figure 21–21. Creating a trough**
Using a flat osteotome, a 7 mm wide trough is created at the base of the tuberosity at the margin of the articular cartilage for the length of the cuff tear. (Modified from Matsen FA, Lippitt SB, Sidles JA, et al [eds]: Practical Evaluation and Management of the Shoulder. Philadelphia: WB Saunders, 1994, p. 139.)

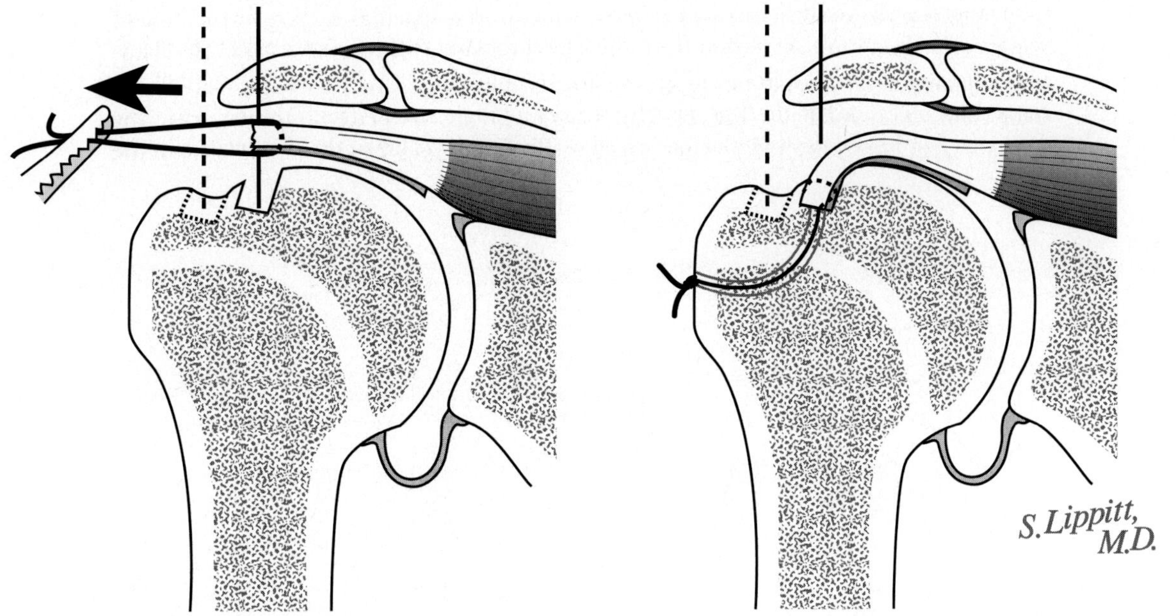


**Figure 21–22. Medializing the trough**
If the tendon will not reach the normal insertion site with the arm in adduction, the trough can be moved medially on the head if this will allow a robust attachment.

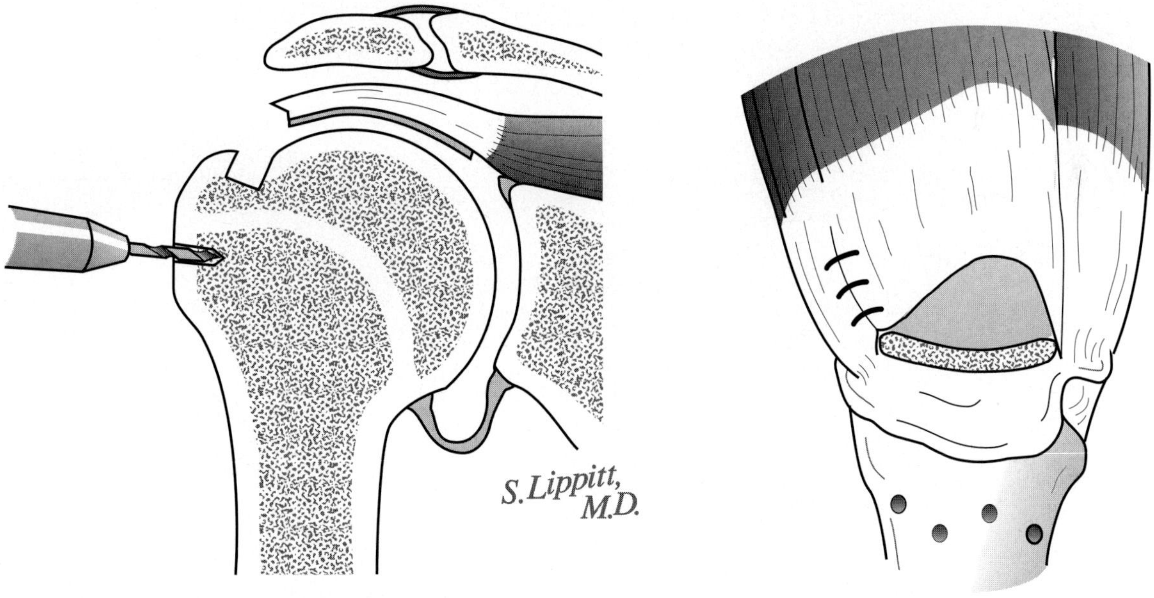


**Figure 21–23. Drilling the greater tuberosity**
Staggered drill holes are made distal to the trough using a 1.8 mm drill.

tuberosity is weak, the drill holes are moved more distally (**Fig. 21–24**). Number 2 braided nonabsorbable sutures are passed from the lateral tuberosity through the most posterior of the holes and into the trough (**Fig. 21–25**). Double sutures are placed through all the remaining holes except the last, which receives a single suture (**Fig. 21–26**). The first suture is then passed through the tendon edge (**Fig. 21–27**). One of the two sutures in the

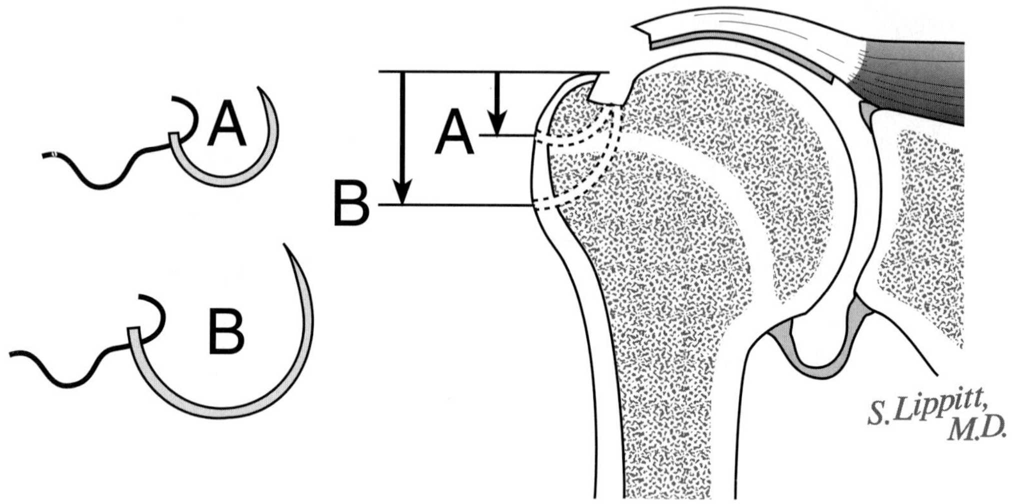


**Figure 21–24. Finding adequate bone**
If the bone of the proximal tuberosity is weak, the holes are made more distally in solid bone.

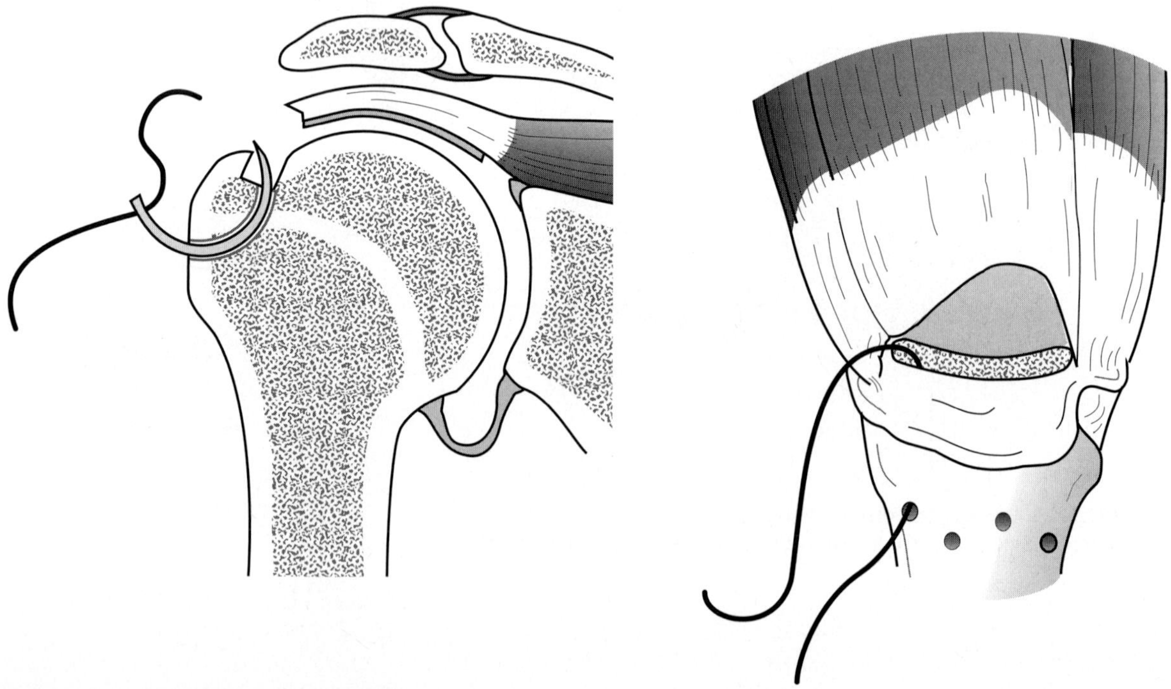

**Figure 21–25. Placement of first suture**
The first suture of #2 braided nonabsorbable suture is passed from the tuberosity into the groove using a #3 trochar needle.

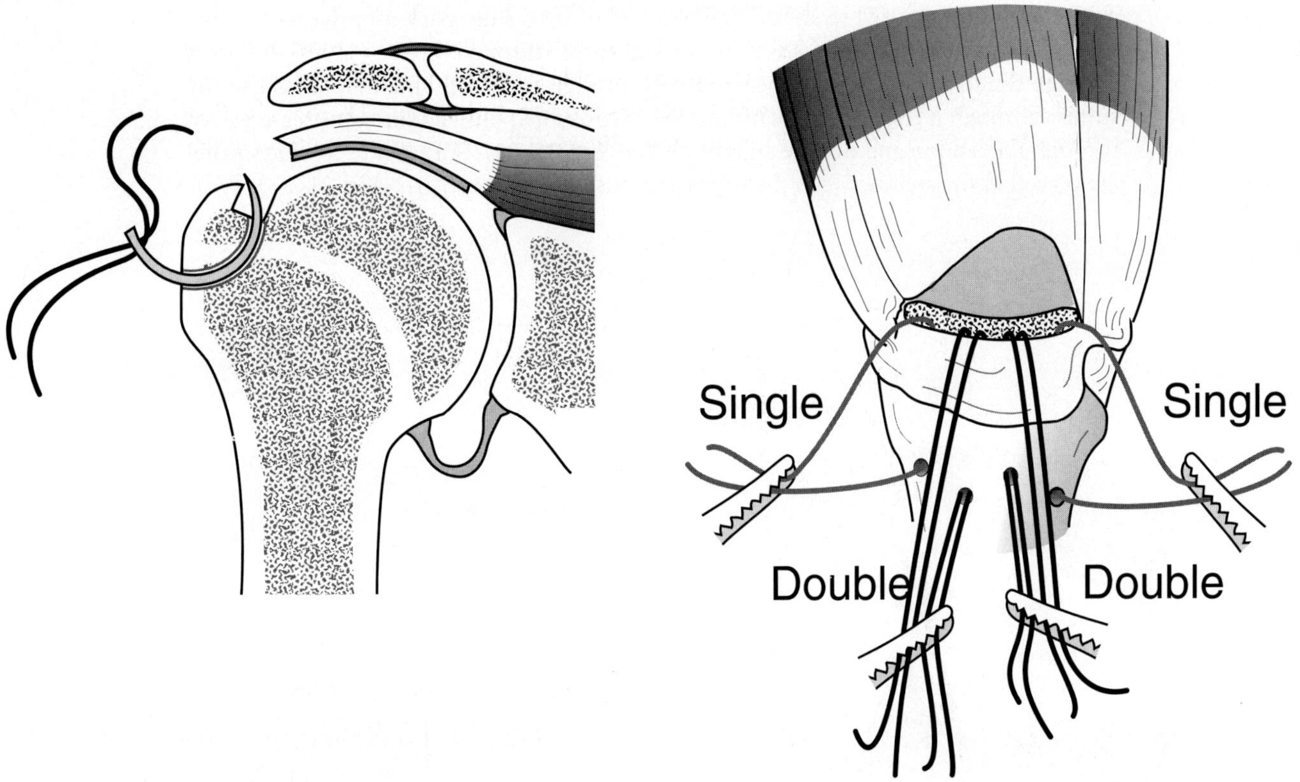


**Figure 21–26. Placement of double sutures**
Double sutures are passed through the remainder of the holes except for the last one.

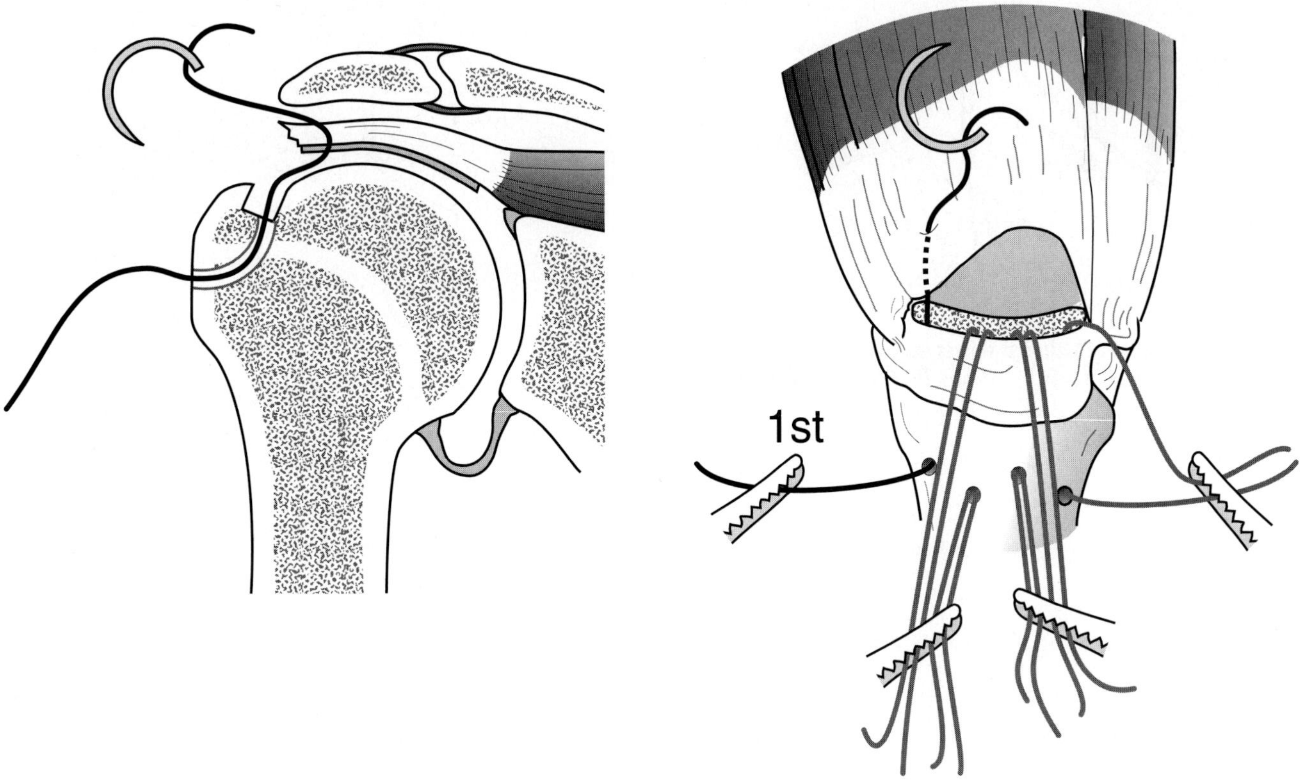


**Figure 21–27. Passing the first suture through tendon**
The first suture is passed through the tendon edge, making sure that the full thickness of the cuff and capsule is included and that the bite is sufficiently medial so that the tissue is robust.

second hole is then used to shuttle the free end of the suture back into the trough and out the adjacent hole (**Fig. 21–28**). The second suture through the second hole is passed through the tendon edge and then shuttled through the third hole by one of the two sutures through it (**Fig. 21–29**). This process is continued until all the sutures are passed through the tendon and out the adjacent holes (**Fig. 21–30**). Buried side-to-side sutures are placed in the split between the supraspinatus and subscapularis (**Fig. 21–31**). Tying

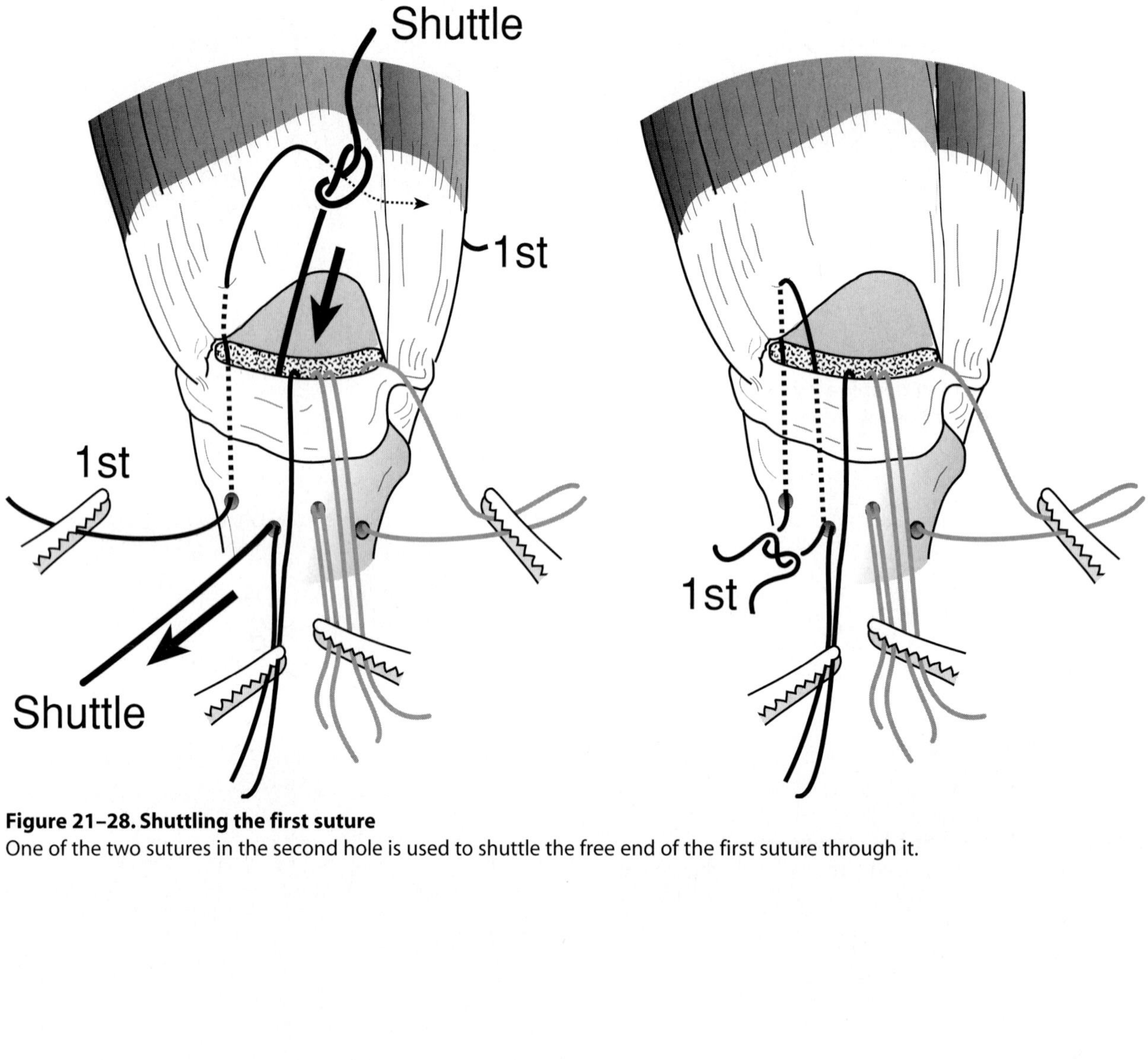


**Figure 21–28. Shuttling the first suture**
One of the two sutures in the second hole is used to shuttle the free end of the first suture through it.

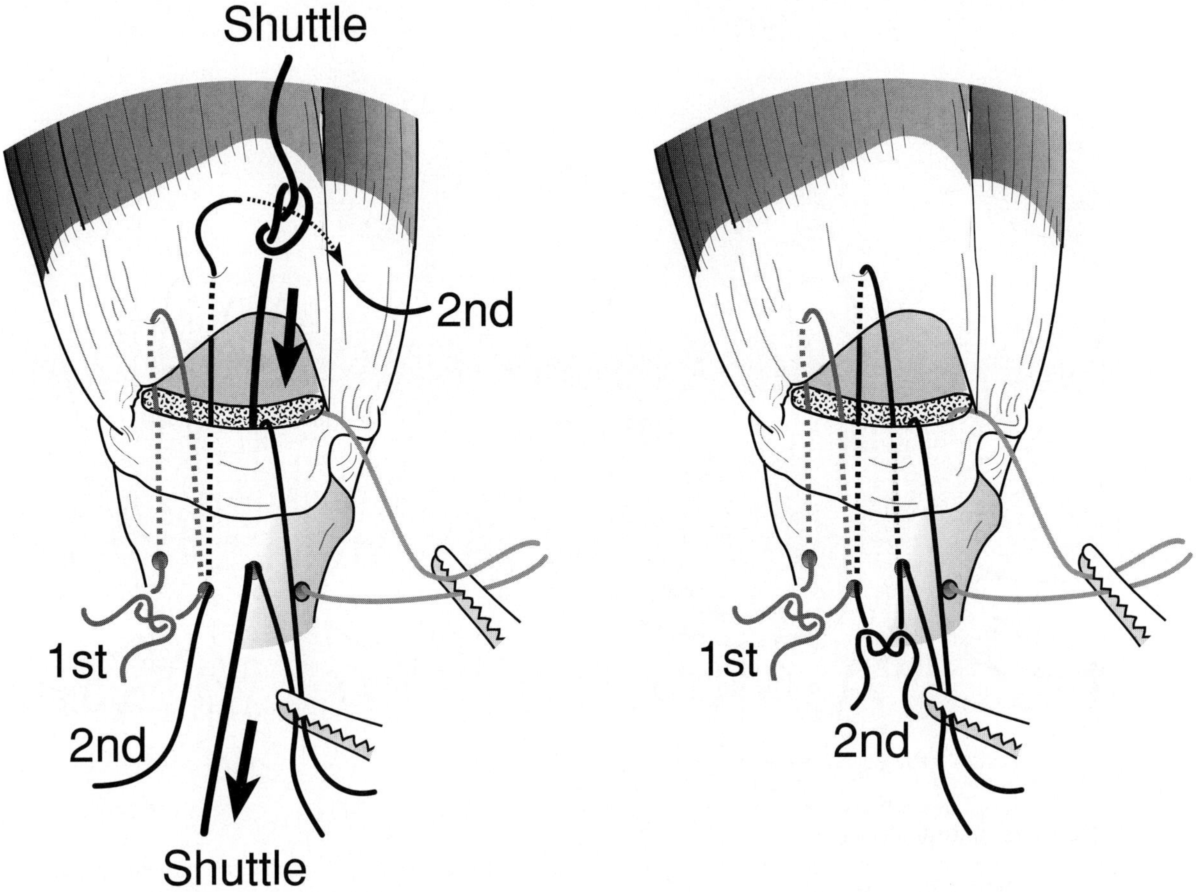


**Figure 21–29. Shuttling the second suture**
The second suture is passed through the tendon and out the adjacent hole.

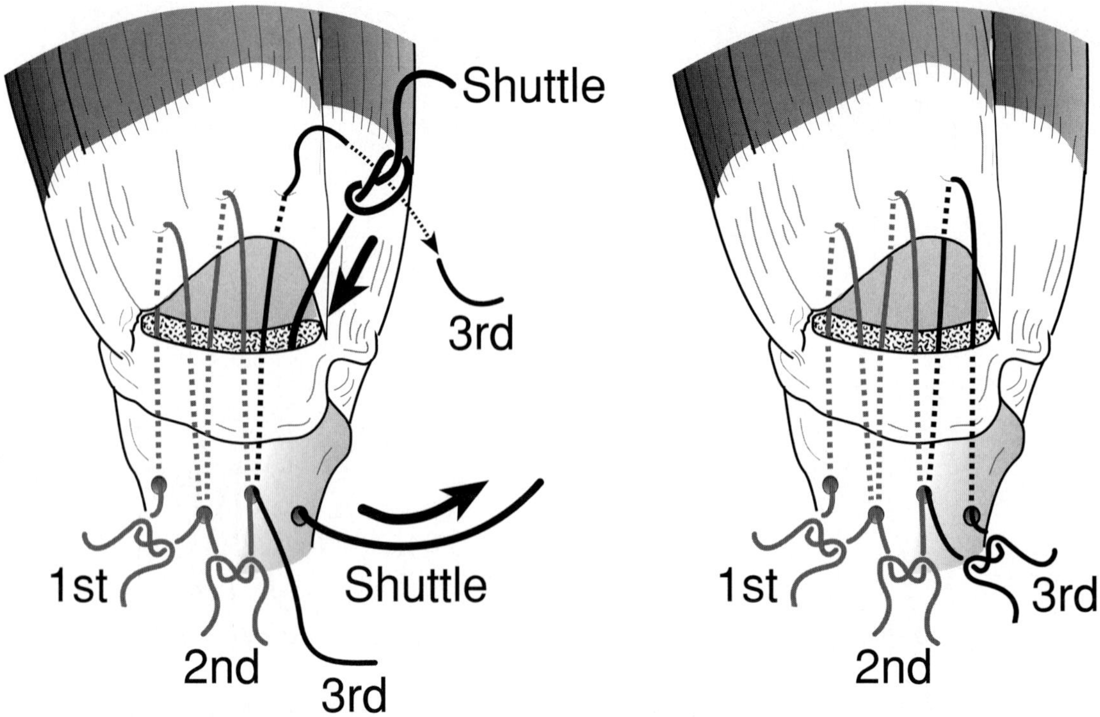


**Figure 21–30. Shuttling the third suture**
The process is continued until the final single suture is used to shuttle the end of the last suture through the last hole.

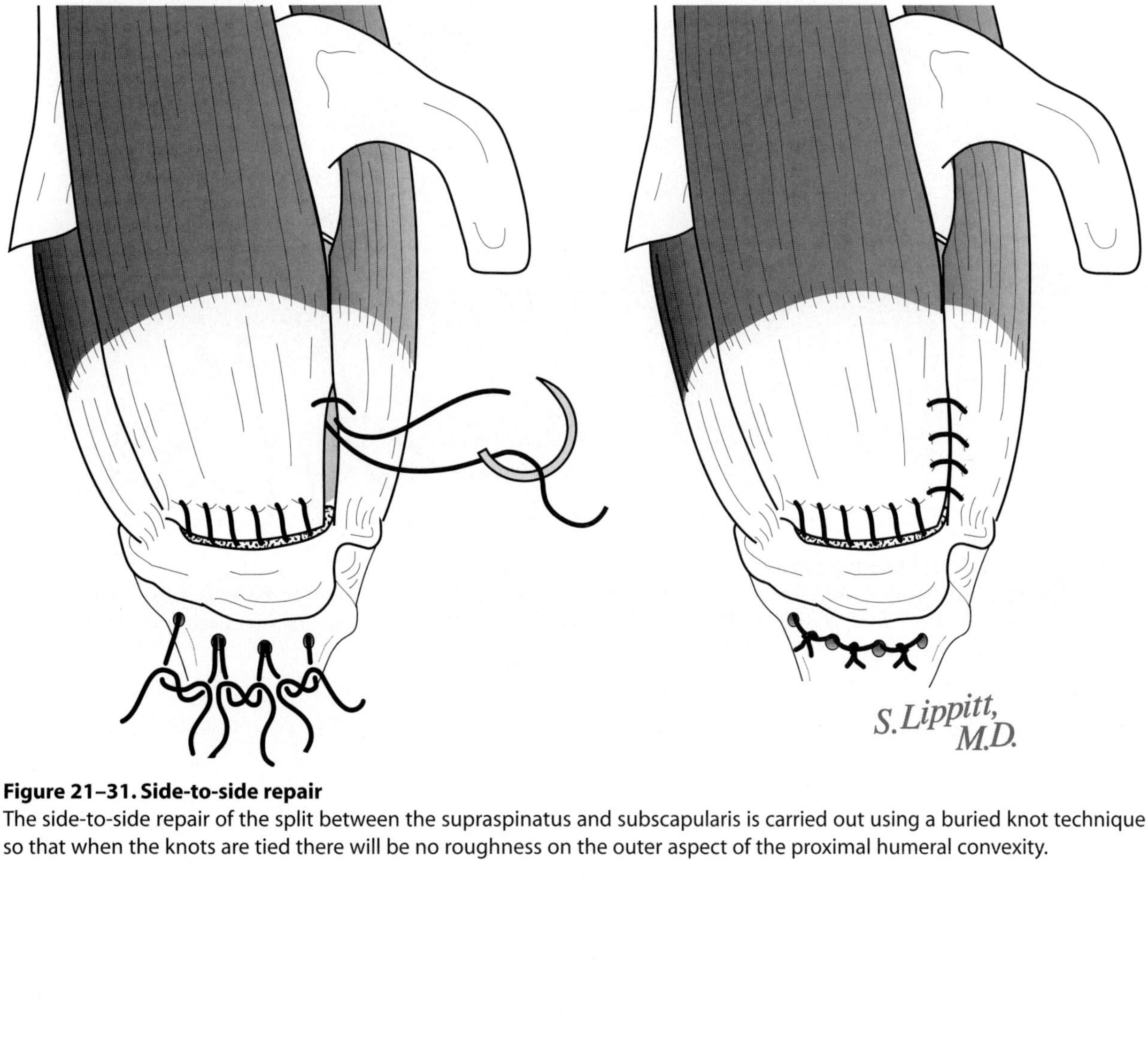


**Figure 21–31. Side-to-side repair**
The side-to-side repair of the split between the supraspinatus and subscapularis is carried out using a buried knot technique so that when the knots are tied there will be no roughness on the outer aspect of the proximal humeral convexity.

these sutures brings the tendon edge into the trough in a tongue-in-groove fashion, leaving a smooth upper surface to articulate beneath the coracoacromial arch and the knots over the lateral tuberosity where they will not catch beneath the coracoacromial arch (**Fig. 21–32**). Any prominence remaining on the greater tuberosity is smoothed using a pinecone burr (**Fig. 21–33**).

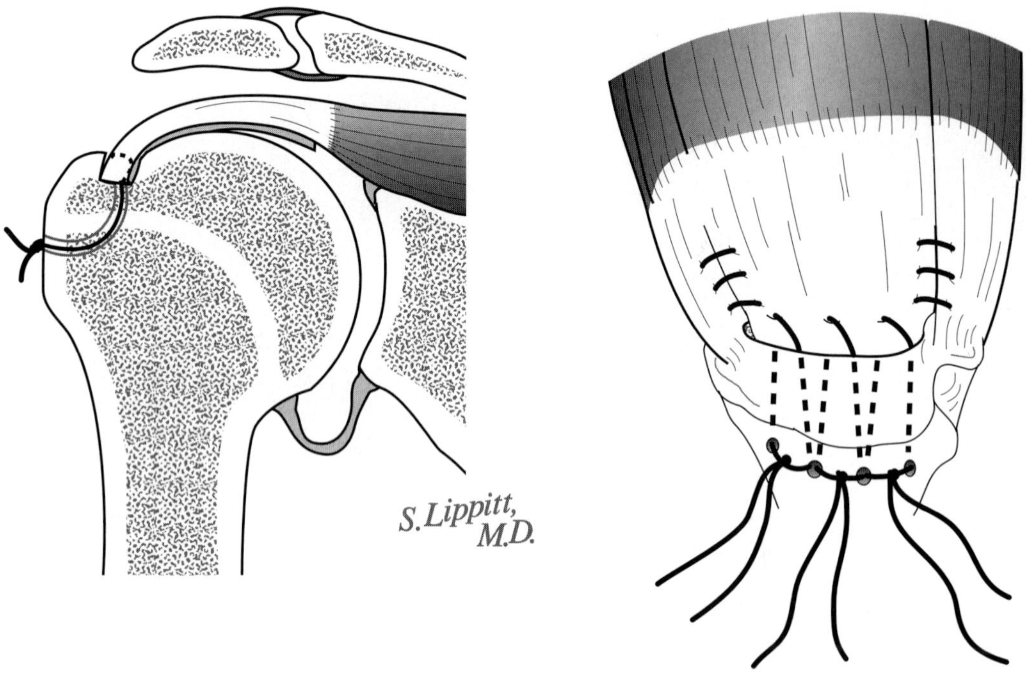


**Figure 21–32. Tying the sutures**
Tying these sutures brings the tendon into the trough and places the knots out of the way of the coracoacromial arch. (Modified from Matsen FA, Lippitt SB, Sidles JA, et al [eds]: Practical Evaluation and Management of the Shoulder. Philadelphia: WB Saunders, 1994, p. 139.)

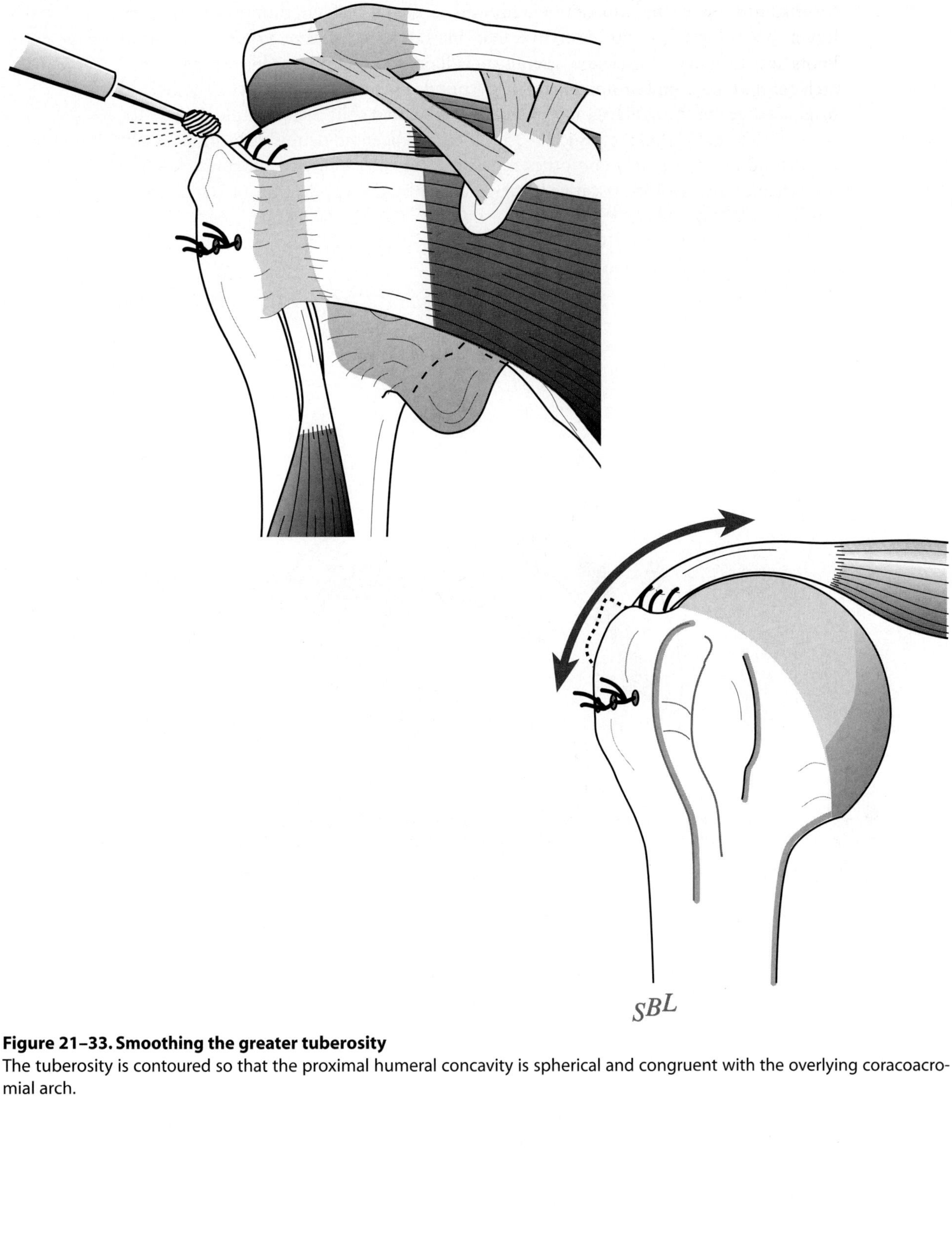


**Figure 21–33. Smoothing the greater tuberosity**

The tuberosity is contoured so that the proximal humeral concavity is spherical and congruent with the overlying coracoacromial arch.

After this repair, the arm can be adducted to the side of the thorax with the cuff under physiologic but not excessive tension. Rotation of the proximal humerus beneath the coracoacromial arch reveals no evidence of crepitance (**Fig. 21–34**).

Hemostasis is seen to be excellent. The wound is thoroughly irrigated. The deltoid origin is intact at the conclusion of the case. The deltoid split is closed side-to-side-to-side with absorbable sutures (**Fig. 21–35**). There has been no deltoid detachment from the deltoid or acromion, so no other repair is needed. A standard subcutaneous and subcuticular skin closure is carried out, followed by the application of sterile paper tape and sterile dressings.

The patient is returned to the recovery room in satisfactory condition, with the arm in continuous passive motion (**Fig. 21–36**).

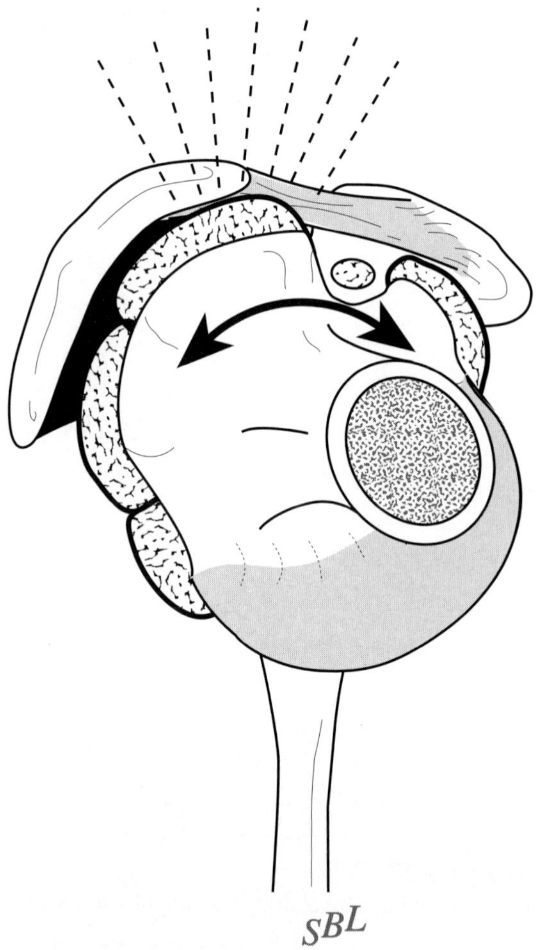


**Figure 21–34. Abrasion test**
After the cuff repair, the repair tendon passes smoothly beneath the coracoacromial arch. (Modified from Matsen FA, Lippitt SB, Sidles JA, et al [eds]: Practical Evaluation and Management of the Shoulder. Philadelphia: WB Saunders, 1994, p. 126.)

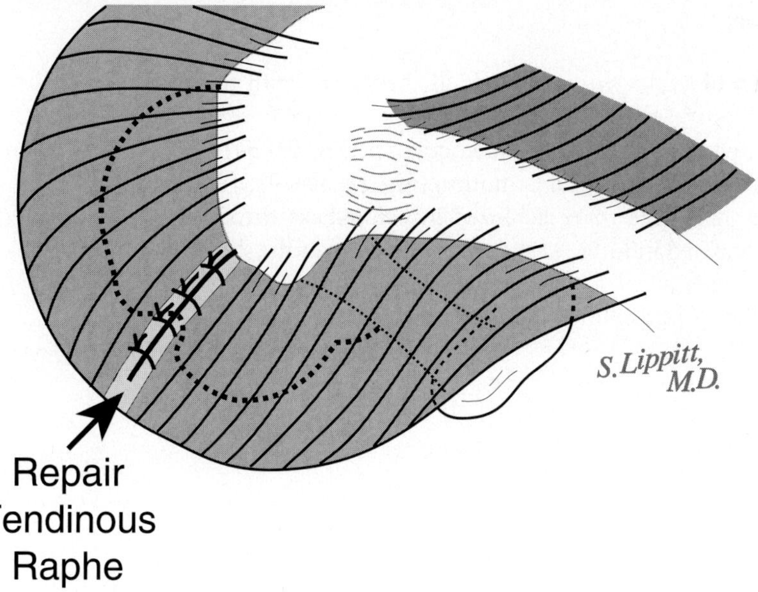


**Figure 21–35. Deltoid split repair**
The tendinous raphe of the deltoid split is repaired, with care taken to ensure that the knots are out of the humeroscapular motion interface and that they are not prominent subcutaneously. (Modified from Matsen FA, Lippitt SB, Sidles JA, et al [eds]: Practical Evaluation and Management of the Shoulder. Philadelphia: WB Saunders, 1994, p. 136.)

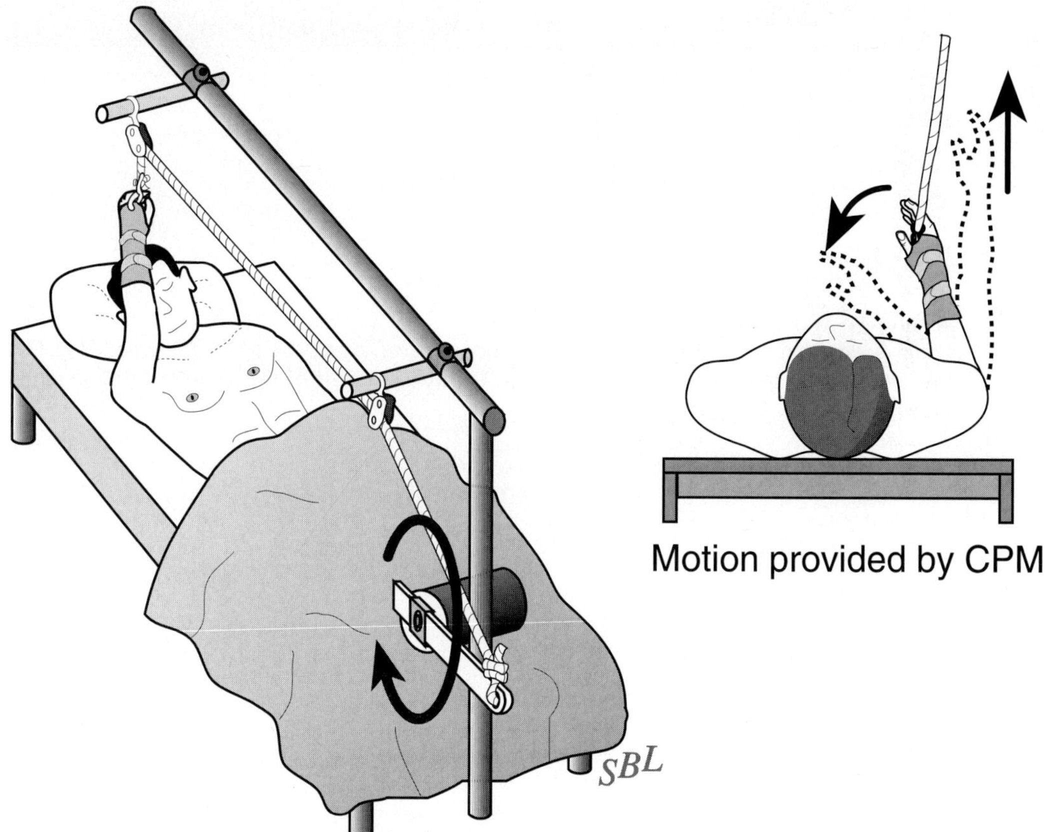


**Figure 21–36. Continuous passive motion**
Continuous passive motion used for the first 36 hours after rotator cuff surgery helps ensure that the healing in the humeroscapular motion interface proceeds in a way that yields smooth articulating surfaces rather than adhesions that can develop rapidly if the shoulder is immobilized during the early healing response after surgery. Continuous passive motion provides mechanical signals to the healing cells, differentiating those that are to heal the tendon to the bone from those that are to facilitate sliding of the cuff surface on the undersurface of the coracoacromial arch. (Modified from Matsen FA, Lippitt SB, Sidles JA, et al [eds]: Practical Evaluation and Management of the Shoulder. Philadelphia: WB Saunders, 1994, p. 50.)

## POSTOPERATIVE PLAN

Our postoperative plan is for the patient to achieve 140 degrees of passive flexion (**Figs. 21–37** and **21–38**) and 40 degrees of passive external rotation (**Fig. 21–39**) prior to discharge. These range of motion goals need to be achieved by the patient before discharge and are continued for a total of 3 months. At that time, activities of the shoulder are resumed progressively.

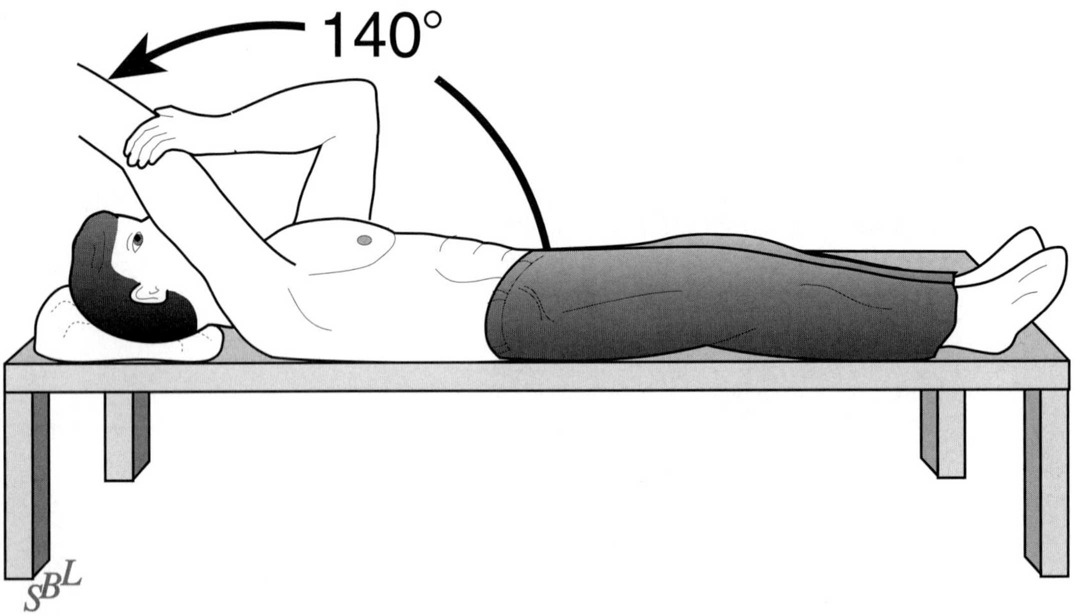


**Figure 21–37. Passive elevation**
Passive elevation is accomplished using the opposite arm as the "therapist." (Modified from Matsen FA, Lippitt SB, Sidles JA, et al [eds]: Practical Evaluation and Management of the Shoulder. Philadelphia: WB Saunders, 1994, p. 46.)

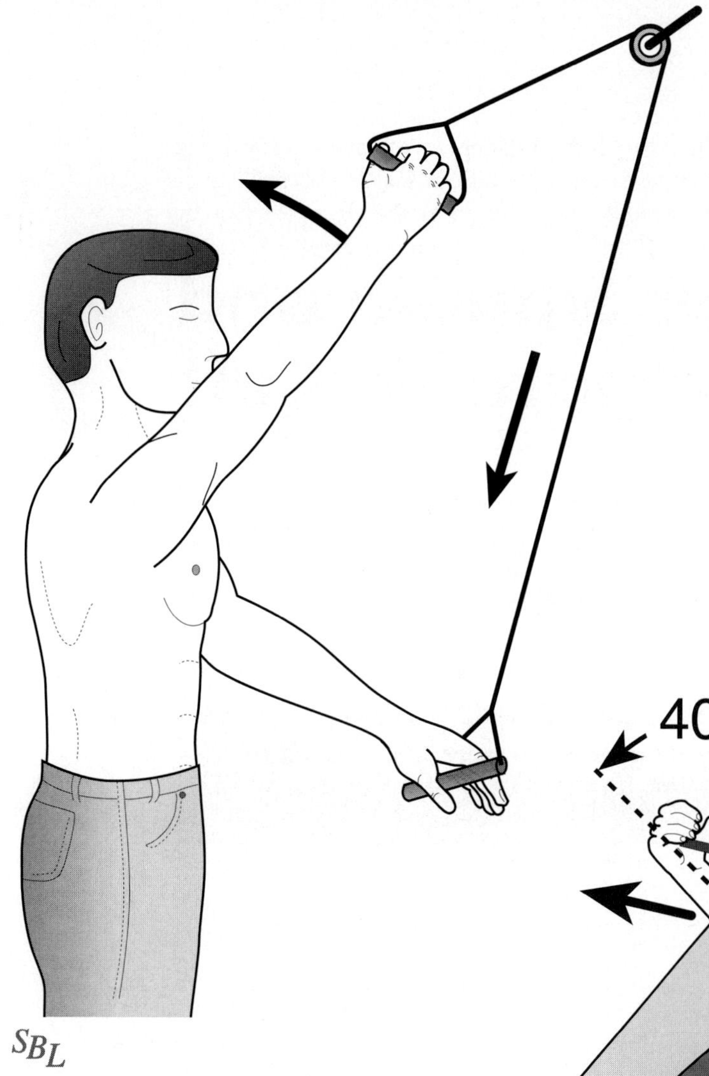


**Figure 21–38. Door pulley**
If the opposite arm is involved, passive flexion can be accomplished using an overhead pulley.

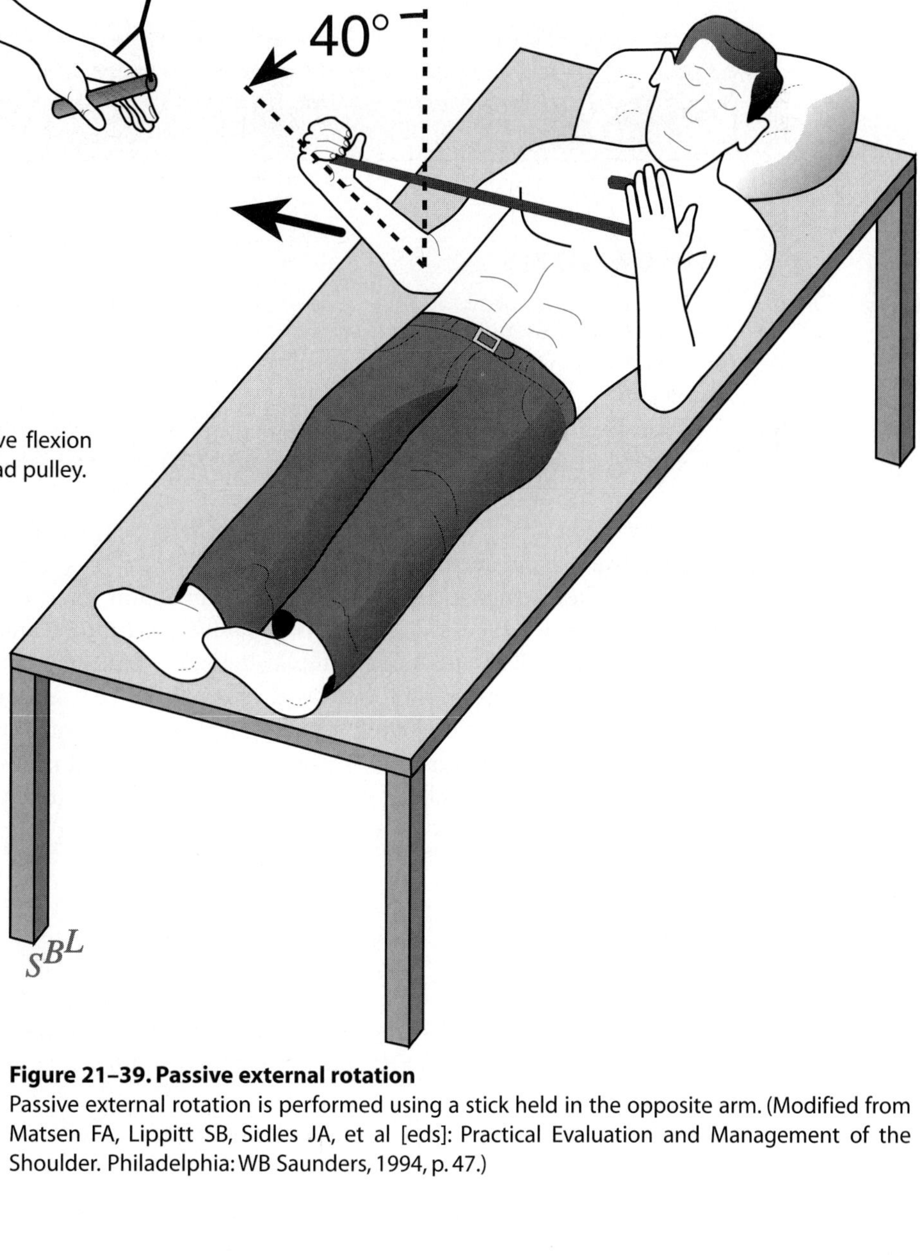


**Figure 21–39. Passive external rotation**
Passive external rotation is performed using a stick held in the opposite arm. (Modified from Matsen FA, Lippitt SB, Sidles JA, et al [eds]: Practical Evaluation and Management of the Shoulder. Philadelphia: WB Saunders, 1994, p. 47.)

CHAPTER 22

# Procedure: Smooth and Move—Irreparable Cuff

***Diagnosis***

***Irreparable rotator cuff tear involving the supraspinatus and infraspinatus tendons ICD9 CODES 840.3 and 840.6***

***Procedure***

***Rotator cuff exploration, lysis of adhesions, resection of bursal tissue, smoothing of greater tuberosity, resection of residual cuff tissue at the tuberosity CPT CODE 23415 or 23130***

## INDICATIONS

The patient has functionally significant crepitance and weakness of his or her shoulder for several years without an identified injury. The patient has been a heavy smoker for many years.

Physical examination reveals atrophy of the supraspinatus and infraspinatus muscles and marked weakness of flexion (**Figs. 22–1** and 22–2) and external rotation (**Fig. 22–3**).

A rotator cuff tear involving the supraspinatus and infraspinatus has been demonstrated by dynamic shoulder ultrasonography. The symptoms have not responded to nonoperative management.

Knowing the alternatives as well as the risks of infection, neurovascular injury, excessive stiffness, pain, weakness, fracture, irreparability, re-rupture, and the need for revision surgery, as well as anesthesia complications, the patient desires to proceed with rotator cuff surgery, including rotator cuff repair if the cuff tendons are of sufficient quantity and quality and including a smoothing without repair if the cuff tissue is of insufficient quantity and quality for repair. The patient recognizes that this procedure cannot be expected to completely restore normal comfort and function to the shoulder. The patient understands his or her critical role in the post-surgical rehabilitation.

## FINDINGS

Examination with the patient under anesthesia reveals substantial crepitance on motion and a palpable defect in the supraspinatus and infraspinatus tendons. Surgical findings include substantial scarring in the humeroscapular motion interface as well as bursal

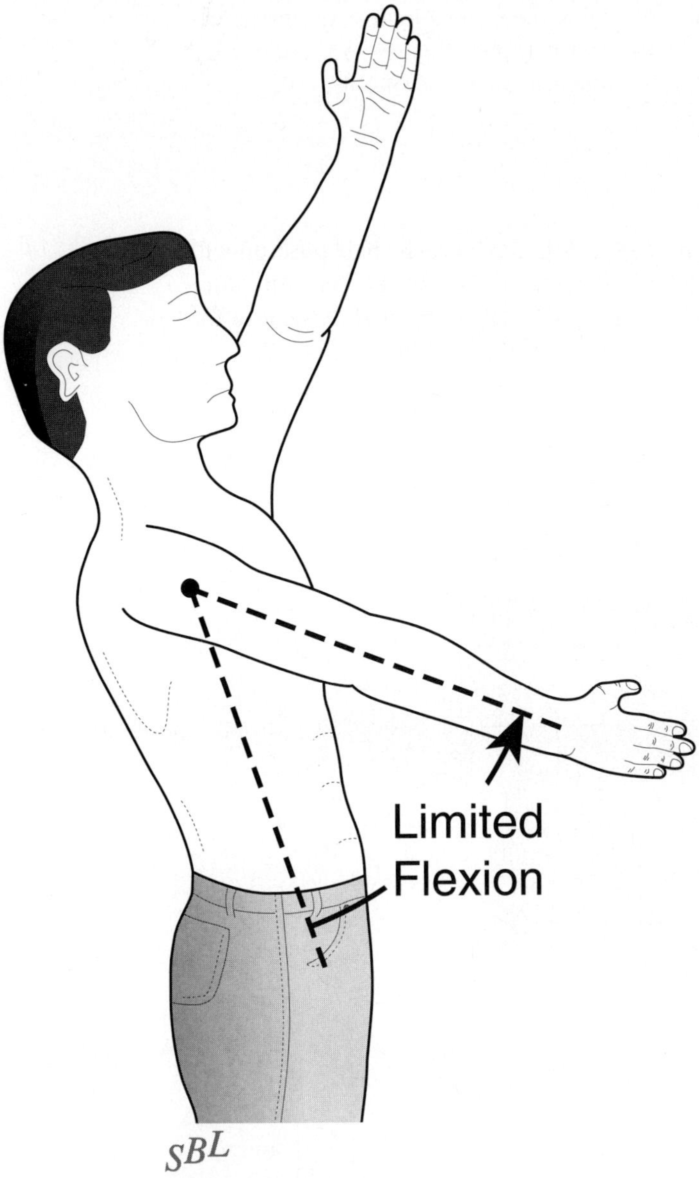


**Figure 22–1. Limited active elevation**
The massive cuff defect results in weakened elevation.

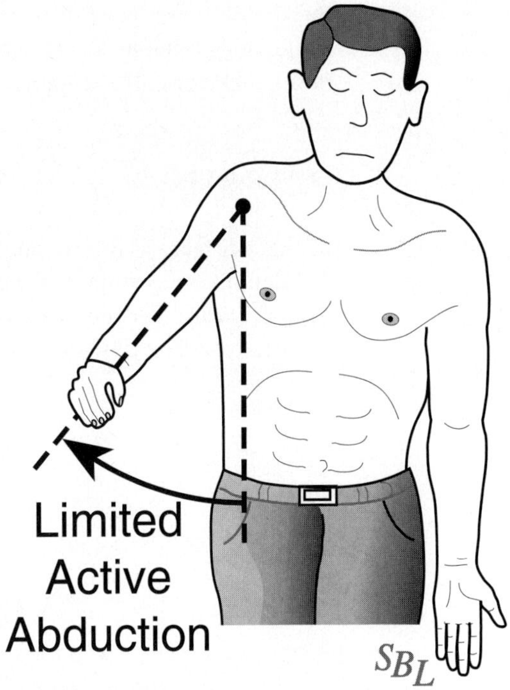


**Figure 22–2. Limited active abduction**
The patient tends to hike up the shoulder to substitute for the deficient cuff.

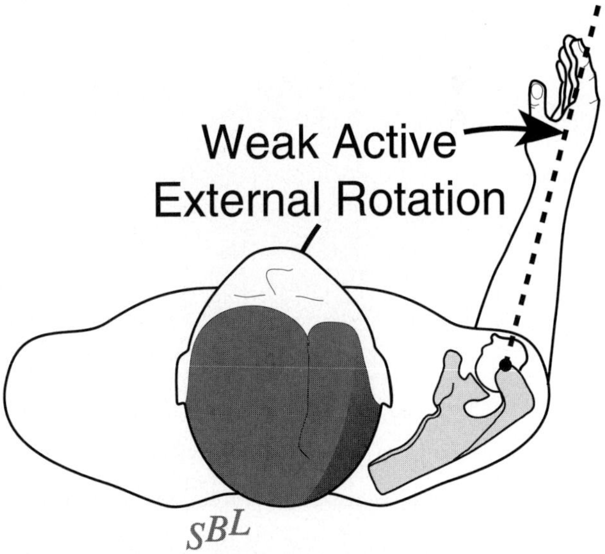


**Figure 22–3. Weak active external rotation**
Isometric external rotation is weak to manual testing.

thickening. There is a full-thickness defect involving the supraspinatus and infraspinatus tendons (see Fig. 22–1). The residual tendons are of poor quality and cannot reach to the tuberosity. The undersurface of the coracoacromial arch is smooth.

## OPERATION

Under satisfactory anesthesia, the patient is placed in a low beach chair position with the glenohumeral joint at the edge of the operating table (**Fig. 22–4**). The entire forequarter is carefully prepped and draped in the usual sterile fashion with the arm free to be moved. The positions associated with crepitance are identified.

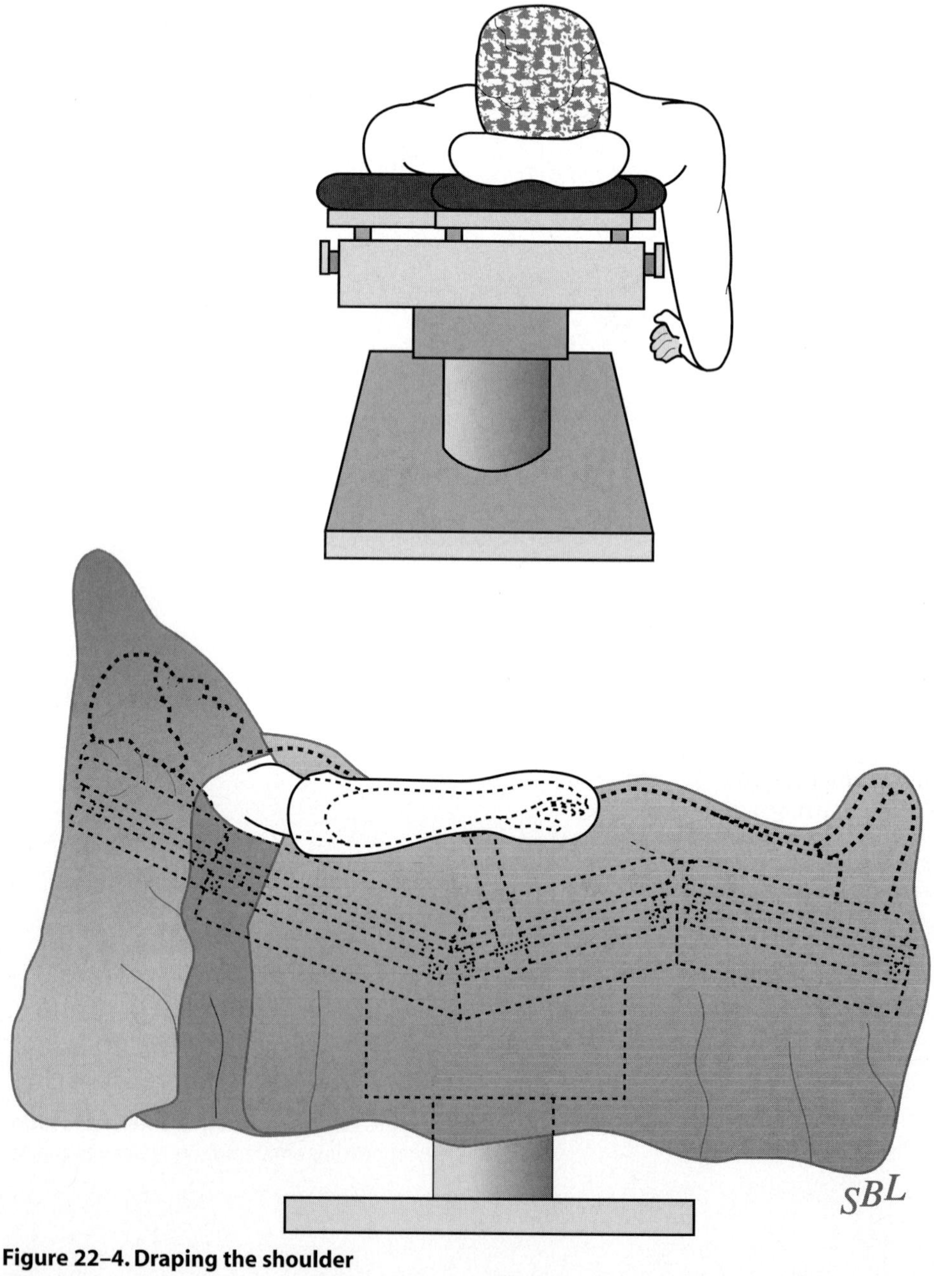


**Figure 22–4. Draping the shoulder**
The patient is placed in beach chair position with the arm draped free. Note that the patient is positioned with the glenohumeral joint at the edge of the table so that the arm can be moved through a full range of motion.

The anterolateral corner of the acromion is identified by palpation. The shoulder is approached through an incision in the skin line crossing the anterior corner of the acromion and perpendicular to the anterolateral fibers of the deltoid (**Fig. 22–5**).

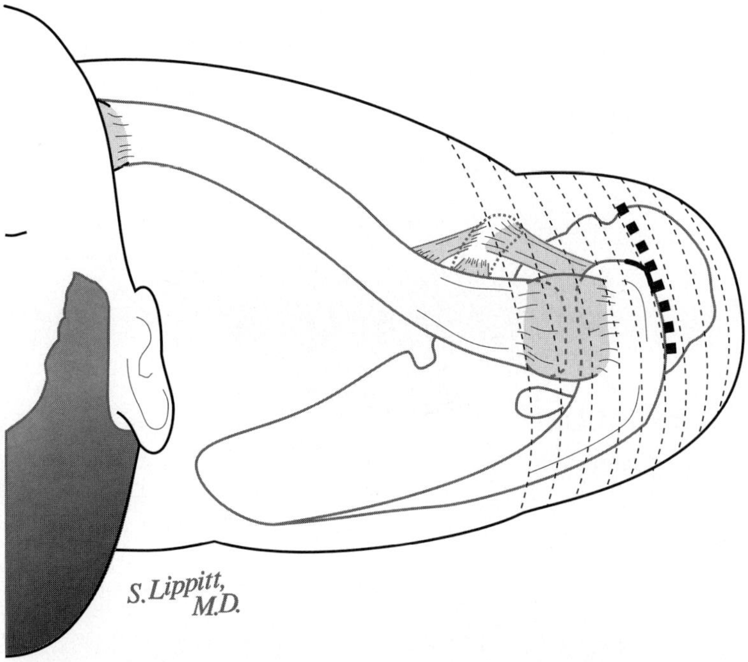


**Figure 22–5. Deltoid-on approach**
The deltoid-on approach, showing the skin incision in Langer's lines.

The major raphe between the anterior and lateral thirds of the deltoid is identified and split sharply so that some "white" remains on either side of the split (**Fig. 22–6**). No deltoid is taken down from the acromion. Once the deltoid raphe has been split, a small smooth elevator is passed beneath the acromion. Rotating this elevator so that it points distally allows the safe incision of the remainder of the bursa attached to its deep surface (**Fig. 22–7**). The total length of the deltoid split is limited to 4 cm from the acromion.

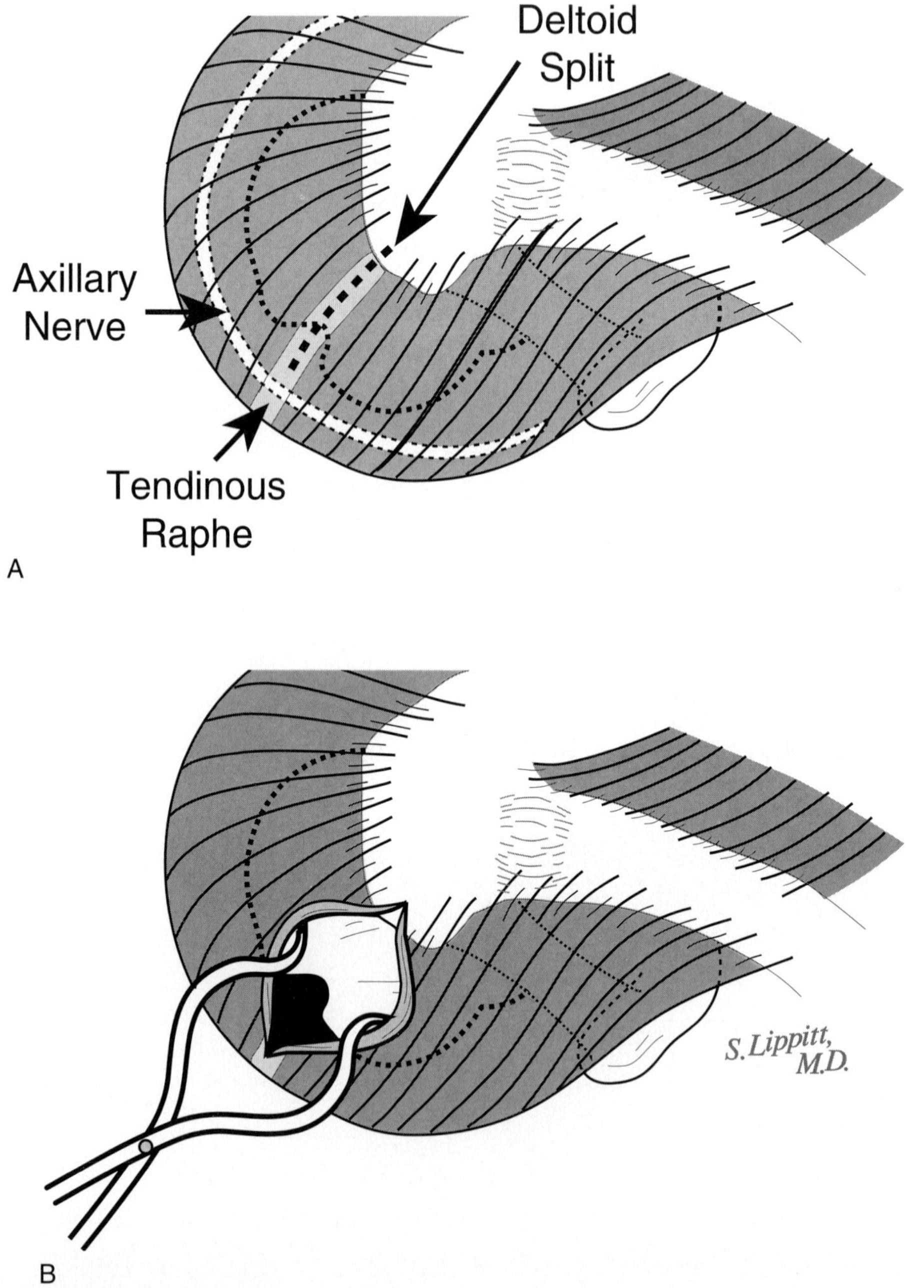


**Figure 22–6. Deltoid split**
The deltoid is split along the raphe between the anterior and lateral thirds of the muscle without any of it being detached from the acromion. (Modified from Matsen FA, Lippitt SB, Sidles JA, et al [eds]: Practical Evaluation and Management of the Shoulder. Philadelphia: WB Saunders, 1994, p. 135.)

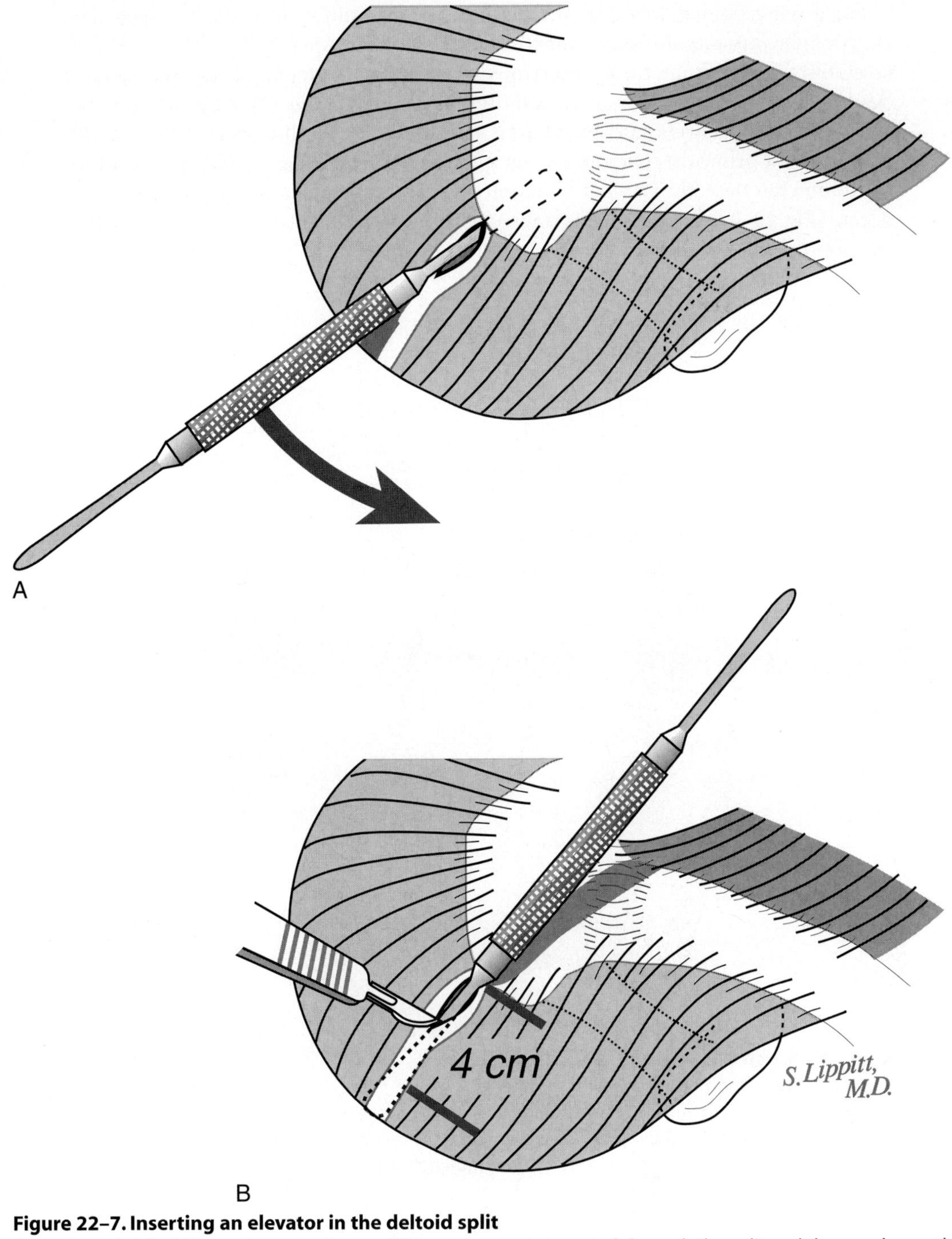


**Figure 22–7. Inserting an elevator in the deltoid split**
Once the subdeltoid bursa is entered, a small blunt elevator is inserted through the split and then underneath the deltoid (**A**). This elevator is then rotated 180 degrees while still in the bursa. The incision in the deltoid and bursa is then extended 4 cm distal from the acromion (**B**).

Small self-retaining retractors are placed in the deltoid split to hold it open. The hypertrophic bursa is differentiated from the underlying cuff by the fact that it does not move with the humerus as the arm is rotated. A nerve-to-nerve release is carried out so that at the conclusion of the resection, the axillary nerve can be palpated in the axilla as it runs across the subscapularis and lateral to the humerus as it traverses around it just below the tuberosities. Since the axillary nerve lies in the humeroscapular motion interface, the fact that it becomes palpable indicates the completeness of the release (**Fig. 22–8**). All of the bursa is resected along with any scar in the humeroscapular motion interface (**Fig. 22–9**).

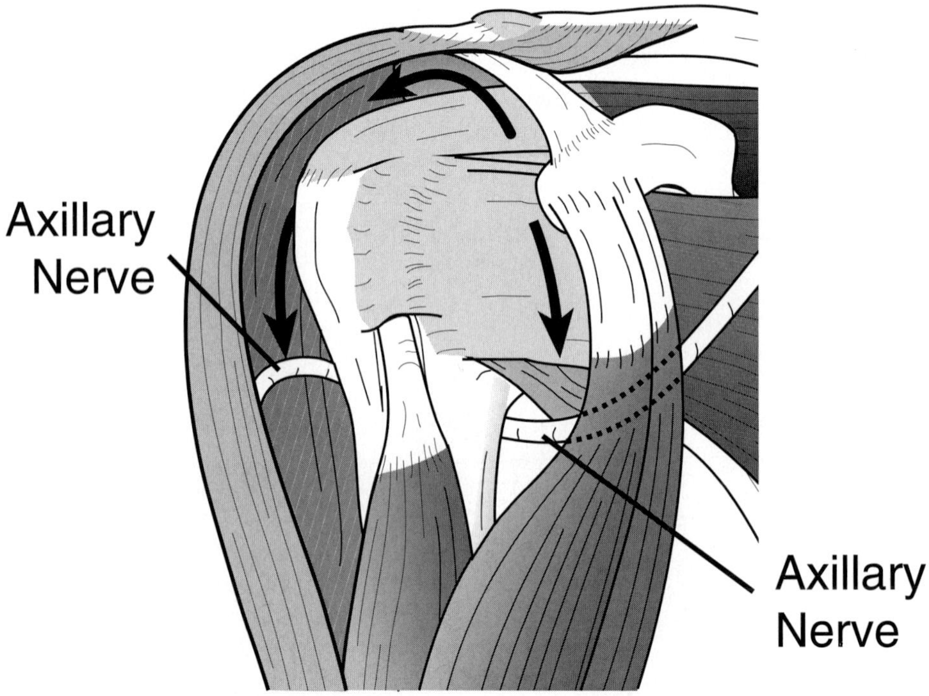


**Figure 22–8. Nerve-to-nerve release**
All scar tissue in the humeroscapular motion interface is released from the axillary nerve medially as it crosses the subscapularis, then under the coracoid, then under the coracoacromial ligament, then under the acromion, and then finally under the deltoid to the axillary nerve posteriorly as it exits the quadrilateral space: the nerve-to-nerve release.

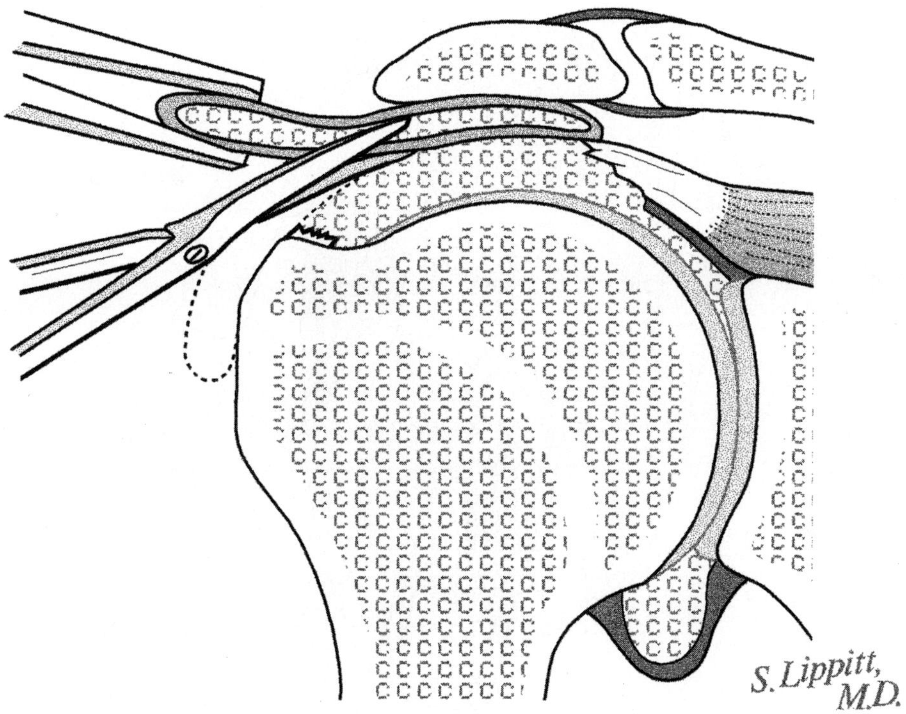


**Figure 22–9. Removal of the bursa**
The hypertrophic bursa is removed by sharp dissection.

The shoulder is gently manipulated to ensure a full range of rotation at the side, rotation at 90 degrees of abduction, flexion, abduction, and cross-body adduction.

This dissection provides excellent exposure of the edge of the torn supraspinatus and infraspinatus tendons; however, the tendon edge is noted to be retracted back to the glenoid lip. Traction sutures are placed in the tendon edge but tear through the tendon with minimal tension (**Fig. 22–10**). Mobilization outside and inside the tendon does not increase the tendon available for repair (**Fig. 22–11**). At this point, it is determined that the cuff is irreparable (**Fig. 22–12**).

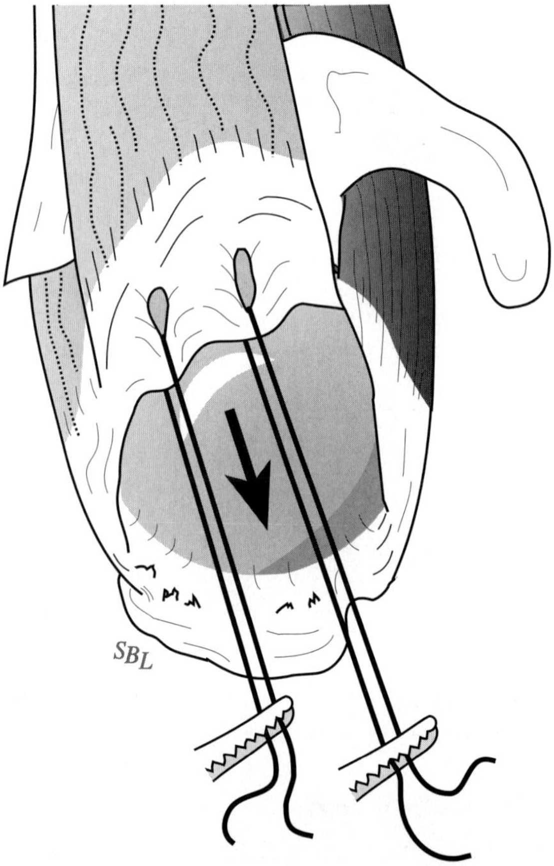


**Figure 22–10. Suture pullout through weak tendon**
Traction sutures pull through the poor-quality tendon.

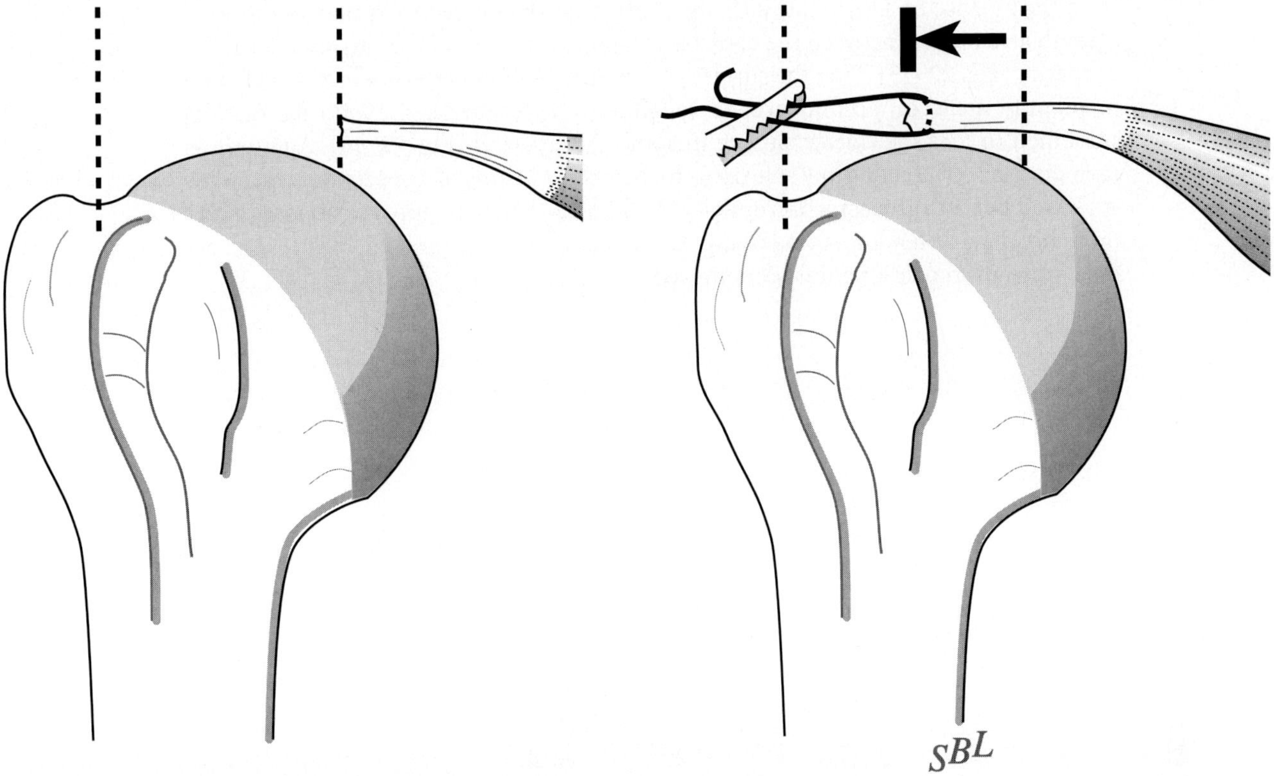


**Figure 22–11. Inadequate tendon length**
Even with extensive mobilization, the cuff tendon edge does not come close to the insertion site with the arm in adduction.

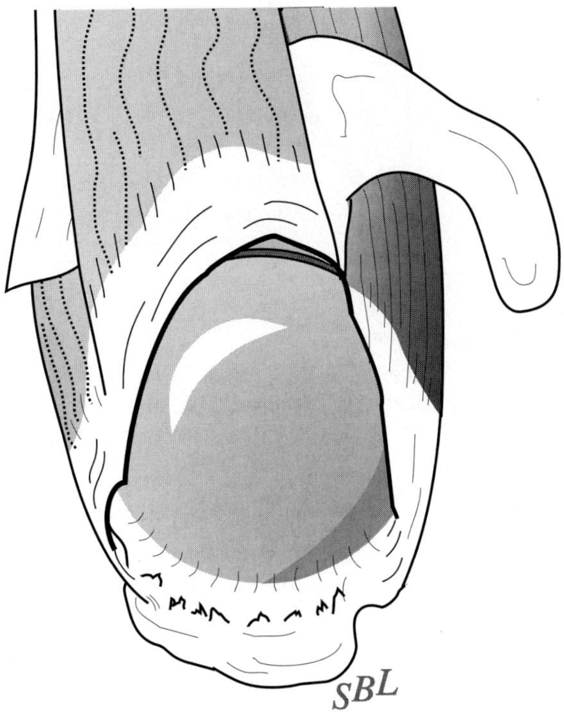


**Figure 22–12. Irreparable cuff**
The tendon edge is too far medial for a repair to be considered.

In the absence of a reparable cuff, the purpose of the procedure is now to restore a smooth articulation between the coracoacromial concavity and the proximal humeral convexity (**Fig. 22–13**). First the surface of the proximal humerus and cuff is palpated to identify areas of prominence or roughness. Any prominence of tuberosity is smoothed so that the convex surface is smoothly spherical (**Fig. 22–14**). Attention is then directed to resecting any soft tissue that causes catching as the proximal humerus is rotated beneath the coracoacromial arch (**Fig. 22–15**). The upper anterior edge of the subscapularis tendon is smoothed. All sutures and any prominent suture anchors from previous repair attempts are removed.

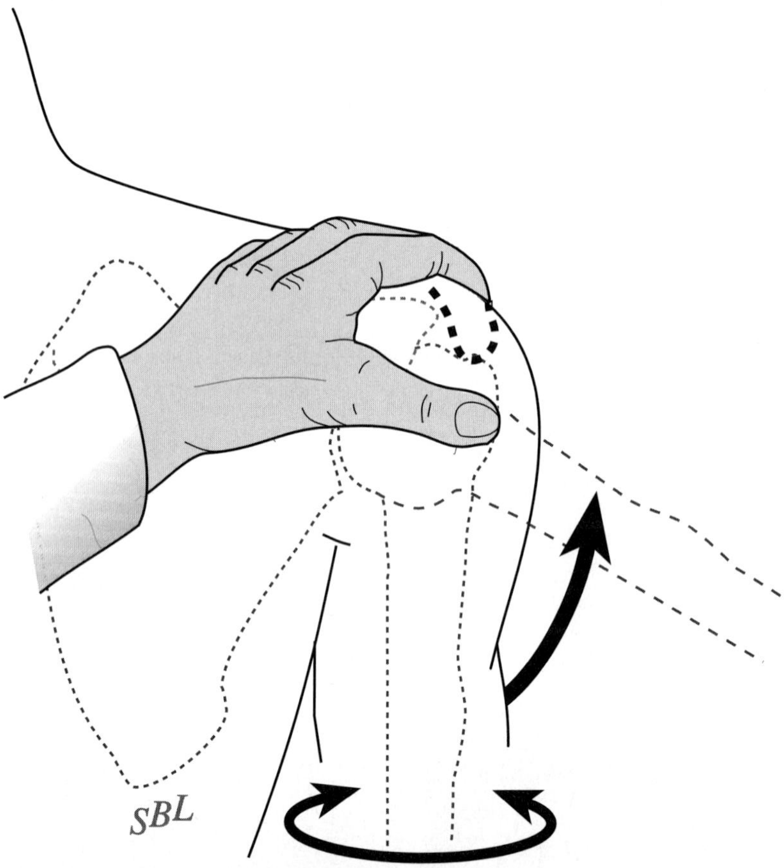


**Figure 22–13. Palpable subacromial crepitance**
The shoulder is rotated and abducted and adducted to identify the positions in which crepitance is produced.

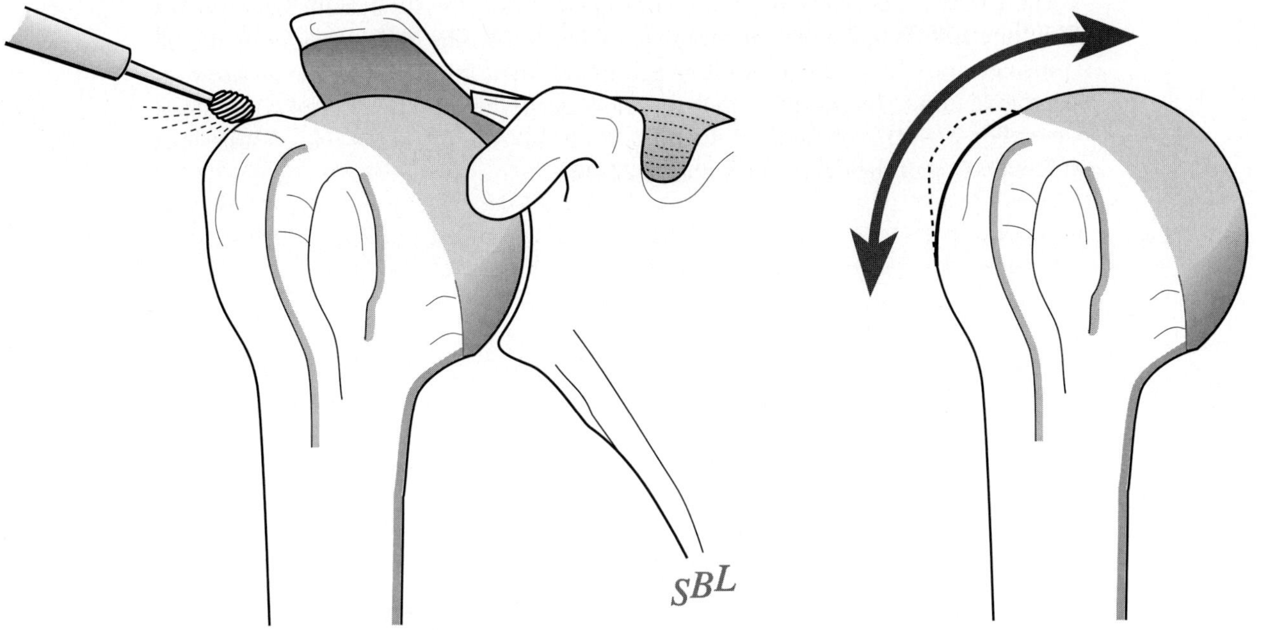


**Figure 22–14. Smoothing the greater tuberosity**
The prominence of the tuberosity is burred down to leave a smooth proximal humeral convexity.

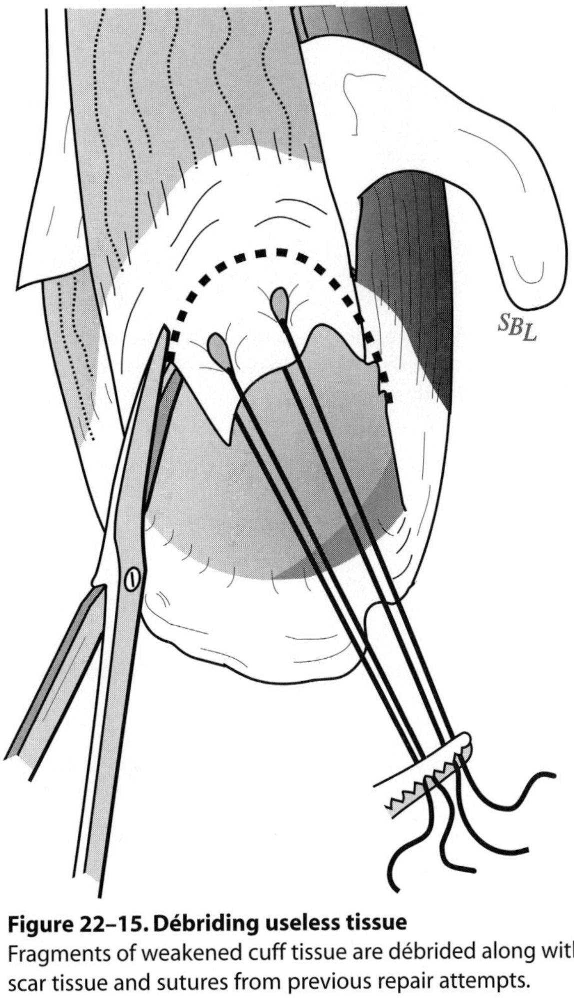


**Figure 22–15. Débriding useless tissue**
Fragments of weakened cuff tissue are débrided along with scar tissue and sutures from previous repair attempts.

The concave undersurface of the coracoacromial arch is palpated to ensure its smoothness. If there is a prominence that encroaches on the cuff, it is smoothed with a pinecone burr (**Fig. 22–16**). Routine acromioplasty is avoided to preserve the coracoacromial concavity so that anterosuperior escape of the humeral head does not occur (**Fig. 22–17**). Avoidance of acromioplasty also minimizes the risk of adhesions and weakening of the deltoid origin (**Fig. 22–18**).

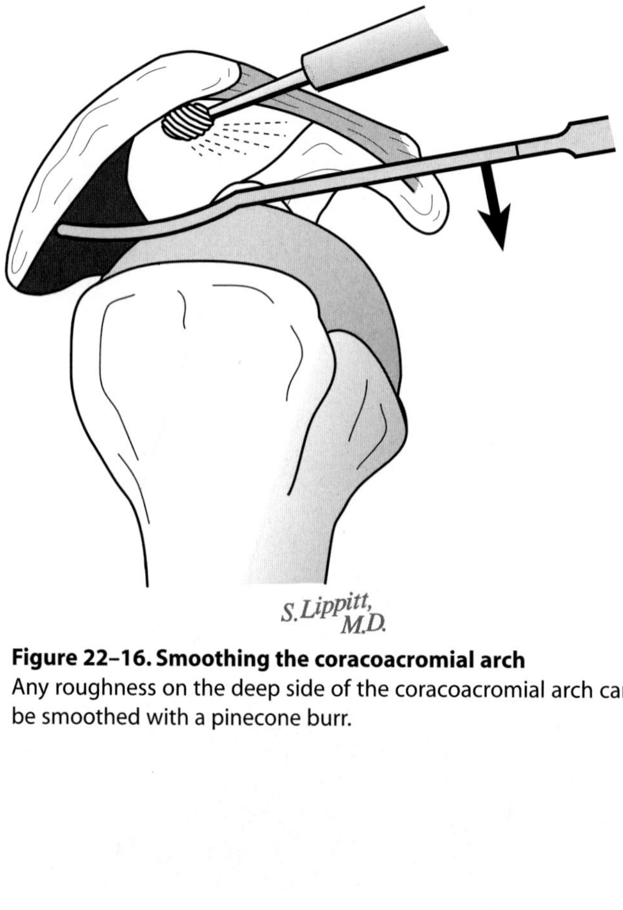


**Figure 22–16. Smoothing the coracoacromial arch**
Any roughness on the deep side of the coracoacromial arch can be smoothed with a pinecone burr.

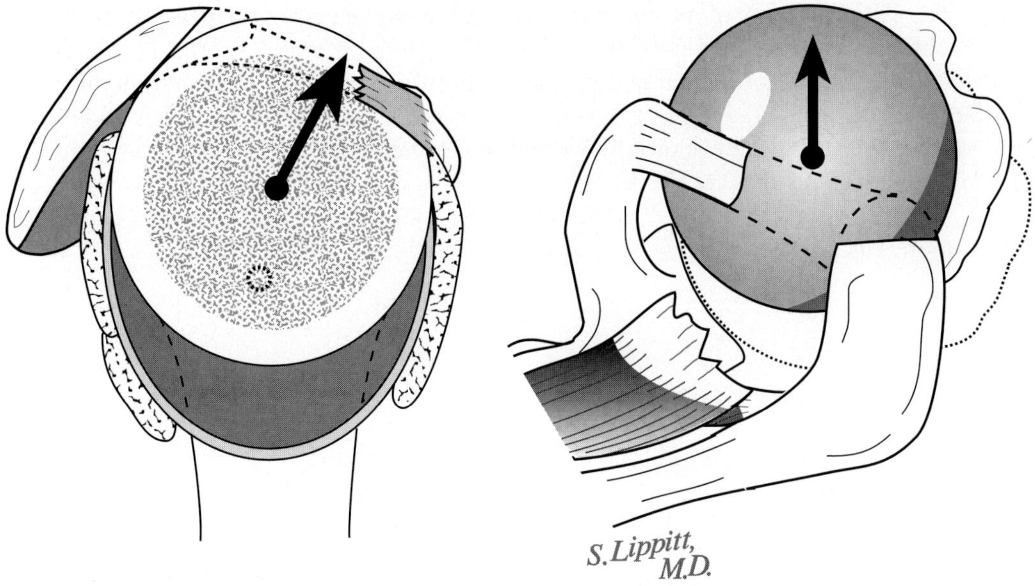


**Figure 22–17. Anterosuperior escape**
The acromion and the coracoacromial ligament are preserved to maintain the deltoid origin and the anterosuperior stability of the glenohumeral joint, avoiding the severe problem of anterosuperior escape.

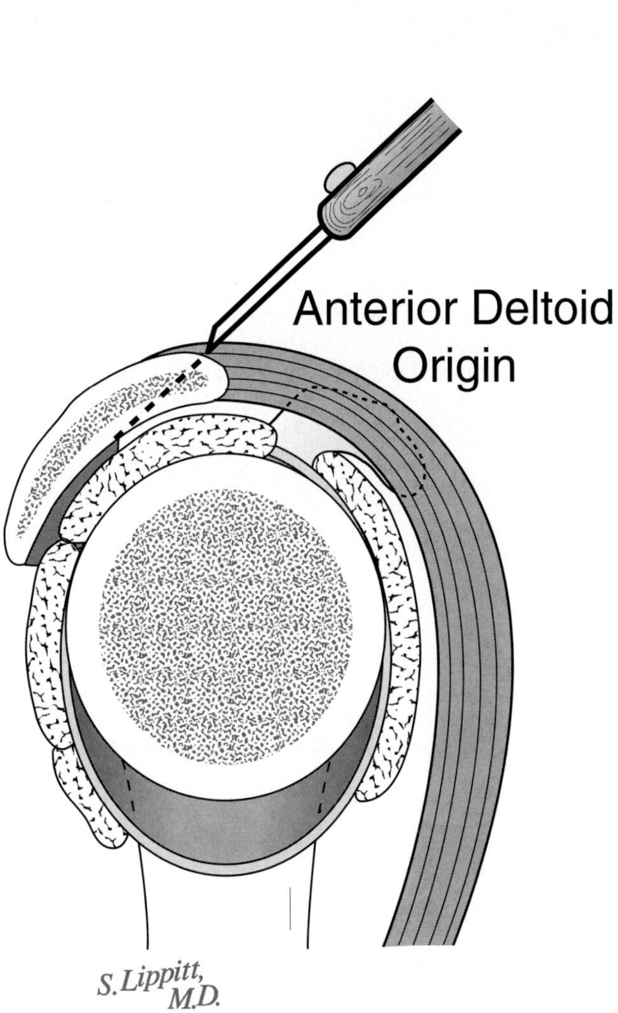


**Figure 22–18. Loss of the deltoid origin**
Acromioplasty sacrifices part of the deltoid origin.

The complete range of motion and lack of crepitance are again verified.

The wound is thoroughly irrigated. The deltoid is closed using absorbable sutures, with care taken to ensure that all knots are out of the humeroscapular motion interface (**Fig. 22–19**).

A subcuticular closure is carried out and reinforced with sterile tapes.

Dry sterile dressings are applied.

The patient is returned to the recovery room with the arm in continuous passive motion (**Fig. 22–20**).

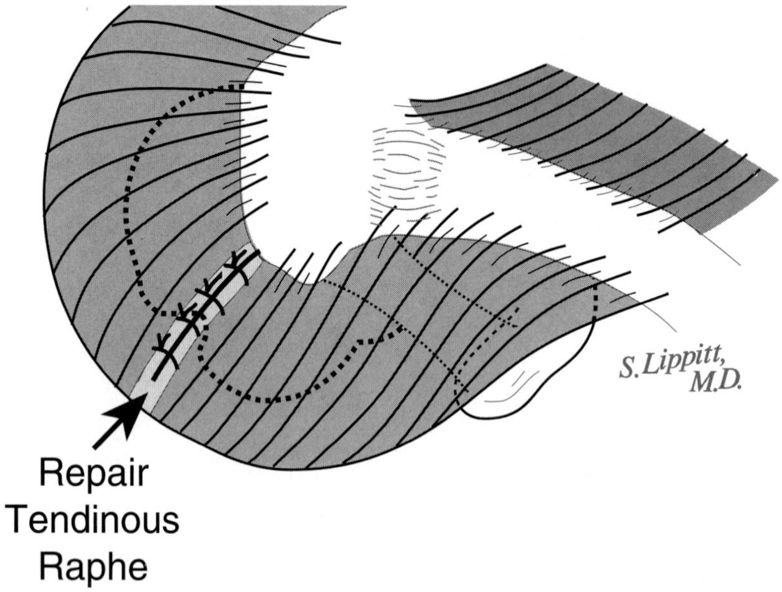


**Figure 22–19. Deltoid split repair**
The tendinous raphe of the deltoid split is repaired, with care taken to ensure that the knots are out of the humeroscapular motion interface and that they are not prominent subcutaneously. (Modified from Matsen FA, Lippitt SB, Sidles JA, et al [eds]: Practical Evaluation and Management of the Shoulder. Philadelphia: WB Saunders, 1994, p. 136.)

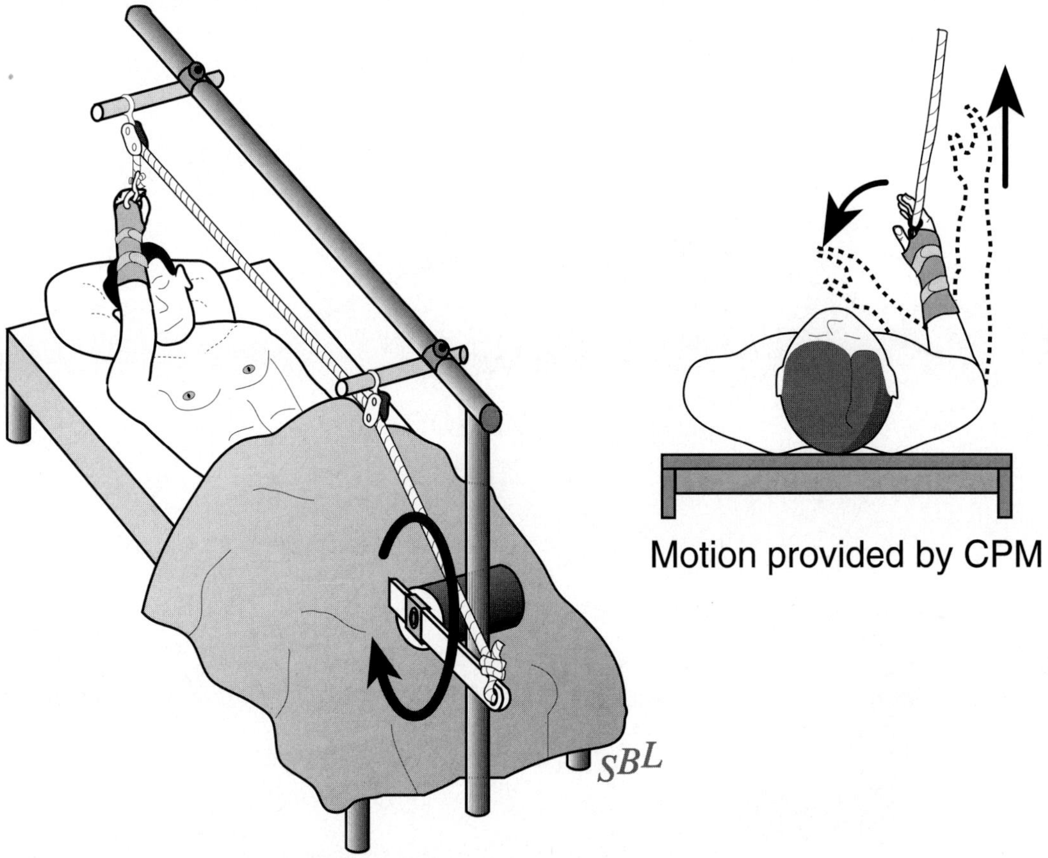


**Figure 22–20. Continuous passive motion**

Continuous passive motion is started immediately in the recovery room and continued while the patient is in the hospital and in bed. It moves the shoulder from adduction and internal rotation to 90 degrees of elevation in neutral rotation using a slow adjustable cam rotating at four cycles per minute. (Modified from Matsen FA, Lippitt SB, Sidles JA, et al [eds]: Practical Evaluation and Management of the Shoulder. Philadelphia: WB Saunders, 1994, p. 50.)

## POSTOPERATIVE PLAN

Continuous passive motion is provided for the first 36 hours whenever the patient is in bed and not doing assisted exercises.

The patient is instructed in a full motion program, including assisted flexion (**Fig. 22–21**), external rotation (**Fig. 22–22**), internal rotation (**Fig. 22–23**), cross-body adduction (**Fig. 22–24**), and internal rotation in abduction. If both shoulders are involved, a pulley may be helpful (**Fig. 22–25**).

The patient is discharged when he or she can flex to 140 degrees and externally rotate to 40 degrees using only the assistance from the opposite arm.

The patient is allowed active use of the shoulder as tolerated, since no deltoid is detached or repaired. The patient is reminded that the key to preventing reformation of scar tissue, adhesions, and crepitance is maintaining full assisted motion.

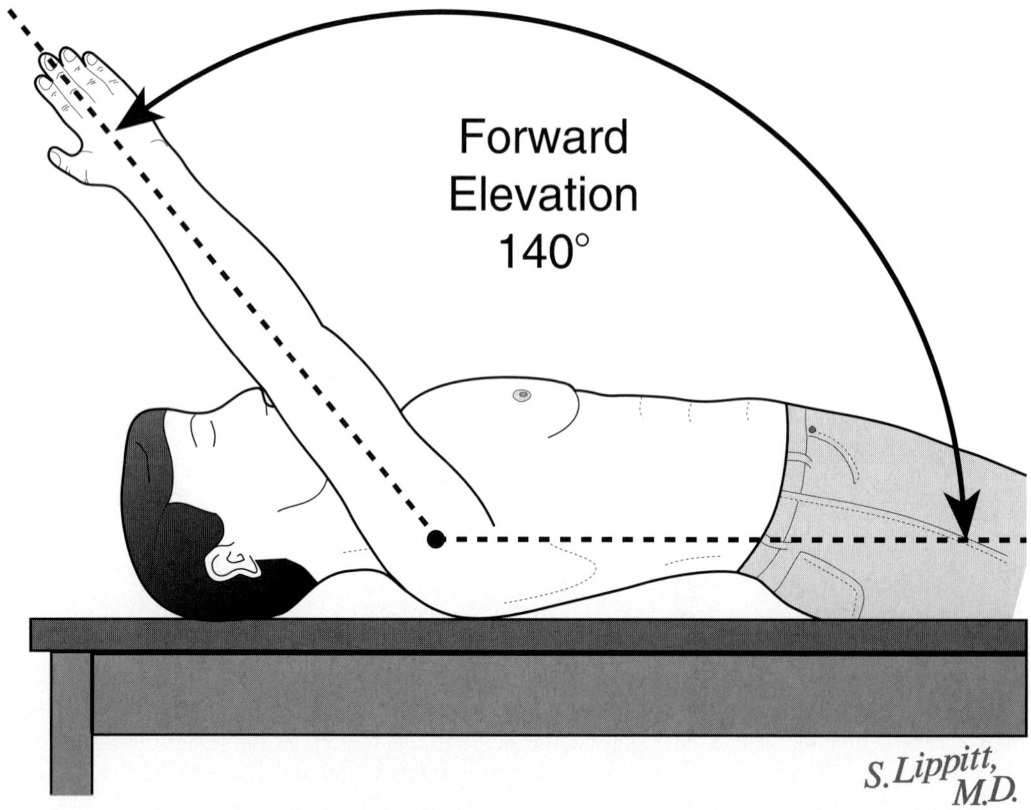


**Figure 22–21. Active assisted forward elevation**
With the assistance of the other hand as necessary, the arm is elevated to 140 degrees.

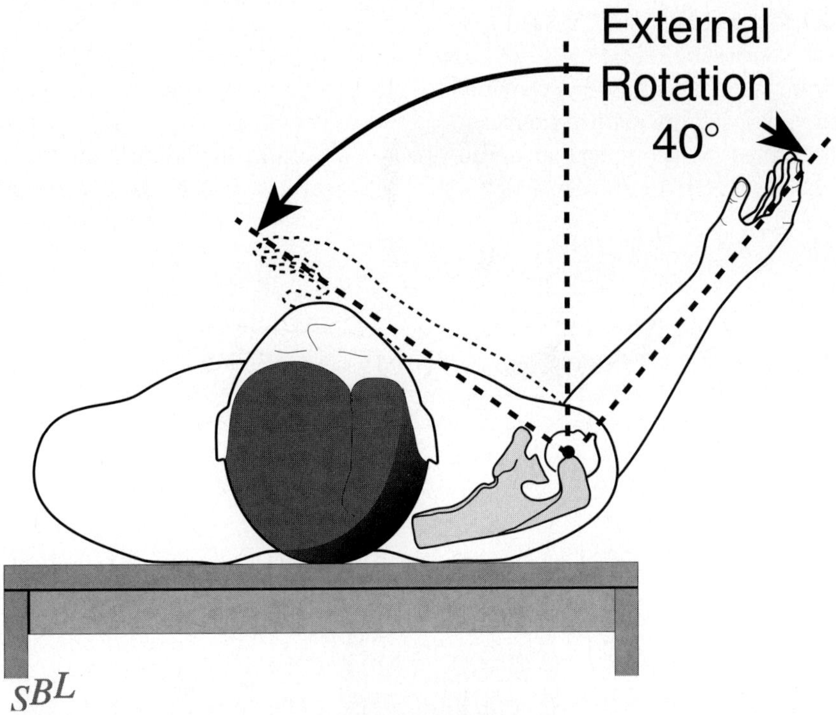


**Figure 22–22. Active assisted external rotation**
With the assistance of the other hand as necessary, the arm is externally rotated to 40 degrees.

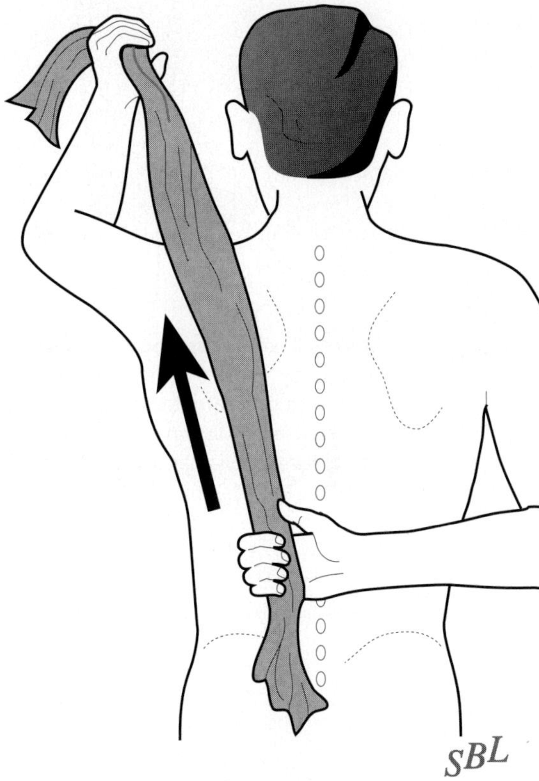


**Figure 22–23. Internal rotation**
Internal rotation up the back is assisted with a towel held in the sound arm. (Modified from Matsen FA, Lippitt SB, Sidles JA, et al [eds]: Practical Evaluation and Management of the Shoulder. Philadelphia: WB Saunders, 1994, p. 48.)

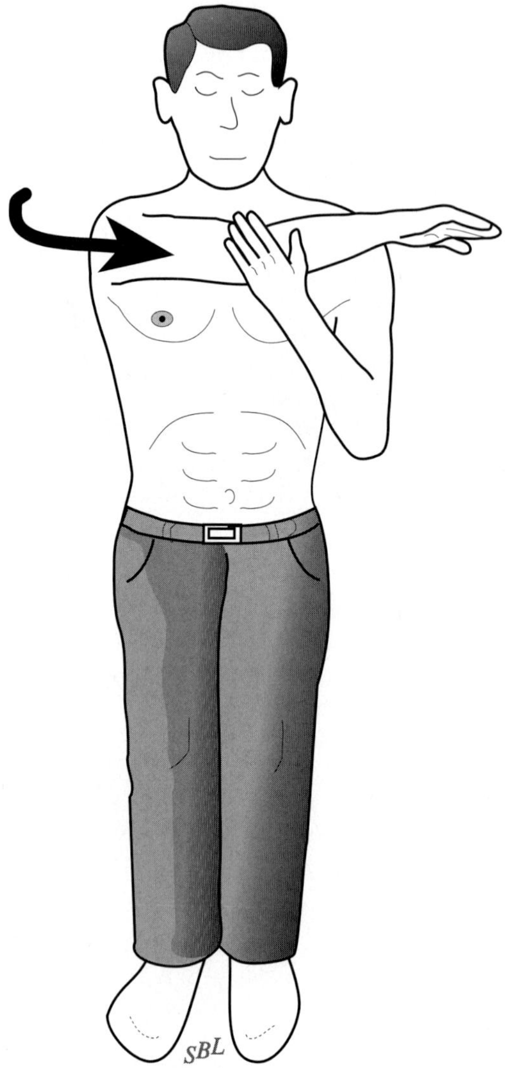


**Figure 22–24. Cross-body adduction**
Cross-body adduction is assisted by the opposite arm drawing the arm toward the opposite shoulder. (Modified from Matsen FA, Lippitt SB, Sidles JA, et al [eds]: Practical Evaluation and Management of the Shoulder. Philadelphia: WB Saunders, 1994, p. 49.)

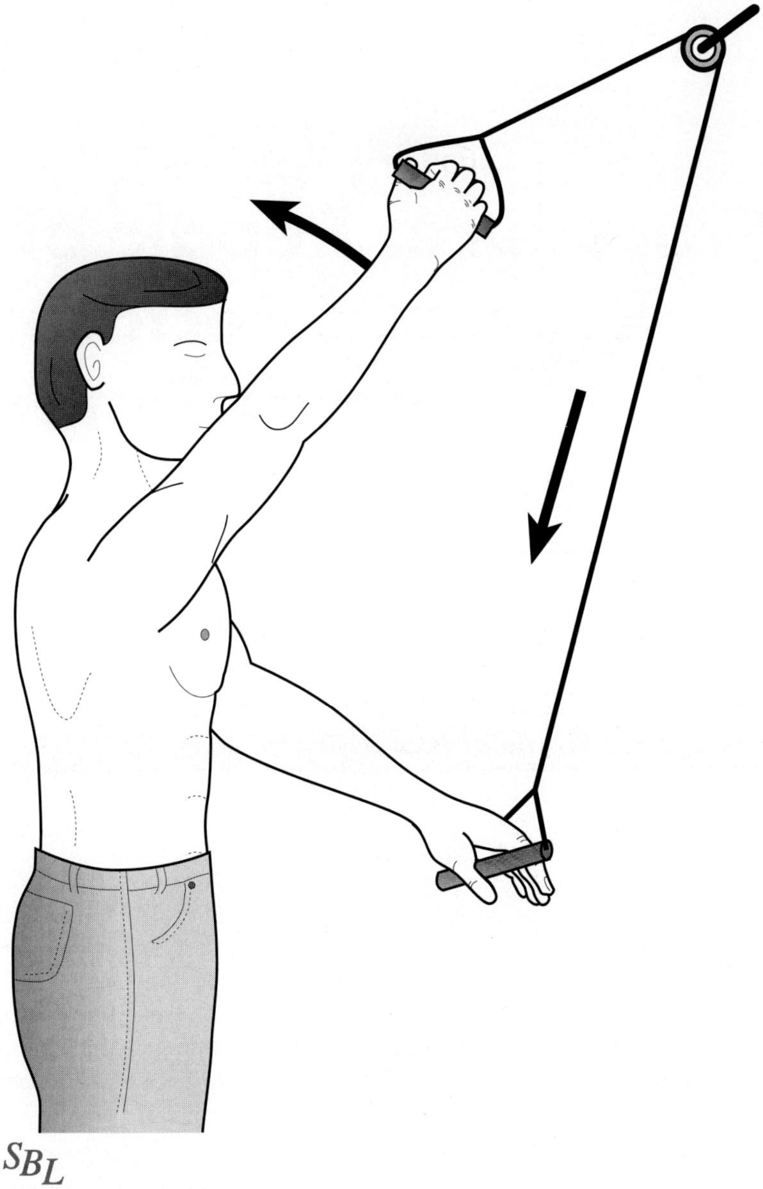

**Figure 22–25. Door pulley**
A pulley mounted on the door can be helpful in achieving elevation, especially when the opposite shoulder is involved.

CHAPTER 23

# Procedure: Repair of a Ruptured Pectoralis Major Tendon

| | |
|---|---|
| ***Diagnosis*** | |
| ***Right pectoralis major rupture*** | ***ICD9 CODE 728.83*** |
| ***Procedure*** | |
| ***Repair of pectoralis major rupture*** | ***CPT CODE 24341*** |

## INDICATIONS

The patient sustained an acute tear of the insertion of the pectoralis major tendon during a bench press. Prior to this injury, the shoulder was strong and asymptomatic.

The physical examination is assisted by knowledge of the normal pectoralis insertion (**Fig. 23–1**). Examination of the patient confirms the absence of the normal insertion of the pectoralis major; the asymmetry becomes particularly obvious when the patient pushes down on his or her waist with his or her hands (**Fig. 23–2**).

The humeral attachment of the clavicular component of the pectoralis is intact. The patient is a nonsmoker and does not take anabolic steroids.

Knowing the alternatives as well as the risks of infection, neurovascular injury, excessive stiffness, pain, weakness, fracture, instability, and the need for revision surgery, as well as anesthetic complications, the patient desires to proceed with the above-described procedure. The patient understands that the purpose of the procedure is to reestablish the attachment of the detached pectoralis tendon to the humerus. The patient recognizes that this procedure cannot be expected to completely restore normal comfort and function to the shoulder. And, lastly, the patient understands his or her critical role in the post-surgical rehabilitation.

## FINDINGS

The pectoralis tendon is retracted and its tendon edges are rounded but strong. Only a small fringe of the original insertion is seen at the lateral lip of the bicipital groove.

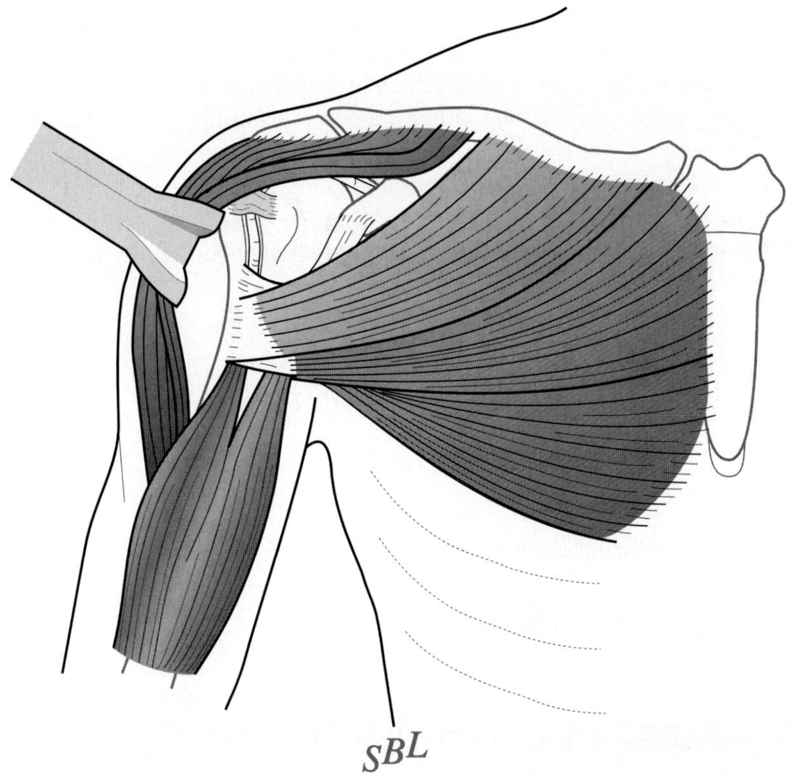

**Figure 23–1. Pectoralis anatomy**
The clavicular head inserts more distally than the sternocostal head of the pectoralis major.

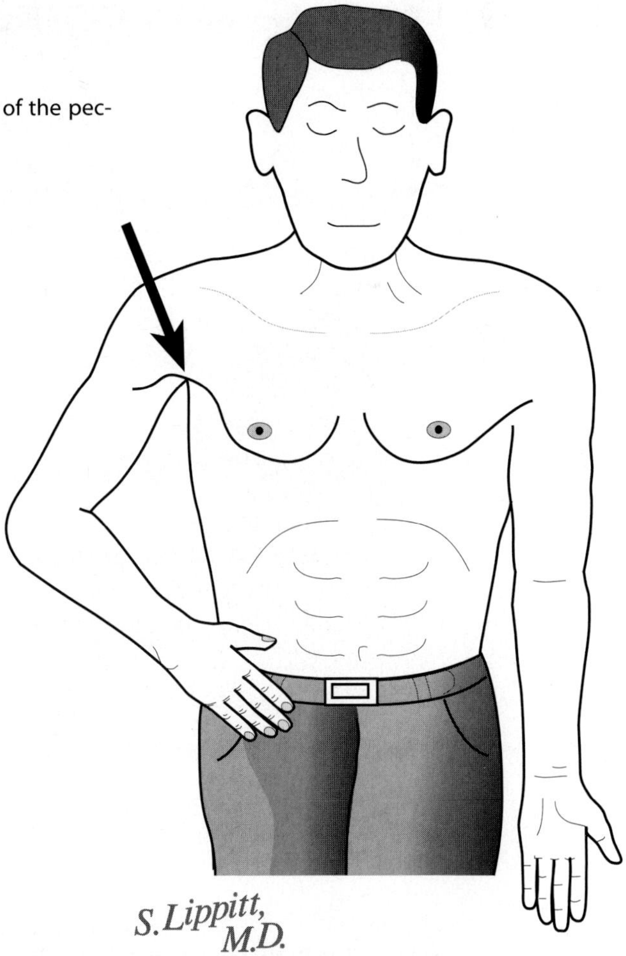

**Figure 23–2. Clinical appearance**
When the patient presses the hand down on the iliac crest, the abnormal contour of the ruptured pectoralis major is accentuated.

## OPERATION

Under satisfactory anesthesia, the patient is placed in a low beach chair position with the arm at the edge of the operating table (**Fig. 23–3**). The shoulder is carefully prepped and draped.

The major axillary crease is marked with a sterile pen. The shoulder is approached through a low anterior axillary incision made in this axillary crease (**Fig. 23–4**). The deltopectoral interval is opened, leaving the cephalic vein on the deltoid laterally. The torn pectoralis major tendon is identified and tagged (**Fig. 23–5**).

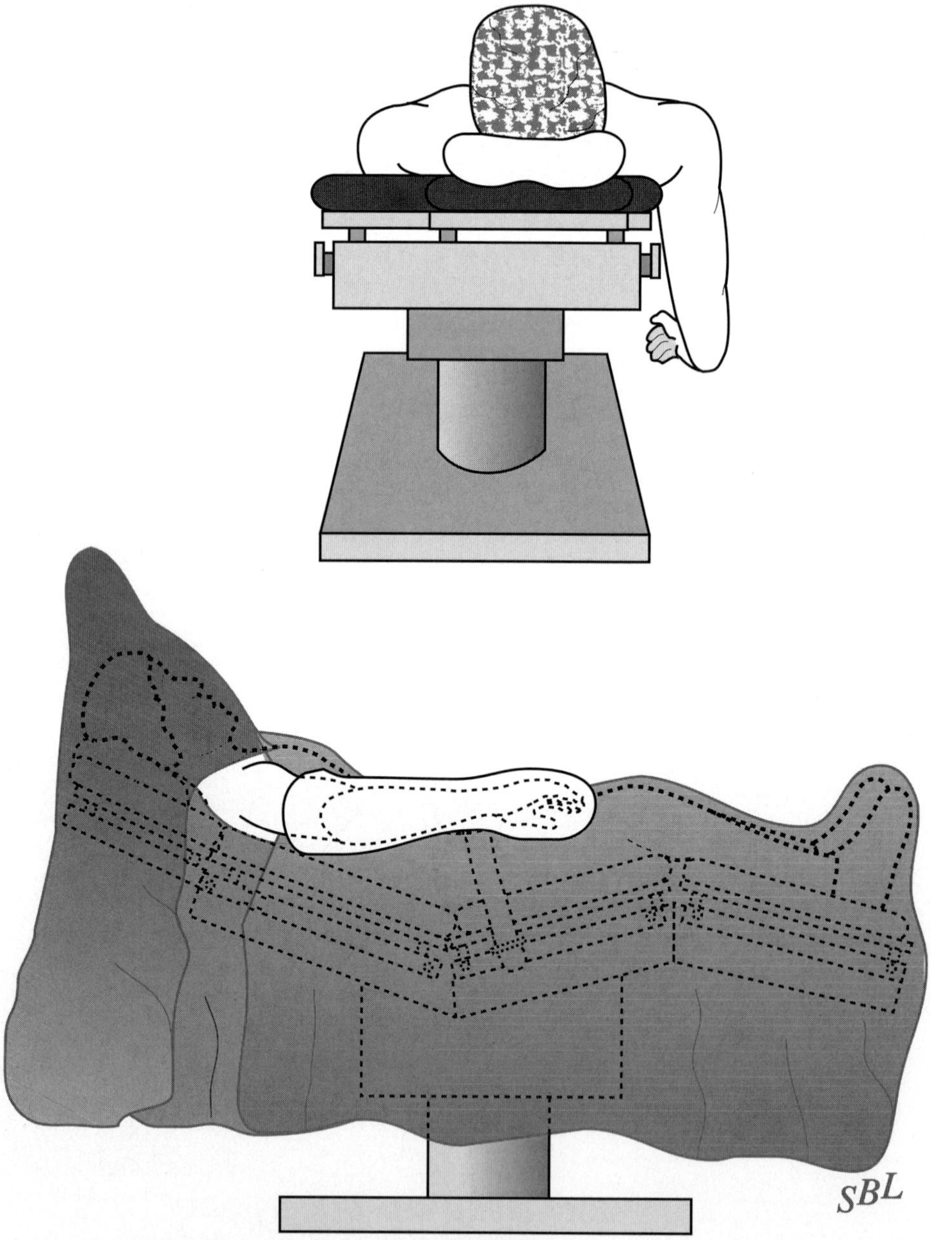


**Figure 23–3. Positioning and draping the shoulder**
The patient is placed in beach chair position with arm draped free. Note that the patient is positioned with the glenohumeral joint at the edge of the table so that the arm can be moved through a full range of motion.

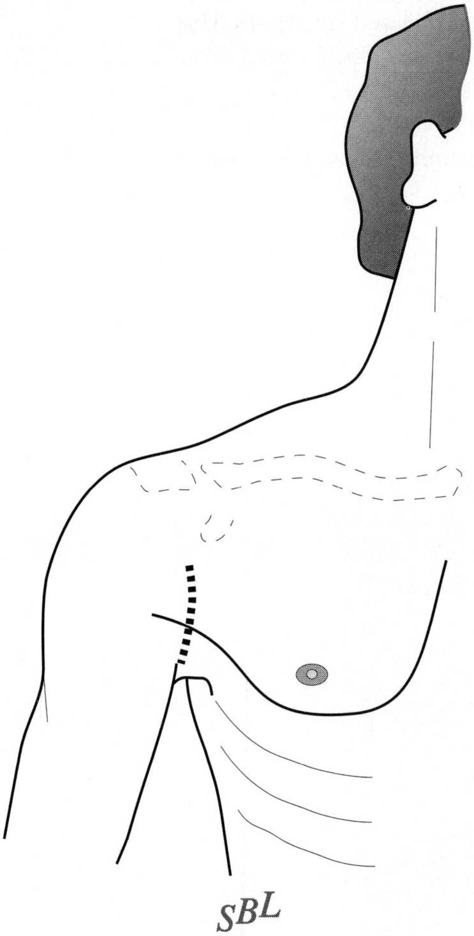


**Figure 23–4. Axillary incision**
The shoulder is approached through a low axillary incision in the major axillary crease. (Modified from Rockwood CA, Matsen FA [eds]: The Shoulder, 2nd ed. Philadelphia: WB Saunders, 1998, p. 704.)

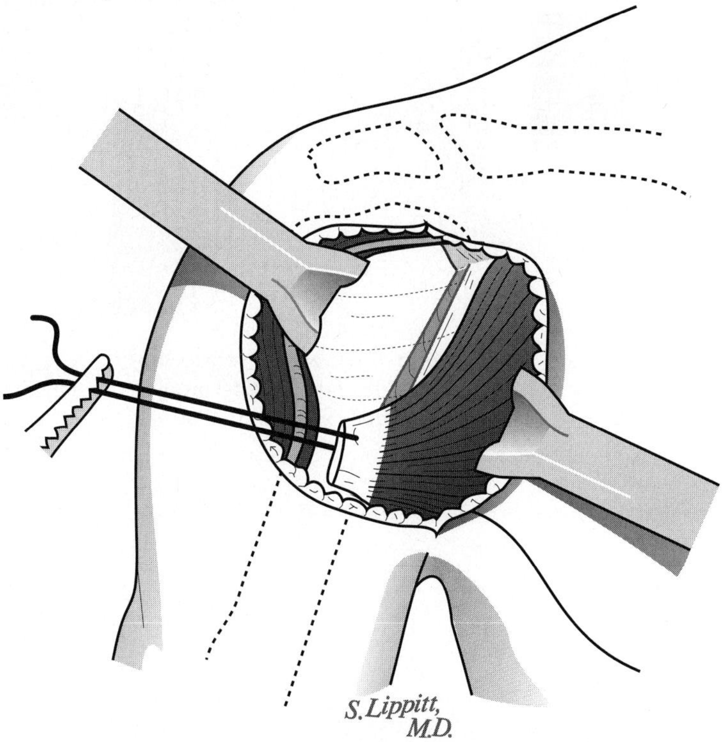


**Figure 23–5. Pectoralis tendon mobilization**
The torn end of the tendon is tagged with sutures. Applying traction to these sutures helps mobilize the tendon.

A groove is created in the humerus just lateral to the bicipital groove (**Fig. 23–6**). Holes of 1.8 mm diameter are drilled lateral to this groove (**Fig. 23–7**). Number 5-0 braided nonabsorbable sutures are passed through each hole, into the groove, then through the mobilized lateral end of the pectoralis major tendon (see Fig. 23–4), and then back into the groove and back out the adjacent hole. Tying these sutures robustly approximates the pectoralis major tendon to the bleeding groove (**Fig. 23–8**). Excellent fixation is achieved. The humerus can be fully externally elevated and rotated without challenging the fixation of the tendon to bone.

The wound is thoroughly irrigated and closed in layers. Dry sterile dressings are applied.

The patient is taken to the recovery room in satisfactory condition with the arm in a sling.

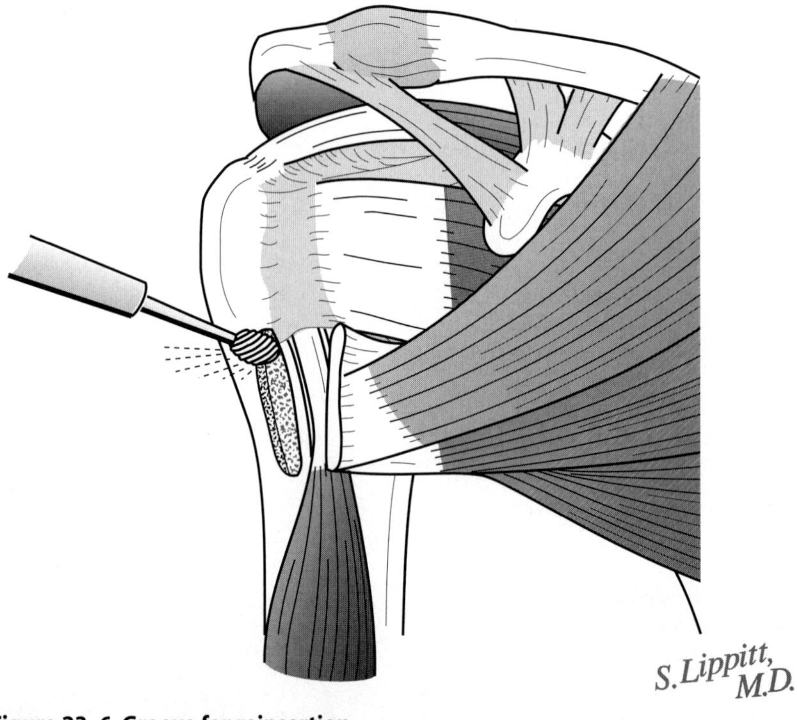


**Figure 23–6. Groove for reinsertion**
The lateral lip of the bicipital groove is identified. A groove is created at the site of avulsion of the pectoralis tendon.

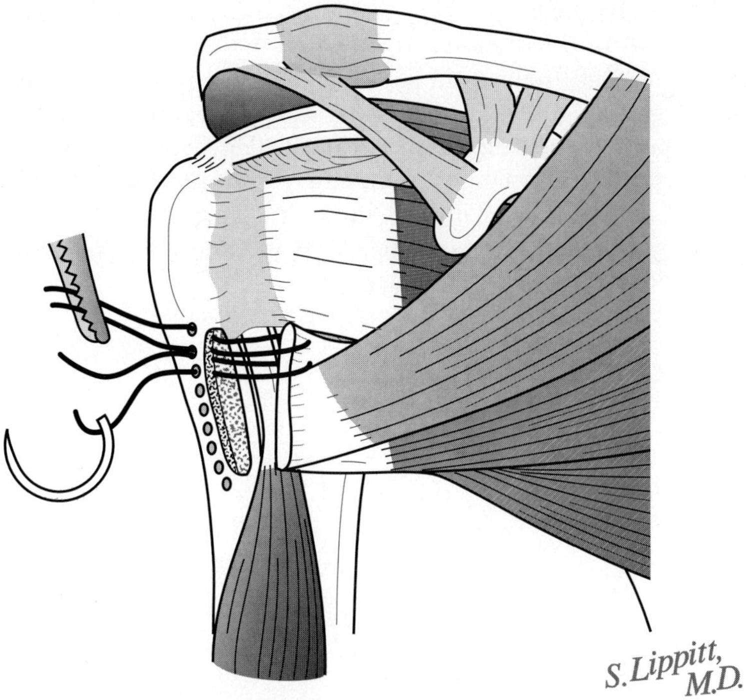


**Figure 23–7. Pectoralis sutures**
Holes are drilled lateral to the groove. Number 5-0 braided sutures are passed through these holes into the groove. These sutures are then passed through the tendon edge, back into the groove, and out the adjacent hole.

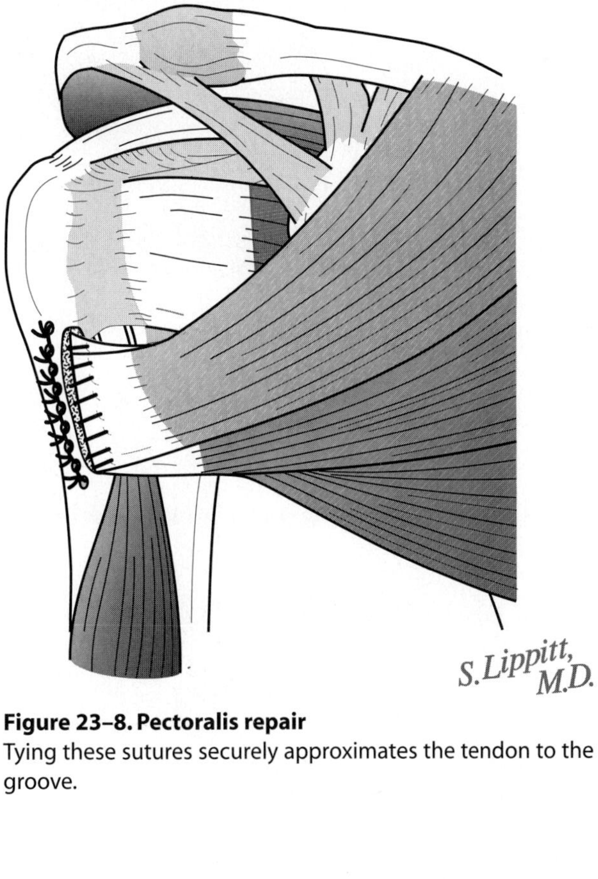


**Figure 23–8. Pectoralis repair**
Tying these sutures securely approximates the tendon to the groove.

## POSTOPERATIVE PLAN

The postoperative plan includes immediate implementation of patient-conducted external rotation to 0 degrees (**Fig. 23–9**) and elevation to 90 degrees (**Fig. 23–10**). As soon as the patient can perform these exercises, the patient is discharged. The patient is encouraged to remove the sling and move the arm actively in the allowed range when functioning in a protected environment. Lifting is limited to 1 pound for 6 weeks.

At 4 weeks after surgery, the patient is instructed to increase external rotation toward 40 degrees and forward elevation to 140 degrees.

Gentle and progressive strengthening exercises are started at 2 months.

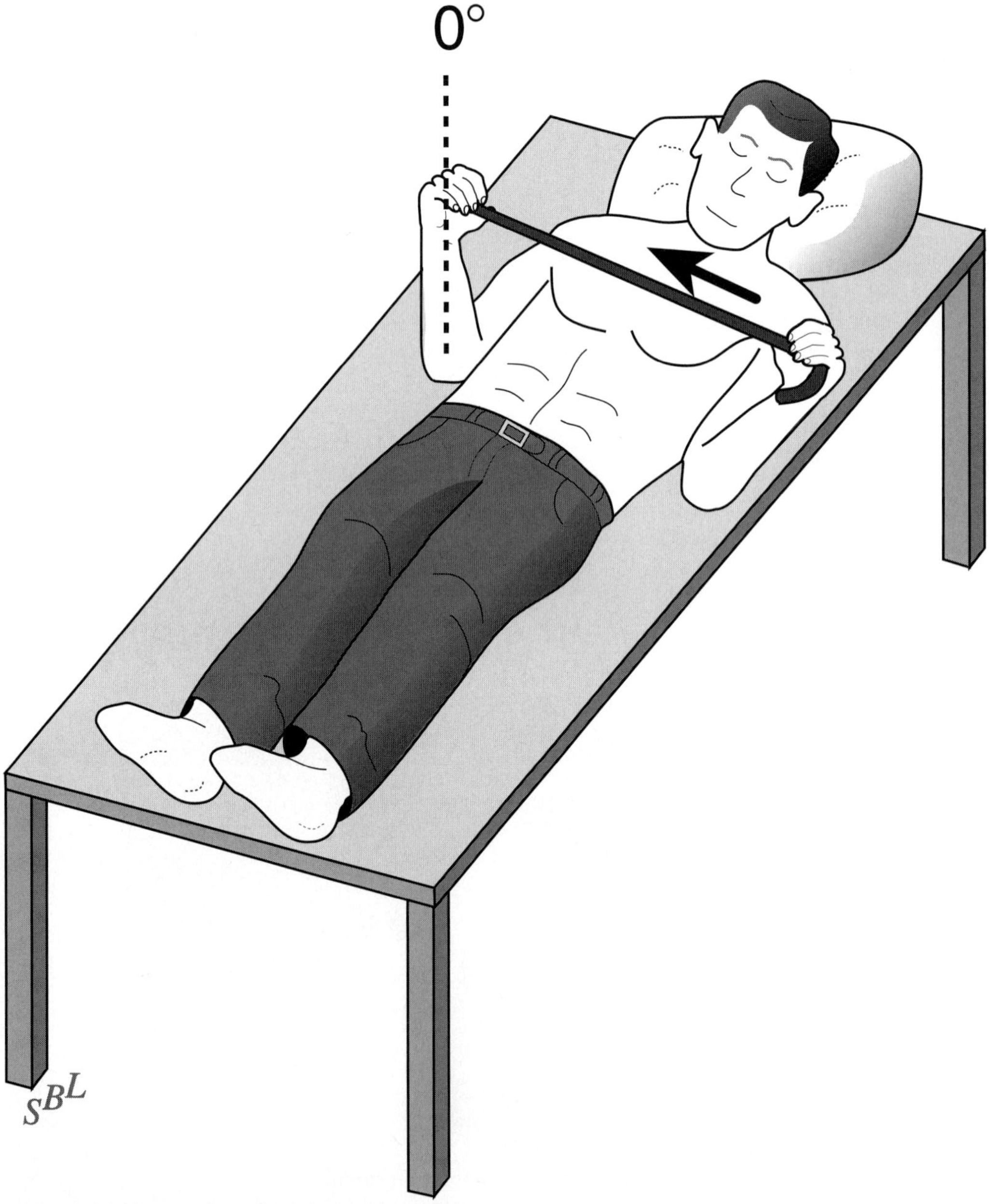


**Figure 23–9. Passive external rotation**
Assisted external rotation to 0 degrees.

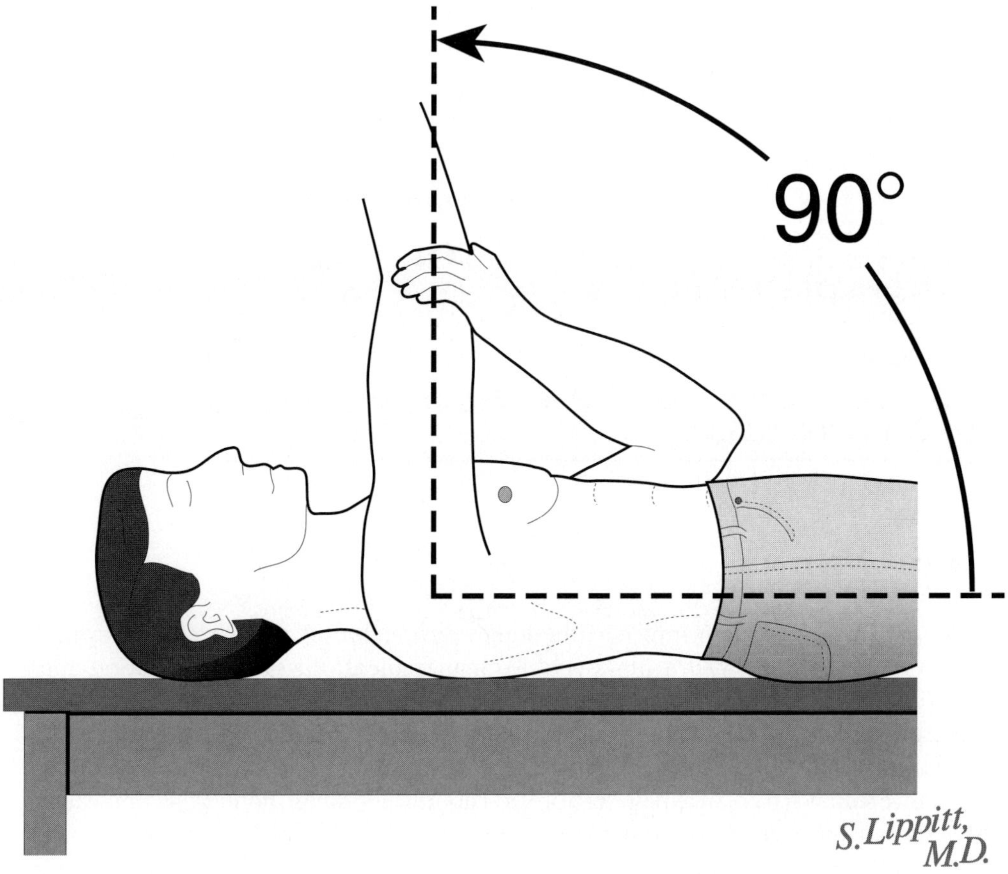


**Figure 23–10. Passive elevation**
Assisted elevation to 90 degrees.

CHAPTER 24

# Procedure: Tenodesis of the Long Head of the Biceps

**Diagnosis**

***Partial tear of the long head tendon of the biceps***
***ICD9 CODE 726.12***
***Rupture of the long head tendon of the biceps***
***ICD9 CODE 727.62***

**Procedure**

***Tenodesis of the long head tendon of the biceps***
***CPT CODE 23430***

## INDICATIONS

The patient sustained an injury to the long head tendon of the biceps. The symptoms have not responded to nonoperative management. Physical examination and tendon imaging indicate a tear in the long head tendon of the biceps. The rotator cuff is unaffected, and plain radiographs indicate no evidence of arthritis.

Knowing in detail the alternatives as well as the risks of infection, neurovascular injury, excessive stiffness, pain, weakness, fracture, re-rupture, nonunion, nonhealing of the tenodesis, instability, arthritis, and the need for revision surgery, as well as anesthetic complications, and knowing that this reconstruction cannot be expected to completely restore the shoulder to its level of comfort and function before the injury, the patient desires to proceed with a tenodesis of the long head of the biceps tendon. The patient understands that a repair of the biceps tendon to restore its normal anatomy is not possible. The patient understands his or her critical role in the post-surgical rehabilitation.

## FINDINGS

The biceps tendon is found torn in the bicipital sheath. A similar procedure would have been performed if the biceps were medially subluxated from its groove beneath the subscapularis tendon.

## SURGICAL PROCEDURE

Under satisfactory anesthesia, the patient is placed in a low beach chair position. The entire forequarter is carefully prepped and draped in the usual sterile fashion with the arm free to be moved.

The shoulder is approached through the deltoid-on incision (see Chapter 21). The frayed, partially torn long head biceps tendon is found in the bicipital groove (**Fig. 24–1**). The tendon is sectioned as far proximally as possible (**Fig. 24–2**).

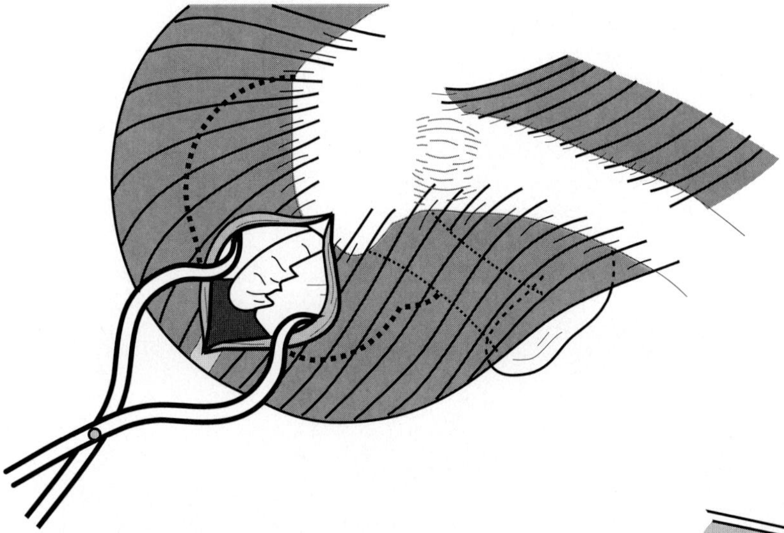

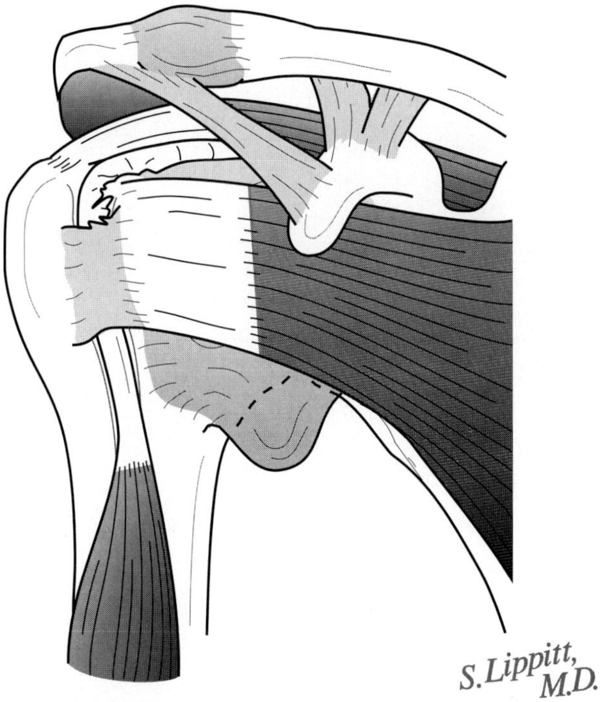


**Figure 24–1. Frayed biceps tendon**
The transverse humeral ligament and the rotator interval are opened to expose the frayed biceps tendon.

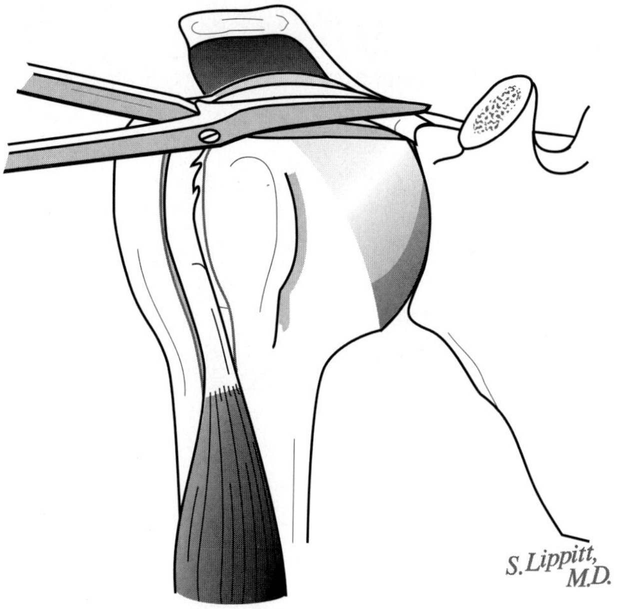


**Figure 24–2. Sectioning the biceps tendon**
The biceps tendon is sectioned proximally and retrieved from the joint.

If the biceps tendon has ruptured at the transverse humeral ligament, the proximal fragment is incised from its origin and discarded. The proximal end of the distal fragment is located by opening the bicipital tendon sheath. If necessary for access to the retracted tendon, a second incision is made vertically over the bicipital groove at the upper edge of the pectoralis major insertion.

The bicipital tendon sheath is opened and the proximal end of strong tendon is identified; weak tendon material is débrided. Number 2 nonabsorbable braided suture is woven through the proximal end of the tendon. With the elbow flexed at 90 degrees, gentle traction is applied to the tendon. Two holes 5 mm in diameter are made in the bicipital groove 1 cm apart (**Fig. 24–3**). The proximal hole in the humerus is located 2 cm distal to the point reached by the proximal end of good quality tendon.

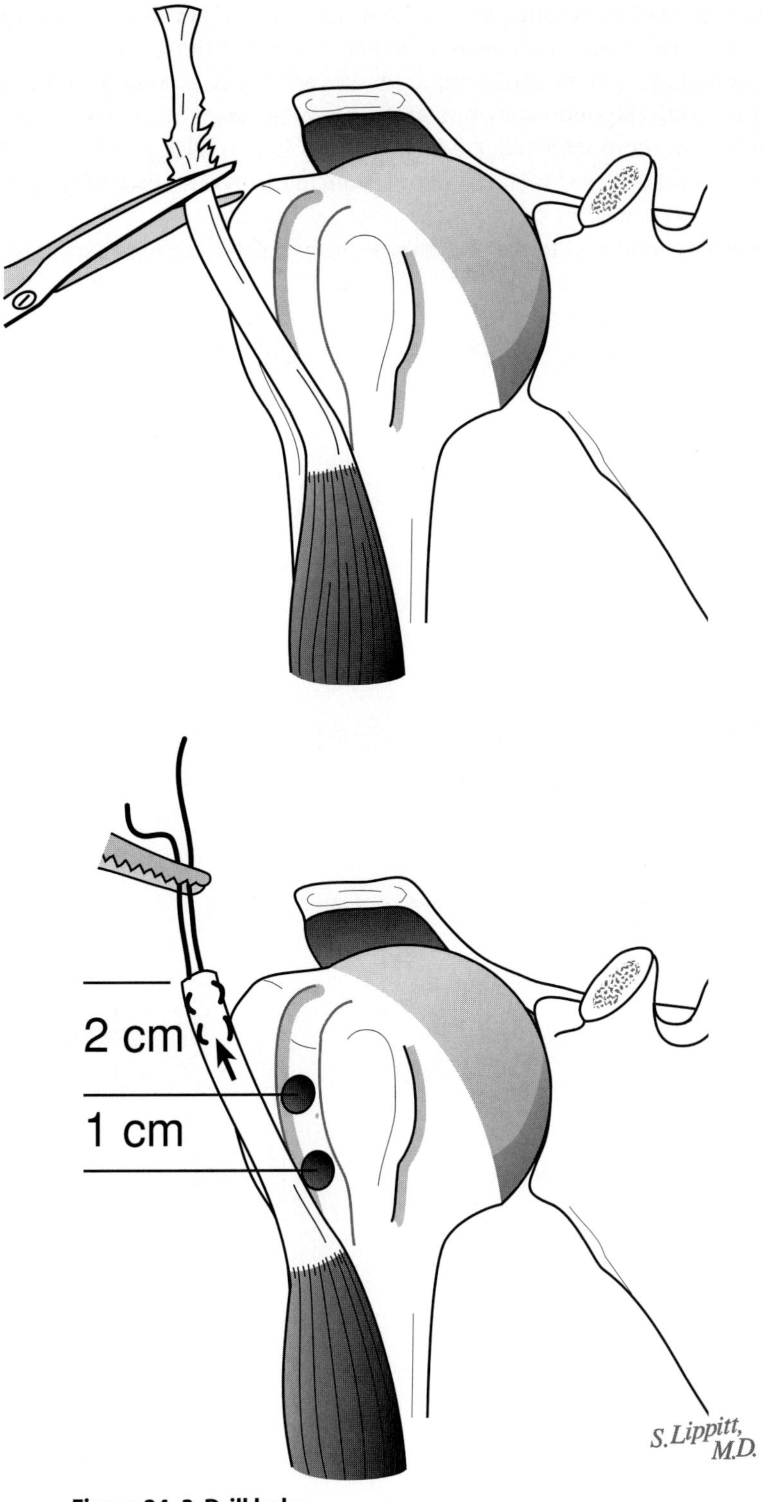


**Figure 24–3. Drill holes**
Friable tendon is débrided from the proximal end of the tendon. Number 2 nonabsorbable suture is woven through the proximal end of the tendon. The proximal of two drill holes in the bicipital groove is made 2 cm distal to the end of the reach of the proximal end of the tendon when tensioned proximally in the groove. This allows sufficient tendon for overlap at the time of suturing. The second hole is made 1 cm more distal, leaving a solid bridge between. The two holes are connected beneath the cortex using an angled curette.

The end of the tendon is brought into the distal hole and out the proximal one (**Fig. 24–4**). The proximal end of the tendon is then sutured to the tendon distal to the distal hole using six #2 nonabsorbable braided sutures. The tendon should be under moderate tension with the elbow flexed at 90 degrees (**Fig. 24–5**).

The wound is thoroughly irrigated. Hemostasis is seen to be excellent.

The incisions are closed with absorbable subcutaneous and subcuticular sutures.

Dry sterile dressings are applied.

The patient is returned to the recovery room in satisfactory condition.

## POSTOPERATIVE PLAN

Our postoperative plan is for assisted elevation up to 140 degrees, avoiding unassisted elbow flexion for 6 weeks.

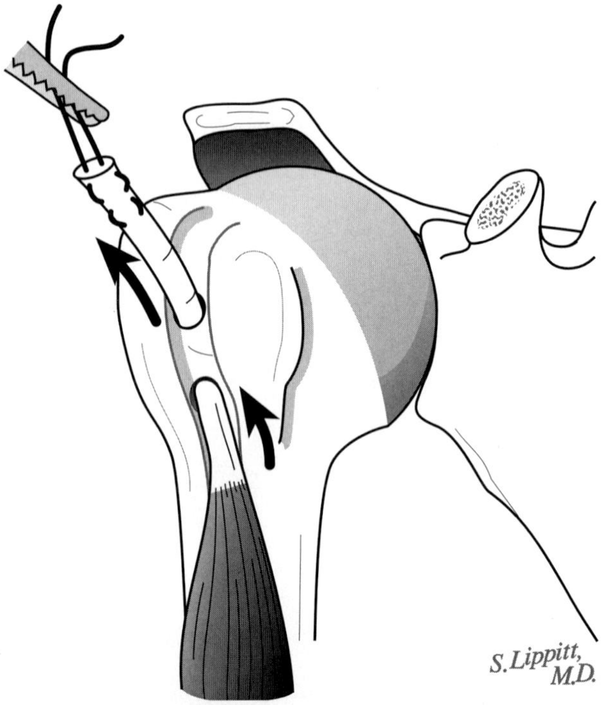


**Figure 24–4. Passing the tendon**
The proximal end of the tendon is passed into the distal hole and out the proximal one.

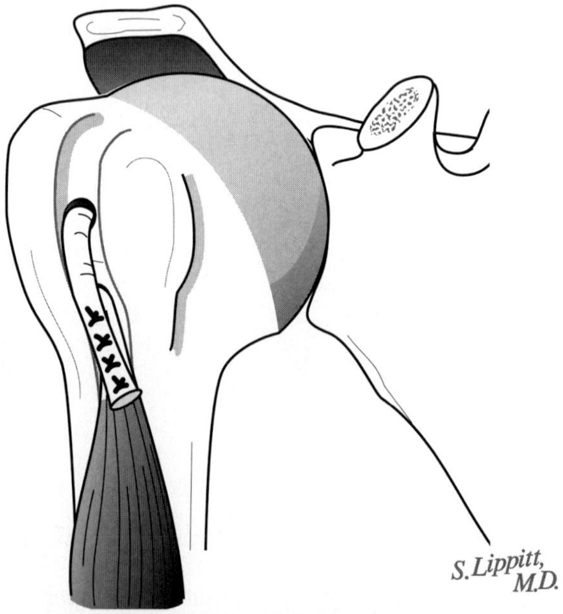


**Figure 24–5. Suturing the tendon**
With the elbow in 90 degrees of flexion and with the tendon under moderate tension, the proximal tendon is folded distally and sutured to the tendon distal to the distal hole with six #2 braided sutures.

# PART V

# SMOOTHNESS

CHAPTER 25

# Principles of Humeroscapular Smoothness

## CONCEPTS

*Humeroscapular smoothness* is the ability of the humerus to move through its allowed range of positions with respect to the scapula without the patient perceiving crepitance, grinding, or irregularities in the movements.

The humeroscapular articulation has two components: the glenohumeral joint and the humeroscapular motion interface. While the glenohumeral joint is well known, the humeroscapular motion interface is less familiar (**Figs. 25–1** and **25–2**). It is composed of the following:

1. A spherical coracoacromial concavity consisting of the deltoid, acromion, coracoacromial ligament, coracoid process, and coracoid muscles (**Fig. 25–3**).

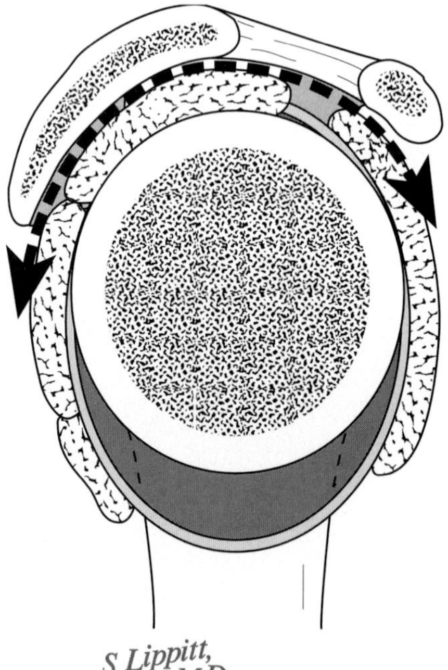


**Figure 25–1. Humeroscapular motion interface**
The external surface of the rotator cuff articulates with the undersurface of the coracoacromial arch. This articulation is part of the humeroscapular motion interface. Smooth, unrestrained movement at this interface is required for normal shoulder function. (Modified from Rockwood CA, Matsen FA [eds]: The Shoulder, 2nd ed. Philadelphia: WB Saunders, 1998, p. 704.)

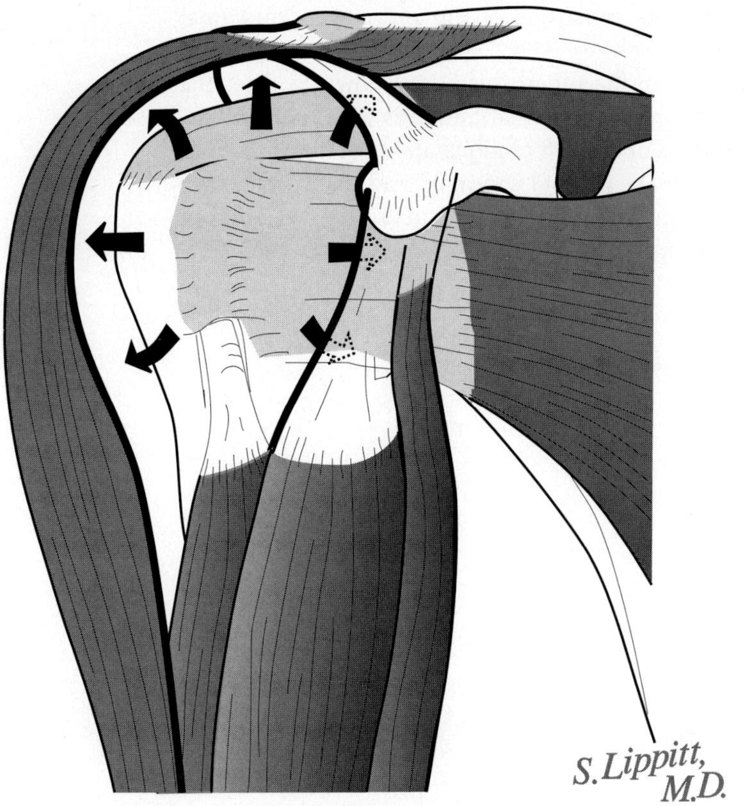


**Figure 25–2. Humeroscapular motion interface**
The humeroscapular motion interface is the set of gliding surfaces between the proximal humerus covered by the rotator cuff tendons and the overlying structures attached to the scapula, including the deltoid, the acromion, the coracoacromial ligament, the coracoid, and the tendons of the coracoid muscles. Approximately 4 cm of motion takes place at this interface in normal shoulder movement. (Modified from Matsen FA, Lippitt SB, Sidles JA, et al [eds]: Practical Evaluation and Management of the Shoulder. Philadelphia: WB Saunders, 1994, p. 34.)

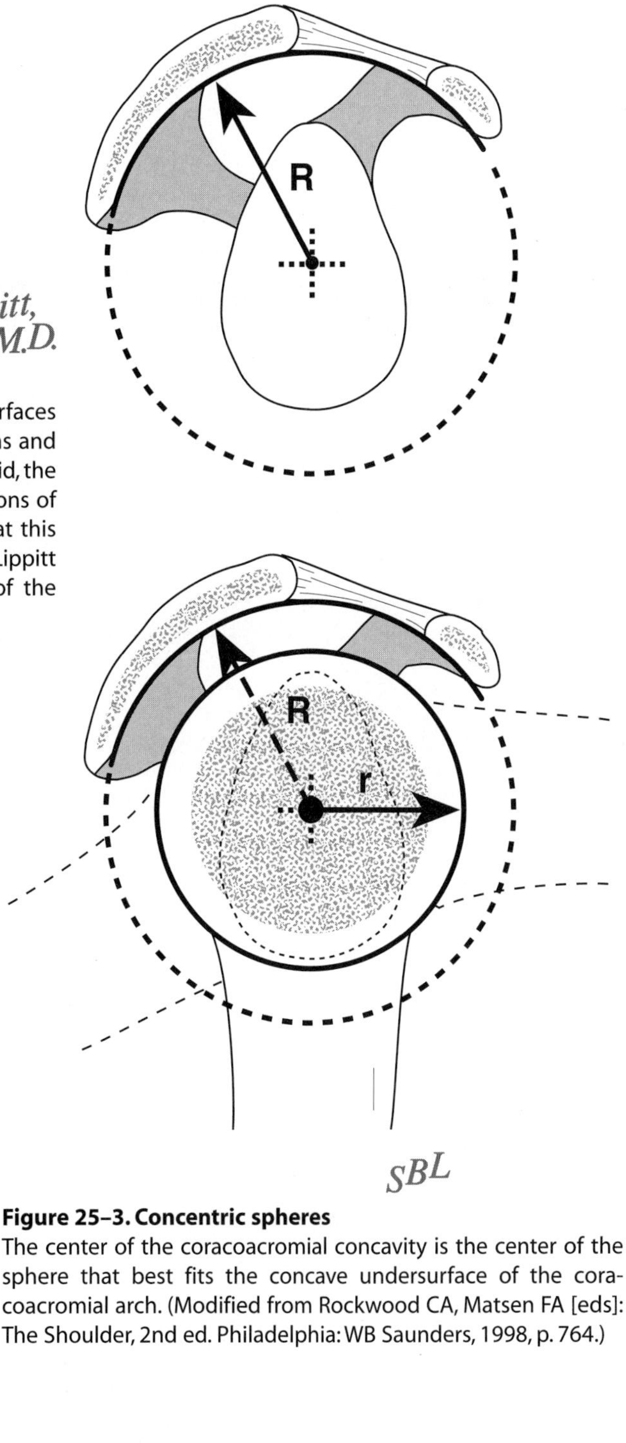


**Figure 25–3. Concentric spheres**
The center of the coracoacromial concavity is the center of the sphere that best fits the concave undersurface of the coracoacromial arch. (Modified from Rockwood CA, Matsen FA [eds]: The Shoulder, 2nd ed. Philadelphia: WB Saunders, 1998, p. 764.)

2. A spherical proximal humeral convexity consisting of the cuff-covered proximal humerus and the long head tendon of the biceps (**Fig. 25–4**). Although radiographs give the impression of a step-off where the tuberosities drop down to meet the articular surface (**Fig. 25–5**), inspection of a proximal humerus with the cuff tendons attached reveals that the thickness of the cuff tendons makes up the difference in radius of curvature between that of the glenoid concavity and that of the coracoacromial concavity. The tendons blend smoothly into the tuberosities, yielding an almost perfect spherical external surface (**Fig. 25–6**).

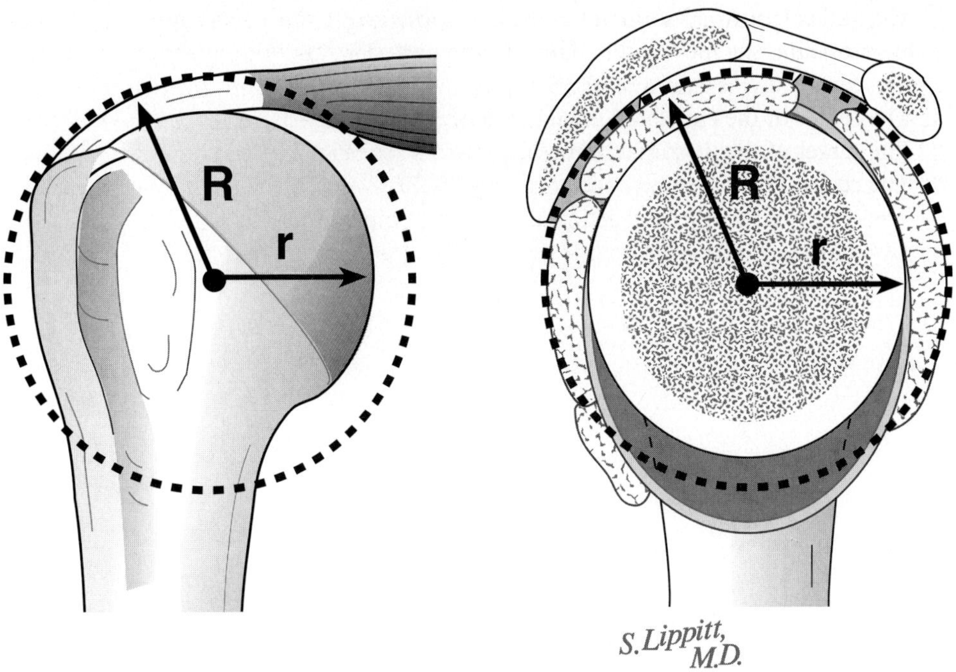


**Figure 25–4. Proximal humeral convexity**
The center of the proximal humeral convexity is the center of the sphere circumscribing the cuff tendons and the tuberosity.

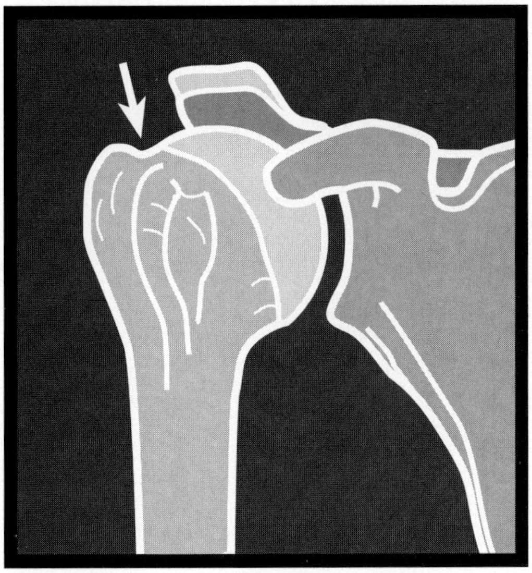

**Figure 25–5. Radiographic impression**
Radiographs suggest that the greater tuberosity is prominent with respect to the humeral articular surface. However, this is not the case if the rotator cuff is intact.

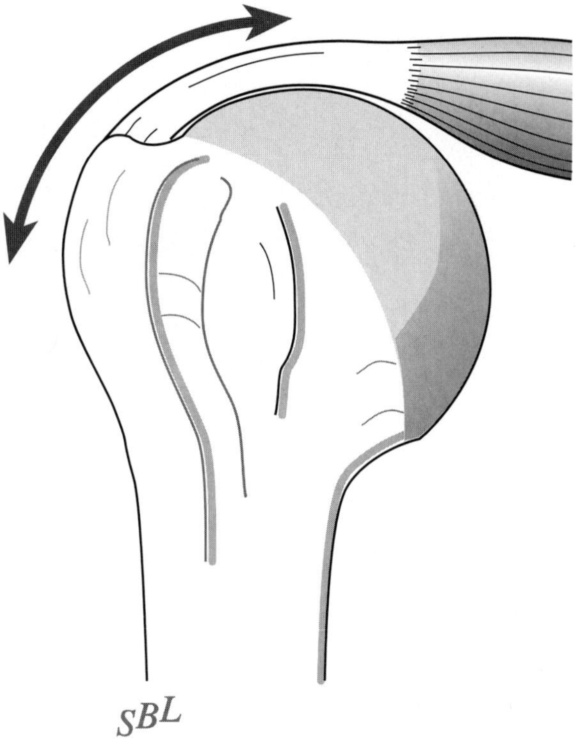


**Figure 25–6. Spherical external surface**
The tendons and tuberosity blend together to form a smooth surface for the proximal humeral convexity.

This articulation is essentially a ball-in-socket with the subacromial-subdeltoid bursa providing the lubrication. Thus, in the perfectly functioning shoulder, the following centers are superimposed:

1. The center of the coracoacromial concavity (see Fig. 25–3)
2. The center of the proximal humeral convexity (see Fig. 25–4)
3. The center of the glenoid concavity **(Fig. 25–7)**
4. The center of the humeral articular convexity **(Fig. 25–8)**

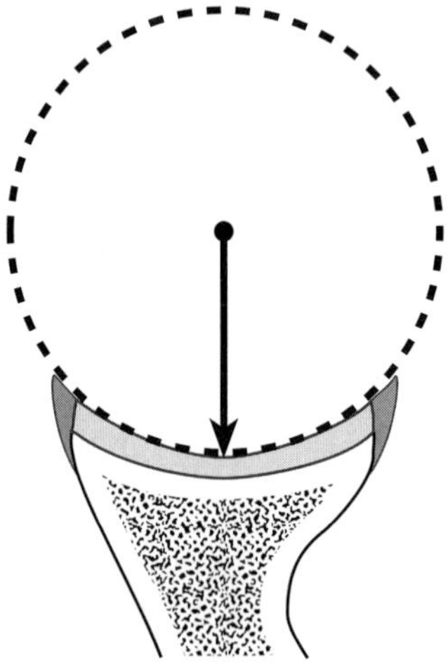

**Figure 25–7. Center of glenoid concavity**
The center of the glenoid concavity is the center of the sphere fit to its articular surface.

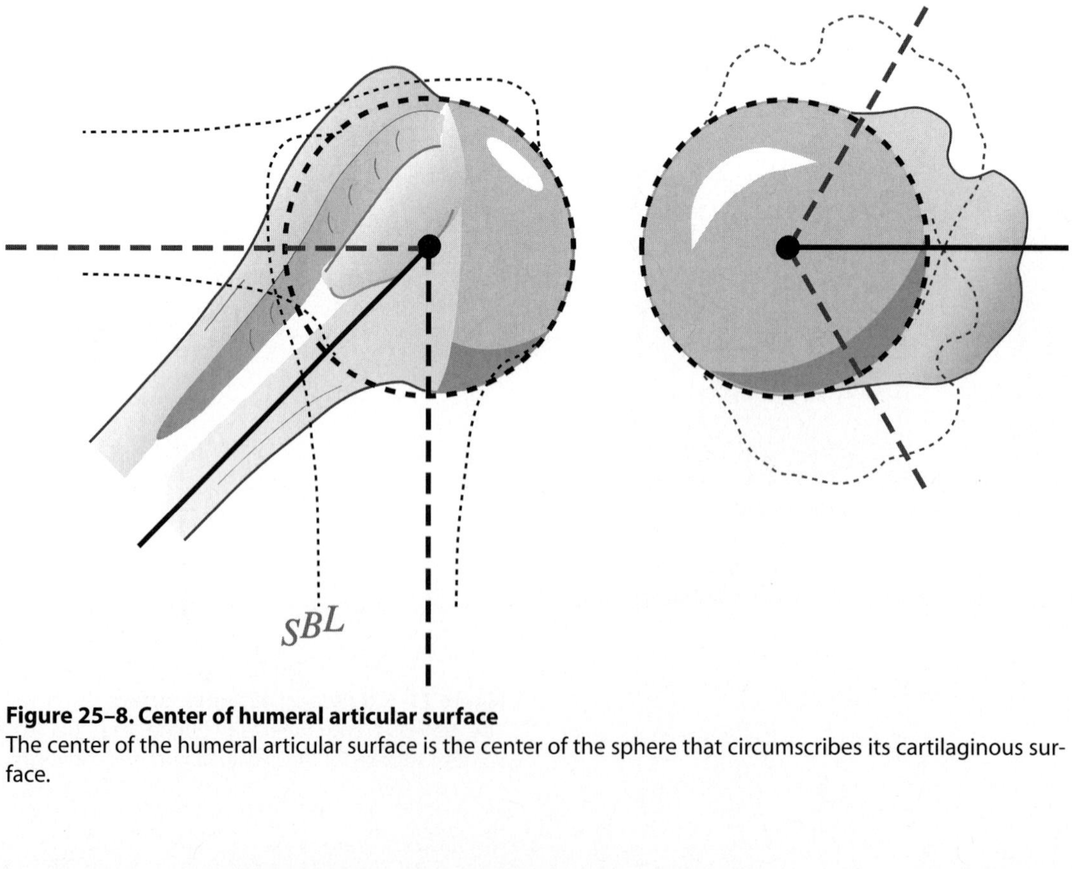


**Figure 25–8. Center of humeral articular surface**
The center of the humeral articular surface is the center of the sphere that circumscribes its cartilaginous surface.

Calcification of the coracoacromial ligament (appearing radiographically as an acromial "spur") does not compromise the congruity of the humeroscapular motion interface (**Fig. 25–9**).

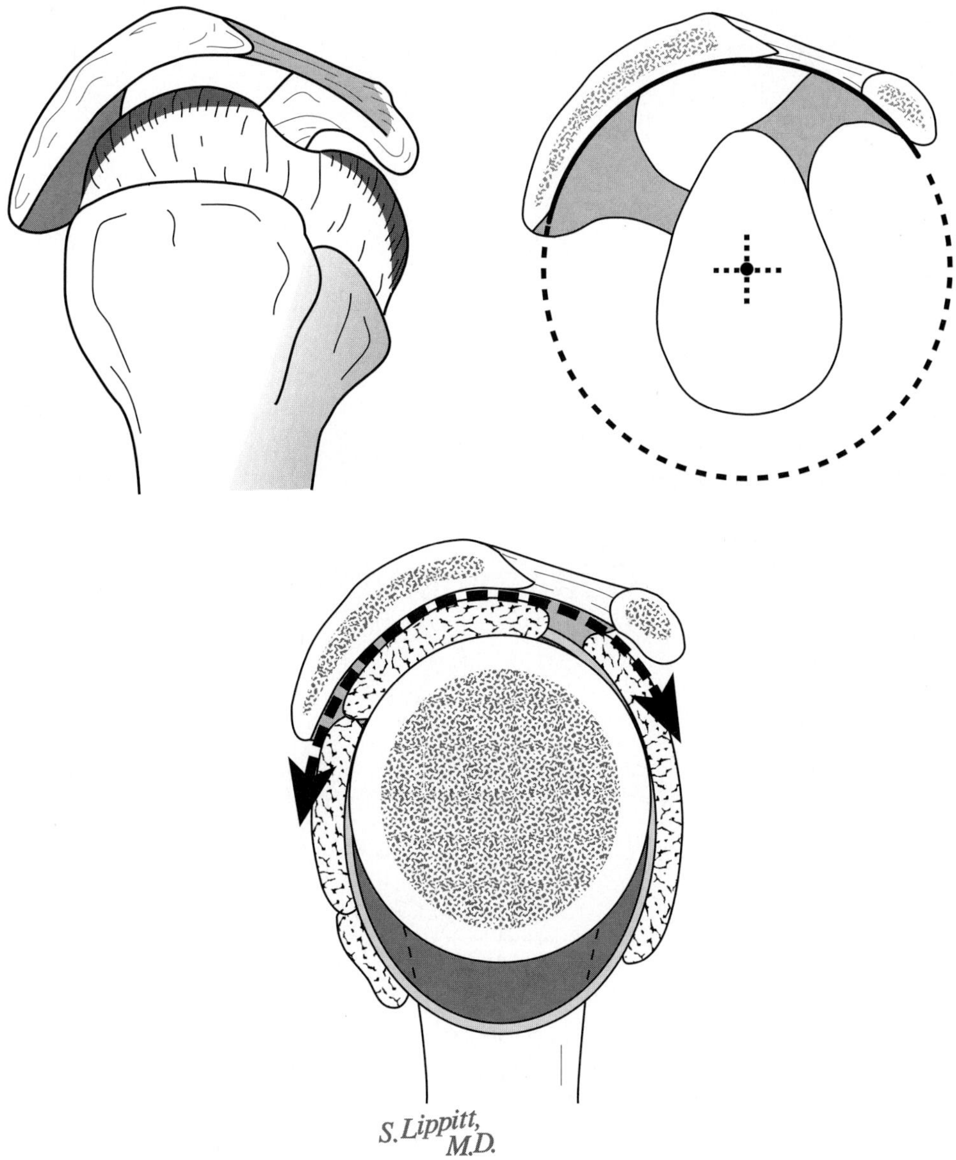


**Figure 25–9. Calcification in coracoacromial ligament**
Calcification in the coracoacromial ligament does not encroach on the rotator cuff.

Loss of humeroscapular smoothness may result when an over-tight anterior or posterior capsule forces the humerus in the opposite direction (obligate translation) (**Fig. 25–10**). Bursal thickening interposed between the proximal humeral convexity and the coracoacromial concavity can interfere with the smooth motion of the two surfaces on each other (**Fig. 25–11**). Loss of humeroscapular smoothness may also result from deviations

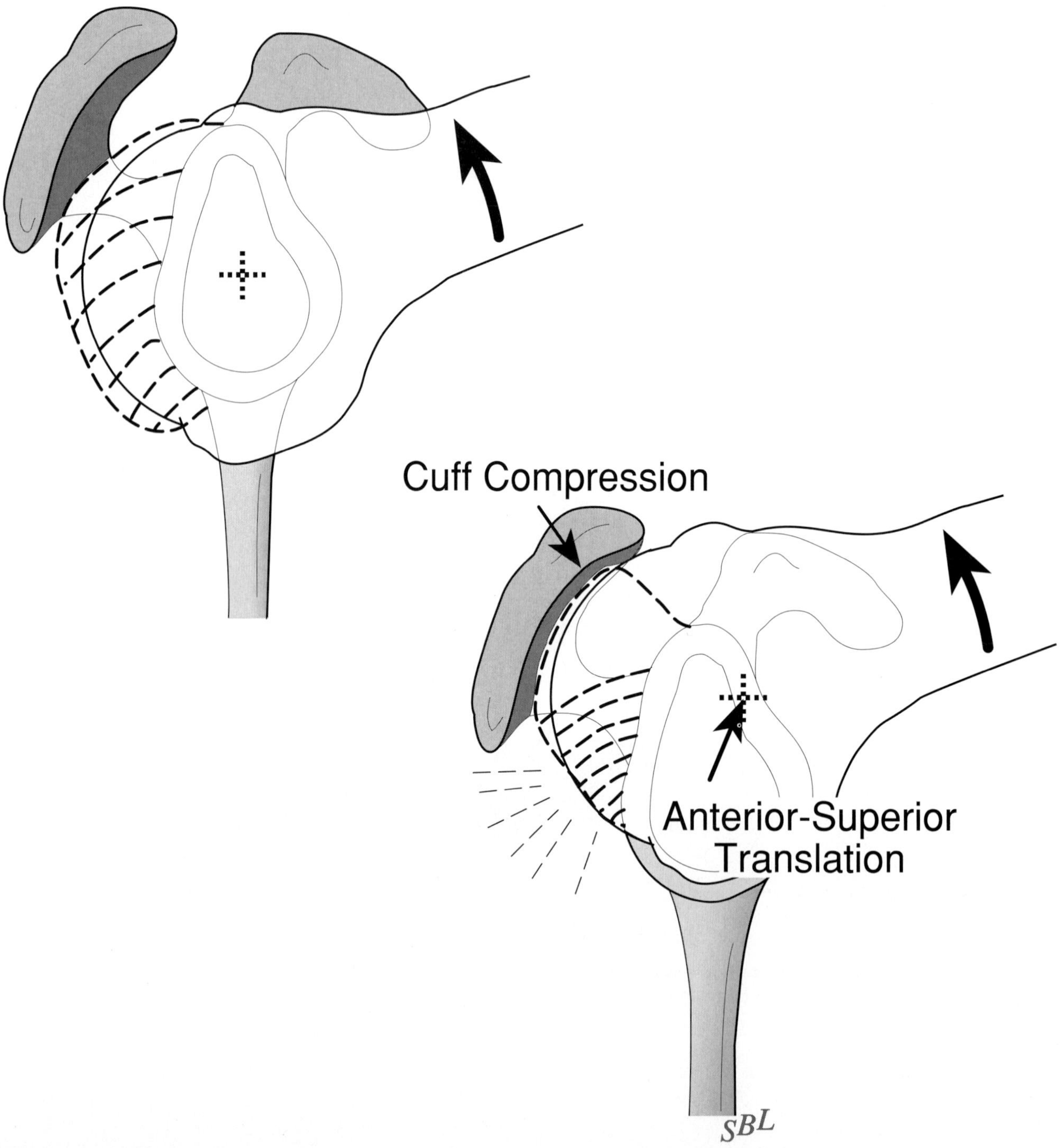


**Figure 25–10. Posterior capsule tightness**
Tightness of the posterior inferior capsule causes obligate anterosuperior translation on flexion. As a result, the centers of the humeral articular surface and proximal humeral convexity are no longer the same as the centers of the coracoacromial arch and the glenoid concavity. (Modified from Matsen FA, Lippitt SB, Sidles JA, et al [eds]: Practical Evaluation and Management of the Shoulder. Philadelphia: WB Saunders, 1994, p. 40.)

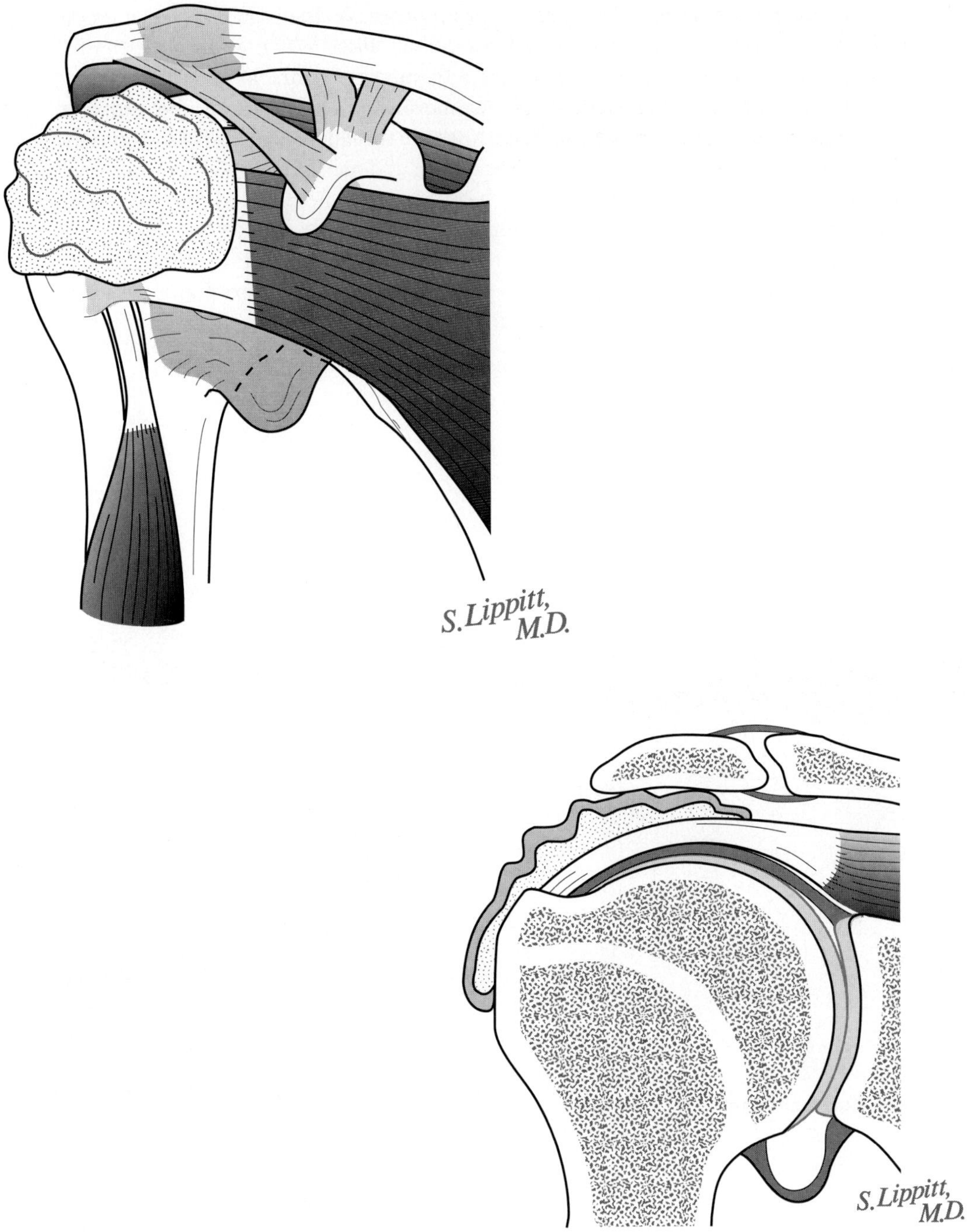


**Figure 25–11. Thick bursa**
Thickened bursa interferes with the smooth articulation of the proximal humeral convexity with the coracoacromial concavity.

from sphericity; this is particularly true for prominences on the proximal humeral side. Such prominences as the edges of torn cuff tendons (**Fig. 25–12**), suture knots on the superior aspect of the rotator cuff (**Fig. 25–13**), suture anchors, large intratendinous calcium deposits, or tuberosities extending beyond the contour of the proximal humeral convexity in the cuff-deficient or prosthetic shoulder (**Fig. 25–14**) can abut the edge of the coracoacromial arch and scrape on the undersurface of the coracoacromial concavity. If the cartilage is lost over the head of the humerus following a cuff tear, roughness can result from cuff tear arthropathy (**Fig. 25–15**).

The goal in managing roughness of the humeroscapular motion interface is to restore smooth articulation between the proximal humeral convexity and the coracoacromial concavity. Some of the useful procedures are described in Chapters 7, 20, and 22.

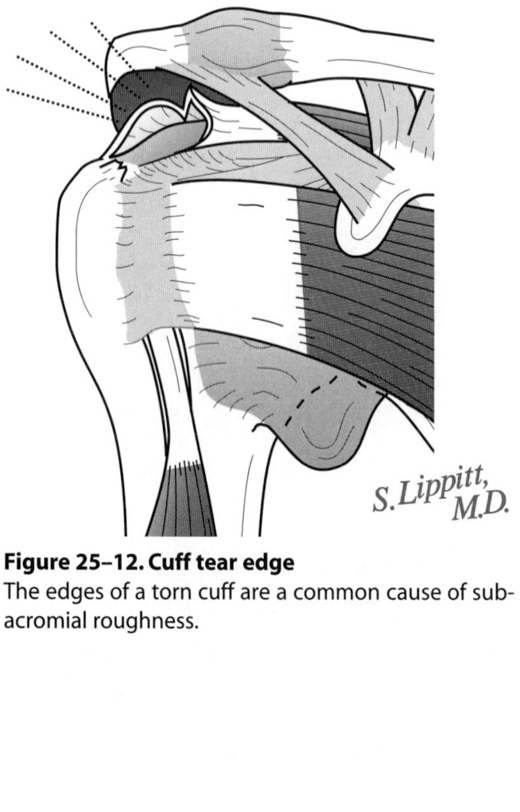


**Figure 25–12. Cuff tear edge**
The edges of a torn cuff are a common cause of subacromial roughness.

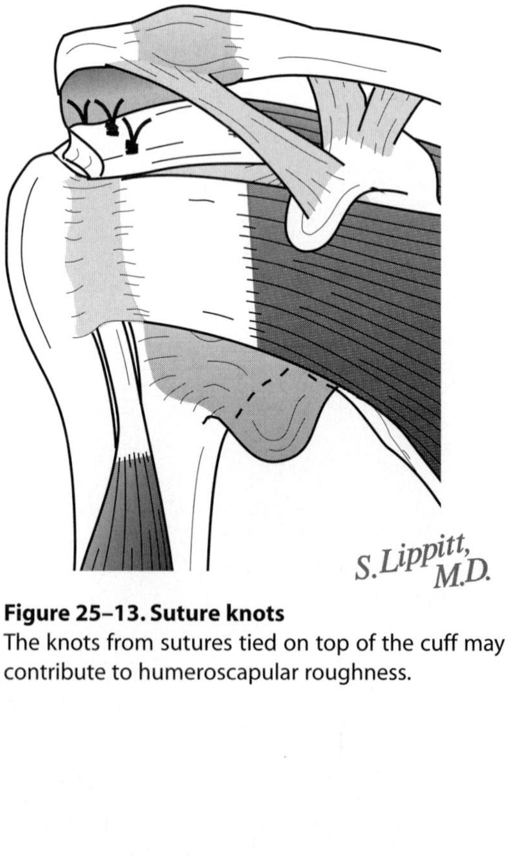


**Figure 25–13. Suture knots**
The knots from sutures tied on top of the cuff may contribute to humeroscapular roughness.

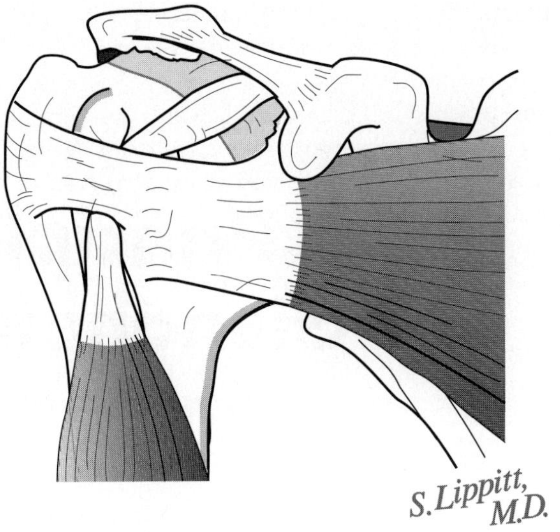


**Figure 25–14. Prominent tuberosity**
When the cuff is absent from its insertion, the tuberosity becomes relatively prominent, disrupting the smoothness of the proximal humeral convexity.

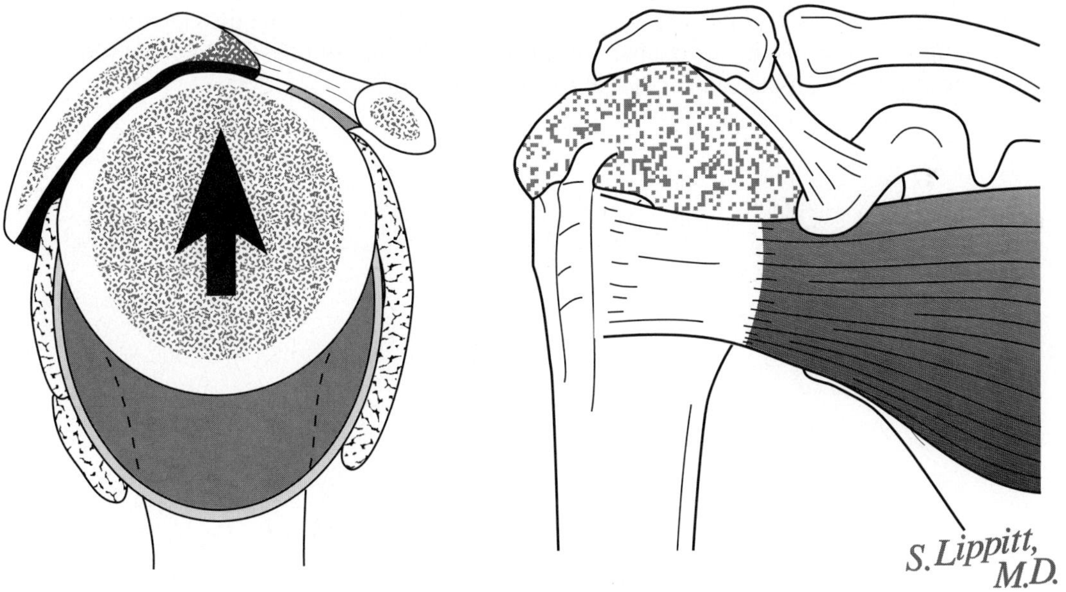


**Figure 25–15. Irreparable cuff**
Loss of the rotator cuff with upward displacement of the humeral head so that it contacts the coracoacromial arch can be followed by the development of cuff tear arthropathy. (Modified from Matsen FA, Lippitt SB, Sidles JA, et al [eds]: Practical Evaluation and Management of the Shoulder. Philadelphia: WB Saunders, 1994, p. 123.)

CHAPTER 26

# Principles of Glenohumeral Smoothness

## CONCEPTS

### Smoothness at the Glenohumeral Joint

The glenohumeral articulation is composed of a spherical convexity (humeral articular surface) **(Fig. 26–1)** and a spherical concavity (the glenoid fossa) **(Fig. 26–2)** that are normally close fitting with essentially identical radii of curvature and with identical centers of rotation. The congruence of the head and glenoid is facilitated by the compliance of the articular cartilage and labrum at the periphery of the articulation. As a result, the loads applied by the humeral head to the glenoid are distributed quite evenly over the maximal possible surface area—this minimizes the joint pressure (force/unit area) and minimizes joint pressure gradients.

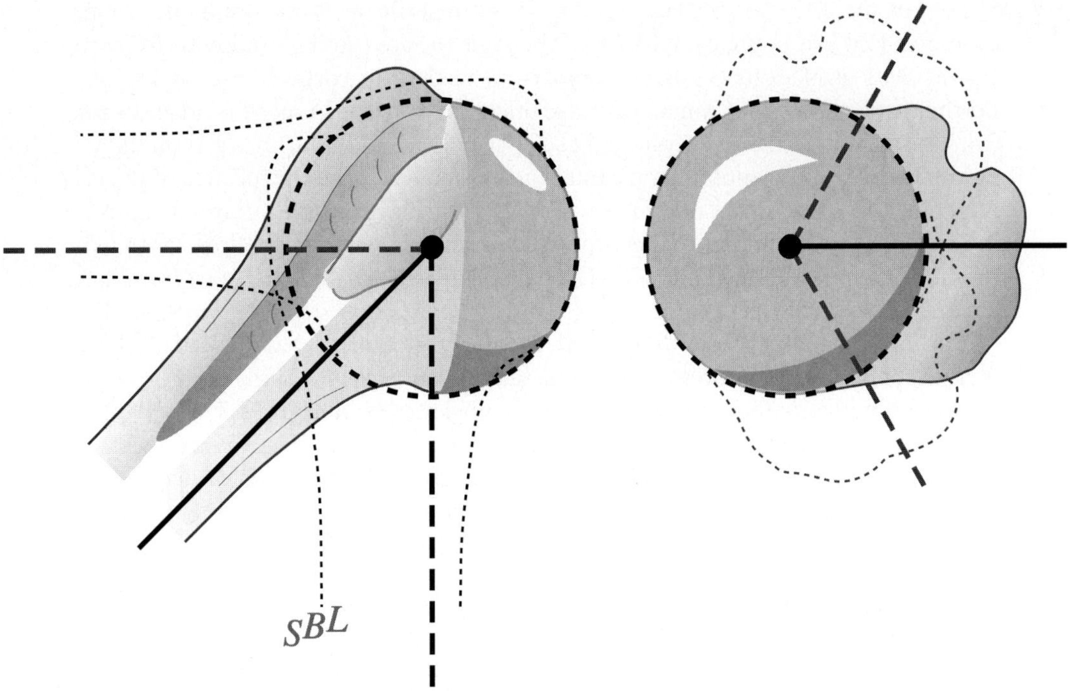


**Figure 26–1. Center of humeral articular surface**
The center of the humeral articular surface is the center of the sphere that circumscribes its cartilaginous surface.

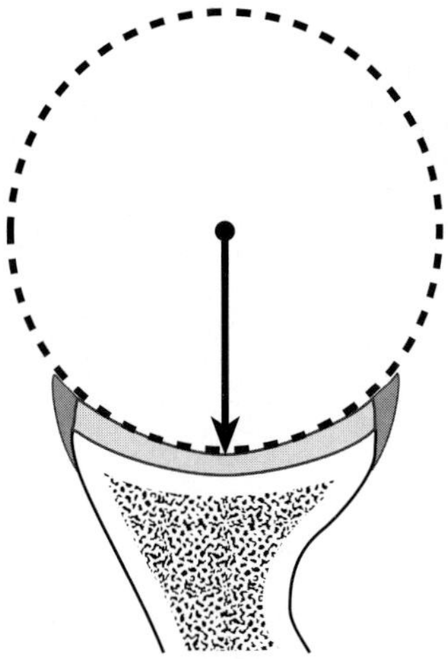

**Figure 26–2. Center of glenoid concavity**
The center of the glenoid concavity is the center of the sphere fit to its articular surface.

Loss of the articular cartilage, locally or throughout the joint, results in a many thousand-fold loss in the compliance of the joint surface (Young's modulus for cartilage is 0.001 gigaPascals (GPa), in comparison to that for cortical bone of 13 GPa). Furthermore, the loss of 1 mm of cartilage thickness from the humeral head and 1 mm from the glenoid results in a 2 mm radial disparity in the fit of the humerus on the glenoid. Therefore, the glenohumeral contact area is reduced from the full area of the glenoid down to a few square millimeters (**Fig. 26–3**). This results in a dramatic increase in local joint pressure and in steep pressure gradients between the loaded and the neighboring unloaded glenoid bone. The pain from arthritis derives in part from these large pressure gradients.

The increased joint pressure contributes to the erosion of any residual cartilage and then to the subchondral bone. In cases of inflammatory arthritis, the pattern of glenoid erosion is commonly central, or occasionally anterior; the humeral articular surface usually remains round (**Fig. 26–4**). In cases of degenerative arthritis and capsulorrhaphy arthropathy, the glenoid erosion is typically posterior, or occasionally central; the humeral articular surface becomes flattened or biconcave (**Fig. 26–5**). In

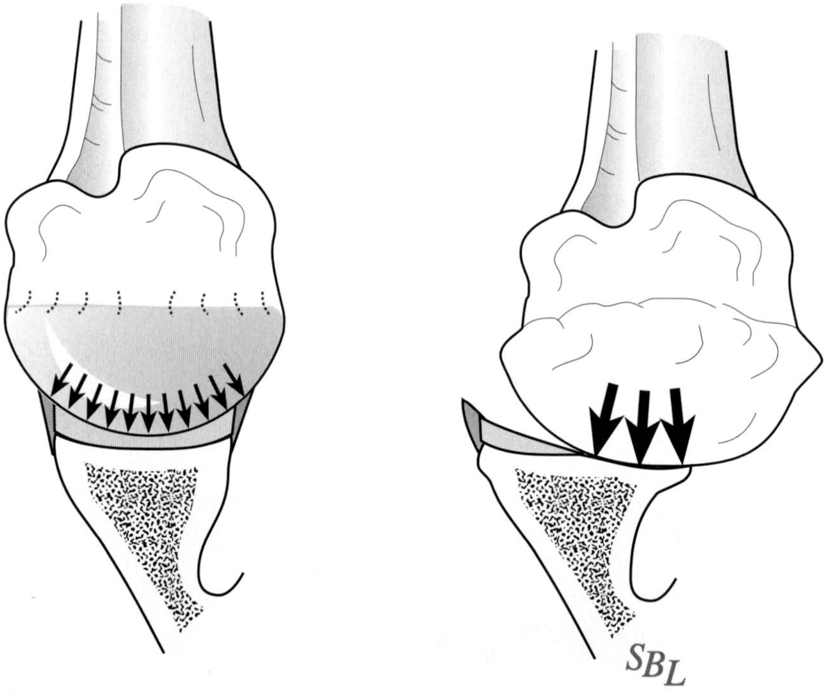


A B

**Figure 26–3. Contact pressure**

Loss of the articular cartilage from the humeral head and glenoid results in loss of the uniform distribution of the humeral joint reaction force over the face of the glenoid. **A,** Normal load transfer. **B,** Load transfer after cartilage loss resulting in locally large joint pressure and in steep pressure gradients between loaded and unloaded glenoid bone.

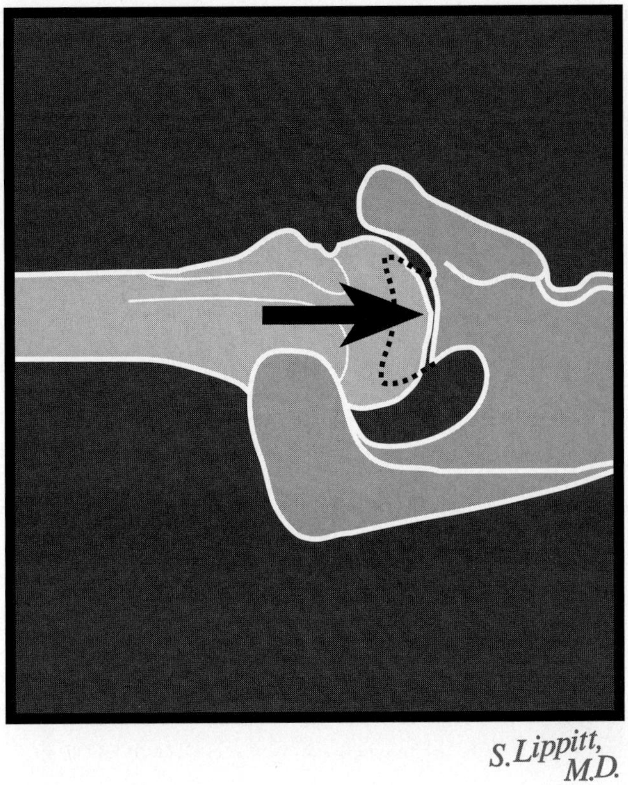


**Figure 26–4. Inflammatory arthritis**
Medial erosion typical of inflammatory arthritis. (From Matsen FA, Lippitt SB, Sidles JA, et al [eds]: Practical Evaluation and Management of the Shoulder. Philadelphia: WB Saunders, 1994, p. 199.)

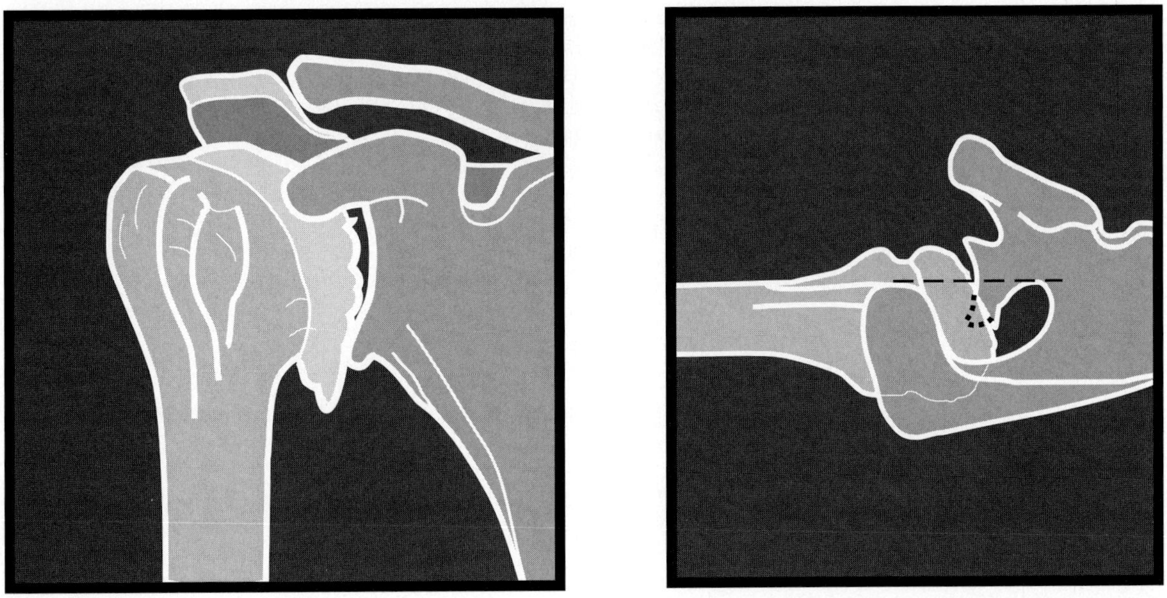

A B

**Figure 26–5. Degenerative arthritis**
Posterior erosion typical of degenerative arthritis and capsulorrhaphy arthropathy. (Modified from Matsen FA, Lippitt SB, Sidles JA, et al [eds]: Practical Evaluation and Management of the Shoulder. Philadelphia: WB Saunders, 1994, p. 199.)

cases of cuff tear arthropathy, the glenoid erosion is typically superior; the loss of the rotator cuff and resultant superior displacement of the humeral head results in a radial mismatch between the coracoacromial arch and the proximal humeral convexity. The result is an increase in the pressure on and the erosion of the undersurface of the coracoacromial arch and the upper rim of the glenoid to the point that a secondary "acetabulum" is formed; the tuberosities are smoothed into congruence with the humeral head ("femoralization") (**Fig. 26–6**).

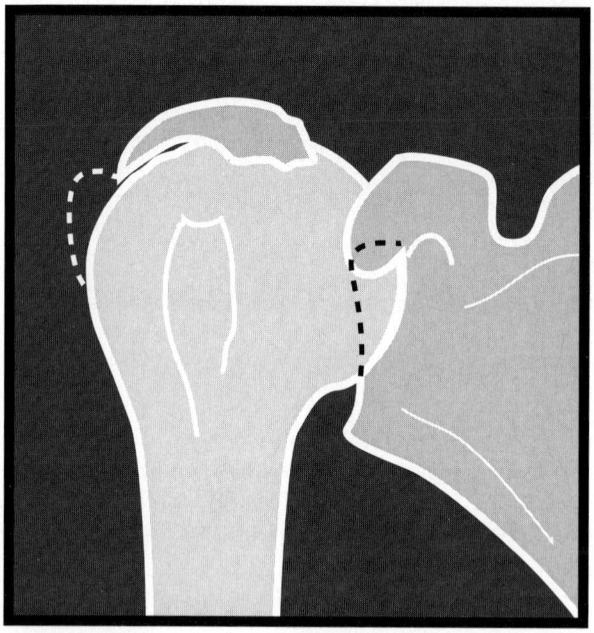

**Figure 26–6. Cuff tear arthropathy**
Superior medial erosion typical of cuff tear arthropathy. (Modified from Matsen FA, Lippitt SB, Sidles JA, et al [eds]: Practical Evaluation and Management of the Shoulder. Philadelphia: WB Saunders, 1994, p. 128.)

CHAPTER 27

# Principles of Humeral Arthroplasty

## CONCEPTS

Doing a humeral arthroplasty just right is challenging. One of the reasons is that there are many different choices that the surgeon needs to manage when replacing a damaged surface with a prosthetic one. When positioning a humeral prosthesis in the humerus, the surgeon must contend with nine interrelated variables: (1) the radius of curvature of the surface, (2) the height of the surface, (3, 4, and 5) the anteroposterior, mediolateral, and superoinferior position of the surface with respect to the bone, as well as (6) the varus/valgus angulation, (7) the flexion/extension, (8) the version of the component relative to the humerus, and (9) the fixation of the prosthetic surface to the bone.

### Radius and Height

The articular part of the humeral head is spherical and is described geometrically as a *spherical cap* (**Fig. 27–1**) with a radius of curvature, a base, a height that is measured along a radius that is perpendicular to the base, and a surface area. The line perpendicular to the base is the *humeral articular center line* (**Fig. 27–2**).

Prosthetic heads are also spherical caps with radii of curvature, bases, heights, and surface areas. Some designs have radii that become smaller at the periphery (**Fig. 27–3**). Such peripheral rounding reduces the amount of the prosthesis that has the desired radius; therefore, the effective area of the spherical cap is diminished. Some prostheses have collars and gaps that separate the spherical cap from the cut surface of the humerus. Because of the limited space in the glenohumeral joint, the height of the collar plus that of the gap must be accommodated by an equivalent reduction in the height of the spherical cap and a proportionate reduction in the effective surface area.

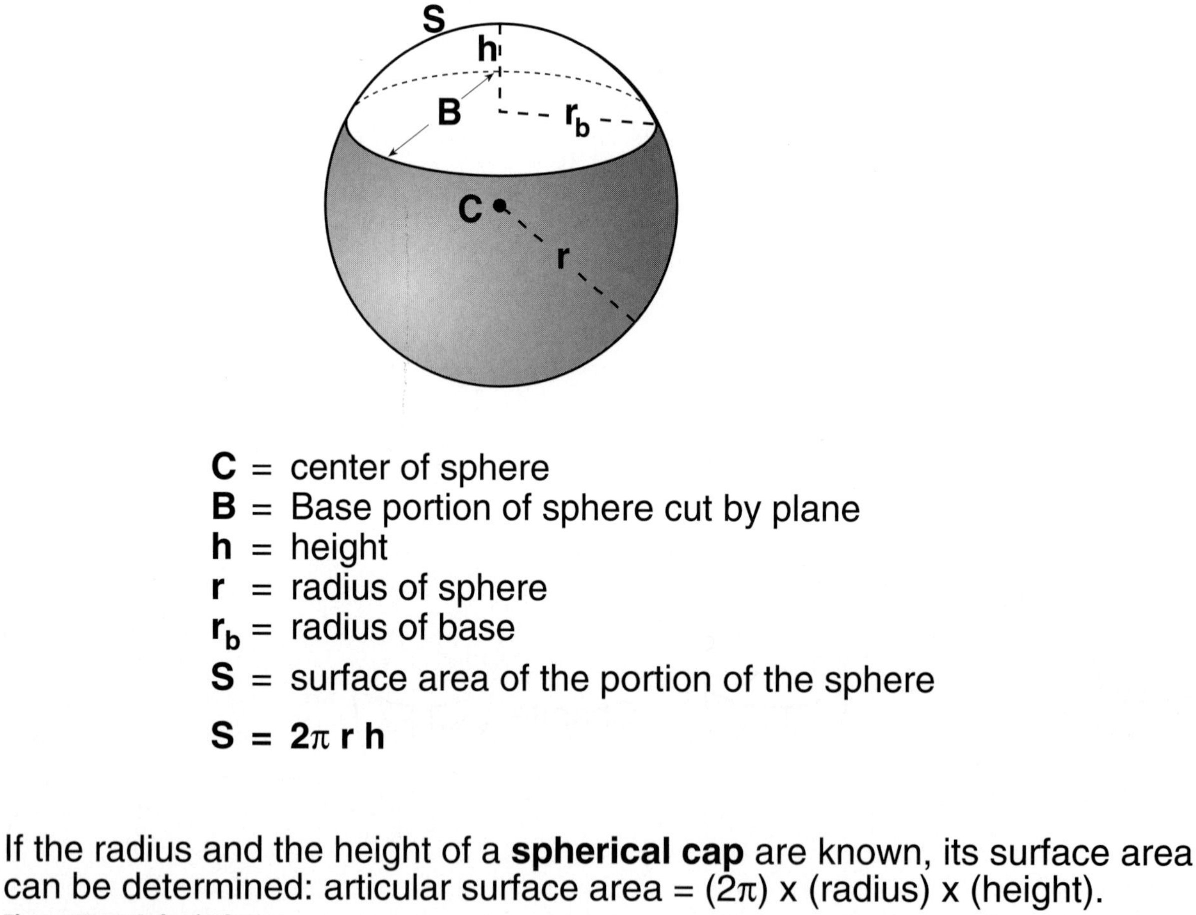


**Figure 27–1. Spherical cap**
The surface area of a spherical cap is $2\pi \times$ radius $\times$ height.

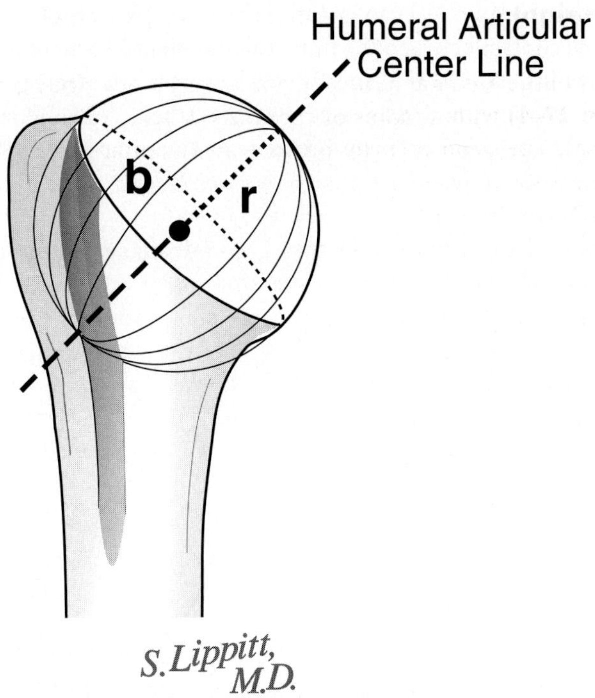


**Figure 27–2. Humeral articular surface**
The humeral articular surface can be described as a spherical cap with a radius of curvature, a base, a height along the humeral articular center line, and a surface area.

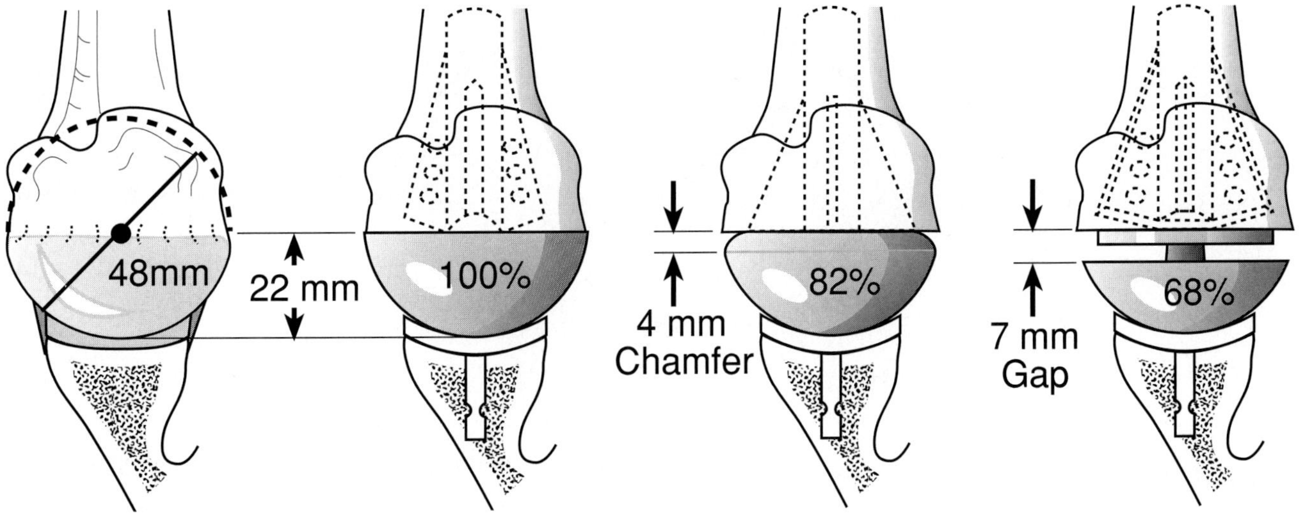


**Figure 27–3. Normal and prosthetic spherical caps**
The prosthetic humeral head is also a spherical cap. Peripheral chamfering or the presence of a collar and gap can reduce the effective articular area by reducing the height of the spherical cap in comparison to the normal biological head.

When the area of the spherical cap is diminished, the arc of motion through which there is full surface contact between the humeral and glenoid articular surfaces is likewise diminished (**Figs. 27–4, 27–5,** and **27–6**). The result is decreased contact area, increased contact pressure, and decreased stability (**Fig. 27–7**). If the height of the prosthetic head and any collar and gap is excessive, the joint is "overstuffed" and the

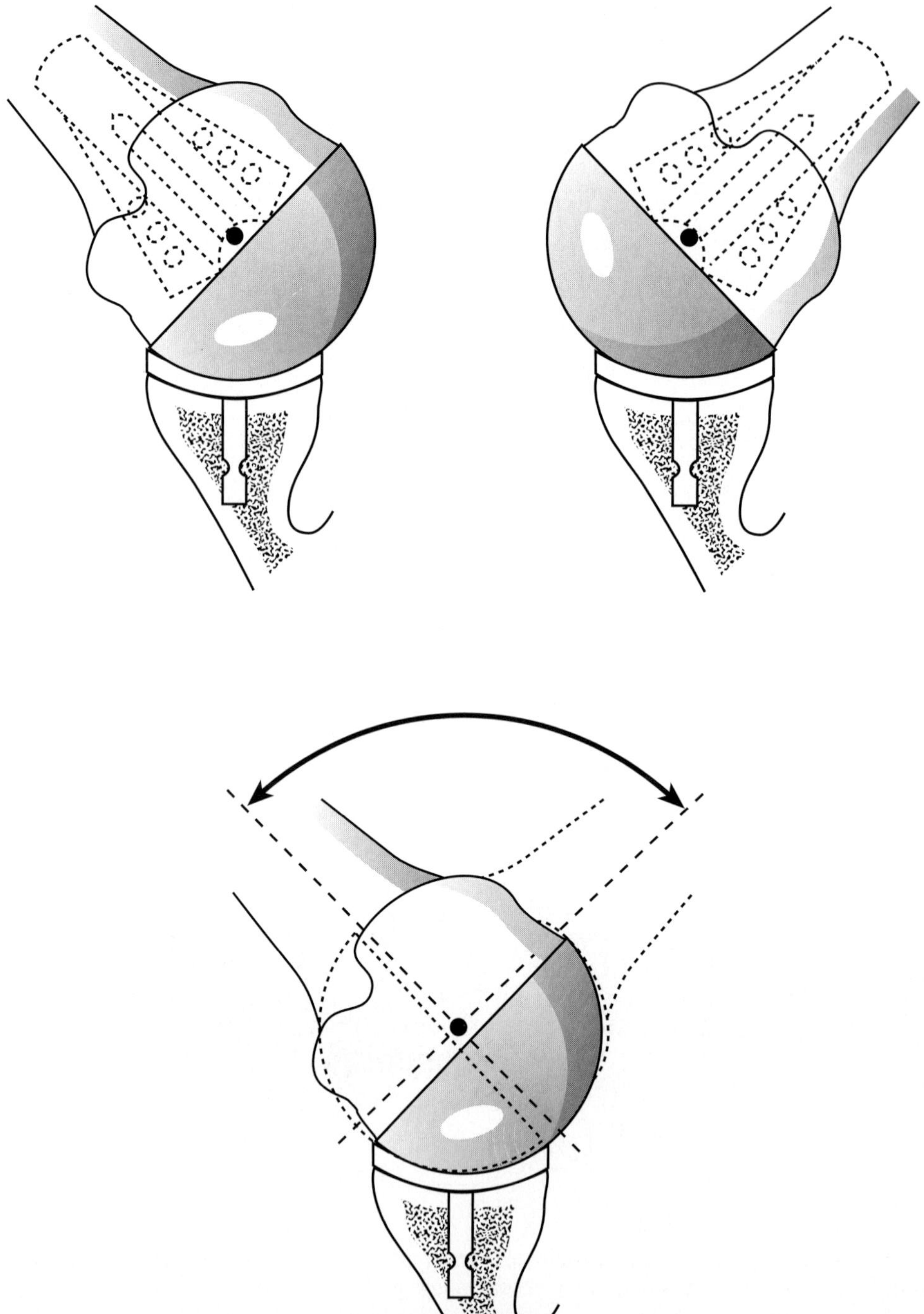

**Figure 27–4. Normal spherical cap**
Restoration of the entire area of the spherical cap maximizes the range of motion with full surface contact between the humeral head and glenoid.

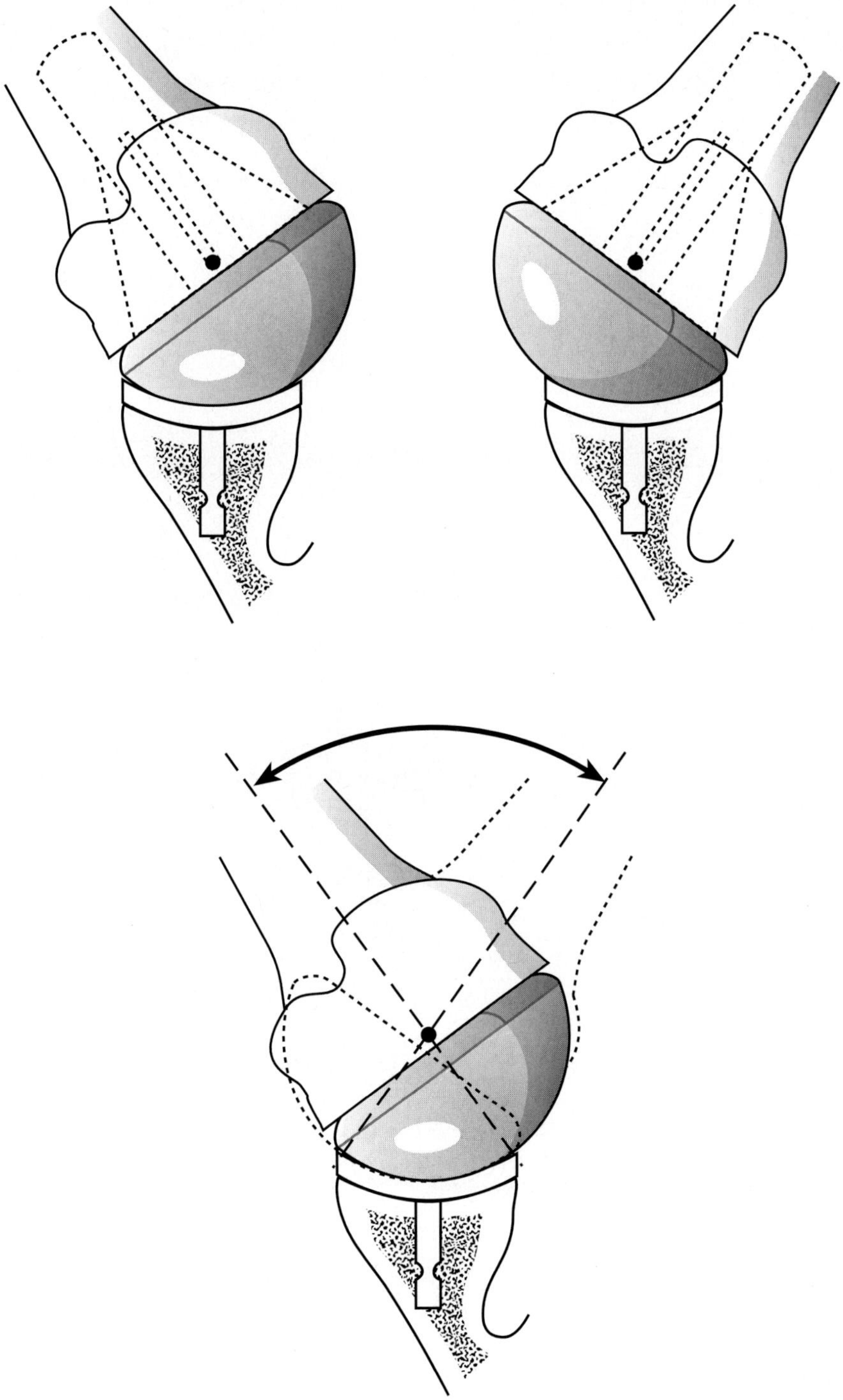

**Figure 27–5. Spherical cap reduced by chamfering**
A chamfered humeral head prosthesis has a reduced height of the spherical cap and range of motion with full surface contact.

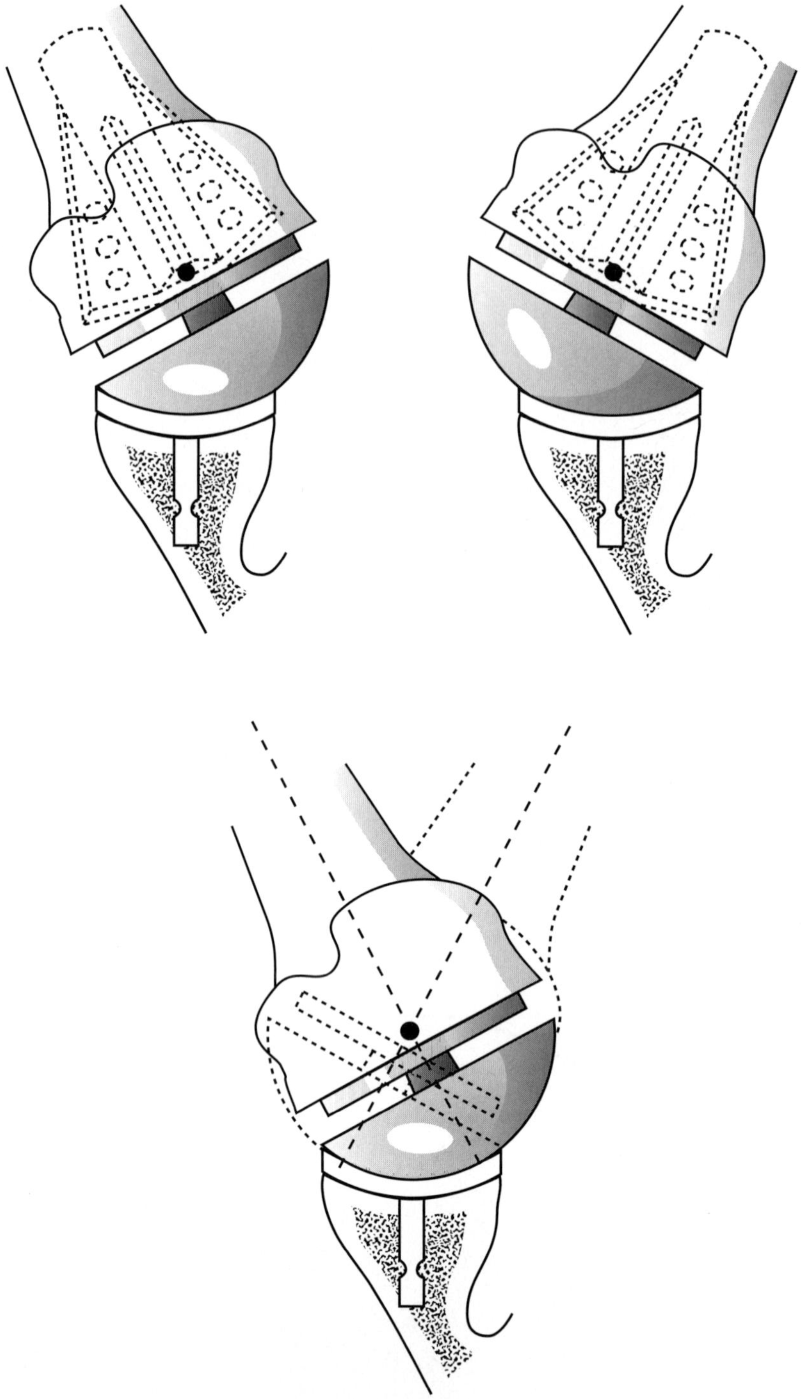

**Figure 27–6. Spherical cap reduced by collar and cap**
A prosthesis with a collar and a gap sacrifices the height of the spherical cap and the range of motion with full surface contact.

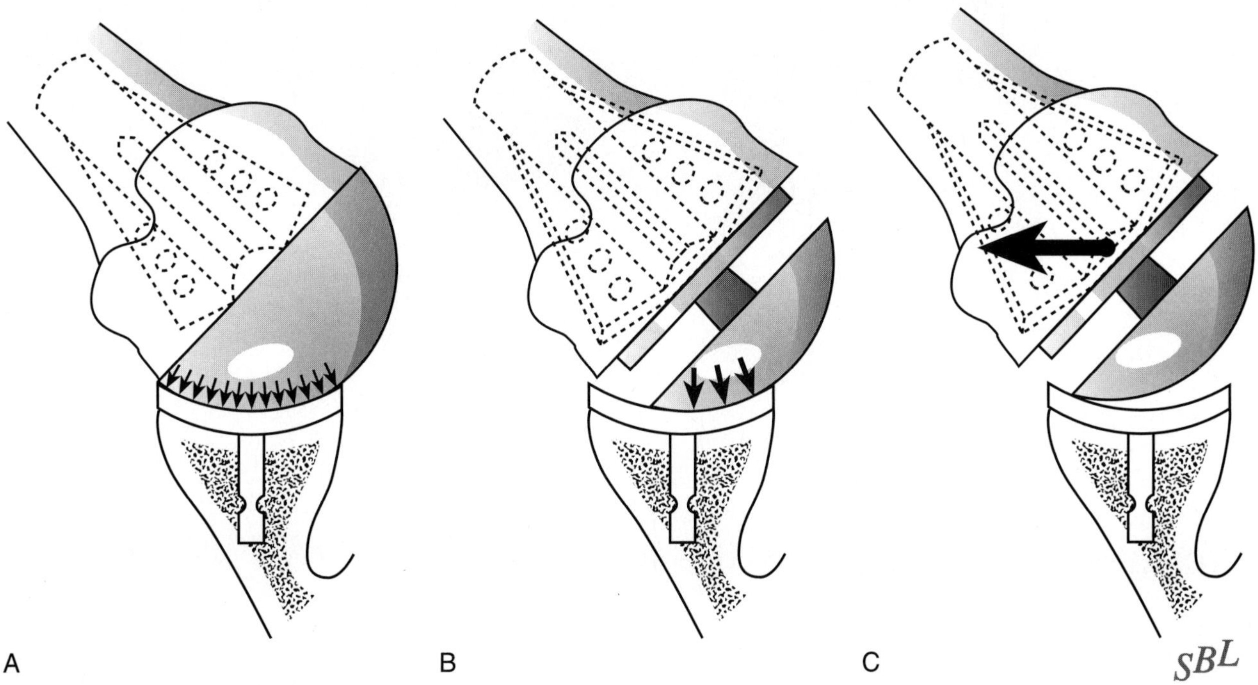


**Figure 27–7. Surface contact**

Full surface contact provides broadly distributed load transfer and maximal joint stability (**A**). When full surface contact is lacking (**B**), the humeral component can be translated in the direction of the empty part of the glenoid (**C**). (Modified from Matsen FA, Lippitt SB, Sidles JA, et al [eds]: Practical Evaluation and Management of the Shoulder. Philadelphia: WB Saunders, 1994, p. 190.)

soft tissues are excessively tightened with risk to the cuff (**Fig. 27–8**) and diminished range of motion. In fact, each 1.25 cm of overstuffing can be predicted to reduce the range of motion in *each* direction by about 28 degrees (12.5 mm of increased height is half a radian for an average humeral head of radius 25 mm; in degrees, half a radian is $0.5 \times 360/2\pi$, or 28 degrees).

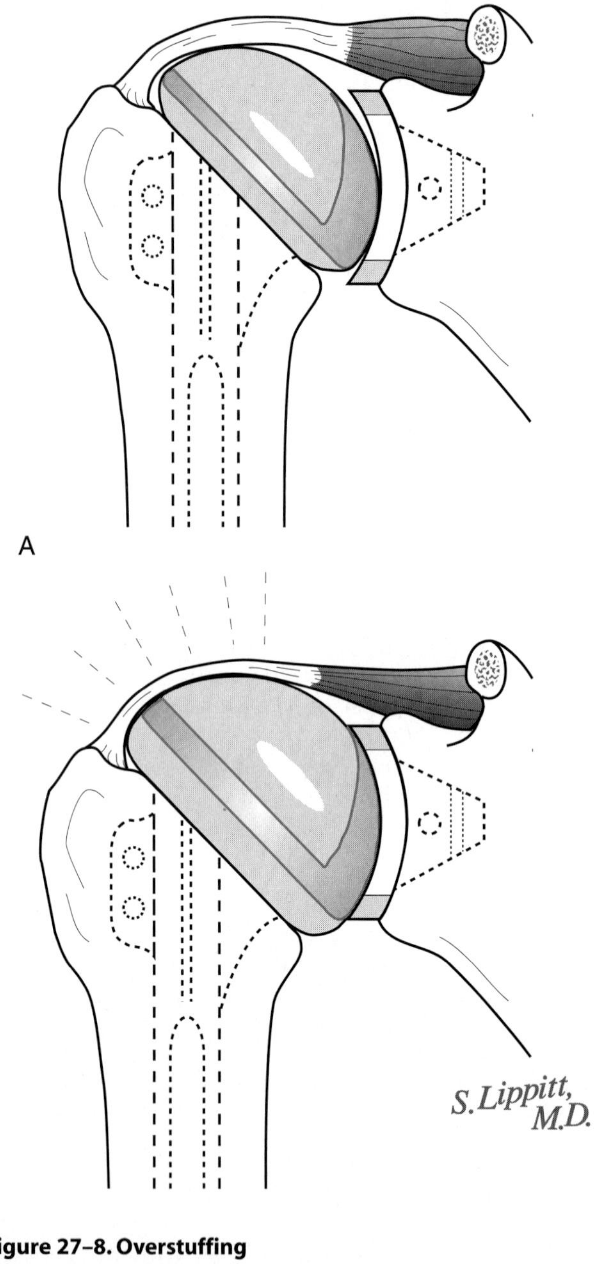


**Figure 27–8. Overstuffing**
As compared to the balanced joint (**A**), an overstuffed joint (**B**) places excessive tension on the cuff when the arm is adducted. (From Matsen FA, Lippitt SB, Sidles JA, et al [eds]: Practical Evaluation and Management of the Shoulder. Philadelphia: WB Saunders, 1994, p. 198.)

When performing a hemiarthroplasty in the presence of a normal glenoid, the surgeon strives to duplicate the curvature of the patient's normal, cartilage-covered biological head to preserve the optimal load transfer at the articulation. If the exact match is not available, the fact that the glenoid is more compliant at its periphery suggests that a slightly too large radius of humeral curvature will achieve greater contact area than a slightly too small one (**Fig. 27–9**).

The same logic does not apply when the humerus articulates with bone or polyethylene. We discuss the effect of the match between the humeral and glenoid radii of curvature on load transfer and stability in the chapter on principles of glenoid arthroplasty (Chapter 28).

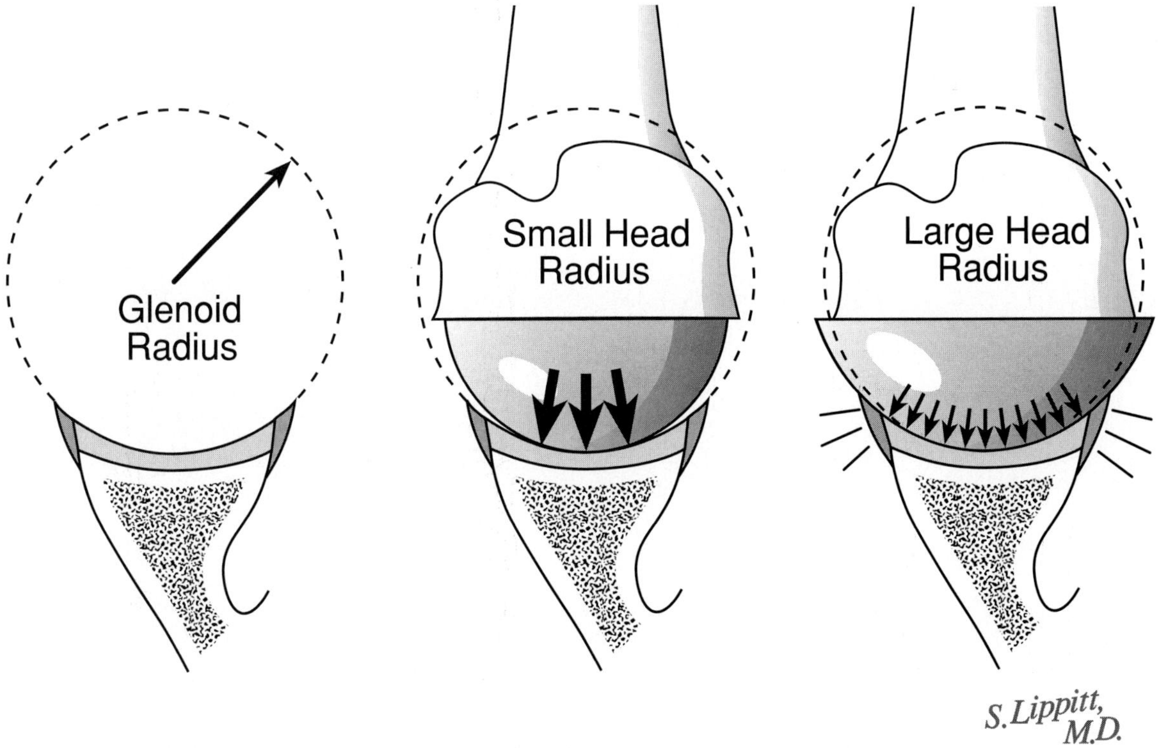


**Figure 27–9. Optimizing head curvature**
In hemiarthroplasty, it is desirable to match the humeral head size to the size of the normal cartilage-covered biological head, so that the prosthesis fits well in the glenoid (*left*). When this cannot be achieved, it is preferable to slightly oversize the head (*right*) because the compliance of the glenoid periphery can accommodate the mismatch. However, if a too-small-head prosthesis is used, the hard center of the glenoid cannot distribute the load that then becomes concentrated on a small amount of the glenoid surface area (*center*).

## Version

Because the humerus is not a straight bone and because the humeral medullary canal has a highly variable shape, its longitudinal axis cannot be rigorously determined in three dimensions from external landmarks or from radiographs. Conveniently, at surgery a unique humeral axis can be determined. In preparing the medullary canal for a humeral prosthesis, the surgeon inserts progressively larger cylindrical reamers until the endosteal surface of the cortex begins to be engaged. The axis of this cylindrical reamer is called the *orthopaedic axis* of the humerus (**Fig. 27–10**). The *plane of the humerus* is defined as the plane containing the orthopaedic axis of the humerus and that is perpendicular to the forearm flexed to a right angle (**Fig. 27–11**). When the relationship of the forearm to the proximal humerus is distorted (for example, because of congenital torsion, a previous humeral fracture, elbow instability, or above-elbow amputation), the plane of the humerus can be estimated as the plane containing the orthopaedic axis of the proximal humerus and perpendicular to a line making a 10-degree angle internal to a line connecting the bicipital groove to the axis of the shaft (**Fig. 27–12**).

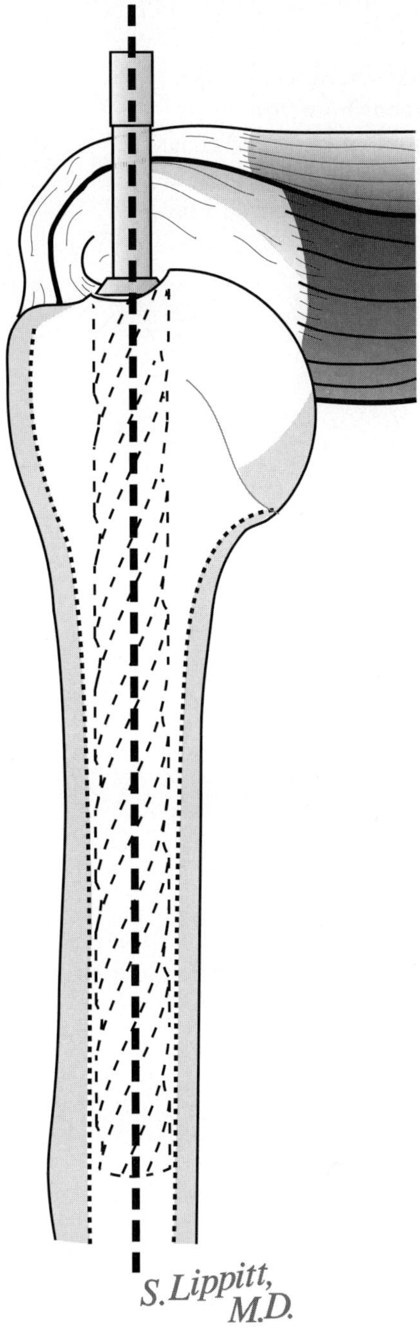


**Figure 27–10. Orthopaedic axis**
The orthopaedic axis is the axis of a cylindrical reamer that just engages the endosteal surface of the humeral shaft.

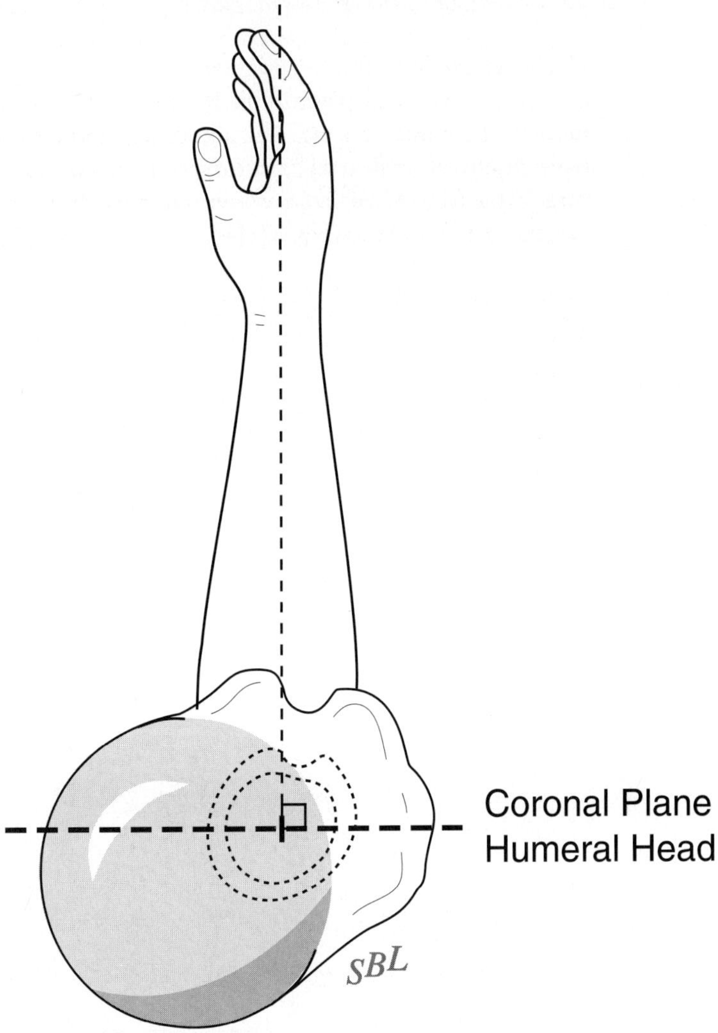


**Figure 27–11. Plane of humerus—forearm reference**
The plane of the humerus contains the orthopaedic axis and is perpendicular to the forearm flexed to 90 degrees.

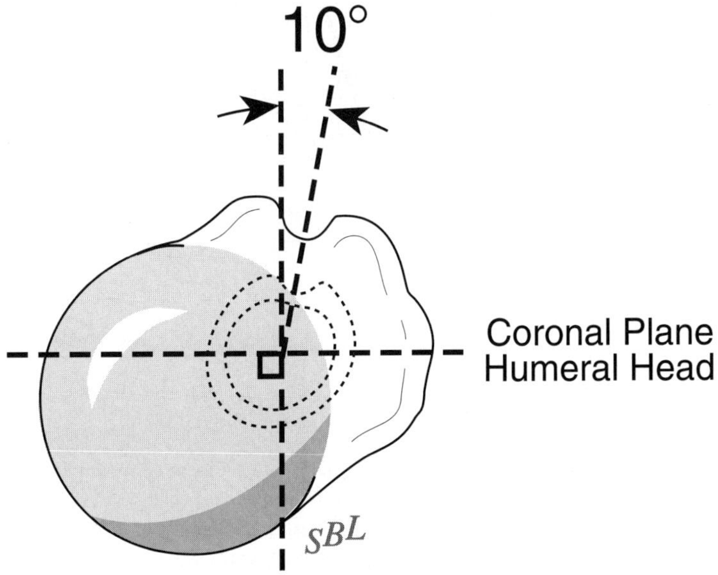


**Figure 27–12. Plane of humerus—biceps reference**
When the distal humeral anatomy is distorted, the plane of the humerus can be defined as the plane containing the orthopaedic axis and perpendicular to a line 10 degrees internal to the bicipital groove.

The *version* of the humeral articular surface is the angle between the humeral articular center line and the plane of the humerus. This angle varies among humeri, but commonly the humeral articular center line points 30 degrees posterior to the humeral plane (commonly referred to as "30 degrees of retroversion") (**Fig. 27–13**). Conveniently, at surgery the humeral articular center line can be observed directly and duplicated by the prosthetic arthroplasty (**Fig. 27–14**).

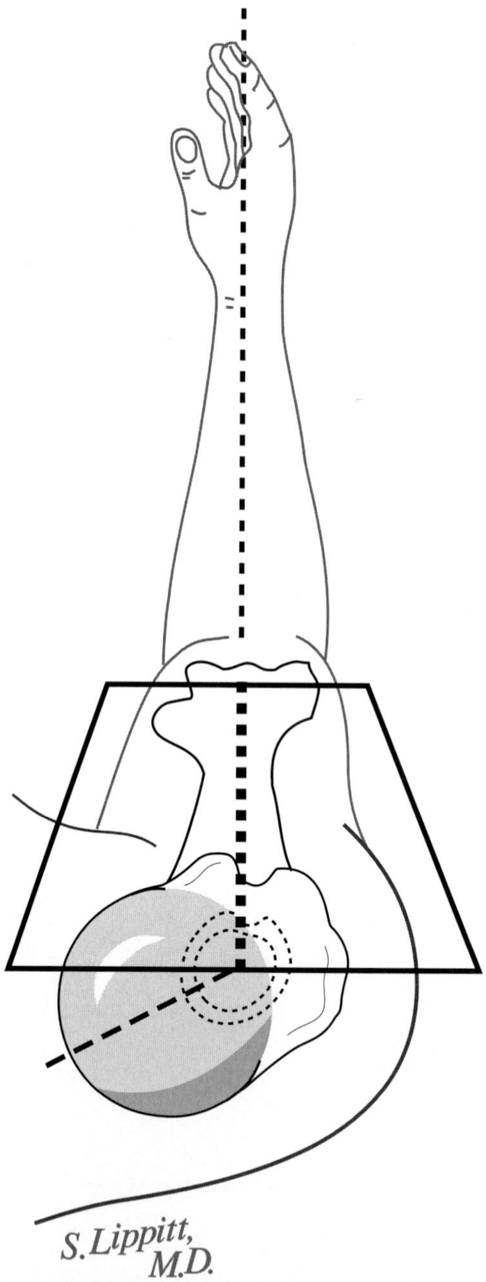


**Figure 27–13. Plane of humerus and humeral center line**
The humeral articular center line usually points posterior and medial to the humeral plane.

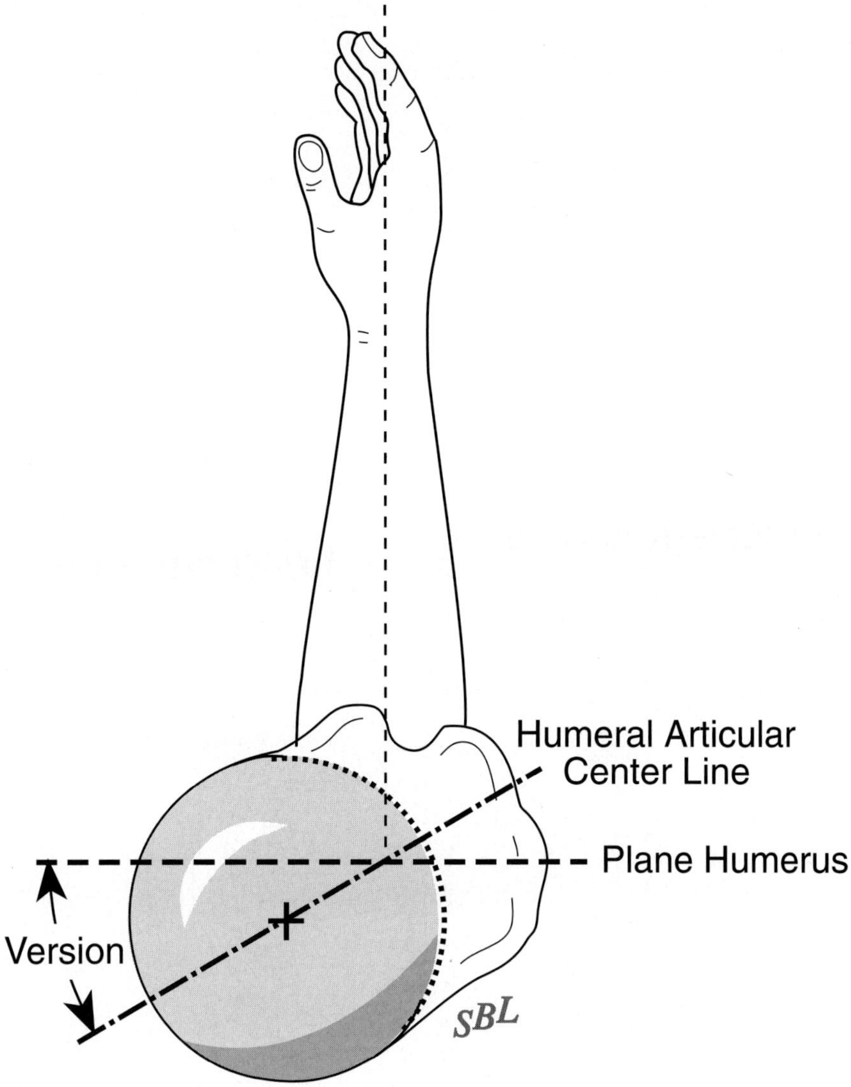


**Figure 27–14. Retroversion**
The amount of this retroversion is usually about 30 degrees.

In prosthetic arthroplasty, the opportunity to alter the version of the humeral component is restricted by the attachments of the rotator cuff anteriorly and posteriorly (**Fig. 27–15**). Furthermore, because the offset between the center of the head and the orthopaedic axis is small, the effect of changes in version on the position of the articular surface is small. This situation is in marked contrast to that in the hip, where there is a major offset between the axis of the femoral canal and the center of rotation of the humeral head (**Fig. 27–16**).

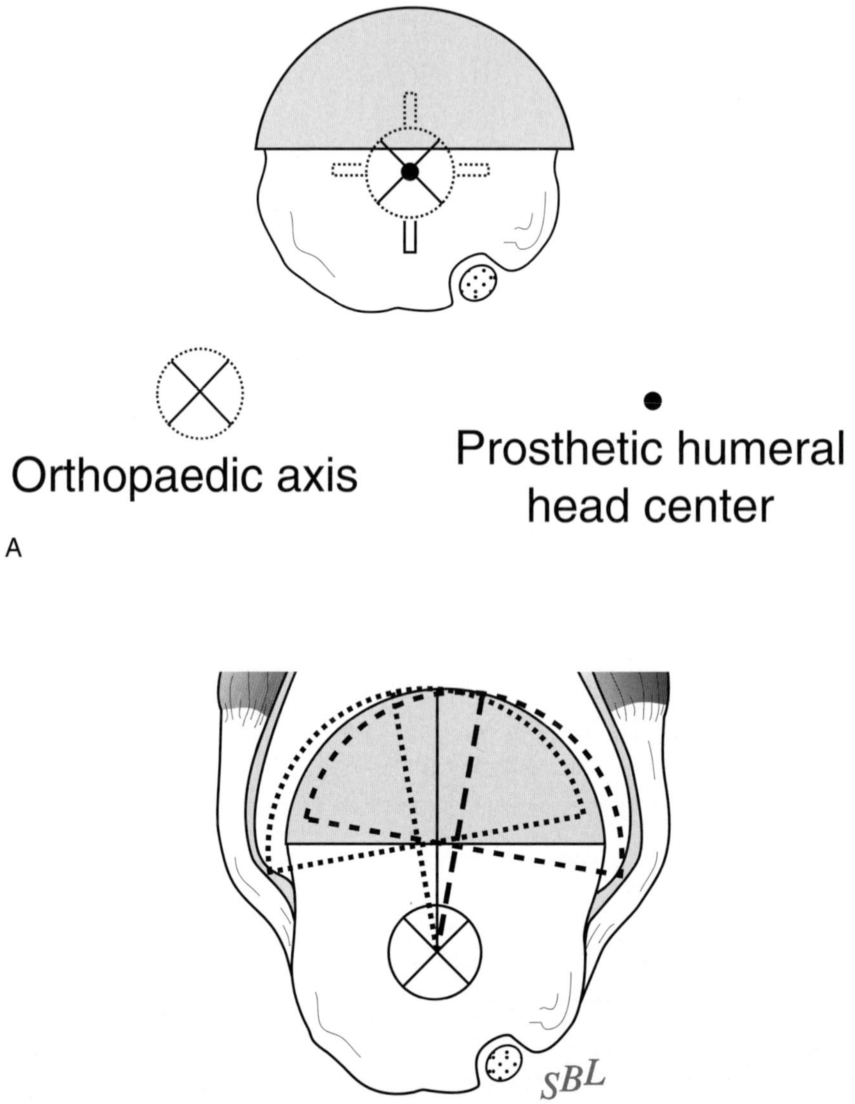


B

**Figure 27–15. Modifying humeral version**
The ability of the surgeon to change the position of the articular surface by changing the humeral component version is restricted by two factors. First, because the offset between the center of rotation of the humeral head and the orthopaedic axis is small, the effect of changing version on the position of the articular surface is small. Second, the amount that the version of the prosthesis can be changed without compromising the cuff insertion is also small. (From Matsen FA, Lippitt SB, Sidles JA, et al [eds]: Practical Evaluation and Management of the Shoulder. Philadelphia: WB Saunders, 1994, p. 188.)

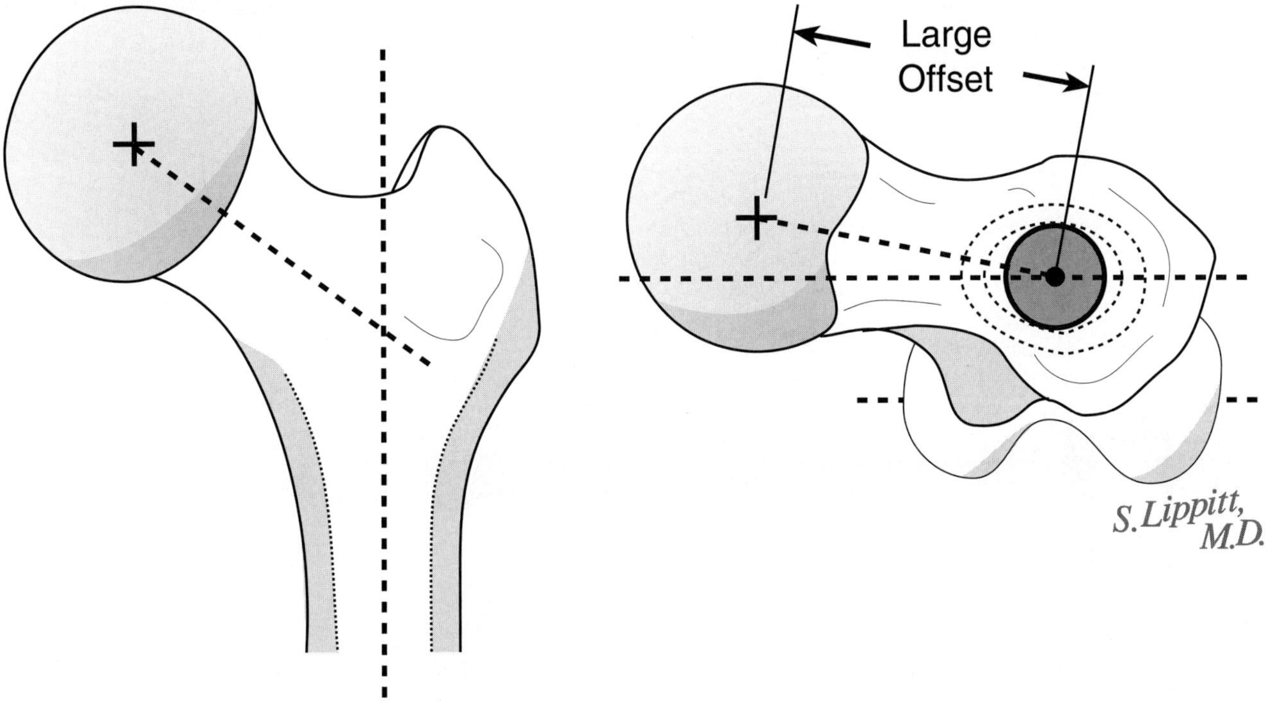


**Figure 27–16. Femoral head center is substantially offset**
By contrast, in the femur, the large offset and the lack of restricting soft tissue attachments allow for a substantial effect of changes in version on articular surface position.

### Anteroposterior Position, Mediolateral Position, and Flexion-Extension

The *offset* is the distance between the spherical center of the head (**Fig. 27–17**) and the axis of the humeral shaft (**Fig. 27–18**). This offset can be resolved into its anteroposterior and mediolateral components. Traditionally, surgeons define offset with respect to the humeral articular center line (**Fig. 27–19**). In these terms, the amount of posterior offset of the center of the humeral head is small. If offset is defined with respect to the plane of the humerus (**Fig. 27–20**), the amount of posterior offset appears much larger due to the retroversion of the articular surface with respect to the humeral plane.

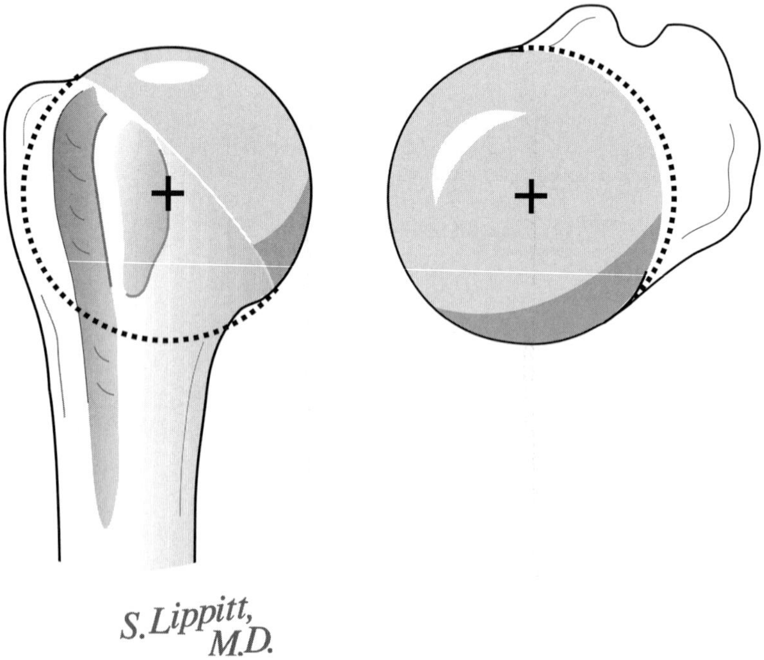


**Figure 27–17. Spherical center of humeral head**
The spherical center of the humeral head is the point at the center of the sphere fit to the articular surface.

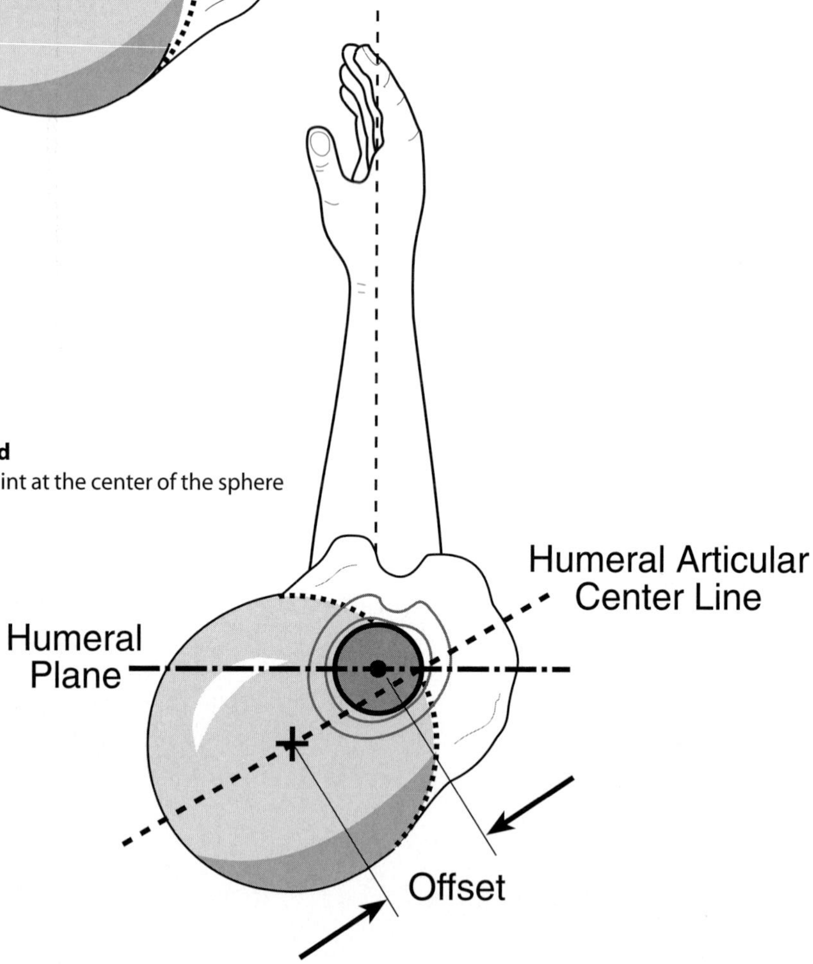


**Figure 27–18. Offset**
The offset of the humeral head is the distance between the orthopaedic axis and the spherical center of the humeral head. When considered in reference to the plane of the humerus, there is a substantial posterior offset of the humeral head. This is actually due to the retroversion of the articular surface.

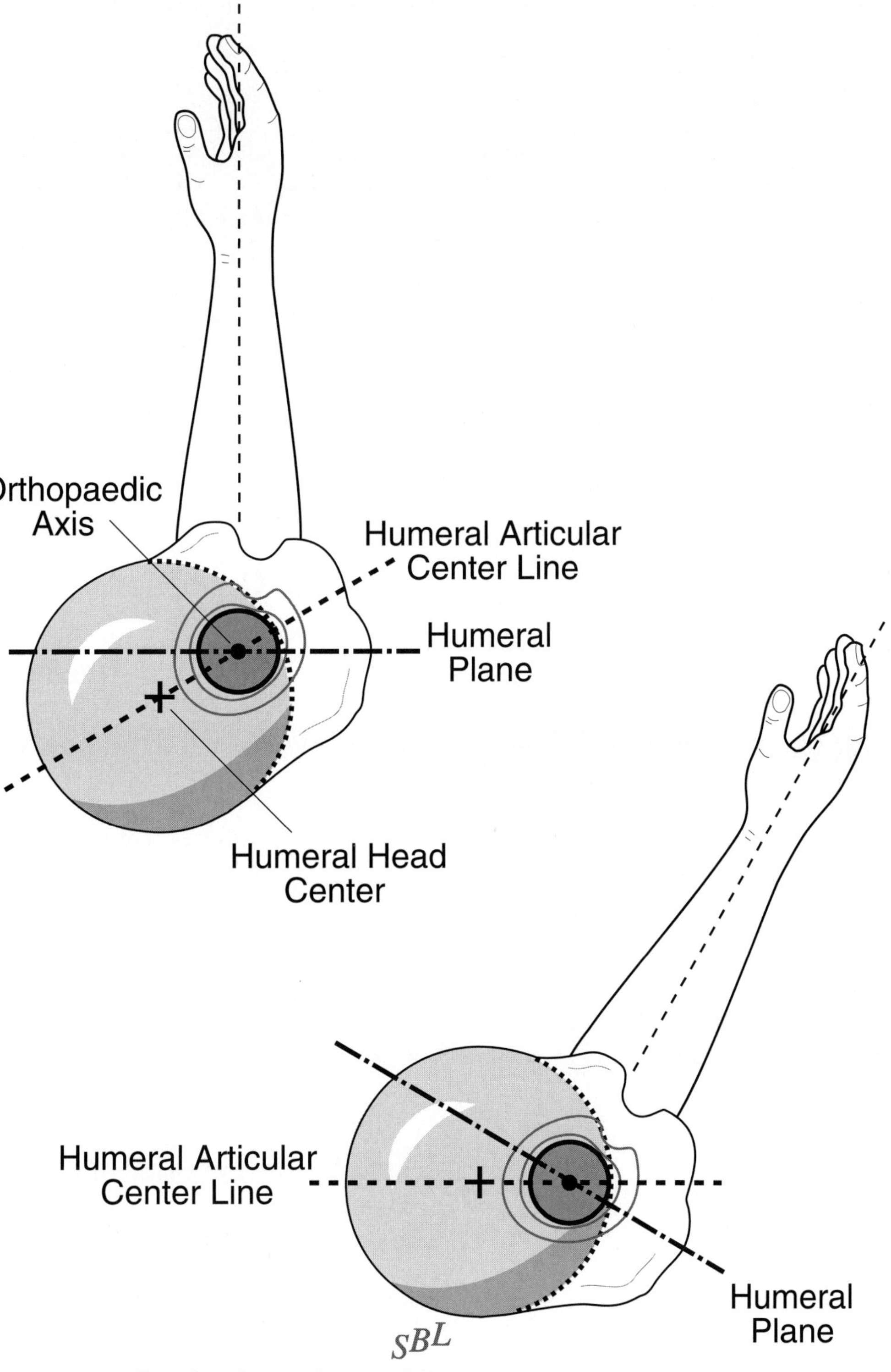


**Figure 27–19. Offset along humeral centrer line**

With reference to the humeral articular center line, the anteroposterior offset is actually quite small. In other words, much of the apparent posterior offset is a manifestation of humeral articular surface retroversion.

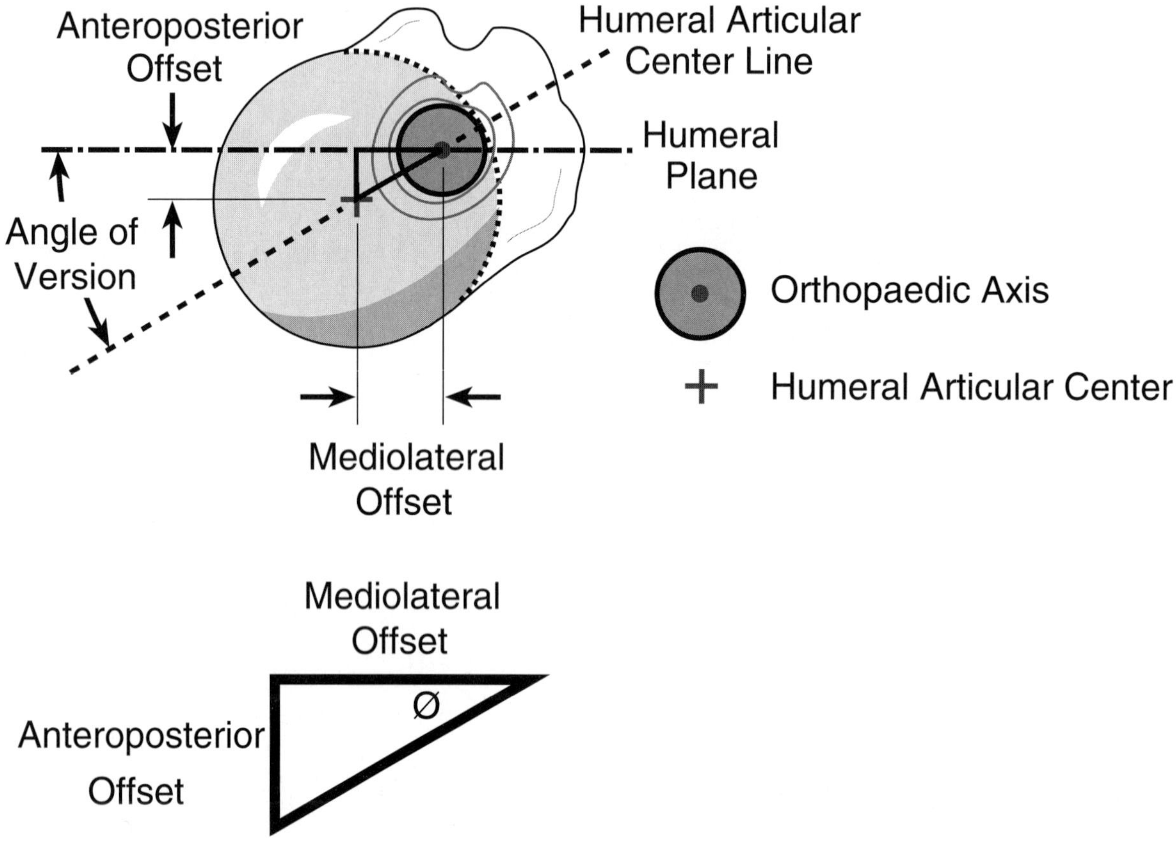


$$\text{Tangent Ø (Angle of version)} = \frac{\text{Anteroposterior Offset}}{\text{Mediolateral Offset}}$$

**Figure 27–20. Offset and version**
The ratio of the anteroposterior offset to the mediolateral offset is the tangent of the angle of retroversion.

The position of a prosthetic head can also be influenced by the anteroposterior and mediolateral position of the prosthetic body in the humeral shaft (**Figs. 27–21** and **27–22**), by flexion or extension angulation of the prosthetic body in the shaft (**Fig. 27–23**), and by the use of prosthetic heads that are offset (**Fig. 27–24**).

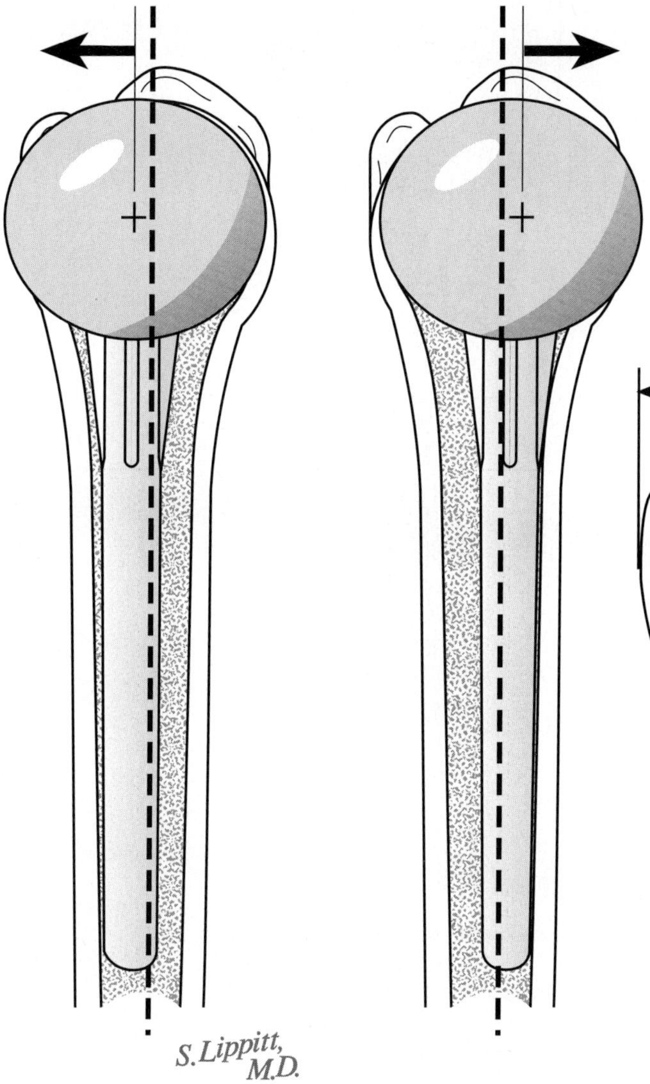


**Figure 27–21. Positioning the prosthetic shaft—anteroposterior**
If the anteroposterior position of the humeral prosthesis is not defined by its fit in the shaft, the position of the prosthesis body may affect the anteroposterior offset of the prosthetic articular surface, giving the impression of posterior or anterior offset of the biological head.

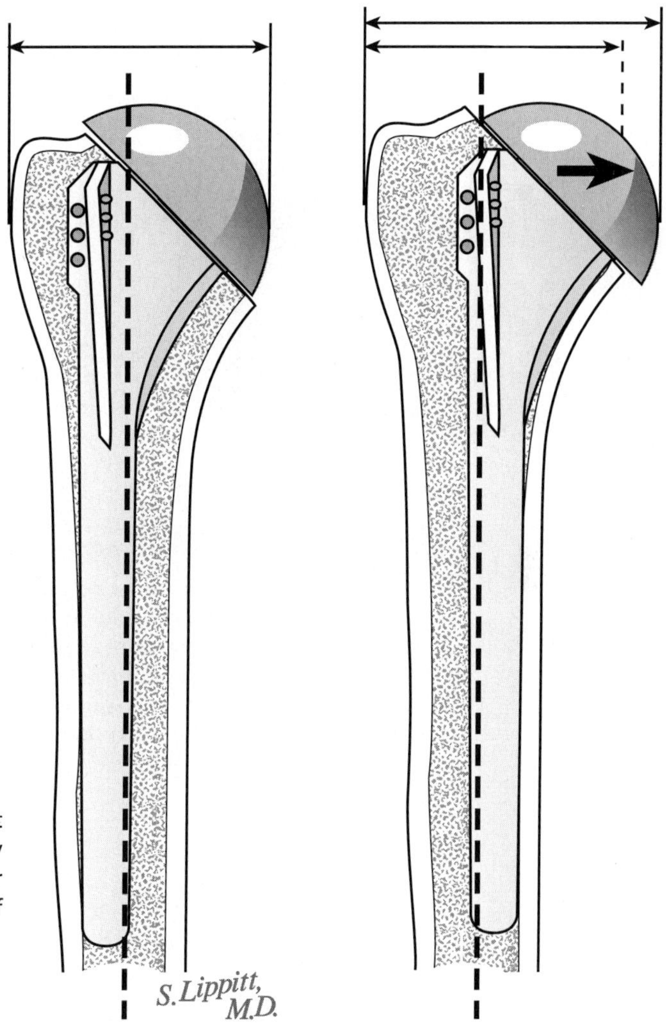


**Figure 27–22. Positioning the prosthetic shaft—medial and lateral**
If the mediolateral position of the humeral prosthesis is not defined by its fit in the shaft, the position of the prosthesis body may affect the offset of the humeral articular surface with respect to the tuberosities, and, therefore, the soft tissue tension.

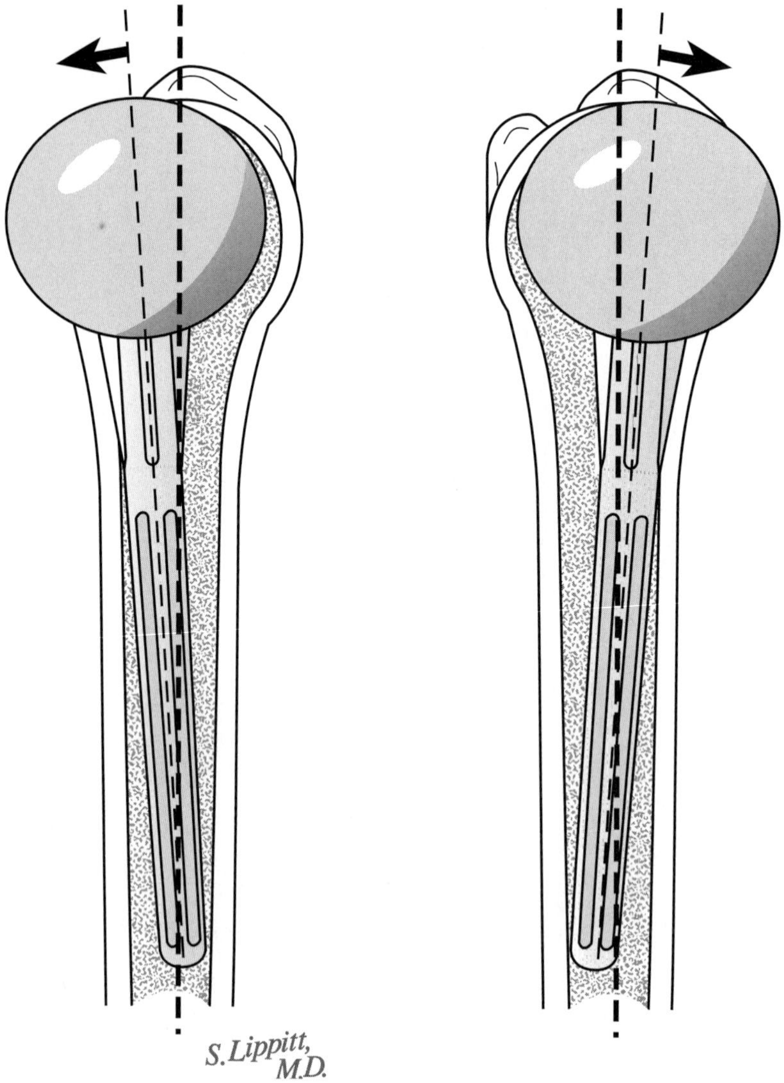


**Figure 27–23. Positioning the prosthetic shaft—flexion and extension**
If the anteroposterior angulation of the prosthetic body is not defined by the humeral canal, the prosthetic head position is not rigorously defined in reference to the humerus. Anterior angulation (*left*) is relatively frequent in humeral arthroplasty because the humerus is approached anteriorly. Such anterior angulation results in anterior position of the humeral prosthesis and gives the impression of posterior offset of the biological head.

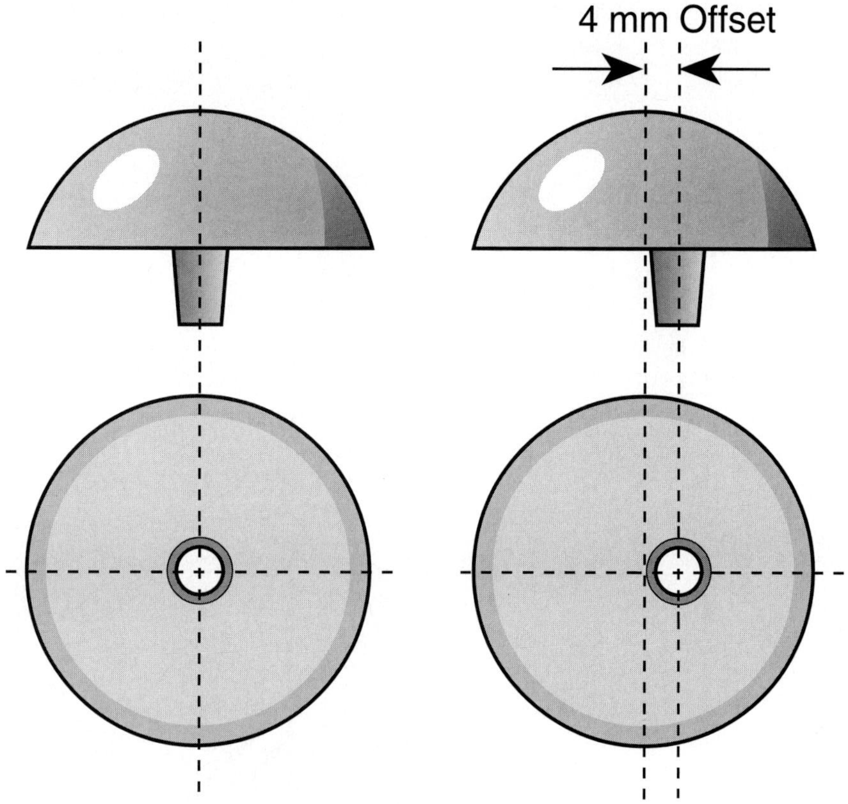


**Figure 27–24. Eccentric head components**

While they may be used to correct for malposition of the prosthetic body, use of eccentric humeral head components may risk offsetting the humeral articular surface of a well-placed prosthetic body into a nonanatomic location.

## Varus/Valgus

The *neck-shaft* angle is the angle between the humeral articular center line and the humeral shaft (**Fig. 27–25**). Although there is variability in this angle among humeri, much of the apparent variability seen in performing arthroplasty is due to the presence of osteophytes at the medial aspect of the humeral neck (**Fig. 27–26**). Fortunately, osteophytes usually do not occur at the superolateral aspect of the articular surface of the humerus near the insertion of the supraspinatus to the greater tuberosity. Thus,

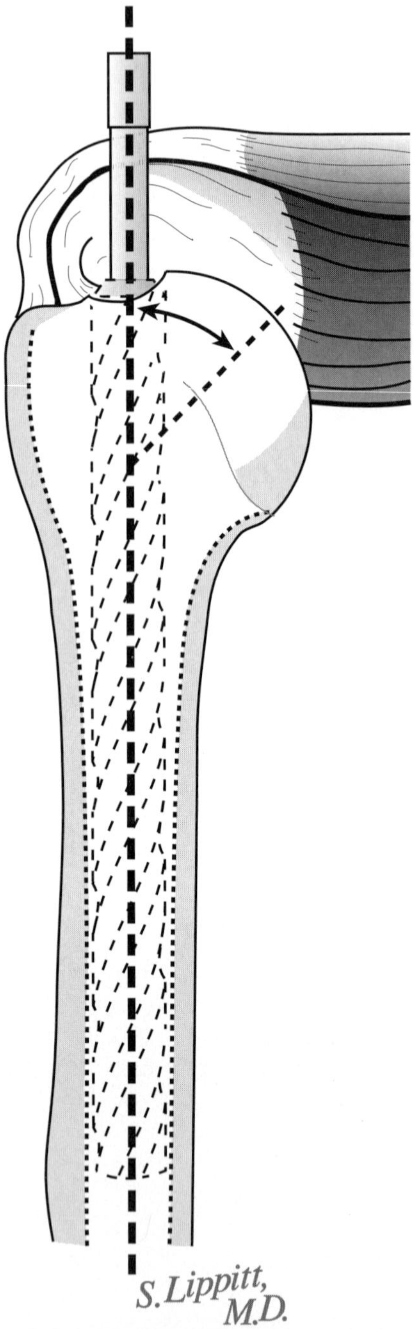


**Figure 27–25. Neck shaft angle**
The neck shaft angle is the angle between the humeral articular center line and the orthopaedic axis.

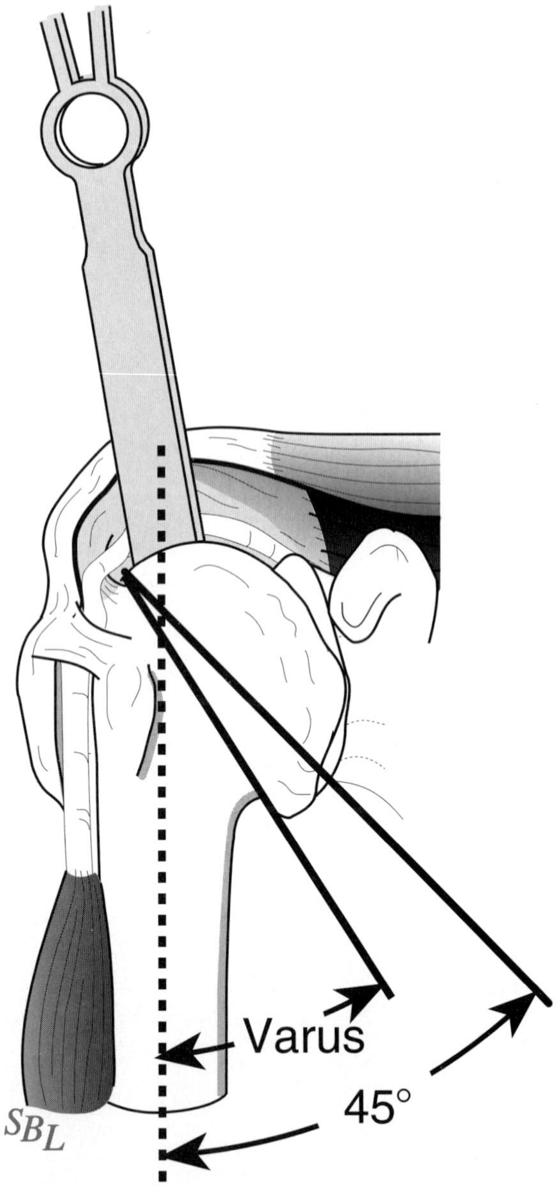


**Figure 27–26. Varus head cut**
Much of the apparent variability of the neck shaft angle is due to the obliteration of the anatomic neck by osteophytes. Cutting below the osteophytes may make an excessively varus humeral head resection. (Modified from Matsen FA, Lippitt SB, Sidles JA, et al [eds]: Practical Evaluation and Management of the Shoulder. Philadelphia: WB Saunders, 1994, p 207.)

this point is a key reference point for making the humeral neck cut. Making a cut just inside the cuff insertion at 45 degrees with the orthopaedic axis of the proximal shaft enables the articular surface to be fit without having to use a prosthesis with variable neck shaft angles (**Fig. 27–27**). While this approach may seem to show disregard for the biological variation in the neck shaft angle, the only consequence is that in those cases in which the anatomic neck shaft angle is more varus than 45 degrees, a small amount

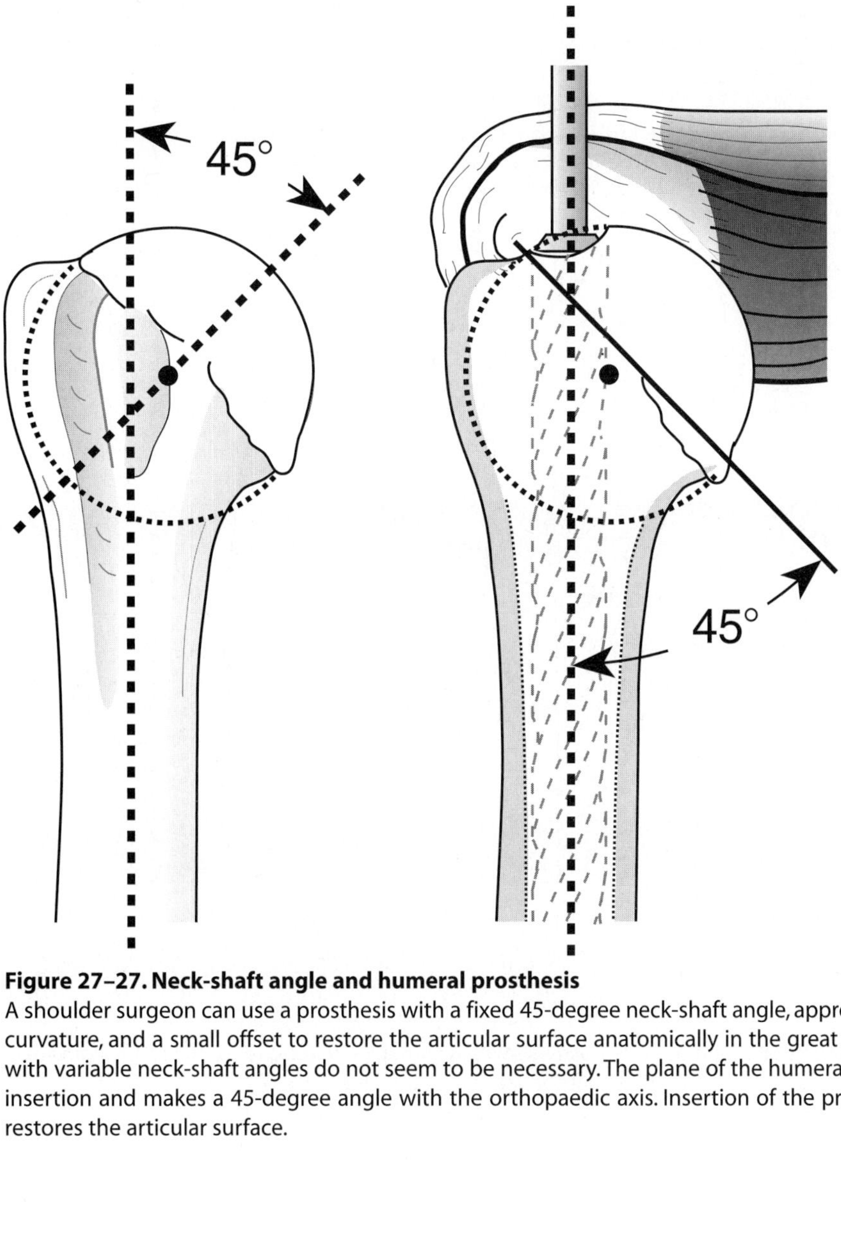


**Figure 27–27. Neck-shaft angle and humeral prosthesis**
A shoulder surgeon can use a prosthesis with a fixed 45-degree neck-shaft angle, appropriate head height and diameter of curvature, and a small offset to restore the articular surface anatomically in the great preponderance of cases. Prostheses with variable neck-shaft angles do not seem to be necessary. The plane of the humeral neck cut passes just inside the cuff insertion and makes a 45-degree angle with the orthopaedic axis. Insertion of the prosthesis along the orthopaedic axis restores the articular surface.

of articular surface may remain inferiorly (**Fig. 27–28**). In those cases in which the anatomic neck shaft angle is more valgus than 45 degrees, a small amount of metaphysis may be resected (**Fig. 27–29**). Neither eventuality would compromise the ability of the prosthesis to resurface the humeral head anatomically. This recognition creates a substantial opportunity for economy in humeral component design.

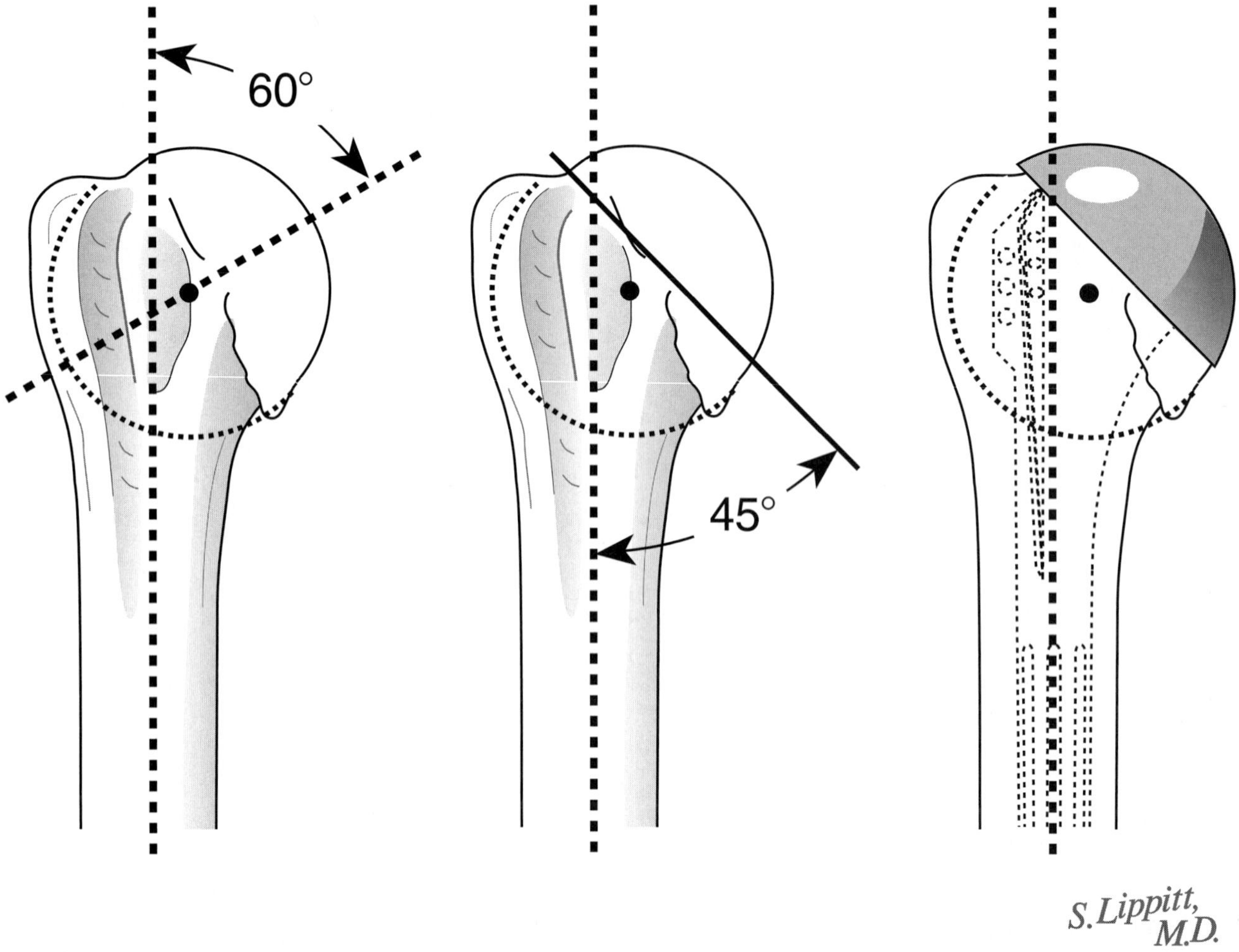


**Figure 27–28. Varus humeral head**
If the biological humeral head is in a more varus configuration, a prosthesis with a 45-degree angle cut can still result in an anatomic restoration of the joint surface by leaving a small amount of the inferior head unresurfaced.

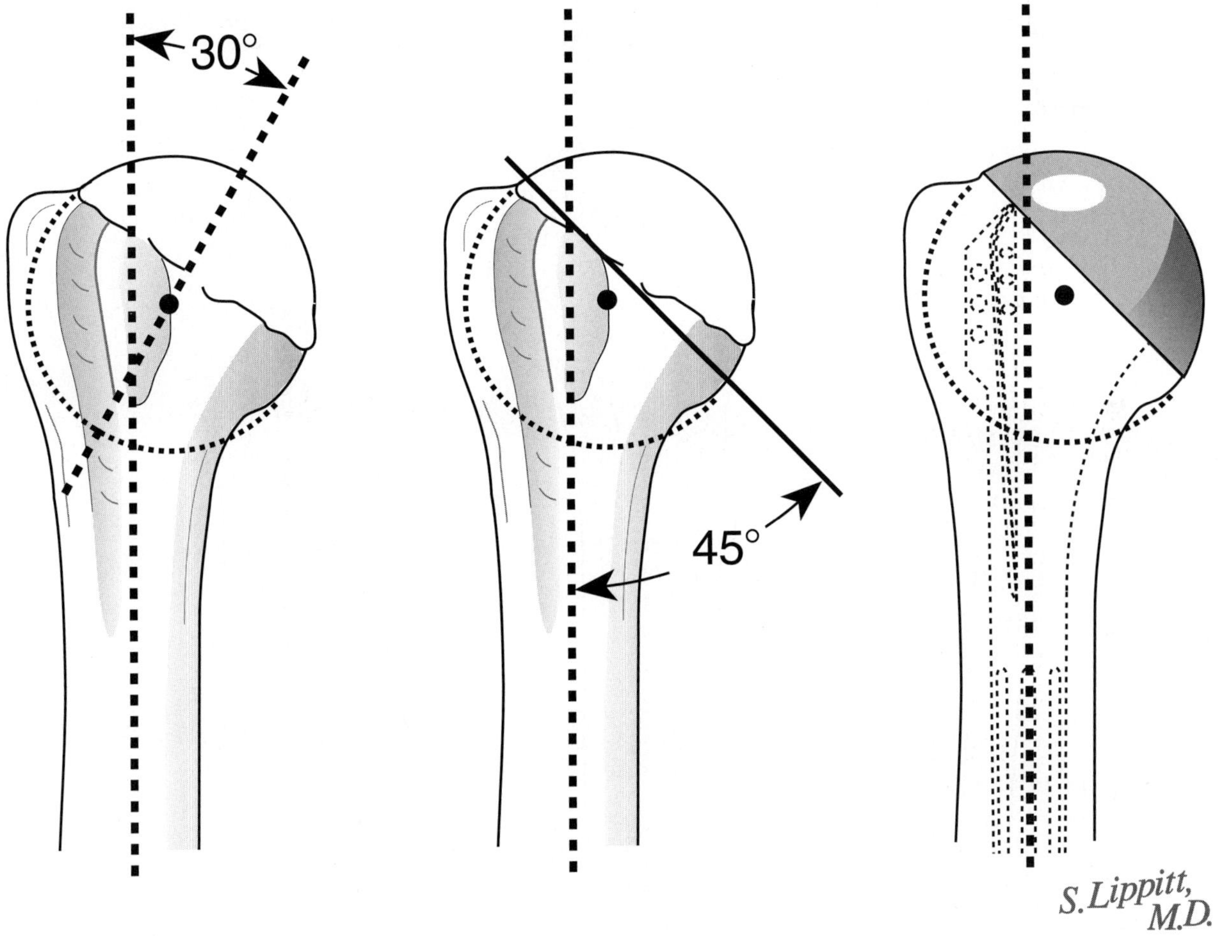


**Figure 27–29. Valgus humeral head**
If the biological humeral head is a more valgus configuration, a prosthesis with a 45-degree angle cut can still result in an anatomic restoration of the joint surface by resecting and resurfacing a small amount of the medial metaphysis.

The varus-valgus position of the prosthetic head can be influenced by the position of the prosthetic body in the humeral shaft (**Fig. 27–30**). It is apparent that these angulations affect not only the angle of the articular surface but also the distance between the lateral tuberosity and the medial aspect of the joint surface. A varus position, for example, can increase the degree of soft tissue tightness and limit the range of motion.

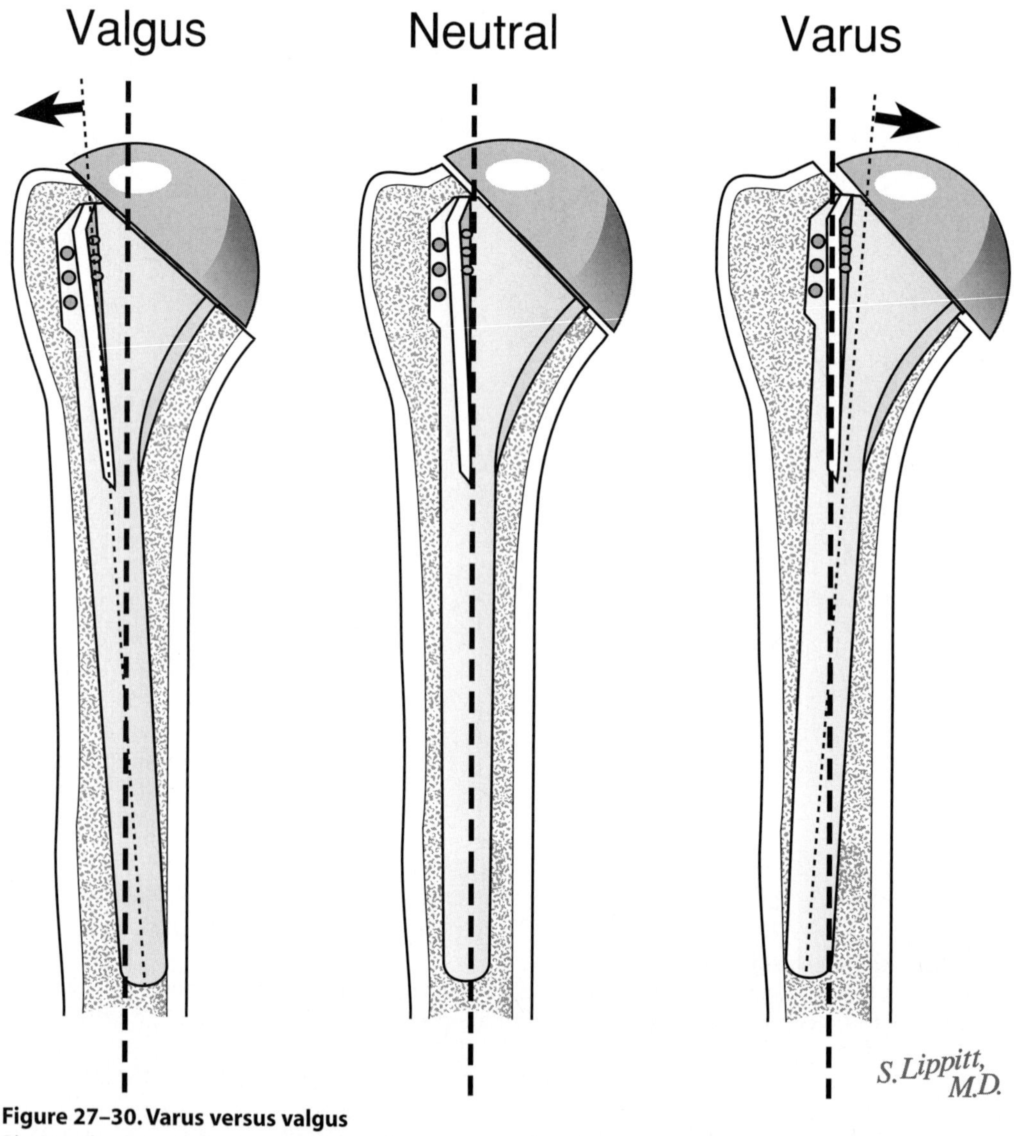


**Figure 27–30. Varus versus valgus**
Placing the humeral component in valgus reduces the effective offset and diminishes the distance between the tuberosity and the medial joint surface. The result is reduced tension on the scapulohumeral soft tissues. Placing the humeral component in varus increases the effective offset and increases the distance between the tuberosity and the medial joint surface. The result is increased tension on the scapulohumeral soft tissues.

### Superoinferior

The humeral articular surface usually extends superiorly about 5 mm above the tuberosity (**Fig. 27–31**). In this position, the long head tendon of the biceps grazes across its superior surface like a tangent. When the humerus is abducted 45 degrees in the plane of the scapula, the humeral articular center line should point to the center of the glenoid.

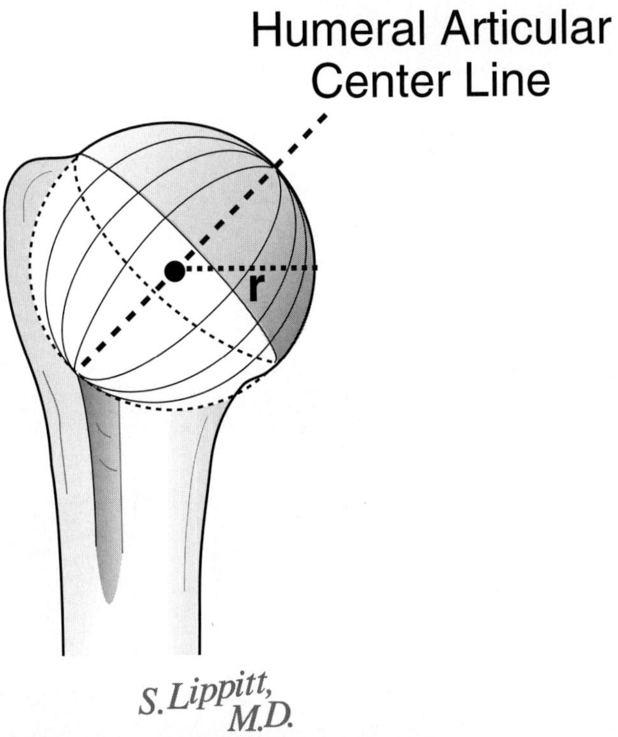


**Figure 27–31. Humeral articular center line**
With the usual height of the humeral articular center line, the top humeral articular surface is about 5 mm above the top of the tuberosity.

In shoulder arthroplasty, if the prosthesis is placed in a too superior position with respect to the tuberosities, the resulting cam effect may place the superior cuff under excessive tension when the arm is adducted **(Fig. 27–32)** and the inferior structures under excessive tension when the arm is abducted **(Fig. 27–33)**.

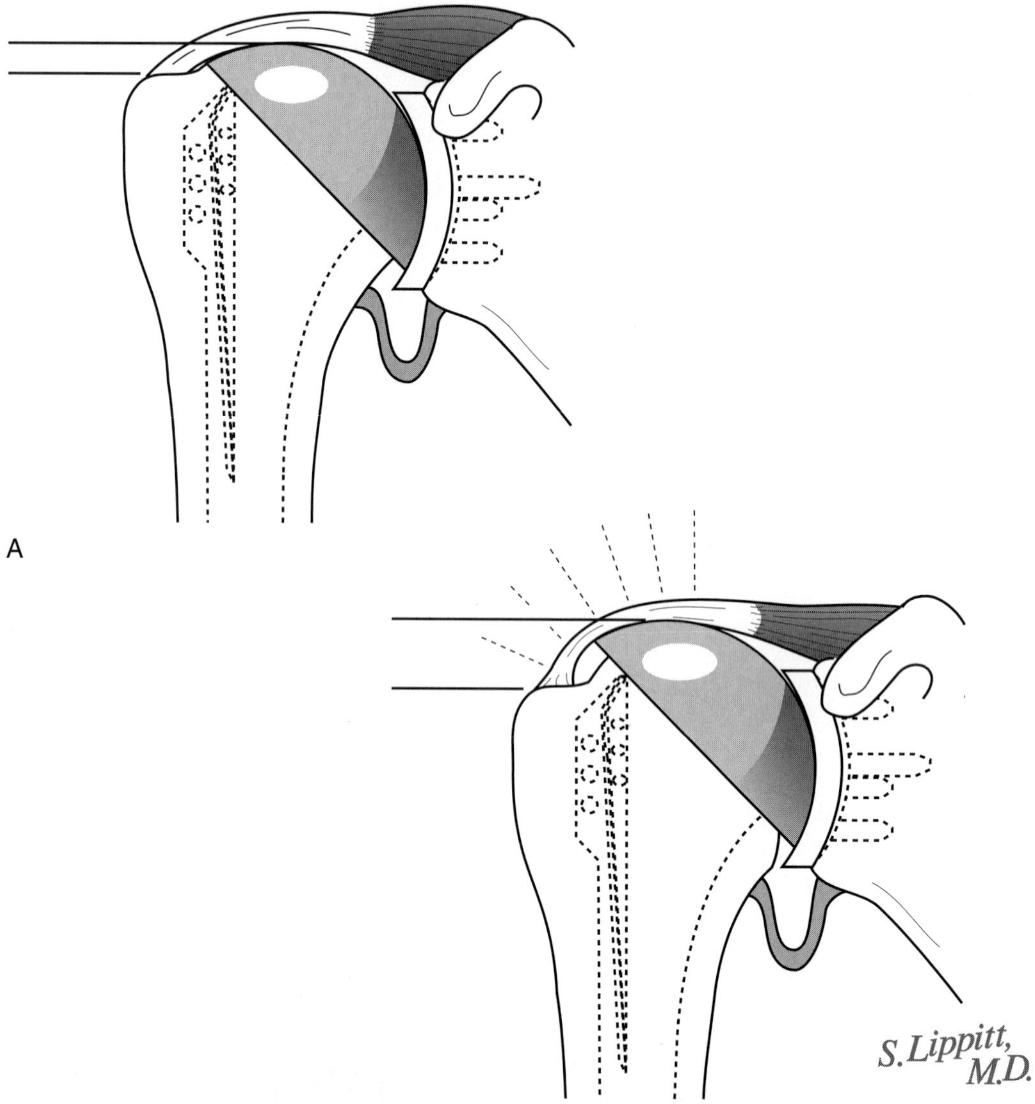


A

B

**Figure 27–32. Head height and adduction**
If the humeral prosthesis is positioned in an excessively superior position, it excessively tensions the superior cuff when the arm is in adduction.

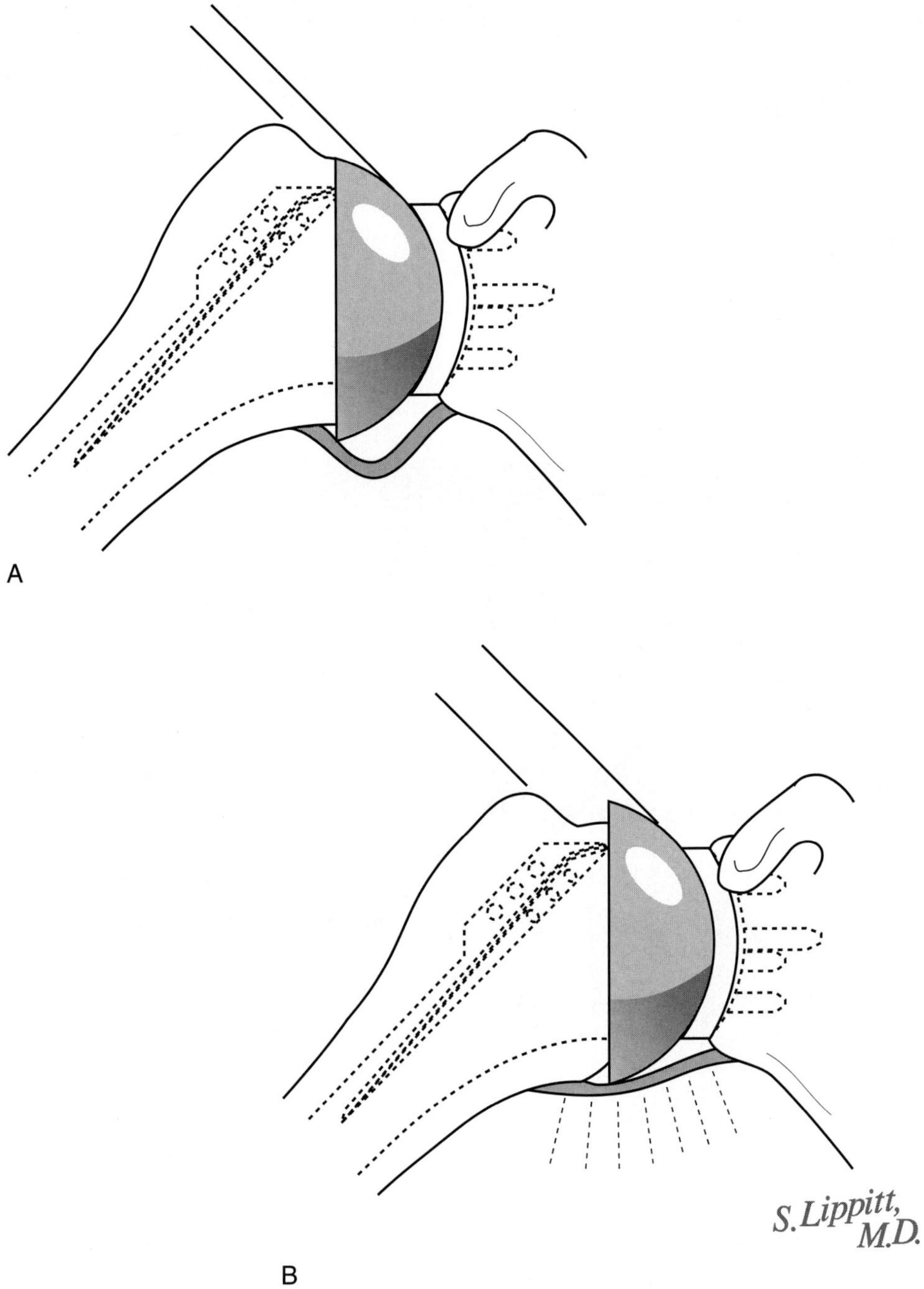


**Figure 27–33. Head height and abduction**

If the humeral prosthesis is positioned in an excessively superior position, it excessively tensions the inferior capsule when the arm is in abduction.

The superoinferior position of the humeral articular surface is constrained by the humeral neck cut (**Fig. 27–34**). The superoinferior position of the articular surface is also affected by the height of the spherical cap of the humeral articular surface and the effective neck length of the humeral prosthesis (**Fig. 27–35**). An example of excessive height of the spherical cap is when the collar and stem of a prosthesis extend the articular surface (**Fig. 27–36**). The superoinferior position can also be altered by the depth of insertion of the prosthesis (**Fig. 27–37**) and by the use of offset heads (**Fig. 27–38**).

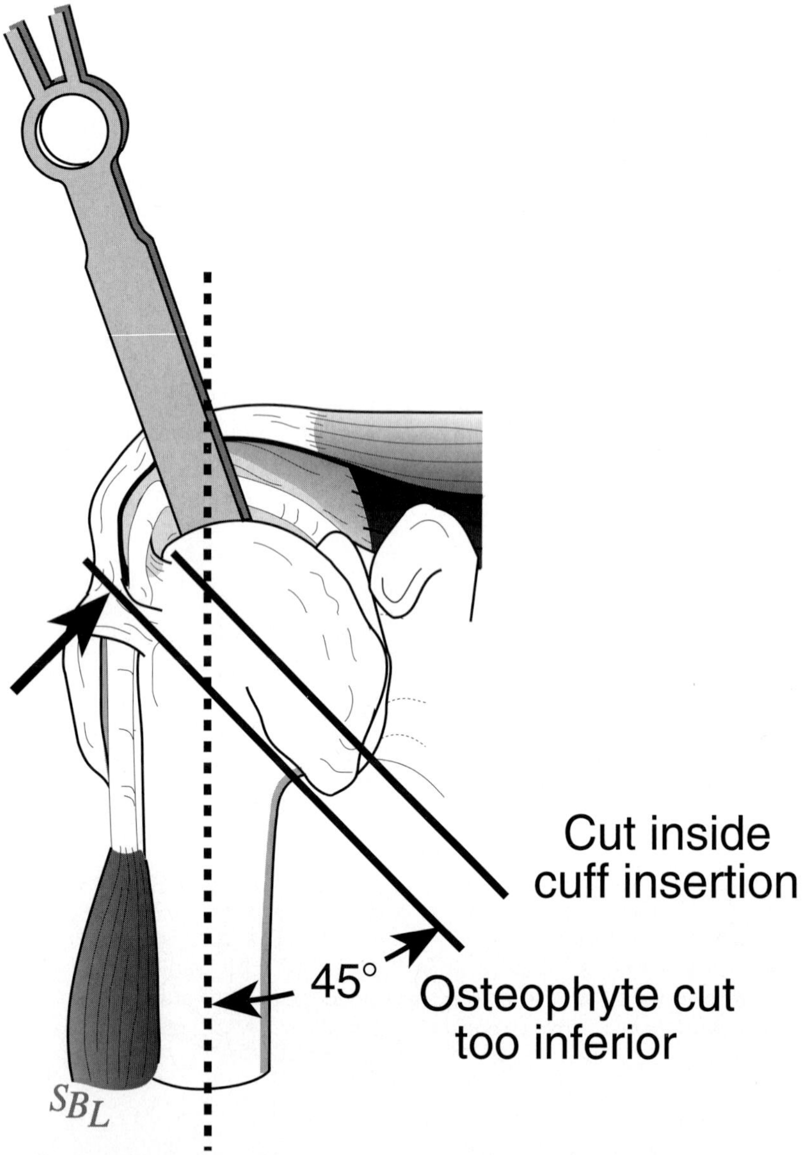


**Figure 27–34. Neck cut height**
The height of the 45-degree neck cut is limited by the cuff insertion. Ideally, the cut plane passes just inside the cuff insertion. A too inferior cut below the level of the osteophyte would endanger the cuff attachment to the tuberosity.

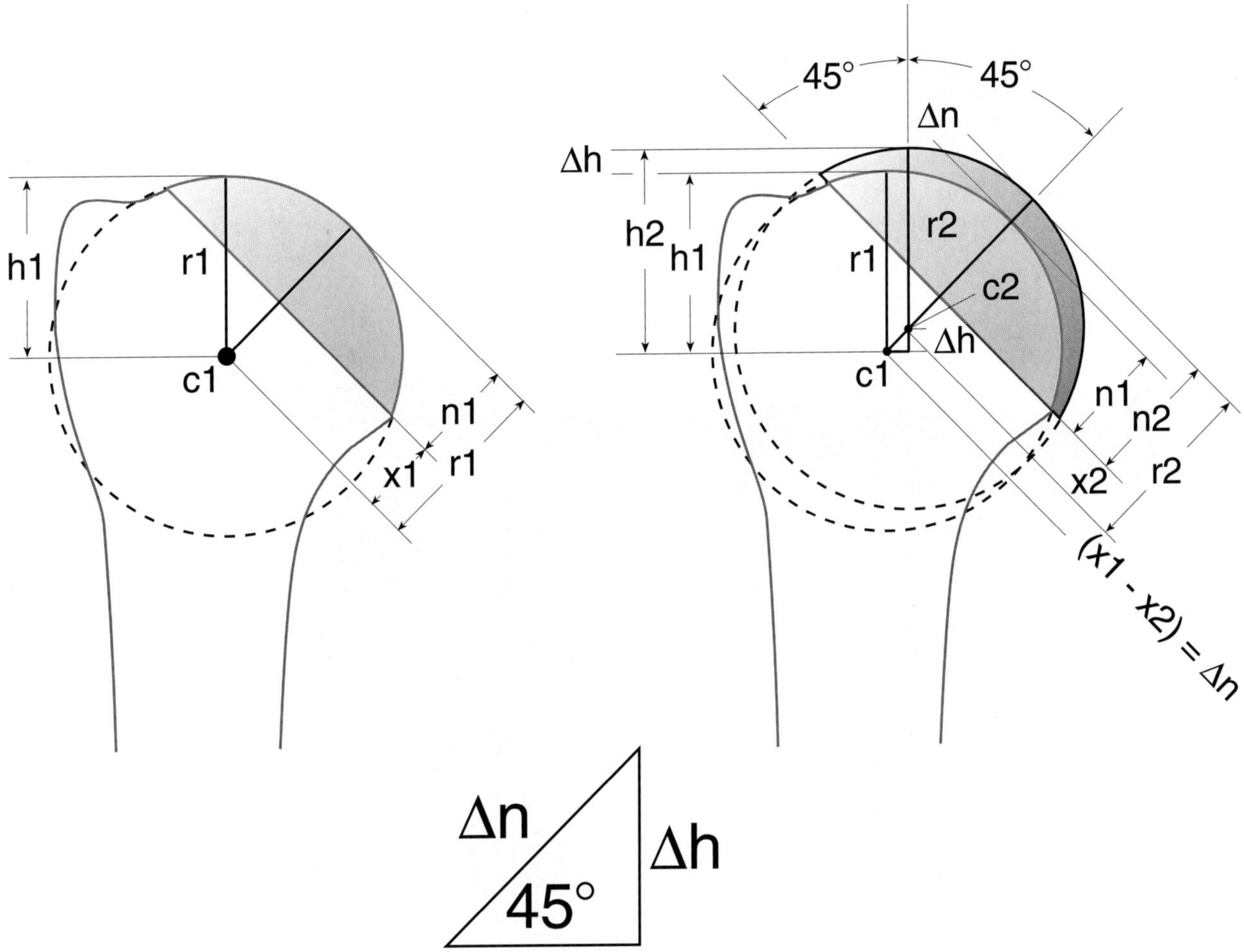


**Figure 27–35. Neck length**
Increasing the neck length (i.e., the height of the articular surface along the humeral articular center line) increases the superior position of the humeral articular surface by an amount equal to the sine 45 degrees × increase in height (or 0.71 × height increase).

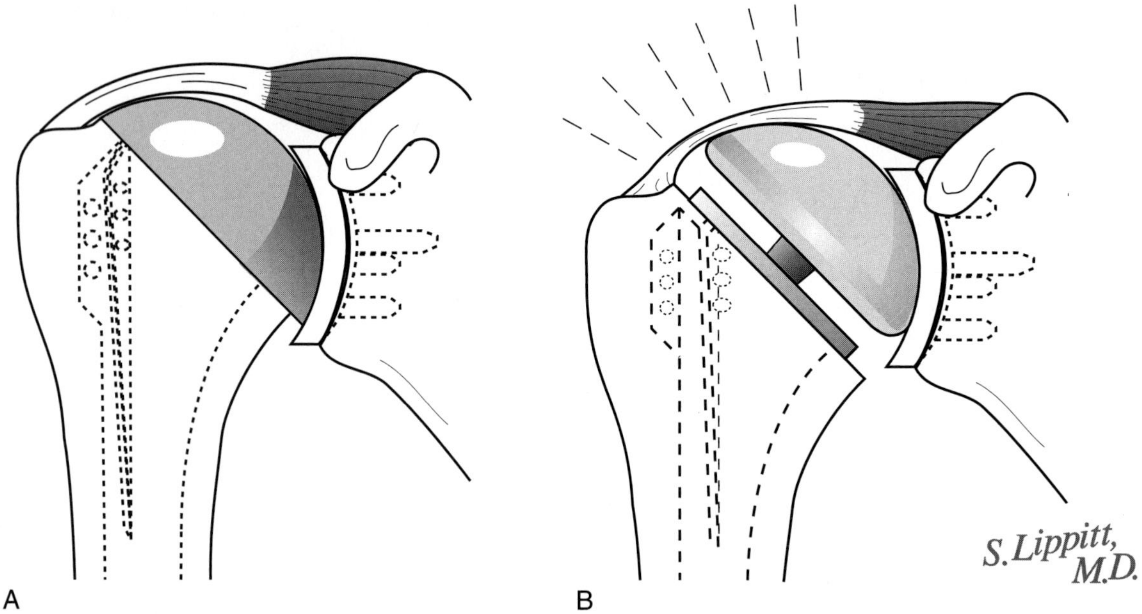


**Figure 27–36. Neck length**
Use of a prosthesis with a collar and gap can increase the effective neck length. (Modified from Matsen FA, Lippitt SB, Sidles JA, et al [eds]: Practical Evaluation and Management of the Shoulder. Philadelphia: WB Saunders, 1994, p. 198.)

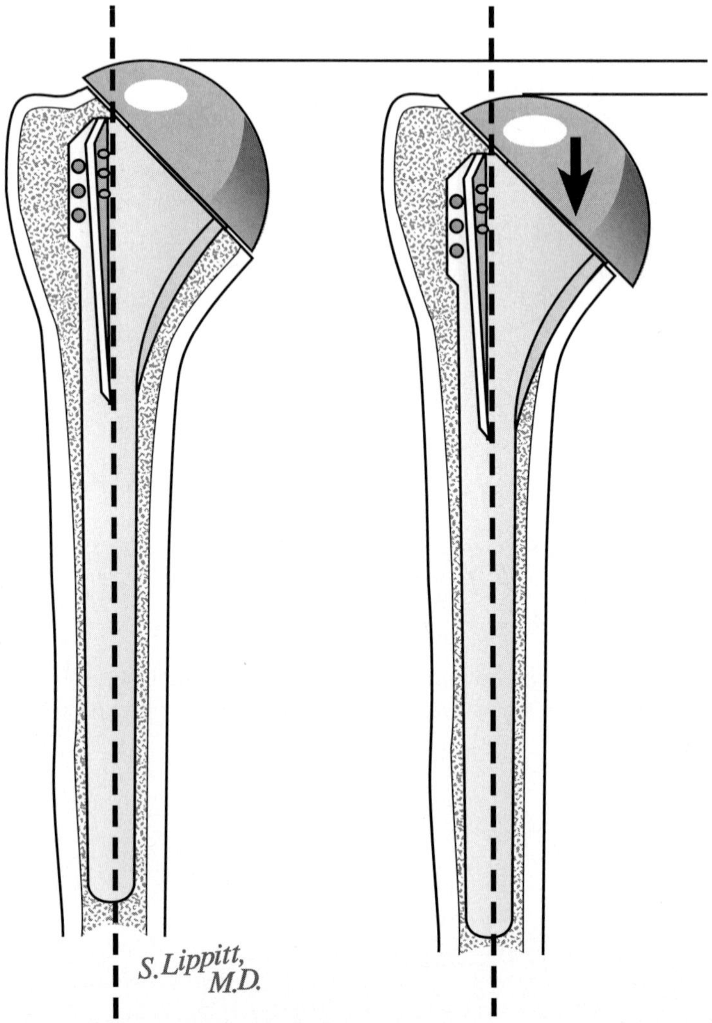


**Figure 27–37. Superoinferior position**
The superoinferior position of the humeral articular surface is affected by the depth to which the component is inserted.

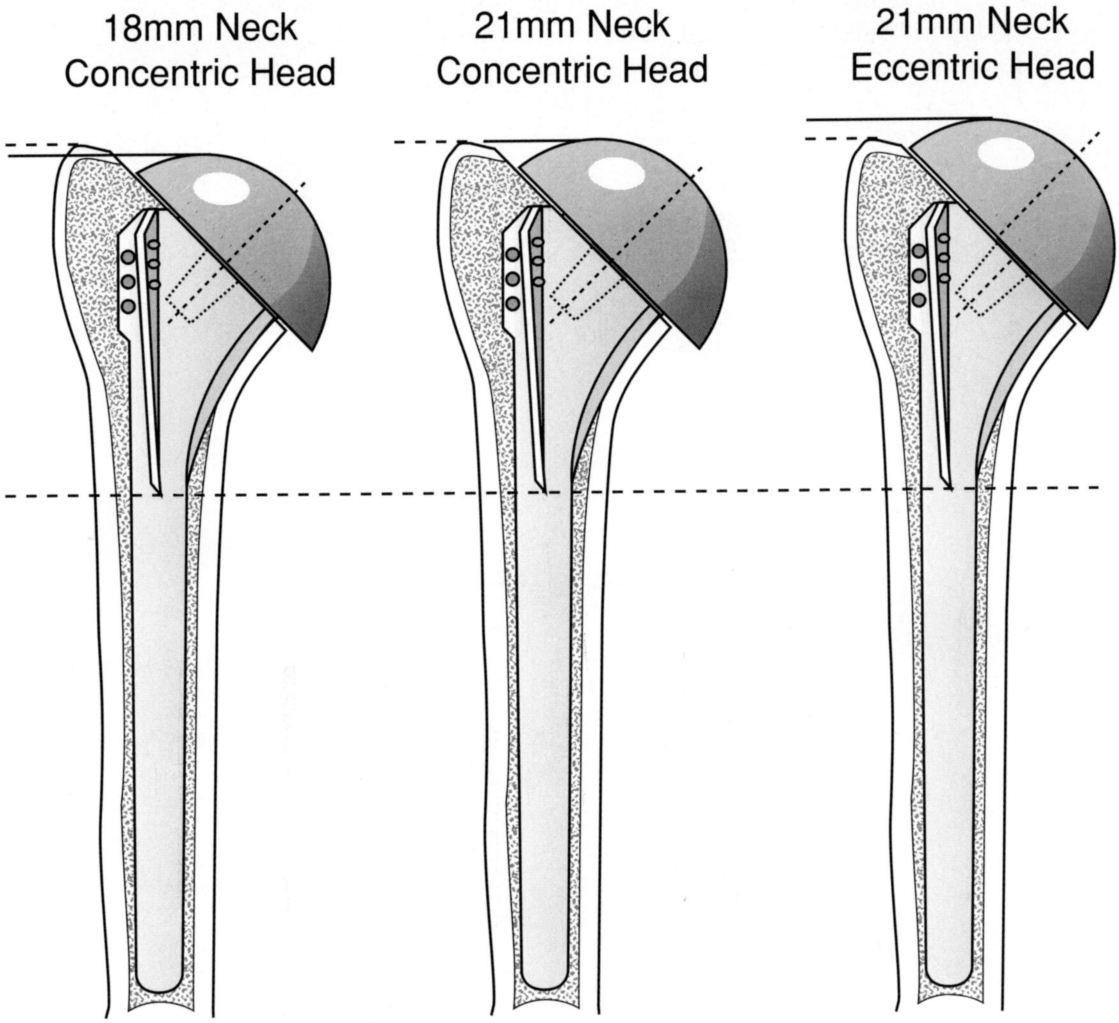


**Figure 27–38. Correcting a low head**
The use and orientation of eccentric heads can affect the superoinferior position of the articular surface. In this example, an eccentric head corrects for an excessively low position of the prosthetic body.

There is another important element of the superoinferior position of the humeral component: the relationship of the humeral articular surface to that of the glenoid; the components must be in proper *register*. If the articular surface of the humeral component does not seat fully in the glenoid fossa, the arthroplasty will lack stability (**Fig. 27–39**). On occasion, the humeral component must be placed in a position that may seem a bit too high or too low relative to the tuberosities to achieve proper register. Ideally, the humeral and glenoid center line will coincide when the arm is abducted 45 degrees in the plane of the scapula (**Fig. 27–40**).

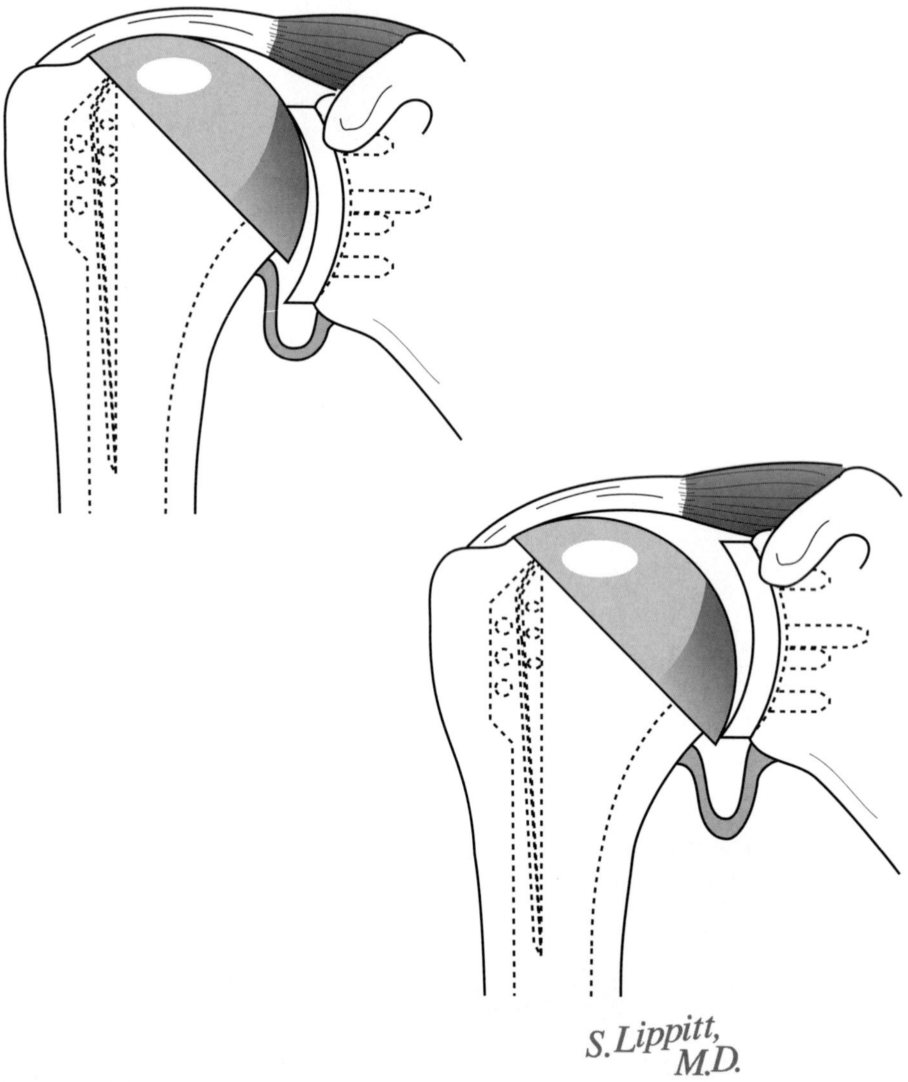


**Figure 27–39. Register**
When the humeral and glenoid components articulate, it is important that they are in proper register. If the humeral articular surface sits too superiorly or too inferiorly with respect to the glenoid, eccentric articulation can jeopardize the durability and stability of the arthroplasty.

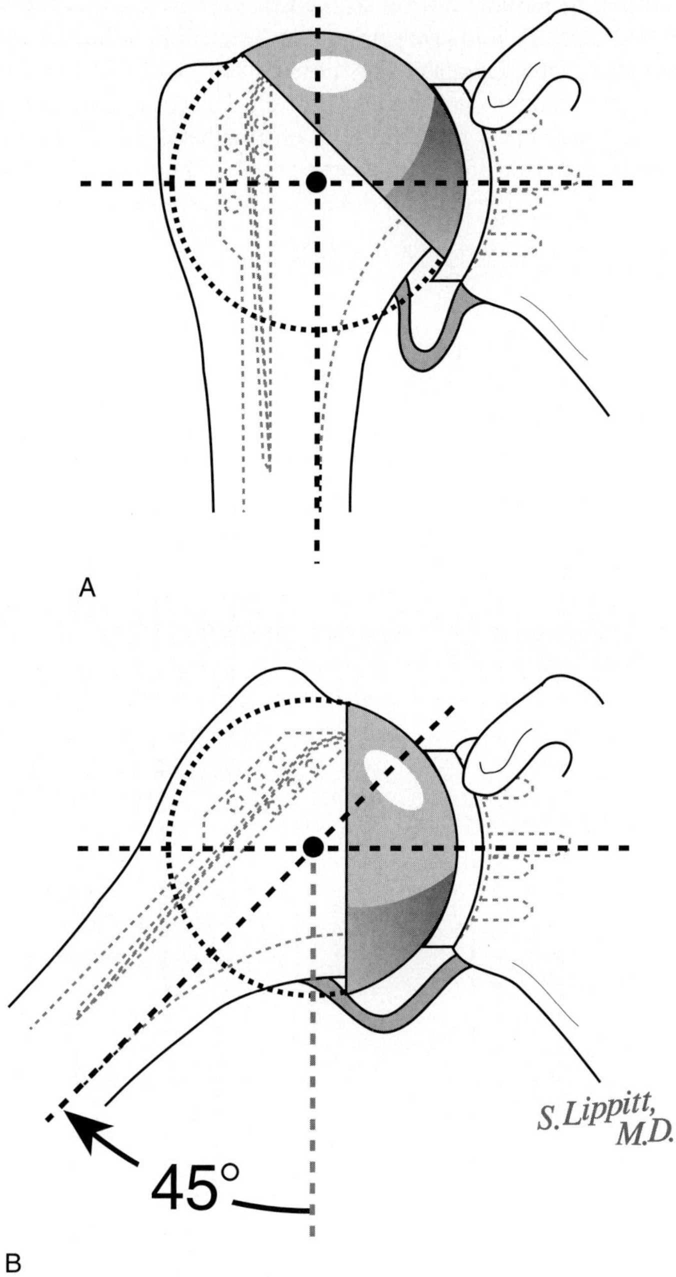


**Figure 27–40. Proper register**

If the components are in proper register, the humeral articular surface should seat fully in the glenoid in adduction and in 45 degrees of abduction.

## Fixation of the Prosthesis to Bone

Humeral arthroplasty requires a method for reliably fixing the humeral component in the medullary canal of the proximal humeral shaft. The ideal fixation system is secure, accommodates the variability in humeral canal shape, and allows for safe revision. Fixation methods using tissue ingrowth and cementing have the disadvantage of complicating the removal of the humeral component for glenoid or humeral revision.

Press fitting of the prosthesis stem to the medullary canal of the humerus is an attractive approach to humeral component fixation. The challenge is fitting a limitless variety of canal shapes with a finite number of prosthetic shapes. Even in the two-dimensional anteroposterior projection, some proximal humeral diaphyses appear to have parallel endosteal borders ("cylindrical"), whereas others converge ("funnel") (**Fig. 27–41**).

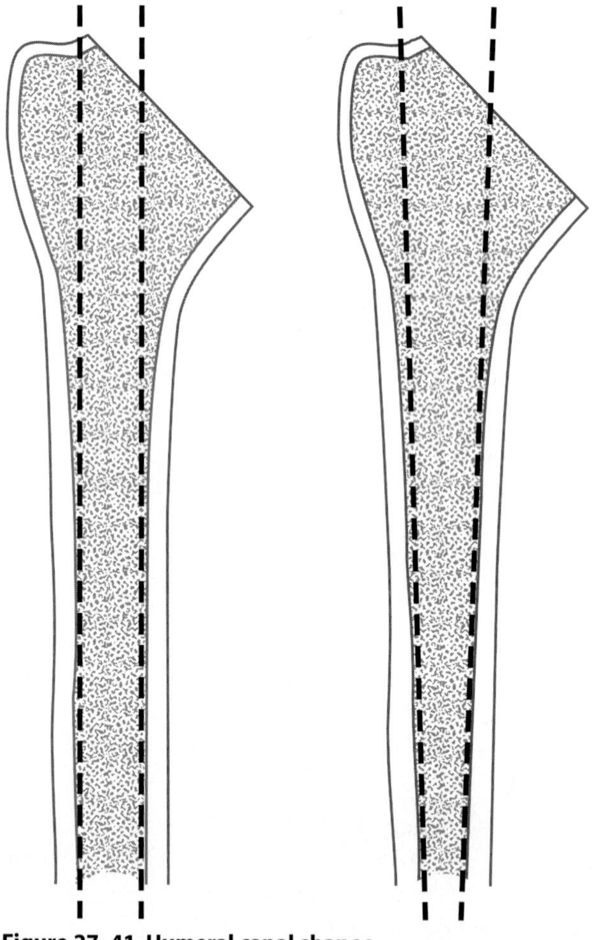

**Figure 27–41. Humeral canal shapes**
There is a wide variety among the shape of humeral medullary canals. Some are more cylindrical (*left*) and some are more funnel-shaped (*right*). It is apparent that a tapered stem would not fit well in the cylindrical canal and that a cylindrical stem would not fit well in the funnel-shaped canal.

It is difficult to achieve a press fit by reaming the canal to a cylindrical shape and inserting a prosthesis with a cylindrical body (**Fig. 27–42**). Reaming a funnel-shaped canal to cylindrical shape runs the risk of weakening the diaphysis distally (**Fig. 27–43**). Press fitting is facilitated by a prosthesis with a tapered metaphyseal section inserted into a tapered metaphyseal canal (**Fig. 27–44**). However, trying to attain a press fit

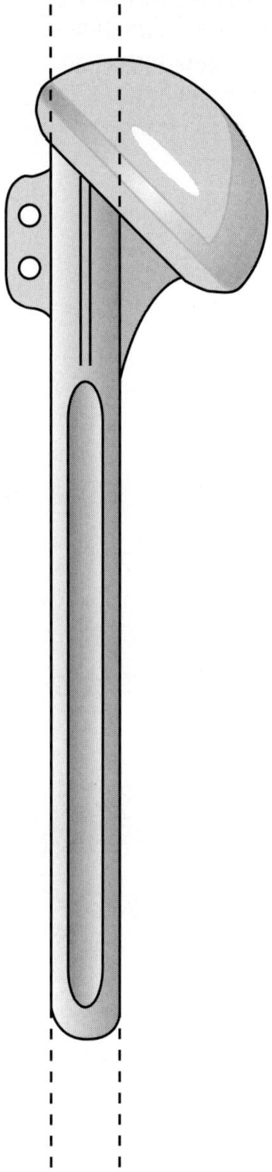

**Figure 27–42. Cylindrical stem**
A cylindrical body can slide within a cylindrical canal. This configuration can allow distal migration of the component.

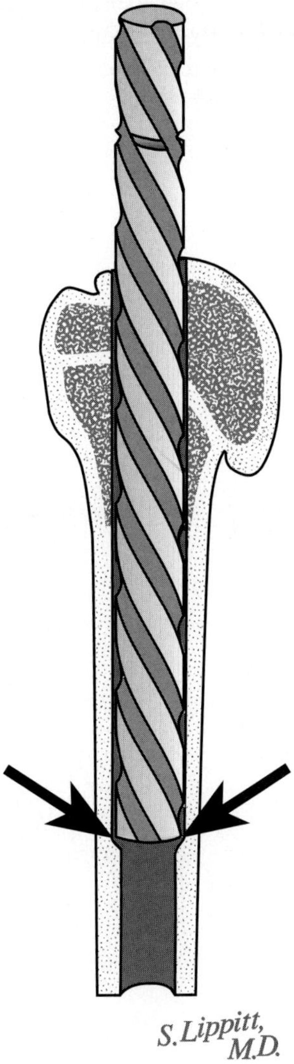


**Figure 27–43. Stress riser from reaming**
Cylindrical reaming of a funnel-shaped canal can create a stress riser distally in the diaphysis.

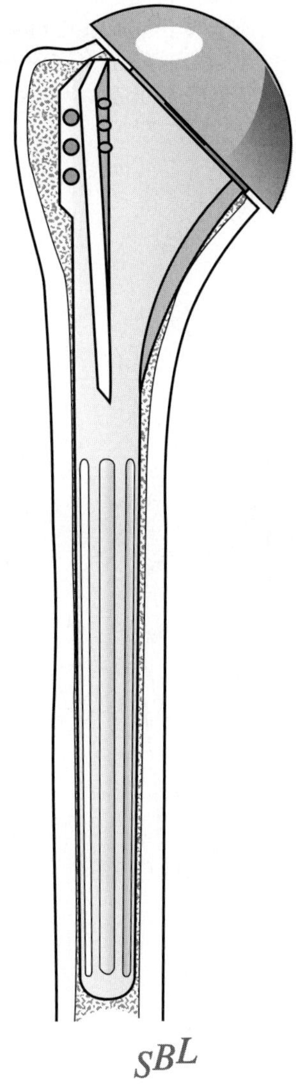


**Figure 27–44. Humeral press fit**
A prosthetic body with a tapered metaphyseal section achieves a press fit in the tapered humeral metaphysis.

against metaphyseal cortex runs the risk of fracture (**Fig. 27–45**). Not only is there substantial variation among individuals with respect to the shape of the canal, but within each humerus the cross-sectional shape of the medullary canal is not uniformly round (**Fig. 27–46**). This high degree of variability means that a predetermined set of prosthetic body geometries cannot be expected to fit the wide variations in endosteal anatomy encountered in clinical practice.

To solve the problem of secure and durable fixation of a limited number of humeral bodies in a limitless variety of humeral medullary canals, we turned for inspiration to Greek mythology, where we meet the innkeeper Procrustes. He kept a house by the side of the road where he offered hospitality to passing strangers, who were invited in for a pleasant meal and a night's rest in his very special bed. Procrustes described it as having the unique property that its length exactly matched whoever lay down upon it.

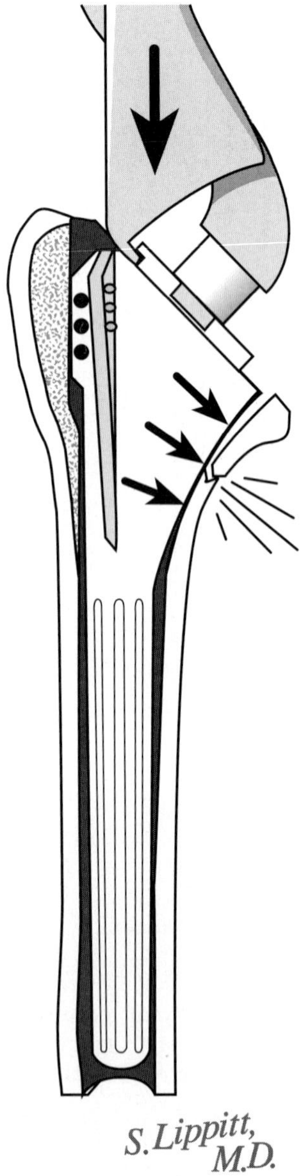


**Figure 27–45. Press fit fracture**
Attempting to achieve a cortical press fit in the metaphysis runs the risk of fracture.

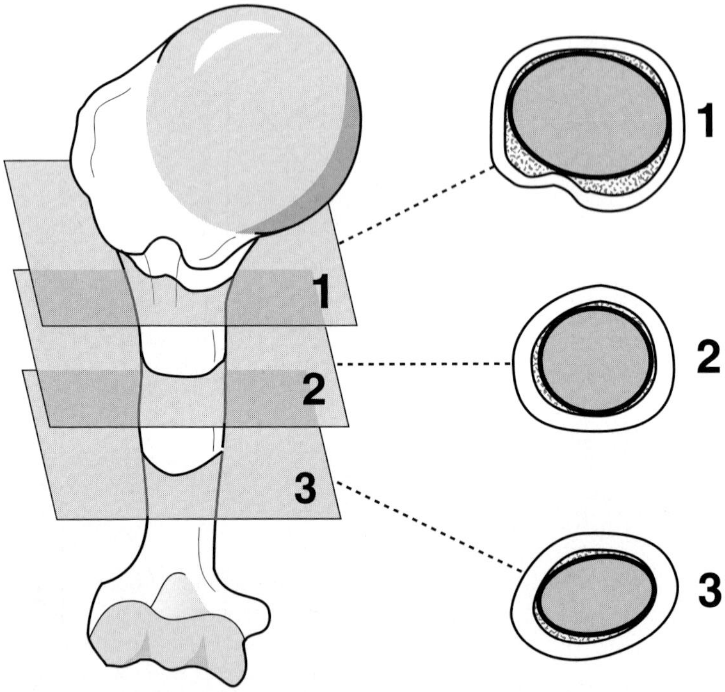


**Figure 27–46. Humerus cross-sections**
The varying shape and orientation of the humeral canal cross-sections along the humerus make it impossible to fit the endosteal surface with a defined shape of the prosthetic body.

What Procrustes did not volunteer was the method by which this "one-size-fits-all" was achieved, namely that as soon as the guest lay down, Procrustes went to work upon him, stretching him on the rack if he was too short for the bed and chopping off his legs if he was too long. In the Procrustean spirit, we fit the humerus to the prosthesis. This is accomplished using autogenous cancellous bone graft harvested from the humeral head. Graft is used to position the component optimally and to achieve a biological fit and fill that prevents instability and loosening by filling the voids between the fixed geometry of the prosthesis and the variable endosteal surface of the bone with fresh autograft. Although trying to achieve a press fit of the prosthesis directly against cortical bone jeopardizes the integrity of the cortical shell, the compliance of cancellous bone graft enables a snug press fit to be achieved that distributes the load evenly and safely to cortical bone (**Fig. 27–47**). In a cadaveric model system, we found that the void volume between a prosthesis and the endosteum is significantly reduced in the proximal and middle regions by Procrustean grafting.

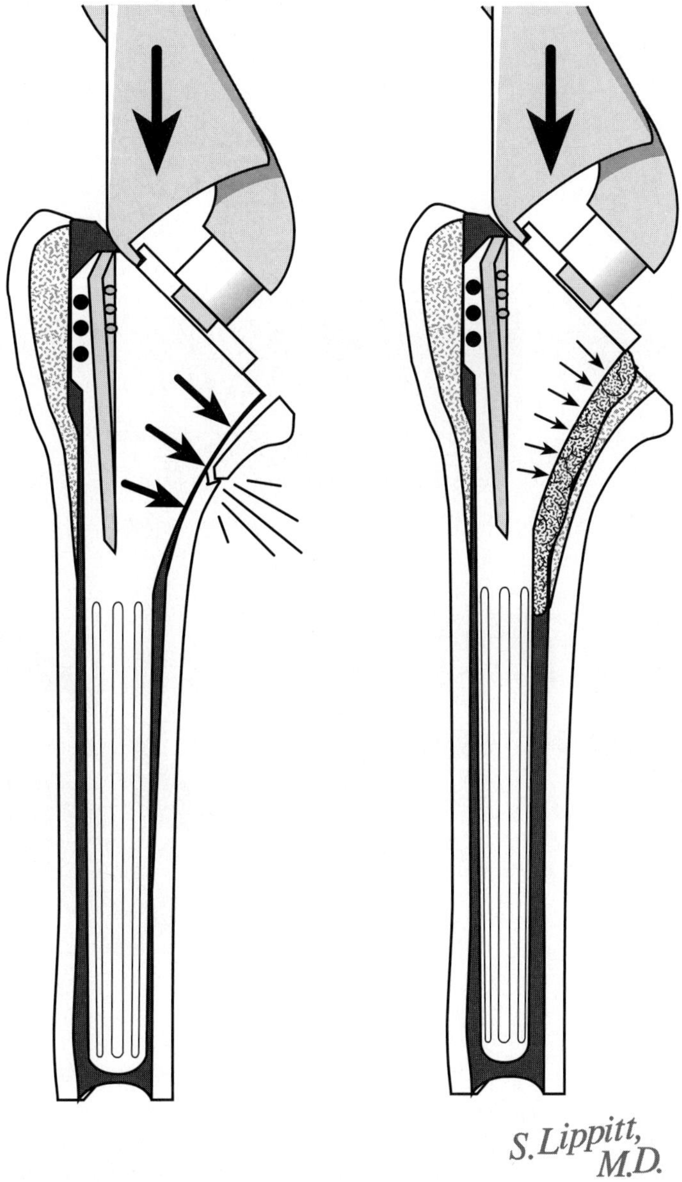


**Figure 27–47. Safety with cancellous grafting**
Impacted cancellous bone fills in the voids and enables more even distribution of loads during press fitting (*right*) and minimizes the risk of fracture (*left*).

## SURGICAL CONSIDERATIONS

### Preoperative Planning

We take a templating x-ray of the humerus **(Fig. 27–48)** to provide a two-dimensional preview of the humeral anatomy. Transparent templates, correcting for magnification, give us advance notice regarding (1) the maximal stem diameter (the endosteal diameter at the distal end of the prosthesis), (2) the amount of taper of the diaphyseal canal, (3) the degree of fill of the medullary canal by a prosthesis with the estimated maximal stem diameter, (4) any eccentricities of proximal humeral anatomy, (5) the estimated starting point for reaming (extrapolation of the orthopaedic axis through the articular surface of the humeral head), (6) the radius of curvature of the biological head, (7) the height of the spherical cap of the biological head, and (8) the position of the assembled humeral prosthesis that will duplicate the location of the biological humeral joint surface **(Fig. 27–49)**.

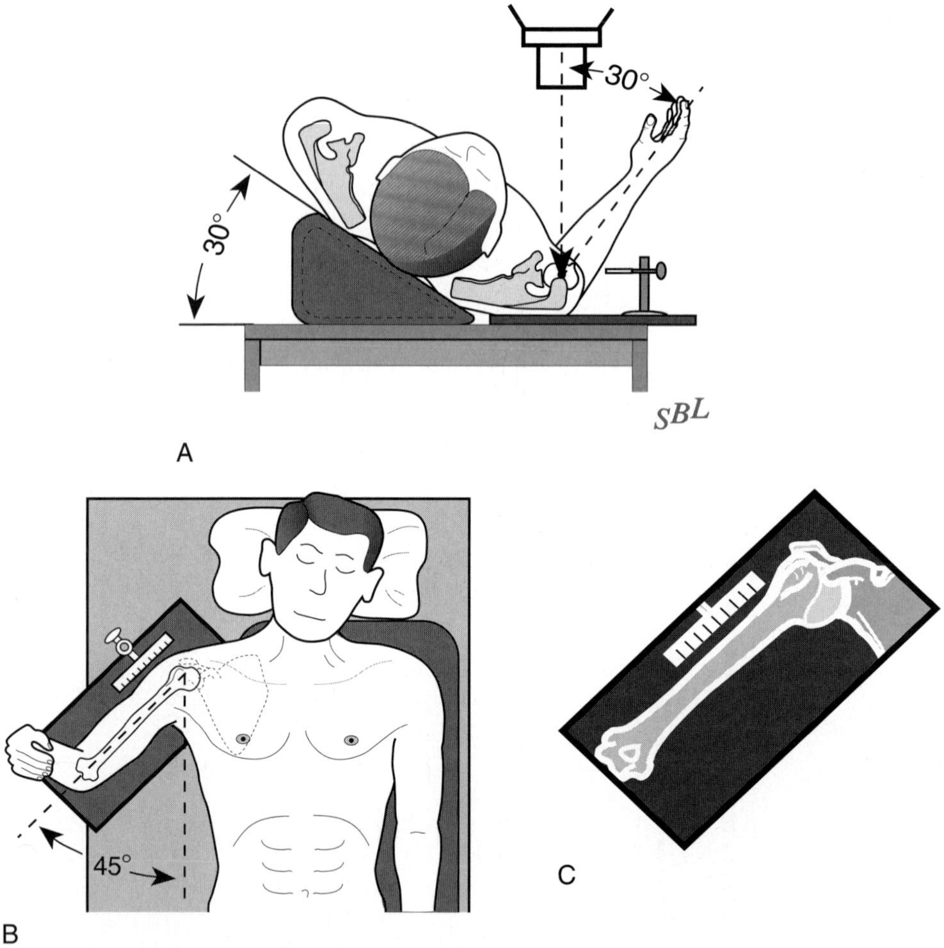


**Figure 27–48. Templating view, the anteroposterior radiograph in the "centered position"**
The humerus is positioned in neutral rotation with respect to the thorax and is abducted 45 degrees. The anteroposterior radiograph in the plane of the scapula is obtained by positioning the scapula flat on the cassette and by aiming the beam at the joint. The beam makes a 30-degree angle with the forearm, and the thorax makes a 30-degree angle with the cassette. A 10 cm marker held adjacent to the lateral humerus indicates the radiographic magnification when templates for various components are compared. The final radiographic appearance is shown in part *C*. (Modified from Matsen FA, Lippitt SB, Sidles JA, et al [eds]: Practical Evaluation and Management of the Shoulder. Philadelphia: WB Saunders, 1994, p 160.)

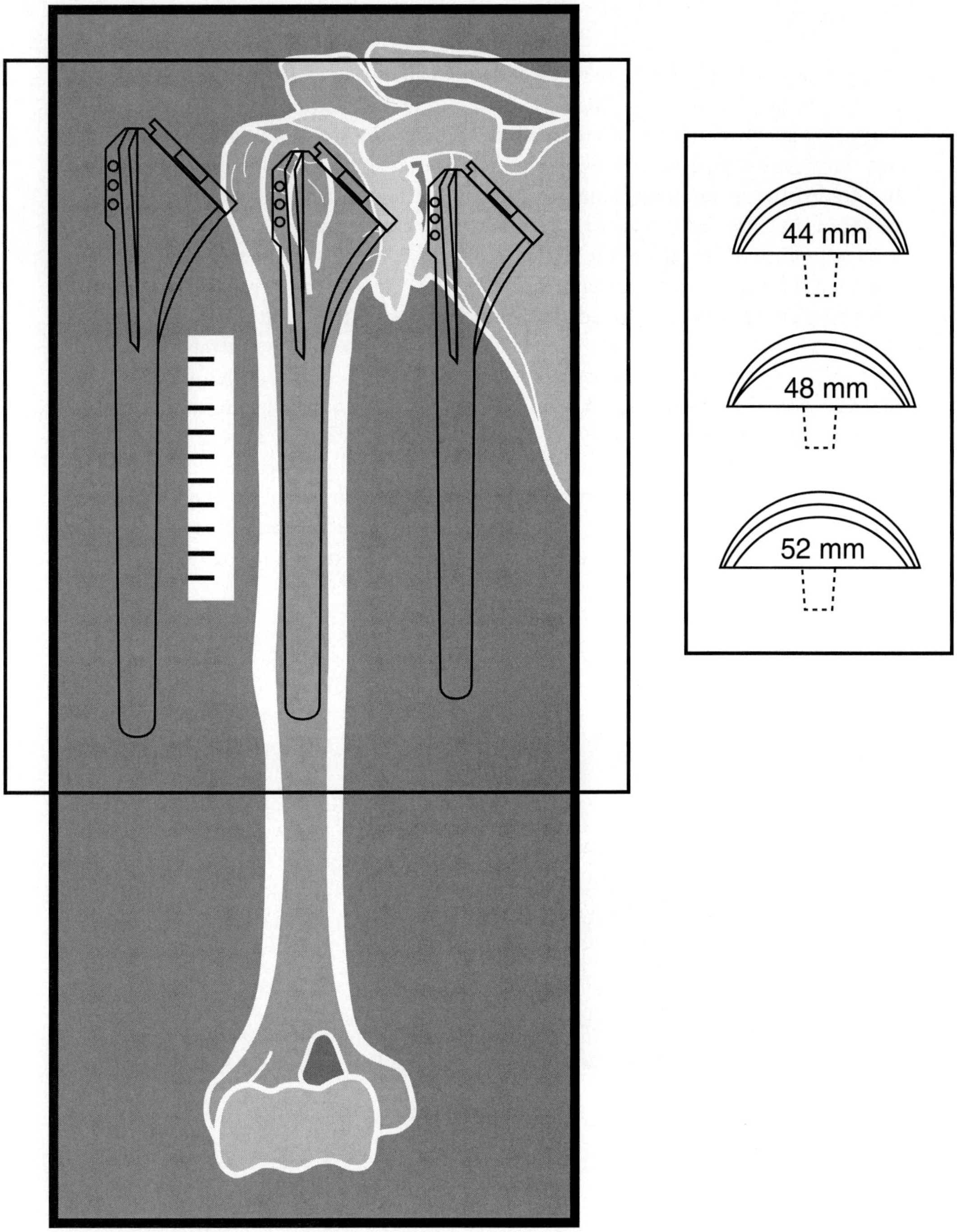


**Figure 27–49. Templating**
Preoperative templating gives the surgeon a preview of the humeral arthroplasty.

### *The Procedure*

Our philosophy is to use the three-dimensional anatomy of the proximal humerus at the time of surgery to guide our efforts to duplicate the position and orientation of the new articular surface. Thus, we do not cut off the biological humeral articular surface until we have extracted as much information from it as possible. First, a line parallel to the humeral articular center line is drawn on the anterior humeral surface, from the center of the articular surface to the lesser tuberosity (**Fig. 27–50**).

Next, a line is drawn from the center of the articular surface superiorly to inferiorly, bisecting the anterior and posterior halves of the articular surface. The starting point for medullary reaming is selected just behind the bicipital groove near the insertion of the supraspinatus to the greater tuberosity along the line drawn midway between the anterior and posterior halves of the humeral articular surface. Special attention is directed toward ensuring that this starting point is far enough posterior, because the surgical exposure may favor a too anterior starting point. A hole is made in the humeral head at the starting point (**Fig. 27–51**). The medullary canal is entered with a straight curette, a tapered reamer, and then cylindrical reamers of sequentially increasing diameters. A slight valgus moment is exerted because the surgical exposure favors a too varus orientation (**Fig. 27–52**). Reamers are inserted only to the depth required

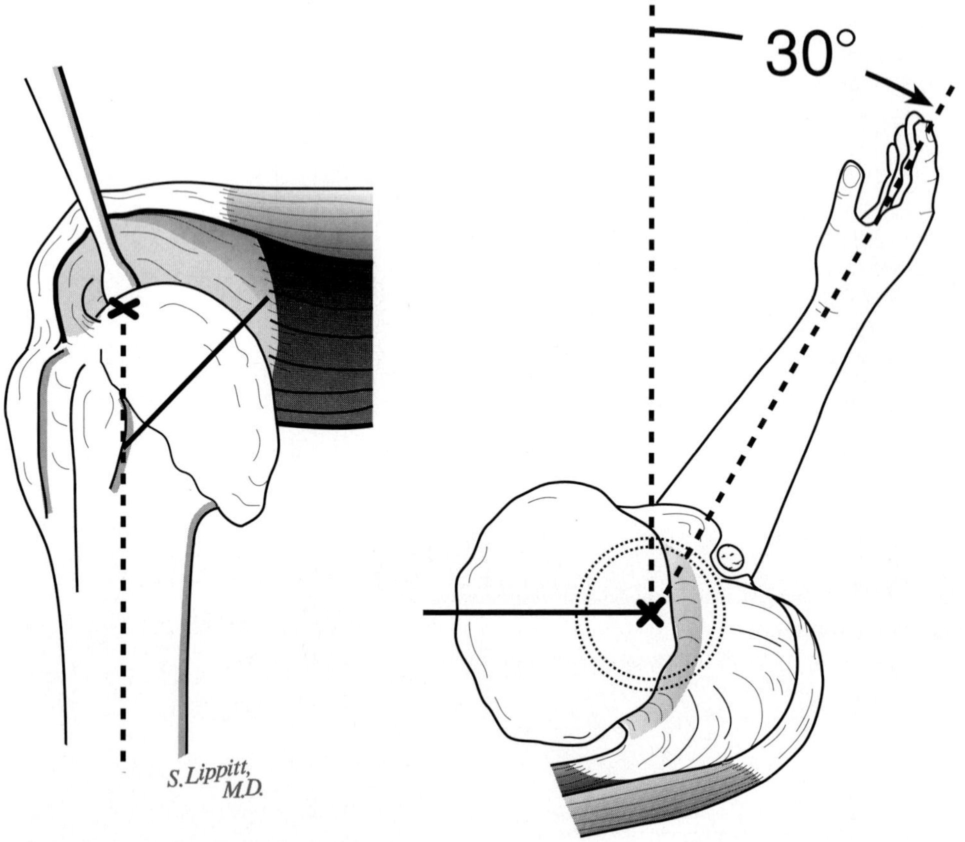


**Figure 27–50. Intraoperative planning**
Two orienting lines are drawn. One is parallel to the humeral articular center line (*left*) and one splits the humeral articular surface into its anterior and posterior halves (humeral bisecting line) (*right*). The starting point for entering the canal is along the bisecting line near the cuff insertion to the tuberosity.

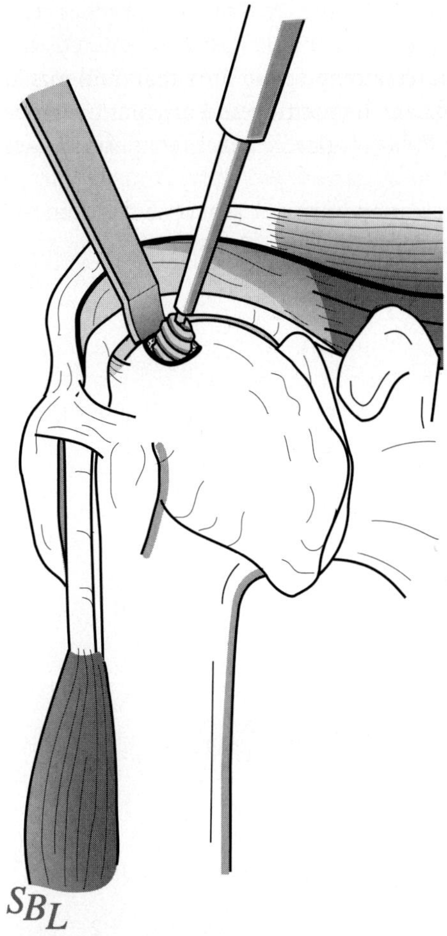

**Figure 27–51. Burr start**
The medullary space of the humeral head is entered at the starting point using a pinecone burr.

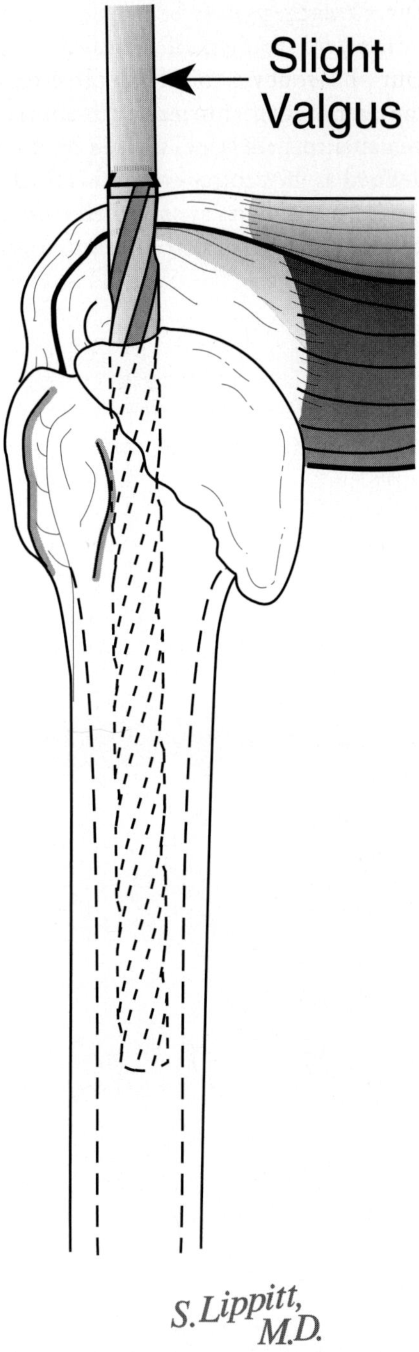


**Figure 27–52. Medullary reaming**
Cylindrical reamers are inserted down to the depth required by the prosthesis, exerting a slight valgus bias.

by the prosthesis to avoid needless reaming of cortical bone. Medullary reaming is continued with reamers of increasing size until a cortical bite is first encountered distally—"love at first bite" (**Fig. 27–53**). The diameter of the prosthetic shaft will match the diameter of this reamer. Reaming with larger diameter reamers would remove valuable cortical bone, weakening the shaft. The orthopaedic axis of the humerus is defined as the central axis of this final reamer.

The osteophytes are removed from the anterior and inferior aspect of the humeral head, using the capsular insertion to the neck as a guide (**Fig. 27–54**).

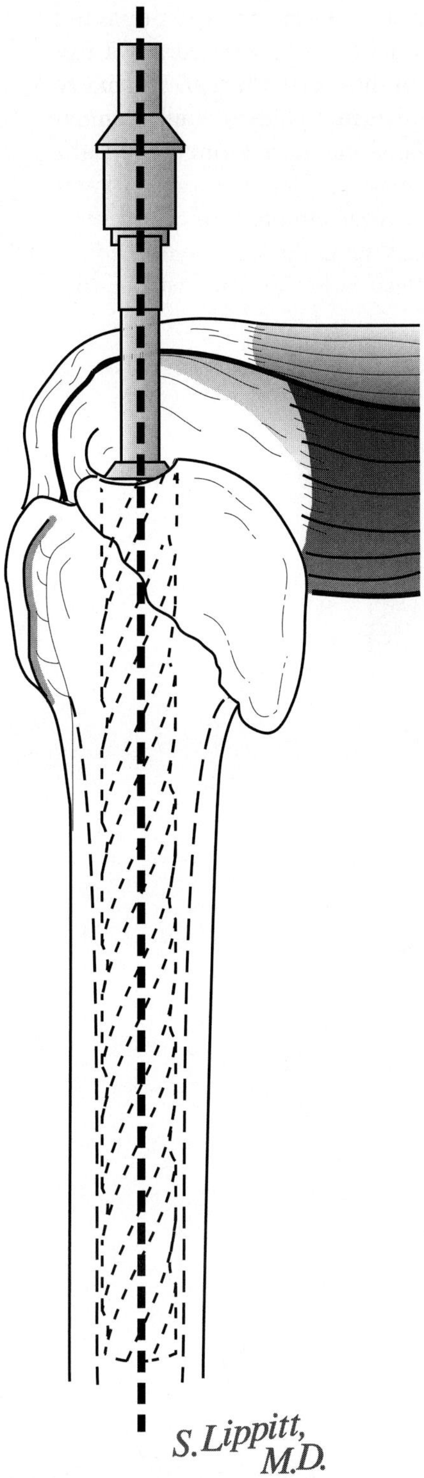


**Figure 27–53. Reaming to the first bite**
Progressively larger reamers are used until the surgeon achieves a bite in the cortex distally. The orthopaedic axis is the central axis of this reamer (*dark dotted line*).

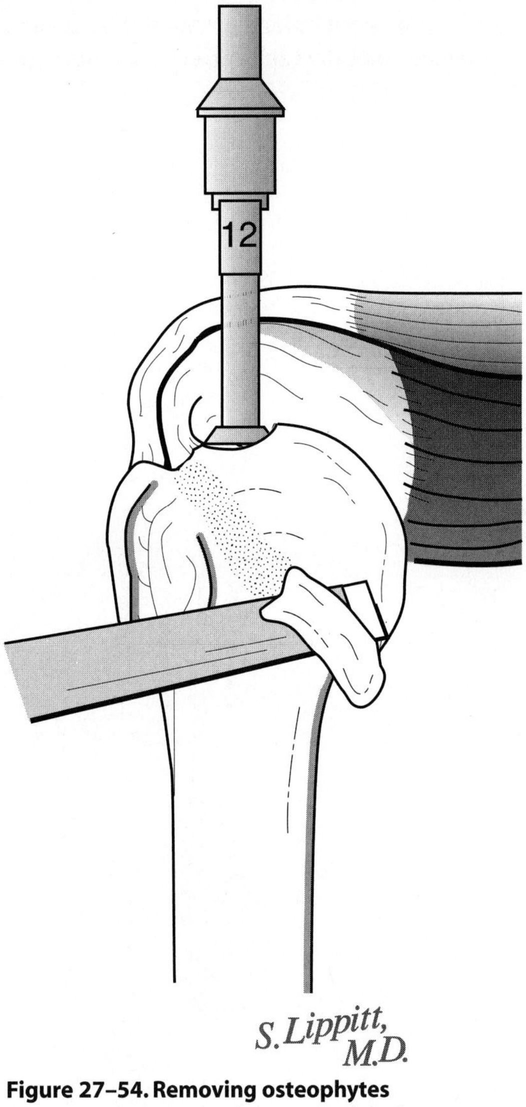


**Figure 27–54. Removing osteophytes**
The osteophytes around the neck of the humerus are removed using a rongeur and an osteotome.

A number of different humeral cutting guides are in current use. Some are extramedullary; that is, a guide is placed on the anterior aspect of the humerus with an angled upper surface indicating the 45-degree neck shaft angle **(Fig. 27–55)**. Some use the medullary canal to orient an extramedullary cutting guide. We use a three-dimensional anatomic orthopaedic axis mask to duplicate the relationship between the stem and the articular surface of the prosthesis. This mask enables the surgeon to preview the position and orientation of the joint surface of different prosthetic head alternatives mounted on a prosthetic body press fit with its stem in the location of the final reamer **(Fig. 27–56)**. The version of the planned cut can be verified by ensuring that

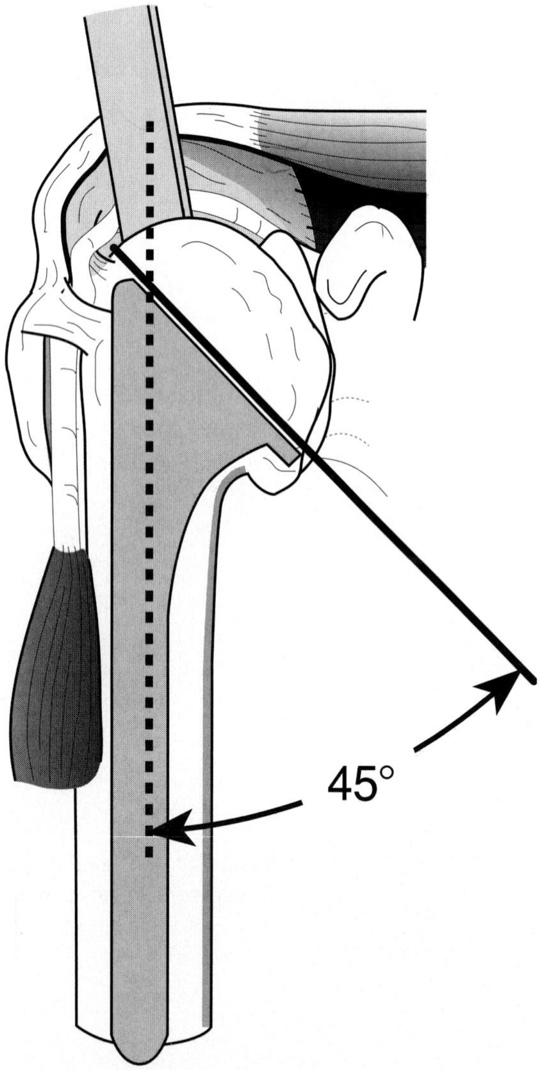


**Figure 27–55. Extramedullary guide**
An extramedullary guide can approximate the desired neck shaft angle, but its accuracy is compromised by the fact that its orientation is not linked to the medullary anatomy of the humerus that guides the position of the component.

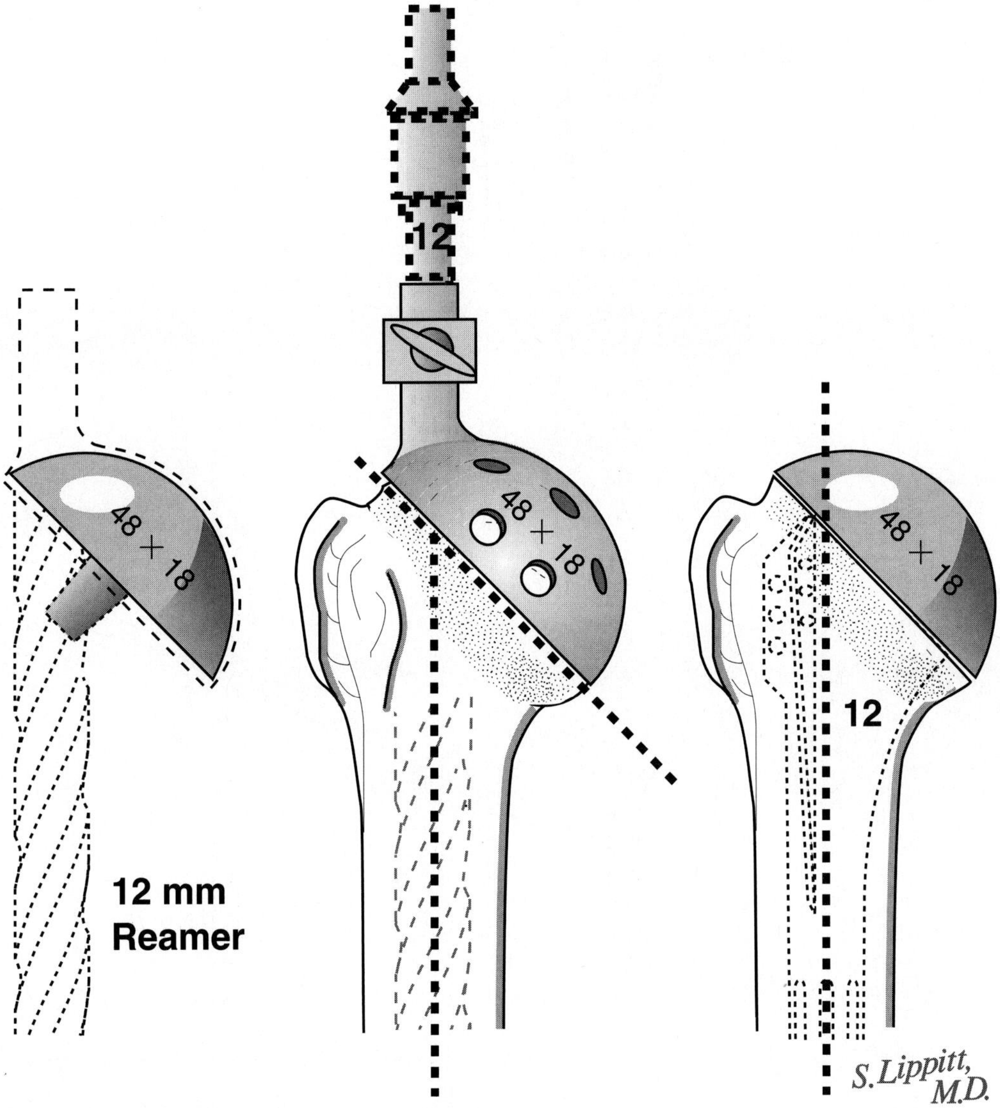


**Figure 27–56. Anatomic orthopaedic axis mask**
A mask can be used that represents the three-dimensional geometrical relationships of the prosthetic articular surface to the prosthetic stem. When the mask is placed on the reamer inserted into the canal, it enables the surgeon to see the resulting position of the articular surface and the location of the plane for humeral head resection *before* committing to a prosthesis size or neck cut.

the posterior edge of the mask is aligned with the humeral bisecting line (**Fig. 27–57**). The anatomic orthopaedic axis template is then used to mark the cut that will result in the anatomic positioning of the definitive prosthesis (**Fig. 27–58**). Care is taken to ensure that the cut plane passes just inside the cuff insertion. The resulting cut respects the version of the particular humerus and is usually in approximately 30 degrees of retroversion (**Fig. 27–59**). In making the cut, extreme care is taken not to make the cut in excessive retroversion, which would jeopardize the cuff insertion (**Fig. 27–60**). Our preference is to make this cut with a broad, sharp osteotome, the edge of which is kept in view so that there is every opportunity to control the osteotomy.

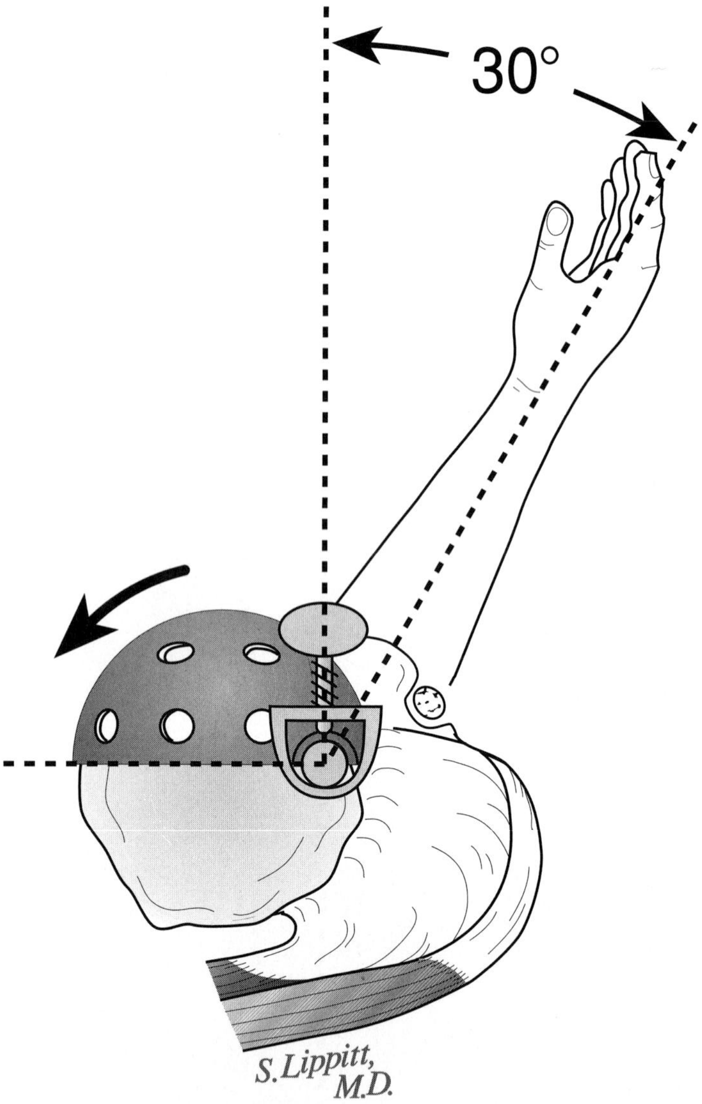


**Figure 27–57. Mask placement**
When in position, the posterior edge of the mask should align along the humeral bisecting line drawn previously.

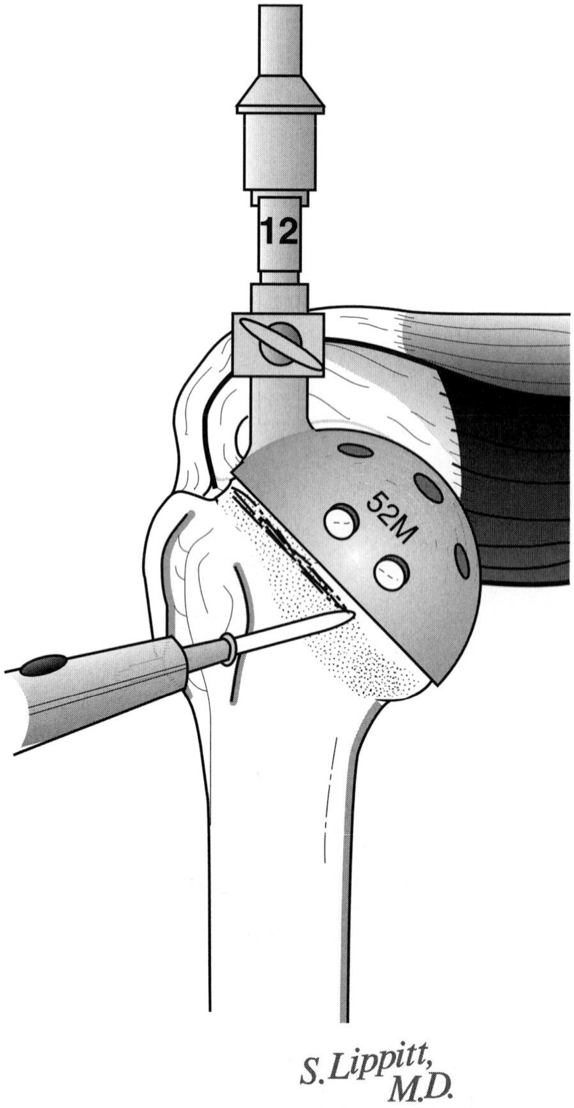


**Figure 27–58. Marking the osteotomy**
Once the position of the mask is determined to be acceptable, the cut plane is marked on the humeral neck with electrocautery.

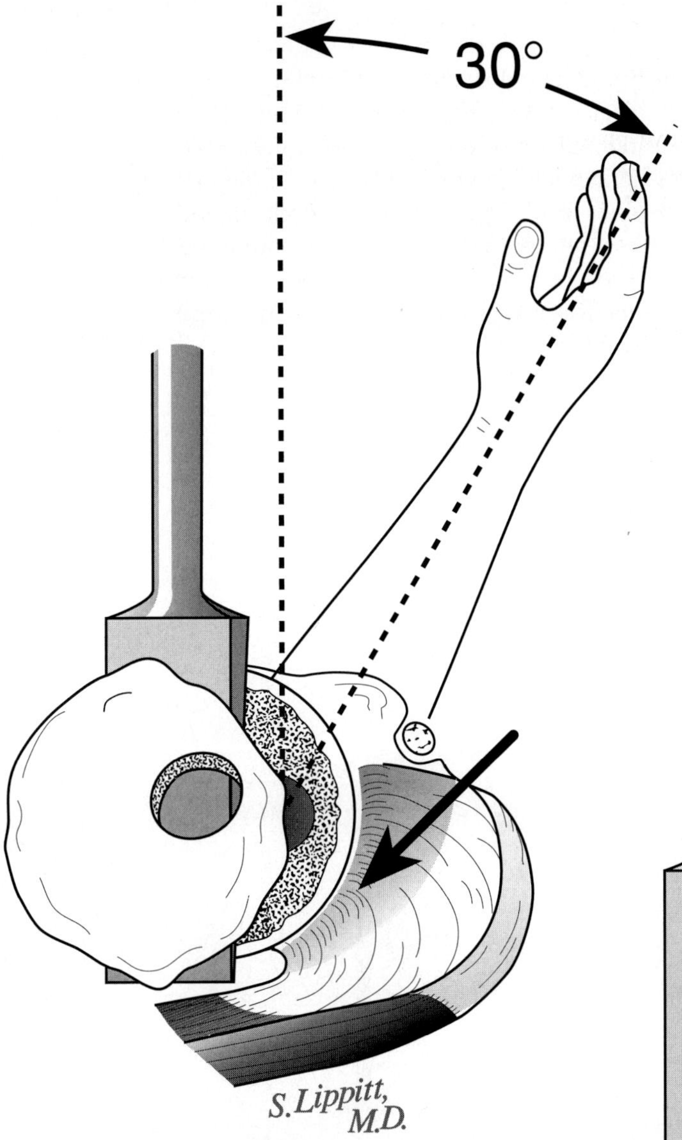


**Figure 27–59. Version of the cut**
The osteotomy passes just inside the cuff insertion.

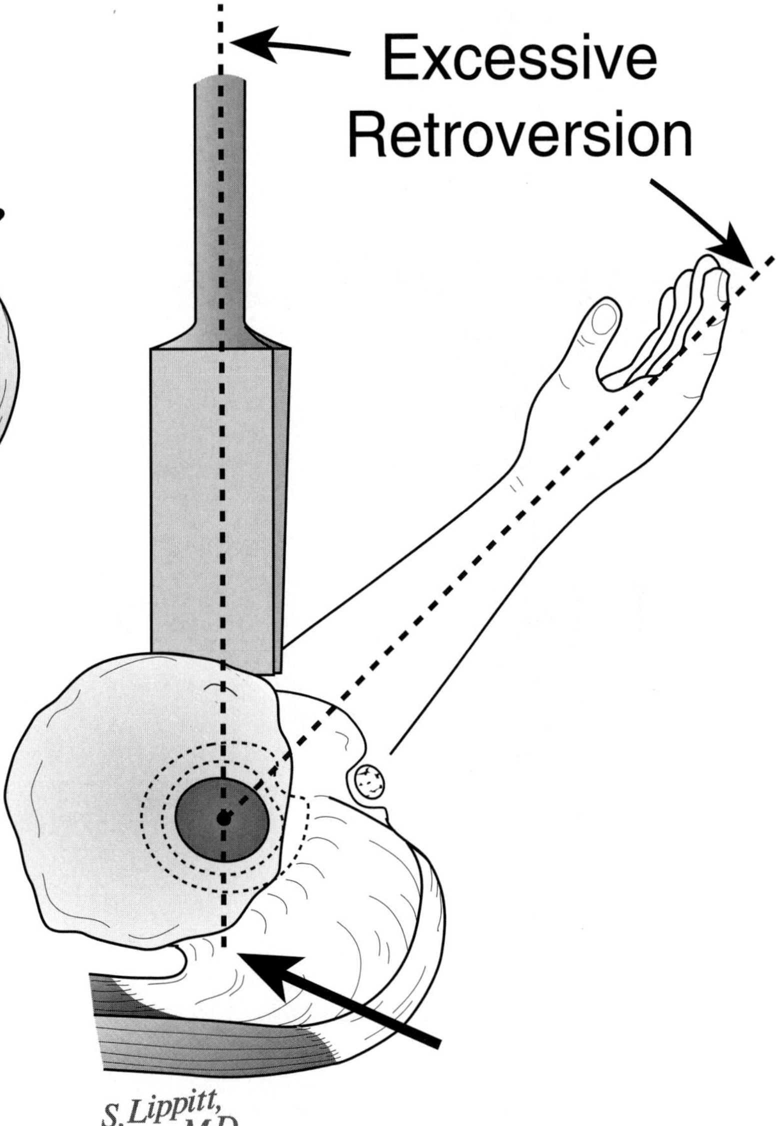


**Figure 27–60. Excessive version of the cut**
Excessive retroversion of the cut jeopardizes the integrity of the tuberosity and the cuff insertion.

The canal is then broached using a broach with a tip diameter corresponding to that of the final reamer. With the broach fully engaged, the position and stability of the broach in the canal is determined. The desired anteroposterior, mediolateral, supero-inferior, and version position of the prosthetic body is established—that is, the one that puts the prosthetic humeral articular center line in the center of the neck cut and parallel to the center line previously drawn on the anterior proximal humerus. Cancellous graft is harvested from the resected humeral head and impacted in the medullary canal (**Figs. 27–61** and **27–62**). Selective graft placement is used to optimize the position of the prosthesis in the center of the neck (**Figs. 27–63** and **27–64**).

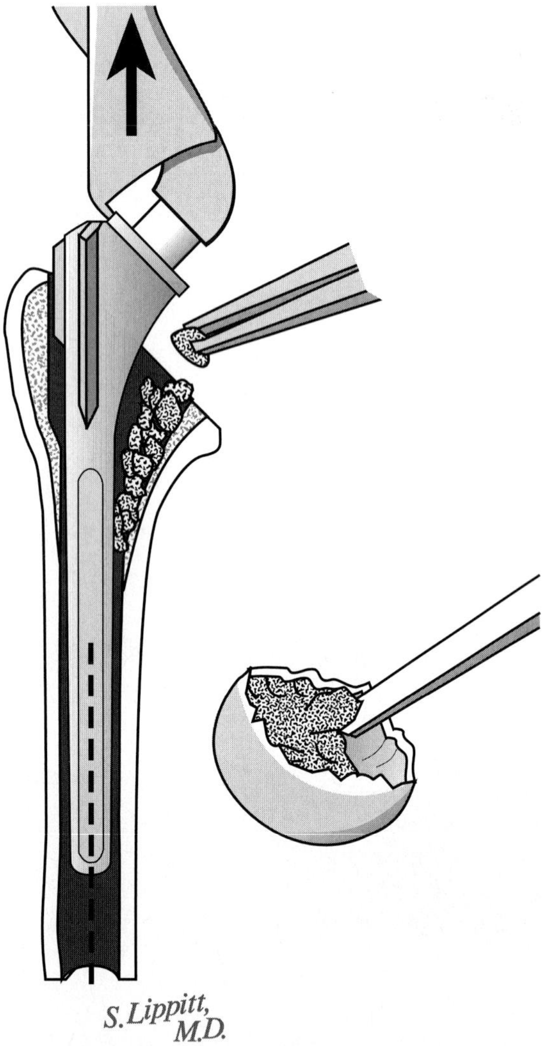


**Figure 27–61. Placing the graft**
Cancellous bone graft is harvested from the humeral head and impacted sequentially in the medullary canal to fill in the voids, to improve the fixation, and to correct any malorientation of the prosthetic body.

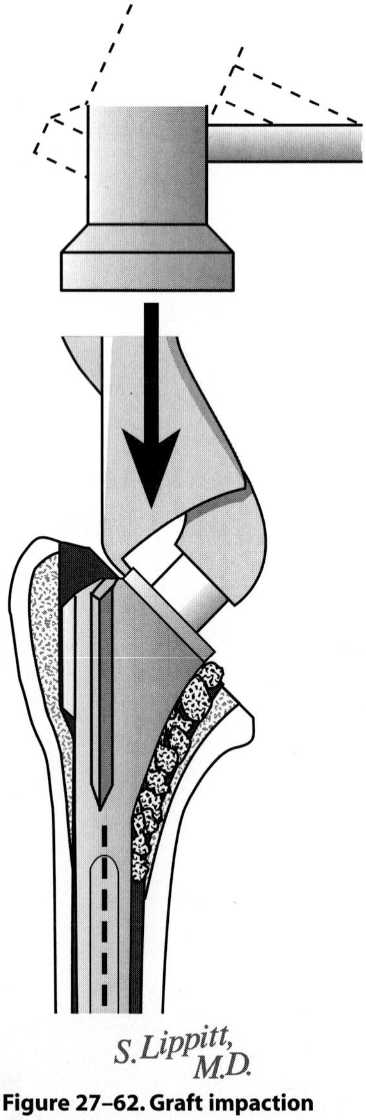


**Figure 27–62. Graft impaction**
Seating the impactor compresses the cancellous graft against the walls of the medullary canal.

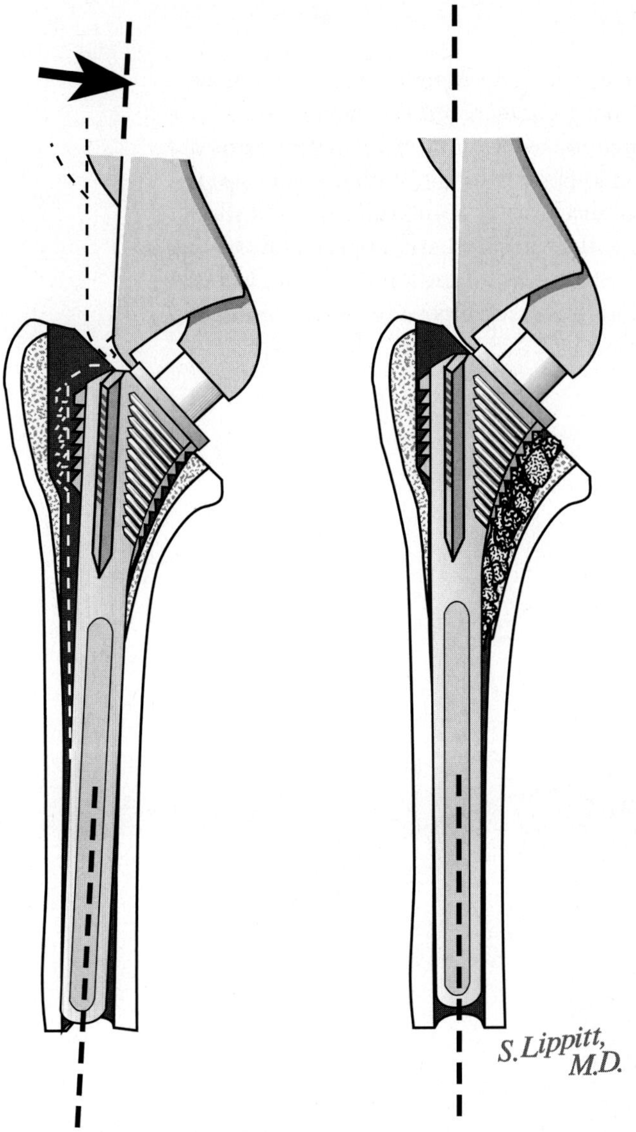


**Figure 27–63. Medial grafting**
Selective medial grafting can eliminate the tendency of the prosthesis to angulate into varus.

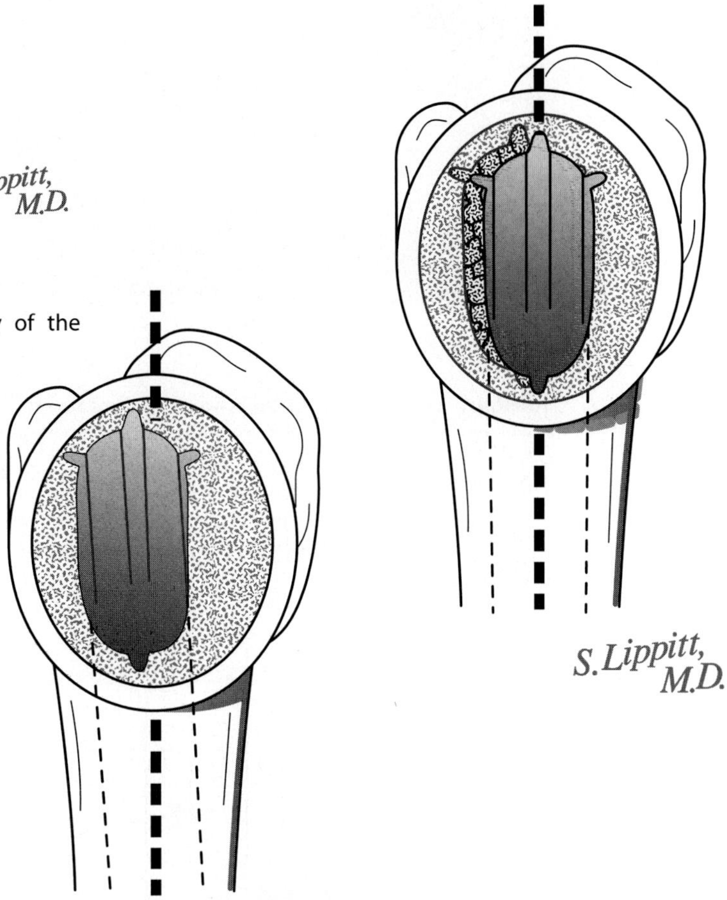


**Figure 27–64. Anterior grafting**
Selective anterior grafting can eliminate the apparent posterior offset of the neck related to anterior inclination of the prosthesis.

At this point in the procedure, the glenoid arthroplasty is performed. The considerations relevant to the glenoid are described in a separate section (Chapter 28).

Once the glenoid arthroplasty has been completed, trial humeral components are used to determine the optimal laxity of the reconstructed joint. With the final size trials in position, the glenohumeral joint should meet the 40, 50, 60 rule; that is, it should allow 40 degrees of external rotation with the subscapularis approximated (**Fig. 27–65**), 50 percent posterior subluxation of the humeral head on the glenoid on the posterior drawer with a spontaneous return to the centered position (**Fig. 27–66**), and

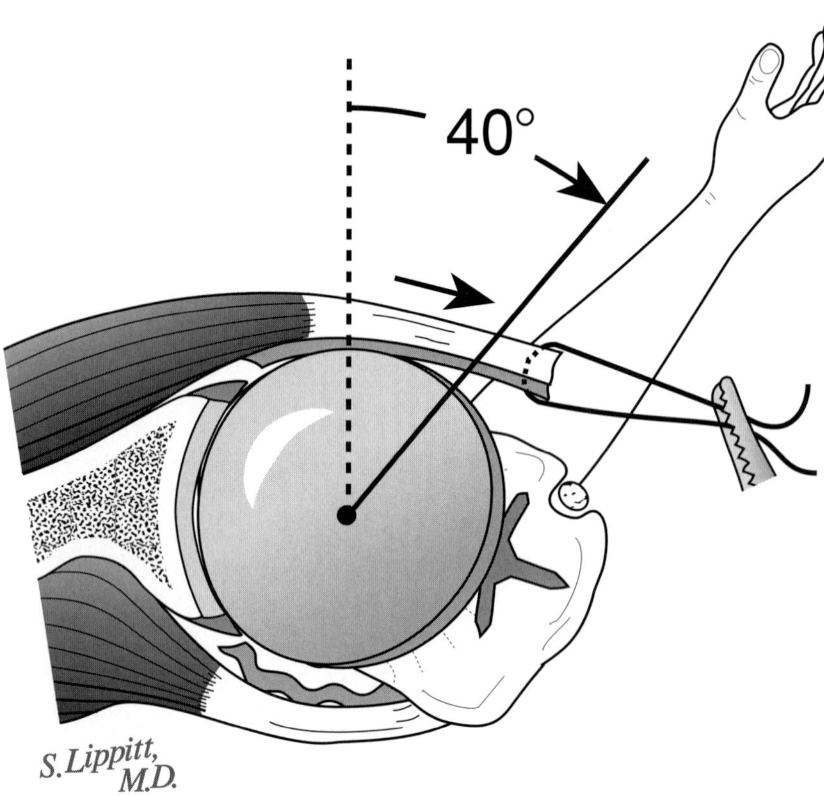


**Figure 27–65. 40, 50, 60 rule—external rotation**
Forty degrees of external rotation with the subscapularis approximated.

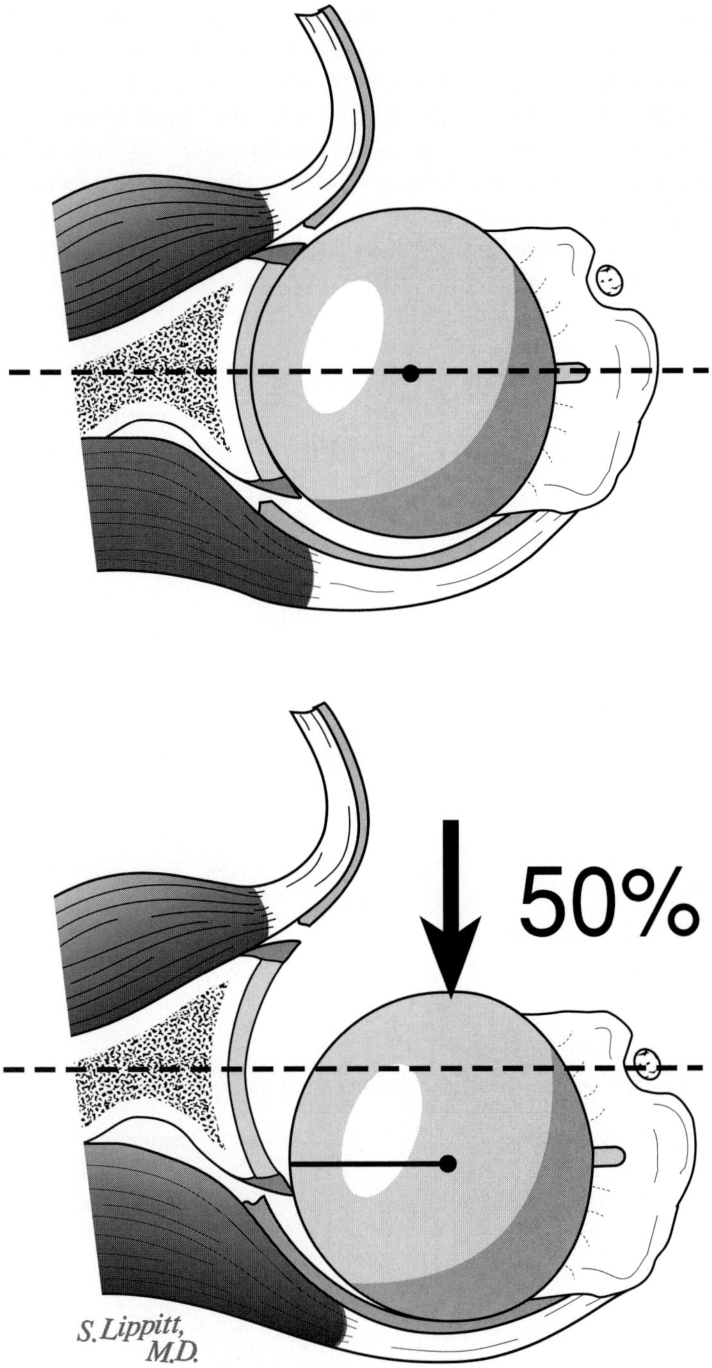


**Figure 27–66. 40, 50, 60 rule—posterior drawer**
Fifty percent posterior subluxation on the posterior drawer test.

60 degrees of internal rotation with the arm in 90 degrees of abduction (**Fig. 27–67**, and see Fig. 27–64). Excessive laxity may call for a prosthetic head with a higher spherical cap. Insufficient laxity may call for more soft tissue release or a shorter spherical cap. For example, lowering the height by 6 mm, from 21 to 15 mm for a head with a radius of 24, would increase the range of motion in *each direction* by 6/24ths or one-quarter radians. One radian is 360/2π or 57 degrees. One quarter radian is therefore about 14 degrees. An important goal is to have the humeral articular surface sit in proper register with the glenoid, so that its center line matches the glenoid center line in 45 degrees of humeral abduction and the humeral articular surface sits concentrically in the glenoid when the humerus is adducted (see Fig. 27–40). If the humeral surface is too high, it may need to be driven distally. If it is too low, it may need to be lifted by the insertion of additional cancellous bone graft in the medial humeral metaphyseal canal. The biceps tendon usually grazes the superior humeral articular surface but is not forced superiorly by it. The superior aspect of the humeral articular surface is usually about 5 mm higher than the greater tuberosity. Procrustean bone grafting allows the surgeon to make necessary modifications in component position prior to final insertion of the prosthesis. If the position and register are not perfect after the initial implantation, the component can be tapped back out, the graft placement modified, more graft added, and the prosthesis reinserted.

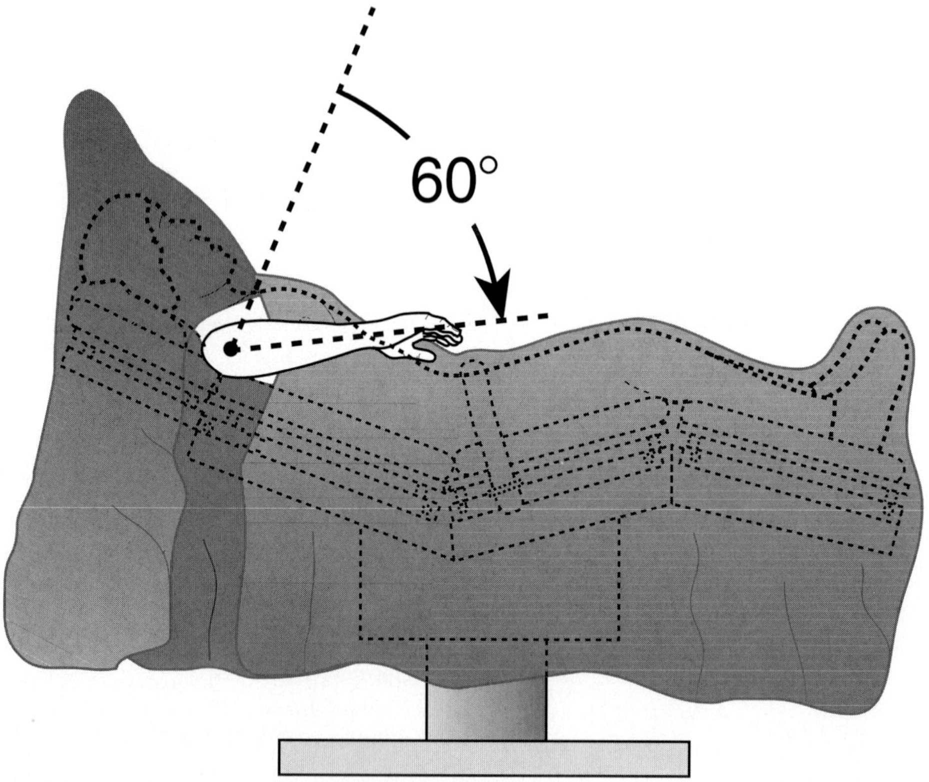


**Figure 27–67. 40, 50, 60 rule—internal rotation**
Sixty degrees of internal rotation of the arm adducted to 90 degrees.

CHAPTER 28

# Principles of Glenoid Arthroplasty

## CONCEPTS

The goal of glenohumeral arthroplasty is to distribute the net humeral joint reaction force evenly and broadly across the glenoid in a way that maintains the stability and mobility of the articulation. The normal glenoid accomplishes this objective using a surface that is relatively compliant, especially toward the periphery **(Fig. 28–1)**.

In reconstructing the glenoid surface, the surgeon has up to 10 variables to control. These include (1) the contact area, (2) the shape of the glenoid surface, (3, 4, and 5) the superoinferior, anteroposterior, and mediolateral positions of the glenoid relative to the scapula, (6 and 7) the superoinferior and anteroposterior tilts of the glenoid surface, (8) the position of the glenoid fossa relative to that of the humeral head, (9) the material on the glenoid articular surface, (10) the thickness of a component placed on the bony glenoid, and (11) the fixation of the glenoid component to bone.

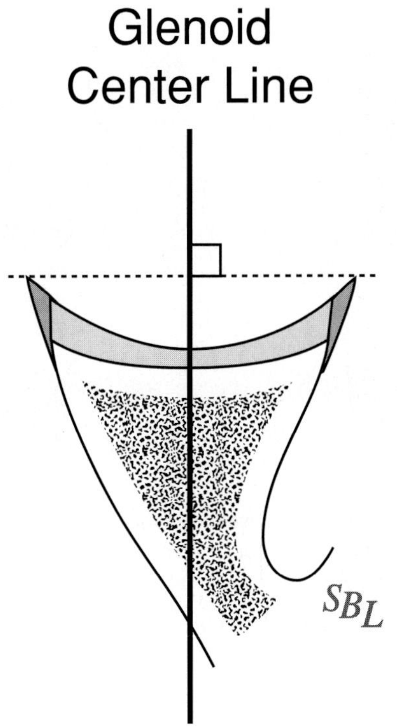


**Figure 28–1. Glenoid center line**
The normal biological glenoid is covered with compliant articular cartilage that is thicker toward its periphery. The edge of the glenoid is covered by even more compliant labrum. The glenoid center line is perpendicular to the center of the glenoid fossa.

## Contact Area

In the normal shoulder, the glenoid articular surface is characterized by its smoothness, its secure fixation to bone, its durability, its concavity (ideally shaped and oriented to provide stability), and its transmission of loads evenly to the underlying subchondral bone. In the arthritic shoulder, all of these characteristics are missing. The smooth cartilage is separated from bone and lost, the shape and orientation of the joint surface become distorted, and the subchondral bone becomes loaded in a nonuniform way **(Fig. 28–2)**. As a simple example, contrast two shoulders subjected to identical glenohumeral loads. In the first shoulder, normal cartilage distributes the load across a contact area with a radius of 10 mm. In the second osteoarthritic shoulder, the humeral head articulates with only part of the glenoid surface with a contact area of 5 mm. The pressure P(r) at a distance r from the center of the contact is $(3F/2\pi\, r_c^{\,2})(1 - r^2/\, r_c^{\,2})^{1/2}$; that is, the pressure is inversely related to the square of the radius of the contact area. Thus, diminishing the radius of the contact area by a factor of 2 increases the pressure by a factor of 4. Furthermore, in the second case there would be a steep pressure gradient between the loaded part of the glenoid and the unloaded part of the glenoid. Both the increased pressure and the increased pressure gradient may be implicated in the shoulder pain of osteoarthritis.

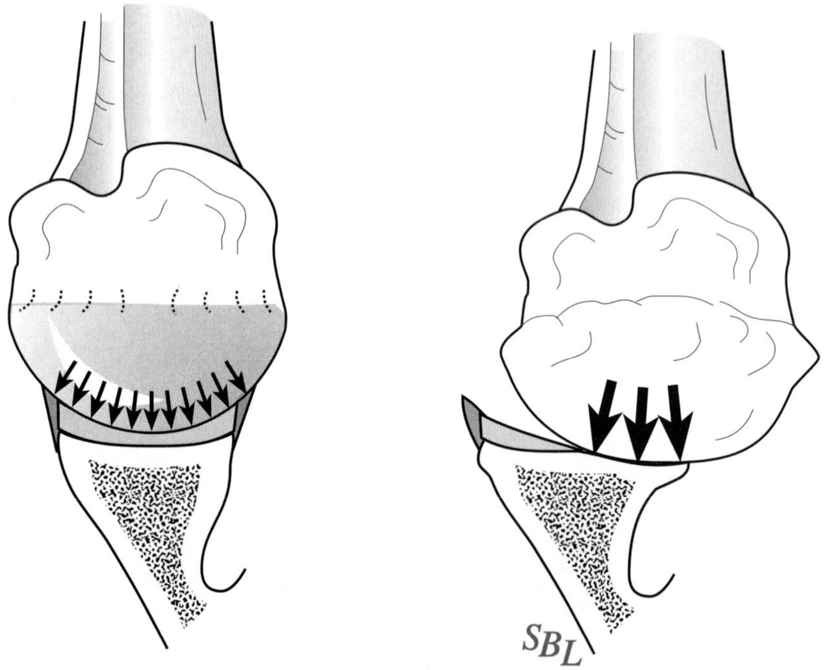


**Figure 28–2. Contact pressure**
In the osteoarthritic shoulder, the normally even distribution of the humeral load across the glenoid is lost. The area of contact becomes small and noncompliant, so the joint pressure, pressure gradient, and susceptibility of the unprotected bone to impact become greater.

## Shape of the Glenoid Surface

If a glenoid surface loses its original shape, the glenoidogram (**Fig. 28–3**), local stability ratios, and balance stability angles are changed (**Fig. 28–4**). If the glenoid pathology is allowed to remain, so will the abnormalities of load distribution and stability (**Fig. 28–5**). Burring down the crest between the normal and pathologic glenoid concavities leaves a retroverted fossa with a diameter of curvature larger than that of the corre-

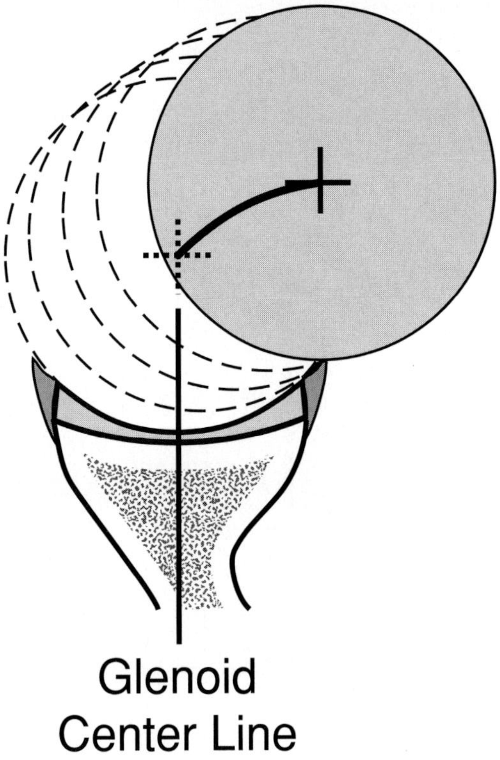


**Figure 28–3. Glenoidogram**
The functional shape of the glenoid surface in a given direction is best characterized by the glenoidogram: the path taken by the head of the humerus as it passes from the center of the glenoid over its rim in that direction. (Modified from Matsen FA, Lippitt SB, Sidles JA, et al [eds]: Practical Evaluation and Management of the Shoulder. Philadelphia: WB Saunders, 1994, p. 66.)

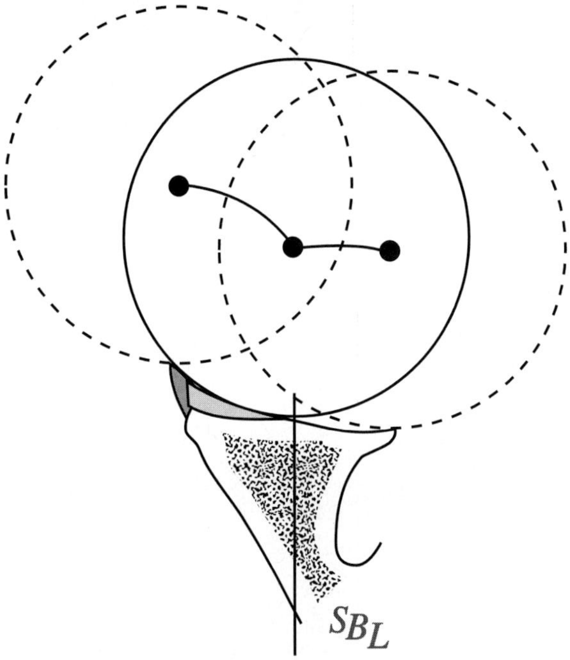


**Figure 28–4. Glenoidogram with posterior erosion**
The normal glenoid concavity creates a glenoidogram that rises dramatically as the humeral head is translated from the center (left half of the curve). When the glenoid is flattened, this rise is lost, indicating a loss of intrinsic stability of the glenoid (right half of the curve).

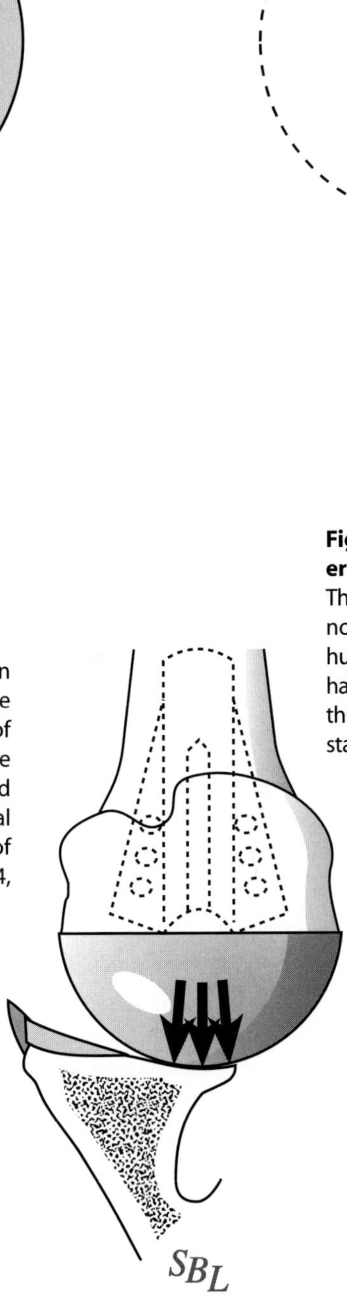


**Figure 28–5. Biconcave glenoid**
Unless the glenoid pathology is addressed at the time of shoulder arthroplasty, the prosthetic humeral head will sit in the abnormal part of the glenoid.

sponding humeral head (**Fig. 28–6**); it does not restore glenoid shape and orientation. Glenoid arthroplasty provides the opportunity to restore the shape, orientation, and stability of the glenoid. The stability is affected by the curvature of the glenoid relative to that of the humeral head (**Figs. 28–7** and **28–8**). If a prosthetic glenoid surface becomes deformed, its stability can be affected as well (**Fig. 28–9**).

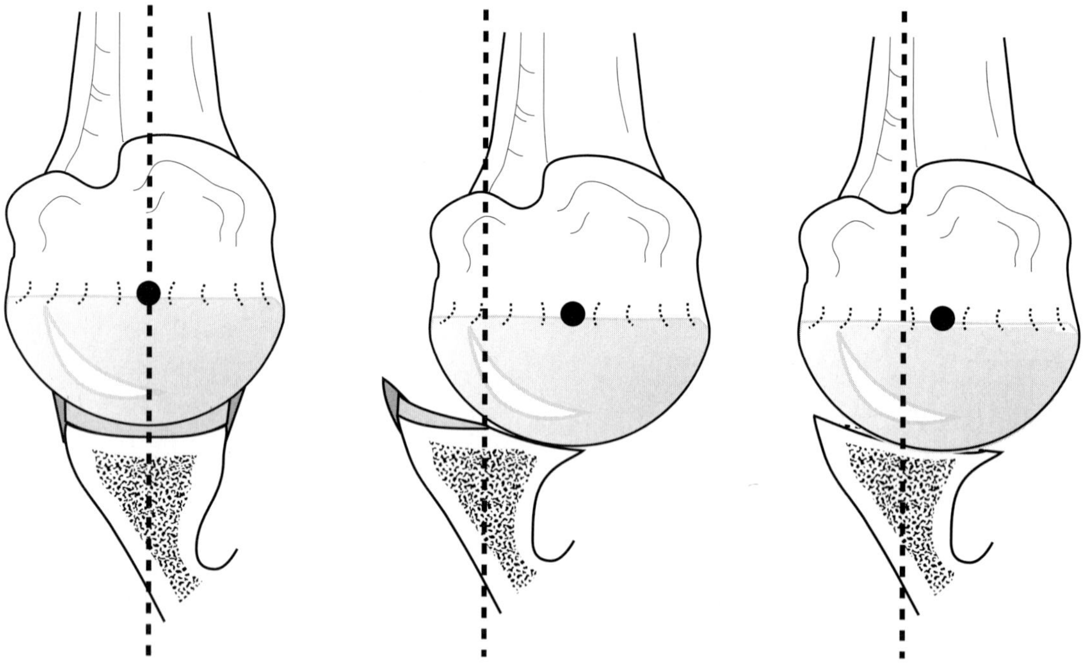

**Figure 28–6. Burring the biconcave glenoid**
Burring down the crest between the normal and abnormal glenoid concavities alone does not restore the glenoid shape or orientation.

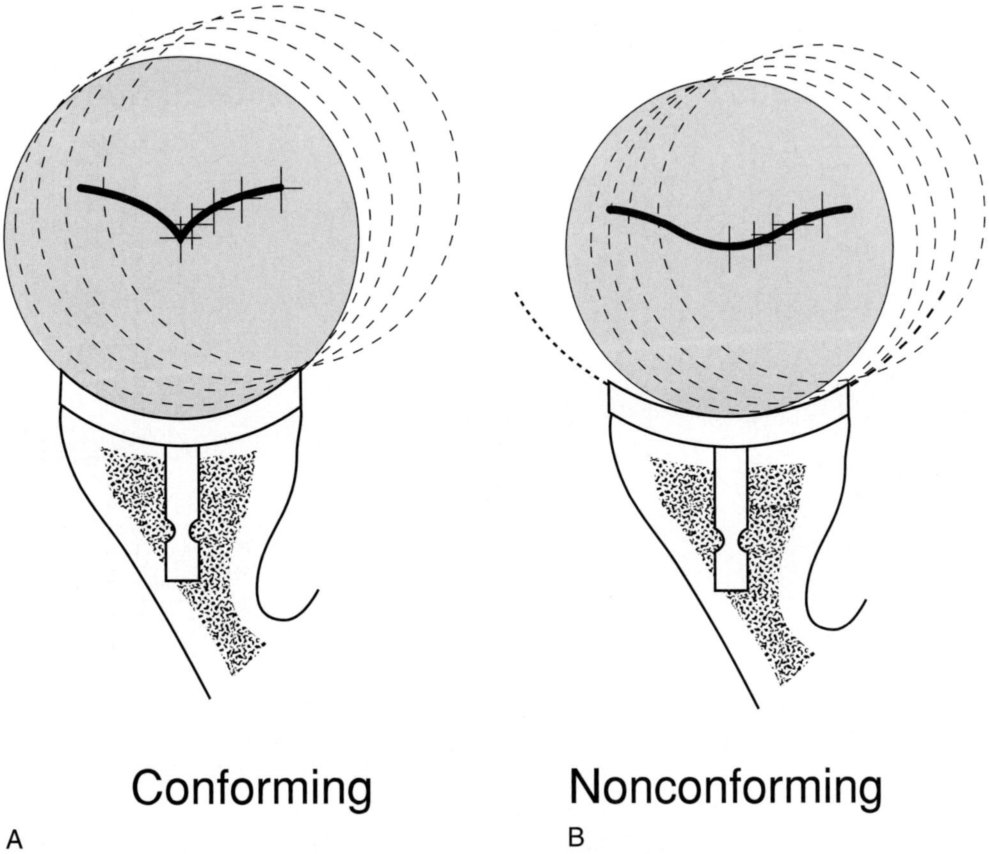


**Figure 28–7. Conforming and noncomforming glenoidograms**

Glenoid arthroplasty offers the opportunity to restore the concavity, orientation, and stability of the glenoid surface. On the left is shown the glenoidogram for a conforming set of glenohumeral joint surfaces. Each of the two convex halves of the glenoidogram has a radius equal to that of the humeral head and each half is centered on the respective glenoid edge. In this situation, the steepest part of each half of the glenoidogram is where the humeral head just begins to leave the center of the glenoid. On the right is shown the glenoidogram for a glenoid surface with a radius of curvature slightly greater than that of the humeral head. In this situation, each of the convex parts of the glenoidogram describes a curve centered on the glenoid edge with a radius equal to that of the humeral head. These two convex parts are connected by a concave segment with a radius equal to the difference between the glenoid and the humeral radius of curvature. The stability against translation in each direction is maximal where the glenoidogram is steepest—a short distance from the glenoid center. This configuration allows some translation of the humeral head in the "well" of the glenoid. (Modified from Matsen FA, Lippitt SB, Sidles JA, et al [eds]: Practical Evaluation and Management of the Shoulder. Philadelphia: WB Saunders, 1994, p. 193.)

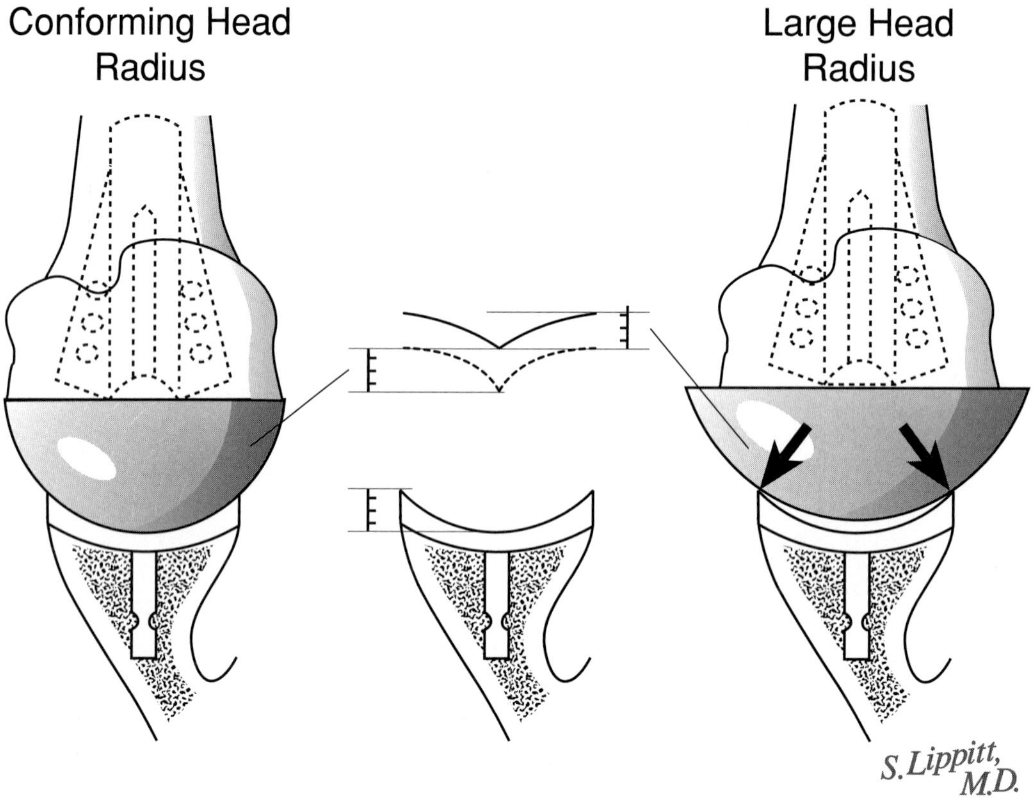


**Figure 28–8. Oversized humeral head**
When the humeral head radius of curvature is larger than that of the glenoid (*right*), the head does not sit fully down in the glenoid; as a result, the height of the glenoidogram is less than the depth of the glenoid concavity. The result is a diminished value for the maximal stability ratio and the balance stability angle, in contrast to the situation in which the glenoid and humeral radii are matching (*left*).

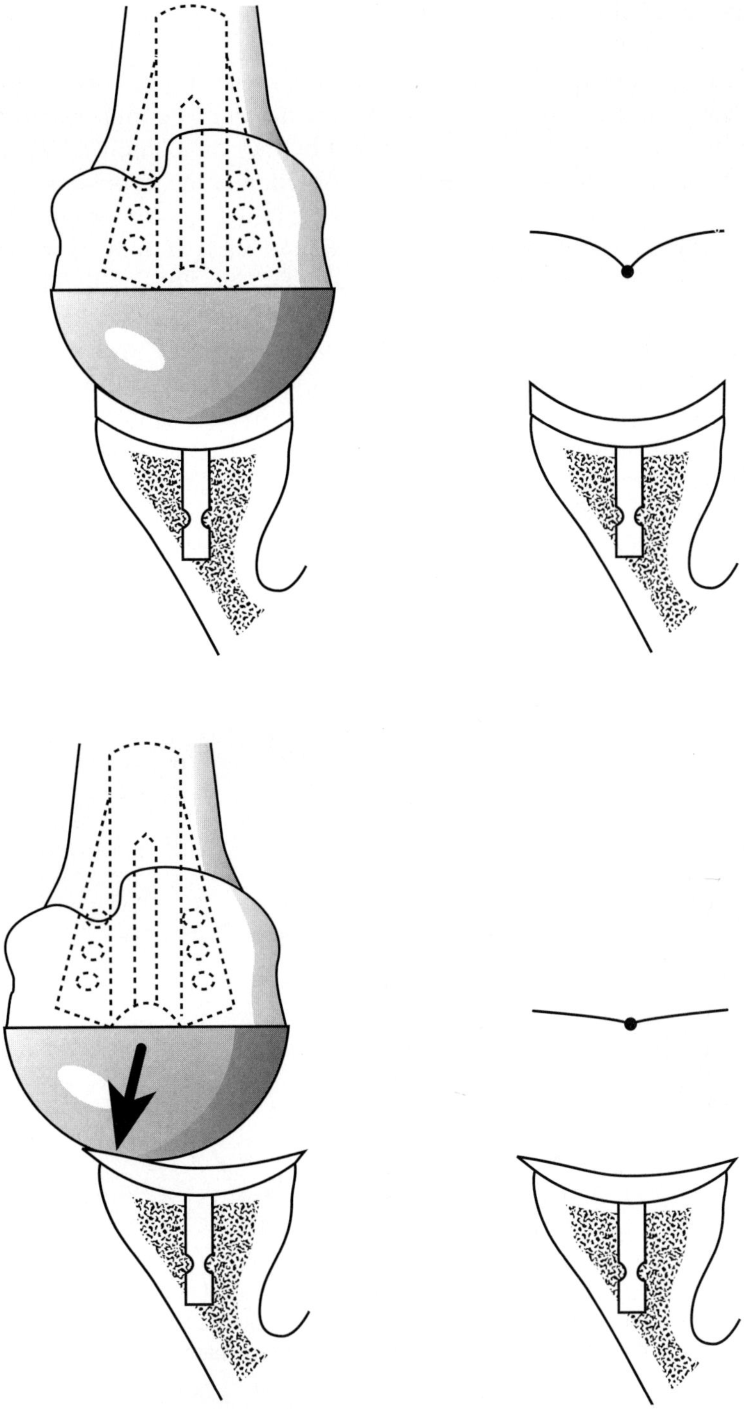

**Figure 28–9. Worn glenoid lips**

In comparison to the situation with the intact glenoid (*top*), cold flow or edge wear can result in loss of the glenoid depth, increased shallowness of the glenoidogram, and loss of intrinsic glenoid stability (*bottom*).

## Orientation of the Glenoid Surface

The characteristics of the glenoid surface must be related to its orientation on the scapula. It is apparent that the direction of the net humeral joint reaction force is determined in large part by the force exerted by the scapulohumeral muscles, particularly the rotator cuff and the deltoid. The direction of the scapulohumeral muscle force vectors is determined by the origin of these muscles on the scapula in relation to their insertion on the humerus. The direction of these vectors is independent of the glenoid surface orientation on the scapula (**Fig. 28–10**). For the glenohumeral joint to be stable, the glenoid articular surface needs to be oriented so that this net humeral joint reaction force falls within the balance stability angles of the glenoid surface. As an example, consider a glenoid with anterior and posterior balance stability angles each equal to 20 degrees (i.e., the net humeral joint reaction force can deviate 20 degrees anterior or posterior to the glenoid center line without instability). If this component is placed in an anatomical orientation, the normal relationship between the muscle force vectors and the glenoid center line are respected. If, however, the glenoid component is placed in 20 degrees of retroversion, the usual net

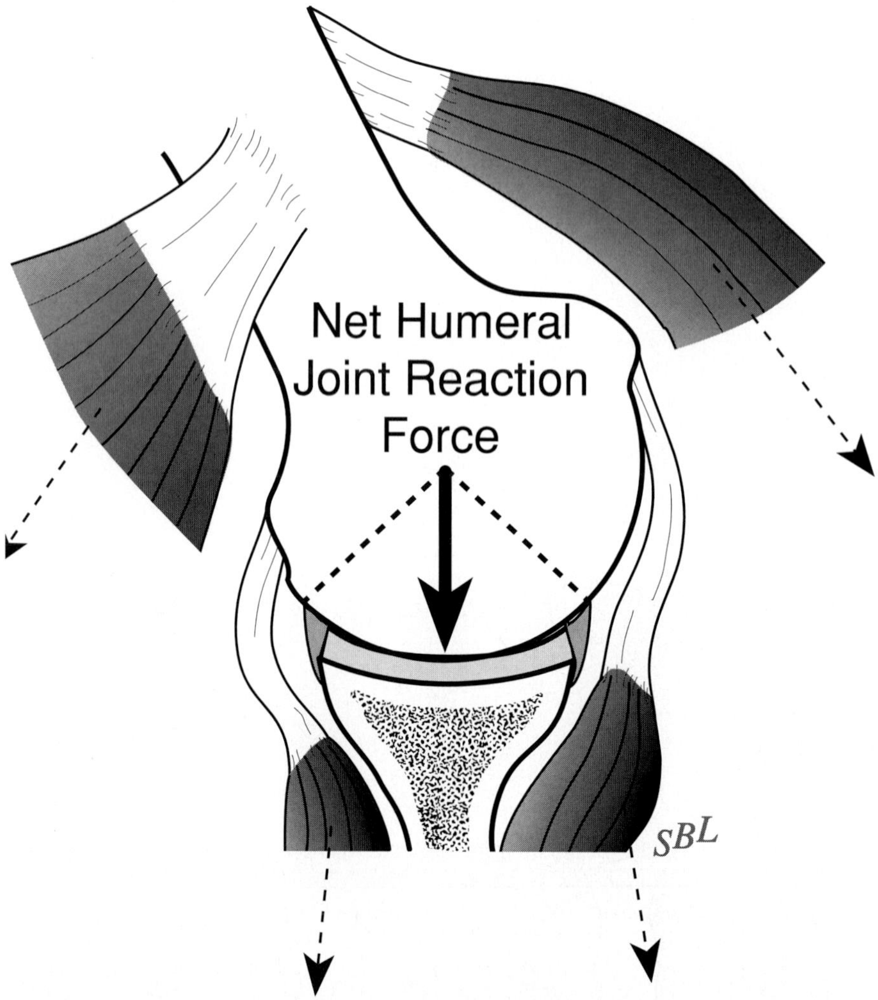


**Figure 28–10. Balanced net forces**
The direction of the forces exerted by the scapulohumeral muscles is determined by their effective attachments to the scapula and humerus. These vectors are independent of the orientation of the glenoid surface on the scapula. (Modified from Matsen FA, Lippitt SB, Sidles JA, et al [eds]: Practical Evaluation and Management of the Shoulder. Philadelphia: WB Saunders, 1994, p. 64.)

humeral joint reaction force will be on the brink of dislocation (**Fig. 28–11**). This analysis suggests the response to the often asked question, "Why can't the surgeon accommodate instability due to glenoid retroversion by humeral anteversion?" The answer is that changing the humeral component version has little effect on the direction of the net humeral joint reaction force, so the adverse effects of glenoid malversion are not accommodated and the glenohumeral joint remains unstable.

For these reasons, the surgeon needs to orient the glenoid concavity with relation to the scapular body. With the patient supine on the operating table, the glenoid center line is usually 20 degrees anterior to the coronal plane (**Fig. 28–12**). Because the plane

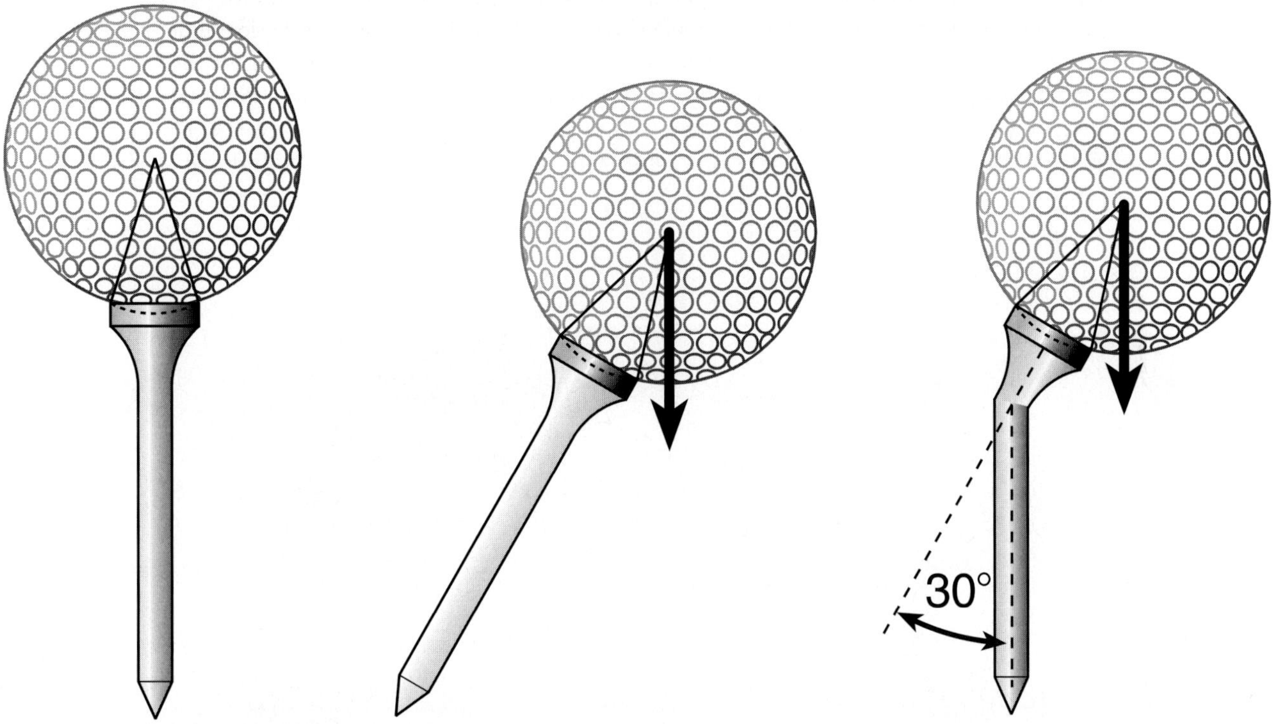


**Figure 28–11. Golf tee analogy**
A golf ball is stabilized in a golf tee when its gravitational force vector passes through the tee (*left*). When the tee is tipped substantially, the force vector passes outside the tee and the ball falls off. Such tipping may occur if the tee is put in the ground in an angled position (*center*) or if the tee is bent (*right*). These situations are analogous to abnormal position and abnormal version, respectively, of the glenoid face.

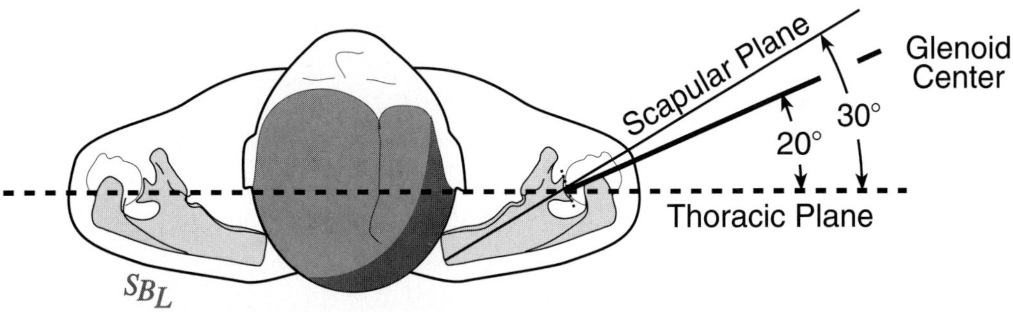


**Figure 28–12. Scapular plane and thoracic plane**
The scapular plane is usually directed about 30 degrees anterior to the thoracic plane. The glenoid center line usually points 10 degrees posterior to the scapular plane. As a result, the glenoid center line characteristically points 20 degrees anterior to the thoracic plane.

of the scapula cannot be rigorously determined at surgery, and because the direction of the glenoid may be distorted (see Fig. 28–2), the normal direction of the glenoid center line can be approximated by reestablishing a glenoid center line as the line connecting the center of the glenoid face to the centering point on the glenoid neck in the subscapularis fossa (**Fig. 28–13**). This line can be drilled (**Fig. 28–14**) and used as a guide for normalizing the glenoid version (**Fig. 28–15**).

### Position of the Glenoid Fossa Relative to that of the Humeral Head

Diminished glenohumeral contact can also result from improper register of the humeral and glenoid articular surfaces (see Figs. 27–39 and 27–40). For example, if the center of the glenoid articular surface is lower than the center of rotation of the humeral head, the humeral articular surface will not seat fully in the glenoid fossa, resulting in an abnormally flat glenoidogram and diminished stability ratios. Furthermore, the glenohumeral contact will be on the glenoid rim, leading to diminished contact area, increased local contact pressure, and rim wear.

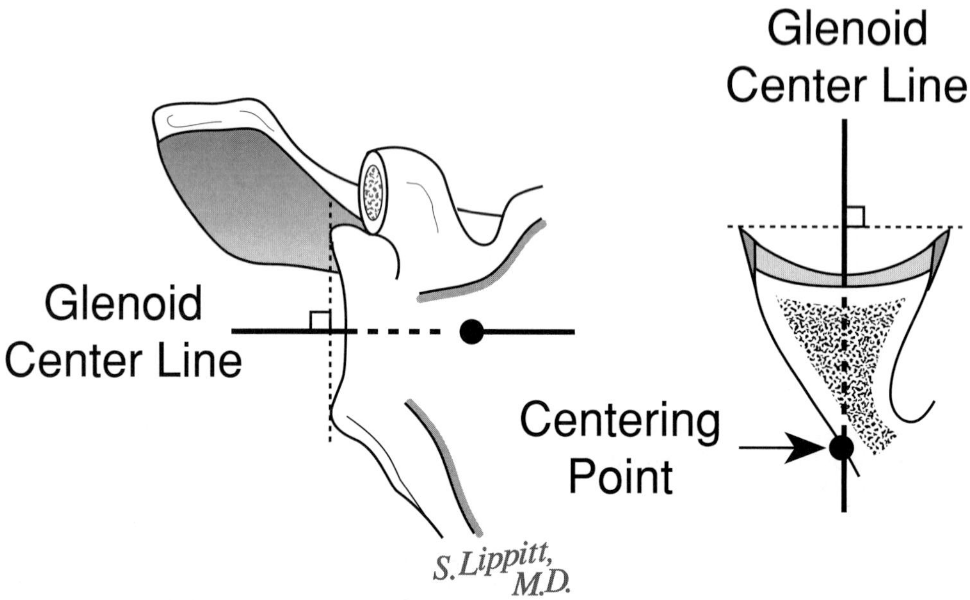


**Figure 28–13. Glenoid centering point**
The normal glenoid center line can be approximated by a line connecting the center of the glenoid face to the centering point in the middle of the anterior neck of the glenoid.

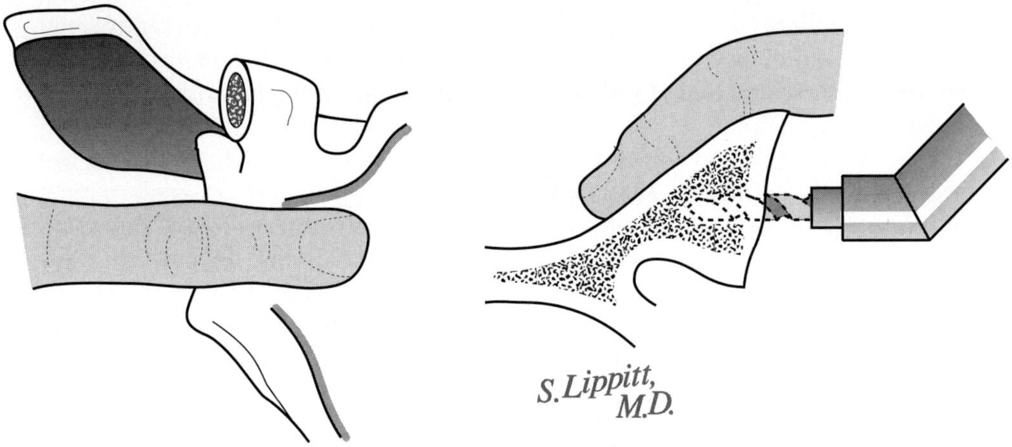


**Figure 28–14. Locating the centering point**
The centering point can be located by palpation with the index finger. The normalized glenoid center line can then be drilled. (Modified from Matsen FA, Lippitt SB, Sidles JA, et al [eds]: Practical Evaluation and Management of the Shoulder. Philadelphia: WB Saunders, 1994, p. 210.)

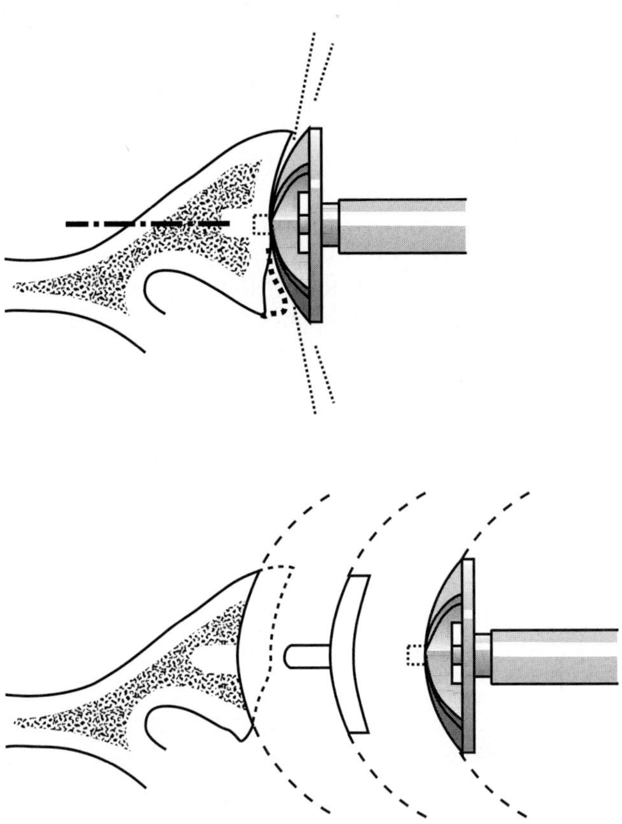

A

B

**Figure 28–15. Glenoid reaming**
Reaming along the normalized glenoid center line normalizes the glenoid version. (Modified from Matsen FA, Lippitt SB, Sidles JA, et al [eds]: Practical Evaluation and Management of the Shoulder. Philadelphia: WB Saunders, 1994, p. 211.)

### Material for the Glenoid Surface

In addition to providing stabilizing orientation and geometry, the surface of the glenoid transfers the humeral joint reaction force to the bone of the glenoid. Because bone is innervated, it is likely that optimizing the distribution of these loads is a major factor in maintaining a painless articulation. Normal articular cartilage is not stiff but rather is compliant enough that the humeral load is distributed across the entire joint surface. One way of quantitating the stiffness is in terms of Young's modulus. Although published values vary, **Table 28–1** lists some approximate values for Young's modulus (in gigaPascals [GPa], or $10^9$ Newtons per meter squared).

It can be seen that cartilage is remarkable in its compliance. When cartilage is lost from a glenoid joint surface, a number of bad things happen. First, the conformity of the joint surfaces is lost, and second, the compliance of the cartilage is lost. As a result, the distribution of the load is transformed from the normal situation, in which compliant cartilage distributes the load evenly over the entire glenoid bone surface, to the abnormal situation, in which the load is concentrated on a much smaller area of noncompliant subchondral cortical bone. The result is a high, and probably painful, loading of a small area of bone (see Fig. 28–2).

The issue of surface stiffness is particularly important when we consider the situation in which the humeral surface radius of curvature is smaller than that of the glenoid, as is the case for many hemiarthroplasties and glenohumeral arthroplasties. To help us get a feeling for these relationships, we can turn to the 1986 book by Landau and Lifshitz on the theory of elasticity. Their equations 9.10–13 enable us to estimate the radius of the contact area, $r_c$, between two surfaces, the humeral head (of radius $R_H$) and the glenoid (of radius $R_G$) pressed together by a force, F, from

$$r_c = ((3F(1\text{-}s^2)\ R_G\ R_H)/(4E(R_G - R_H)))^{1/3}$$

where *E* is Young's modulus and *s* is Poisson's ratio (which is a measure of how much thinner a material gets when you pull on it—think of chewing gum having a high Poisson's ratio). Poisson's ratio is about 0.3 for most materials that we encounter in orthopaedics. Note that the radius of the contact area increases dramatically as the radius of the humeral head approaches that of the glenoid. Note also that as the glenoid surface becomes less stiff (Young's modulus gets smaller), the contact area increases. The result is intuitive: a surgeon can increase contact area by increasing the congruence of the joint surfaces and/or by increasing the compliance of the glenoid joint surface (**Fig. 28–16**).

If the humerus translates so that it contacts the glenoid rim, the contact area drops dramatically (**Fig. 28–17**), with a correspondingly dramatic increase in contact pressure. In the case of a polyethylene glenoid arthroplasty, this increase in contact area would substantially increase the risk of cold flow and wear. Thus, in polyethylene glenoid arthroplasty, the surgeon must minimize the risk of rim contact (which would argue for a radial mismatch) on one hand and maximize contact area (which would argue for no radial mismatch) on the other.

**Table 28–1**

**Approximate Values for Young's Modulus***

| Material | Young's Modulus (GPa) |
|---|---|
| Cartilage | 0.001 |
| Polyethylene | 0.2 |
| Cancellous bone | 1 |
| Cortical bone | 13 |
| Steel | 200 |

*Modulus in GigaPascals (Gpa), or $10^9$ Newtons per meter squared.

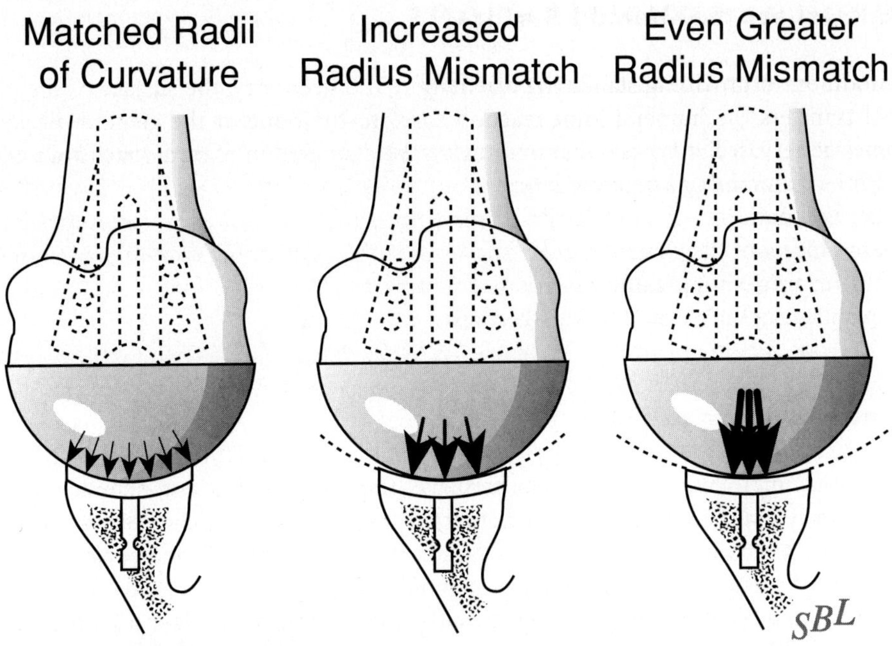


**Figure 28–16. Diameter mismatch**
With greater degrees of mismatch between the radius of curvature of the glenoid and that of the humeral head, there is a decreased contact area, increased contact pressure, and increased pressure gradient between the loaded and unloaded polyethylene. (Modified from Matsen FA, Lippitt SB, Sidles JA, et al [eds]: Practical Evaluation and Management of the Shoulder. Philadelphia: WB Saunders, 1994, p. 191.)

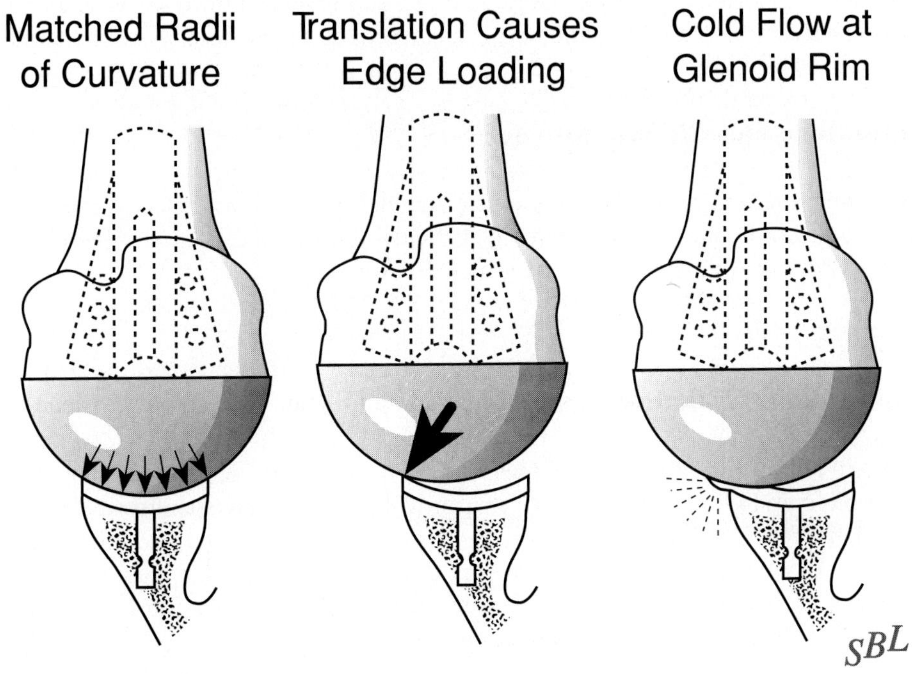


**Figure 28–17. Glenoid rim load**
If the humeral head translates from the center to a position where it is up on the glenoid rim, the contact area becomes very small (including only the sharp edge of the polyethylene) so that the contact pressure becomes very high, risking polyethylene cold flow and wear. (Modified from Matsen FA, Lippitt SB, Sidles JA, et al [eds]: Practical Evaluation and Management of the Shoulder. Philadelphia: WB Saunders, 1994, p. 191.)

## SURGICAL CONSIDERATIONS

### Details of the Glenoid Arthroplasty

There are at least five types of glenoid surface encountered in shoulder arthroplasty:
1. Preserving intact glenoid cartilage
2. Leaving damaged glenoid cartilage unmodified
3. Smoothing of the glenoid surface
4. Performing a nonprosthetic glenoid arthroplasty
5. Resurfacing the glenoid with a prosthesis

### Intact Glenoid Cartilage

In the face of totally intact glenoid cartilage, the load bearing and stability of the arthroplasty can be optimized by a humeral prosthesis that matches or just slightly exceeds that of the biological humeral head. An undersized humeral prosthesis will preferentially load the hard center of the glenoid while a slightly oversized one will load the more compliant periphery of the glenoid—the labrum and thicker peripheral cartilage. For this reason, retention of the labrum is important and all capsular releases should be performed extralabrally.

### Leaving Damaged Glenoid Cartilage Unmodified

If a glenoid loses its cartilage, the diameter of the bony concavity is greater than that of the original concavity, and the surface is irregular (see Fig. 28–2). Replacing the humeral head with a metal prosthesis without changing the glenoid contour does not change the abnormal loading of the glenoid (see Fig. 28–5). Abnormalities of glenoid version and any resulting instability are not corrected if the glenoid is left unaltered.

### Smoothing the Glenoid Surface

Removing residual cartilage and removing irregularities (such as the crest in between the two glenoid concavities) flattens the articular surface and decreases the contact area between the humeral head and the glenoid. Abnormalities of glenoid version and any resulting instability are not corrected (see Fig. 28–6).

### Nonprosthetic Glenoid Arthroplasty

The goal of this procedure (see Chapter 30) is to take an arthritic glenoid and reestablish a biological glenoid joint surface that provides appropriate stability and contact area. This is accomplished by optimizing (1) the glenoid orientation, (2) the glenoid diameter of curvature that will produce the desired stability, (3) the diameter of curvature of the humeral component relative to that of the glenoid, and (4) the relative positions of the humeral and glenoid components.

*Orientation*

The osteoarthritic glenoid surface is usually retroverted and biconcave **(Fig. 28–18)**. The new glenoid articular surface needs to be oriented with respect to the normal glenoid center line so that it will have the optimal relationship to the force vectors of the scapulohumeral muscles. The glenoid center line is the line connecting the center of the glenoid face with the centering point in the middle of the glenoid neck as it joins with the subscapularis fossa **(Fig. 28–19)**. The centering point can be identified by palpation of the glenoid neck. When the glenoid is eroded posteriorly (e.g., in osteoarthri-

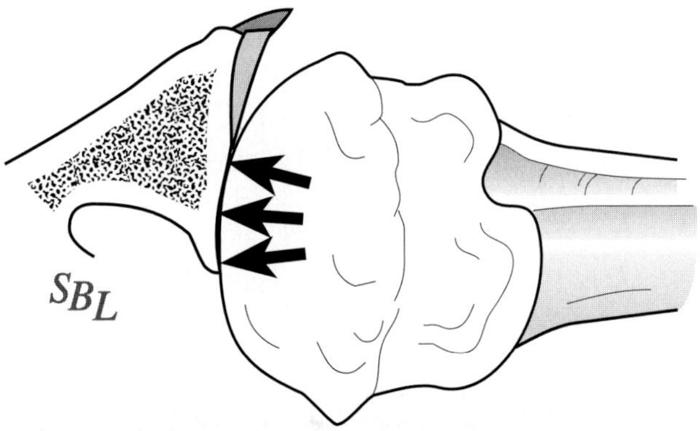


**Figure 28–18. Osteoarthritic glenoid surface**
A glenoid configuration that is typical of osteoarthritis or capsulorrhaphy arthropathy.

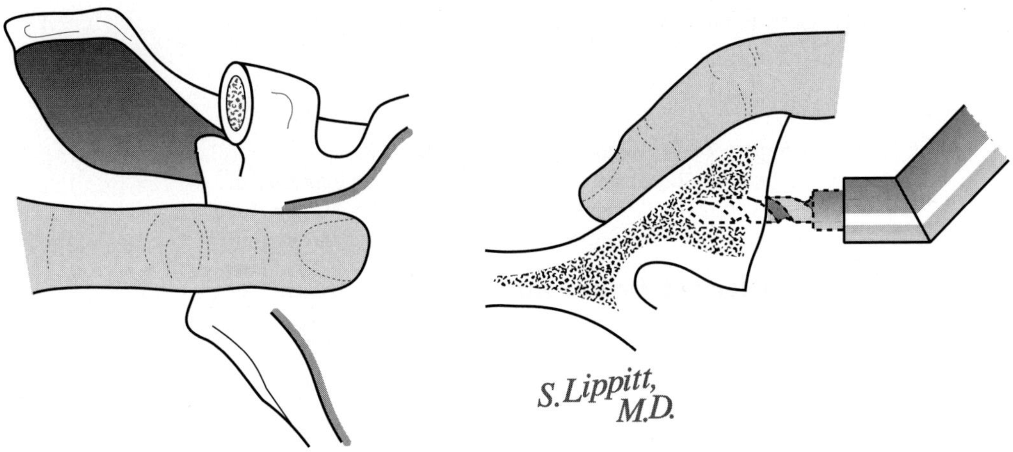


**Figure 28–19. Glenoid center line**
The normalized glenoid center line is identified and drilled. (Modified from Matsen FA, Lippitt SB, Sidles JA, et al [eds]: Practical Evaluation and Management of the Shoulder. Philadelphia: WB Saunders, 1994, p. 210.)

tis of capsulorrhaphy arthropathy), the anteroposterior position of the center of the glenoid face must be extrapolated from cues such as the preserved anterior glenoid rim. Once the center of the normal glenoid face and the centering point in the subscapularis fossa are identified, the glenoid center line is drilled to orient the reamers. Because it is difficult to alter the center line once it has been drilled, considerable care is applied to selecting its position and orientation (**Figs. 28–20** and **28–21**).

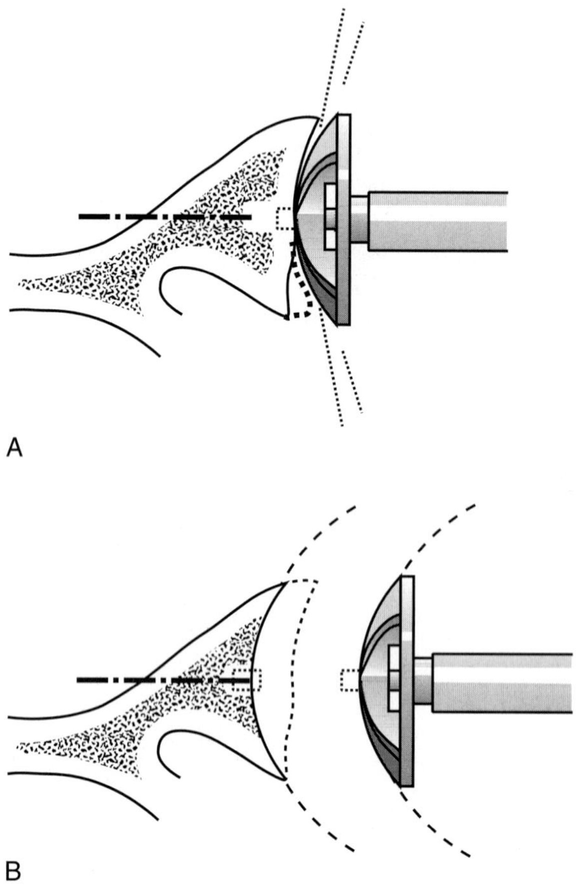


**Figure 28–20. Reaming of glenoid bone**
The glenoid bone is reamed to the desired diameter of curvature and orientation. (Modified from Matsen FA, Lippitt SB, Sidles JA, et al [eds]: Practical Evaluation and Management of the Shoulder. Philadelphia: WB Saunders, 1994, p. 211.)

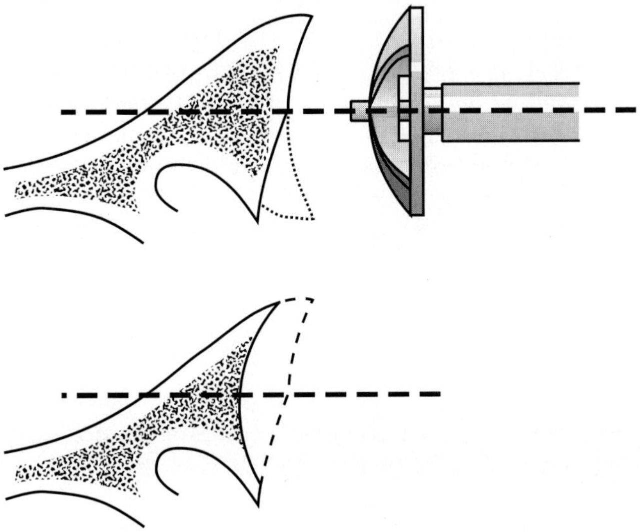

A

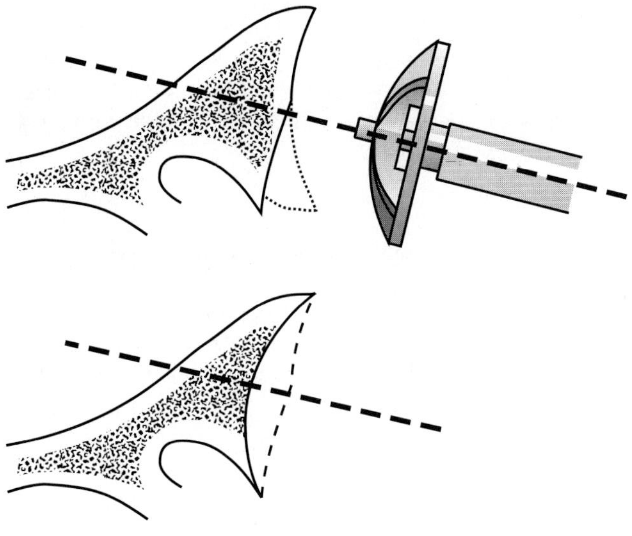

B

**Figure 28–21. Glenoid reaming with posterior deficiency**
**A,** It is important that there is sufficient bone stock to provide an adequate posterior and anterior glenoid concavity after reaming. **B,** When there is insufficient bone stock posteriorly, an adequate posterior concavity cannot be achieved and there is a risk of posterior instability if the glenoid is reamed in retroversion. In this situation, it may be preferable to convert to a prosthetic glenoid arthroplasty in an attempt to augment the effective posterior concavity.

### *Glenoid Diameter of Curvature Relative to the Size of the Bony Glenoid*

The maximal angle that the net humeral joint reaction force can make with the glenoid center line before dislocation occurs is the balance stability angle (**Fig. 28–22**). Ideally, the shape of the glenoid articular surface will provide balance stability angles of at least 20 degrees in each direction. If the glenoid surface has a radius curvature of R and the width from the glenoid center line to the glenoid lip is W, the sine of the balance stability angle is W/R, or, if we know the effective width and the radius, the balance stability angle is the arc sine of W/R (see Fig. 28–22). This analysis demonstrates why it is necessary to have reamers of differing diameters of curvature for nonprosthetic glenoid arthroplasty. The spherical reamer commonly used with prosthetic glenoid arthroplasty has a diameter of curvature of 60 mm. If such a reamer is used on a glenoid with a width of 7 mm, the resulting nonprosthetic glenoid arthroplasty would provide anterior and posterior balance stability angles of only 57.3 × 7 mm/30 or 13 degrees: less than the desired 20 degrees. A glenoid this narrow would require a reamer with a diameter of 40 mm to offer the desired 20-degree balance stability angle in a nonprosthetic glenoid arthroplasty.

### *Diameter of Curvature of the Humeral Component Relative to that of the Glenoid*

Since this procedure places a metal prosthetic head in contact with reamed cancellous bone, and since cancellous bone is much stiffer than polyethylene, a closer match between the diameters of curvature of the humerus and glenoid is necessary to achieve contact areas similar to those of prosthetic glenoid arthroplasties. In prosthetic glenoid arthroplasty, the glenoid diameter of curvature is commonly 6 mm greater than that of the humerus. In nonprosthetic glenoid arthroplasty, we have used a 2 mm diametral mismatch; that is, a 48 mm diameter humeral head is paired with a bony glenoid reamed to a diameter of curvature of 50 mm (**Fig. 28–23**). This is because bone is substantially stiffer than polyethylene (Young's modulus is 13 GPa for cortical bone, 1 GPa for cancellous bone, and only 0.2 GPa for polyethylene), so that a smaller degree of mismatch is necessary to achieve reasonable contact areas when a humeral prosthesis articolates with bone.

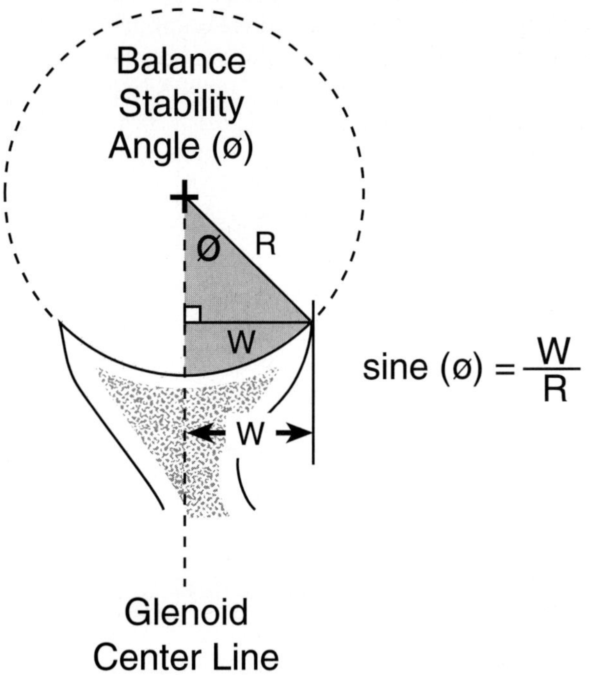


**Figure 28–22. Calculating the balance stability angle**

The predicted balance stability angle in a specified direction for a spherical glenoid is given by the arc sine of the ratio of the glenoid width in the direction of interest (the distance from the glenoid center to the reamed edge) and the radius of curvature for the reamed glenoid. BSA = arc sin W/R. Since for small angles (less than 30 degrees, for example), the sine and the tangent are about equal and since for small angles (again less than 30 degrees) the tangent is approximately equal to the angle expressed in radians, and recalling that a radian is approximately 57.3 degrees, we come up with the convenient rule of thumb that the balance stability angle in degrees is about 57.3 × W/R. For a normally directed glenoid concavity, the desired stability angle is at least 20 degrees. So if the glenoid width from the center to the edge is W, the reamed radius should be less than three times the width (20 = 57.3 × W/R or R = 3 × W) or the diameter should be less than six times the width from the center to the edge. Thus, a glenoid with a width of 10 mm would have the desired intrinsic stability if it were reamed to a properly oriented concavity with a diameter of less than 60 mm, whereas a glenoid with a width of 7 mm would need to be reamed to a diameter of less than 42 mm.

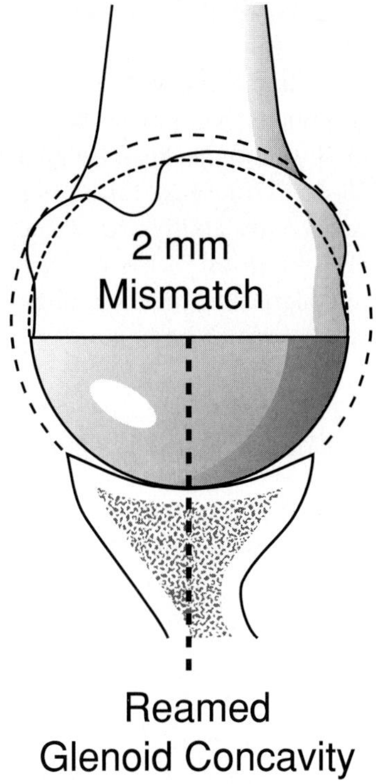


**Figure 28–23. Mismatch for nonprosthetic arthroplasty**

For nonprosthetic glenoid arthroplasty, we usually select a humeral head diameter of curvature that is 2 mm smaller than the glenoid that will articulate with it. In this situation, we choose a smaller amount of mismatch than the 6 mm mismatch we use with a prosthetic arthroplasty because of the fact that reamed bone is less compliant than polyethylene. Thus, to achieve a larger contact area, a smaller amount of mismatch is needed.

### *Relative Position of the Humeral and Glenoid Articular Surfaces*

Because the reamed bony glenoid is less compliant than polyethylene and much less compliant than normal articular cartilage, it is important that the center of curvature of the humeral head be aligned with the center of the reamed glenoid fossa (**Fig. 28–24**). Otherwise, the humeral component will not be fully seated in the glenoid concavity and stability and contact area will be compromised. If, after glenoid reaming and after insertion of the trial humeral components, the glenohumeral joint surfaces do not align congruently, adjustments of humeral articular surface height or anteroposterior position may be necessary to achieve a full concentric reduction.

### *Limitations of the Method*

In cases in which there has been severe anterior or posterior glenoid erosion or in the face of substantial glenoid dysplasia, there may be insufficient glenoid bone for reestablishing needed wall height. In glenoids that have a small anteroposterior dimension, there may be insufficient bone to create adequate glenoid depth in a reasonable diameter of curvature (see Fig. 28–22).

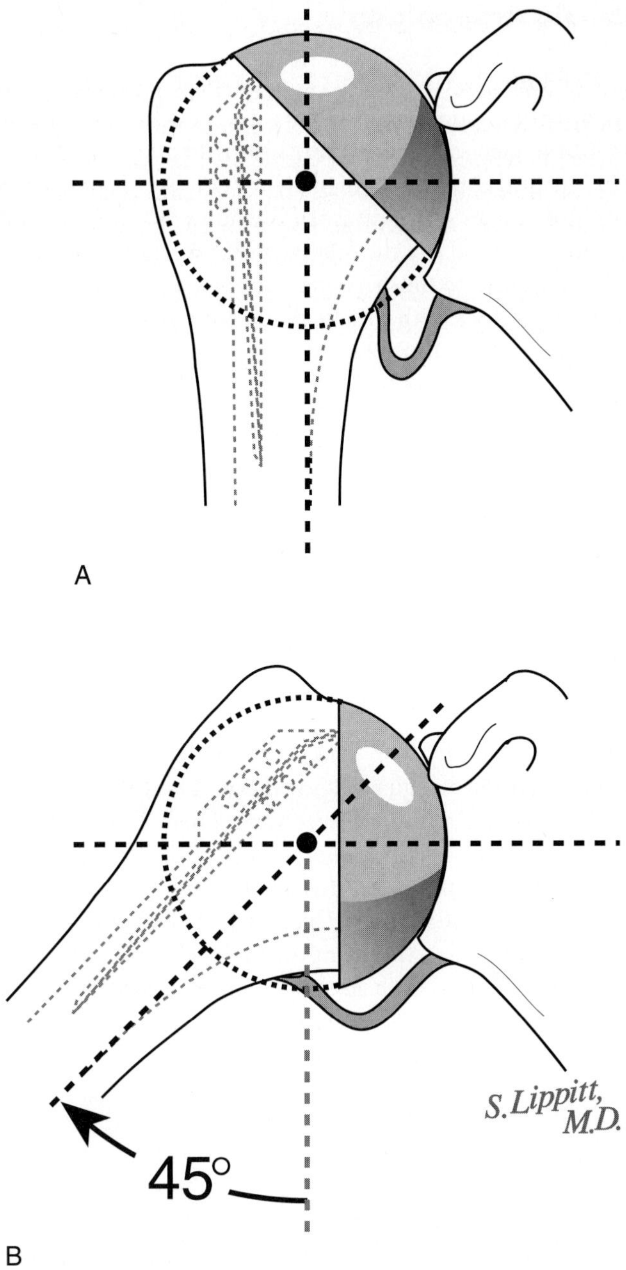


**Figure 28–24. Proper register**
Because of the lack of compliance of reamed bone, the nonprosthetic glenoid arthroplasty is less forgiving; thus, proper register (i.e., the alignment of the humeral and glenoid centers) is critical for comfort and stability.

## Prosthetic Glenoid Arthroplasty

The goal of this procedure (see Chapter 31) is to establish a durable prosthetic glenoid joint surface that provides appropriate stability and contact area and that is durably fixed to the bone of the glenoid. The concerns regarding (1) the glenoid component orientation, (2) the glenoid component diameter of curvature relative to the size of the bony glenoid, (3) the diameter of curvature of the humeral component relative to that of the glenoid component, and (4) the relative positions of the humeral and glenoid components are all analogous to those for the nonprosthetic glenoid arthroplasty. Two additional considerations arise with prosthetic glenoid arthroplasty: the thickness of the glenoid component and the fixation of the component to bone.

### *Orientation*

The prosthetic glenoid component is oriented to the glenoid center line in a manner identical to the nonprosthetic glenoid arthroplasty. The same strategies are used for orienting and drilling the glenoid center line (see Figs. 28–12, 28–13, and 28–14).

### *Glenoid Diameter of Curvature Relative to the Size of the Bony Glenoid*

Although it is commonplace to first determine the diameter of curvature of the humeral head and then choose the glenoid prosthetic curvature accordingly, there may be circumstances in which the primary choice should be based on the size of the bony glenoid. An example is where the anteroposterior dimension of the glenoid bone is small (**Fig. 28–25**). In this circumstance, it is a consideration to ensure that the prosthetic glenoid surface has an adequate articular surface curvature based on the rule of thumb described previously for the nonprosthetic glenoid arthroplasty (see Fig. 28–22) and to ensure that there is both adequate bony support for the component and a sufficient balance stability angle and then select the appropriate humeral diameter for that glenoid surface.

### *Diameter of Curvature of the Humeral Component Relative to that of the Glenoid*

This relationship is established by the manufacturer of the components. Different degrees of glenohumeral diametral mismatch may be built into the design of different components (**Fig. 28–26**).

### *Relative Position of the Humeral and Glenoid Components*

On occasion, in spite of attention to the details of glenoid and humeral component placement, trial reduction indicates that the humerus and glenoid are not in proper register: the humeral component may sit too high or too low on the glenoid component, contacting the rim rather than the depth of the concavity (see Fig. 27–39). Unless the joint reduces easily with gentle compression, this misalignment may cause rim contact, rim wear, and loss of stability. At this point in the procedure, it is easier to change the humeral articular surface position by adjusting the position of the entire prosthesis or through the use of modular eccentric head components, rather than adjusting the position of the glenoid.

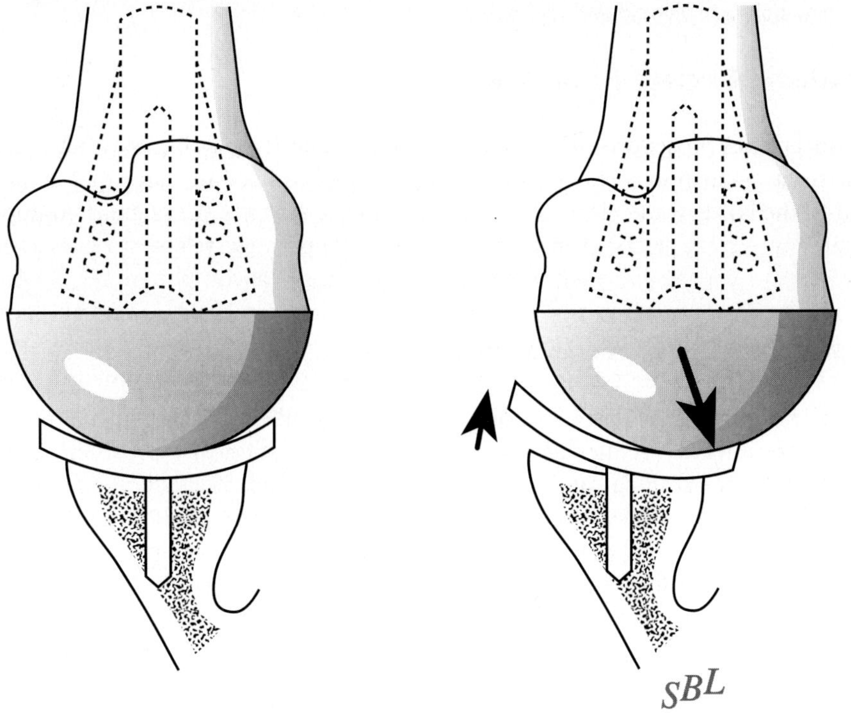


**Figure 28–25. Glenoid overhang**
If the edges of the prosthetic glenoid are unsupported by bone, there is an increased risk of loosening when rim loading occurs.

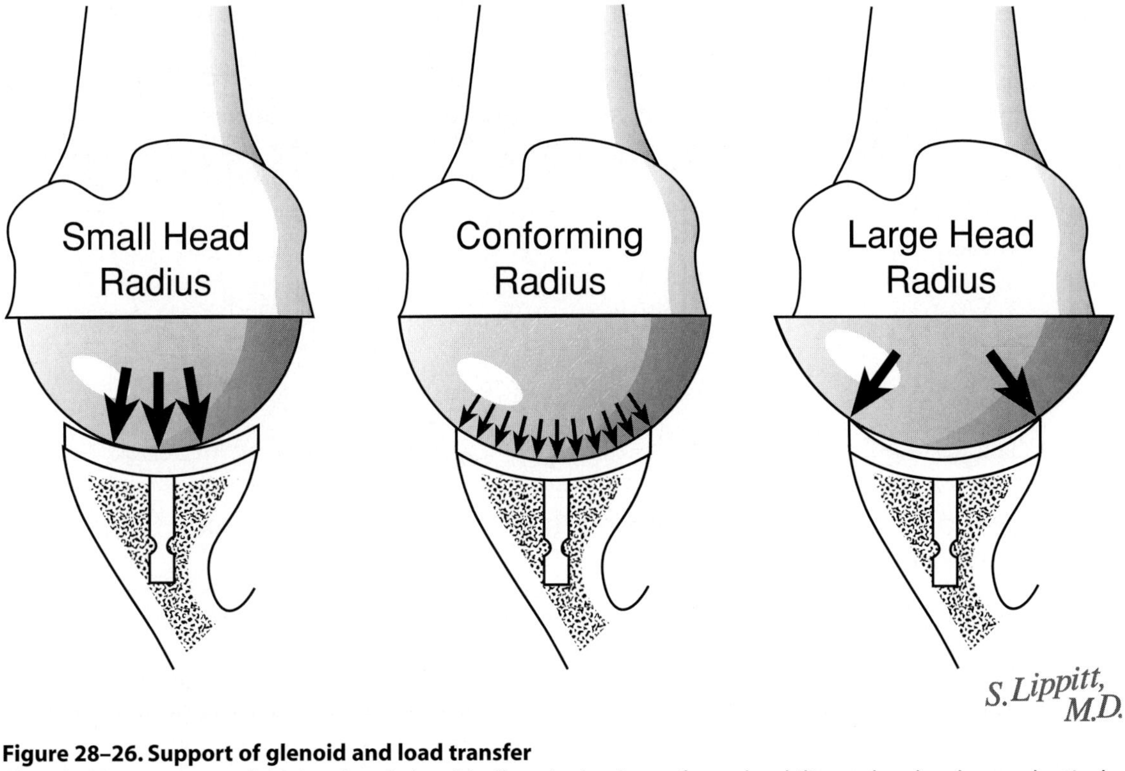


**Figure 28–26. Support of glenoid and load transfer**
The relative curvatures of the head and glenoid affect the load transfer and stability at the glenohumeral articulation. If the radius of curvature of the head is smaller than that of the glenoid (*left*), there is focal loading in the center of the glenoid and the opportunity for small amounts of translation before rim loading. If the head conforms to the glenoid (*center*), the load is evenly distributed and no translation can occur without rim loading. If the head is larger than the glenoid (*right*), the load is concentrated on the glenoid rim, subjecting it to cold flow and wear; furthermore, the humeral head does not seat completely in the glenoid—a situation that reduces glenohumeral stability. Laboratory and clinical experience suggest that for a polyethylene glenoid component, the relationships are optimized when the diameter of glenoid curvature is 6 mm greater than that of the humeral head articulating with it.

### *Thickness of the Glenoid Component*

Normal glenoid cartilage is only a few millimeters thick. In arthritis, the loss of cartilage is accompanied by a contracture of the surrounding soft tissues. Thus, when the lost cartilage thickness is "replaced" with a prosthesis, the thickness of the component may compromise motion by relatively overstuffing it **(Fig. 28–27)**.

### *Fixation of the Glenoid Surface to Bone*

Normal cartilage is well fixed to bone, with collagen fibers anchoring the matrix at microscopic intervals. Achieving secure and durable fixation of a prosthetic glenoid component to the scapula can be difficult. The use of methylmethacrylate in glenoid component fixation can lead to high bone temperatures, particularly since the glenoid is relatively avascular and polyethylene is an excellent insulator. Living bone is considered to be at risk for thermal necrosis if the temperature exceeds 133°F, is greater than 122°F for 1 minute, or is greater than 117°F for 5 minutes. The heat applied to the glenoid bone has been shown to be directly related to the amount of cement used. Thus glenoid cementing techniques should minimize the volume of cement by optimizing the fit of the bone to the component **(Figs. 28–28** and **28–29)**.

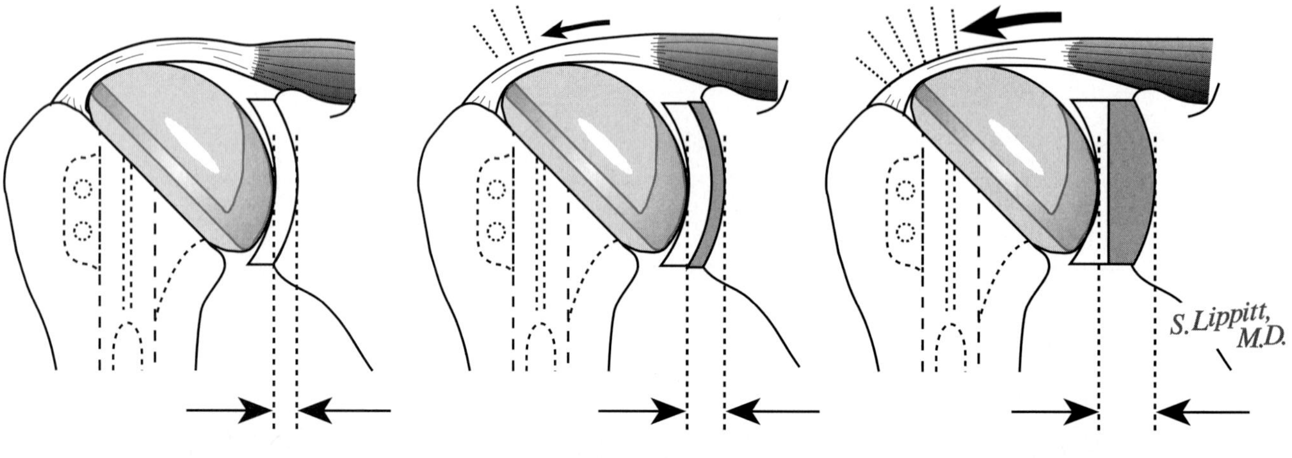


**Figure 28–27. Glenoid thickness**
The glenoid thickness contributes to the relative stuffing of the joint. This is particularly an issue with some metal-backed components, where a minimum thickness of 3 to 4 mm of polyethylene must be superimposed on a metal base. As a result, some components are up to 1.25 cm thick. Insertion of such a component can be predicted to reduce the range of rotation in *each* direction by about 28 degrees (12.5 mm of increased thickness is half a radian for an average humeral head of radius 25 mm; in degrees, a half a radian is 0.5 $\times$ 360/2$\pi$, or 28 degrees). Thus, the restoration of motion to an arthritic shoulder may require a combination of soft tissue releases and avoidance of the insertion of a thick glenoid component. (Modified from Matsen FA, Lippitt SB, Sidles JA, et al [eds]: Practical Evaluation and Management of the Shoulder. Philadelphia: WB Saunders, 1994, p. 190.)

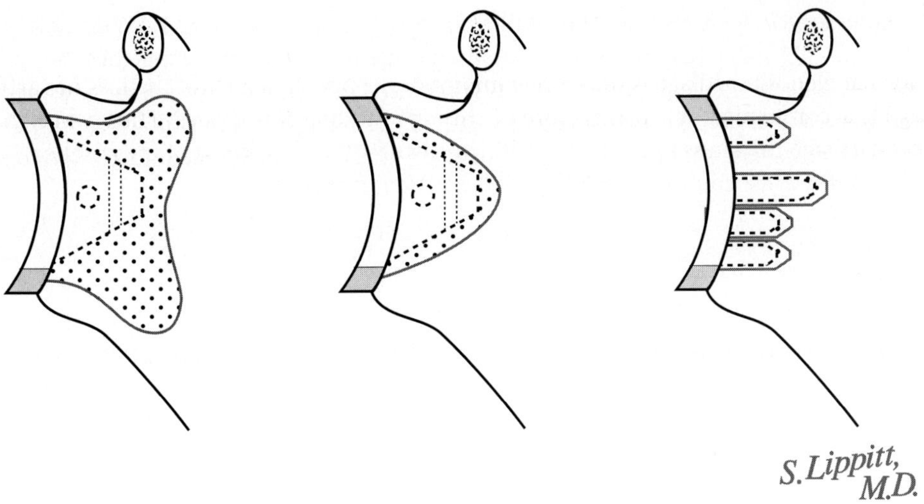


**Figure 28–28. Cement volume**
Certain glenoid fixation techniques involve the use of substantial amounts of polymethyl methacrylate (*left*), putting the surrounding bone at risk for thermal necrosis. Other methods (*right*) use geometrical precision in glenoid preparation to minimize the amount of cement needed to fill the voids.

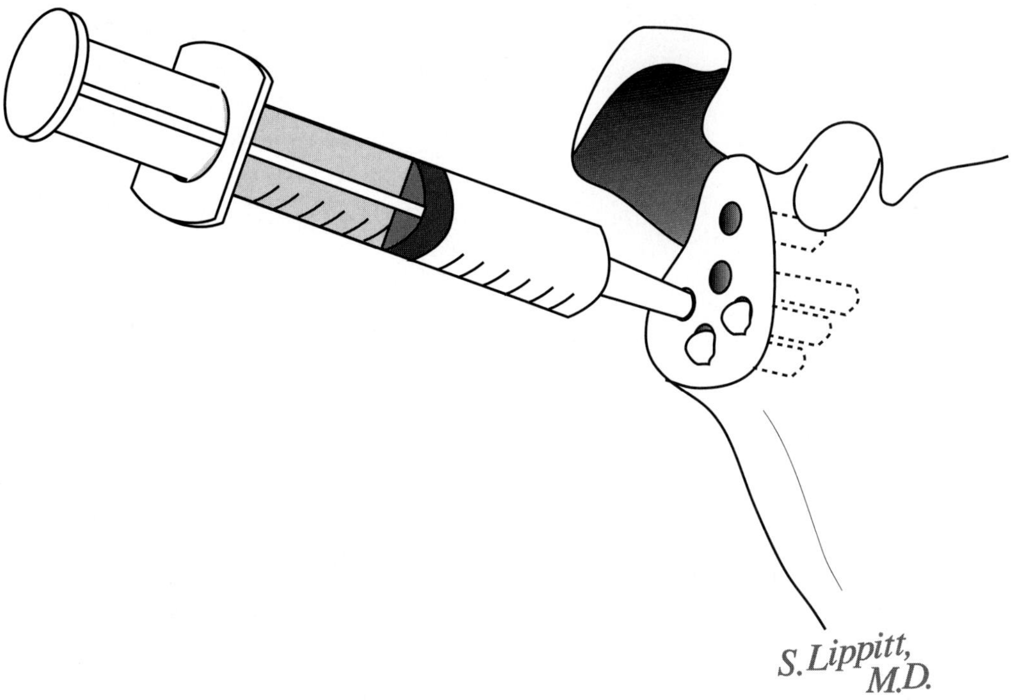


**Figure 28–29. Glenoid minimization cement**
Drilling precisely oriented glenoid fixation holes that are only slightly larger than the pegs enables the surgeon to minimize the amount of cement used. (Modified from Pearl ML, Lippitt SB: Shoulder arthroplasty with a modular prosthesis. Techniques Orthop 8:159, 1993.)

One approach to reproducibly achieving this precision of fit and secure fixation combines (1) spherically reaming the glenoid bone so that it exactly matches the convex back of a glenoid component, avoiding the need for cement between the prosthesis and the reamed glenoid surface (**Fig. 28–30**); (2) using a precision drill guide to make fixation holes just slightly larger than pegs on the back of the glenoid component;

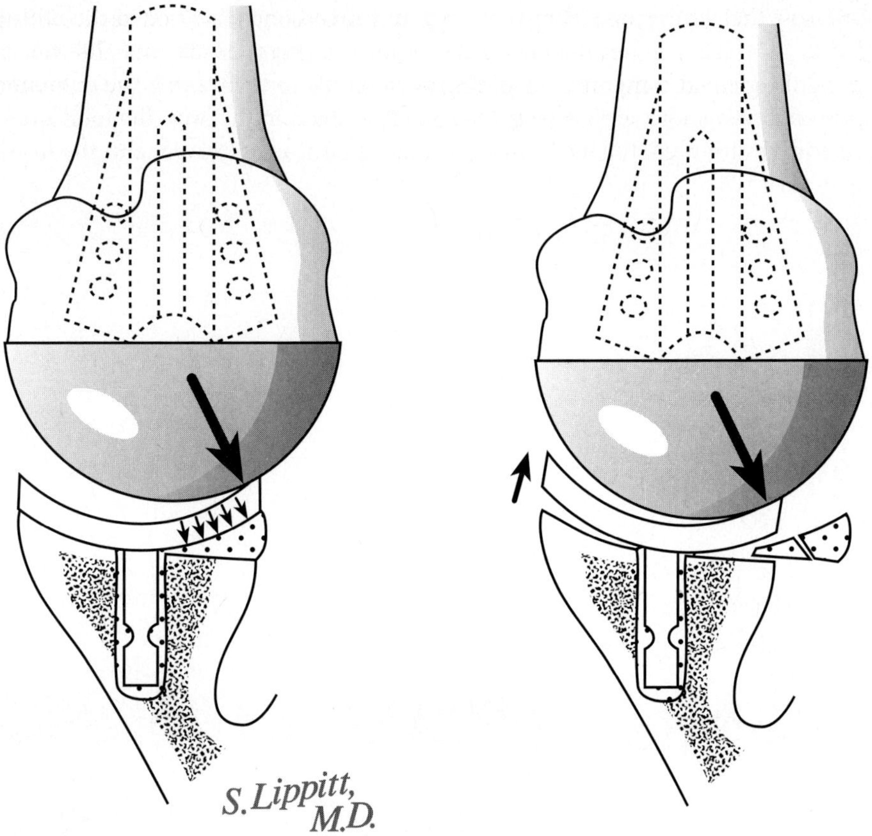


**Figure 28–30. Posterior glenoid cement problem**
If the glenoid bone is not reamed to conform to the back of the glenoid component, the resulting interposed cement wedge is at risk for cracking out, leaving the component unsupported.

(3) ensuring that at least one of the pegs is anterior and one posterior to the mid-glenoid line to prevent anterior and posterior lift-off (**Figs. 28–31** and **28–32**); and (4) using the glenoid center line as an alignment guide to ensure that the component sits concentrically and completely on the reamed surface. In this way, the total amount of cement is minimized, the maximum amount of bone is preserved, and the fixation is enhanced.

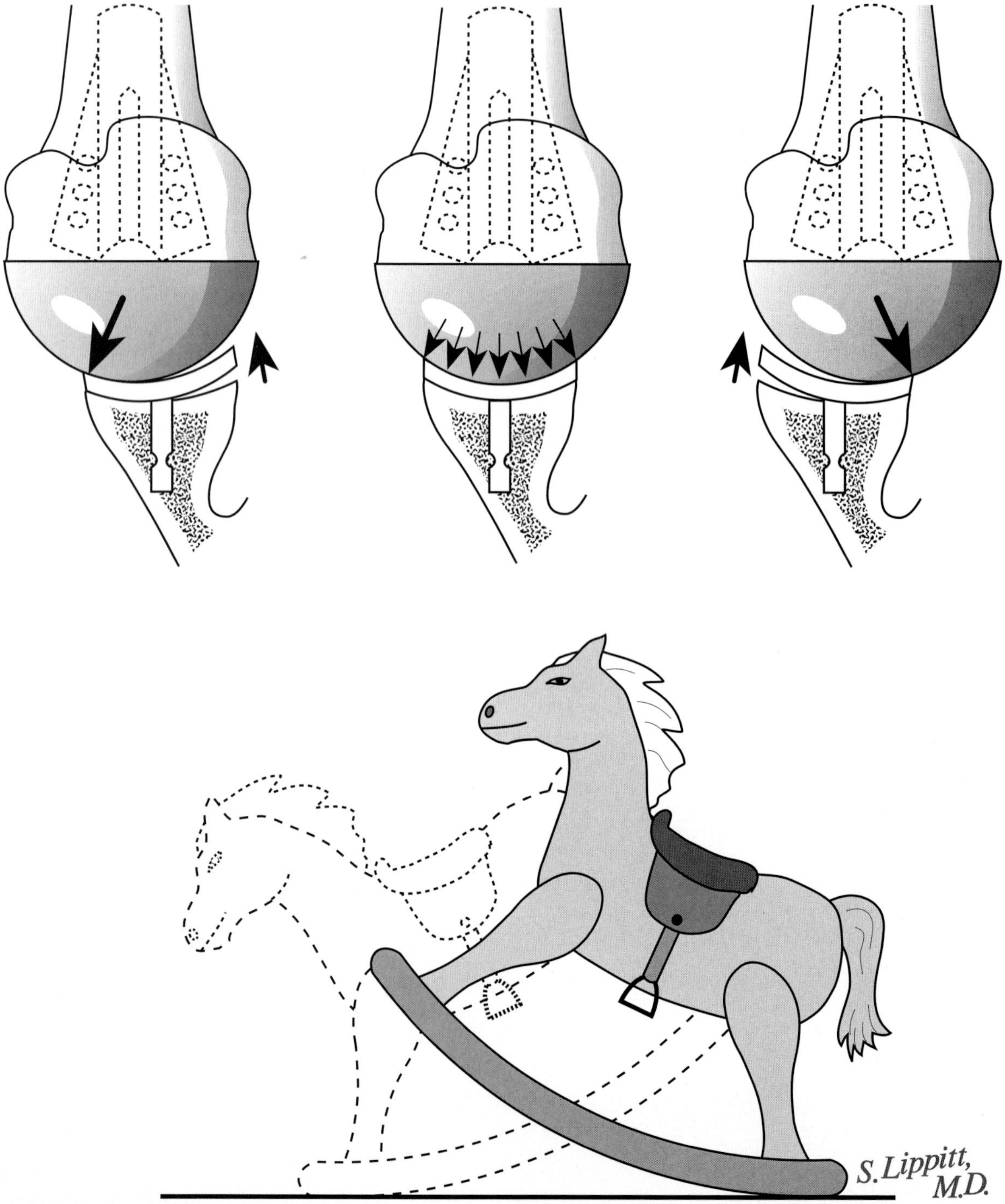


**Figure 28–31. Rocking horse mechanism**

Eccentric loading of the glenoid exposes it to risk via the "rocking horse" mechanism. (Modified from Matsen FA, Lippitt SB, Sidles JA, et al [eds]: Practical Evaluation and Management of the Shoulder. Philadelphia: WB Saunders, 1994, p. 190.)

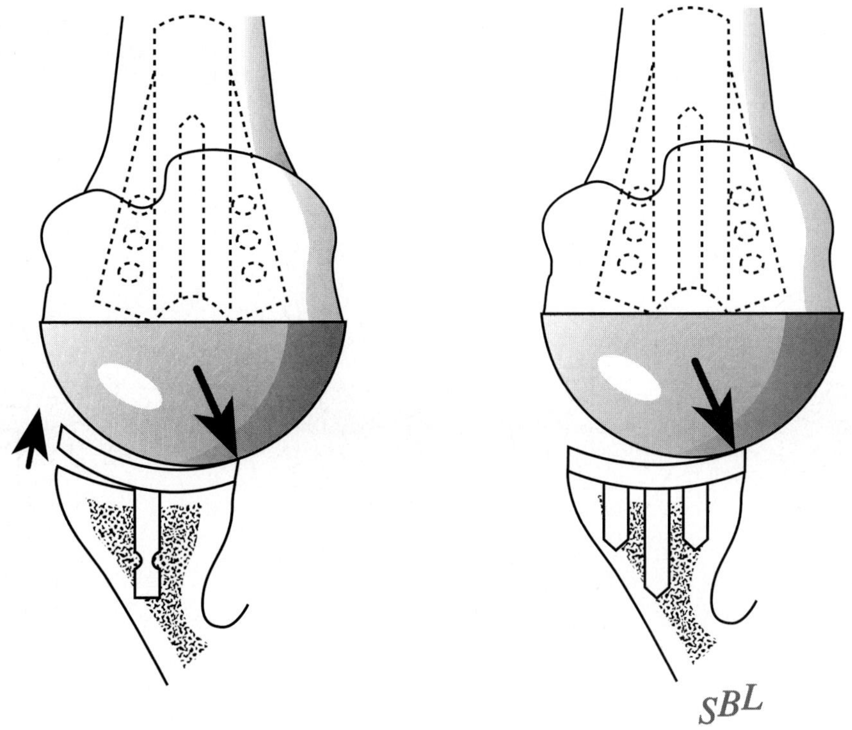


**Figure 28–32. Peg fixation**
A glenoid fixation design that has a peg anterior and posterior to the glenoid midline helps minimize the problem of "lift-off" with eccentric loading.

The precision of the glenoid bone preparation has a substantial effect on the quality of the glenoid component fixation (**Fig. 28–33**).

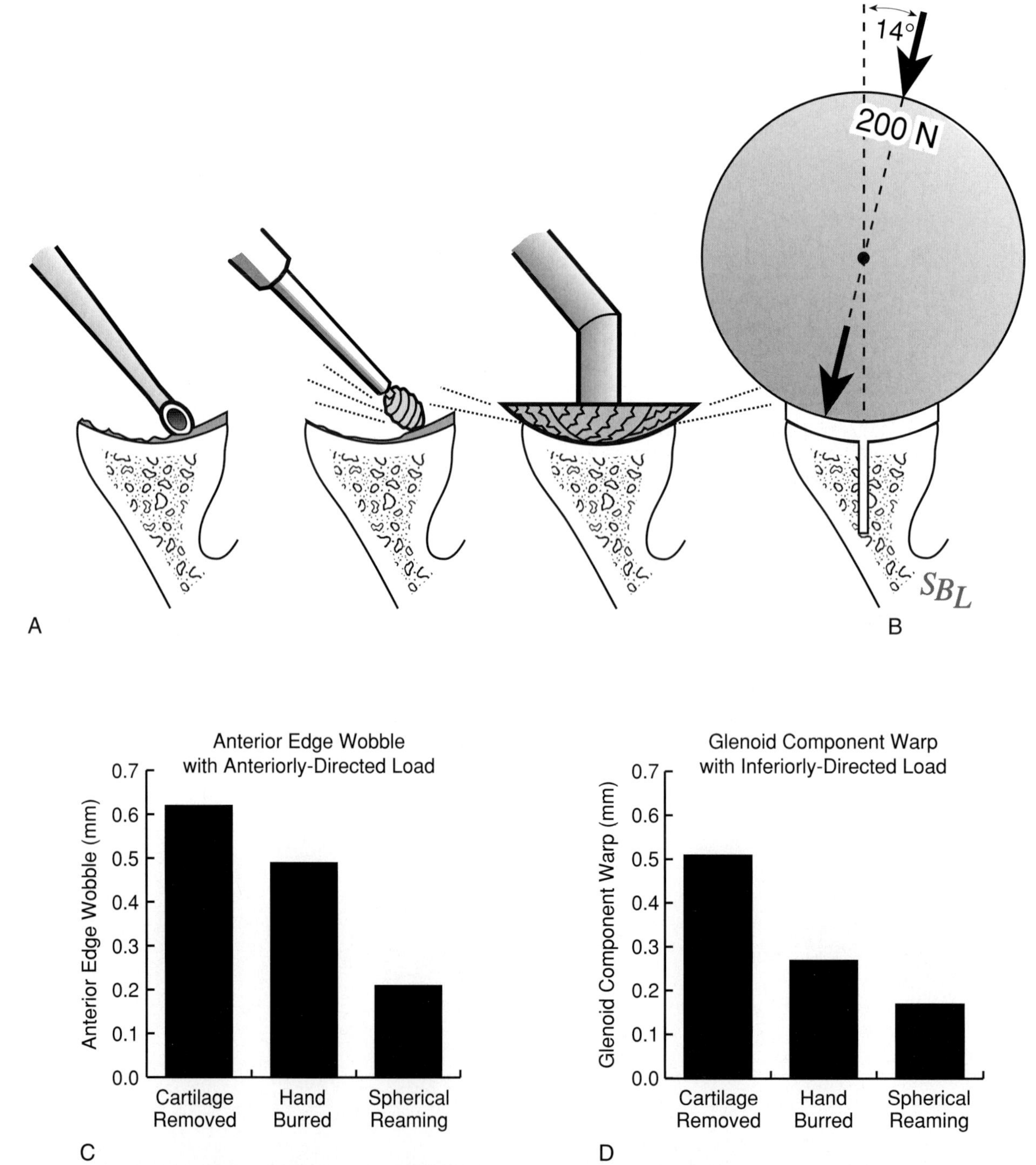


**Figure 28–33. The effect of glenoid bone preparation on component stability**

**A,** Three methods of bone preparation were compared: curettage, hand burring, and spherical reaming. **B,** Loads of 200 N were applied through a metal ball at an angle of 14 degrees with respect to the glenoid center line. The glenoid was fixed only with a single uncemented flexible central peg. Displacement transducers measured the change in position of the edges of the glenoid component. **C** and **D,** Data on the stability of a glenoid component with three different types of glenoid surface preparation. Spherical reaming of the glenoid along the glenoid center line significantly reduced the wobble (**C**) and warp (**D**) of the glenoid component and thus provided more glenoid component stability than did curettage or hand burring. (From Matsen FA, Lippitt SB, Sidles JA, et al [eds]: Practical Evaluation and Management of the Shoulder. Philadelphia: WB Saunders, 1994, p. 196.)

CHAPTER 29

# Procedure: Humeral Arthroplasty

**Diagnosis**

***Rheumatoid arthritis   ICD9 CODE 714.0***
***or***
***Osteoarthritis   ICD9 CODE 715.11***
***or***
***Traumatic arthritis   ICD9 CODE 716.11***
***or***
***Avascular necrosis   ICD9 CODE 733.41***

**Procedure**

***Humeral arthroplasty (combined with nonprosthetic or prosthetic glenoid arthroplasty)   CPT CODE 23929 or 23472.52***

## INDICATIONS

The patient has primary or secondary glenohumeral arthritis that limits the comfort and function of the shoulder. The shoulder has not responded to nonoperative management.

Preoperative radiographs reveal loss of the normal humeral contour and radiographic joint space. These views are used for templating the arthroplasty (**Fig. 29–1**).

Knowing the alternatives as well as the risks of infection, neurovascular injury, excessive stiffness, pain, weakness, fracture, instability, component loosening, and the need for revision surgery, as well as anesthetic complications, the patient desires to proceed with the above-described procedure. The patient understands that the purpose of the procedure is to restore a smooth, round, well-fixed humeral articular surface that is of appropriate size, location, and orientation. The patient recognizes that this procedure cannot be expected to completely restore normal comfort and function to the shoulder. And, lastly, the patient understands his or her critical role in the postsurgical rehabilitation.

## FINDINGS

Examination under anesthesia reveals that range of glenohumeral motion is limited in all directions and there is bony crepitance on glenohumeral motion.

Surgical findings include loss of normal humeral articular cartilage with the central area worn down to bone. The remaining cartilage is in the process of dissolution. There are substantial osteophytes around the articular surface. The humeral articular surface has lost its normal smoothness and roundness.

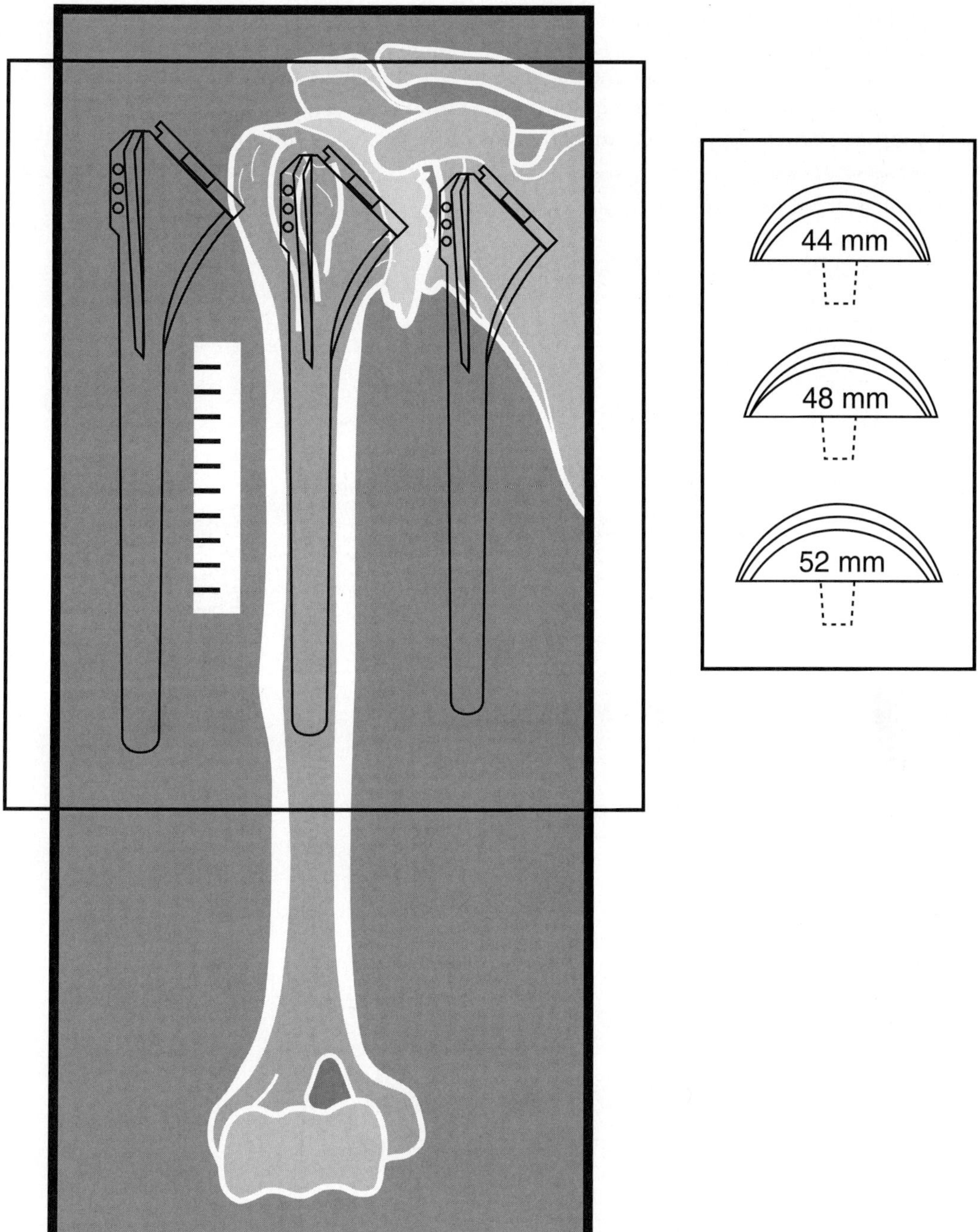


**Figure 29–1. Template x-ray**
The template view enables the surgeon to preview the procedure and estimate the component size and fit.

## OPERATION

Under satisfactory anesthesia, the patient is placed in a low beach chair position with the glenohumeral joint at the edge of the operating table (**Fig. 29–2**). The entire forequarter is doubly prepped and draped in the usual sterile fashion with the arm free to be moved.

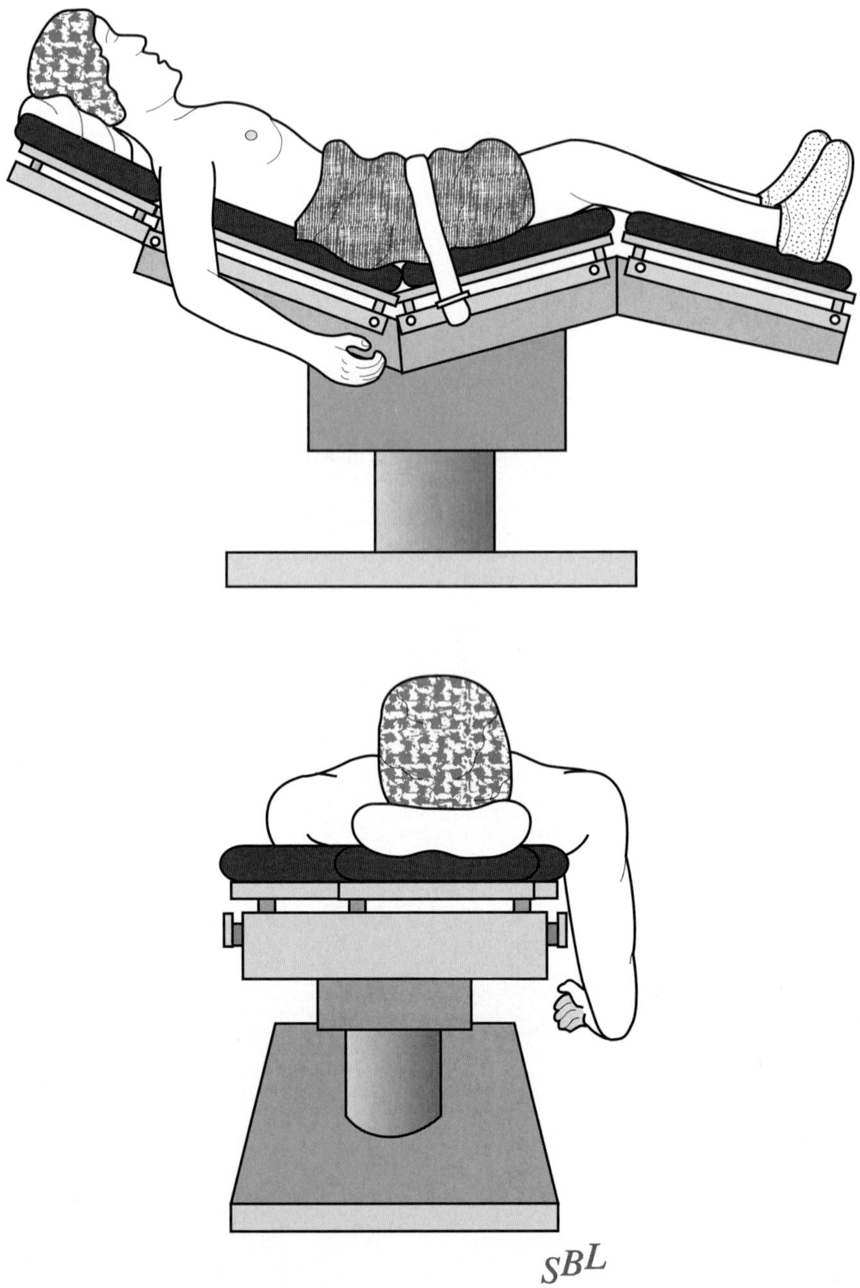


**Figure 29–2. Positioning the patient**
The patient is placed in a comfortable position as in a beach chair with the thorax angled 30 degrees above the horizontal. The neck is in a neutral position. The glenohumeral joint is at the edge of the table and the arm is completely free. Compressive stockings (not shown here) are applied to the legs.

The shoulder is approached through a standard deltopectoral incision along a line connecting the mid-clavicle to the mid-lateral humerus at the deltoid tubercle (**Fig. 29–3**). The deltopectoral interval is opened, and the cephalic vein is retracted laterally (**Fig. 29–4**). The clavipectoral fascia is opened just lateral to the coracoid muscles (**Fig. 29–5**).

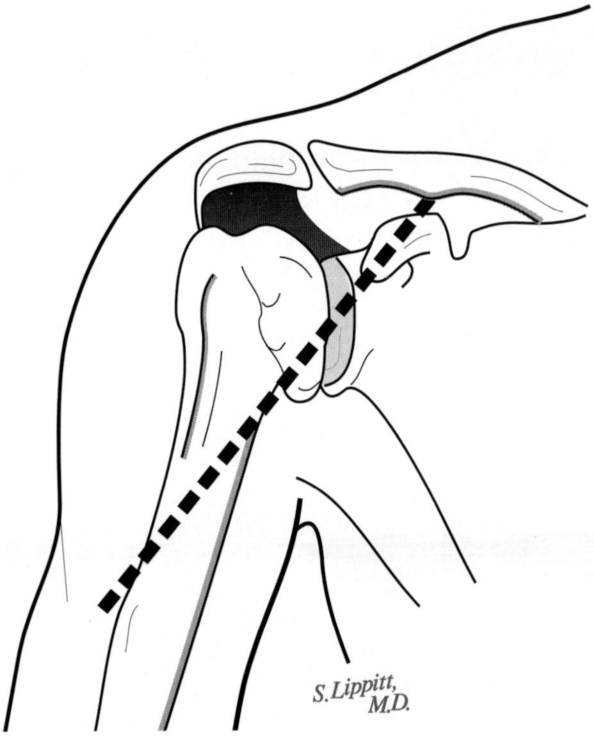


**Figure 29–3. Incision**
The skin incision for the extended deltopectoral approach utilizes the mid-clavicle, the tip of the coracoid process, and the deltoid tuberosity of the mid-humerus as landmarks. It is important that the incision avoids the axillary crease; otherwise, painful scarring may result.

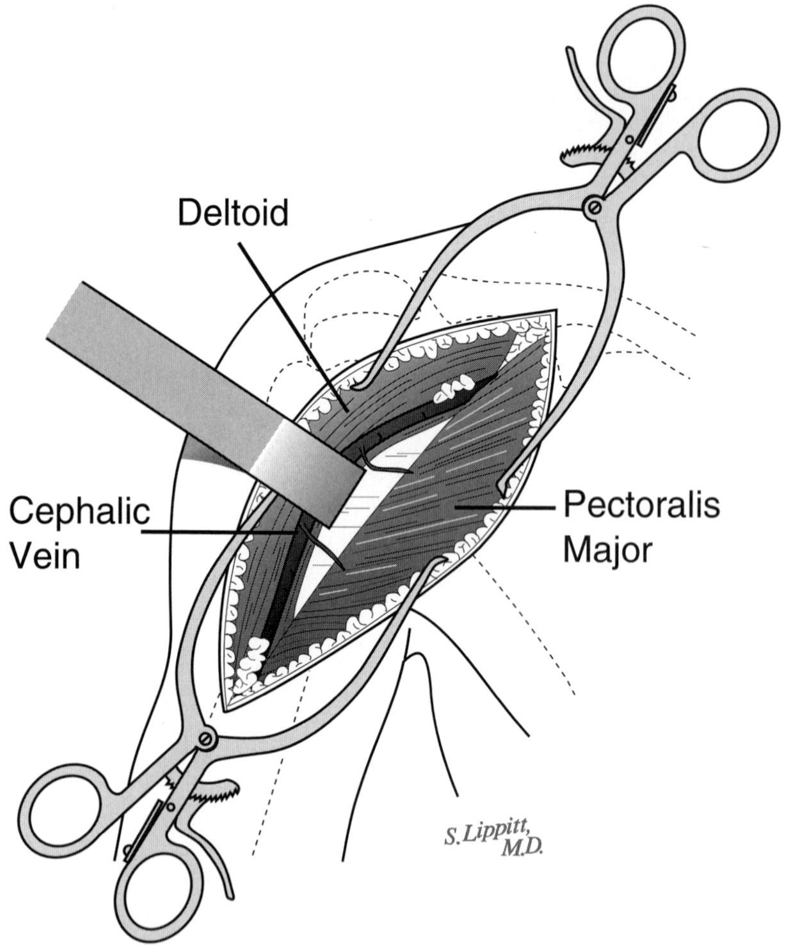


**Figure 29–4. Cephalic vein**
The cephalic vein is identified in the deltopectoral groove. It is retracted laterally along with the deltoid to expose the clavipectoral fascia. (From DePuy Global Fx, Warsaw, IN.)

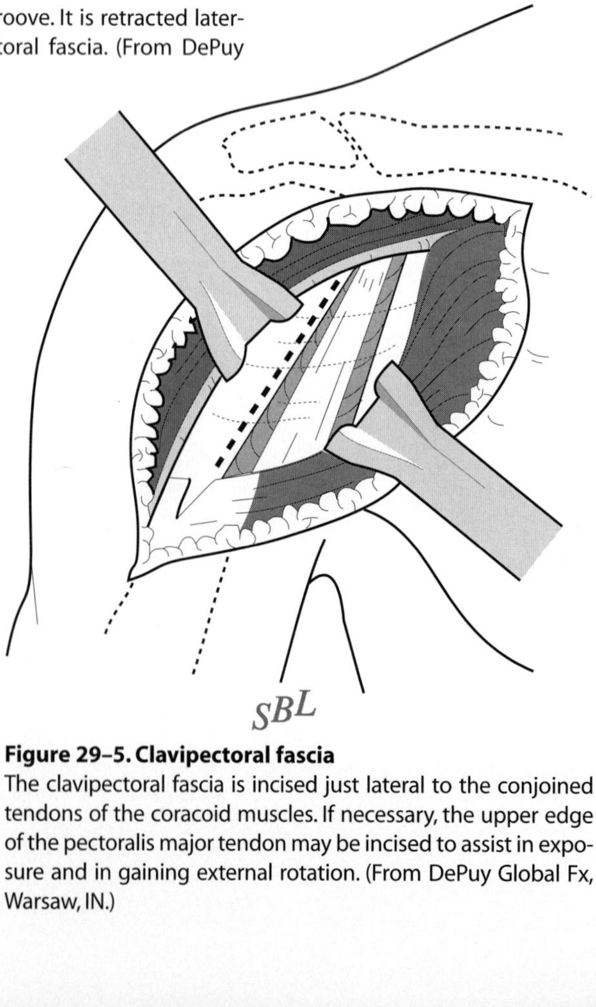


**Figure 29–5. Clavipectoral fascia**
The clavipectoral fascia is incised just lateral to the conjoined tendons of the coracoid muscles. If necessary, the upper edge of the pectoralis major tendon may be incised to assist in exposure and in gaining external rotation. (From DePuy Global Fx, Warsaw, IN.)

The humeroscapular motion interface is mobilized. The axillary nerve is palpated medially as it crosses the subscapularis and laterally as it exits the quadrilateral space (**Fig. 29–6**). It is protected throughout the case. A self-retaining retractor is placed with one blade underneath the coracoid muscles and one blade beneath the deltoid (**Fig. 29–7**).

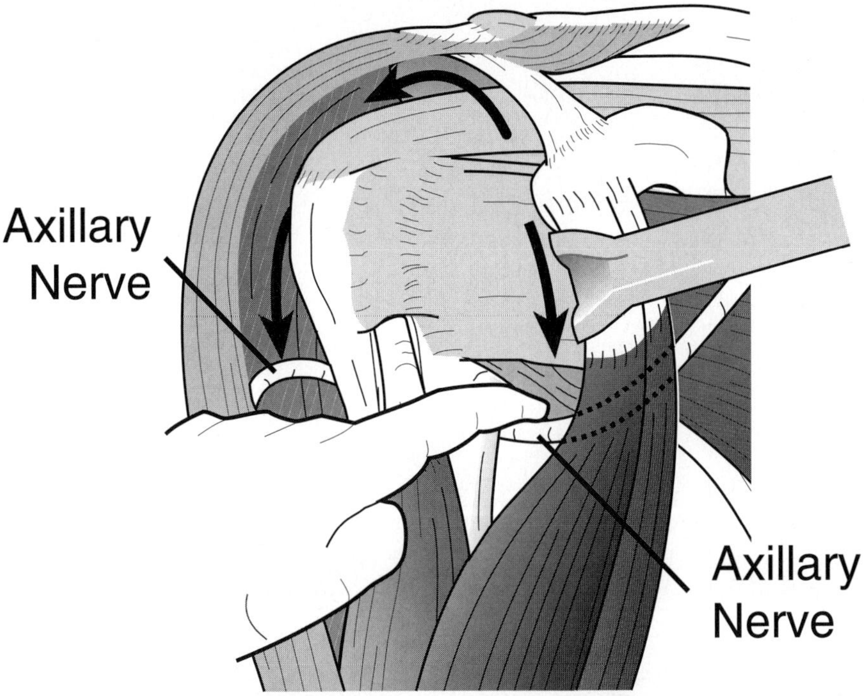


**Figure 29–6. Nerve-to-nerve release**
All scar tissue in the humeroscapular motion interface is released from the axillary nerve medially as it crosses the subscapularis, then under the coracoid, then under the coracoacromial ligament, then under the acromion, and then finally under the deltoid to the axillary nerve posteriorly as it exits the quadrilateral space: the nerve-to-nerve release.

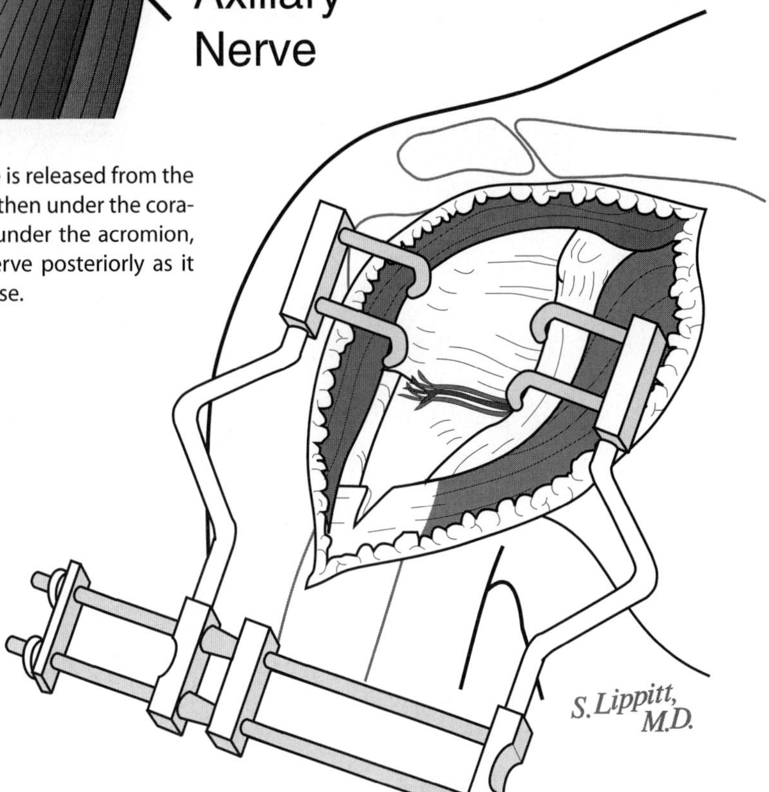


**Figure 29–7. Self-retaining retractor**
A self-retaining retractor is placed below the conjoined tendons medially and the deltoid muscle laterally. The subscapularis is now seen with the anterior humeral circumflex vessels marking its inferior border. (From Pearl ML, Lippitt SB: Shoulder arthroplasty with a modular prosthesis. Techniques Orthop 8:151–162, 1994.)

The subscapularis and subjacent capsule are incised from their insertion to the lesser tuberosity, leaving all possible tendon length with the muscle (**Fig. 29–8**). A 360-degree release of the subscapularis is performed (**Fig. 29–9**), incising the coraco-humeral ligament and incising any connections of the anterior capsule to the glenoid (**Figs. 29–10** and **29–11**). The capsule is left on the deep side of the subscapularis to reinforce the tendon for its reattachment at the conclusion of the case.

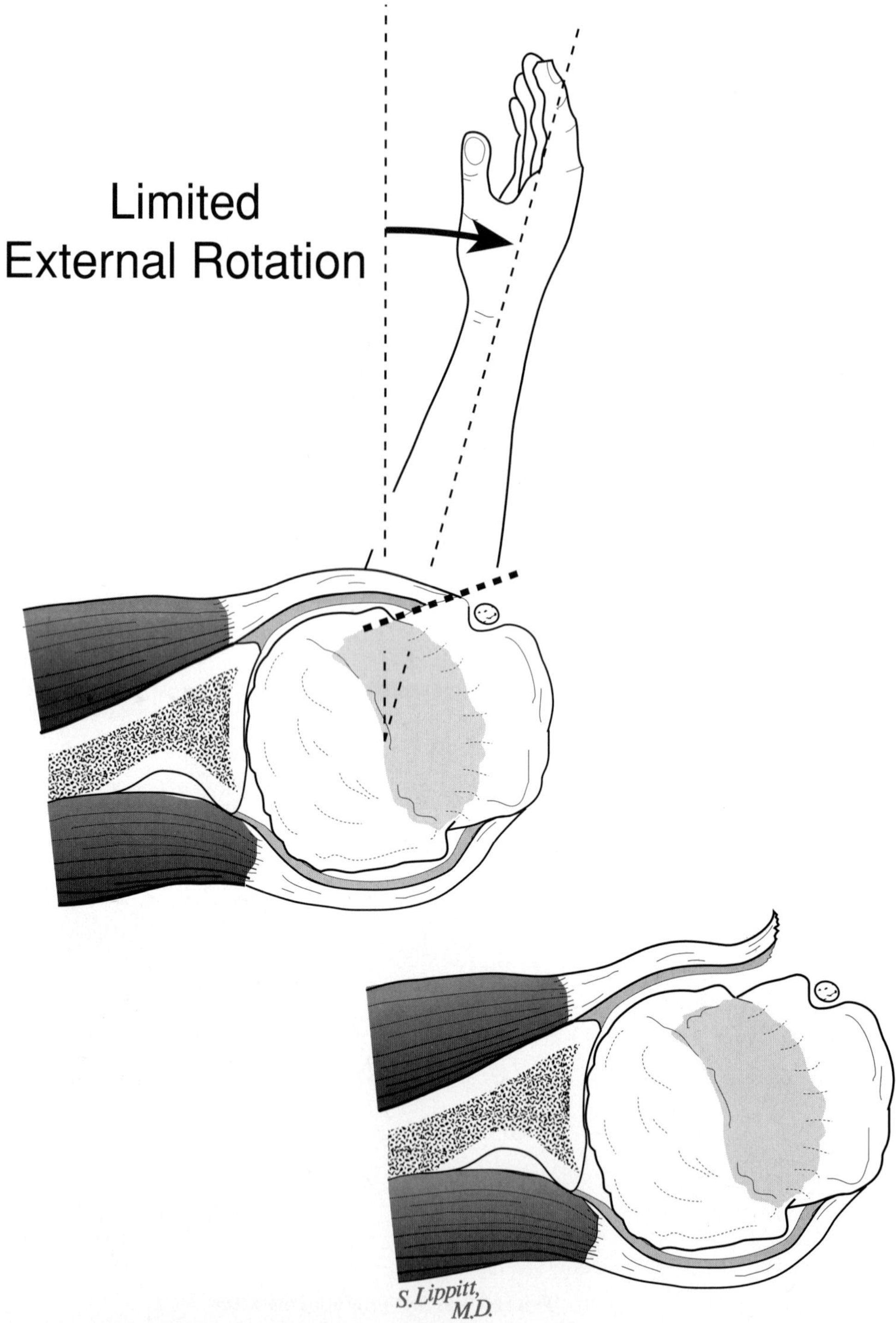


**Figure 29–8. Incising the subscapularis**
The subscapularis and the subjacent capsule are incised directly from the lesser tuberosity, striving for maximal length of the tendon so that external rotation can be regained. (Modified from Matsen FA, Lippitt SB, Sidles JA, et al [eds]: Practical Evaluation and Management of the Shoulder. Philadelphia: WB Saunders, 1994, p. 203.)

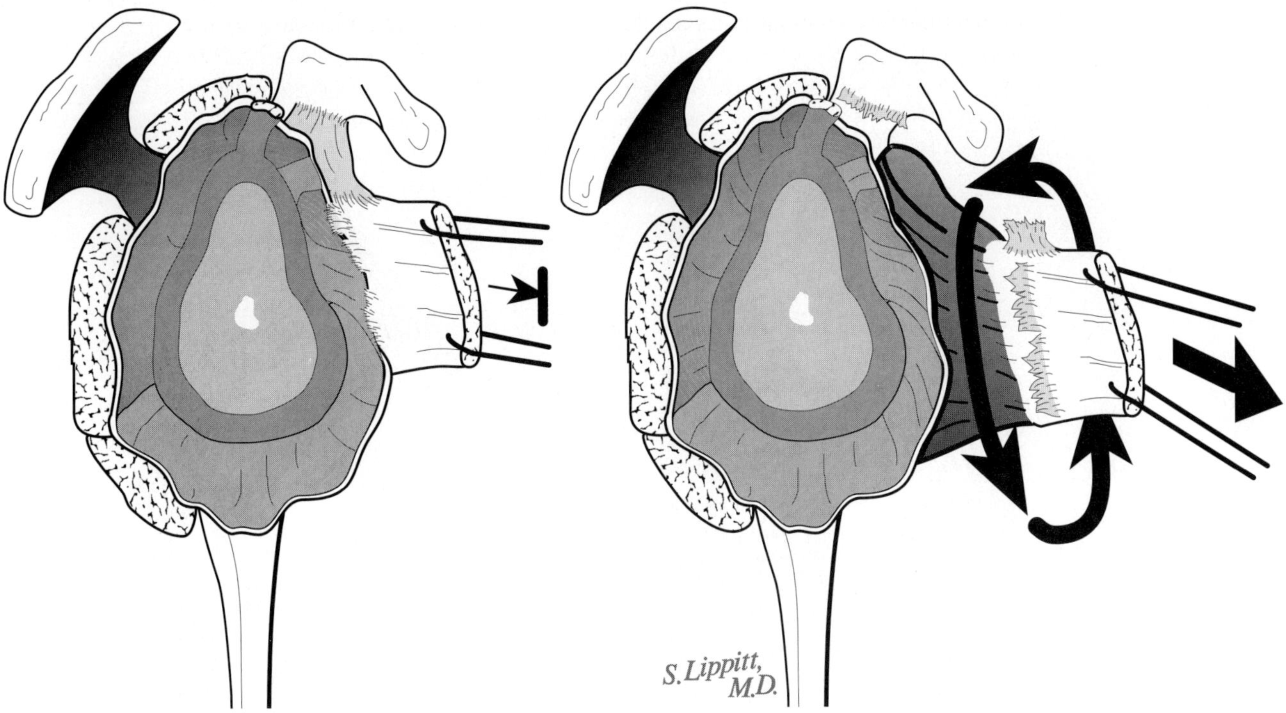


**Figure 29–9. Releasing the subscapularis**
The subscapularis is released circumferentially, freeing it from the coracoid, the anterior glenohumeral capsule, the axillary nerve, and the coracoid muscles.

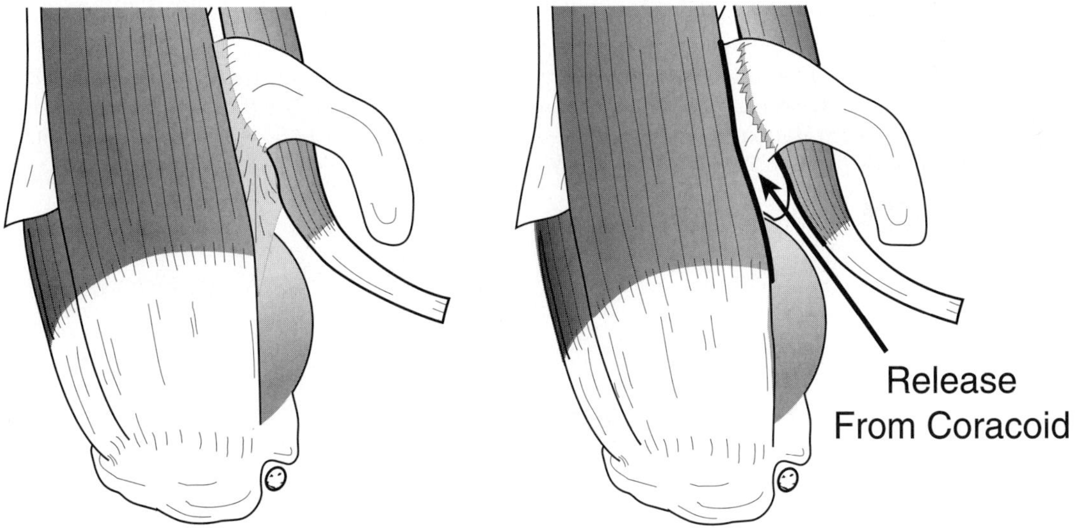


**Figure 29–10. Releasing the coracohumeral ligament**
The coracohumeral ligament is released from the base of the coracoid process, allowing unrestricted gliding of the supraspinatus as well as the subscapularis. (Modified from Matsen FA, Lippitt SB, Sidles JA, et al [eds]: Practical Evaluation and Management of the Shoulder. Philadelphia: WB Saunders, 1994, p. 138.)

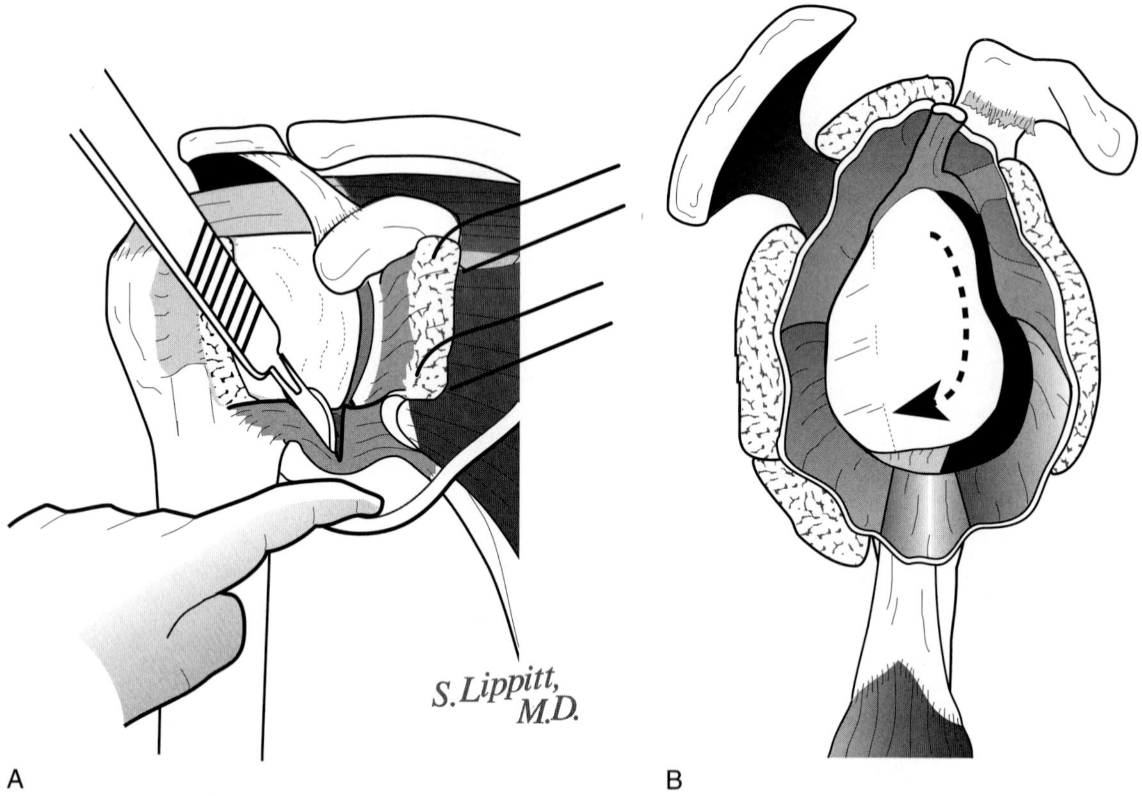


**Figure 29–11. Releasing the anterior capsule**
Release of the anterior capsule from the glenoid under direct vision while the axillary nerve is protected. In cases of osteoarthritis and capsulorrhaphy arthropathy, the capsular release extends just past the origin of the long head of the triceps to ensure sectioning of the anterior and posterior bands of the inferior glenohumeral ligament. (Modified from Matsen FA, Lippitt SB, Sidles JA, et al [eds]: Practical Evaluation and Management of the Shoulder. Philadelphia: WB Saunders, 1994, p. 205.)

The capsule is released from the humeral neck anteriorly and inferiorly. The humerus is exposed by gentle external rotation and extension of the arm, with a smooth broad elevator inserted into the depths of the joint to ease the passage of the posterior humeral osteophytes onto the glenoid (**Fig. 29–12**). This elevator is then placed behind the humeral head to bring the proximal humerus into full view (**Fig. 29–13**).

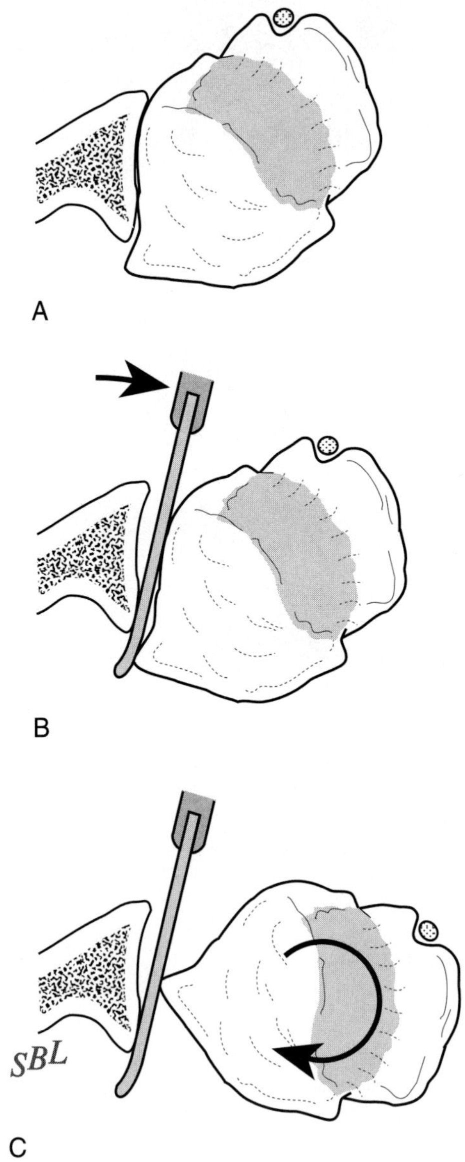


**Figure 29–12. Osteophytes**
Large posterior humeral osteophytes can form a barrier to external rotation and dislocation of the humeral head. Reduction of the osteophytes onto the joint face can usually be accomplished by placing a broad smooth retractor through the joint while the humerus is in internal rotation and then gently externally rotating the humerus. (Modified from Matsen FA, Lippitt SB, Sidles JA, et al [eds]: Practical Evaluation and Management of the Shoulder. Philadelphia: WB Saunders, 1994, p. 206.)

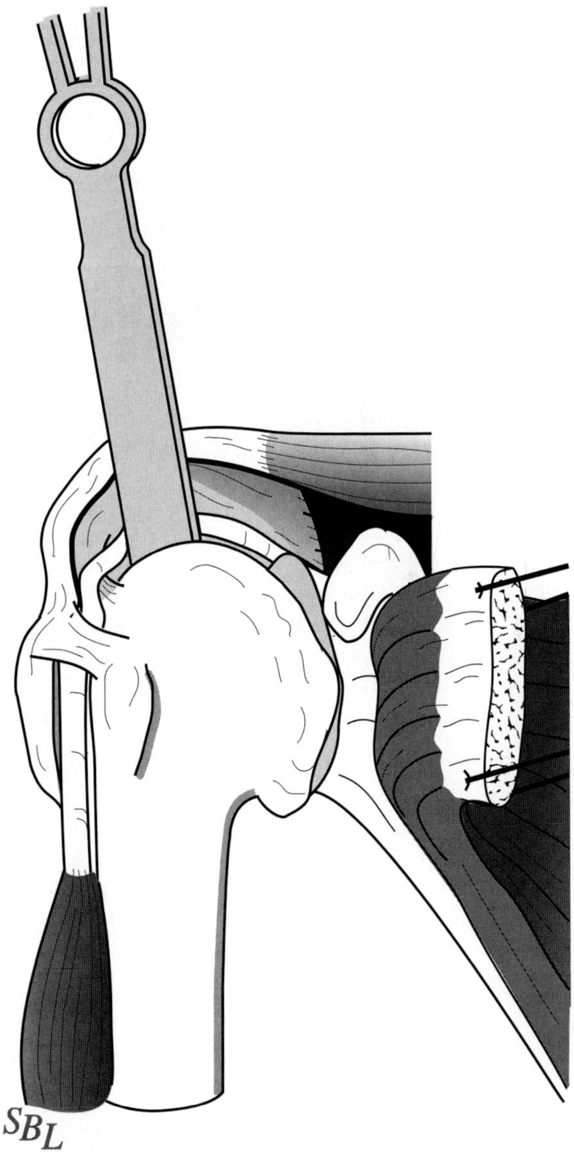


**Figure 29–13. Exposing the humeral head**
A broad smooth retractor is inserted beneath the supraspinatus and levers gently against the deltoid and acromion to expose the proximal humerus. (Modified from Matsen FA, Lippitt SB, Sidles JA, et al [eds]: Practical Evaluation and Management of the Shoulder. Philadelphia: WB Saunders, 1994, p. 207.)

The center of the articular surface is marked with the cautery. A vertical line is drawn upward and downward from this point, dividing the humeral articular surface into its anterior and posterior halves. A second line, starting at the center point and extending parallel to the humeral center line, is drawn on the anterior surface of the humeral head and lesser tuberosity **(Fig. 29–14)**. The starting point for reaming is the point where the center of the humeral shaft projects through the superior articular surface of the humerus along the vertical line bisecting the head. This is usually at the most superior aspect of the humeral head, just posterior to the bicipital groove, 1 cm from the cuff insertion, and halfway between the anterior and posterior margins of the humeral head.

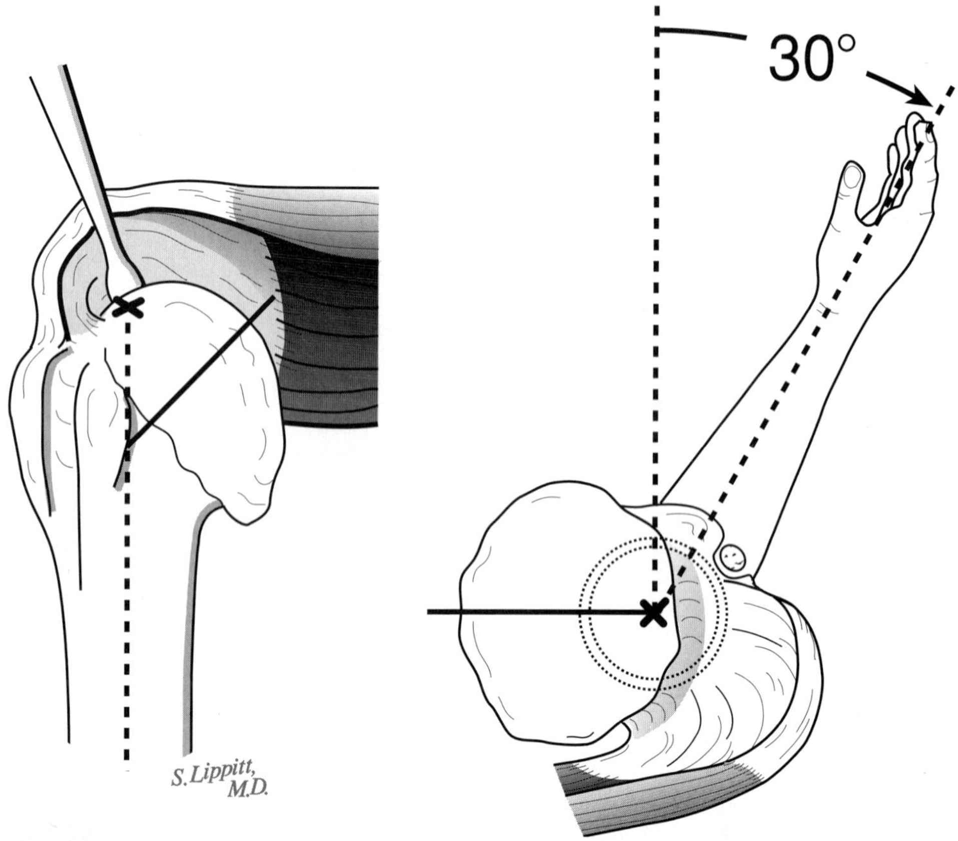


**Figure 29–14. Intraoperative planning**
Two orienting lines are drawn. One is parallel to the humeral articular center line (*left*) and one splits the humeral articular surface into its anterior and posterior halves (humeral bisecting line) (*right*). The starting point for entering the canal is along the second line near the cuff insertion to the tuberosity.

A pinecone burr is used to open the medullary canal at this point (**Fig. 29–15**). A straight curette held in the surgeon's dominant hand is passed through this hole and down the medullary canal while the elbow is held in the nondominant hand, guiding the direction of the curette and positioning the humerus. Next, a straight tapered reamer is used to increase the size of the hole, again being guided by the surgeon's nondominant hand at the elbow. This and all subsequent medullary instruments are inserted with a gentle valgus bias (**Fig. 29–16**).

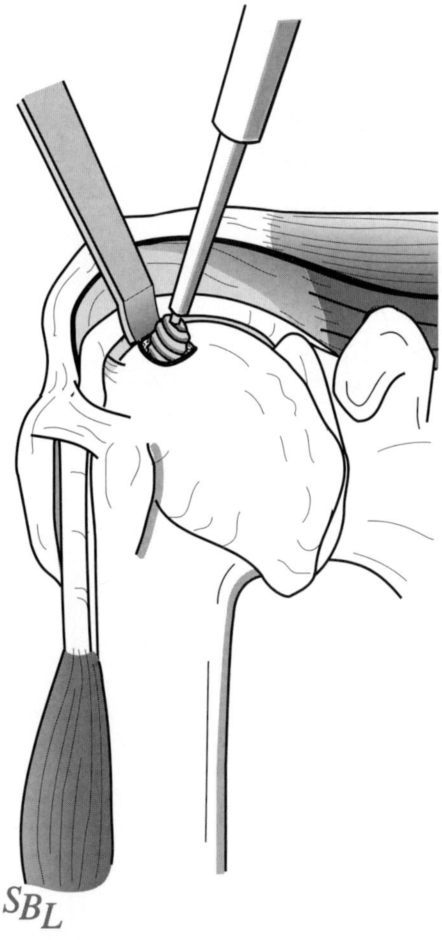


**Figure 29–15. Burr start**
The medullary space of the humeral head is entered at the starting point using a pinecone burr.

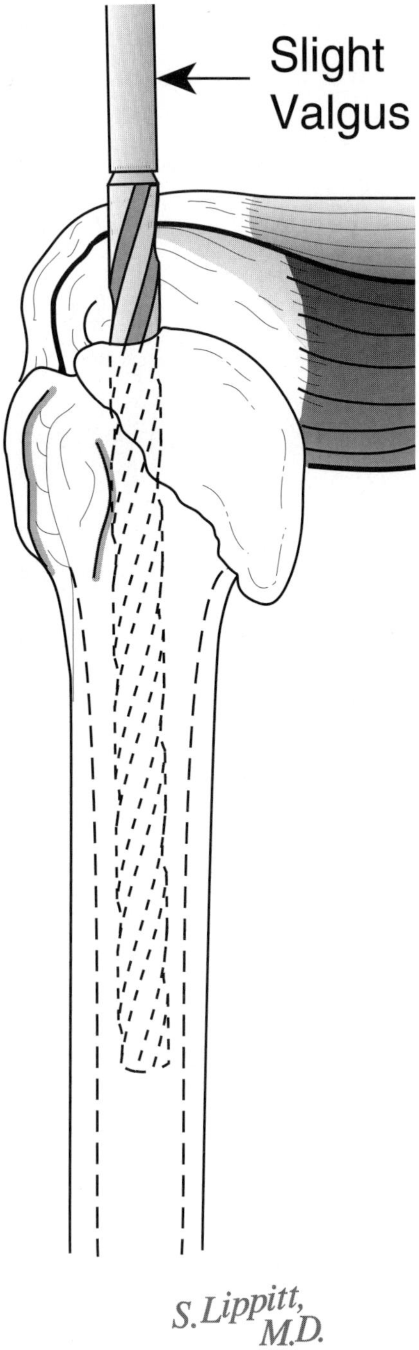


**Figure 29–16. Medullary reaming**
Cylindrical reamers are inserted down to the depth required by the prosthesis, with a slight valgus bias exerted.

Next, successively larger medullary reamers are inserted down the canal to the depth required by the prosthesis, but no further (**Fig. 29–17**). The largest reamer that can be fully inserted without cortical reaming is selected as the final reamer; its axis is the orthopaedic axis of the humerus.

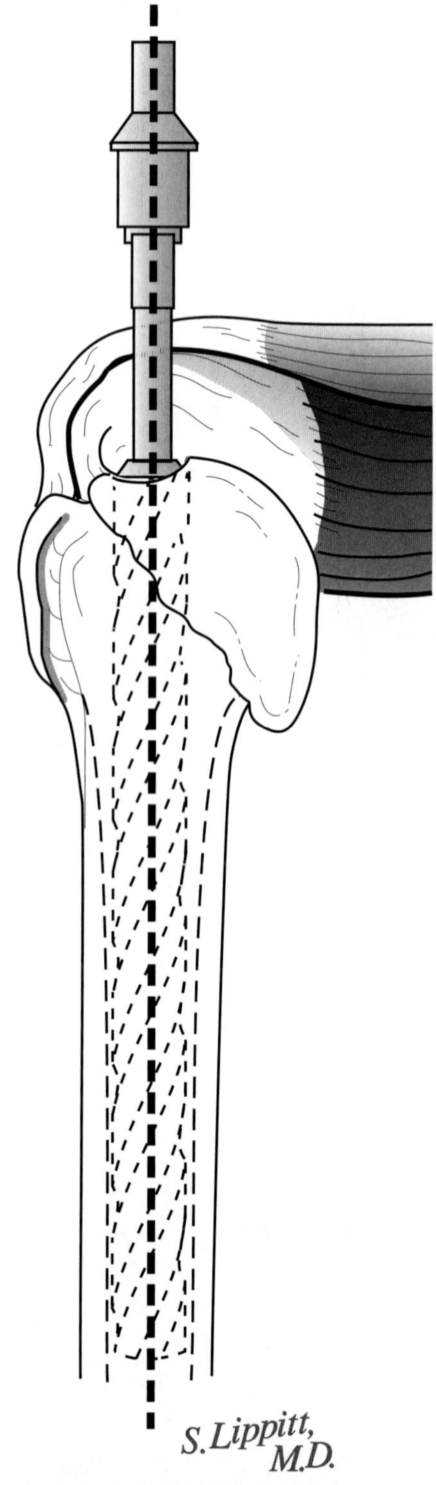


**Figure 29–17. Medullary reaming**
Progressively larger reamers are used until one achieves a bite in the cortex distally. The orthopaedic axis is the central axis of this reamer (*dark dotted line*).

Osteophytes are removed from the humeral neck (**Fig. 29–18**). Although an extramedullary cutting guide can approximate in the orientation of the humeral osteotomy plane (**Fig. 29–19**), such a system cannot be referenced to the medullary anatomy of the humerus that will determine the position of the implant. Instead, we prefer an intraoperative templating method that reveals the three-dimensional relationship between the orthopaedic axis of the medullary canal, the articular surface that would be provided by different prosthetic heads, and the cut plane. Such a system links the geometry of the medullary canal to that of the head and cut using a mask that fits onto

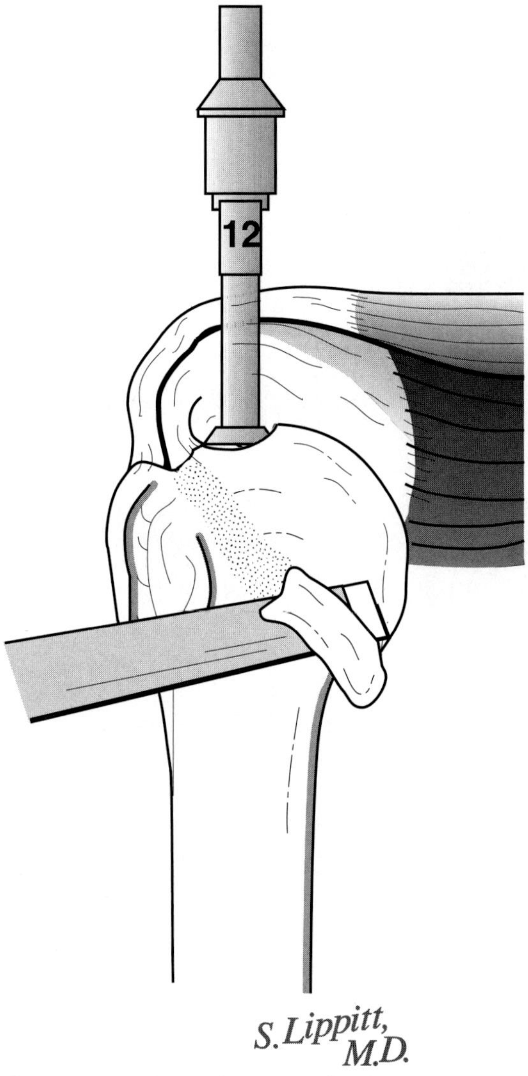


**Figure 29–18. Removing osteophytes**
The osteophytes around the neck of the humerus are removed with a rongeur and an osteotome.

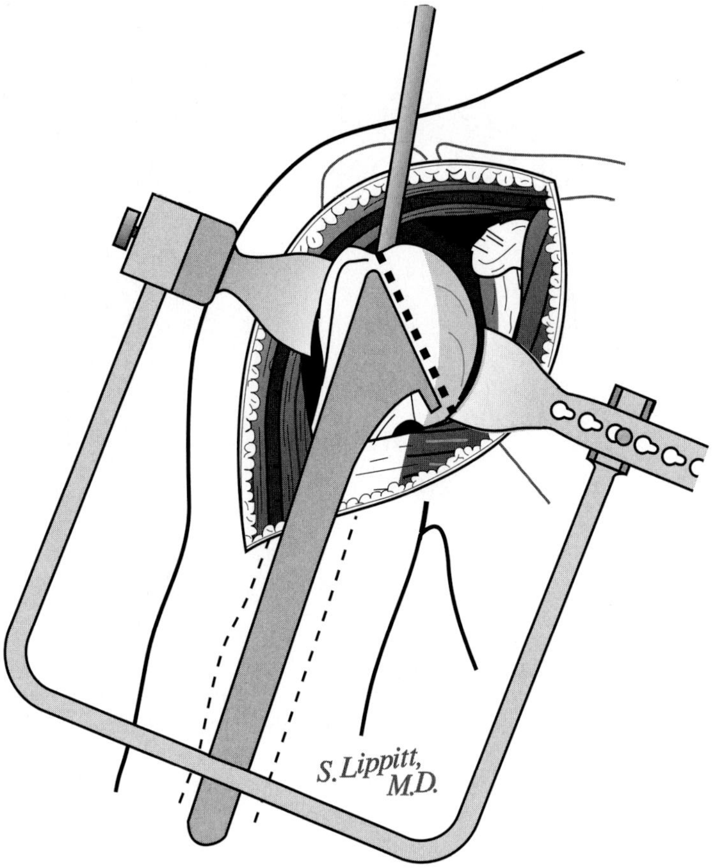


**Figure 29–19. Extramedullary cutting guide**
An extramedullary guide can approximate the desired neck shaft angle, but its accuracy is compromised by the fact that its orientation is not linked to the medullary anatomy of the humerus that guides the position of the component.

the reamer. The mask is selected that most closely matches the diameter of curvature and height of the humeral head (**Fig. 29–20**). When placed on the medullary reamer, this construct has the same basic geometry as the definitive prosthesis with the selected diameter stem, head diameter, and head height. The mask is then mounted on the medullary reamer that has been inserted into the humeral canal and oriented to respect the version of the biological head—its superior edge should bisect the humeral head along the line previously drawn (**Fig. 29–21**).

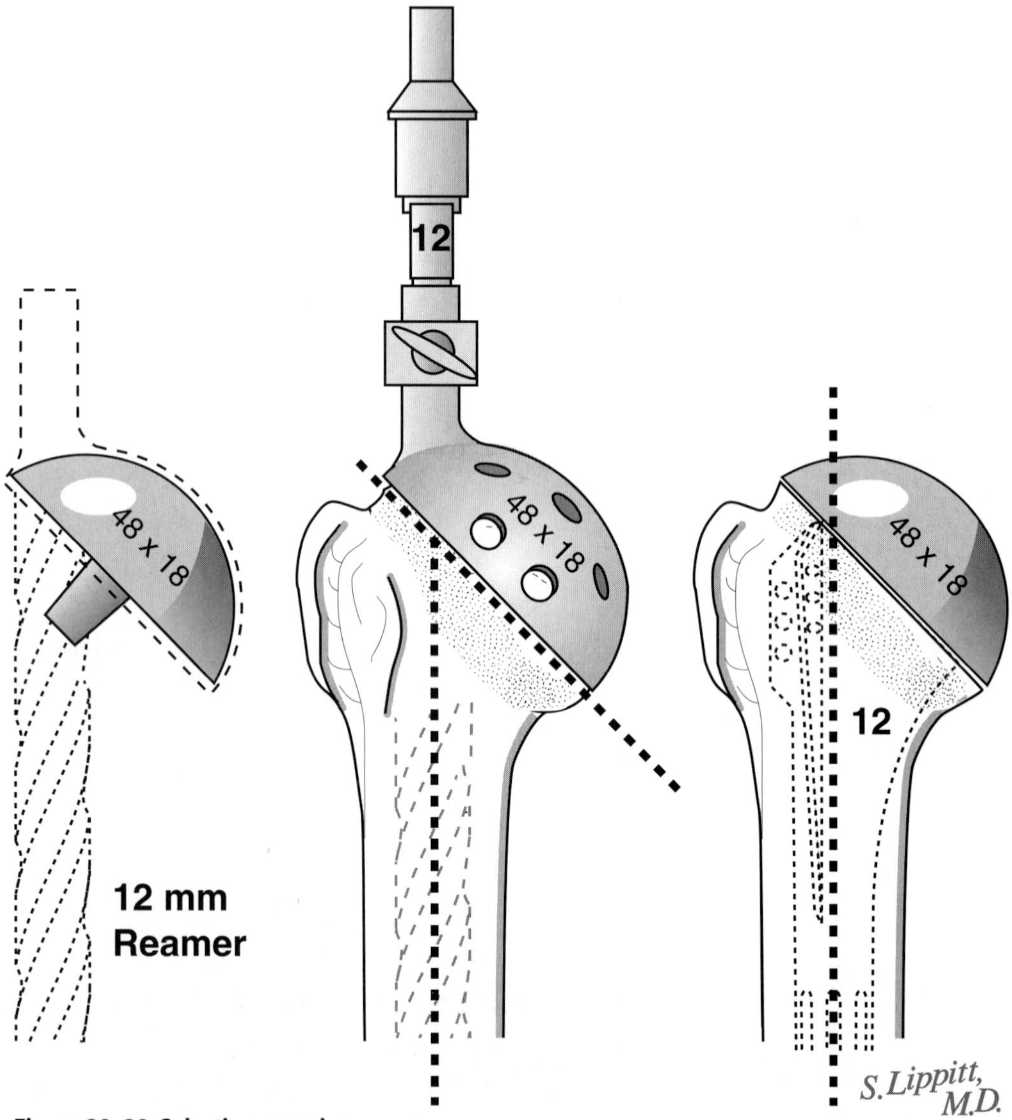


**Figure 29–20. Selecting a mask**
A mask can be used that represents the three-dimensional geometrical relationships of the prosthetic articular surface to the prosthetic stem. When the mask is placed on the reamer inserted into the canal, it enables the surgeon to see the resulting position of the articular surface and the location of the plane for humeral head resection *before* committing to a prosthesis size or neck cut.

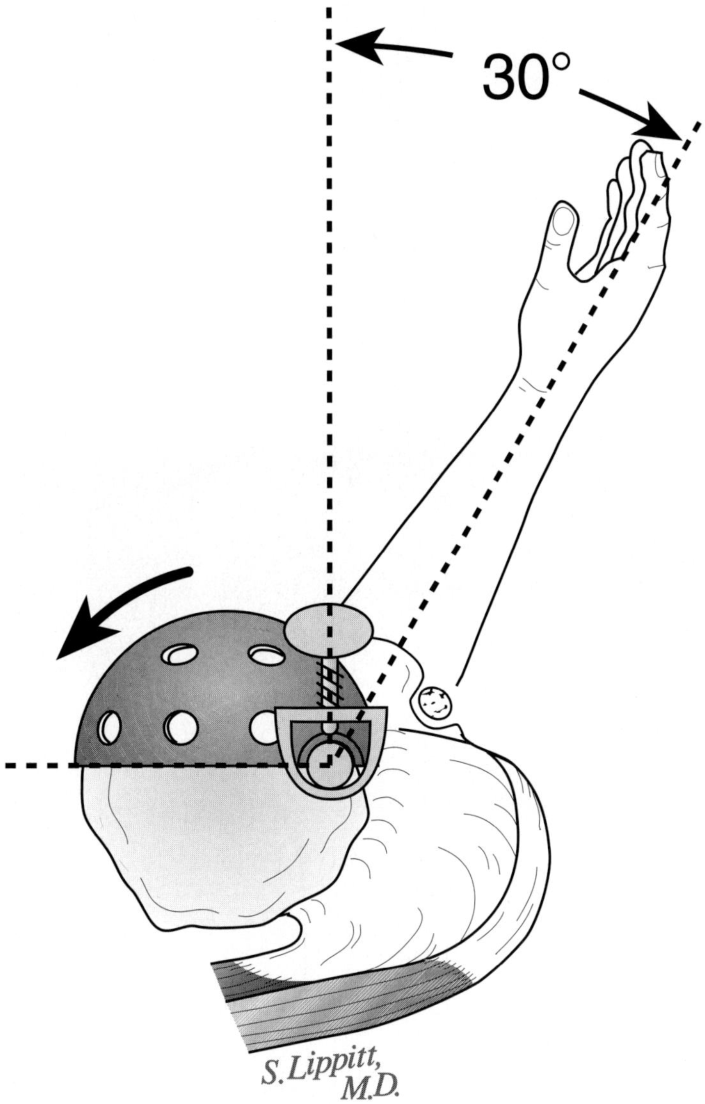


**Figure 29–21. Position of the mask**
When in position, the posterior edge of the mask should align along the humeral bisecting line drawn previously.

Using the mask, the anterior neck cut is marked with the electrocautery (**Fig. 29–22**). This line should run perpendicular to the humeral center line drawn on the proximal humerus. The mask and medullary reamer are removed and the cut line is extrapolated posteriorly, passing just inside the cuff attachment to the base of the tuberosity (**Fig. 29–23**).

Using a sharp, broad, flat osteotome, the humeral head is resected along the cut marks. The cut plane is in approximately 30 degrees of retroversion and at a 45-degree angle with the long axis of the shaft. Excessive retroversion of the cut is carefully avoided (**Fig. 29–24**). Any remaining superior humeral neck is resected down to the level of the cuff insertion.

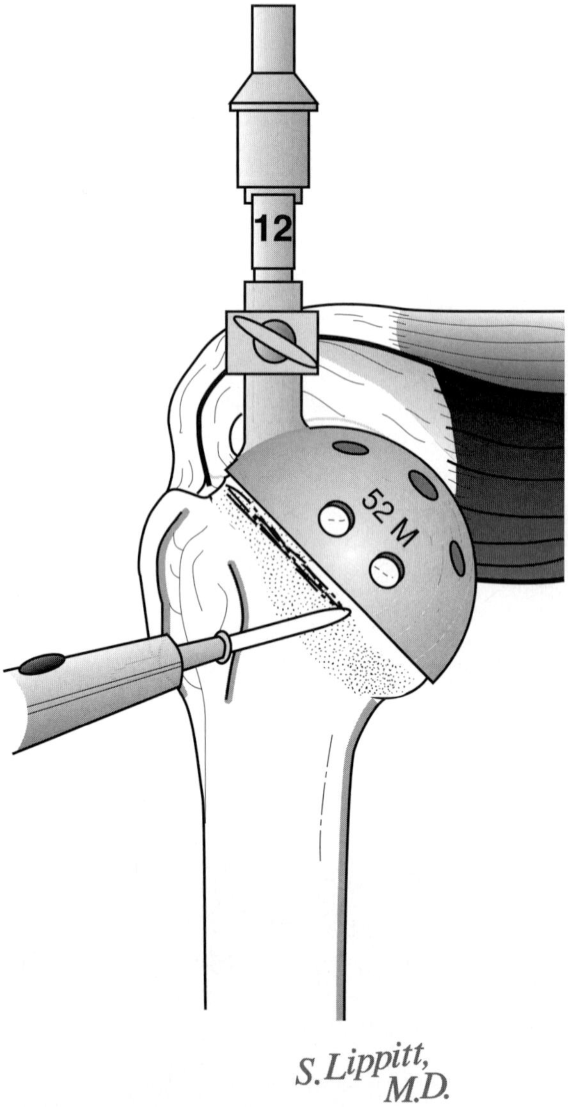


**Figure 29–22. Marking the osteotomy**
Once the position of the mask is determined to be acceptable, the cut plane is marked on the humeral neck with electrocautery.

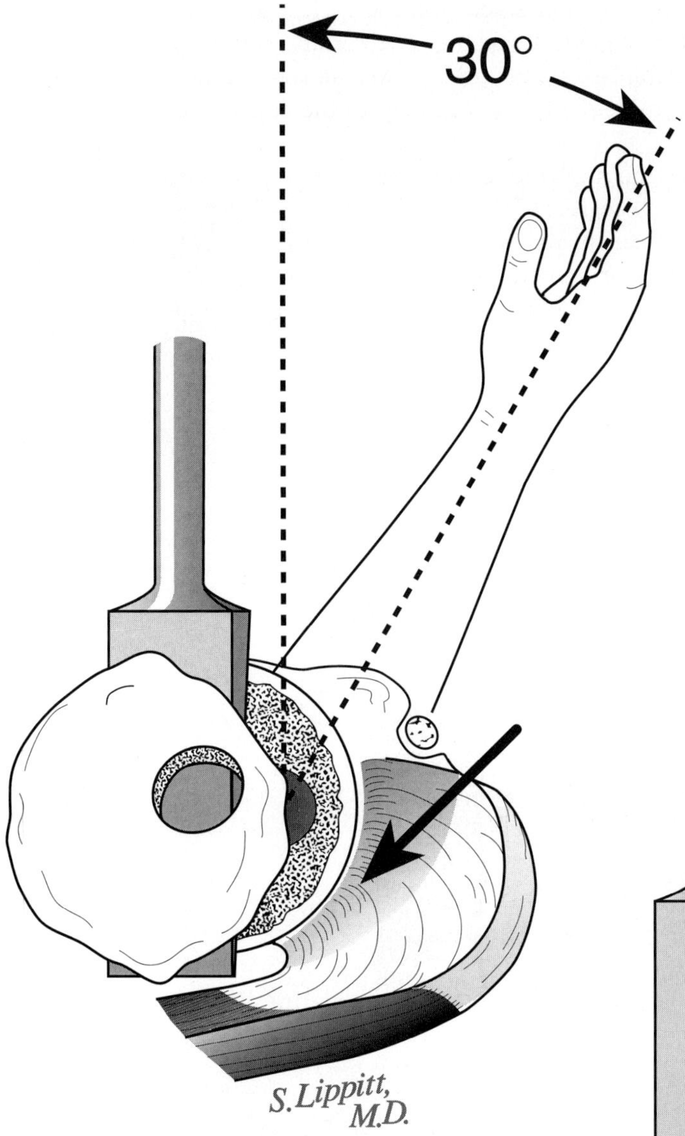


**Figure 29–23. Extending the cut line**
The osteotomy passes just inside the cuff insertion.

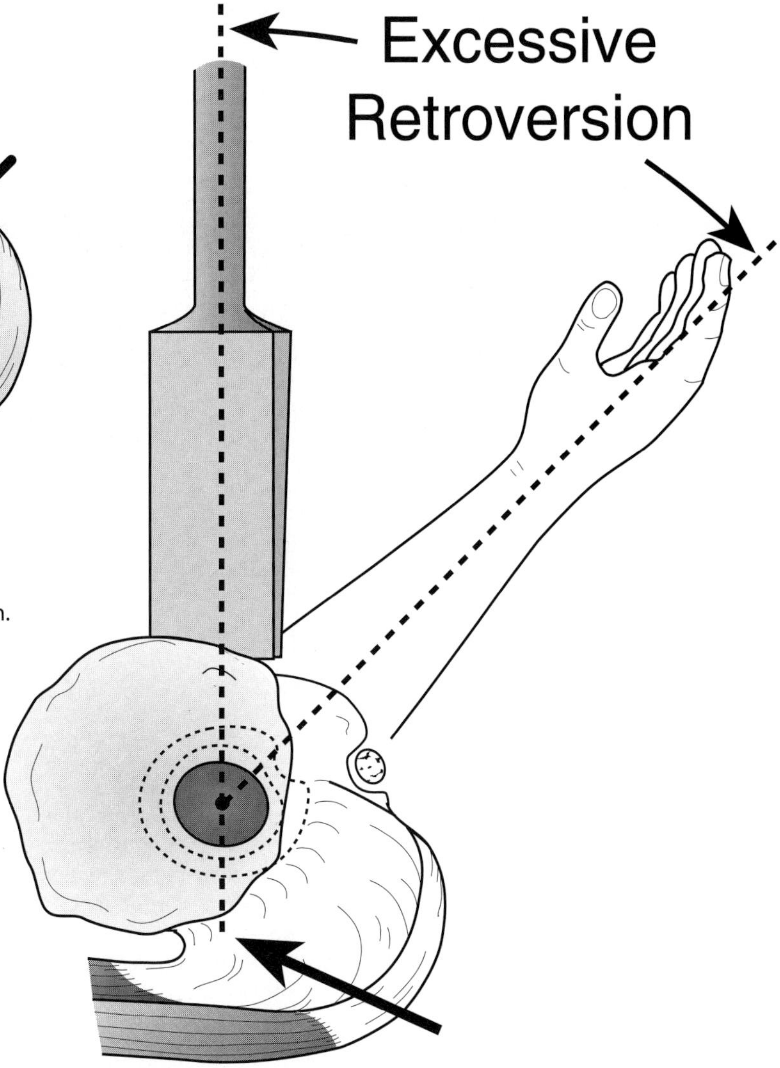


**Figure 29–24. Retroversion of the cut**
Excessive retroversion of the cut jeopardizes the integrity of the tuberosity and the cuff insertion.

While ensuring the desired version, the surgeon drives a broach osteotome corresponding to the size of the final medullary reamer into the cancellous bone at the neck cut, marking the location of the fins and the metaphyseal body (**Fig. 29–25**). The lateral and anterior fins should straddle the bicipital groove. The lateral and medial fins should parallel the bisecting line previously drawn on the humerus. The cancellous bone within the outline of the broach is removed (**Fig. 29–26**). The medullary broach

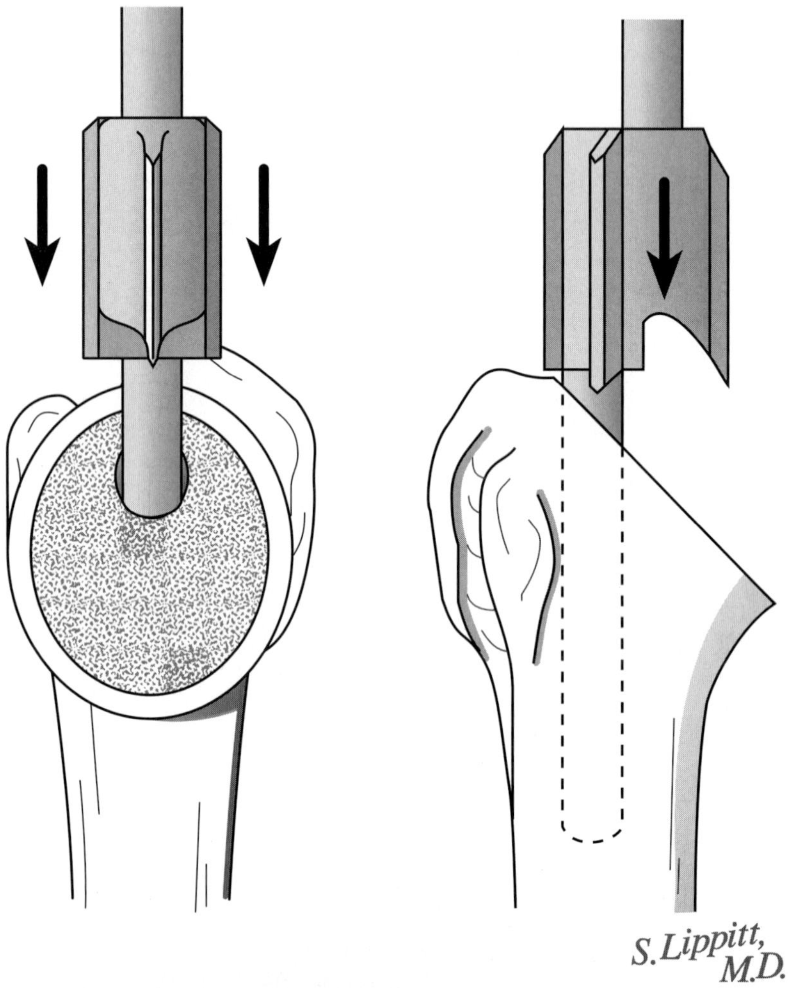


**Figure 29–25. Orienting the humeral osteotome**
A broach osteotome, or "cookie cutter," is placed down the medullary canal so that it is centered in the anteroposterior direction and held with a valgus bias so that the lateral bone will not force it into varus. Its rotation is oriented so that it is aligned with the neck and so that the anterior and lateral fins straddle the bicipital groove. This osteotome is then driven into the metaphysis to mark the resection of the metaphyseal bone.

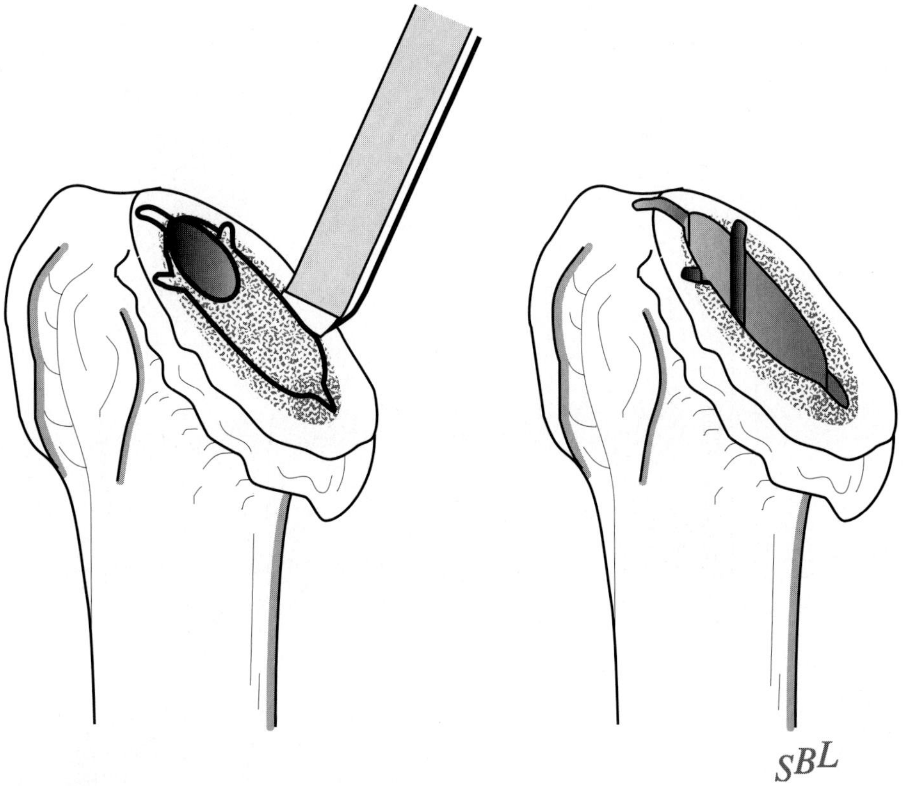


**Figure 29–26. After body sizing**
A 1/4 inch osteotome is used to remove the bone outlined by the cookie cutter.

is selected that corresponds to the final reamer diameter. The broach is advanced down the canal in the same orientation as the broach osteotome—in approximately 30 degrees of retroversion (**Fig. 29–27**). Anterior angulation of the broach is avoided (**Fig. 29–28**). The broach is used as a guide to resect the marginal osteophytes anteriorly, medially, and posteriorly. This ensures that osteophytes will not block external rotation by abutting against the posterior glenoid (**Fig. 29–29**).

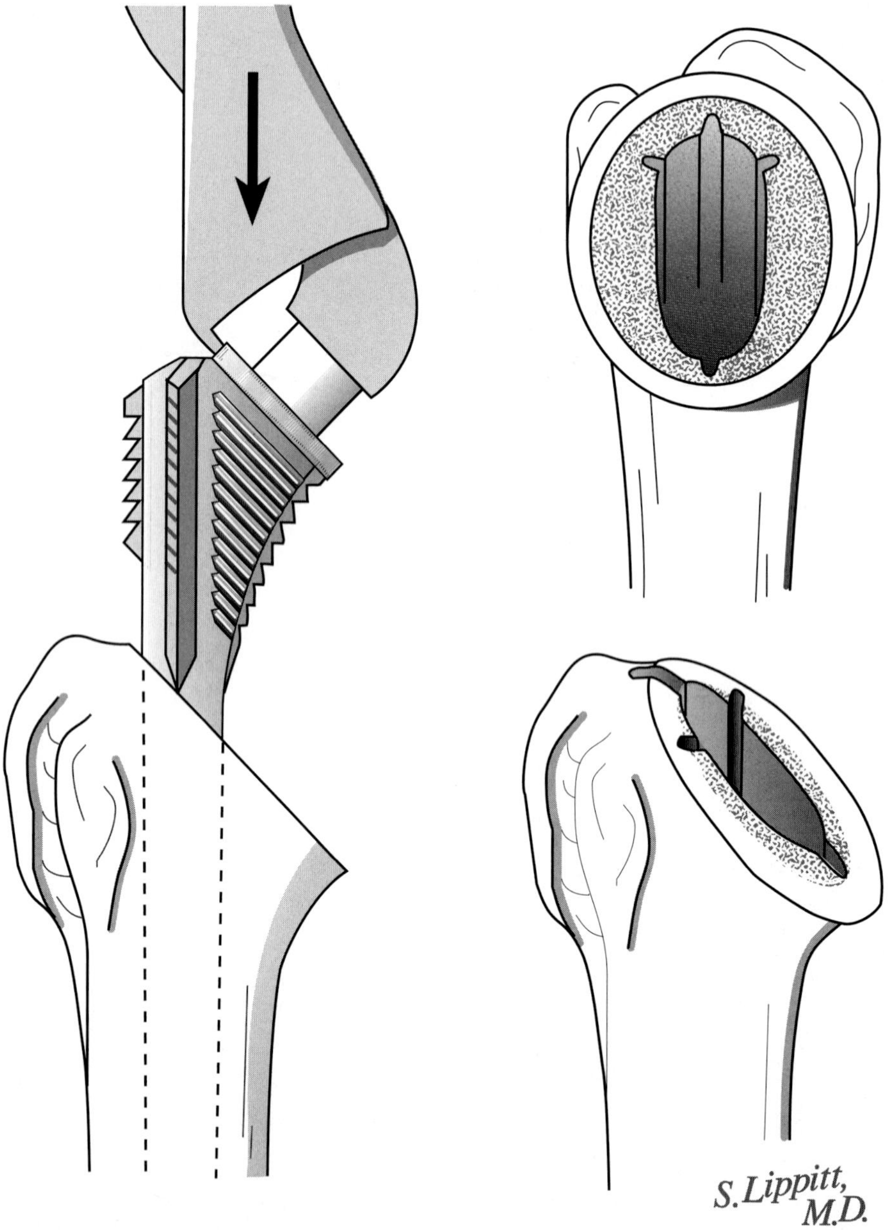


**Figure 29–27. Medullary broach**
The medullary broach corresponding to the size of the medullary reamer is inserted in proper retroversion, with care taken that the center of the broach is positioned in the center of the neck cut.

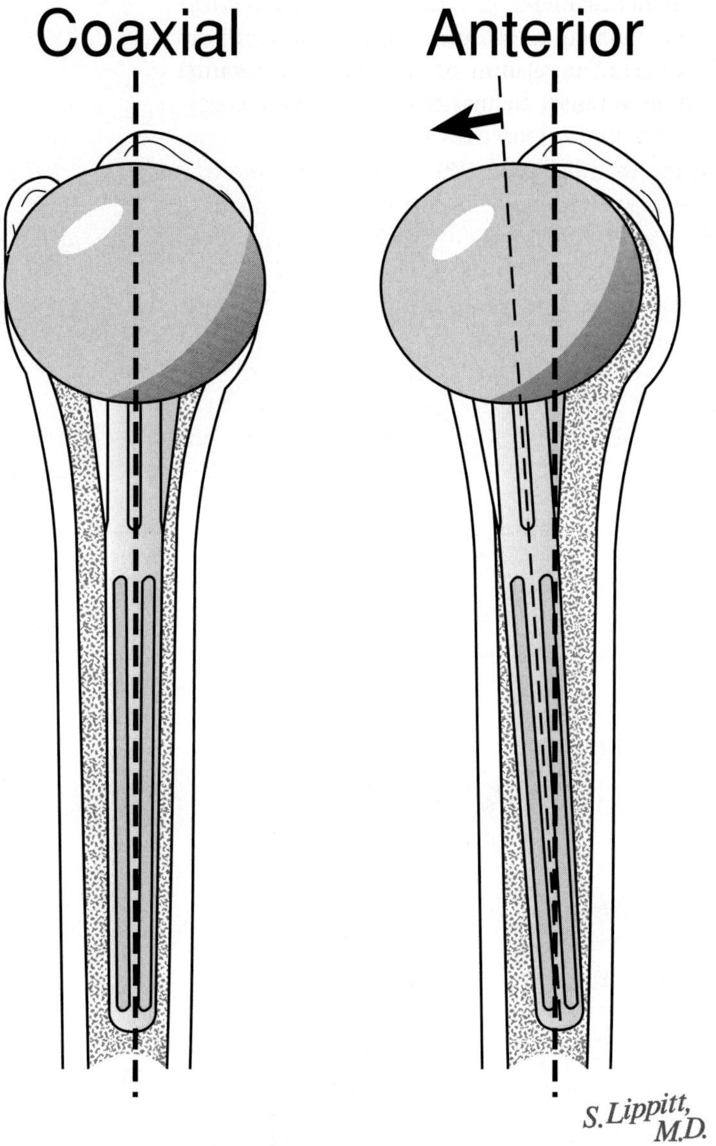


**Figure 29–28. Positioning the broach**
Particular care is needed to keep the broach coaxial with the medullary canal (*left*) rather than being inserted with its upper end too far anterior (*right*). Such anterior angulation gives the false impression of posterior offset of the humeral neck.

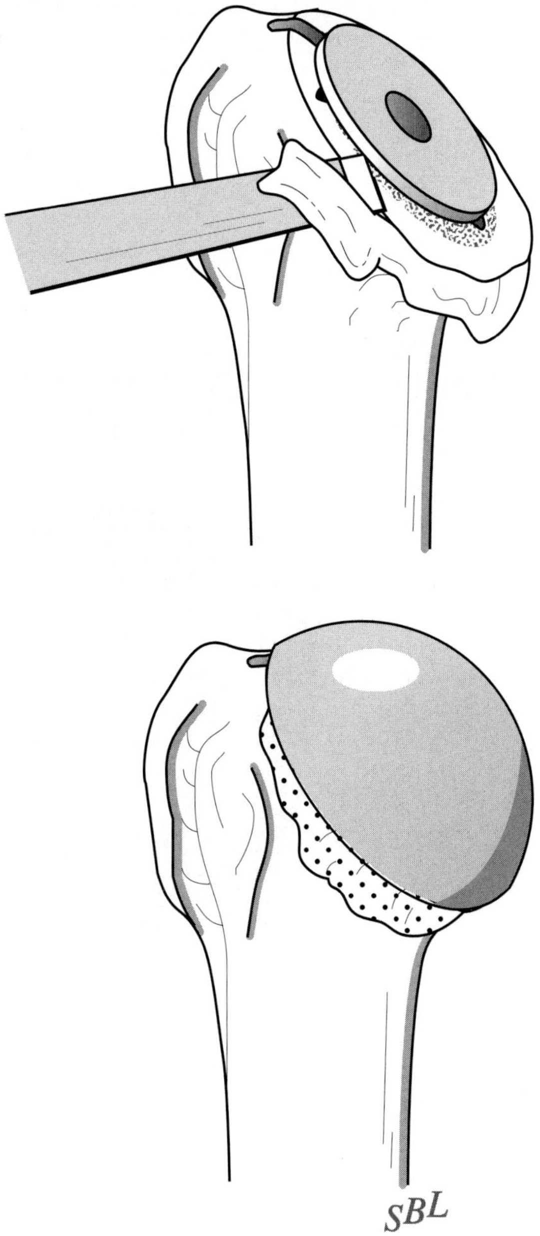


**Figure 29–29. Osteophyte removal**
The osteophytes are removed from around the neck using the centered humeral broach as a reference. Placing a trial humeral head on the broach may help guide this resection.

At this point, the nonprosthetic or prosthetic glenoid arthroplasty is carried out (see Chapters 30 and 31). Note is taken of the diameter of curvature of the humeral head that will be appropriate for the glenoid arthroplasty (2 mm smaller than the curvature of a nonprosthetic glenoid arthroplasty and 6 mm smaller than the curvature of a prosthetic glenoid arthroplasty).

Following the glenoid arthroplasty, the medullary broach (which is also the trial body) is reinserted in the medullary canal. The set of trial heads with the diameter of curvature appropriate for the glenoid are selected. Starting by inserting the trial head with the smallest head height, the laxity for each head possibility is examined until the head height is found that allows 40 degrees of external rotation with the subscapularis approximated (**Fig. 29–30**), 50% posterior translation on the posterior drawer test (**Fig. 29–31**), and 60 degrees of internal rotation with the arm in 90 degrees of abduction (**Fig. 29–32**). These are the 40, 50, 60 guidelines. The height of the trial head providing these mechanics is checked to be sure that it lies in proper relationship to the humerus and the glenoid (**Fig. 29–33**).

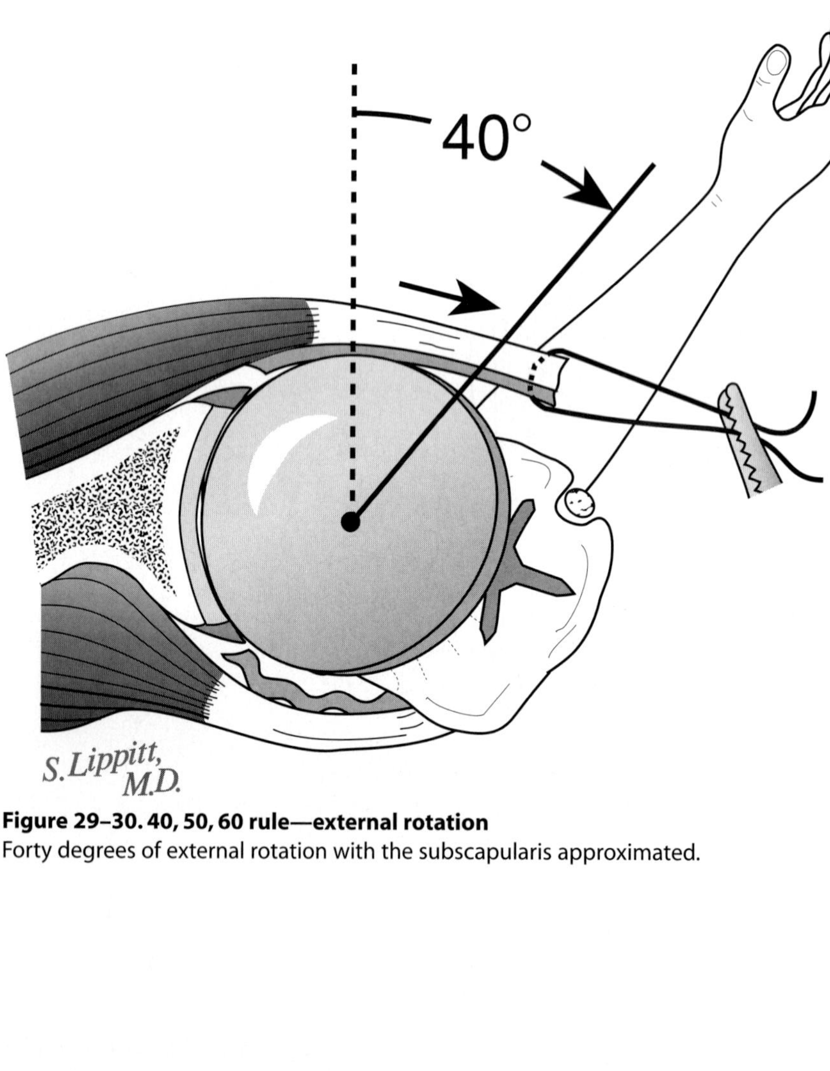


**Figure 29–30. 40, 50, 60 rule—external rotation**
Forty degrees of external rotation with the subscapularis approximated.

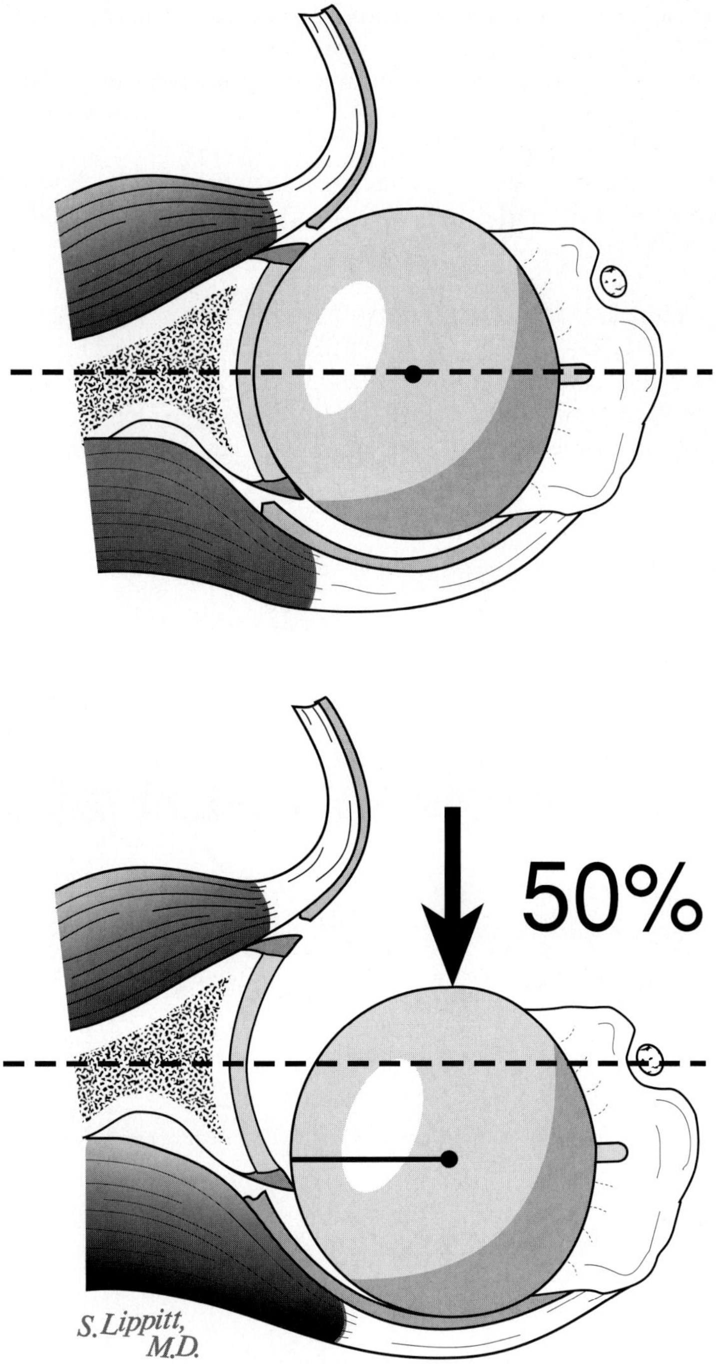


**Figure 29–31. 40, 50, 60 rule—posterior drawer**
Fifty percent posterior subluxation on the posterior drawer test.

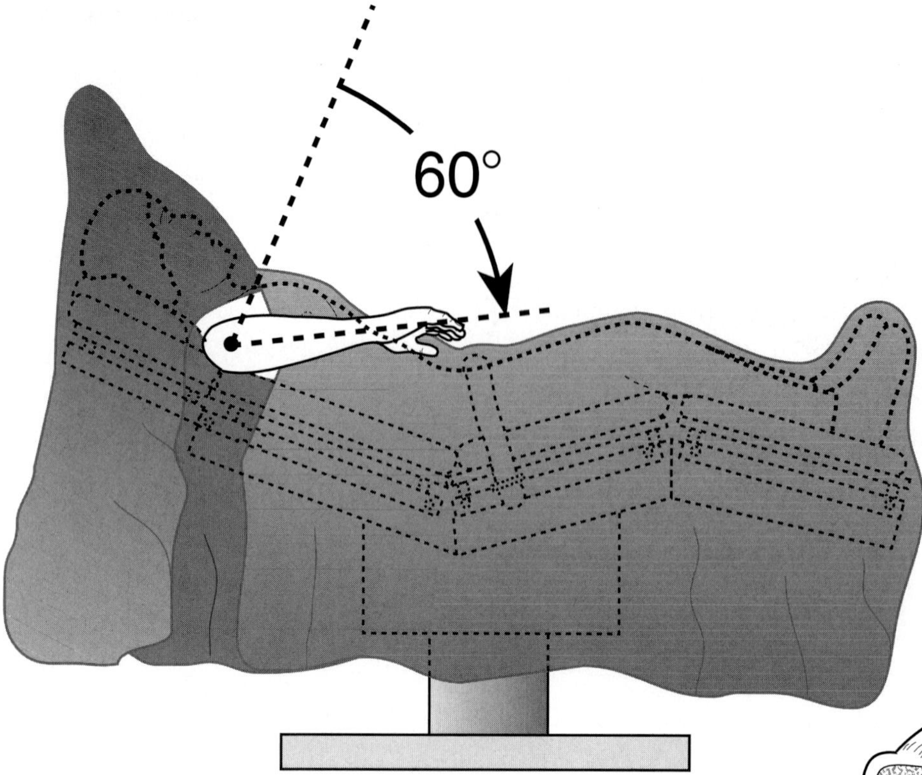


**Figure 29–32. 40, 50, 60 rule—internal rotation**
Sixty degrees of internal rotation with the arm adducted to 90 degrees.

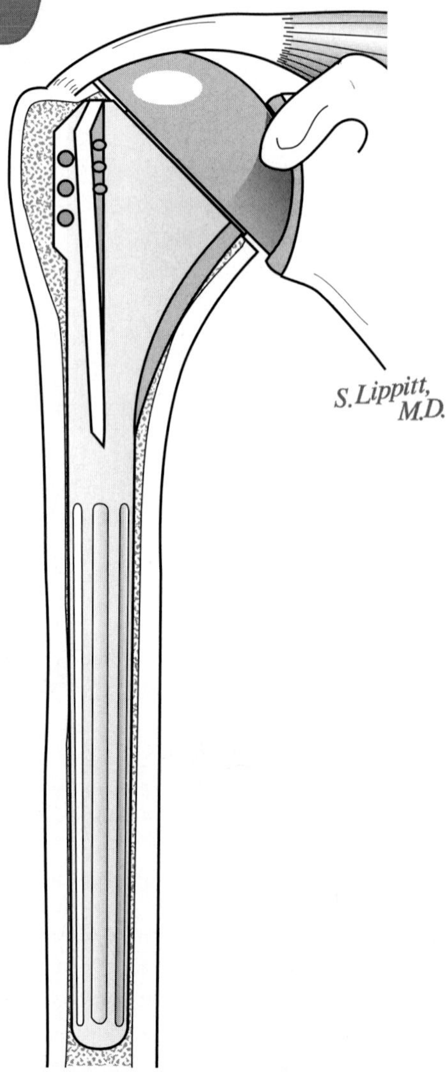


**Figure 29–33. Humeral arthroplasty**
The articular surface of the trial component should align anatomically with the tuberosity and with the glenoid.

Procrustean grafting of the humeral canal is now carried out. Small bits of cancellous bone harvested from the resected humeral head are impacted against the walls of the medullary canal using a smooth impactor with the same medullary geometry as the definitive humeral prosthesis (**Figs. 29–34** and **29–35**). Graft is added selectively to manage any tendency for the impactor to incline medially (**Fig. 29–36**) or anteriorly (**Fig. 29–37**). Selective anterior grafting can eliminate the apparent posterior offset of the neck related to anterior inclination of the prosthesis. Grafting is continued by adding and impacting successive bits of graft until the impactor cannot be removed by hand without a tap of a mallet.

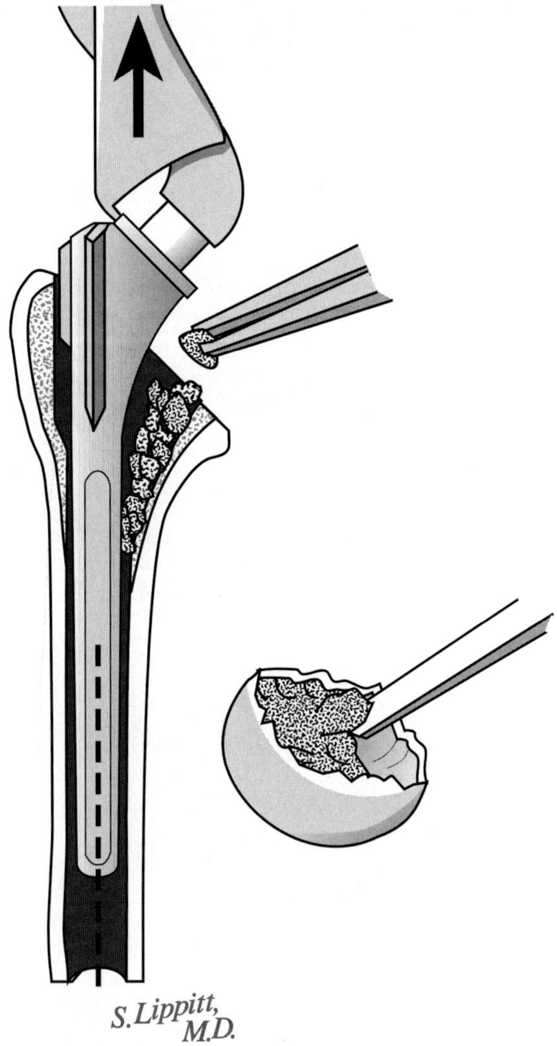


**Figure 29–34. Placing the graft**
Cancellous bone graft is harvested from the humeral head and impacted sequentially in the medullary canal to fill in the voids, to improve the fixation, and to correct any malorientation of the prosthetic body.

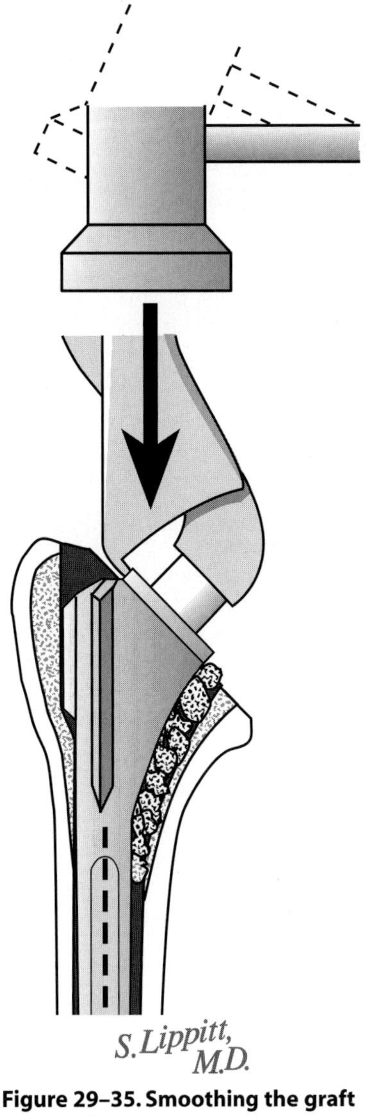


**Figure 29–35. Smoothing the graft**
Seating the impactor compresses the cancellous graft against the walls of the medullary canal.

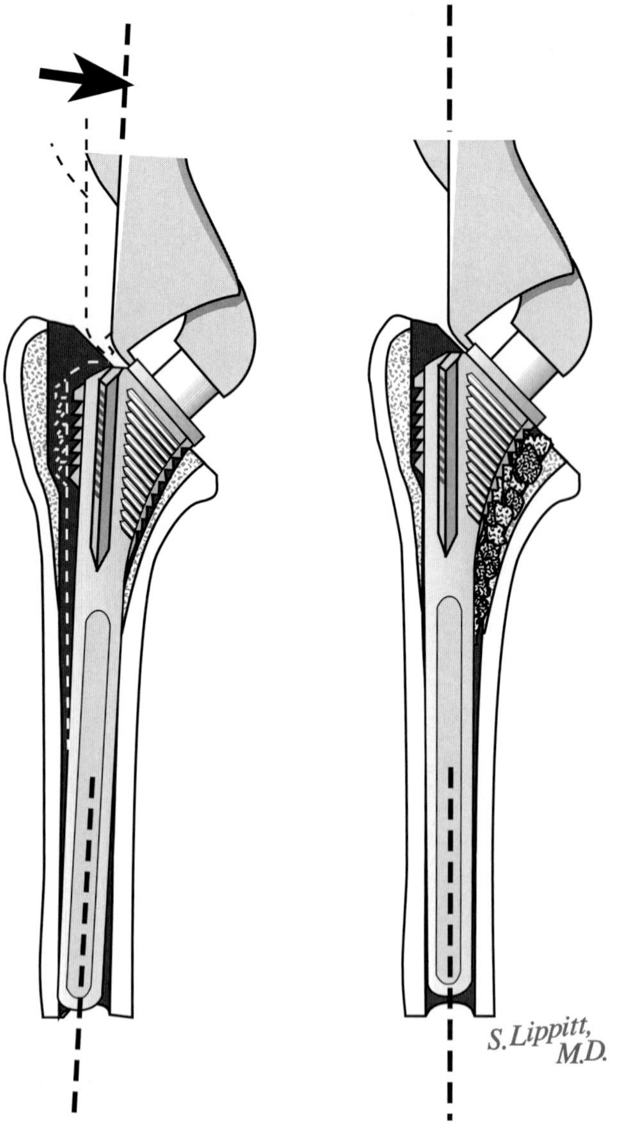


**Figure 29–36. Medial grafting**
Selective medial grafting can eliminate the tendency of the prosthesis to angulate into varus.

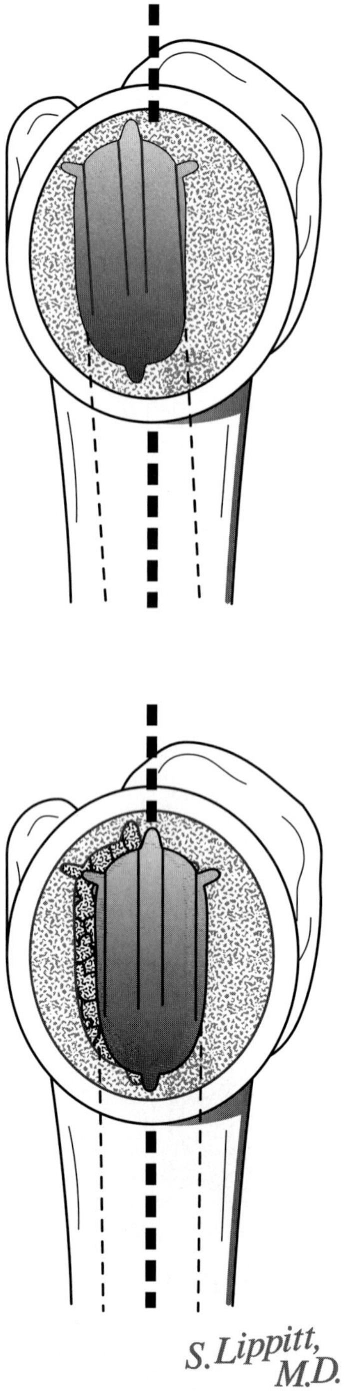


**Figure 29–37. Anterior grafting**
Selective anterior grafting can eliminate the apparent posterior offset of the neck related to anterior inclination of the prosthesis.

At least six 1.8 mm drill holes are placed along the anterior aspect of the humeral neck cut starting near the biceps tendon superiorly. Number 2 braided nonabsorbable sutures are passed through each of these holes for later reattachment of the subscapularis (**Fig. 29–38**).

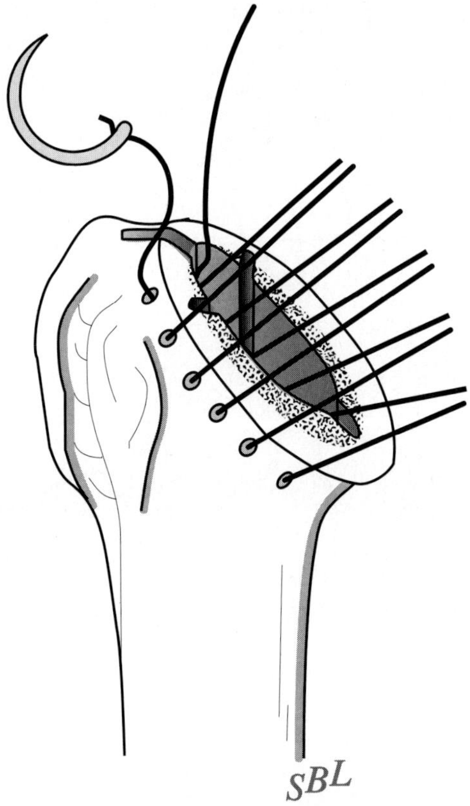


**Figure 29–38. Subscapular sutures**
At least six #2 braided nonabsorbable sutures are placed through drill holes in the anterior neck for reattachment of the subscapularis. Moving the subscapularis insertion from the lesser tuberosity to the neck gains about 1 cm in subscapularis length or about a 20-degree increase in external rotation. (Modified from Rockwood CA, Matsen FA [eds]: The Shoulder, 2nd ed. Philadelphia: WB Saunders, 1998, p. 919.)

If there is a cuff tear with good-quality tendon that can be approximated to the greater tuberosity under physiologic tension with the trial component in position and the arm at the side, it is repaired to the bone of the tuberosity at this point (**Fig. 29–39**).

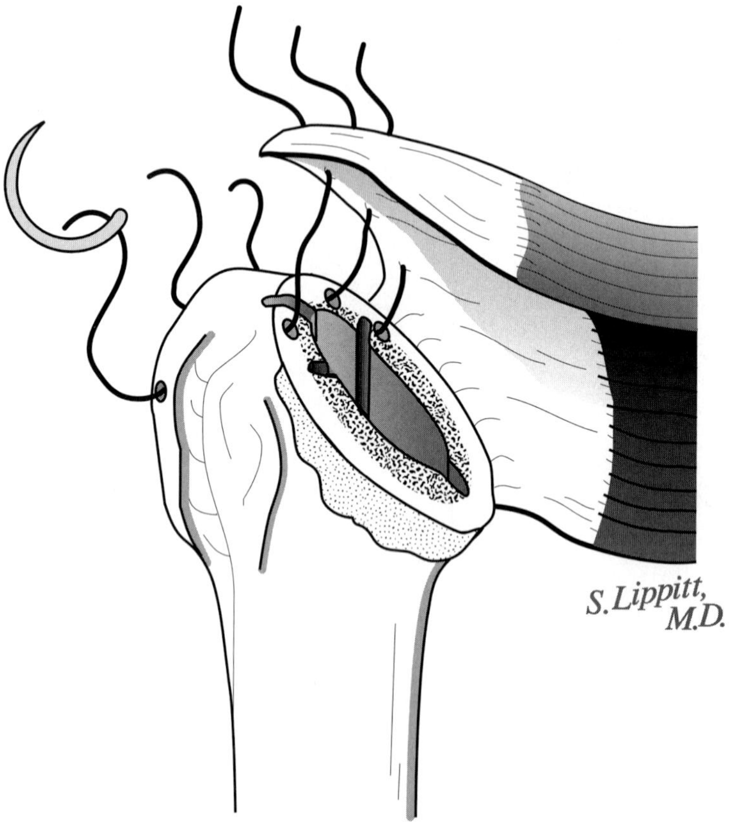


**Figure 29–39. Cuff repair**
If there is a rotator cuff tear and if the cuff tendon tissue is of sufficient quality and quantity for a durable rotator cuff repair, drill holes are placed in the tuberosity for cuff attachment before the insertion of the definitive humeral component. (Modified from Matsen FA, Lippitt SB, Sidles JA, et al [eds]: Practical Evaluation and Management of the Shoulder. Philadelphia: WB Saunders, 1994, p. 209.)

The definitive humeral prosthesis with the desired canal diameter, medullary size, head diameter of curvature, and height is selected. A small amount of additional cancellous bone graft is inserted (**Fig. 29–40**). The definitive prosthesis is inserted in the same orientation as the impactor.

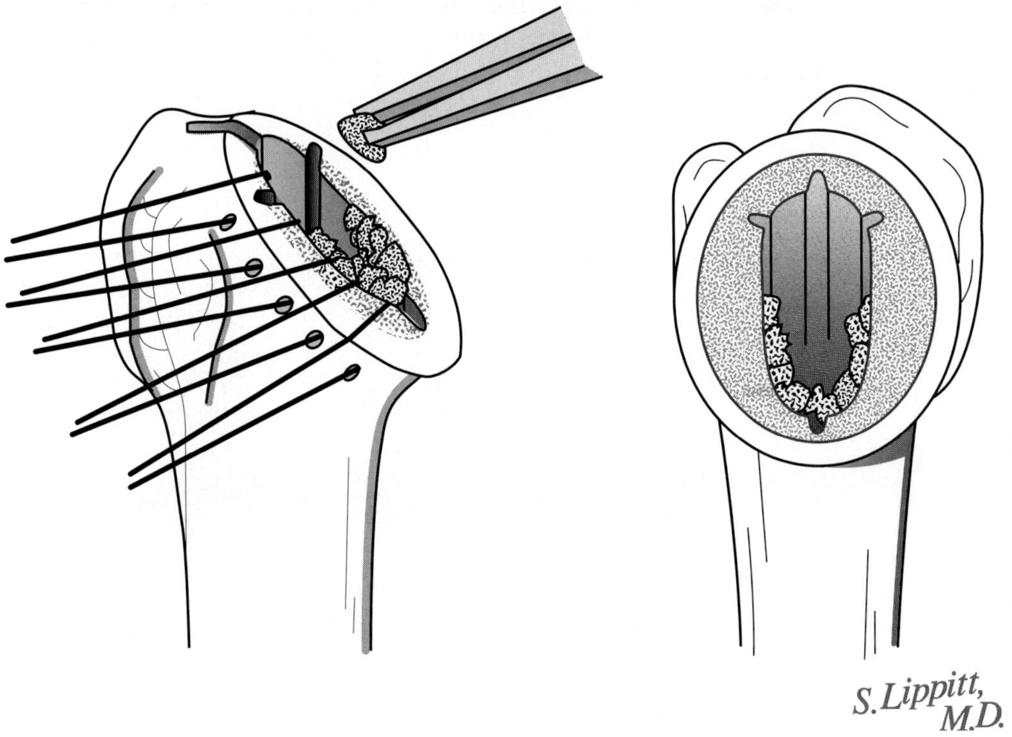


**Figure 29–40. Placement of graft**
Additional cancellous bone graft is placed in the medullary canal immediately prior to the insertion of the definitive prosthesis.

The humeral prosthesis is driven down distally until it is positioned in proper register with the glenoid; that is, the center of the head is aligned with the center of the glenoid. The arm is placed in maximal adduction while the humerus is rotated to be sure that there is no abutment between the humeral bone and the inferior glenoid (**Fig. 29–41**). The security of the humeral fixation is verified in that it cannot be budged by hand. Excellent fixation has been achieved.

The desired laxity of the shoulder is again verified (40 degrees of external rotation, 50% posterior translation, and 60 degrees of internal rotation in abduction). The humerus is externally rotated in different angles of elevation to be sure that there is no bone abutting posteriorly against the glenoid. Such posterior abutment is signaled by levering open a gap between the humeral and glenoid joint surfaces as the arm is externally rotated (**Fig. 29–42**).

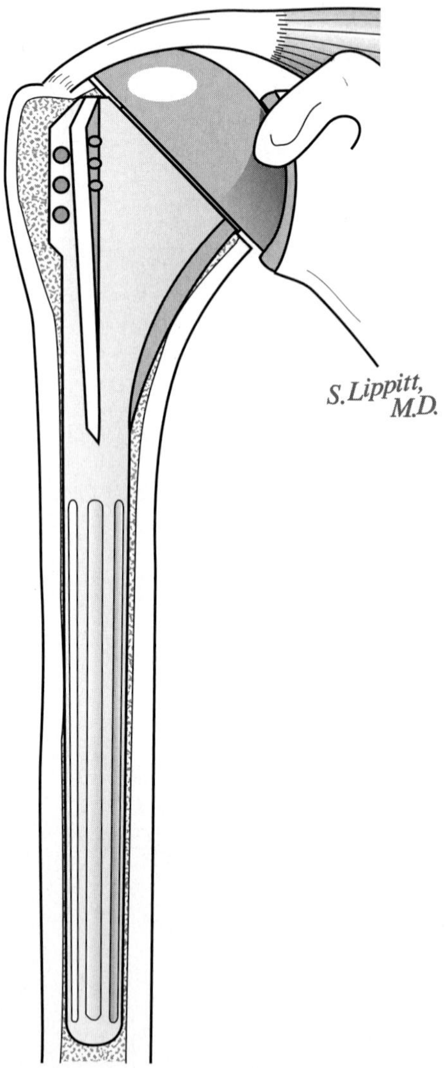


**Figure 29–41. Humeral arthroplasty with ideal register**

The articular surface of the humeral component should align anatomically with the tuberosity and with the glenoid.

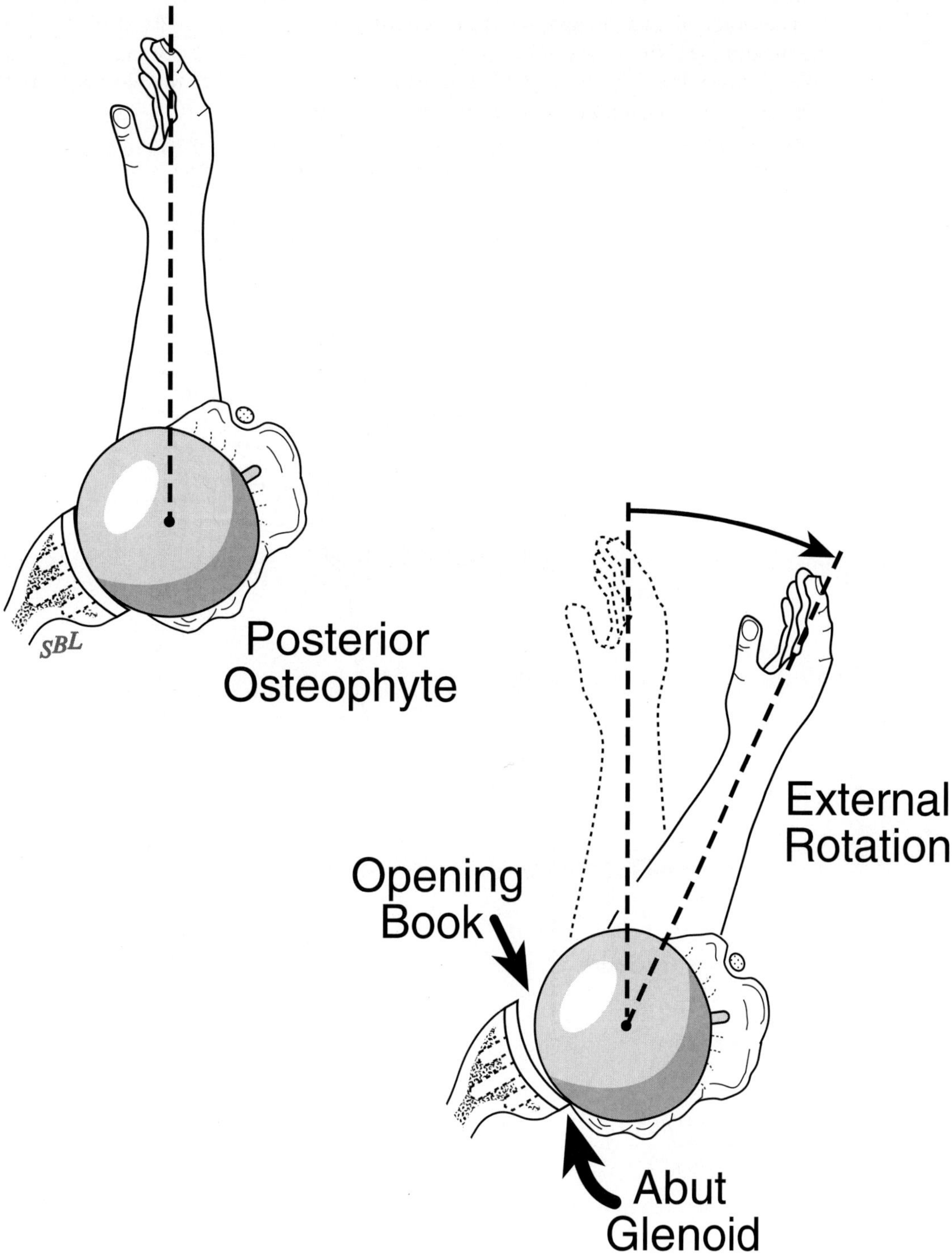


**Figure 29–42. Posterior abutment**
Bone extending beyond the contour of the humeral head posteriorly can abut the posterior glenoid, causing the shoulder to "open book" on external rotation.

The wound is thoroughly irrigated to remove any remaining bits of bone or debris.

The subscapularis is then repaired to the sutures previously placed at the anterior neck cut. Particular attention is directed at securing the upper border of the tendon (**Fig. 29–43**). If additional subscapularis length had been needed, an "inside-out" Z-plasty would have been considered (**Fig. 29–44**). An excellent subscapularis repair is achieved.

The wound is again irrigated and closed in layers over a drain. Interrupted closures are used in the skin to allow for drainage.

Dry sterile dressings are applied, and the patient is returned to the recovery room with the arm in continuous passive motion.

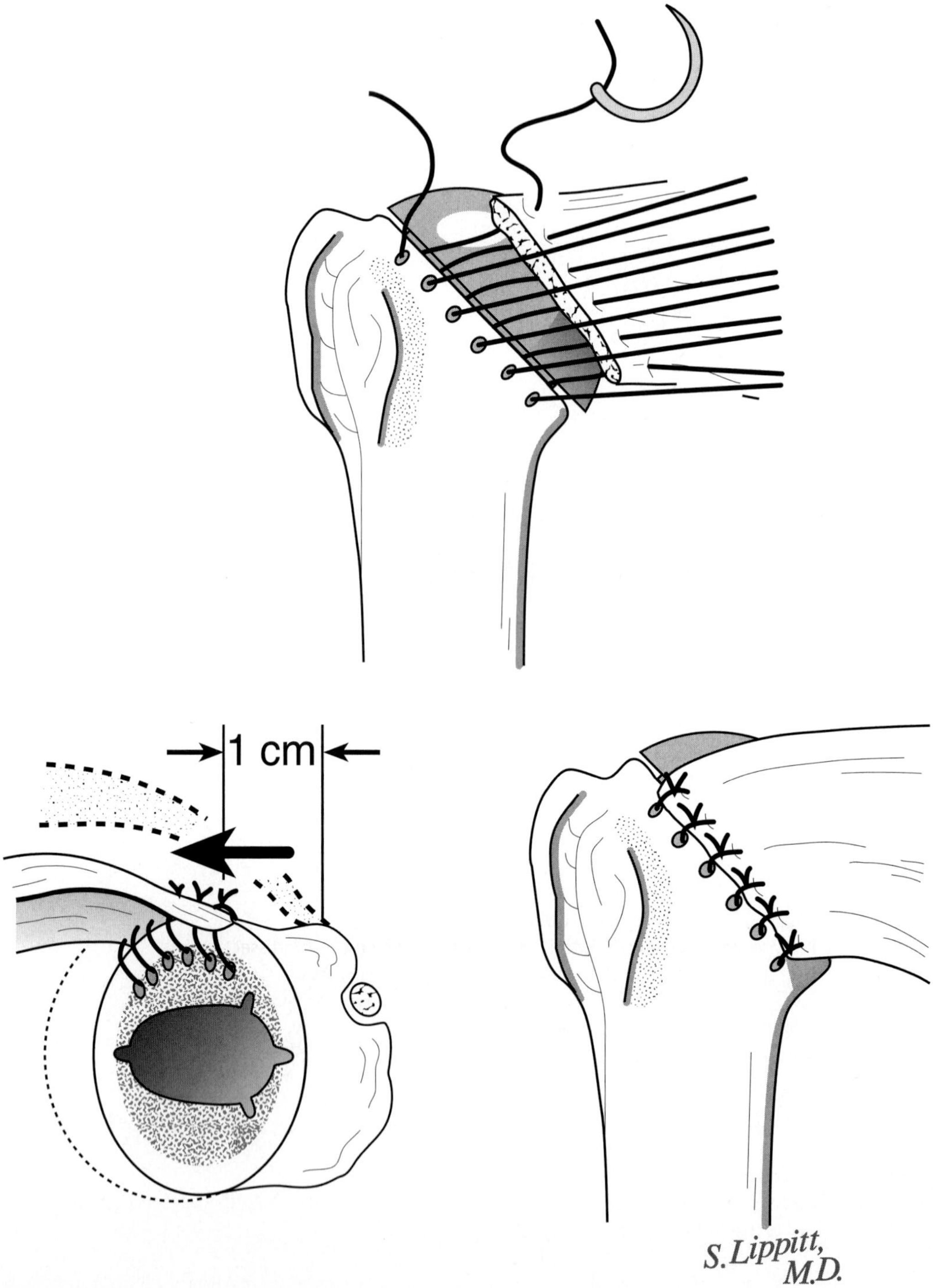


**Figure 29–43. Repair subscapularis**
The subscapularis is repaired to the anterior humeral neck cut. (Modified from Matsen FA, Lippitt SB, Sidles JA, et al [eds]: Practical Evaluation and Management of the Shoulder. Philadelphia: WB Saunders, 1994, p. 204.)

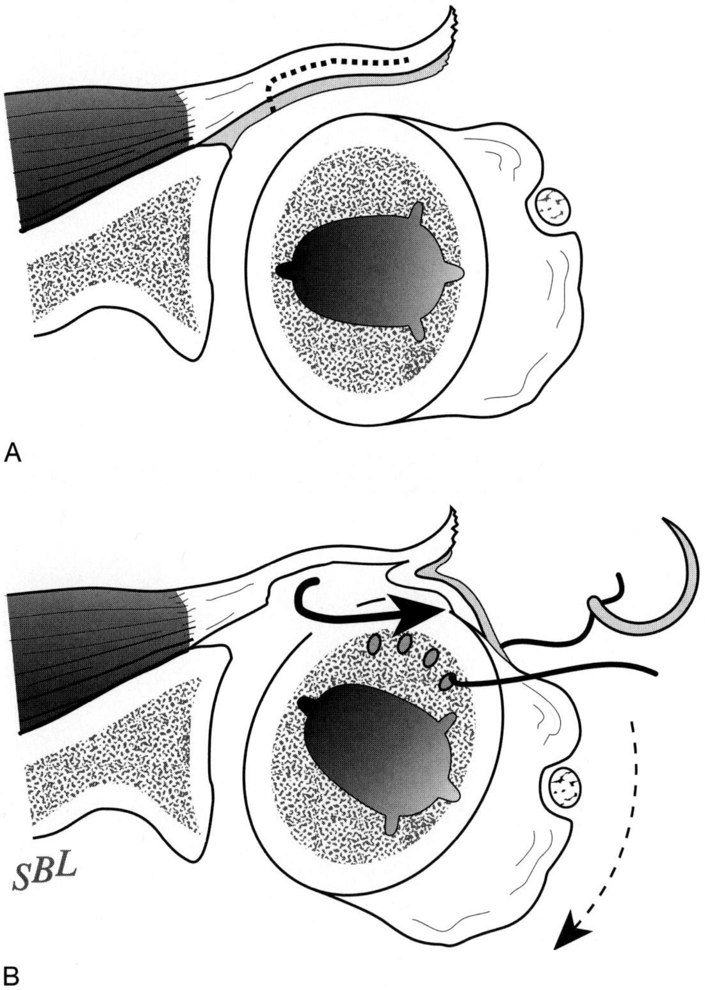


B

**Figure 29–44. Inside-out subscapularis Z-plasty**

If more subscapularis length is needed, the capsule can be dissected medially from the deep side of the subscapularis tendon, leaving their connection laterally, and swung out for attachment to the lesser tuberosity. (Modified from Matsen FA, Lippitt SB, Sidles JA, et al [eds]: Practical Evaluation and Management of the Shoulder. Philadelphia: WB Saunders, 1994, p. 204.)

## POSTOPERATIVE PLAN

Continuous passive motion is continued while the patient is in bed for the first 36 hours after surgery (**Fig. 29–45**). It is removed when the patient is in a chair or ambulating.

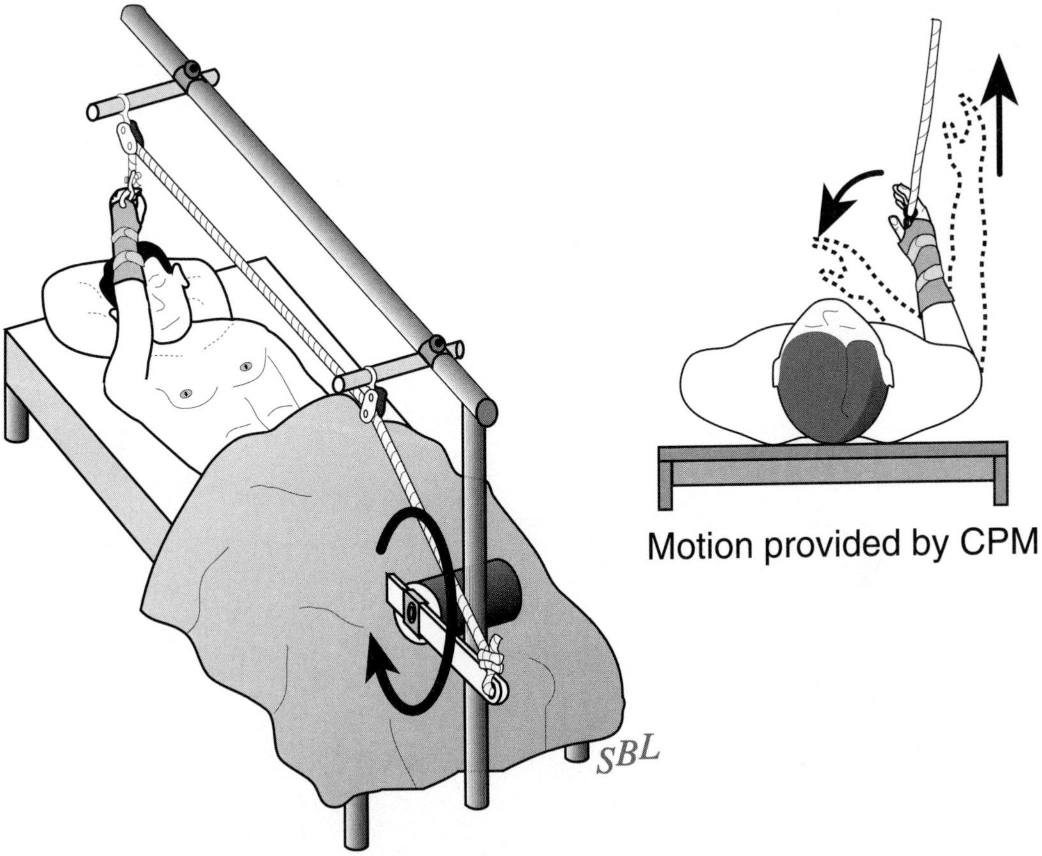


**Figure 29–45. Continuous passive motion**

Continuous passive motion for the first 36 hours after surgery helps ensure that the healing in the humeroscapular motion interface proceeds in a way that yields smooth articulating surfaces rather than adhesions, which can develop rapidly if the shoulder is immobilized during the early healing response after surgery. Continuous passive motion provides mechanical signals to the healing cells, differentiating those that are to heal the subscapularis tendon to the bone from those that are to facilitate sliding of the proximal humeral convexity on the undersurface of the coracoacromial arch. (Modified from Matsen FA, Lippitt SB, Sidles JA, et al [eds]: Practical Evaluation and Management of the Shoulder. Philadelphia: WB Saunders, 1994, p. 50.)

On the day of surgery, the patient begins assisted flexion to 140 degrees and assisted external rotation to 40 degrees (**Figs. 29–46, 29–47,** and **29–48**).

Activities of daily living are encouraged, but the patient should avoid lifting more than 1 pound for 6 weeks.

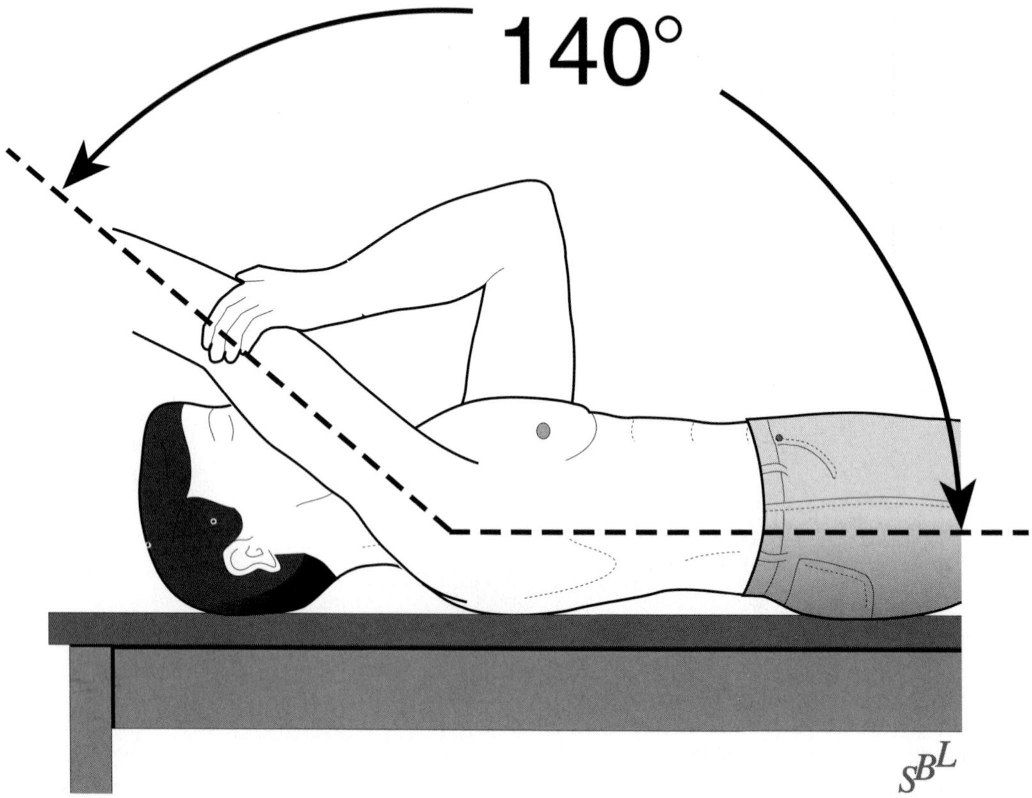


**Figure 29–46. Postoperative exercise—elevation**

Using the opposite arm as necessary for assistance, the patient works to elevate the arm to 140 degrees. (Modified from Matsen FA, Lippitt SB, Sidles JA, et al [eds]: Practical Evaluation and Management of the Shoulder. Philadelphia: WB Saunders, 1994, p. 46.)

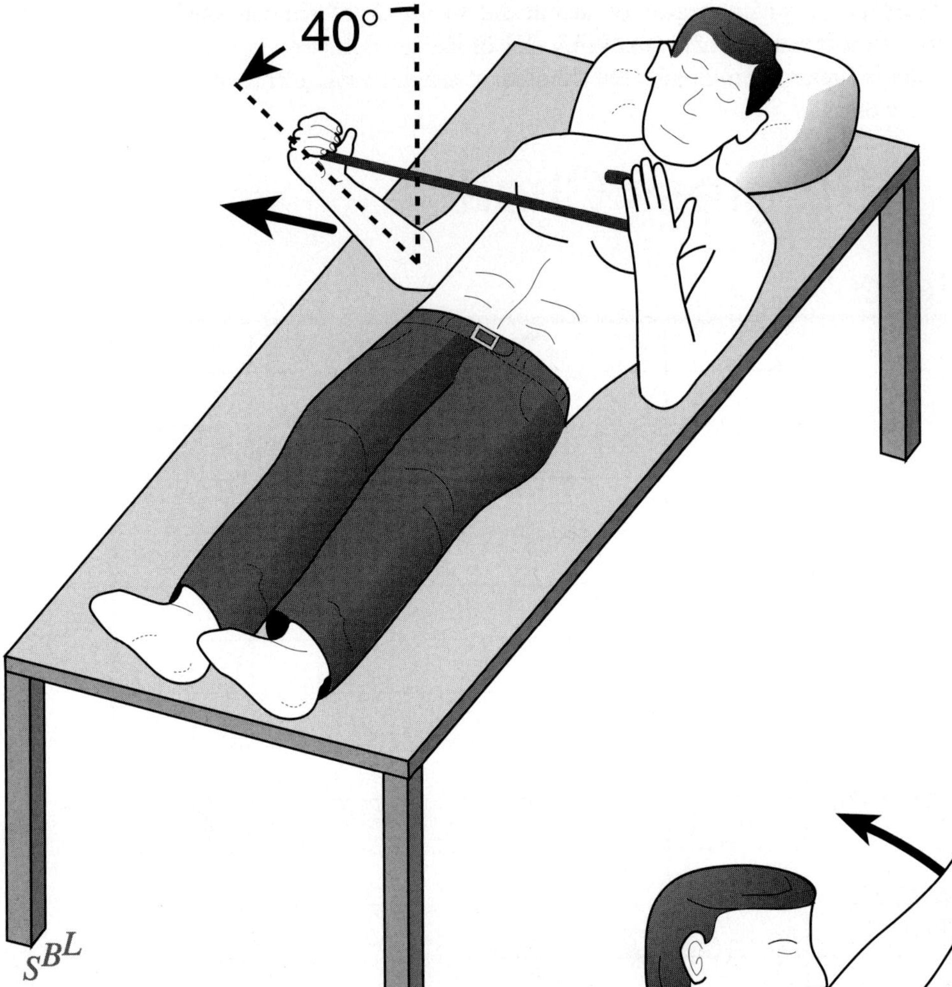


**Figure 29–47. Postoperative exercise—external rotation**
Using the opposite arm as necessary for assistance, the patient works to externally rotate the arm to 40 degrees. (Modified from Matsen FA, Lippitt SB, Sidles JA, et al [eds]: Practical Evaluation and Management of the Shoulder. Philadelphia: WB Saunders, 1994, p. 47.)

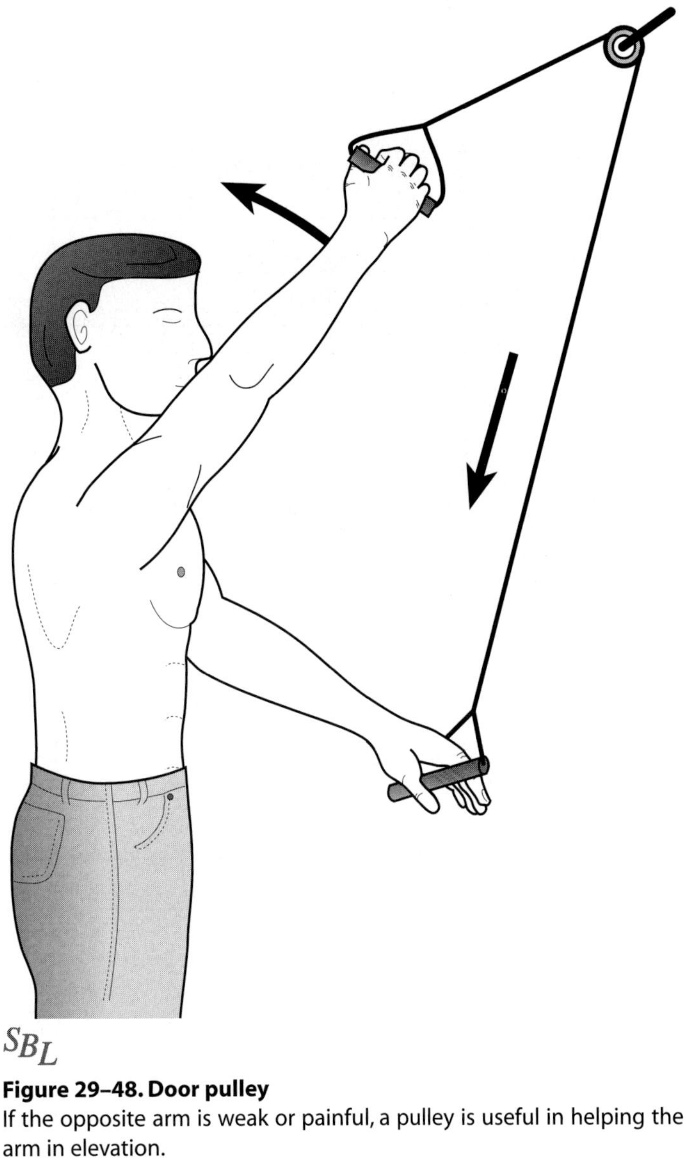


**Figure 29–48. Door pulley**
If the opposite arm is weak or painful, a pulley is useful in helping the arm in elevation.

As soon as assisted motion of 140 degrees of flexion and 40 degrees of external rotation is achieved, the patient is discharged to continue his or her rehabilitation at home (**Fig. 29–49**). Emphasis is placed on moving the shoulder through its range of motion at least five times per day.

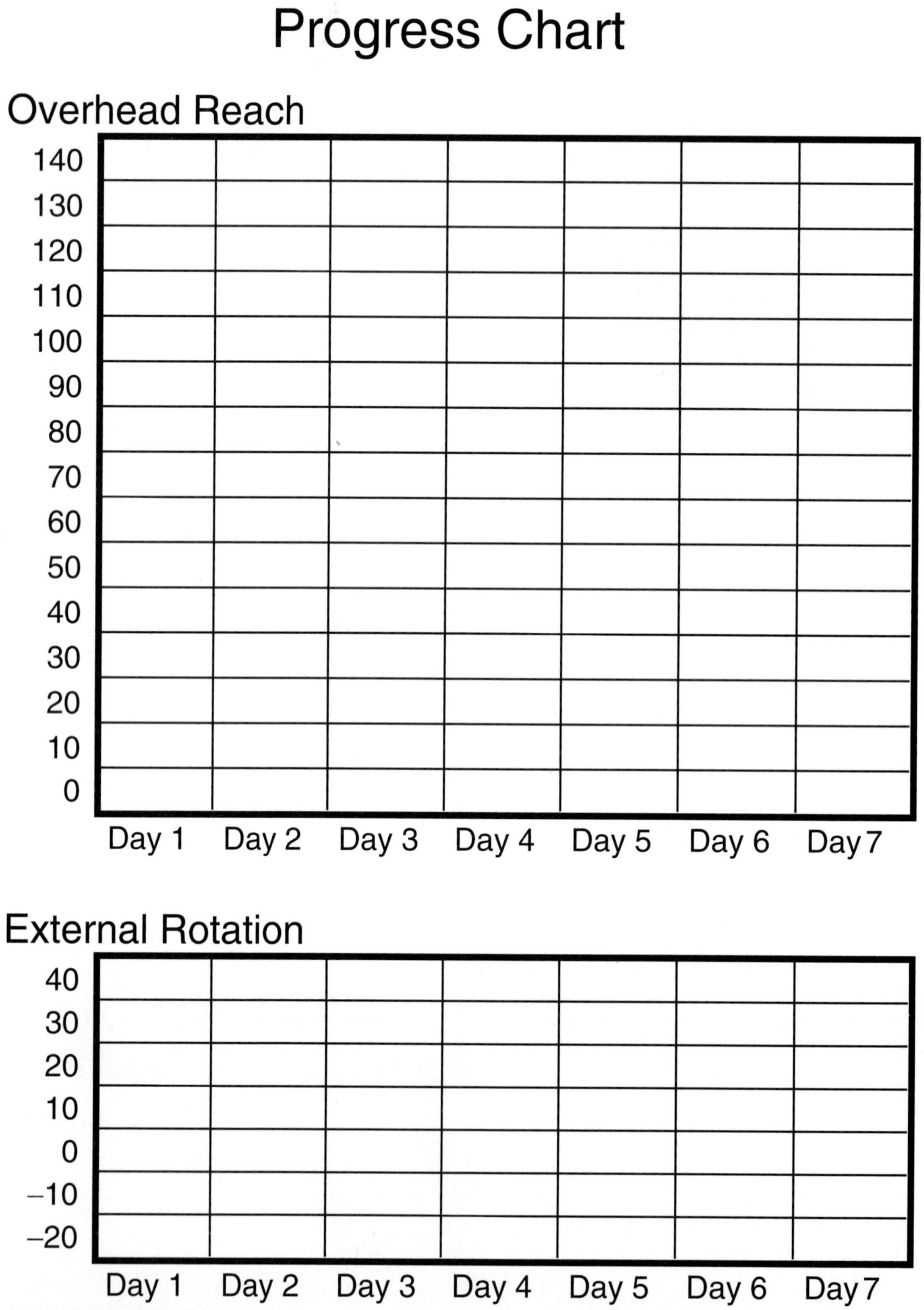


**Figure 29–49. Wall chart**
The patient's daily progress in the hospital is marked on a wall chart so that visitors and staff can provide positive feedback. (Modified from Matsen FA, Lippitt SB, Sidles JA, et al [eds]: Practical Evaluation and Management of the Shoulder. Philadelphia: WB Saunders, 1994, p. 56.)

After 6 weeks, progressively more activity is allowed as long as these activities are comfortable. Additional stretching exercises are started at this time (**Figs. 29–50, 29–51, 29–52,** and **29–53**).

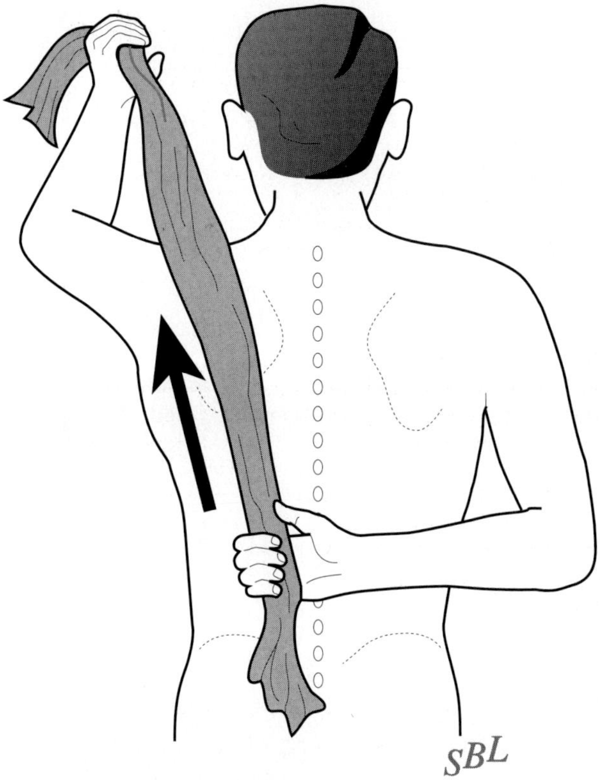

**Figure 29–50. Stretching exercise—internal rotation**
With the assistance of the other hand as necessary, the hand of the involved arm is brought up the back, stretching internal rotation in adduction. (Modified from Matsen FA, Lippitt SB, Sidles JA, et al [eds]: Practical Evaluation and Management of the Shoulder. Philadelphia: WB Saunders, 1994, p. 48.)

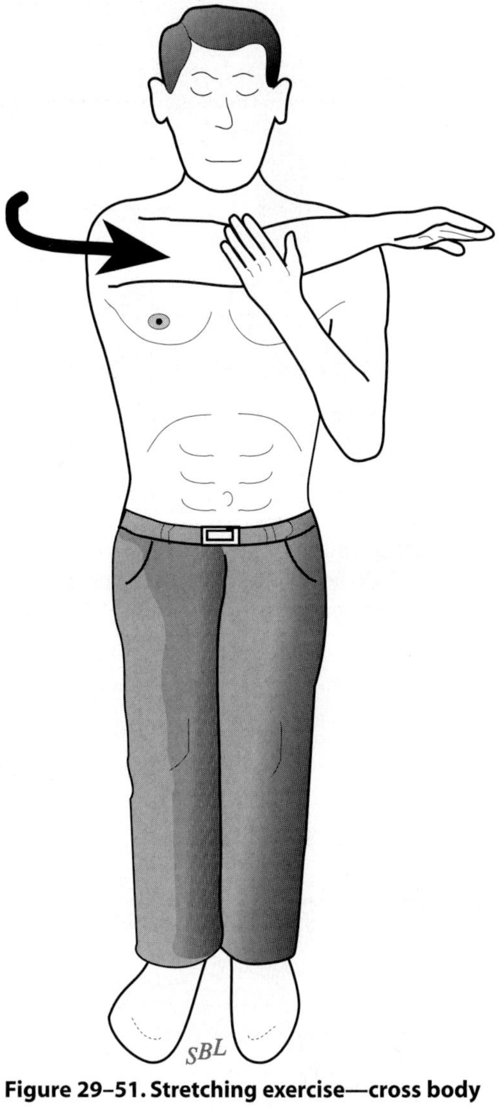

**Figure 29–51. Stretching exercise—cross body**
With the assistance of the other hand as necessary, the involved arm is brought across the body toward the opposite shoulder, stretching in cross-body adduction. (Modified from Matsen FA, Lippitt SB, Sidles JA, et al [eds]: Practical Evaluation and Management of the Shoulder. Philadelphia: WB Saunders, 1994, p. 49.)

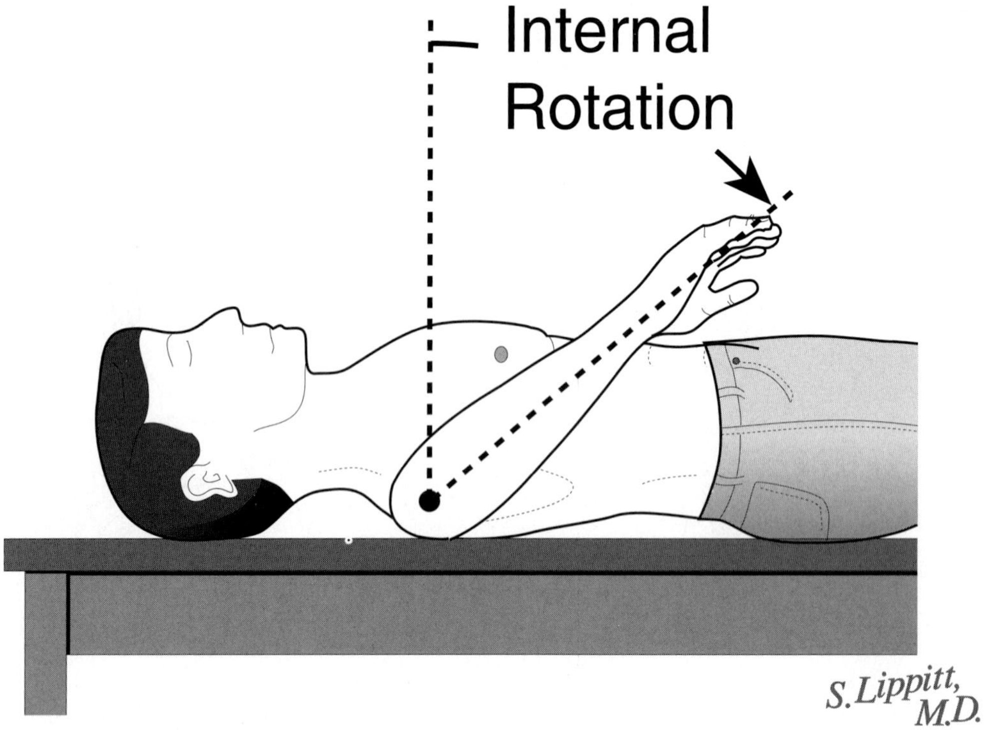


**Figure 29–52. Stretching exercise—internal rotation in abduction**
With the arm abducted to 90 degrees, the involved arm is internally rotated using the opposite arm or with the help of a friend, stretching internal rotation in abduction. (Modified from Rockwood CA, Matsen FA [eds]: The Shoulder, 2nd ed. Philadelphia: WB Saunders, 1998, p. 1083.)

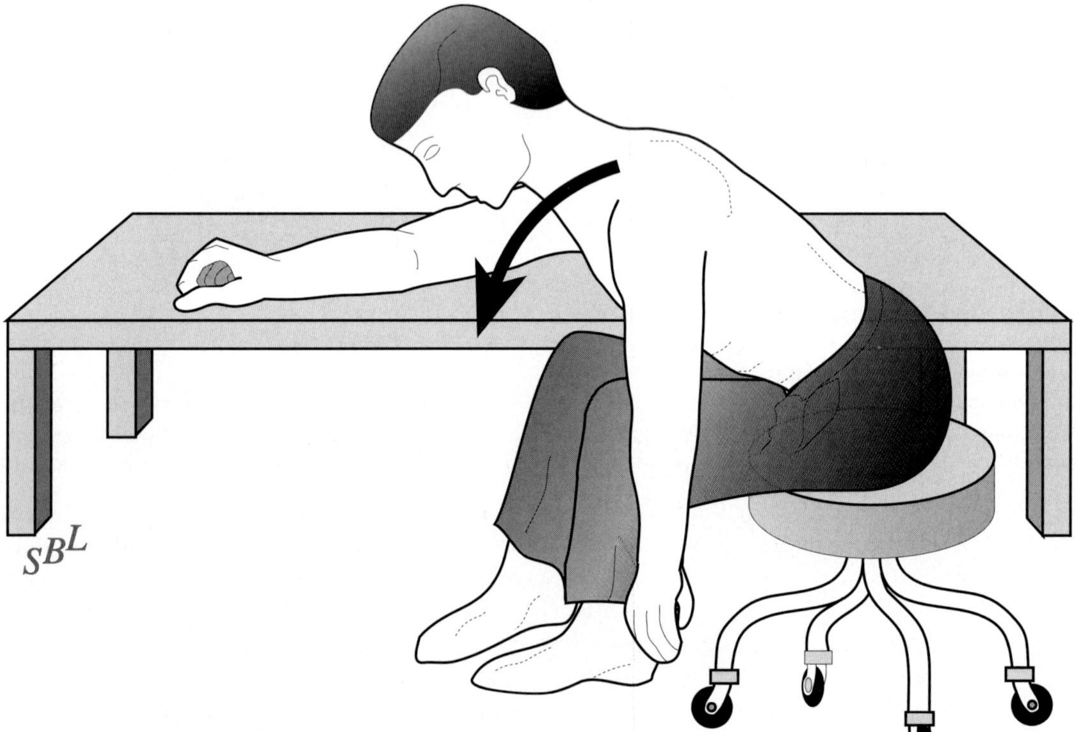


**Figure 29–53. Stretching exercise—forward lean**
Advanced stretching in forward flexion can be achieved by this forward-leaning exercise. (Modified from Matsen FA, Lippitt SB, Sidles JA, et al [eds]: Practical Evaluation and Management of the Shoulder. Philadelphia: WB Saunders, 1994, p. 46.)

CHAPTER 30

# Procedure: Reconstruction of the Glenoid Surface Using a Nonprosthetic Glenoid Arthroplasty

***Diagnosis***

***Rheumatoid arthritis ICD9 CODE 714.0***
***or***
***Osteoarthritis ICD9 CODE 715.11***
***or***
***Traumatic arthritis ICD9 CODE 716.11***
***or***
***Avascular necrosis ICD9 CODE 733.41***

***Procedure***

***Nonprosthetic glenoid arthroplasty CPT CODE 23929***
***Performed with humeral hemiarthroplasty***
***CPT CODE 23470.22 or 23472.52***

## INDICATIONS

The patient has glenohumeral arthritis that limits the comfort and function of the shoulder. It has not responded to nonoperative management.

Preoperative radiographs reveal loss of the normal glenoid concavity.

The patient desires an alternative to prosthetic glenoid arthroplasty to avoid the potential problems related to polyethylene and polymethylmethacrylate.

Knowing the alternatives as well as the risks of infection, neurovascular injury, excessive stiffness, pain, weakness, fracture, instability, glenoid arthritis, and the need for revision surgery, as well as anesthetic complications, the patient desires to proceed with the above-described procedure. The patient understands that the purpose of the procedure is to recreate a functional glenoid concavity without the use of polyethylene or bone cement. The patient accepts the fact that the postoperative course is not expected to be as rapid or as comfortable as with a prosthetic glenoid arthroplasty. The patient recognizes that this procedure cannot be expected to completely restore normal comfort and function to the shoulder. And, lastly, the patient understands his or her critical role in the post-surgical rehabilitation.

## FINDINGS

Examination under anesthesia reveals a range of glenohumeral motion that is limited in all directions and bony crepitance on glenohumeral motion.

Surgical findings include loss of normal glenoid articular cartilage with some areas worn down to bone. Much of the cartilage is fibrillated and in the process of dissolution.

The bone is of good quality and there is sufficient bone anteriorly and posteriorly for the establishment of anterior and posterior wall height.

## OPERATION

Under satisfactory anesthesia, the patient is placed in a low beach chair position with the glenohumeral joint at the edge of the operating table (see Fig. 29–2). The shoulder is doubly prepped and draped so that the arm is free to be moved. The shoulder is approached through a deltopectoral incision along a line connecting the mid-clavicle to the deltoid tubercle (see Figs. 29–3, 29–4, and 29–5).

The humeroscapular motion interface is mobilized (see Fig. 29–6). The axillary nerve is identified and protected throughout the case. The subscapularis and subjacent capsule are incised from their insertion to the lesser tuberosity (see Figs. 29–7 and 29–8). A 360-degree subscapularis release is performed (see Fig. 29–9 and 29–10).

The proximal humerus is prepared for a humeral arthroplasty as described in the previous procedure description (see Chapter 29).

The capsule is released from the anterior and inferior glenoid, with the labrum left attached to the bone. This dissection is carried just past the origin of the long head of the triceps, incising the anterior and posterior bands of the inferior glenohumeral ligaments (**Fig. 30–1**). This release is usually sufficient for cases of primary osteoarthritis and capsulorrhaphy arthropathy, because the posterior capsule is often stretched in these conditions. However, if the posterior capsule is tight, it can be released from the posterior glenoid labrum. In performing a posterior capsular release, the surgeon places the capsule under tension by rotating the humeral head retractor away from the glenoid, first inferiorly and then superiorly (**Fig. 30–2**). These releases provide excellent exposure of the glenoid (**Fig. 30–3**).

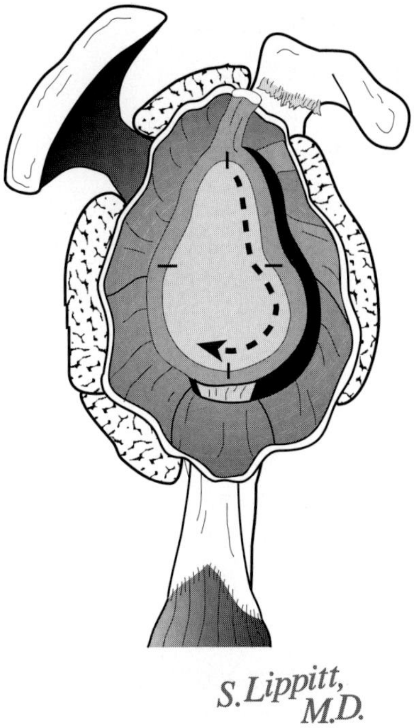


**Figure 30–1. Anterior capsule release**
The anterior capsule is released, with the labrum left intact to the glenoid so that its fossa-deepening effect is retained. The release is carried down and through the anterior and posterior bands of the inferior glenohumeral ligament. (Modified from Matsen FA, Lippitt SB, Sidles JA, et al [eds]: Practical Evaluation and Management of the Shoulder. Philadelphia: WB Saunders, 1994, p. 205.)

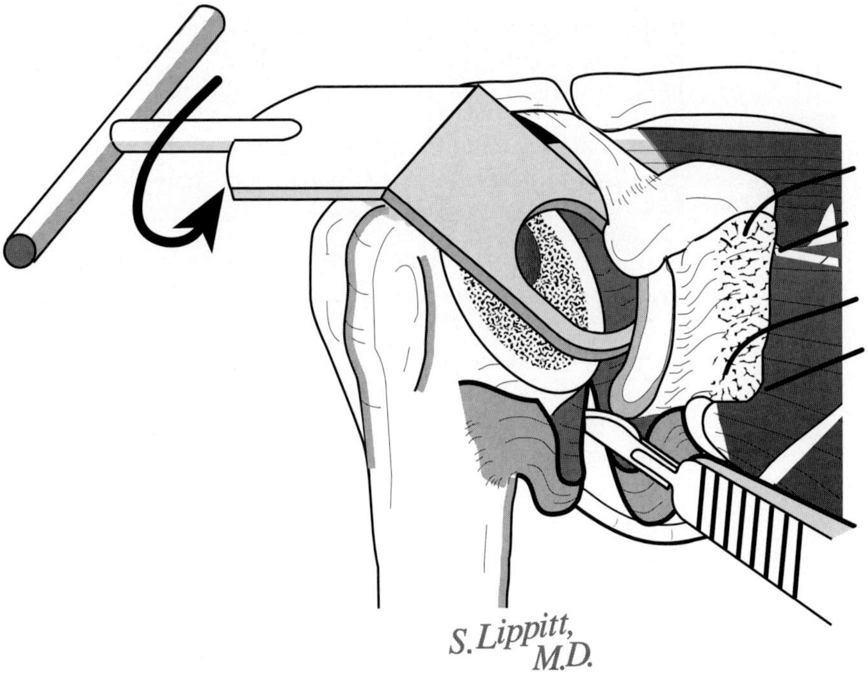


**Figure 30–2. Posterior capsule release**
If the posterior capsule is tight, it can be released under direct vision. The surgeon puts the capsule under tension by rotating the inferior aspect of the retractor away from the glenoid and by gently internally rotating the humerus. (Modified from Matsen FA, Lippitt SB, Sidles JA, et al [eds]: Practical Evaluation and Management of the Shoulder. Philadelphia: WB Saunders, 1994, p. 209.)

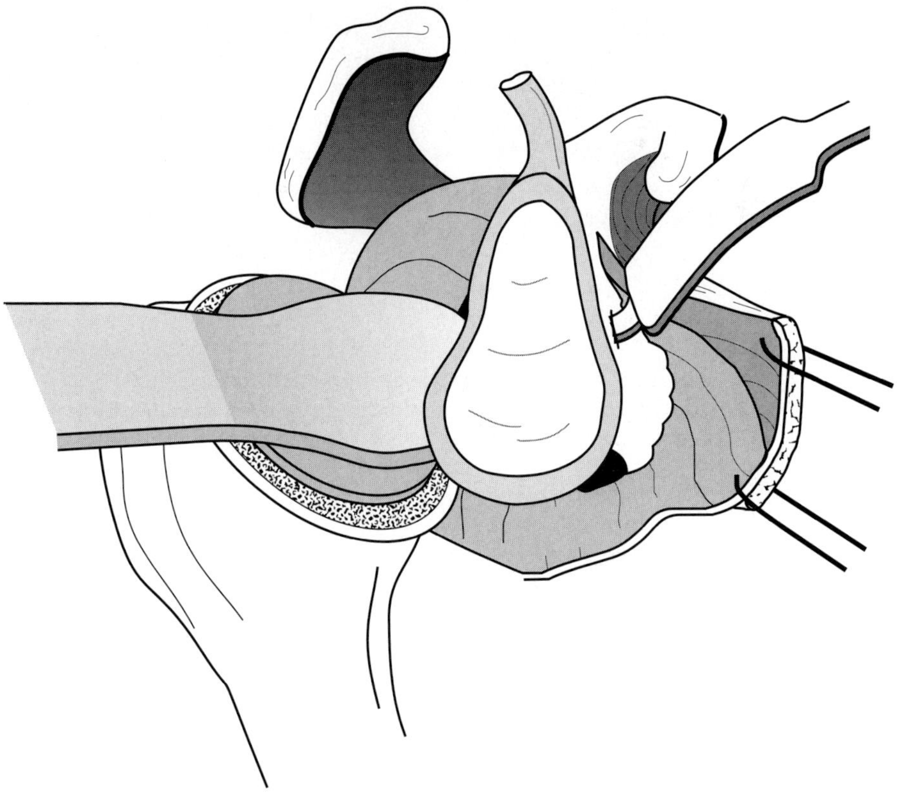

**Figure 30–3. Glenoid exposure**
By placing a broad smooth retractor behind the glenoid and a spiked retractor anteriorly, the surgeon can achieve an excellent exposure of the glenoid.

The fibrillated cartilage is curetted away (**Fig. 30–4**). The anterior and posterior rims of the bony glenoid are identified. The center of the glenoid is marked with cautery (**Fig. 30–5**), and a pinecone burr is used to create a small drill-centering hole in the glenoid surface (**Fig. 30–6**). An index finger is placed in the subscapularis fossa at the centering point on the anterior neck of the glenoid (**Fig. 30–7**). A 6 mm drill is then used to establish the normal glenoid center line by drilling from the centering hole on the face of the glenoid toward the centering point on the anterior neck (**Fig. 30–8**).

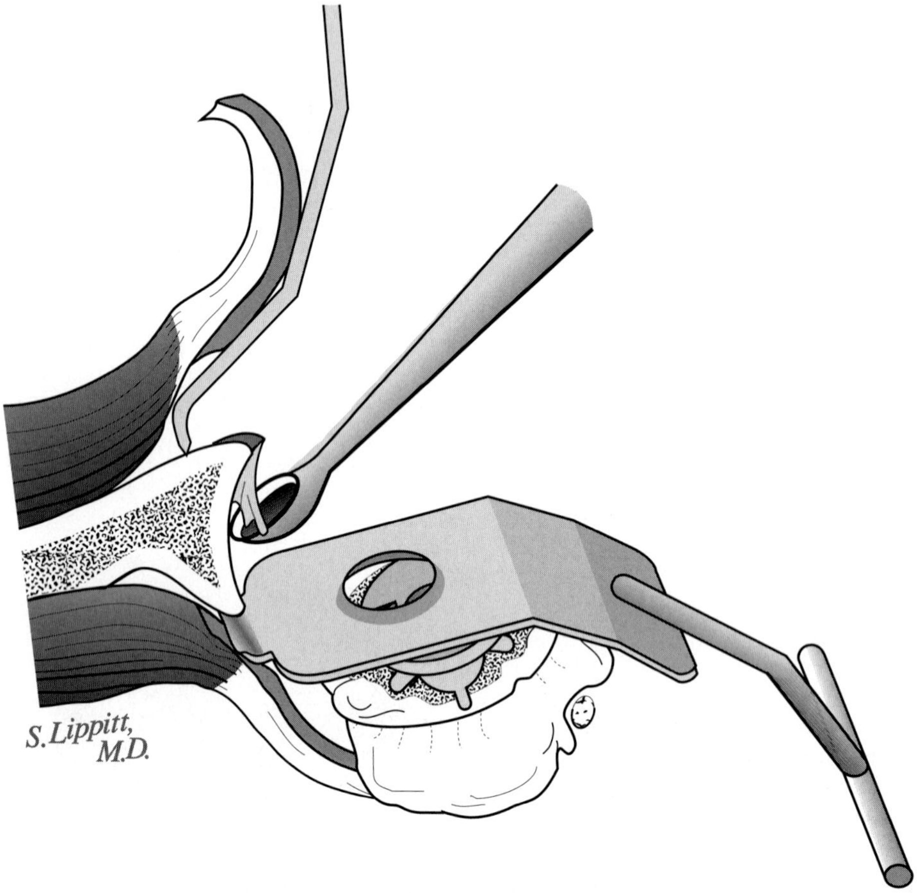


**Figure 30–4. Curettage of the glenoid cartilage**
Any remaining cartilage is curetted away to reveal the underlying bony anatomy and to facilitate reaming.

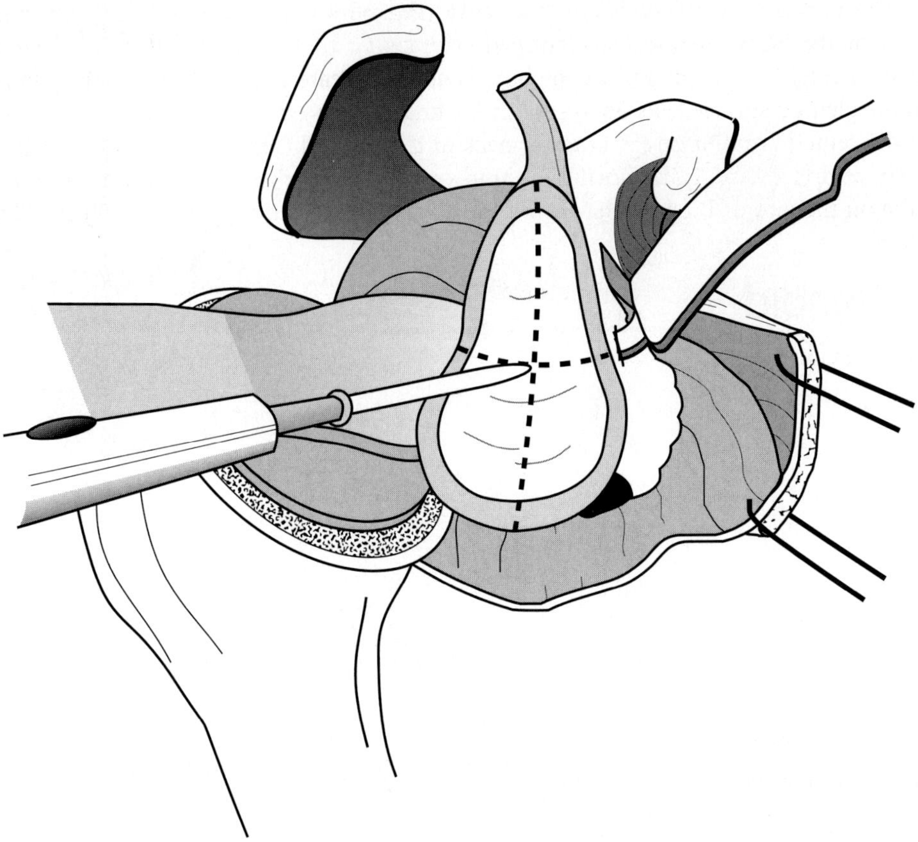

**Figure 30–5. Cautery of glenoid center**
The center of the glenoid is marked with electrocautery.

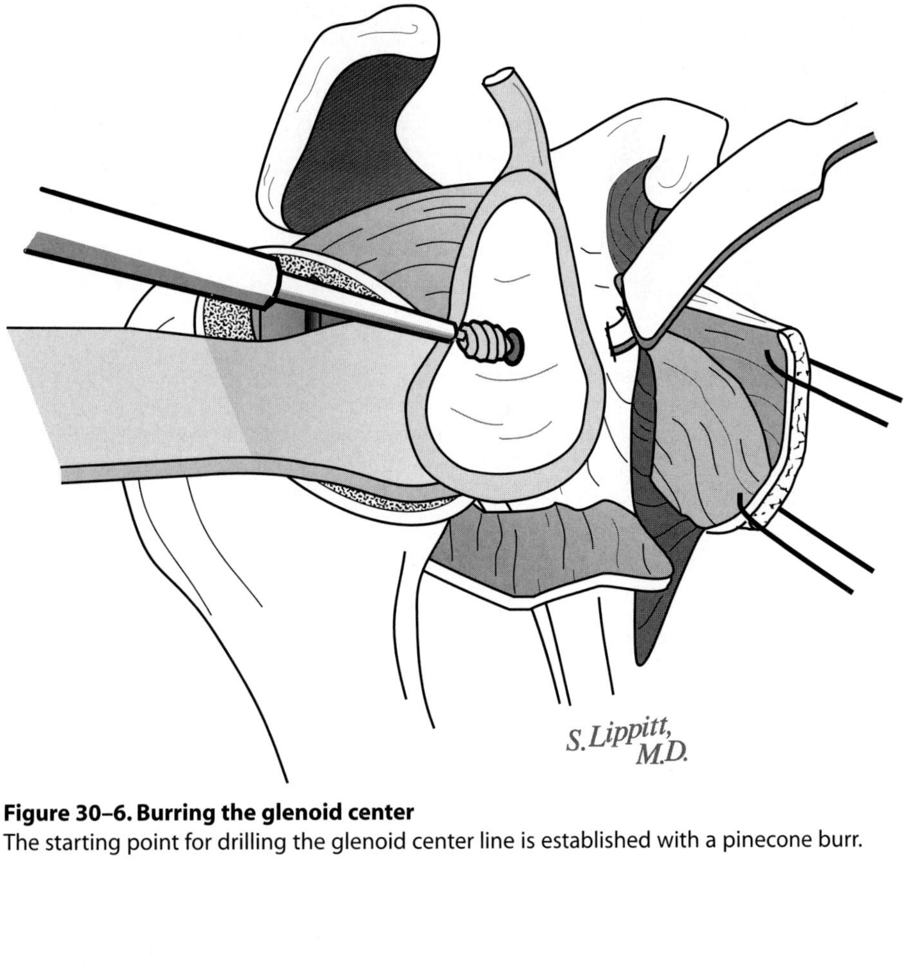


**Figure 30–6. Burring the glenoid center**
The starting point for drilling the glenoid center line is established with a pinecone burr.

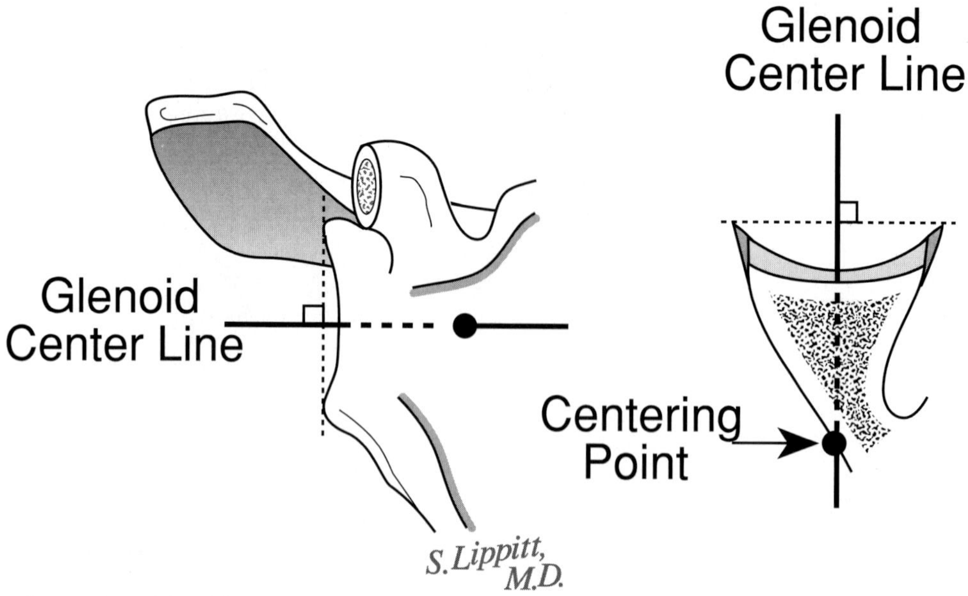


**Figure 30–7. Glenoid center point**
The centering point lies on the mid-anterior glenoid neck.

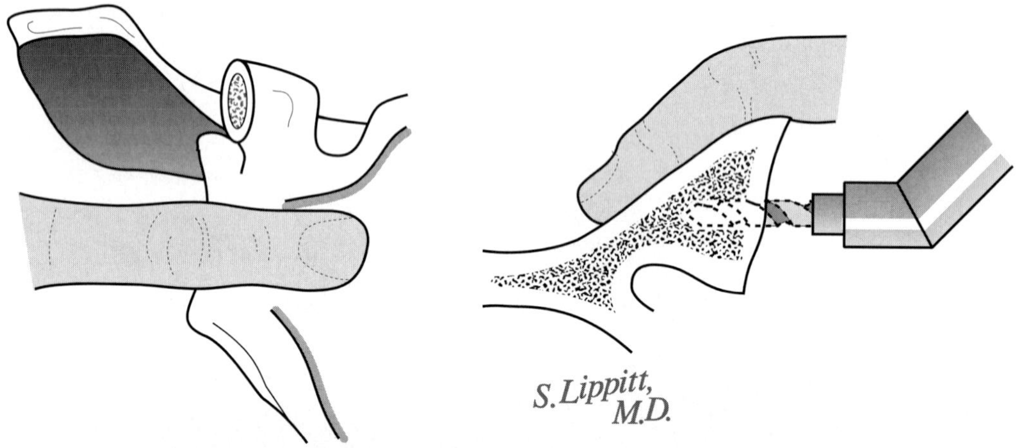


**Figure 30–8. Glenoid centering point—palpation**
The centering point can be palpated with a finger (*left*). The normalized glenoid center line is then drilled, connecting the center of the glenoid face with the centering point. (Modified from Matsen FA, Lippitt SB, Sidles JA, et al [eds]: Practical Evaluation and Management of the Shoulder. Philadelphia: WB Saunders, 1994, p. 210.)

We note that the glenoid width from the center of the hole to the posterior lip is 10 mm and use this measurement to predict the desired glenoid surface diameter of curvature (**Fig. 30–9**). From the relationship: Balance Stability Angle = 57.3 × Width/Radius of Glenoid Curvature, we note that a radius of curvature of 25 mm will yield an anterior and posterior balance stability angle of 23 degrees when the width is 10 mm. We also note that a glenoid radius of curvature of 25 mm (diameter = 50 mm) will yield the desired 2 mm mismatch with a 48 mm diameter humeral head (**Fig. 30–10**). We verify that there is sufficient glenoid bone anteriorly and posteriorly to allow for the necessary reaming. If this were not the case, a prosthetic glenoid arthroplasty with the appropriate diameter of curvature would be considered.

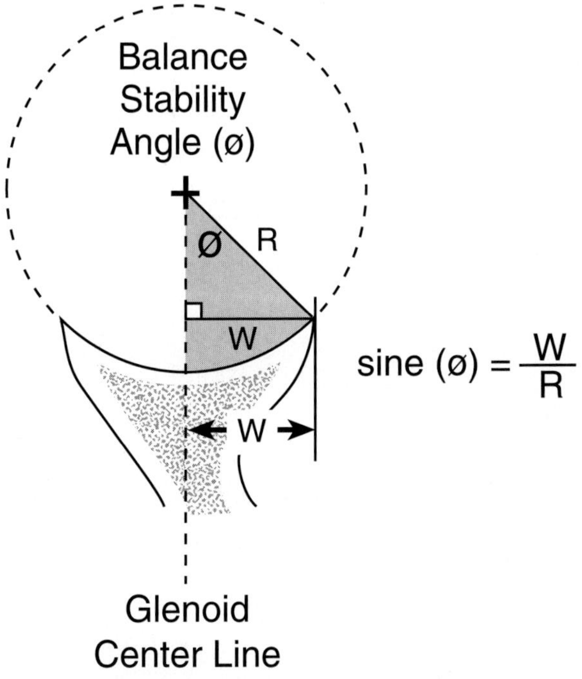


**Figure 30–9. Stability angle**
The predicted balance stability angle in a specified direction for a spherical glenoid is given by the arc sine of the ratio of the glenoid width in the direction of interest (the distance from the glenoid center to the reamed edge) and the radius of curvature for the reamed glenoid. BSA = arc sin W/R. Since for small angles (less than 30 degrees, for example), the sine and the tangent are about equal (see Section III on stability) and since for small angles (again less than 30 degrees) the tangent is approximately equal to the angle expressed in radians, and recalling that a radian is approximately 57.3 degrees, we come up with the convenient rule of thumb that the balance stability angle in degrees is about 57.3 × W/R. For a normally directed glenoid concavity, the desired stability angle is at least 20 degrees. So, if the glenoid width from the center to the edge is W, the reamed radius should be less than three times the width (20 = 57.3 × W/R or R = 3 × W) or the diameter should be less than six times the width from the center to the edge. Thus, a glenoid with a width of 10 mm would have the desired intrinsic stability if it were reamed to a properly oriented concavity with a diameter of less than 60 mm, whereas a glenoid with a width of 7 mm would need to be reamed to a diameter of less than 42 mm.

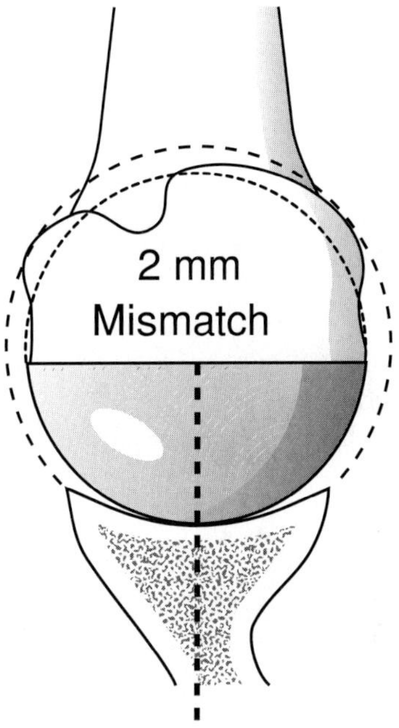


**Figure 30–10. Head mismatch for nonprosthetic glenoid arthroplasty**
For nonprosthetic glenoid arthroplasty, we usually select a humeral head diameter of curvature that is 2 mm smaller than the glenoid that will articulate with it. In this situation, we choose a smaller amount of mismatch than the 6 mm mismatch we use with a prosthetic arthroplasty because of the fact that reamed bone is less compliant than polyethylene. Thus, to achieve a larger contact area, a smaller amount of mismatch is needed.

The surgeon reams the glenoid in physiologic version with the spherical reamer using the normalized glenoid center line as a guide (**Fig. 30–11**). Exposure for reaming is achieved by the appropriate placement of retractors (**Fig. 30–12**). Reaming is continued until there is a concentric glenoid surface in normal glenoid version. Concentricity is verified by a transparent template with a diameter of curvature equal to that of the reamer and ensuring smooth contact throughout the reamed area. Care is taken not to compromise the anterior or posterior extent of the glenoid by reaming. At the conclusion of the reaming, the glenoid should have the desired curvature, width, version, and smoothness.

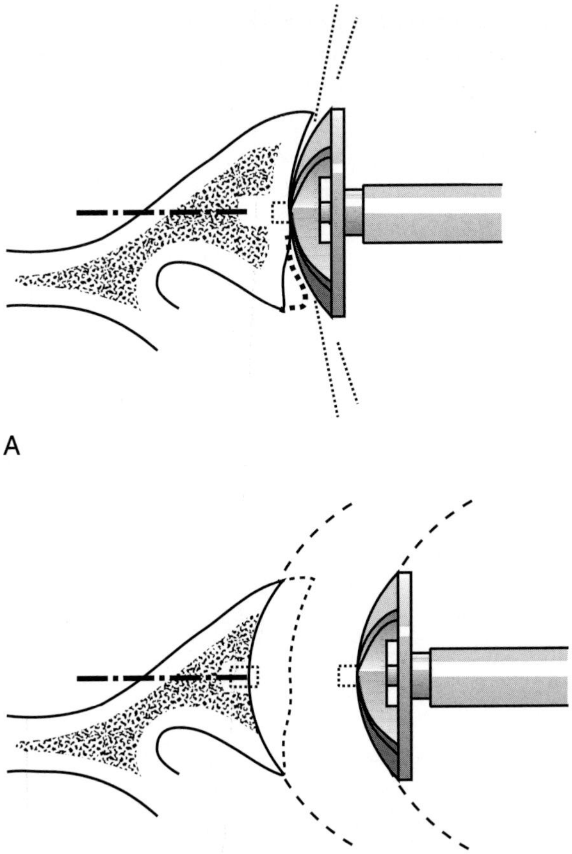

A

B

**Figure 30–11. Glenoid reaming—nonprosthetic glenoid arthroplasty**
The bony glenoid is reamed in the desired version until the full anterior and posterior extent of the surface has the desired spherical contour. (Modified from Matsen FA, Lippitt SB, Sidles JA, et al [eds]: Practical Evaluation and Management of the Shoulder. Philadelphia: WB Saunders, 1994, p. 211.)

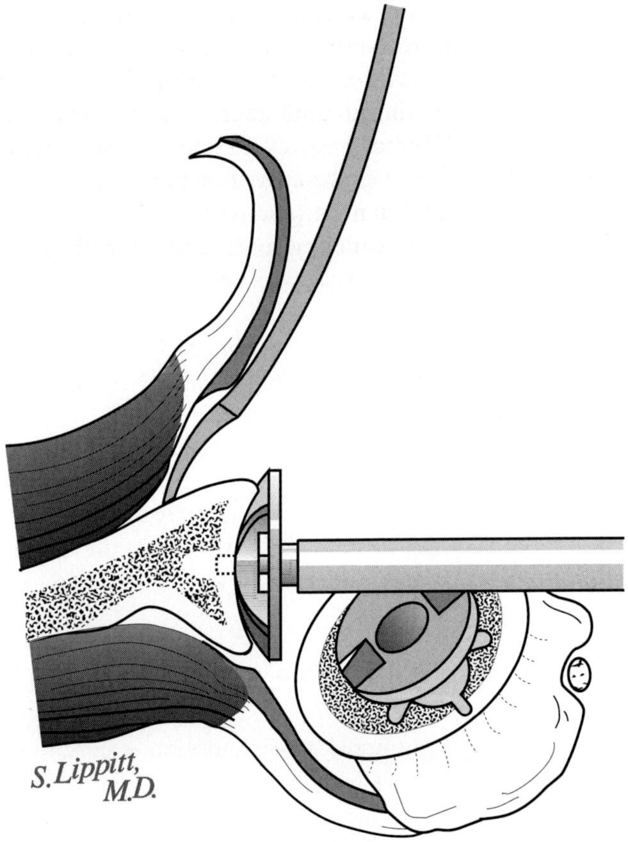


**Figure 30–12. Exposure of the glenoid for reaming**
Exposure for reaming is gained by a combination of retractors and a straight (shown here) or an angled reamer handle. (Modified from Rockwood CA, Matsen FA [eds]: The Shoulder, 2nd ed. Philadelphia: WB Saunders, 1998, p. 918.)

The surgeon verifies the stability offered by the reamed glenoid by performing a load and shift test (**Fig. 30–13**) with a trial modular humeral head with a radius of curvature 2 mm less than the radius of curvature of the glenoid.

The humeral arthroplasty is completed, with particular care taken to ensure that the humeral head sits centered in the glenoid and that (1) the humerus can be smoothly externally rotated 40 degrees with the subscapularis approximated, (2) the humeral head can be posteriorly subluxated 50% of the glenoid width with a spontaneous return to the glenoid center (Springbok), and (3) that the humerus can be internally rotated 60 degrees with the arm in 90 degrees of abduction: the 40, 50, 60 guidelines (see Figs. 29–30, 29–31, and 29–32).

The joint is examined to be sure that there is no abutment of the adducted humerus against the glenoid inferiorly (see Fig. 29–41) and to ensure that there is no posterior abutment (**Fig. 30–14**).

The wound is thoroughly irrigated. The subscapularis is repaired to the sutures at the anterior humeral neck cut (see Figs. 29–38 and 29–43).

The wound is again irrigated and closed in layers. Dry sterile dressings are applied, and the patient is returned to the recovery room with the arm in continuous passive motion (see Fig. 29–45).

## POSTOPERATIVE PLAN

Continuous passive motion is continued while the patient is in bed for the first 36 hours after surgery. It is removed when the patient is in a chair or ambulating.

On the day of surgery, the patient begins assisted flexion to 140 degrees and assisted external rotation to 40 degrees (see Figs. 29–46, 29–47, and Fig. 29–48).

The patient is encouraged to perform activities of daily living but to avoid lifting more than 1 pound for 6 weeks.

As soon as assisted motion of 140 degrees of flexion and 40 degrees of external rotation is achieved, the patient is discharged to continue his or her rehabilitation at home (see Fig. 29–49). Emphasis is placed on putting the shoulder through its range of motion at least five times per day.

After 6 weeks, progressively more activity is allowed as long as these activities are comfortable. Additional stretching exercises are started (see Figs. 29–50, 29–51, 29–52, and 29–53).

During this period, the emphasis is on assisted motion and comfort.

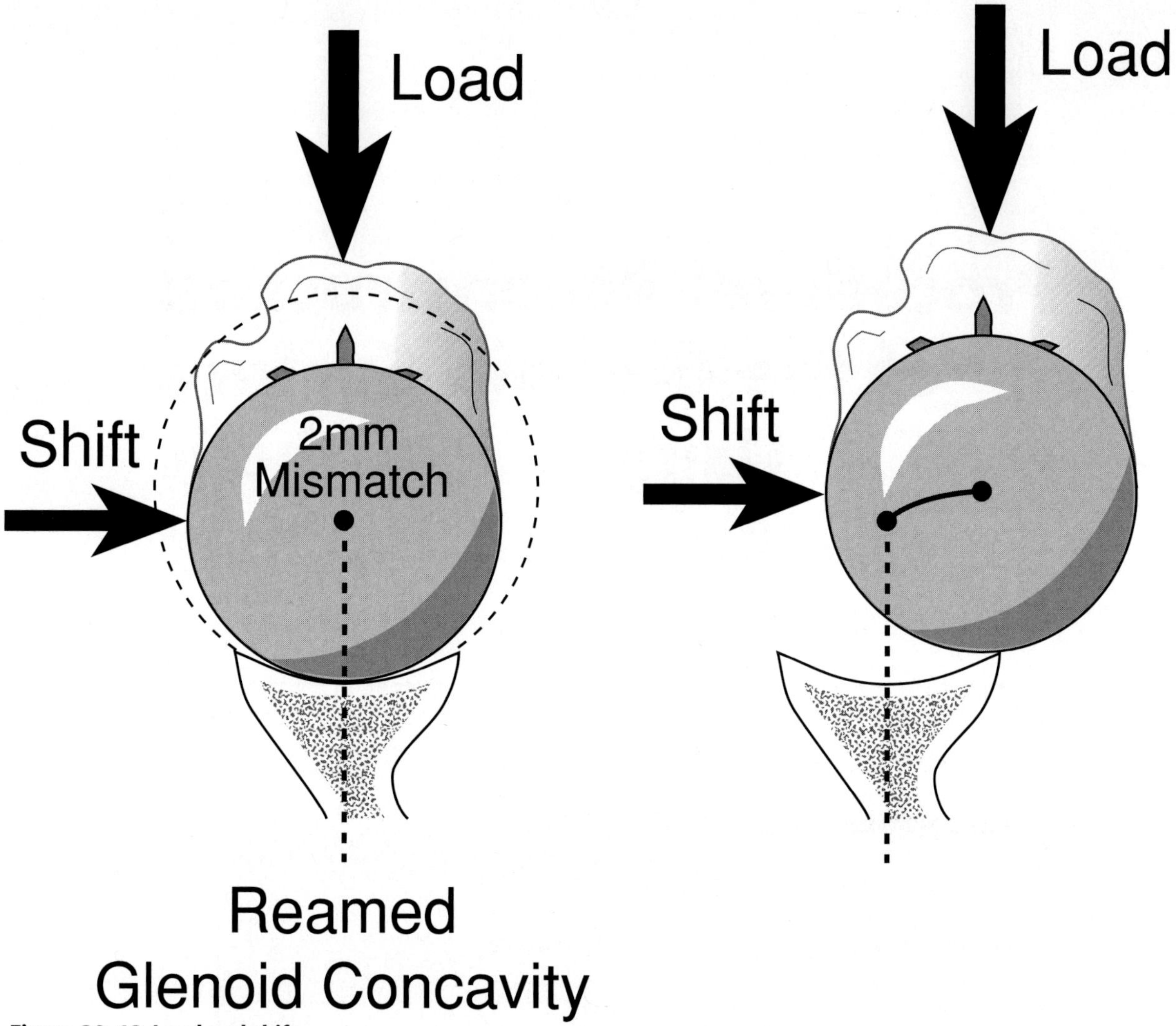


**Figure 30–13. Load and shift**
The intrinsic stability of the reamed glenoid can be determined by pressing the prosthetic head into the concavity and then verifying that there is substantial resistance to humeral head translation.

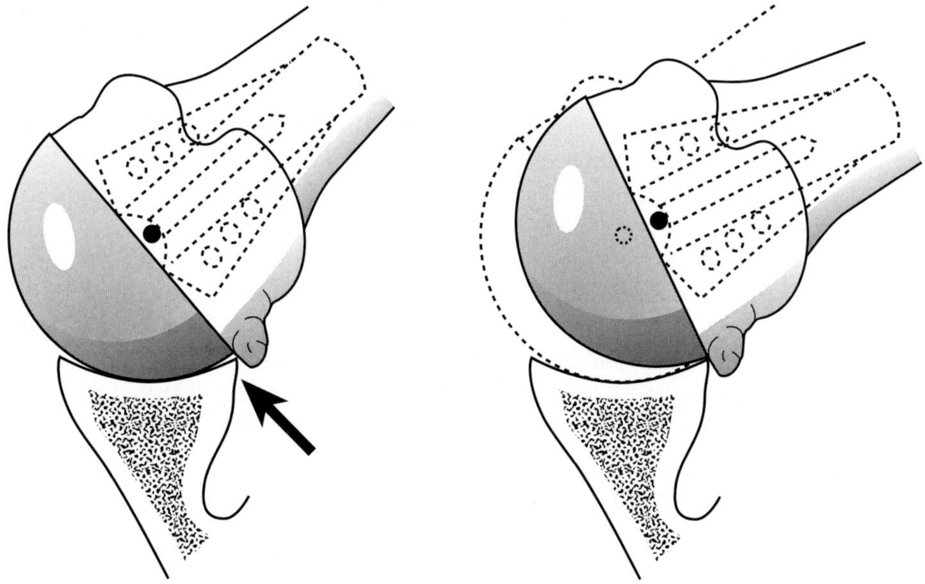

**Figure 30–14. Posterior open book**
The shoulder is carefully examined to be sure that posterior abutment does not cause the joint to "open book" in external rotation.

CHAPTER 31

# Procedure: Reconstruction of the Glenoid Surface Using a Prosthetic Glenoid Arthroplasty

| |
|---|
| ***Diagnosis*** |
| ***Rheumatoid arthritis    ICD9 CODE 714.0*** |
| ***or*** |
| ***Osteoarthritis    ICD9 CODE 715.11*** |
| ***or*** |
| ***Traumatic arthritis    ICD9 CODE 716.11*** |
| ***or*** |
| ***Avascular necrosis    ICD9 CODE 733.41*** |
| ***Procedure*** |
| ***Prosthetic glenoid arthroplasty performed with humeral hemiarthroplasty    CPT CODE 23472*** |

## INDICATIONS

The patient has glenohumeral arthritis that limits the comfort and function of the shoulder. The condition has not responded to nonoperative management.

Preoperative radiographs reveal loss of the normal glenoid concavity with posterior erosion producing a biconcave glenoid.

Knowing the alternatives as well as the risks of infection, neurovascular injury, excessive stiffness, pain, weakness, fracture, instability, component loosening, component wear, and the need for revision surgery, as well as anesthetic complications, the patient desires to proceed with the above-described procedure. The patient understands that the purpose of the procedure is to recreate a functional glenoid concavity. The patient recognizes that this procedure cannot be expected to completely restore normal comfort and function to the shoulder. And, lastly, the patient understands his or her critical role in the post-surgical rehabilitation.

## FINDINGS

Examination under anesthesia reveals that the range of glenohumeral motion is limited in all directions and there is bony crepitance on glenohumeral motion.

Surgical findings include loss of normal glenoid articular cartilage with some areas worn down to bone. Much of the cartilage is fibrillated and in the process of dissolution.

The posterior glenoid is eroded to form a biconcave glenoid.

The bone is of good quality.

## OPERATION

Under satisfactory anesthesia, the patient is placed in a low beach chair position with the glenohumeral joint at the edge of the operating table (see Fig. 29–2). The shoulder is doubly prepped and draped so that the arm is free to be moved. The shoulder is approached through a standard deltopectoral incision along a line connecting the mid-clavicle to the deltoid tubercle (see Figs. 29–3, 29–4, and 29–5).

The humeroscapular motion interface is mobilized (see Fig. 29–6). The axillary nerve is identified and protected throughout the case. The subscapularis and subjacent capsule are incised from their insertion to the lesser tuberosity (see Figs. 29–7 and 29–8). A 360-degree subscapularis release is performed (see Figs. 29–9 and 29–10).

The proximal humerus is prepared for a humeral arthroplasty as described in a separate procedure description (see Chapter 29).

The capsule is released from the anterior and inferior glenoid just past the origin of the long head of the triceps incising the anterior and posterior bands of the inferior glenohumeral ligament (see Fig. 29–11). This release is usually sufficient for cases of primary osteoarthritis and capsulorrhaphy arthropathy because the posterior capsule is often stretched in these conditions. However, if the posterior capsule is tight, it can be released from the posterior glenoid labrum. The surgeon places the capsule under tension by rotating the humeral head retractor away from the glenoid, first inferiorly and then superiorly (see Fig. 29–12). These releases provide excellent exposure of the glenoid **(Fig. 31–1)**. The labrum is sequentially dissected away from the anterior glenoid lip **(Fig. 31–2)**. The fibrillated cartilage is curetted away.

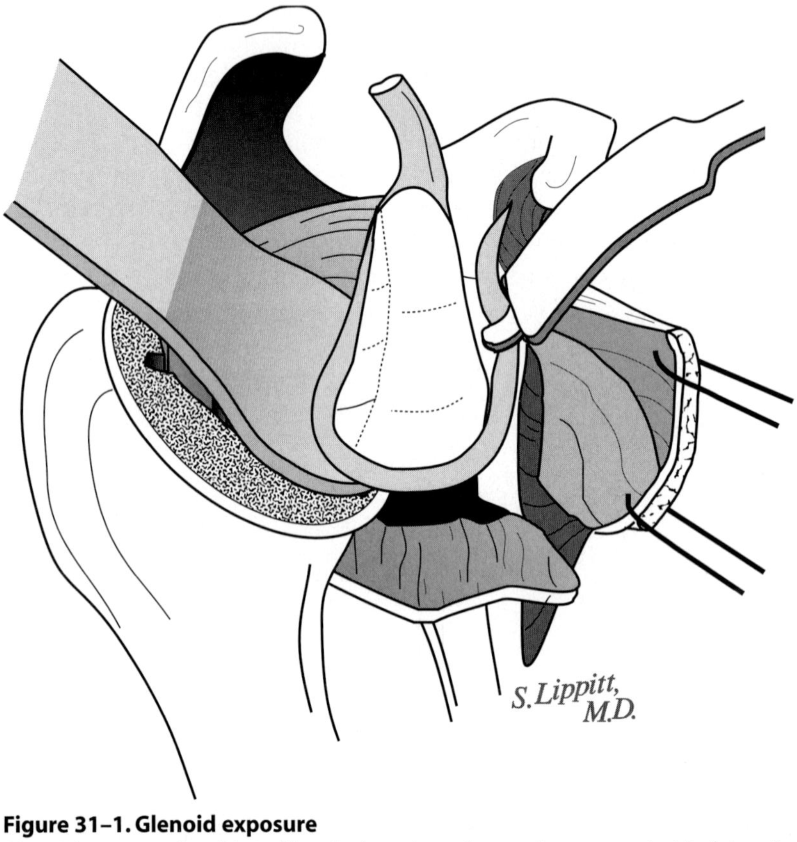


**Figure 31–1. Glenoid exposure**
Glenoid exposure is achieved by placing a broad smooth retractor behind the glenoid, pushing the proximal humerus posteriorly. A sharp-tipped retractor is placed on the glenoid neck beneath the labrum.

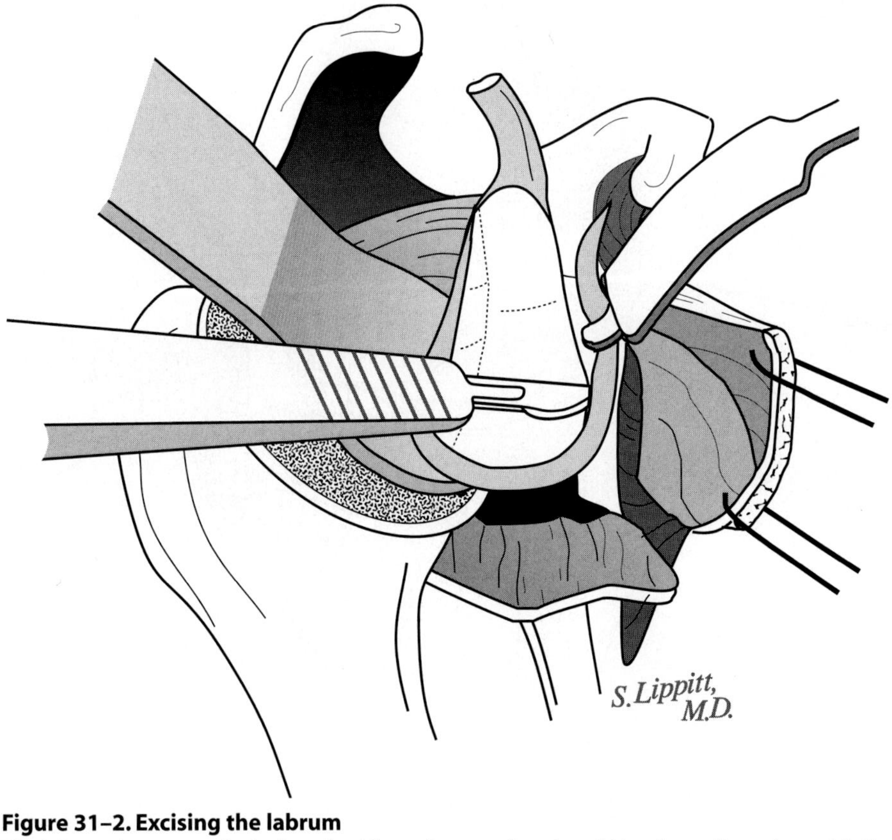


**Figure 31–2. Excising the labrum**
The labrum is progressively detached from the anterior glenoid by sharp dissection, with the sharp-tipped retractor moved inferiorly beneath the detached labrum in small successive steps.

The anterior and posterior rims of the bony glenoid are identified. The center of the glenoid is marked with cautery (**Fig. 31–3**), and a pinecone burr is used to create a small drill-centering hole in the glenoid surface (**Fig. 31–4**). An index finger is placed in the subscapularis fossa at the centering point on the anterior neck of the glenoid (**Fig. 31–5**). A 6 mm drill is then used to establish the normal glenoid center line by

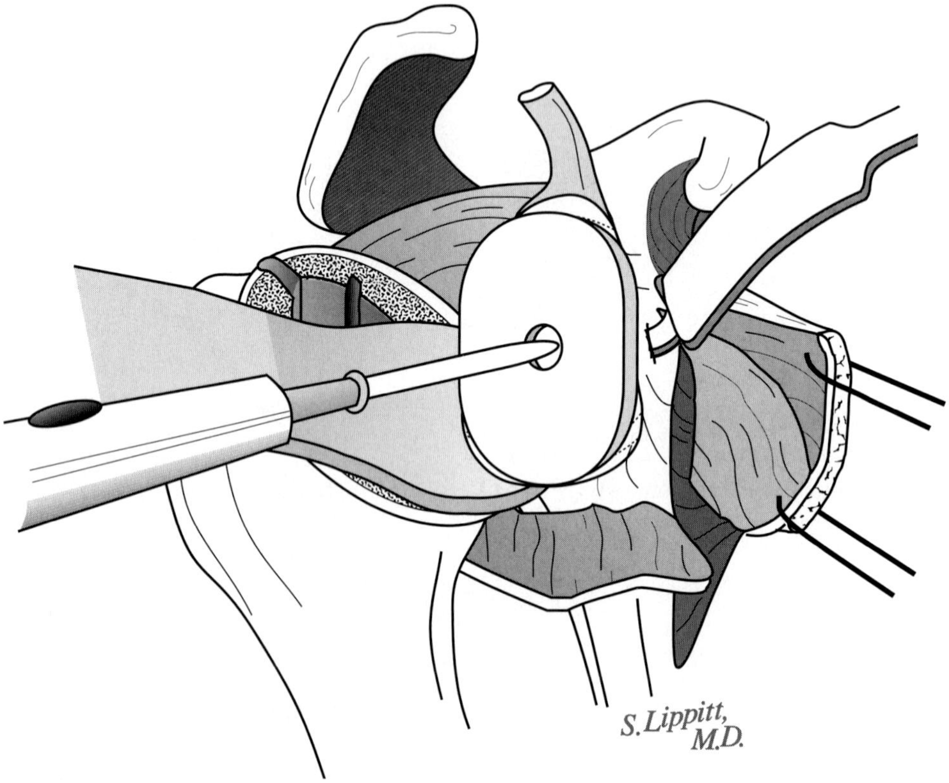


**Figure 31–3. Cautery of the glenoid center**
The center of the glenoid is marked with electrocautery.

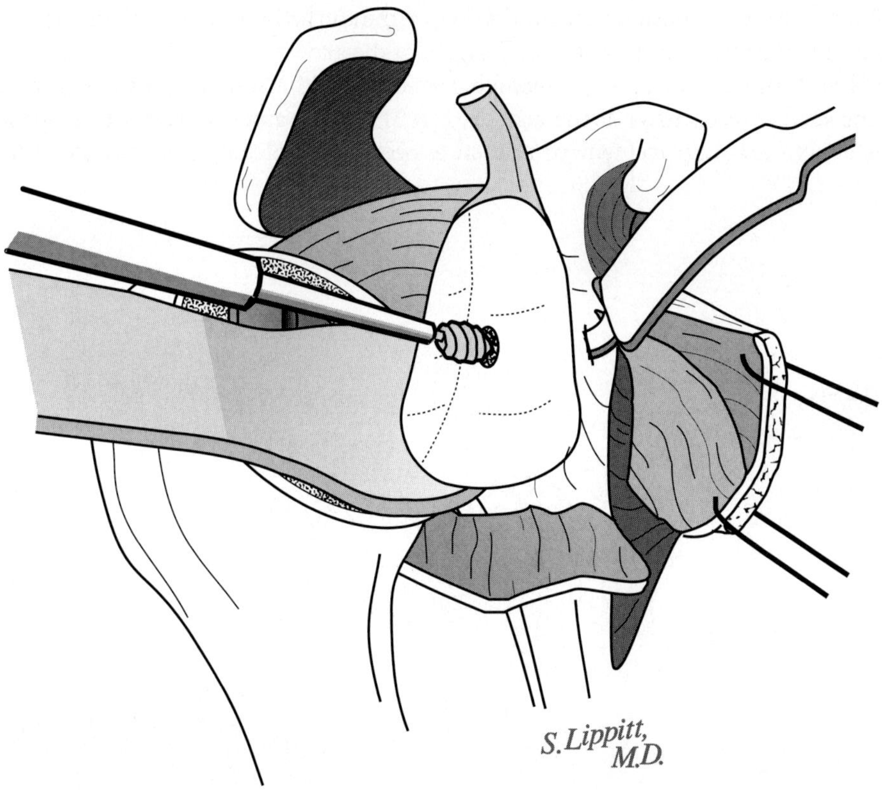


**Figure 31–4. Burring the glenoid center**
The starting point for drilling the glenoid center line is established with a pinecone burr.

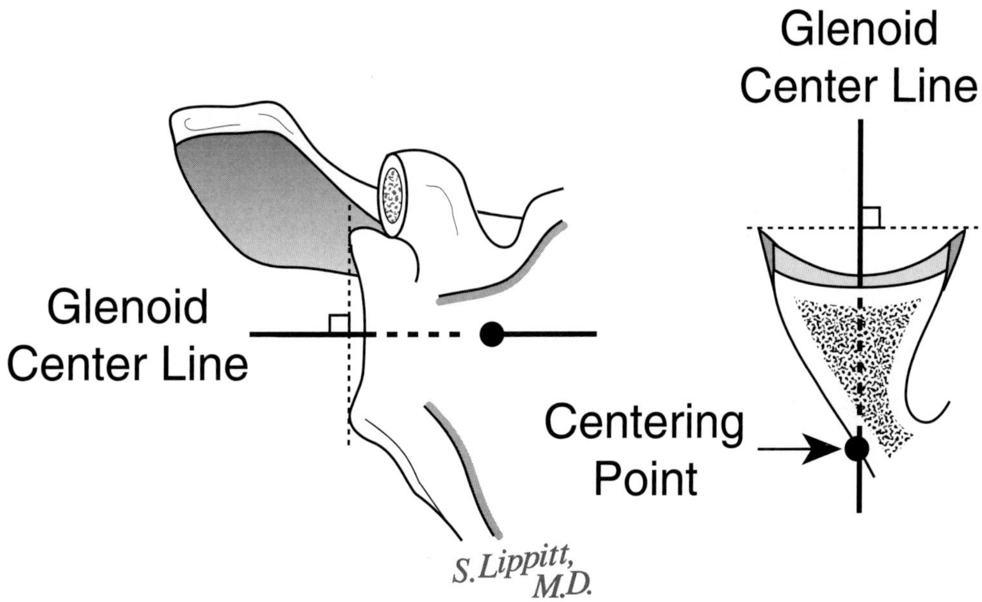


**Figure 31–5. Glenoid center point**
The centering point lies on the mid-anterior glenoid neck.

drilling from the centering hole on the face of the glenoid toward the centering point on the anterior neck (**Fig. 31–6**).

The glenoid is reamed in physiologic version with the spherical reamer using the normalized glenoid center line as a guide (**Fig. 31–7**). Exposure for reaming is achieved by the appropriate placement of retractors (**Fig. 31–8**). Reaming is continued until

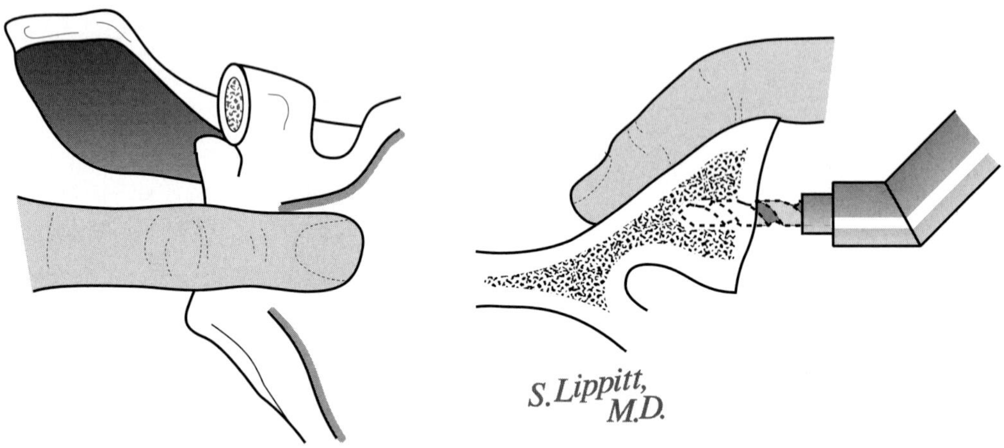


**Figure 31–6. Palpating the glenoid center point**
The centering point can be palpated with a finger (*left*). The normalized glenoid center line is then drilled, connecting the center of the glenoid face with the centering point. (Modified from Matsen FA, Lippitt SB, Sidles JA, et al [eds]: Practical Evaluation and Management of the Shoulder. Philadelphia: WB Saunders, 1994, p. 210.)

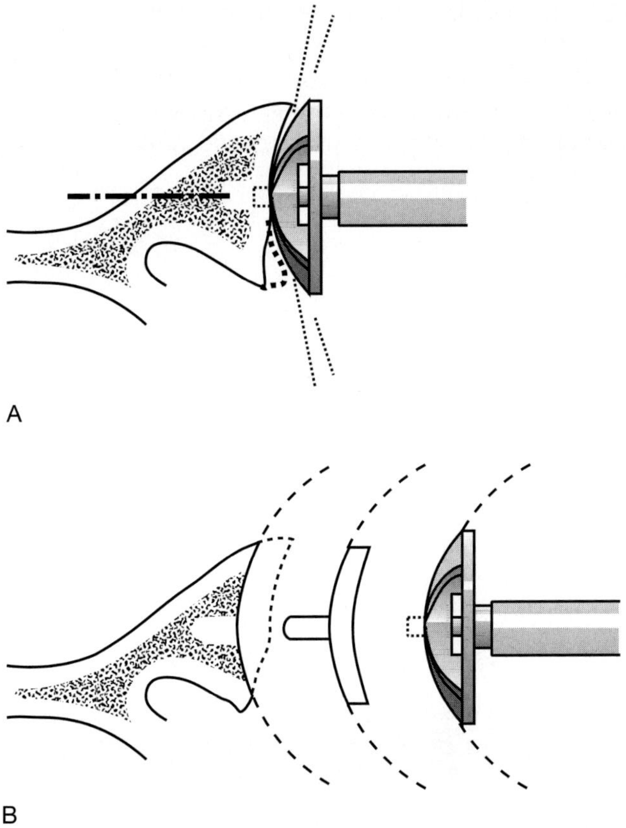


**Figure 31–7. Glenoid reaming**
The glenoid bone is spherically reamed to a diameter of curvature matching the back of the prosthetic glenoid. (Modified from Matsen FA, Lippitt SB, Sidles JA, et al [eds]: Practical Evaluation and Management of the Shoulder. Philadelphia: WB Saunders, 1994, p. 211.)

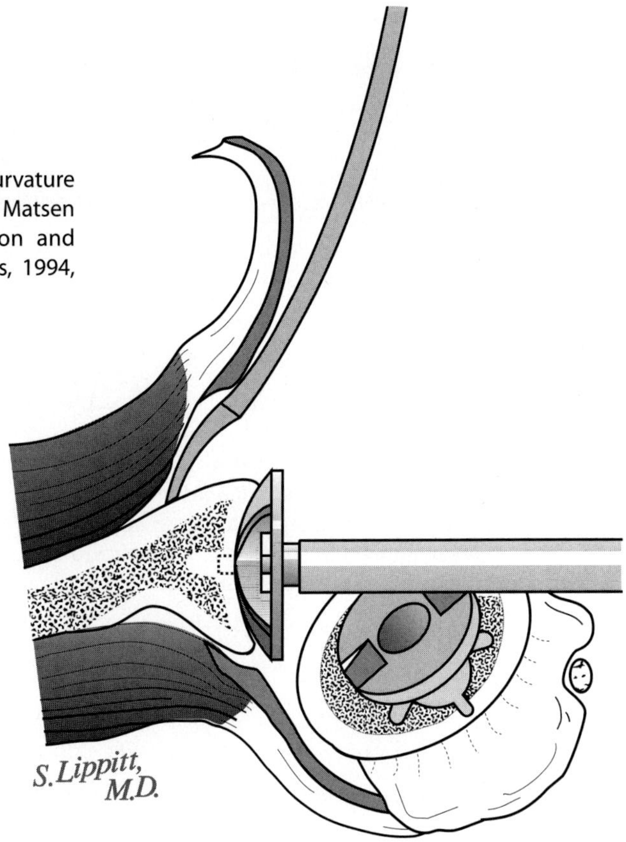


**Figure 31–8. Exposure of the glenoid for reaming**
Exposure for glenoid reaming is provided by a sharp-tipped retractor on the anterior glenoid neck and by allowing the handle of the reamer to push the proximal humerus posteriorly. In this illustration, a straight reamer handle is used. In many cases, a 45-degree angled reamer handle works well. (Modified from Rockwood CA, Matsen FA [eds]: The Shoulder, 2nd ed. Philadelphia: WB Saunders, 1998, p. 918.)

there is a concentric glenoid surface in normal glenoid version (**Fig. 31–9**). Concentricity is verified using a transparent template with a diameter of curvature equal to that of the reamer and ensuring smooth contact throughout the reamed area (**Fig. 31–10**). Care is taken not to compromise the anterior or posterior extent of the glenoid by reaming. At the conclusion of the reaming, the glenoid surface should have the desired curvature, width, version, and smoothness.

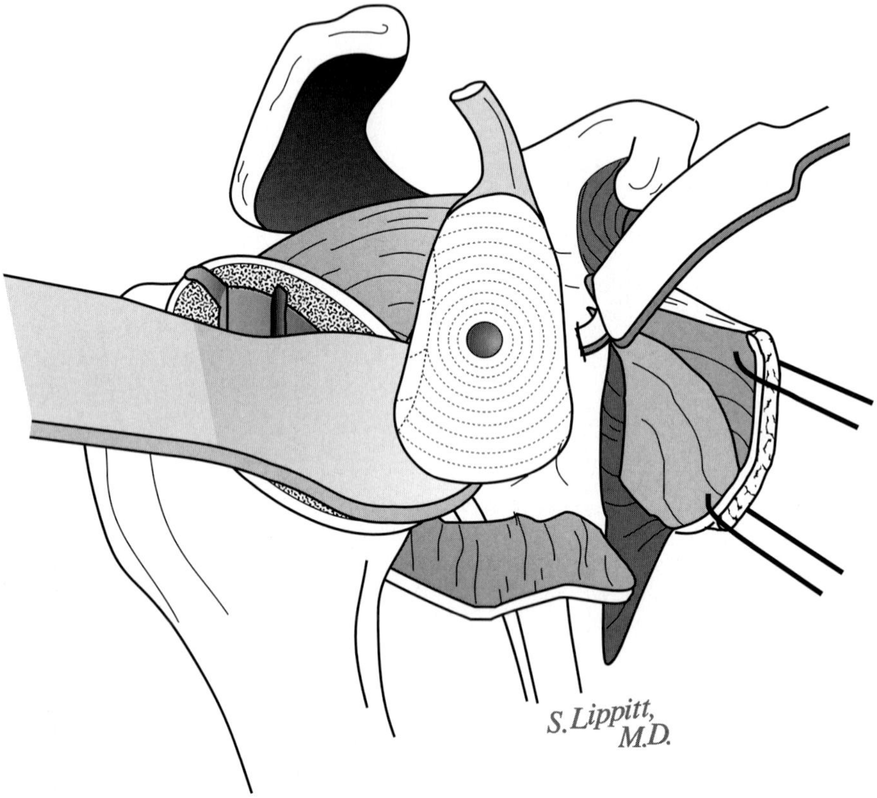


**Figure 31–9. Reamed glenoid**
Reaming is continued until the smooth reamed surface extends to the anterior and posterior margins of the glenoid. Often concentric circular marks are left by the reamer, indicating the extent of the reamed surface.

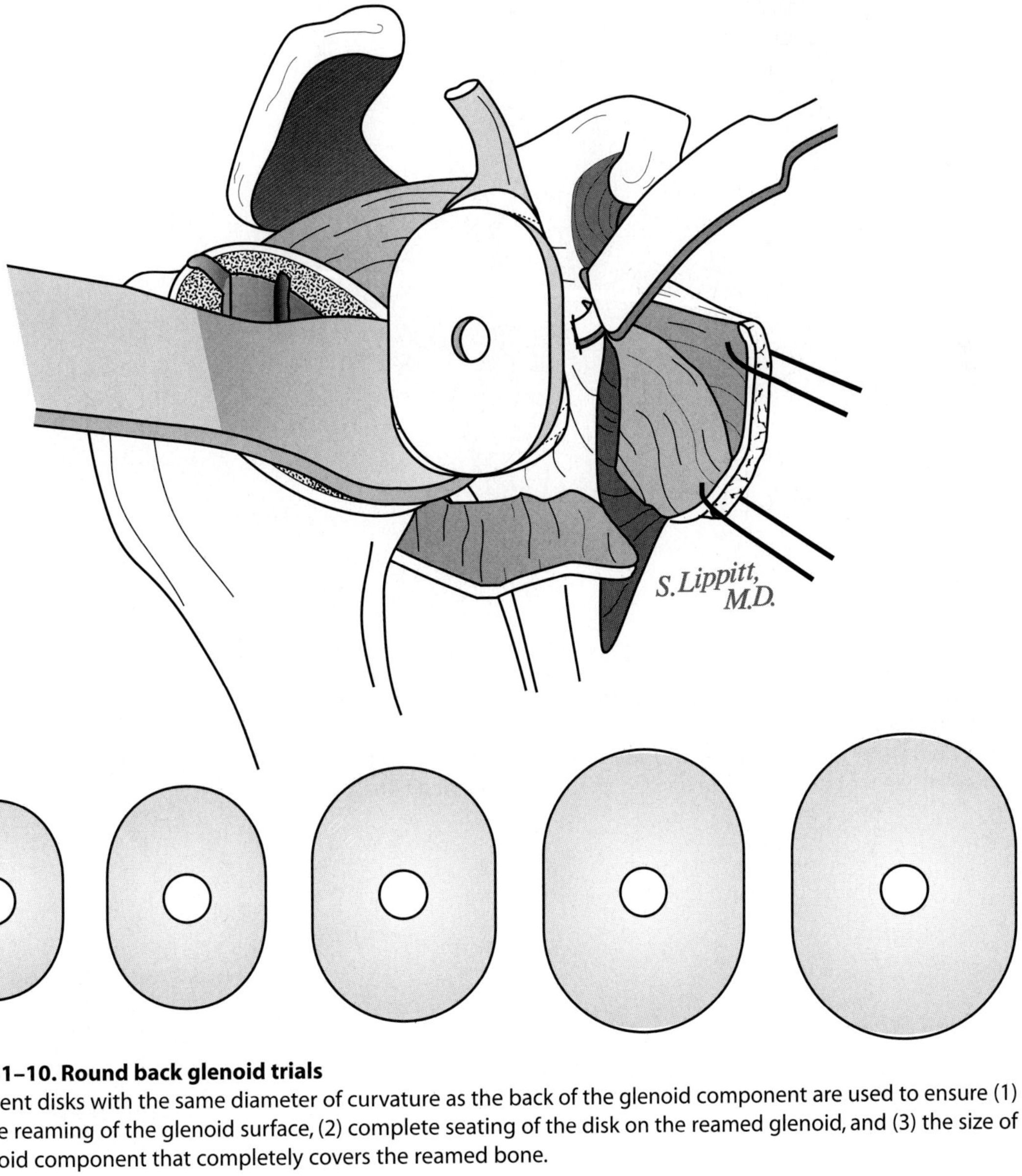


**Figure 31–10. Round back glenoid trials**
Transparent disks with the same diameter of curvature as the back of the glenoid component are used to ensure (1) complete reaming of the glenoid surface, (2) complete seating of the disk on the reamed glenoid, and (3) the size of the glenoid component that completely covers the reamed bone.

A drill guide is then used to orient the drilling of the four peripheral drill holes for fixation of the pegged glenoid component (**Figs. 31–11, 31–12, 31–13, 31–14,** and **31–15**). The pegged trial component is inserted and the excellence of the fit is verified by the absence of wobble when a trial glenoid component is subjected to peripheral loading anteriorly, posteriorly, superiorly, and inferiorly (**Fig. 31–16**). The trial glenoid is removed. A sterile saline spray irrigation is used to remove particulate debris from the

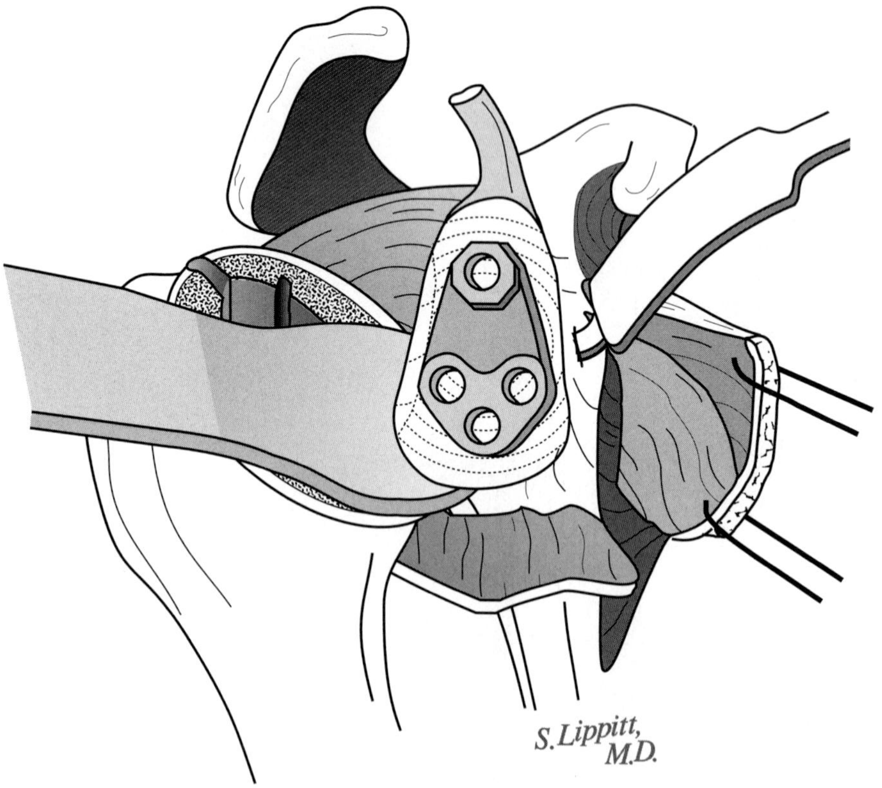


**Figure 31–11. Peg hole guide**
A drill guide with the central peg on its backside is inserted into the central hole and rotated until the superior and inferior holes lie in the long axis of the glenoid. Spikes on the back of the glenoid are driven into the glenoid bone to maintain its rotational orientation. Care is taken to ensure that the drill guide is fully seated on the reamed bone surface.

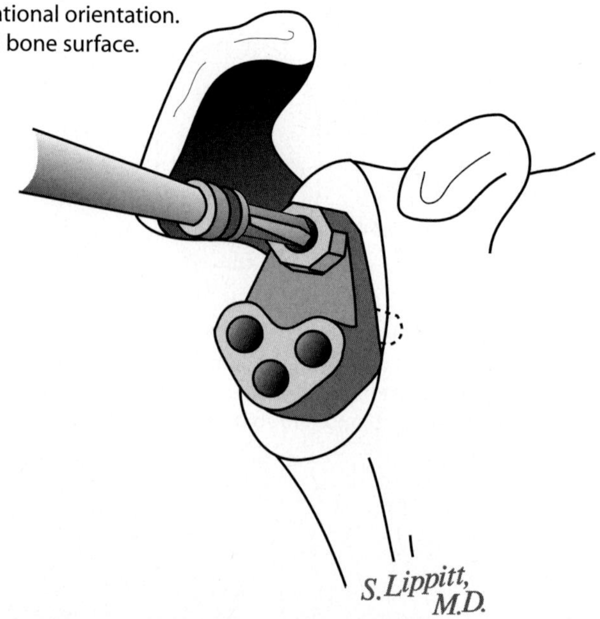


**Figure 31–12. Drilling the superior hole**
The superior hole is drilled while the drill guide is stabilized on the glenoid face.

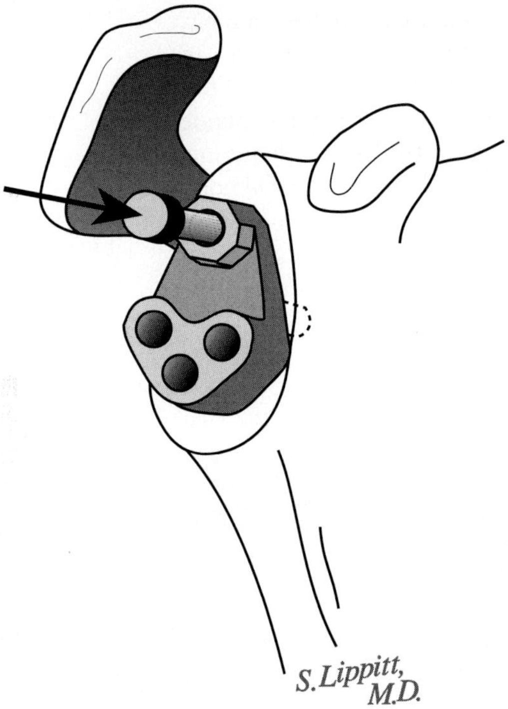


**Figure 31–13. Push pin**
A push pin is fully inserted through the superior hole in the drill guide into the drilled bone.

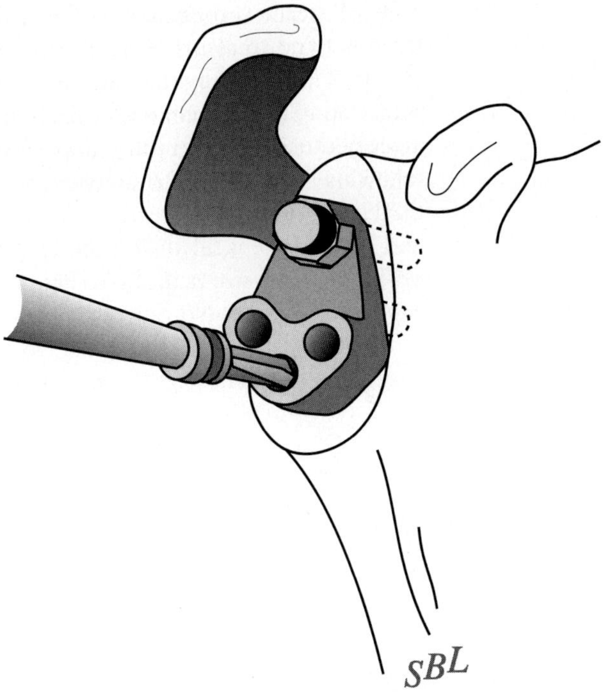


**Figure 31–14. Drilling the inferior peg hole**
The inferior hole is drilled while the drill guide is stabilized to the glenoid.

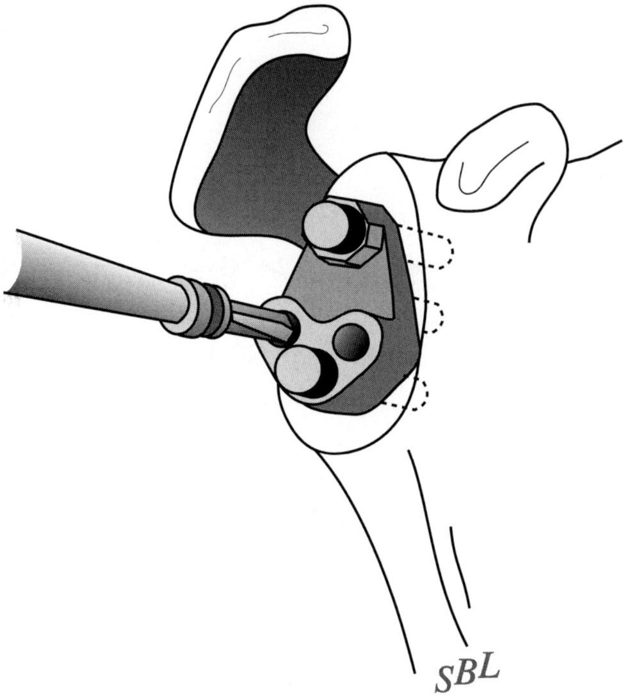


**Figure 31–15. Drilling the posterior and anterior peg holes**
A push pin is fully inserted through the inferior hole and into drilled bone. The posterior and anterior holes are then drilled.

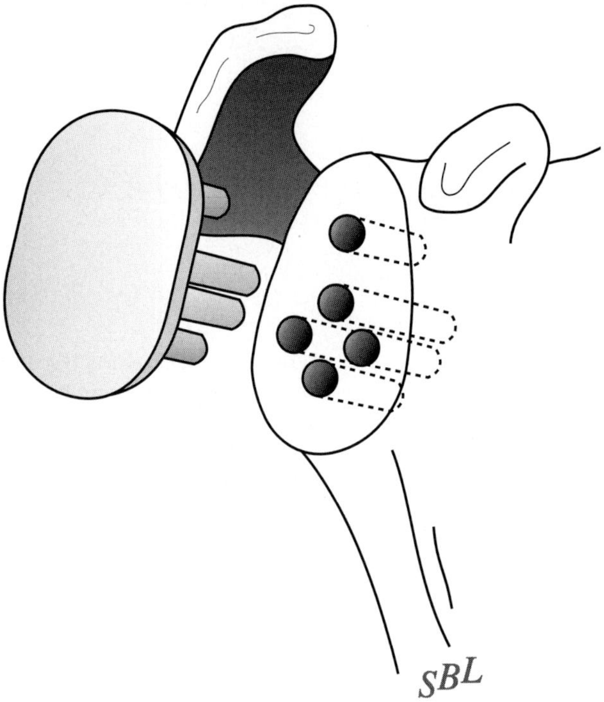


**Figure 31–16. Trial glenoid component**
The seating and stability of a trial glenoid component are verified.

holes. A sterile carbon dioxide jet spray is used to check for penetration of each of the holes and to assure their dryness before cement is inserted (**Fig. 31–17**). If penetration is identified by the leakage of bubbles around the glenoid, the leaky hole will be subjected to less cement pressurization. There is no need to avoid cement or to cut off a peg because of penetration. Each of the drill holes is cemented sequentially with the following steps in rapid succession: (1) the hole is irrigated with a saline spray, (2) the fluid is aspirated from the hole, (3) the hole is dried using a sterile carbon dioxide spray, and (4) the hole is filled with cement under moderate pressure using a syringe with an orifice the same size as the hole (**Fig. 31–18**). Excess cement is removed with a small elevator (**Fig. 31–19**). No cement is placed on the face of the glenoid. The total volume of cement used is less than 2 $cm^3$ to minimize the heat generated by the exothermic curing reaction. The pegs of the glenoid prosthesis are inserted into the cemented holes

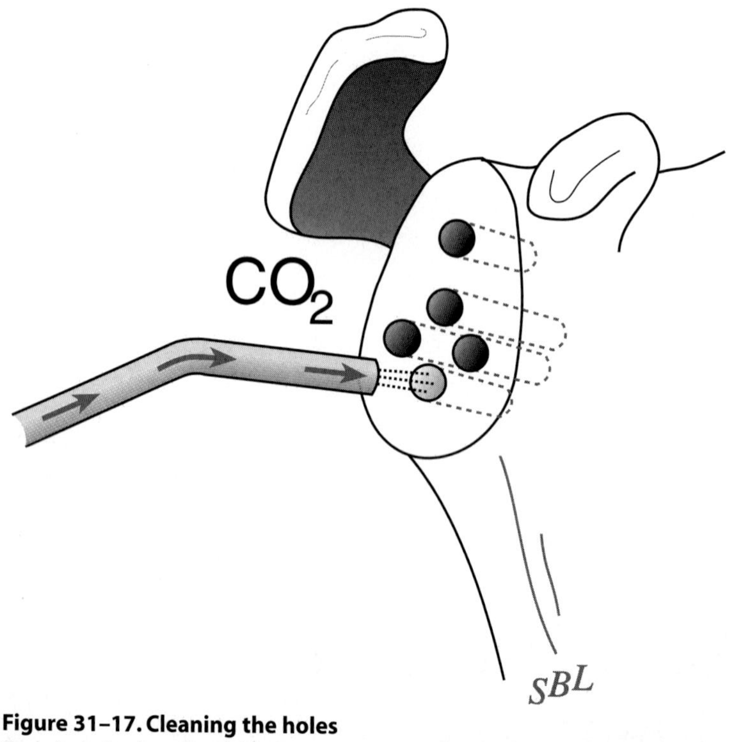


**Figure 31–17. Cleaning the holes**
Each hole in the glenoid bone is cleaned with a saline spray irrigator and then dried with a sterile carbon dioxide jet spray immediately prior to insertion of the cement in that hole. The carbon dioxide spray also reveals any leaks from the holes into the area around the glenoid that may have resulted from penetration by the drill.

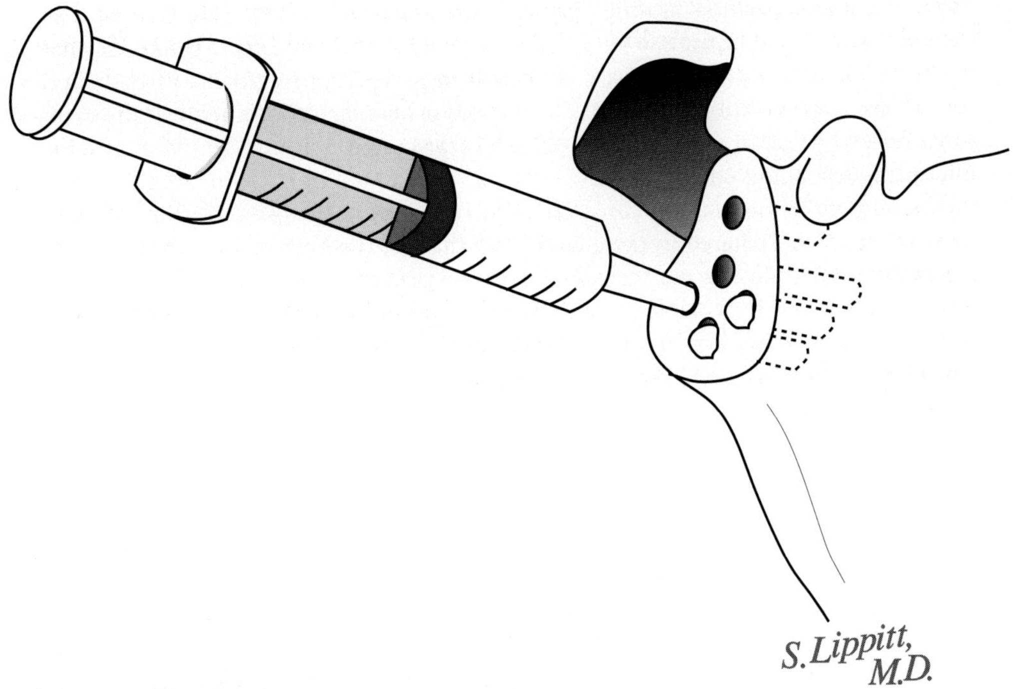


**Figure 31–18. Injecting the cement**
Cement is pressured into each hole immediately after that hole has been dried with the carbon dioxide spray. (From Pearl ML, Lippitt SB: Shoulder arthroplasty with a modular prosthesis. Techniques Orthop 8:151–162, 1994.)

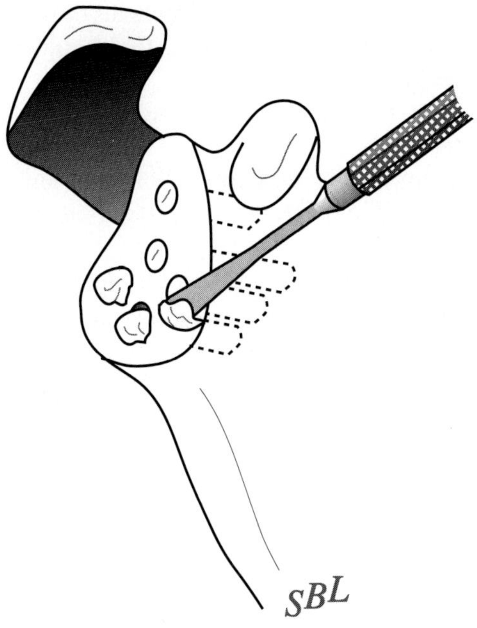


**Figure 31–19. Removing the excess cement**
All cement on the face of the glenoid is removed with a small elevator.

and impacted into its final seating position with a ball-ended tamp (**Fig. 31–20**). The humerus is retracted laterally with a bone hook and slightly internally rotated so that the posterior recesses of the joint can be well inspected. All fragments of bone and cement are removed from the joint. The glenoid is held in position with steady pressure exerted by the unyielding thumb of the surgeon and irrigated until the exothermic curing reaction is complete.

The humeral arthroplasty is completed, with particular care taken to ensure that the humeral head sits centered in the glenoid and that (1) the humerus can be smoothly externally rotated 40 degrees with the subscapularis approximated, (2) the humeral head can be posteriorly subluxated 50% of the glenoid width with a spontaneous return to the glenoid center (Springbok), and (3) the humerus can be internally rotated 60 degrees with the arm in 90 degrees of abduction: the 40, 50, 60 guidelines (see Figs. 29–30, 29–31, and 29–32).

The joint is examined to be sure that there is no abutment of the adducted humerus against the glenoid inferiorly (see Fig. 29–41) and that there is no posterior abutment (**Fig. 31–21**).

The wound is thoroughly irrigated. The subscapularis is repaired to the sutures at the anterior humeral neck cut (see Figs. 29–38 and 29–43).

The wound is again irrigated and closed in layers. Dry sterile dressings are applied, and the patient is returned to the recovery room with the arm in continuous passive motion (see Fig. 29–45).

## POSTOPERATIVE PLAN

Continuous passive motion is continued while the patient is in bed for the first 36 hours after surgery. It is removed when the patient is in a chair or ambulating.

On the day of surgery, the patient begins assisted flexion to 140 degrees and assisted external rotation to 40 degrees (see Figs. 29–46, 29–47, and 29–48).

As soon as assisted motion of 140 degrees of flexion and 40 degrees of external rotation is achieved, the patient is discharged to continue his or her rehabilitation at home (see Fig. 29–49). Emphasis is placed on putting the shoulder through its range of motion at least five times per day.

Activities of daily living are encouraged, but the patient should avoid lifting more than 1 pound for 6 weeks.

After 6 weeks, progressively more activity is allowed as long as these activities are comfortable. Additional stretching exercises are started (see Figs. 29–50, 29–51, 29–52, and 29–53).

During this period, the emphasis is on range of motion and comfort.

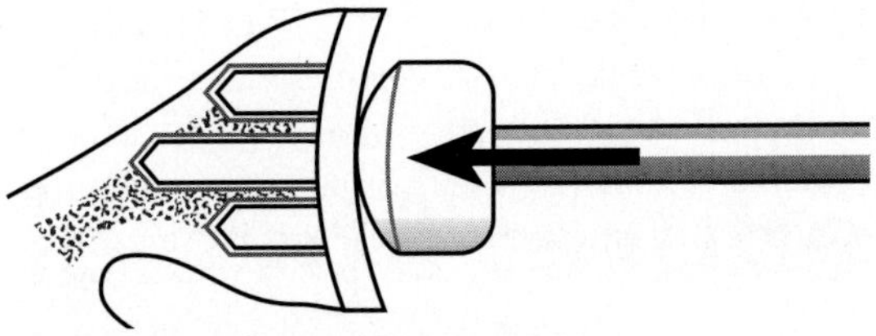

**Figure 31–20. Impacting the glenoid**
The final component is impacted into the prepared glenoid with a smooth impactor.

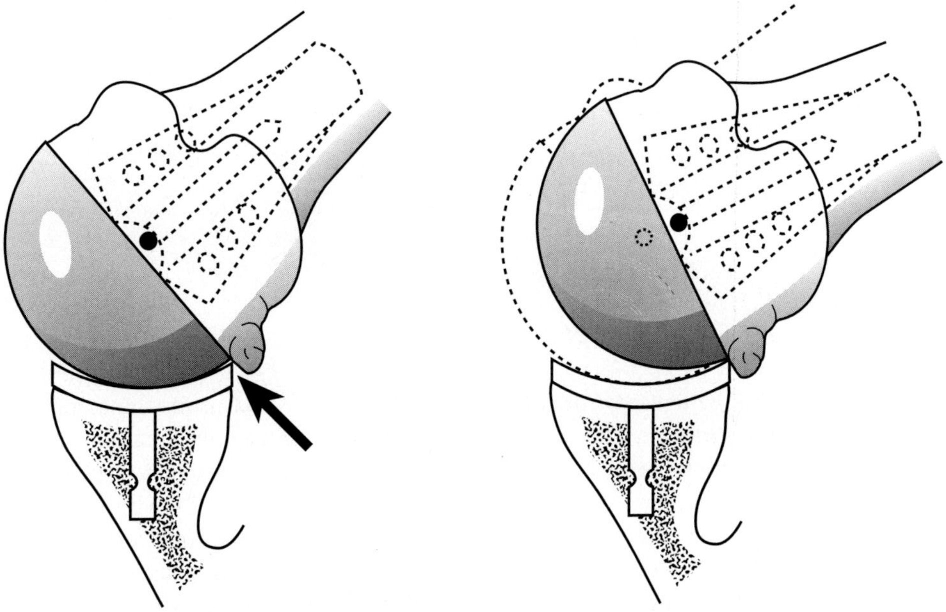

**Figure 31–21. Posterior open book**
If the posterior nonarticular humerus abuts the posterior corner of the glenoid, the joint will "open book" on external rotation.

CHAPTER 32

# Procedure: Special Hemiarthroplasty for Cuff Tear Arthropathy

| |
|---|
| ***Diagnosis*** |
| ***Rotator cuff tear arthropathy    ICD9 CODE 716.91*** |
| ***Procedure*** |
| ***Special humeral hemiarthroplasty for cuff tear arthropathy    CPT CODE 23470.22*** |

## INDICATIONS

The patient has rotator cuff tear arthropathy that limits the comfort and function of the shoulder. The shoulder has not responded to nonoperative management.

Preoperative radiographs reveal loss of the normal humeral contour and radiographic joint space as well as upward displacement of the humeral head into the coracoacromial arch (**Fig. 32–1**). Special views are taken for templating the arthroplasty (see Fig. 29–1).

Knowing the alternatives as well as the risks of infection, neurovascular injury, excessive stiffness, pain, weakness, fracture, instability, component loosening, and the need for revision surgery, as well as anesthetic complications, the patient desires to proceed with the above-described procedure. The patient recognizes that the shoulder has irreparable rotator cuff deficiency and that the procedure cannot restore the strength of the rotator cuff to the shoulder. The patient understands that the purpose of the procedure is to restore a smooth, round, well-fixed humeral articular surface that is of appropriate size, location, and orientation. The patient recognizes furthermore that this procedure cannot be expected to restore normal comfort and function to the shoulder. And, lastly, the patient understands his or her critical role in the post-surgical rehabilitation.

## FINDINGS

Examination under anesthesia reveals that range of glenohumeral motion is limited in all directions and there is bony crepitance on glenohumeral and subacromial motion.

Surgical findings include substantial bursal thickening and a substantial bursal effusion. The tendons of the upper subscapularis, supraspinatus, and infraspinatus muscles are totally absent, offering no possibility of repair. There is loss of normal humeral

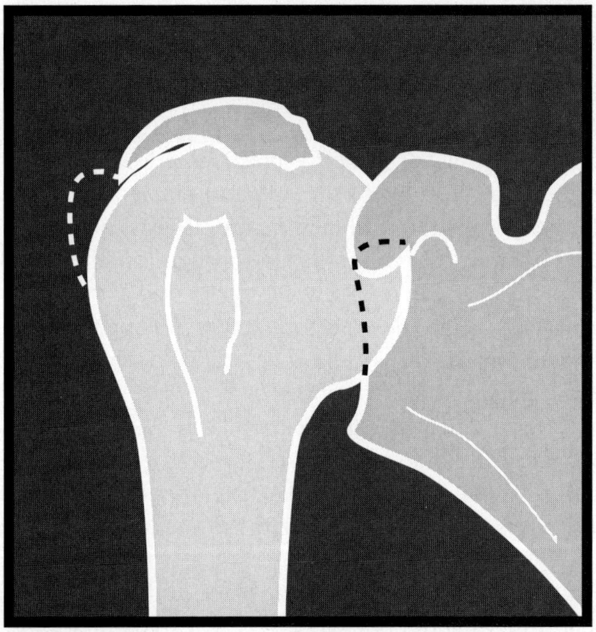

**Figure 32–1. Cuff tear arthropathy**
In cuff tear arthropathy, the radiographs reveal femoralization of the proximal humerus and acetabularization of the coracoacromial/glenoid arch. (Modified from Matsen FA, Lippitt SB, Sidles JA, et al [eds]: Practical Evaluation and Management of the Shoulder. Philadelphia: WB Saunders, 1994, p. 128.)

articular cartilage over the upper medial aspect of the humeral head. The remaining cartilage is in the process of dissolution. There are substantial osteophytes around the articular surface. The humeral articular surface has lost its normal smoothness and roundness. The acromion is thinned. The undersurface of the coracoacromial arch is smooth. The upper glenoid cartilage is eroded with a concavity congruent to that of the coracoacromial arch.

## OPERATION

Under satisfactory anesthesia, the patient is placed in a low beach chair position with the glenohumeral joint at the edge of the operating table (see Fig. 29–2). The entire forequarter is doubly prepped and draped in the usual sterile fashion with the arm free to be moved. The shoulder is approached through a standard deltopectoral incision along a line connecting the mid-clavicle to the mid-lateral humerus at the deltoid tubercle (see Fig. 29–3). The deltopectoral interval is opened, and the cephalic vein retracted laterally (see Fig. 29–4). The clavipectoral fascia is opened just lateral to the coracoid muscles (see Fig. 29–5).

The humeroscapular motion interface is mobilized. Substantial scar and thickened bursa are resected from the motion interface. Resecting the bursa helps prevent re-accumulation of the effusion after surgery. The axillary nerve is palpated medially as it crosses the subscapularis and laterally as it exits the quadrilateral space (see Fig. 29–6). It is protected throughout the case.

A self-retaining retractor is placed with one blade underneath the coracoid muscles and one blade beneath the deltoid (see Fig. 29–7). The remaining subscapularis tendon and subjacent capsule are incised from their insertion to the lesser tuberosity, leaving all possible tendon length with the muscle (see Fig. 29–8).

A 360-degree release of the subscapularis (see Fig. 29–9) is performed, incising the coracohumeral ligament and incising any connections of the anterior capsule to the glenoid (see Figs. 29–10 and 29–11). The capsule is left on the deep side of the subscapularis to reinforce the tendon for its reattachment at the conclusion of the case.

The capsule is released from the humeral neck anteriorly and inferiorly. The humerus is exposed by gentle external rotation and extension of the arm, inserting a smooth broad elevator into the depths of the joint to ease passage of the posterior humeral osteophytes onto the glenoid (see Fig. 29–12). This elevator is then placed behind the humeral head to bring the proximal humerus into full view (see Fig. 29–13). Care is taken to avoid excessive pressure on the fragile acromion.

The center of the humeral articular surface is marked with the cautery. A vertical line is drawn upward and downward from this point, dividing the humeral articular surface into its anterior and posterior halves. A second line, starting at the center point and extending parallel to the humeral center line, is drawn on the anterior surface of the humeral head and lesser tuberosity (see Fig. 29–14). The starting point for reaming is the point where the center of the humeral shaft projects through the superior articular surface of the humerus along the vertical line bisecting the head. This is usually at the most superior aspect of the humeral head, just posterior to the bicipital groove, 1 cm from the cuff insertion, and halfway between the anterior and posterior margins of the humeral head.

A pinecone burr is used to open the medullary canal at this point (see Fig. 29–15). A straight curette held in the surgeon's dominant hand is passed through this hole and down the medullary canal while the elbow is held in the nondominant hand, guiding the direction of the curette and positioning the humerus. Next, a straight tapered reamer is used to increase the size of the hole, again being guided by the surgeon's nondominant hand at the elbow. This and all subsequent medullary instruments are inserted with a gentle valgus bias (see Fig. 29–16).

Next, successively larger medullary reamers are inserted down the canal to the depth required by the prosthesis, but no further (see Fig. 29–17). The largest reamer that can be fully inserted without cortical reaming is selected as the final reamer; its axis is the "orthopaedic axis of the medullary canal of the humerus."

Osteophytes are removed from the humeral neck (see Fig. 29–18). An extramedullary cutting guide can approximate in the orientation of the humeral osteotomy plane (see Fig. 29–19), but such a system cannot be referenced to the medullary anatomy of the humerus that will determine the position of the implant. Instead, we prefer an intraoperative templating method that reveals the three-dimensional relationship between the orthopaedic axis of the medullary canal, the articular surface that would be provided by different prosthetic heads, and the cut plane. Such a system links the geometry of the final reamer to that of the head and cut, using a mask that fits onto the reamer. This is particularly important in the case of cuff tear arthropathy, in which the goal is to anatomically resurface the humeral articular cartilage so that it can articulate with the "acetabulum" sculpted out of the coracoacromial arch and the upper glenoid. The mask is selected that most closely matches the diameter of curvature and height of the humeral head (see Fig. 29–20). When placed on the medullary reamer, this construct has the same basic geometry as the definitive prosthesis with the selected diameter stem, head diameter, and head height. The mask is then mounted on the medullary reamer that has been inserted into the humeral canal and oriented to respect the version of the biological head—its superior edge should bisect the humeral head along the line previously drawn (see Fig. 29–21).

Using the mask, the anterior neck cut is marked with the electrocautery (see Fig. 29–22). This line should run perpendicular to the humeral center line drawn on the proximal humerus. The mask and medullary reamer are removed and the cut line is extrapolated posteriorly, passing just inside what was formerly the attachment of the cuff to the base of the tuberosity.

Using a sharp, broad, flat osteotome, the humeral head is resected along the cut marks. The cut plane is in approximately 30 degrees of retroversion and at a 45-degree angle with the long axis of the shaft.

The diameter of curvature is measured with a cutout template **(Fig. 32–2)**. While ensuring the desired version, a broach osteotome corresponding to the size of the final medullary reamer is driven into the cancellous bone at the neck cut, marking the location of the fins and the metaphyseal body (see Fig. 29–25). The lateral and anterior fins should straddle the bicipital groove. The lateral and medial fins should parallel the bisecting line previously drawn on the humerus.

The cancellous bone within the outline of the broach is removed (see Fig. 29–26). The medullary broach is selected that corresponds to the final reamer diameter. The broach is advanced down the canal in the same orientation as the broach osteotome—in approximately 30 degrees of retroversion (see Fig. 29–27). Anterior angulation of the broach is avoided (see Fig. 29–28). The broach is used as a guide to resect the marginal osteophytes anteriorly, medially, and posteriorly (see Fig. 29–29). This ensures that osteophytes will not block external rotation by abutting the posterior glenoid **(Fig. 32–3)**.

All scar tissue is removed from under the coracoacromial arch, but the arch itself is carefully preserved to avoid the problem of anterosuperior escape **(Fig. 32–4)**.

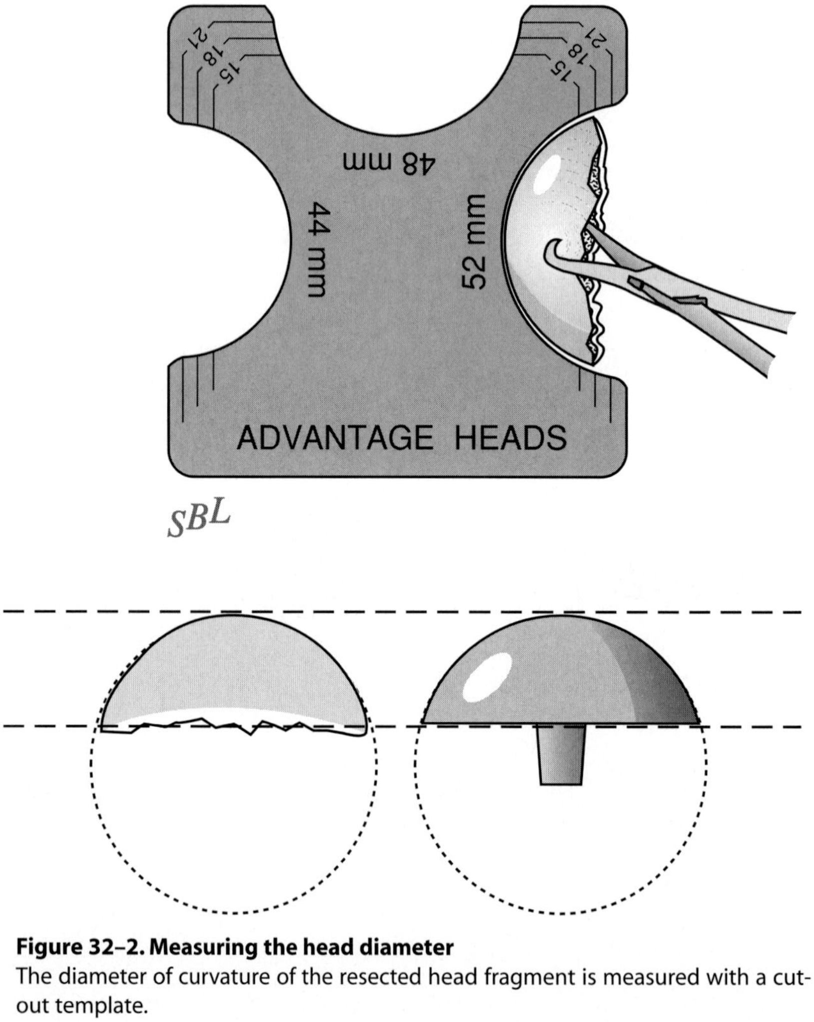


**Figure 32–2. Measuring the head diameter**
The diameter of curvature of the resected head fragment is measured with a cut-out template.

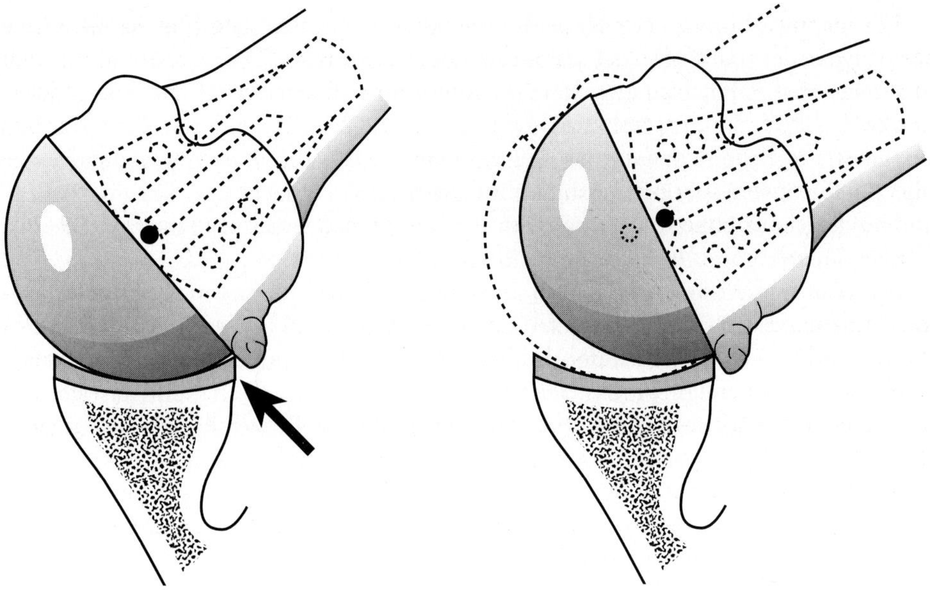

**Figure 32–3. Posterior open book**
Care is taken to be sure that the posterior humeral head does not abut the posterior glenoid in external rotation, causing the joint to "open book" anteriorly.

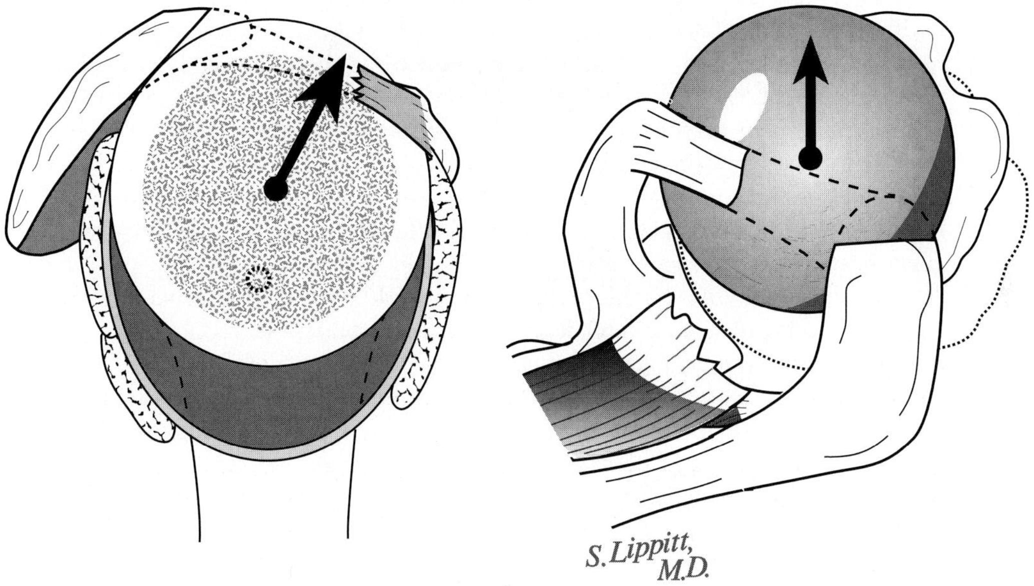


**Figure 32–4. Anterosuperior escape**
If the coracoacromial arch is compromised by acromioplasty and coracoacromial arch section, the humeral head is at risk for anterosuperior escape.

The medullary broach (which is also the trial body) is reinserted in the medullary canal. The set of trial heads that are selected have a diameter of curvature equal to that of the resected biological head. Starting by inserting the trial head with the smallest height, the laxity for each head possibility is examined until the head height is found that allows 40 degrees of external rotation with the subscapularis approximated (see Fig. 29–30), 50% posterior translation on the posterior drawer test (see Fig. 29–31), and 60 degrees of internal rotation with the arm in 90 degrees of abduction (see Fig. 28–32). These are the 40, 50, 60 guidelines.

Procrustean grafting of the humeral canal is now carried out. Small bits of cancellous bone harvested from the resected humeral head are impacted against the walls of the medullary canal using a smooth impactor with the same medullary geometry as the definitive humeral prosthesis (see Figs. 29–34 and 29–35). Graft is added selectively to manage any tendency for the impactor to incline medially (see Fig. 29–36) or anteriorly (see Fig. 29–37). Selective anterior grafting can eliminate the apparent posterior offset of the neck related to anterior inclination of the prosthesis. Grafting is continued by adding and impacting successive bits of graft until the impactor cannot be removed by hand without the tap of a mallet.

At least six 1.8 mm drill holes are placed along the anterior aspect of the humeral neck cut starting near the biceps tendon superiorly. Number 2 braided nonabsorbable sutures are passed through each of these holes for later reattachment of the subscapularis (see Fig. 29–38).

The definitive humeral prosthesis with the desired canal diameter, medullary size, head diameter of curvature, and height is selected. A small amount of additional cancellous bone graft is inserted (see Fig. 29–40). The definitive prosthesis is inserted in the same orientation as the impactor.

The humeral prosthesis is driven down distally until it is positioned in proper register with the glenoid; that is, the center of the head is aligned with the center of the glenoid. The arm is placed in maximal adduction while the humerus is rotated to ensure that there is no abutment between the humeral bone and the inferior glenoid. It is also essential to be sure that the tuberosity is smoothed so that it does not extend beyond the surface curvature of the prosthetic articular surface (**Fig. 32–5**) and that it does not abut the coracoacromial arch in abduction or rotation (**Figs. 32–6** and **32–7**).

The security of the humeral fixation is verified in that it cannot be budged by hand. Excellent fixation has been achieved.

The desired laxity of the shoulder is again verified (40 degrees of external rotation, 50% of posterior translation, and 60 degrees of internal rotation in abduction).

The wound is thoroughly irrigated to remove any remaining bits of bone or debris.

The subscapularis is then repaired to the sutures previously placed at the anterior neck cut. Particular attention is directed at securing the upper border of the tendon (see Fig. 29–43). An excellent subscapularis repair is achieved.

The wound is again irrigated and closed in layers over a drain. Interrupted closures are used in the skin to allow for drainage.

Dry sterile dressings are applied as the patient is returned to the recovery room with the arm in continuous passive motion.

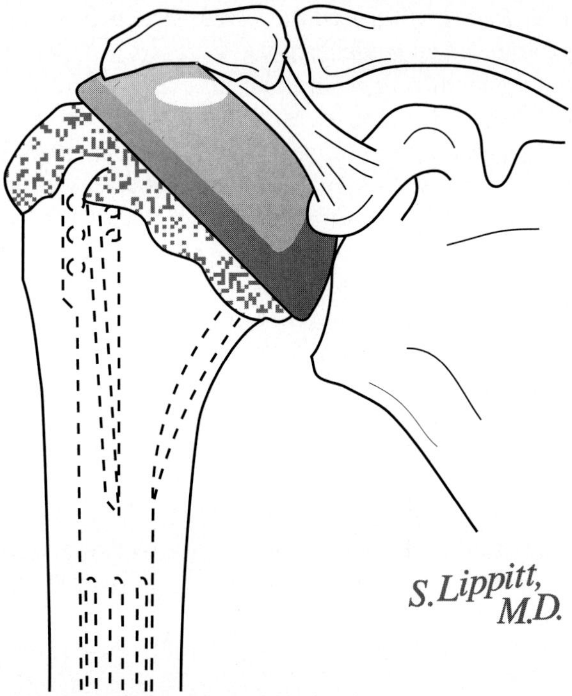


**Figure 32–5. Prominent tuberosity**
The tuberosity is inspected to be sure that no bone extends beyond the contour of the humeral articular surface.

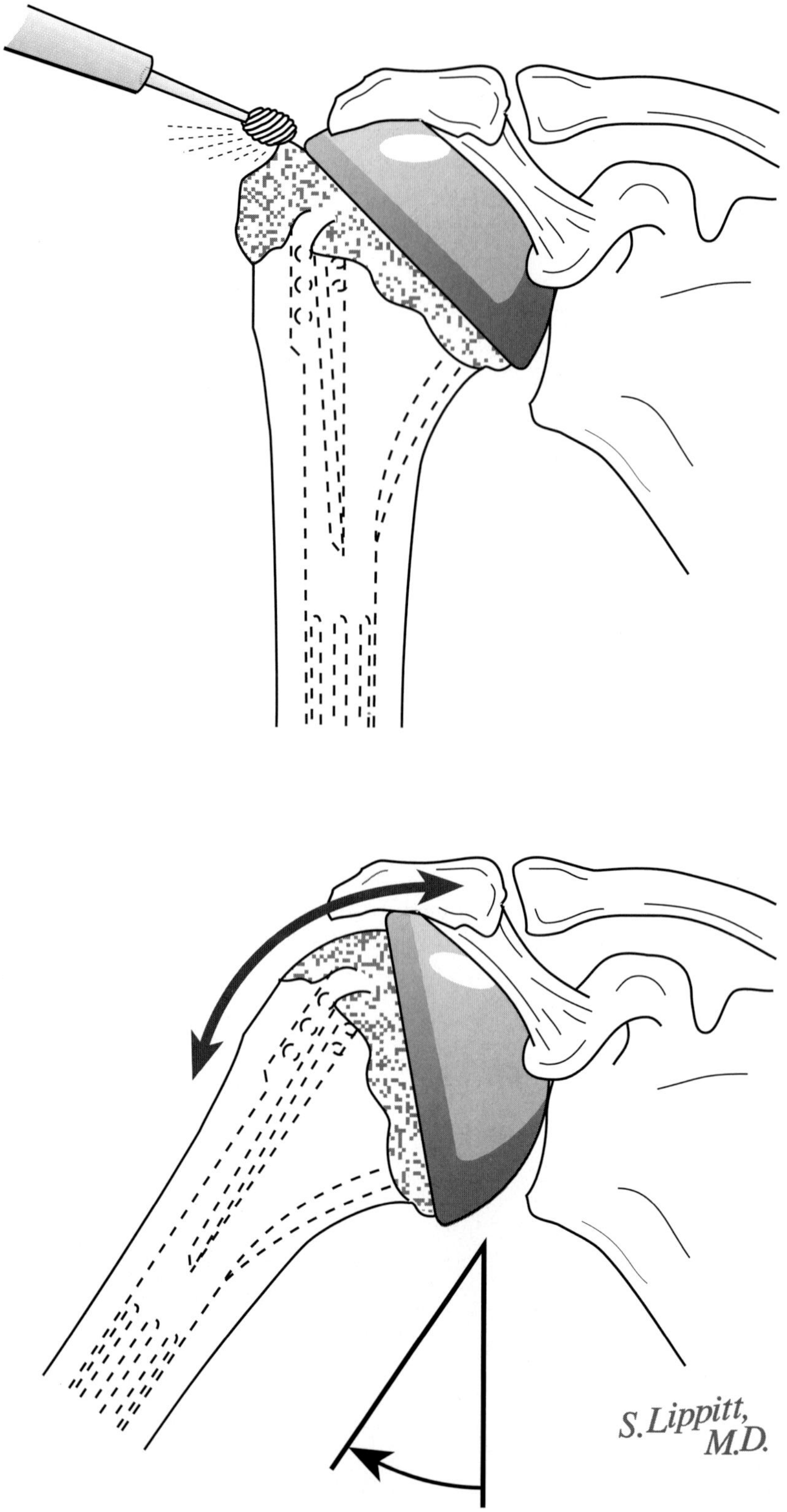


**Figure 32–6. Smoothing the greater tuberosity**
The adequacy of the sculpting of the greater tuberosity is verified by ensuring that there is no contact between the smoothed tuberosity and the coracoacromial arch when the arm is abducted.

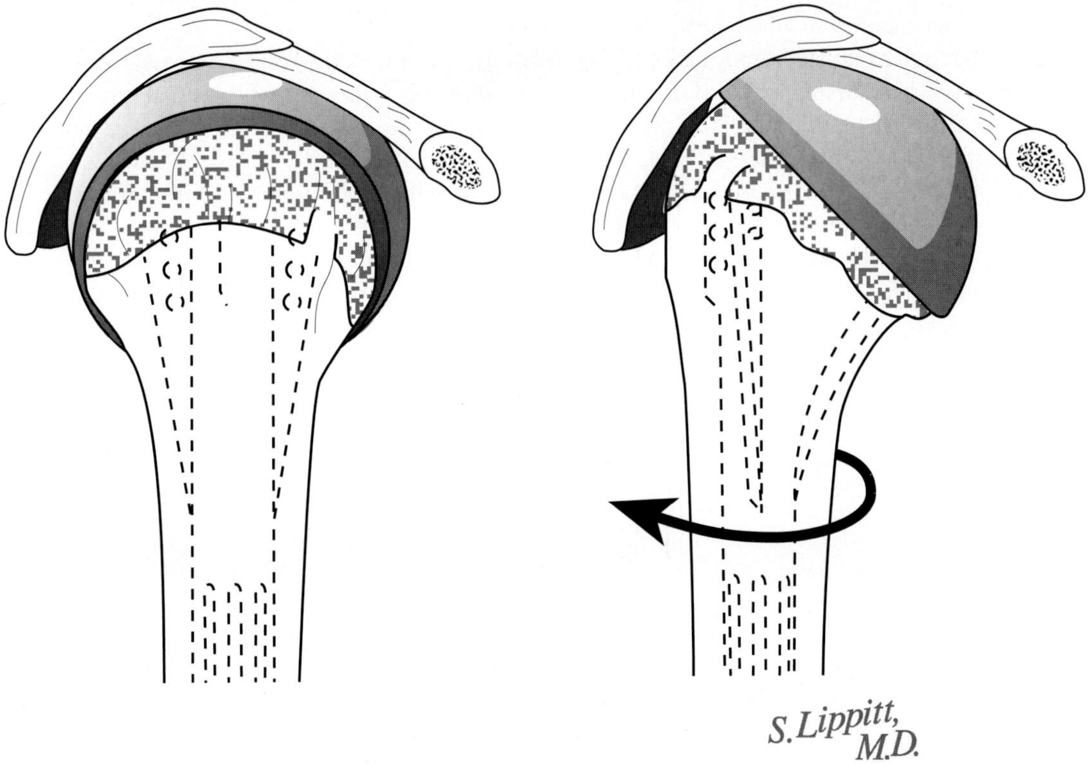


**Figure 32–7. Verifying the smoothness of the greater tuberosity**
It is important to verify that there is no contact between the tuberosity and the coracoacromial arch when the arm is rotated.

## POSTOPERATIVE PLAN

Continuous passive motion is continued while the patient is in bed for the first 36 hours after surgery (see Fig. 29–45). It is removed when the patient is in a chair or ambulating.

On the day of surgery, the patient begins assisted flexion to 140 degrees and assisted external rotation to 40 degrees (see Figs. 29–46, 29–47, and 29–48).

As soon as assisted motion of 140 degrees of flexion and 40 degrees of external rotation is achieved, the patient is discharged to continue his or her rehabilitation at home (see Fig. 29–49). Emphasis is placed on putting the shoulder through its range of motion at least five times per day.

Activities of daily living are encouraged, but the patient should avoid lifting more than 1 pound for 6 weeks.

After 6 weeks, progressively more activity is allowed as long as these activities are comfortable. Additional stretching exercises are started at this time (see Figs. 29–50, 29–51, 29–52, and 29–53).

PART VI

# FRACTURES

CHAPTER 33

# Principles of Proximal Humeral Fracture Management

## CONCEPTS

The goal of the surgical management of fractures is to achieve a reconstruction that (1) heals; (2) maintains functional position of the bone fragments; (3) avoid problems such as avascular necrosis, hardware failure, arthritis, and sepsis; and (4) ideally enables early motion and use of the arm.

We will not devote time here to the management of fractures that can be reduced and held by closed manipulation or by percutaneous pinning. Instead we will focus on (1) the unstable subtuberous fracture (see Chapter 34), (2) the un-united subtuberous fracture (see Chapter 35), and (3) the displaced four-part proximal humeral fracture to be treated by reconstruction around a proximal humeral prosthesis (see Chapter 36).

We recognize that the substantial excursion of the deltoid muscle can accommodate substantial shortening in the subtuberous area; however, because of the smaller excursion of the cuff muscles and the need for the upper surface of the cuff and tuberosities to articulate smoothly with the undersurface of the coracoacromial arch, displacement of the tuberosities can produce weakness, stiffness, and roughness. Thus, secure, smooth, and anatomic fixation of the tuberosities to the shaft of the humerus is one of the highest priorities in proximal humeral fracture fixation.

The quality of proximal humeral bone is a key consideration in the management of proximal humeral fractures. High-energy fractures through strong bone can be managed by interfragmentary lag screw fixation, intramedullary nails with interlocking screws, or conventional plate fixation **(Fig. 33–1)**. Even with these methods of fixation, care must be taken to respect the anatomical constraints of the region **(Fig. 33–2)**. However, the fractures that present major surgical challenges are those in which bone quality is compromised by age, disease, or disuse; as a result, conventional fracture fixation methods cannot be applied **(Fig. 33–3)**. With fractures through osteopenic bone, a substantial part of the fixation needs to derive from compression of the bone fragments against each other. Allowance needs to be made for compaction or resorption of the soft bone at the fracture site; thus, "tension band" plate and suture configurations can be helpful.

A particular challenge with proximal humeral fractures is that of rotational control. It is apparent that the rotator cuff muscles attach to the tuberosities and that most of the important fractures occur at the subtuberous level. The distal fragment of these fractures includes the humeral shaft and the remainder of the upper extremity, including the elbow. When active external rotation is attempted, for example in opening a car door, the force is applied at a distance of approximately 50 cm from the axis of the shaft. Let us say, for example, that the force exerted on the car door handle is

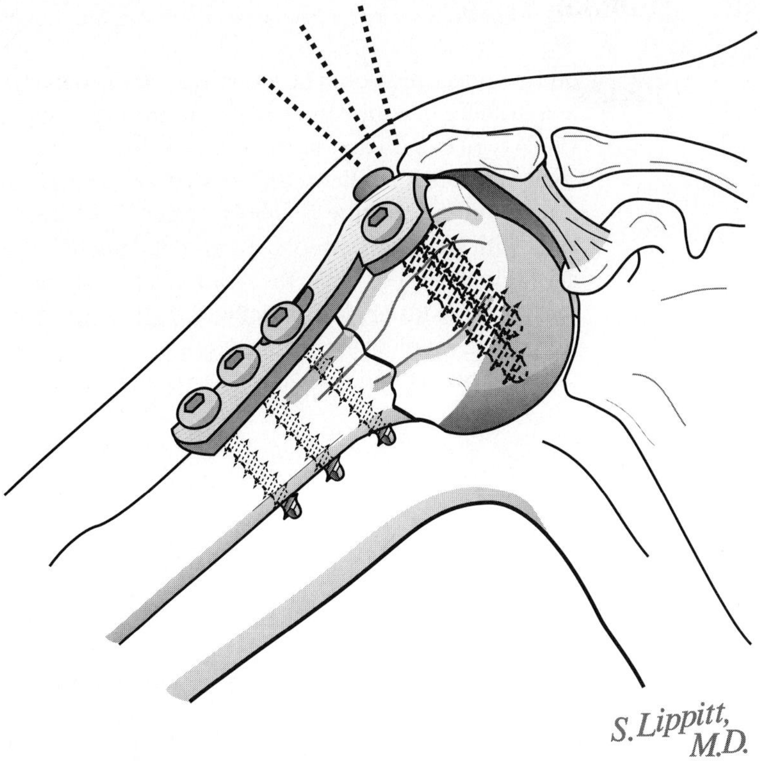


**Figure 33–2. Plate abutment**
If the plate is placed superiorly on the proximal fragment in an attempt to optimize fixation, it may abut the coracoacromial arch when the arm is abducted.

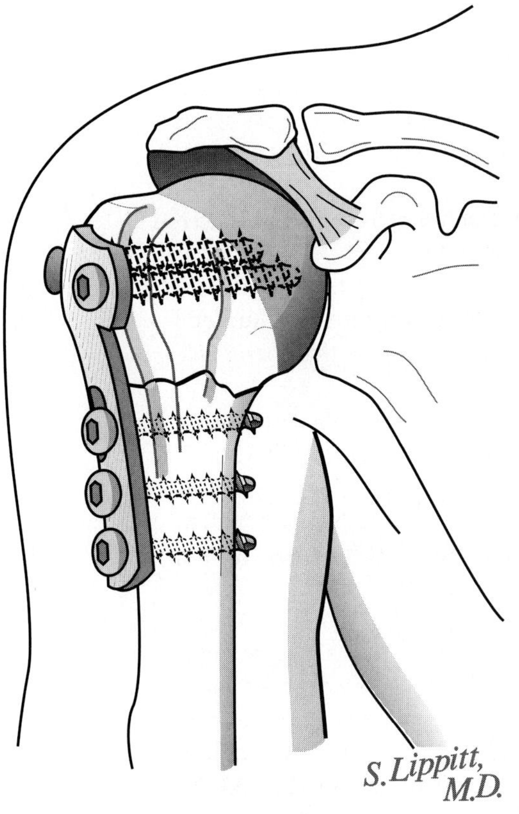


**Figure 33–1. Plating a subtuberous fracture**
Conventional plating of subtuberous fractures depends on screws getting a secure bite in the proximal fragment. Such a bite may not be possible when the head is osteopenic.

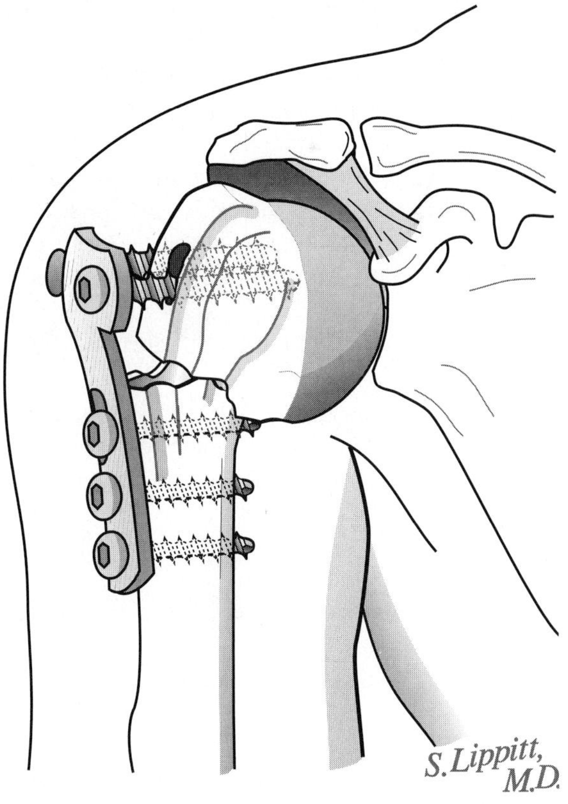


**Figure 33–3. Screw pullout**
While fixation in the distal fragment can almost always be achieved, screw fixation in the proximal fragment is often precarious, allowing the head to fall in varus or to fail in rotation.

50 Newtons (this would be a very easy door to open). The external rotator muscles act at a distance of approximately 2.5 cm from the shaft and thus a force of 1000 Newtons (50 N × 50 cm/2.5 cm) must be resisted by the fixation of the greater tuberosity to the shaft **(Fig. 33–4)**. Patients are advised not to perform activities such as opening a car door until the fracture is solidly healed. The same force multiplier effect is in place even with seemingly minor activities of daily living, such as lifting the bedcovers when getting out of bed. Thus, the fixation of proximal humeral fractures must anticipate these large loads applied directly to the fracture site. It is also of note that these rotational loads applied to the tuberosities may produce displacements that are difficult to see on standard radiographs.

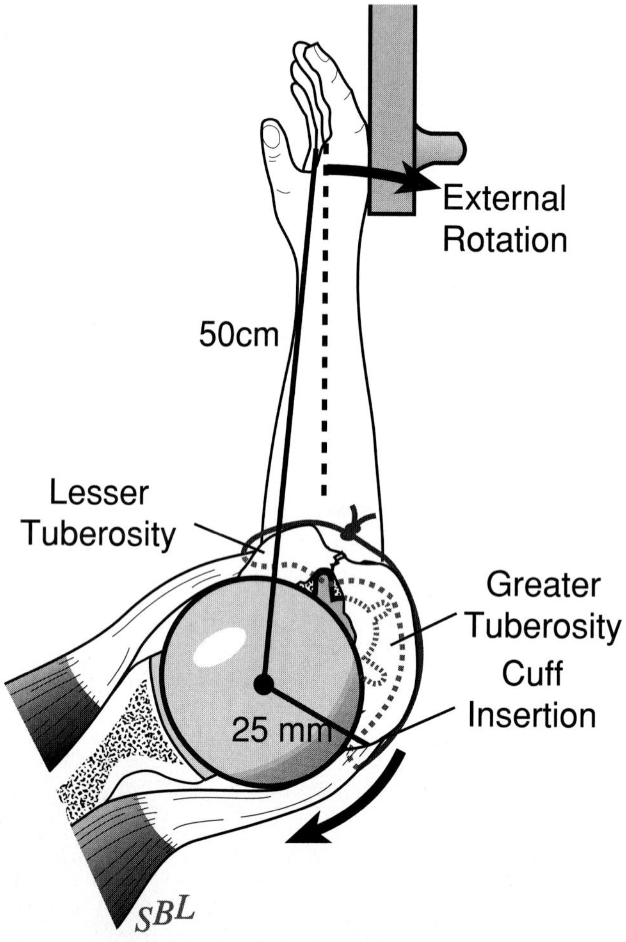


**Figure 33–4. Greater tuberosity torque**
The fixation of the external rotators to the humerus has a moment arm of only 25 mm, while a load applied by the hand may have a moment arm of 500 mm. Thus, the force challenging the fixation of the tuberosities may be 20 times as high as the force applied by the hand.

Another special challenge is related to the fact that proximal humeral fractures often take place through osteopenic bone, where special methods of fixation must be considered (**Fig. 33–5**).

Finally, because fractures and fracture fixation can be followed by unanticipated complications, the incisions used for fracture surgery must preserve the deltoid and must allow for an extensile approach down the arm as necessary. Thus, we use a long anterior deltopectoral incision for almost all proximal humeral fracture surgery. If, for example, conversion of fracture fixation to a proximal humeral replacement is necessary, the secondary approach is not compromised by an awkwardly placed prior incision.

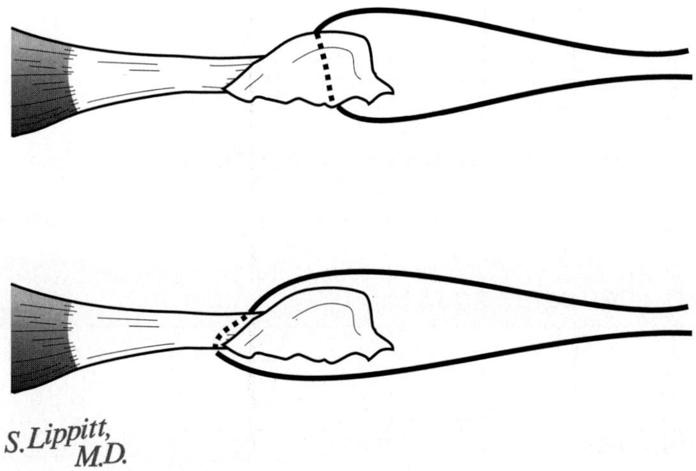


**Figure 33–5. Suturing**
The bone of fractured tuberosities is soft and often comminuted. For these reasons, fixation is optimized by passing sutures around the tuberosities rather than through them.

CHAPTER 34

# Procedure: Pinning of an Unstable Subtuberous Fracture

***Diagnosis***

***Unstable subtuberous fracture    ICD9 CODE 812.01***

***Procedure***

***Closed reduction and percutaneous pinning under fluoroscopic control    CPT CODE 23611***

## INDICATIONS

The patient sustained a fracture of the humerus below the level of the tuberosities. Closed reduction can be accomplished but cannot be maintained with a sling or splint.

Physical examination reveals medial displacement of the proximal humeral shaft and motion at the fracture site.

Radiographs show that the proximal end of the humeral shaft is significantly displaced medially to the distal end of the proximal fragment.

Knowing the alternatives as well as the risks of infection, neurovascular injury, excessive stiffness, pain, weakness, fracture, instability, nonunion, and the need for revision surgery as well as anesthetic complications, the patient desires to proceed with the above-described procedure. The patient understands that the purpose of the procedure is to align the humeral shaft with the proximal fragment. The patient understands that the pinning will not provide rigid internal fixation and that the arm will need to be protected in a sling until healing has occurred. The patient recognizes that this procedure cannot be expected to completely restore normal comfort and function to the shoulder. And, lastly, the patient understands his or her critical role in rehabilitation after the fracture has healed.

## FINDINGS

Examination with the patient under anesthesia reveals discontinuity of the humeral shaft below the level of the tuberosities (**Fig. 34–1**). Fluoroscopy indicates that the fracture can be reduced by the application of lateral traction to the proximal shaft while the arm is adducted. One can accomplish this by pulling anterolaterally on the proximal shaft using a towel passed through the proximal axilla (**Fig. 34–2**).

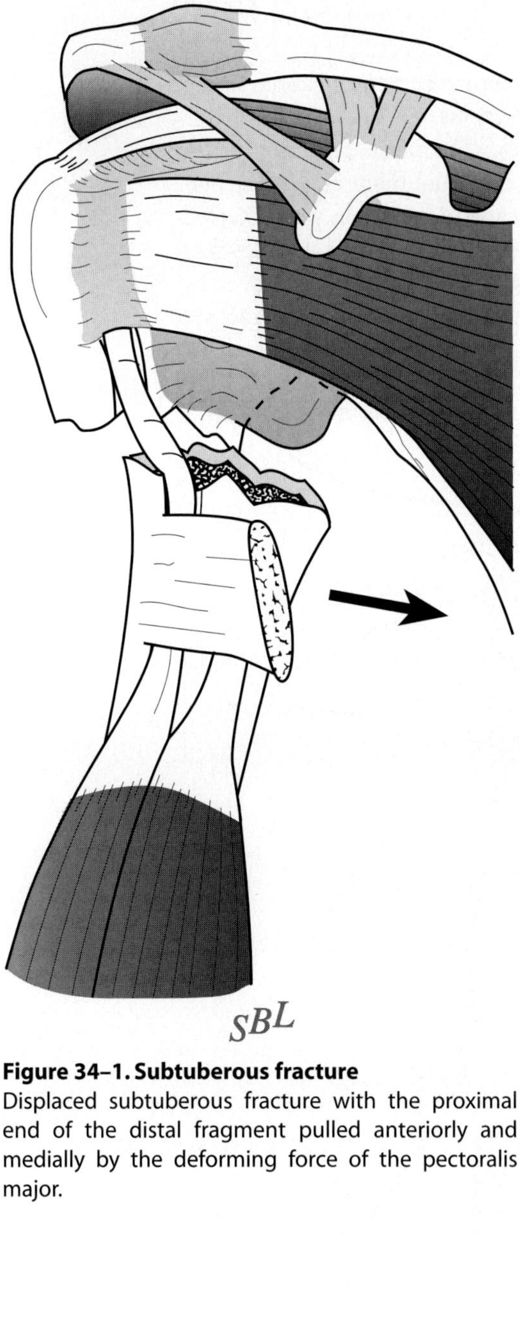


**Figure 34–1. Subtuberous fracture**
Displaced subtuberous fracture with the proximal end of the distal fragment pulled anteriorly and medially by the deforming force of the pectoralis major.

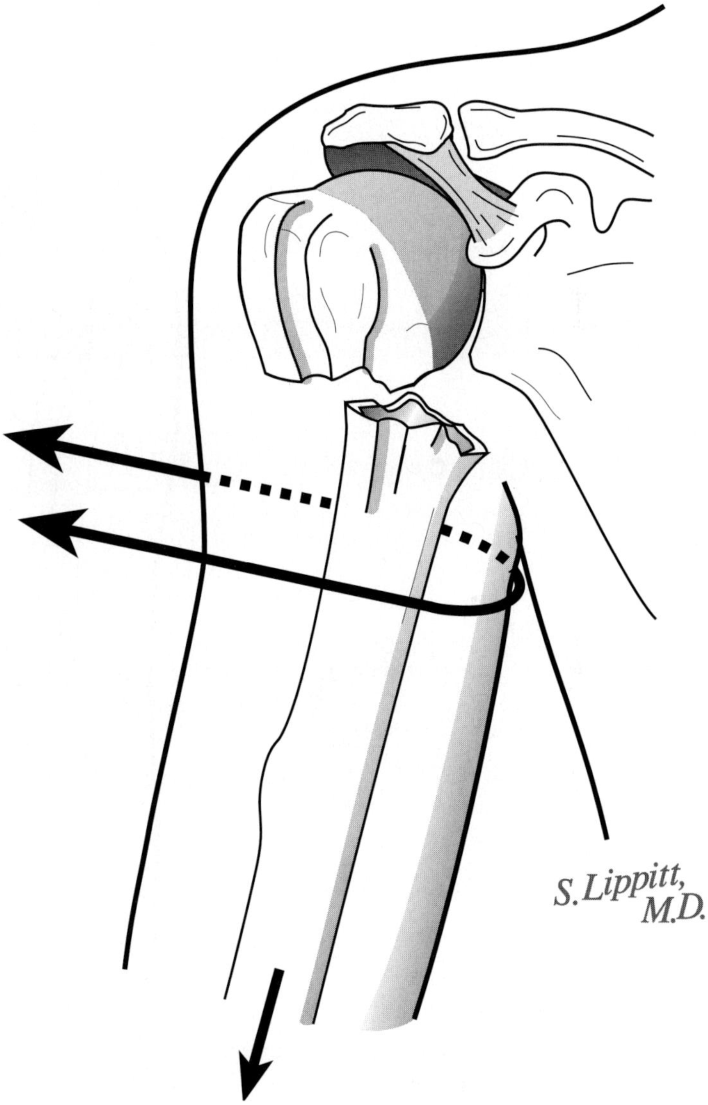


**Figure 34–2. Reduction**
Lateral traction with a towel in the axilla and adduction of the arm reduces the fracture.

## OPERATION

Under satisfactory anesthesia, the patient is placed supine on an operating table set up for fluoroscopy in the anteroposterior and axillary projections.

The reduction maneuver is practiced under fluoroscopy before the arm is prepped.

The arm is then thoroughly prepped and draped in the usual manner. A skin incision is made over the deltoid tubercle. A 3 mm fully threaded Steinmann pin is started at the deltoid tubercle, and then passed upward in the medullary canal to the level of proximal extent of the shaft fragment (**Figs. 34–3** and **34–4**). The fracture is reduced by application of traction with a sterile towel. The pin is then driven across the fracture

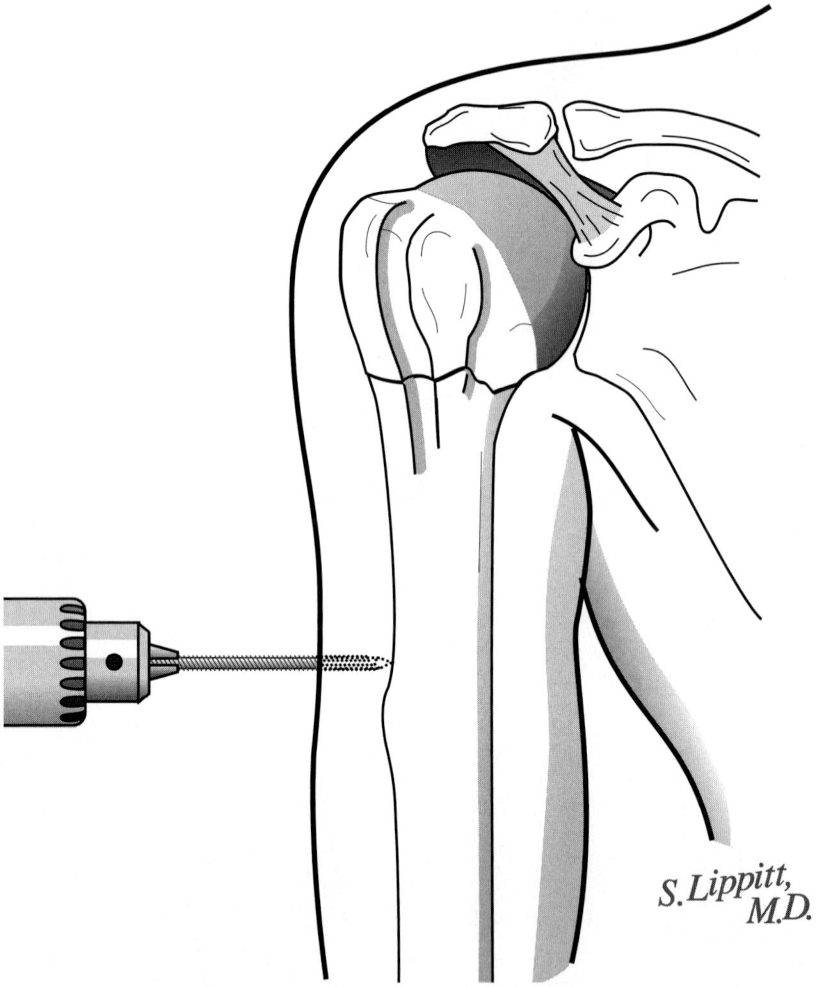


**Figure 34–3. Inserting the pin**
A 3 mm threaded pin is inserted percutaneously starting at the deltoid tubercle.

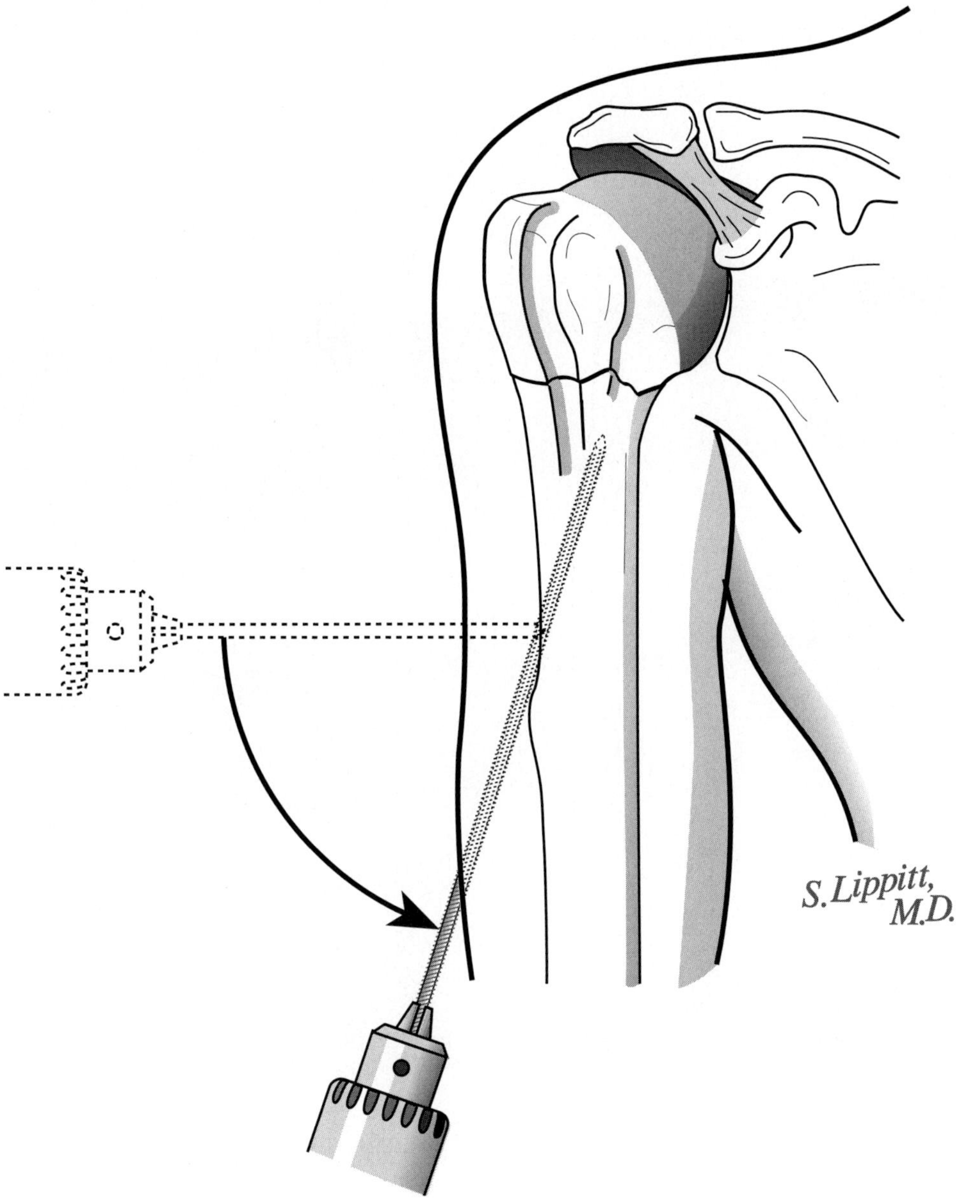


**Figure 34–4. Advancing the pin**
The pin is advanced up the medullary canal of the humerus along its medial endosteal wall.

site, into the humeral head, and 3 mm out the articular surface (**Fig. 34–5**). Excellent reduction is achieved as verified by fluoroscopy in the anteroposterior and axillary projections. The pin is cut off subcutaneously and the wound is closed loosely.

Dry sterile dressings are applied, and the patient is returned to the recovery room with the arm in a sling.

## POSTOPERATIVE PLAN

The arm is kept in a sling until callus is visible on radiographs. While in the sling, the patient is encouraged to look after his or her axillary hygiene and to use the hand for gripping and light activities in the sling position. Rotation from the sling position is avoided.

At 6 weeks, follow-up radiographs are taken to verify that healing is occurring. The pin is then removed with the patient under local anesthesia and light sedation.

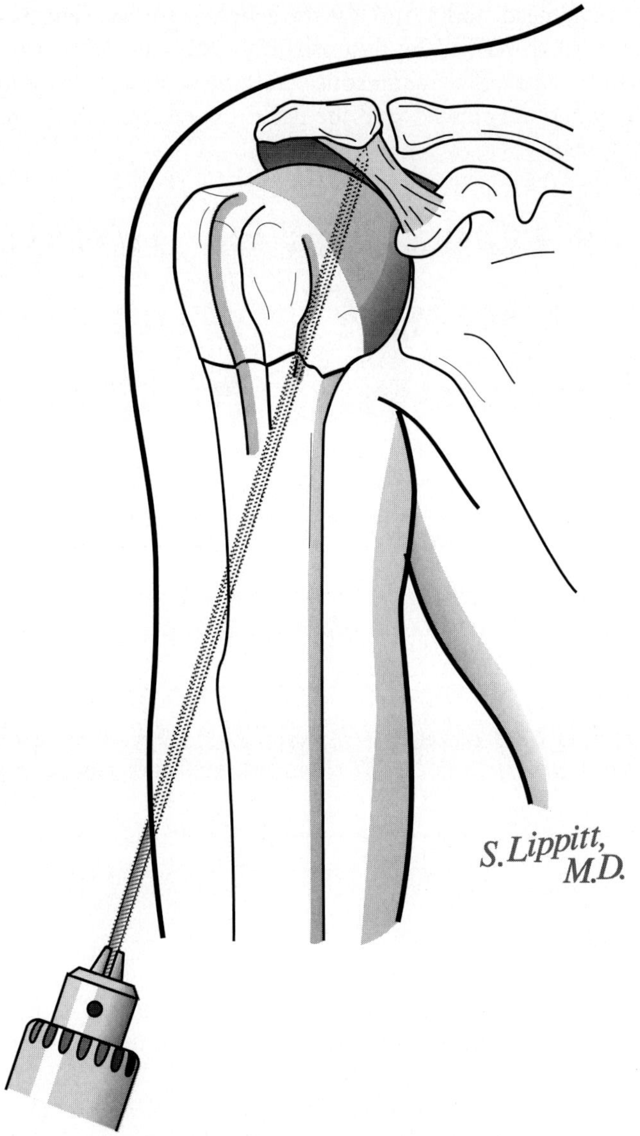


**Figure 34–5. Pinning the deltoid tubercle**

The fracture is reduced under C-arm control while the pin is advanced across the fracture until it extends 3 mm beyond the articular surface. This degree of advancement is desired to achieve maximal purchase on the subchondral bone of the humeral head. Because the pin will be removed before motion is started, it should not produce problems at the glenohumeral joint.

CHAPTER 35

# Procedure: Triangle Plate Fixation of a Subtuberous Nonunion

**Diagnosis**

***Nonunion/pseudoarthrosis of a subtuberous fracture of the proximal humerus ICD9 CODE 733.82***

**Procedure**

***Open reduction and custom triangle plate fixation of a subtuberous nonunion, with iliac cancellous autograft CPT CODE 23615.20900***

## INDICATIONS

The patient sustained a subtuberous fracture of the humerus. The fracture has not healed with nonoperative management and has resulted in loss of comfort and function from the nonunion.

Radiographs show that the tuberosities and humeral head are all intact to each other. There is a varus angulation between the proximal humerus and the humeral shaft. The proximal end of the shaft has excavated a cup-shaped defect in the distal end of the proximal fragment. There is minimal callus. Fluoroscopy has demonstrated substantial rotational instability at the fracture site. The patient's neurovascular status is intact. The patient is a nonsmoker in good nutritional and general health.

Knowing in detail the alternatives as well as the risks of infection, neurovascular injury, excessive stiffness, pain, weakness, nonunion, problems related to the plate fixation, and the possible need for revision surgery as well as the need for and potential complications of iliac crest autograft harvest and anesthetic complications, the patient desires to proceed with the above-described procedure. The patient recognizes that this procedure cannot be expected to completely restore normal comfort and function to the shoulder. The patient understands his or her critical role in the post-surgical rehabilitation.

## FINDINGS

There is a mature pseudoarthrosis of the subtuberous fracture, with joint fluid and fibrocartilage as well as gross motion at the fracture site (**Fig. 35–1**). There is no

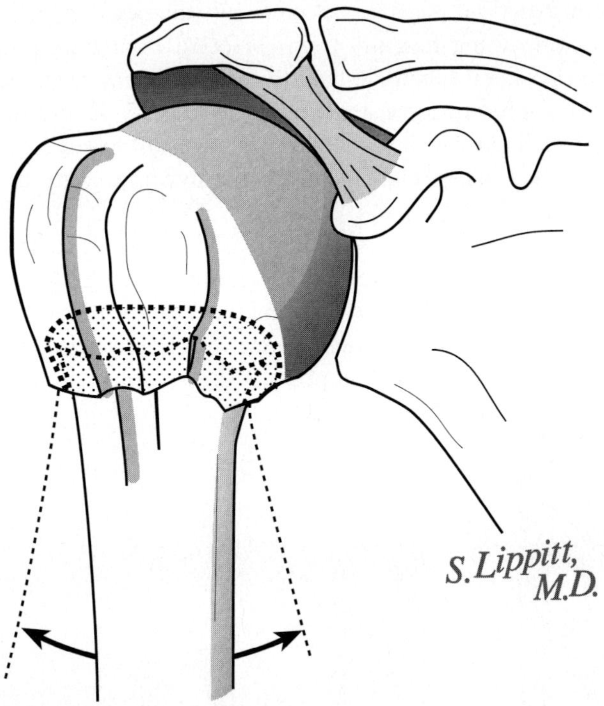


**Figure 35–1. Subtuberous nonunion**
An established subtuberous nonunion with gross motion at the fracture site.

evidence that the fracture would have healed without surgical intervention. The rotator cuff and axillary nerve are intact.

## OPERATION

A 4.5 mm reconstruction plate is selected for the reconstruction (**Fig. 35–2**). Preoperative planning using magnification-corrected radiographs suggests that the distance between the lateral tuberosity and the articular surface will safely accommodate three holes of a 4.5 mm reconstruction plate (**Fig. 35–3**) and that an additional five holes will be required to achieve at least six secure cortices of fixation in the proximal shaft (**Fig. 35–4**). Thus, an eight-hole, 4.5 mm dynamic compression reconstruction plate is anticipated.

Under satisfactory anesthesia, the patient is placed supine on an operating table that allows C-arm fluoroscopy in the anteroposterior and axillary projections. Positioning of the C arm is verified before the prep and draping. The entire forequarter is carefully prepped and draped in the usual sterile fashion with the arm free to be moved. The ipsilateral anterior iliac crest is also prepped and draped for the bone graft harvest.

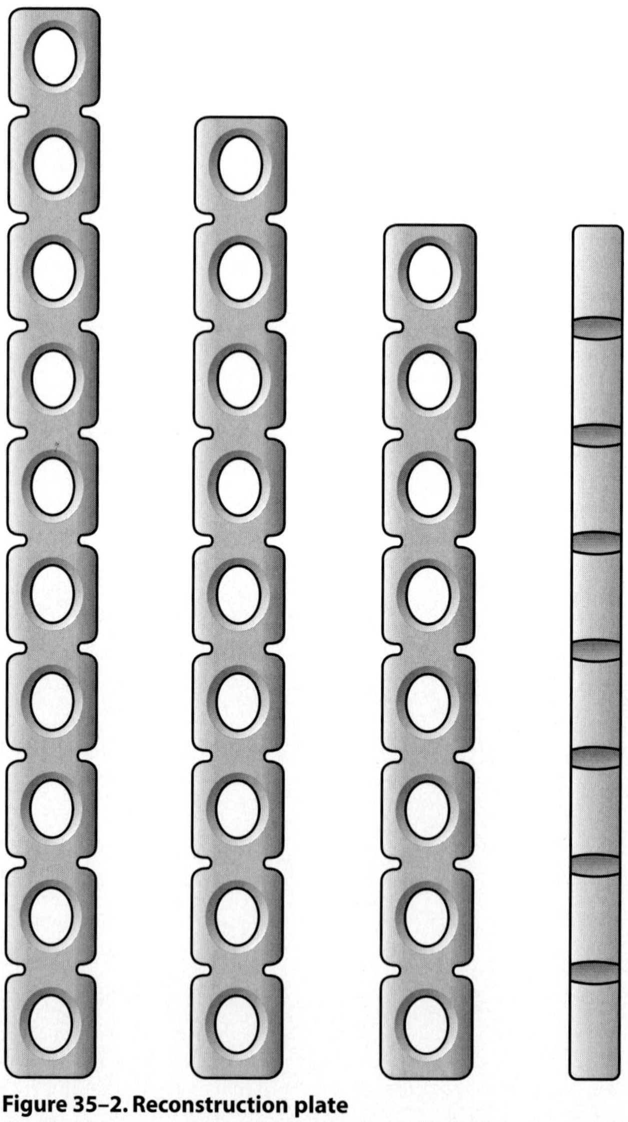

**Figure 35–2. Reconstruction plate**
A 4.5 mm reconstruction plate is usually well suited to the reconstruction.

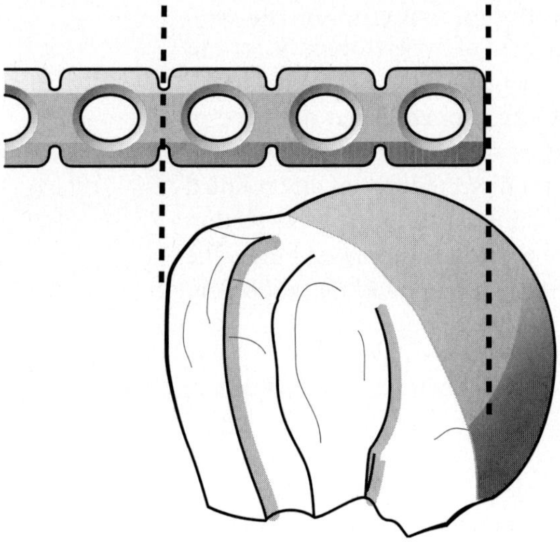

**Figure 35–3. Appropriate head fit**
In this example, the head will accommodate three holes of a 4.5 mm reconstruction plate.

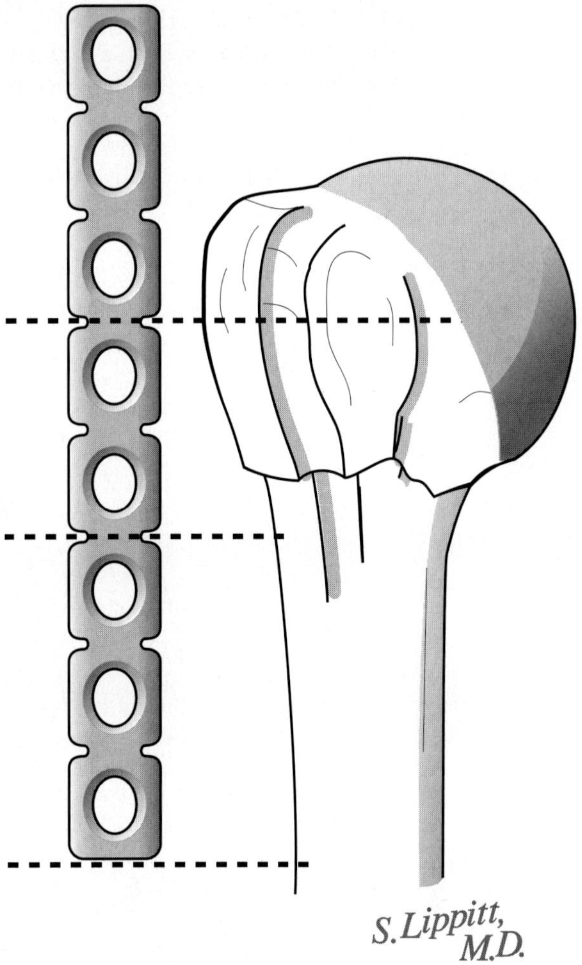


**Figure 35–4. Appropriate shaft fit**
An additional five holes will be required to secure the plate to the lateral shaft.

The shoulder is approached through a long anterior deltopectoral incision (**Fig. 35–5**). The humeroscapular motion interface is cleared of hypertrophic bursa and scar (**Fig. 35–6**) The long head tendon of the biceps is identified in the intertubercular groove and followed to the fracture site. The fracture site is opened and débrided of fibrous and cartilaginous tissue so that bare bone is exposed at the intended union site. The proximal end of the shaft is inspected, opened, and dissected free of any residual fibrous tissue and cartilage (**Fig. 35–7**). It is then shaped into an elliptical cross section with a burr or rongeur in a manner that preserves the maximal amount of bone. The long head tendon of the biceps is used as a guide to ensure correct rotational alignment

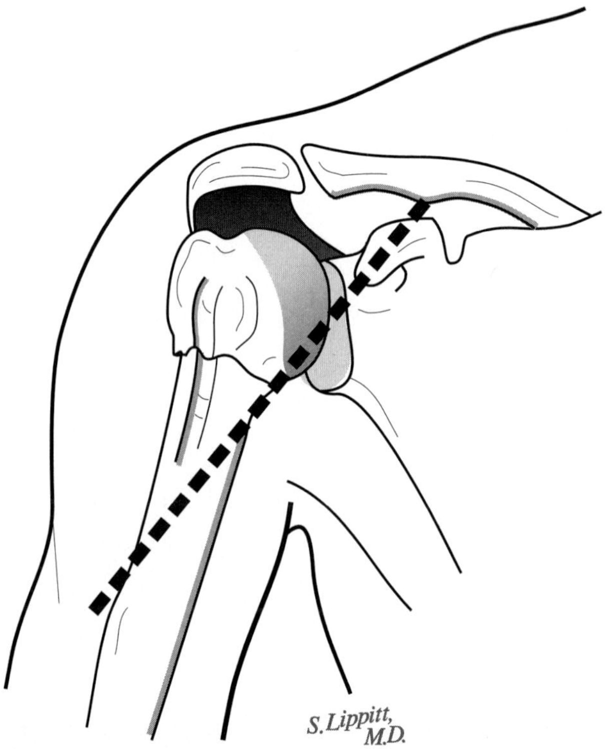


**Figure 35–5. Incision**
The fracture is approached through a long deltopectoral incision.

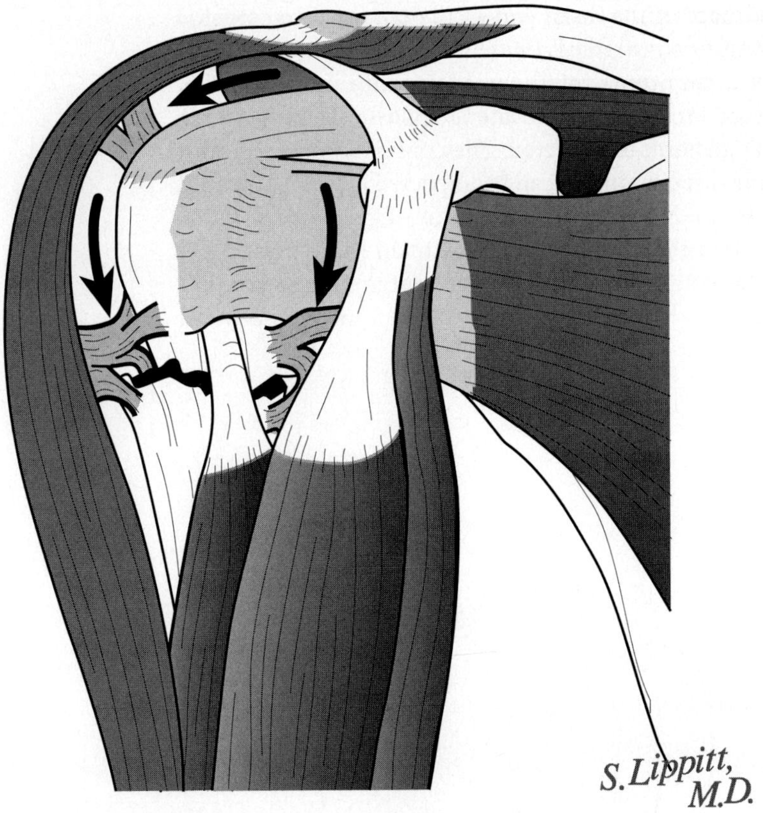


**Figure 35–6. Adhesions**
The humeroscapular motion interface is cleared of scar tissue.

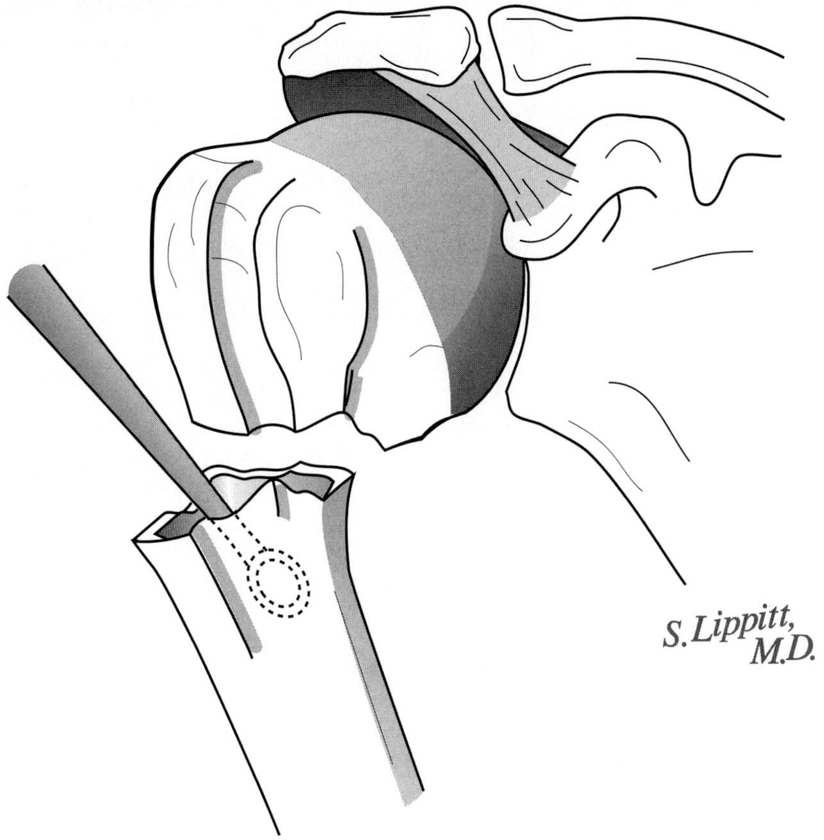


**Figure 35–7. Preparing the shaft**
The proximal end of the shaft fragment is opened with a curette.

of the fragments. The medullary space of the distal end of the proximal fragment is opened with a curette and burr to leave an elliptical slot that will receive the elliptically shaped proximal end of the shaft when proper rotational alignment is imposed (**Fig. 35–8**). The lateral contour of the tuberosities and the lateral contour of the shaft are aligned to ensure that the varus angulation is corrected. The configuration is checked to be sure that the upper end of the distal fragment can be impacted into the hollowed area in the proximal fragment with a slight valgus configuration (**Fig. 35–9**).

An arthrotomy incision is made in the rotator interval between the subscapularis and supraspinatus tendons (**Fig. 35–10**). This arthrotomy is just large enough to admit an index finger, so that the depth and orientation of the plate can be controlled

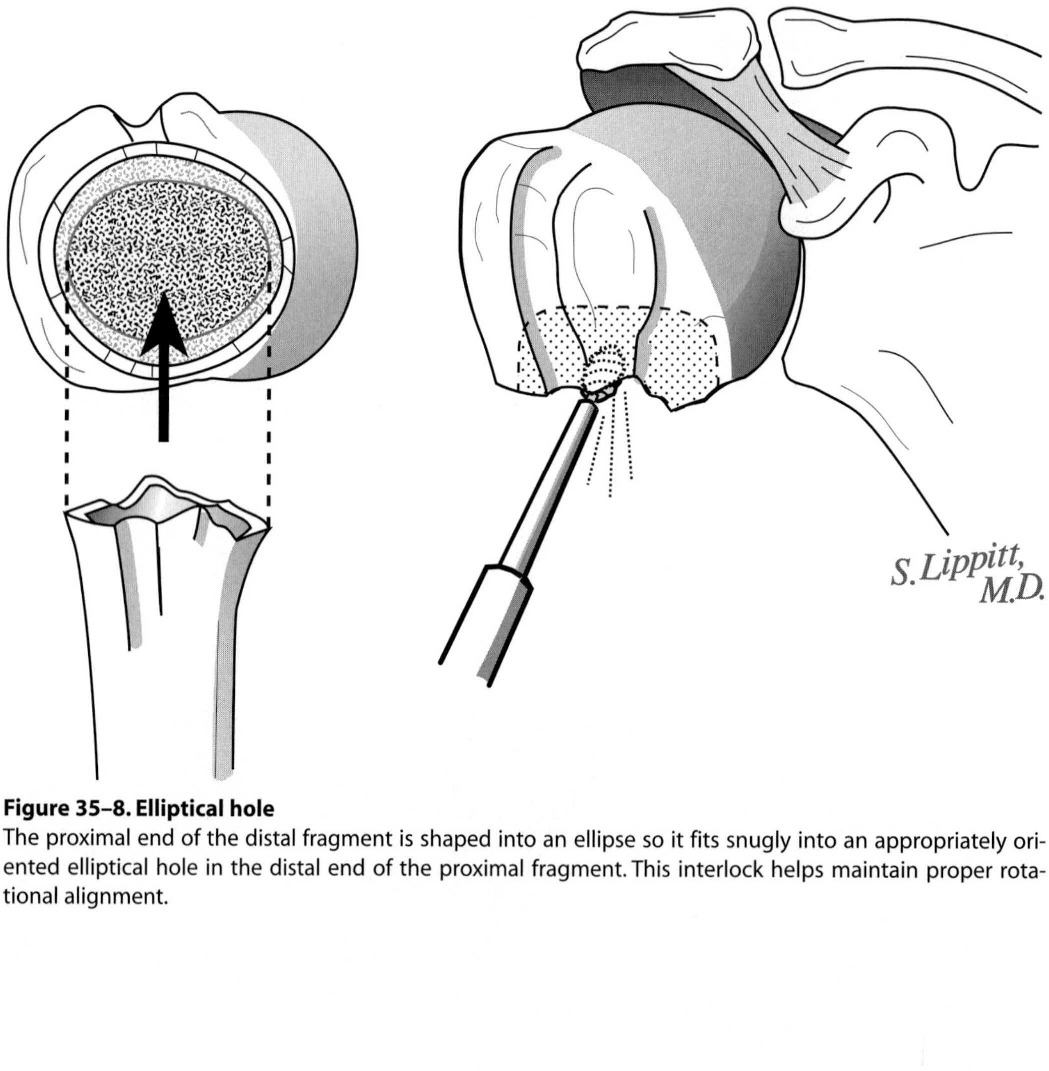


**Figure 35–8. Elliptical hole**
The proximal end of the distal fragment is shaped into an ellipse so it fits snugly into an appropriately oriented elliptical hole in the distal end of the proximal fragment. This interlock helps maintain proper rotational alignment.

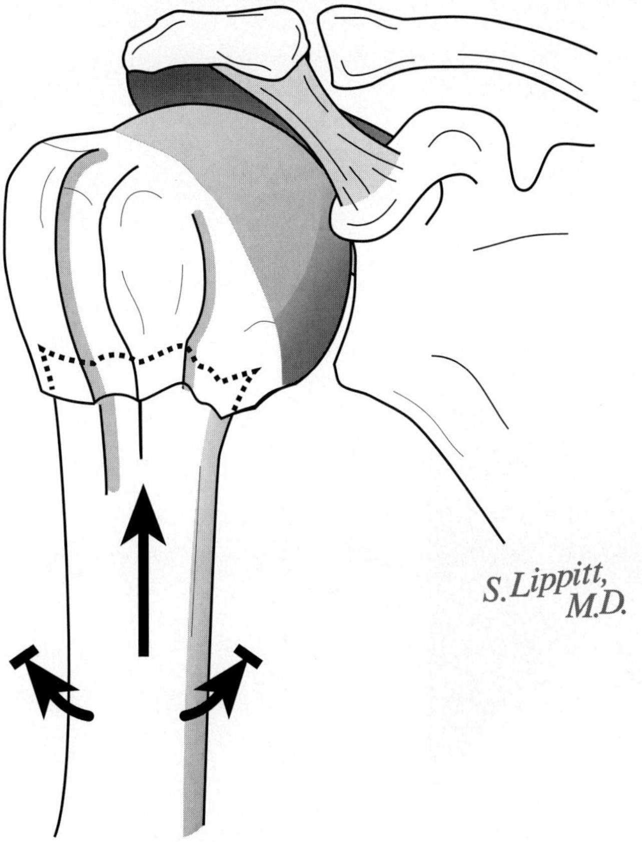


**Figure 35–9. Impact of the shaft**
The contouring is checked to be sure that the bone ends can be impacted into a slightly valgus configuration with good rotational control.

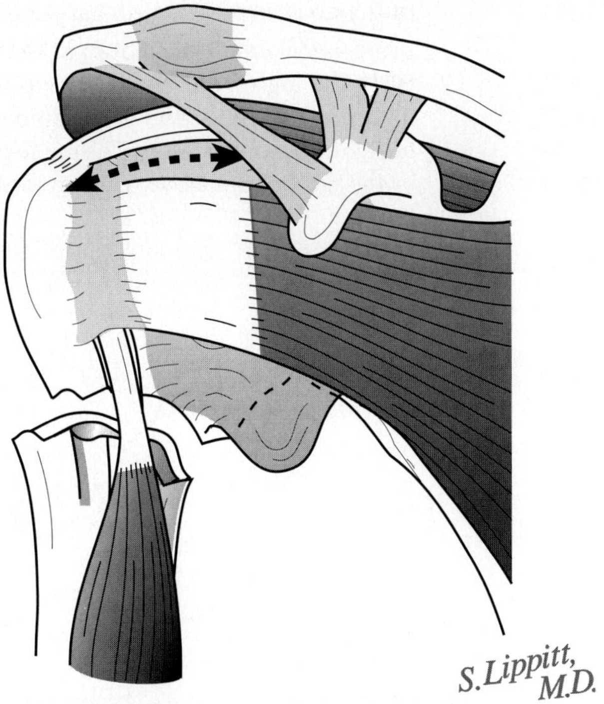


**Figure 35–10. Open rotator interval**
An arthrotomy is made through the rotator interval between the supraspinatus and the subscapularis.

**(Fig. 35–11)**. The orientation of the proximal humeral fragment is determined, and a 2 mm guide pin is drilled from a point just posterior to the biceps tendon, 1.5 cm distal to the top of the greater tuberosity, perpendicular to the lateral tuberosity, and toward the central aspect of the humeral articular surface, as indicated by the intraarticular finger **(Fig. 35–12)**. The guide pin is advanced gently by hand until it is stopped by the subchondral bone. The intraosseous length of the pin is measured **(Fig. 35–13)**.

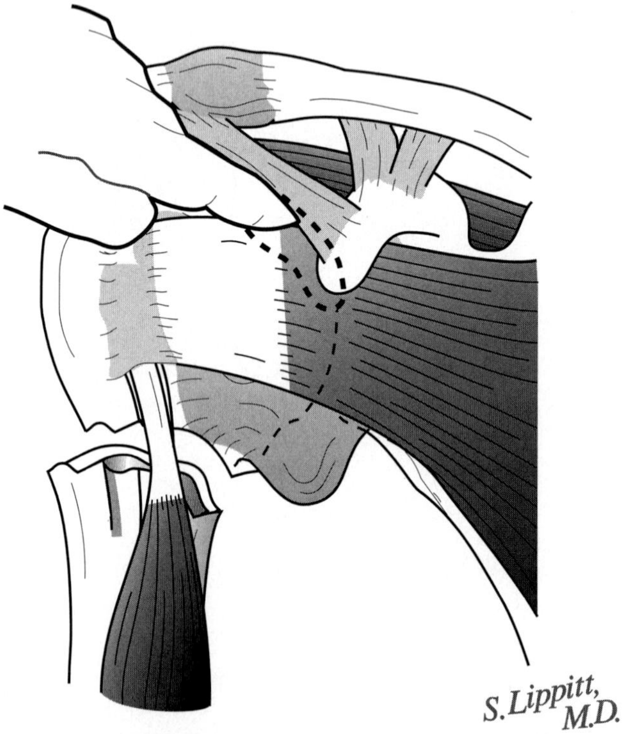


**Figure 35–11. Palpating the head**
The location and the orientation of the articular surface are verified by direct palpation. The arthrotomy allows the surgeon to control the depth and orientation of the guide pin, osteotome, and plate fixation.

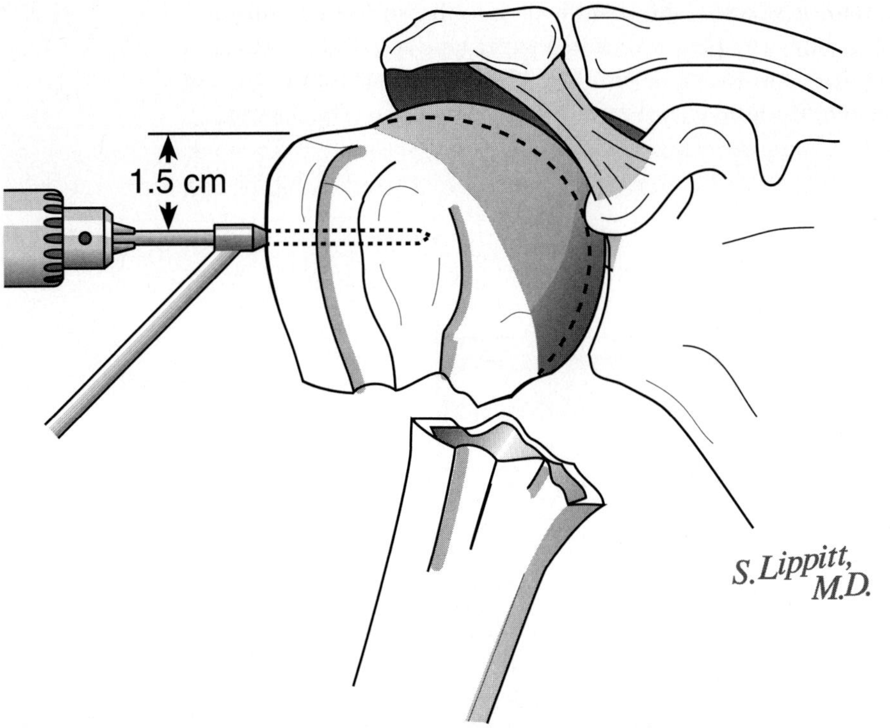


**Figure 35–12. Guide pin**
A 2 mm guide pin is started 1.5 cm below the top of the tuberosity, just behind the bicipital groove, and directed toward the middle of the articular surface. It is advanced by hand perpendicular to the long axis of the humerus until it is stopped by the subchondral bone of the head medially.

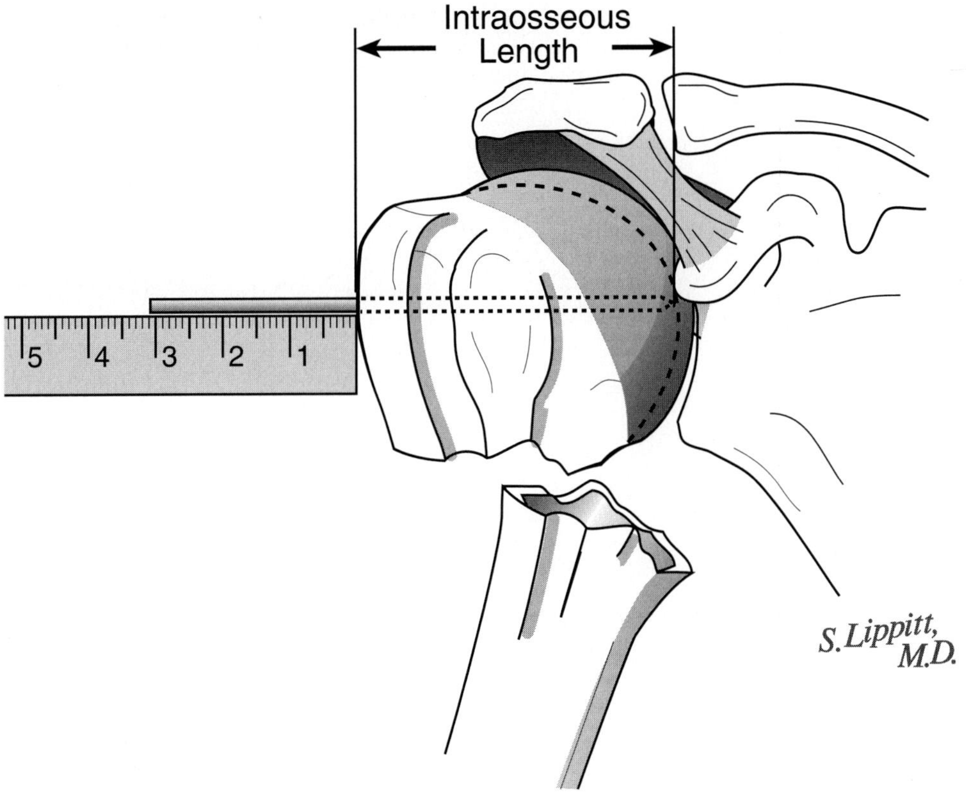


**Figure 35–13. Measuring the pin**
The intraosseous length of the guide pin is determined by measuring the length of the pin protruding from the bone and then subtracting this length from the total length of the pin.

A straight flat osteotome is selected with a width close to that of the 4.5 mm compression plate. The osteotome is marked with sterile paper tape at a distance equal to 80% of the intraosseous length of the guide pin (**Fig. 35–14**). The osteotome is driven into the head to this depth just distal to and parallel to the guide pin (**Fig. 35–15**).

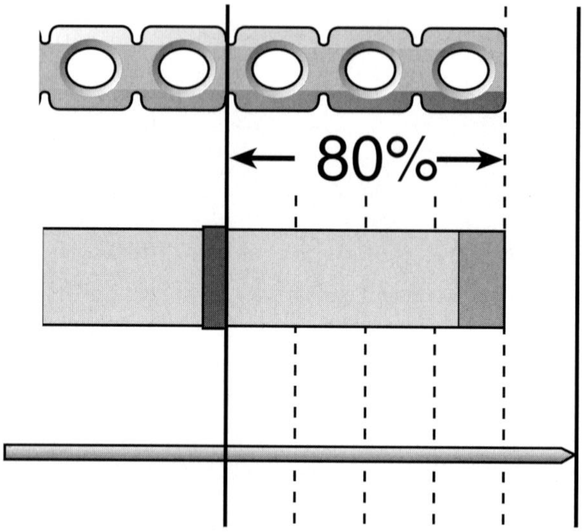


**Figure 35–14. Marking the osteotome**
A flat osteotome with the same width as the plate (4.5 mm) is marked with sterile paper tape at a distance from the sharp end equal to 80% of the measured intraosseous length of the pin.

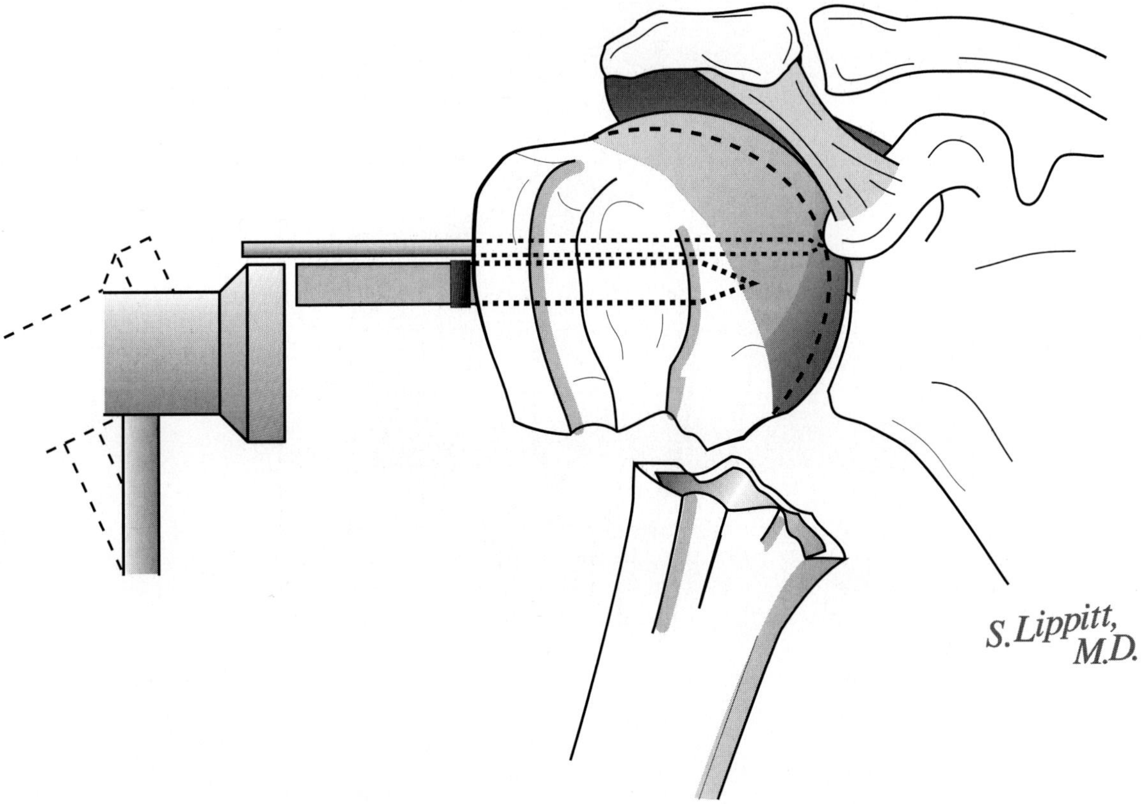


**Figure 35–15. Impacting the osteotome**
The osteotome is driven into the humeral head just distal to and parallel to the guide pin and perpendicular to the long axis of the humerus.

An eight-hole, 4.5 mm reconstruction plate is bent at a right angle, with the bend at the same distance from one end as the depth of the osteotome **(Fig. 35–16)**. The plate is further contoured as necessary so that it will fit the side of the humerus when the fracture is reduced. Once the plate has been contoured, a cortical screw is selected of a length that will enable it to pass obliquely from one of the lateral holes of the plate and just exit the last hole in the bent aspect of the plate (the one closest to the articular surface) **(Fig. 35–17)**. This maneuver is practiced to identify the optimal lateral hole and the angle of passage relative to the lateral aspect of the plate before the plate is inserted.

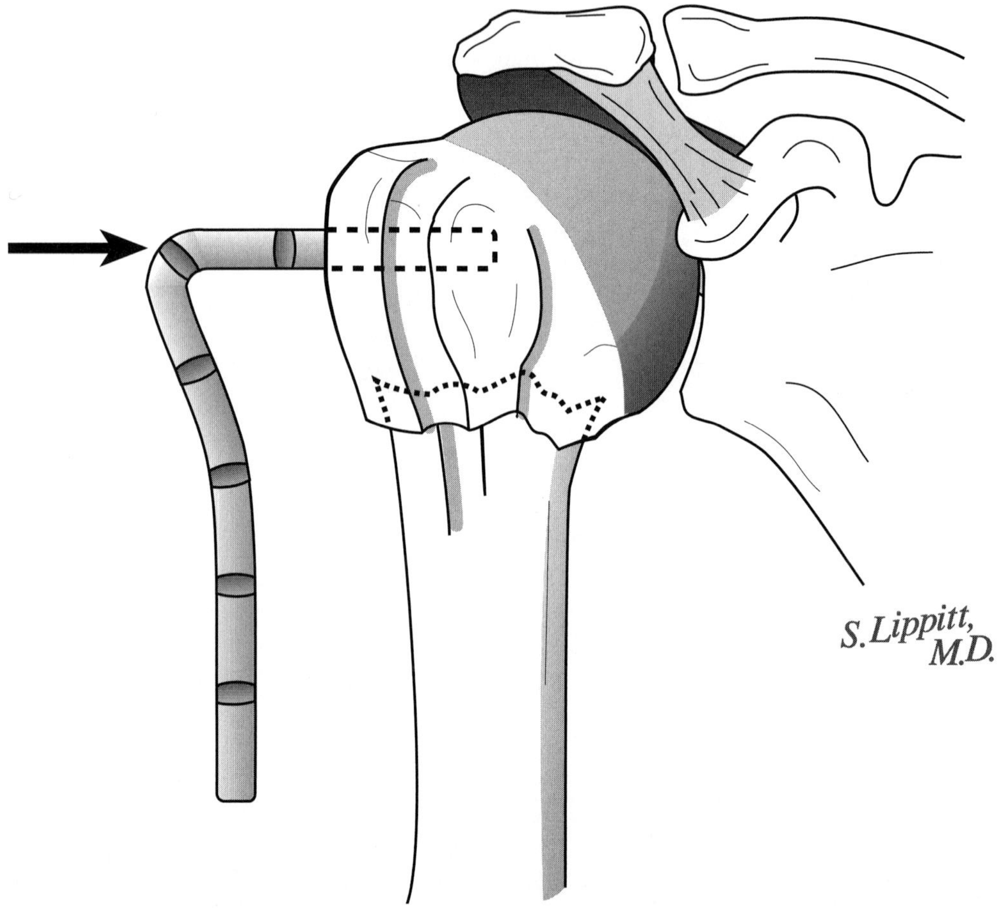


**Figure 35–16. Contouring the plate**
The 4.5 mm reconstruction plate is bent at a 90-degree angle so that the transverse segment has a length equal to 80% of the intraosseous length of the guide pin and so that the longitudinal segment is contoured to fit the side of the impacted humerus.

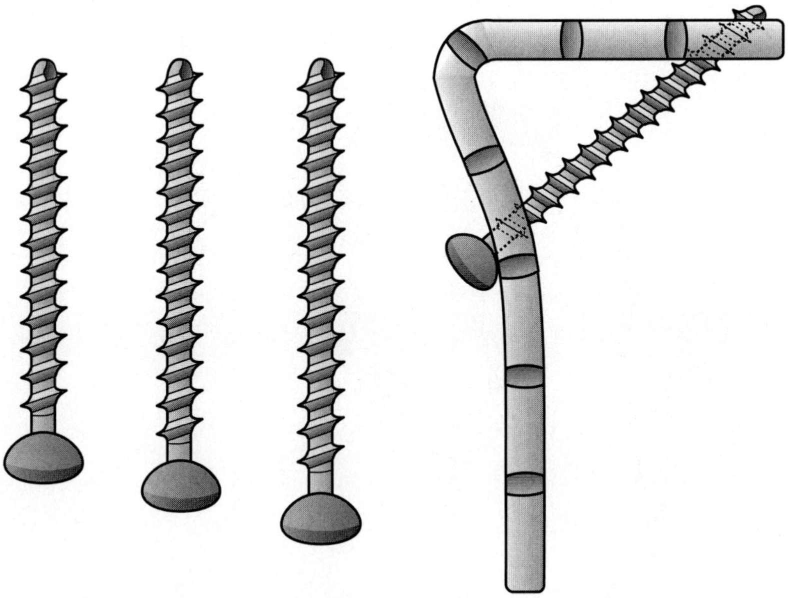

**Figure 35–17. Practicing screw placement**

An assortment of long 3.5 mm self-tapping cortical screws is needed to ensure the availability of the proper length for triangulation. A screw is selected that, when inserted through one of the upper lateral holes in the plate at an angle of 45 degrees, will extend 2 mm beyond the superior aspect of the most medial hole of the transverse segment of the plate. The hole through which the screw should be inserted and the angle of screw insertion are determined and practiced.

The osteotome is then removed from the proximal fragment and the bent aspect of the plate is driven down the path of the osteotome while the position and orientation are monitored by an intraarticular finger (**Fig. 35–18**). The hole for the triangulation screw is drilled (**Fig. 35–19**) and the oblique screw is placed, starting at an angle slightly steeper than that identified during the ex vivo practice. This allows the screw to "walk" toward the target hole, rather than risking its walking away from it. The joint is checked again at this point to be sure that the plate and screw have not penetrated the joint surface. The position of the plate and screw are verified by fluoroscopy. The locking screw binds against the walls of the last hole in the plate and is tightened securely (**Fig. 35–20**).

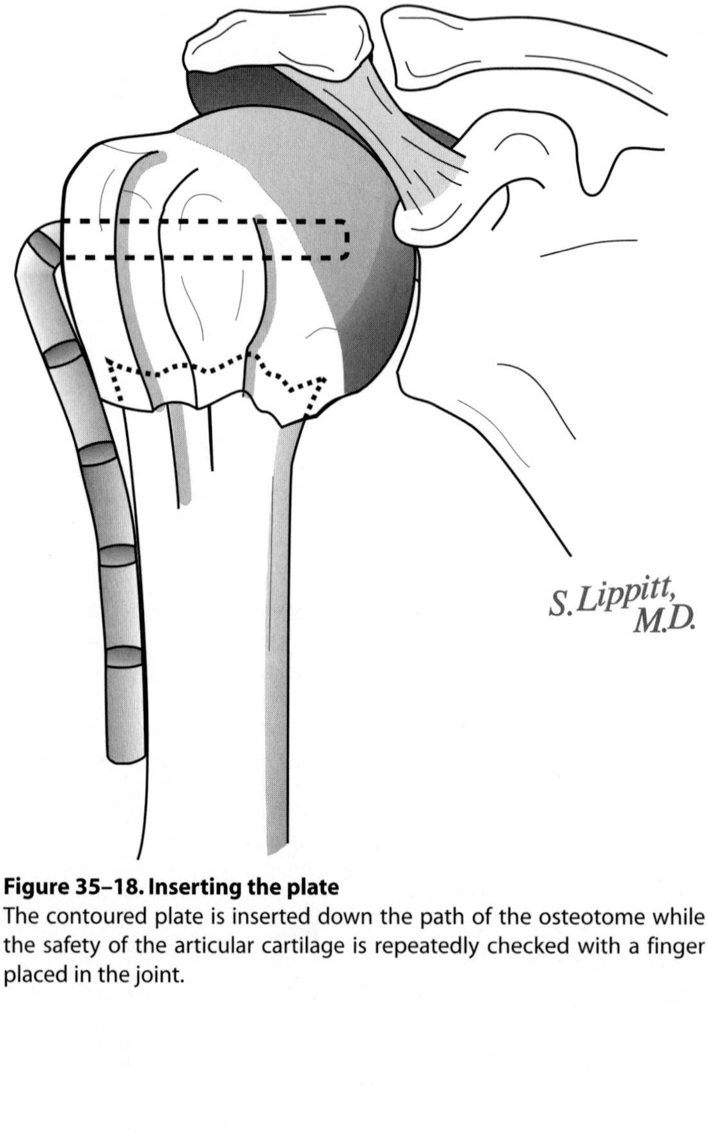


**Figure 35–18. Inserting the plate**
The contoured plate is inserted down the path of the osteotome while the safety of the articular cartilage is repeatedly checked with a finger placed in the joint.

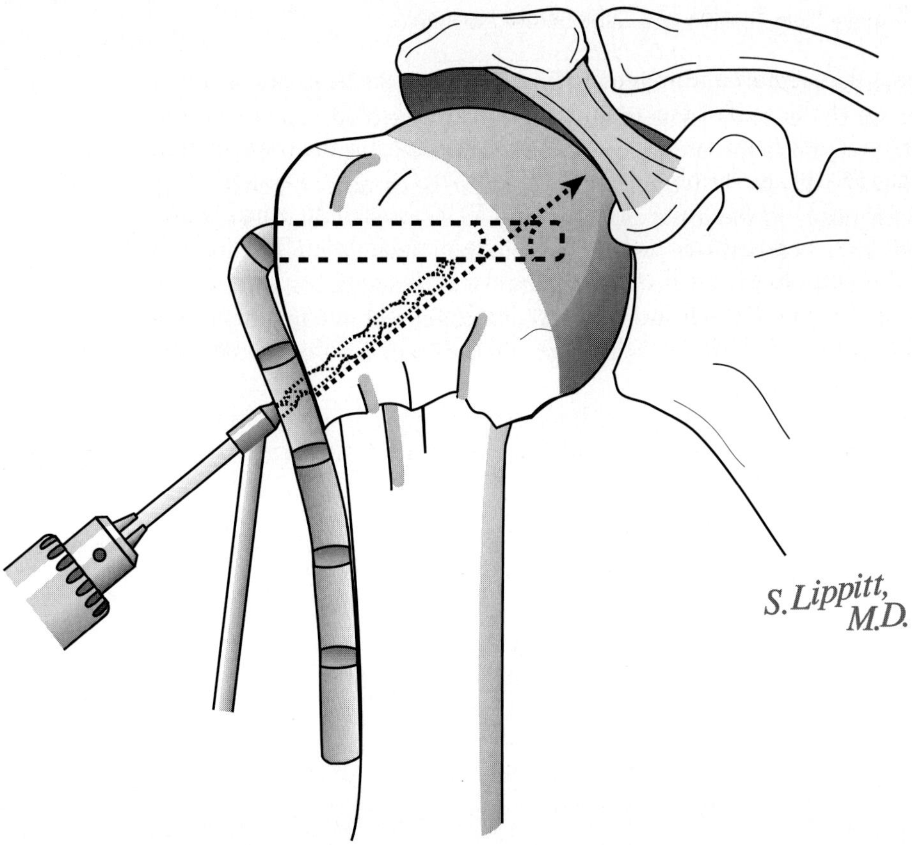


**Figure 35–19. Drilling for the triangulation screw**
The lateral cortical hole is drilled for the triangulation screw.

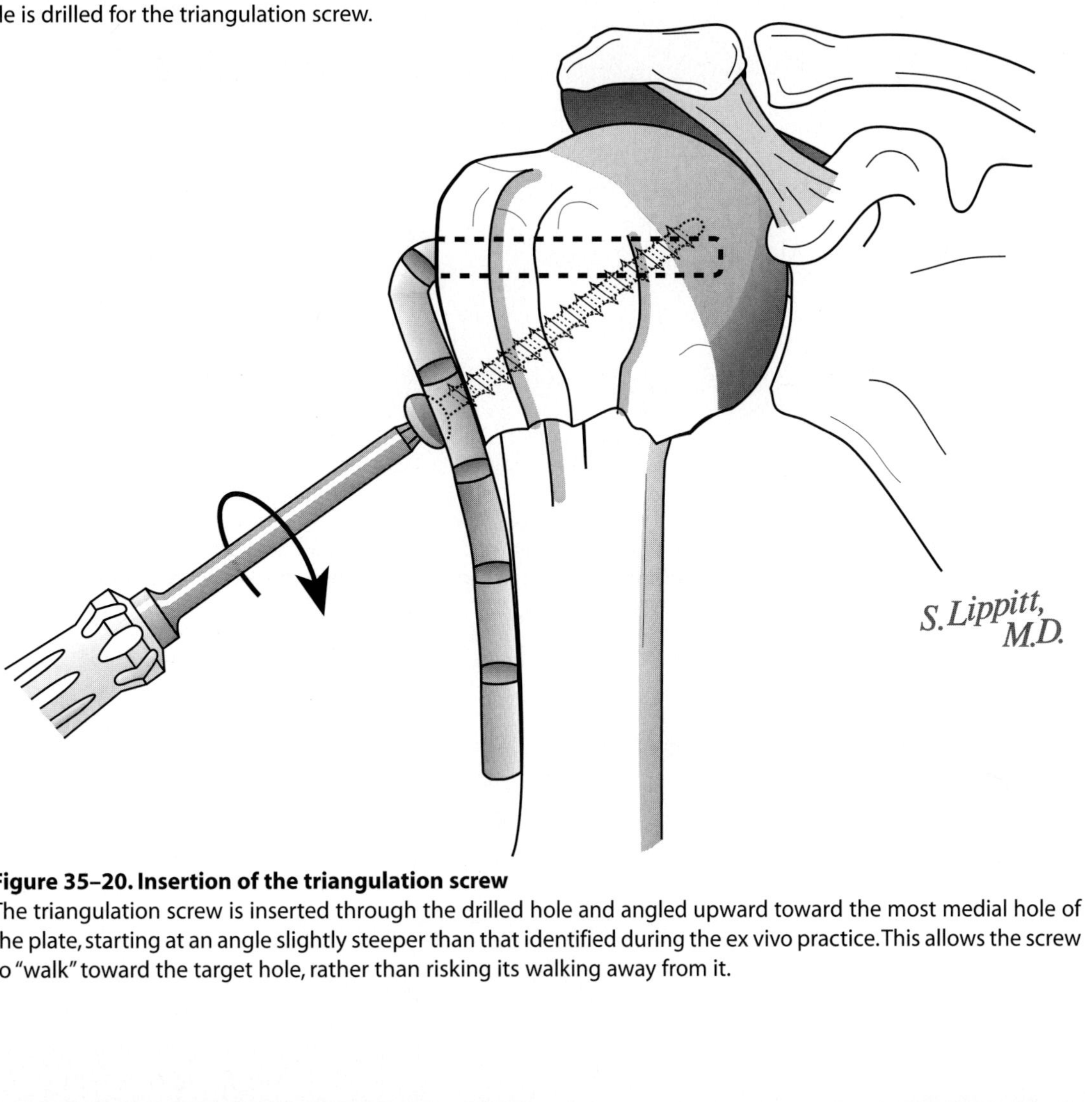


**Figure 35–20. Insertion of the triangulation screw**
The triangulation screw is inserted through the drilled hole and angled upward toward the most medial hole of the plate, starting at an angle slightly steeper than that identified during the ex vivo practice. This allows the screw to "walk" toward the target hole, rather than risking its walking away from it.

The shaft is then reduced to the proximal fragment and held in position with a bone-holding clamp. The fit of the plate to the lateral shaft is verified. Adjustments to the plate configuration and to the lateral cortex of the proximal fragment are made as necessary (**Fig. 35–21**). The plate is fixed in compression to the cortex of the shaft using screws placed eccentrically in the distal aspects of the plate's holes (**Figs. 35–22** and **35–23**). At least six secure cortical bites are achieved in the humeral shaft.

The security of the fixation is verified. Intraoperative anteroposterior and axillary x-rays document the quality of the reduction, the contact between the fragments, the depth of penetration of the bent aspect of the plate into the head, and the desired position of the oblique locking screw.

The range of motion allowed by the shoulder is determined by gentle examination under anesthesia. This range of motion will guide the early postoperative exercise program.

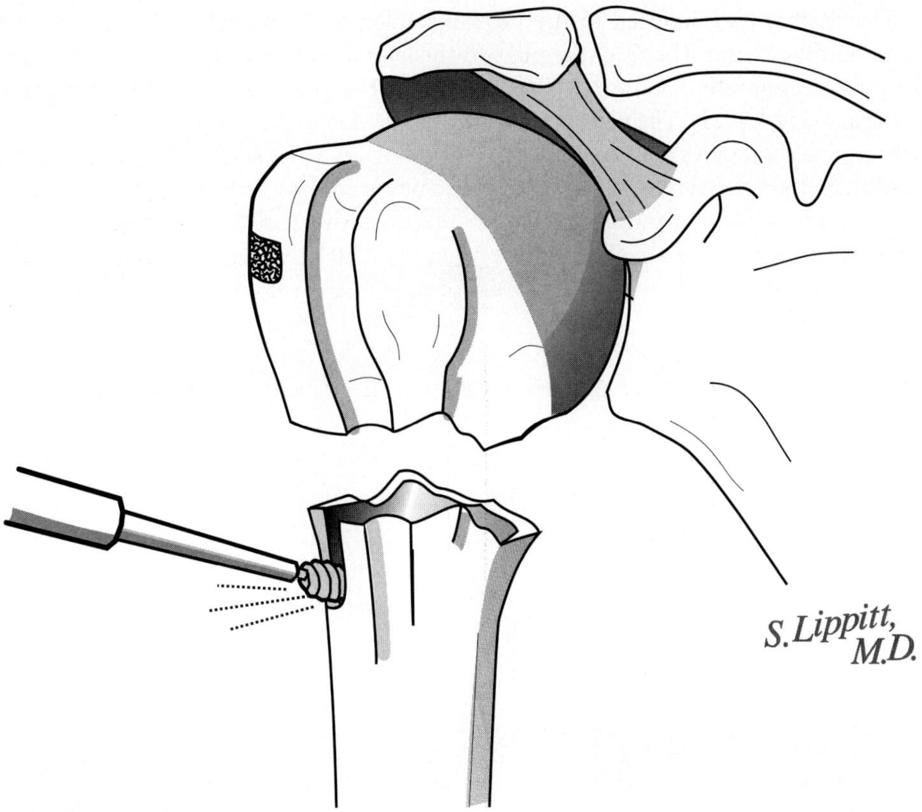


**Figure 35–21. Notching the lateral shaft**
If necessary, the proximal end of the distal fragment is notched laterally to make sure that the triangulation screw does not interfere with the reduction of the fracture.

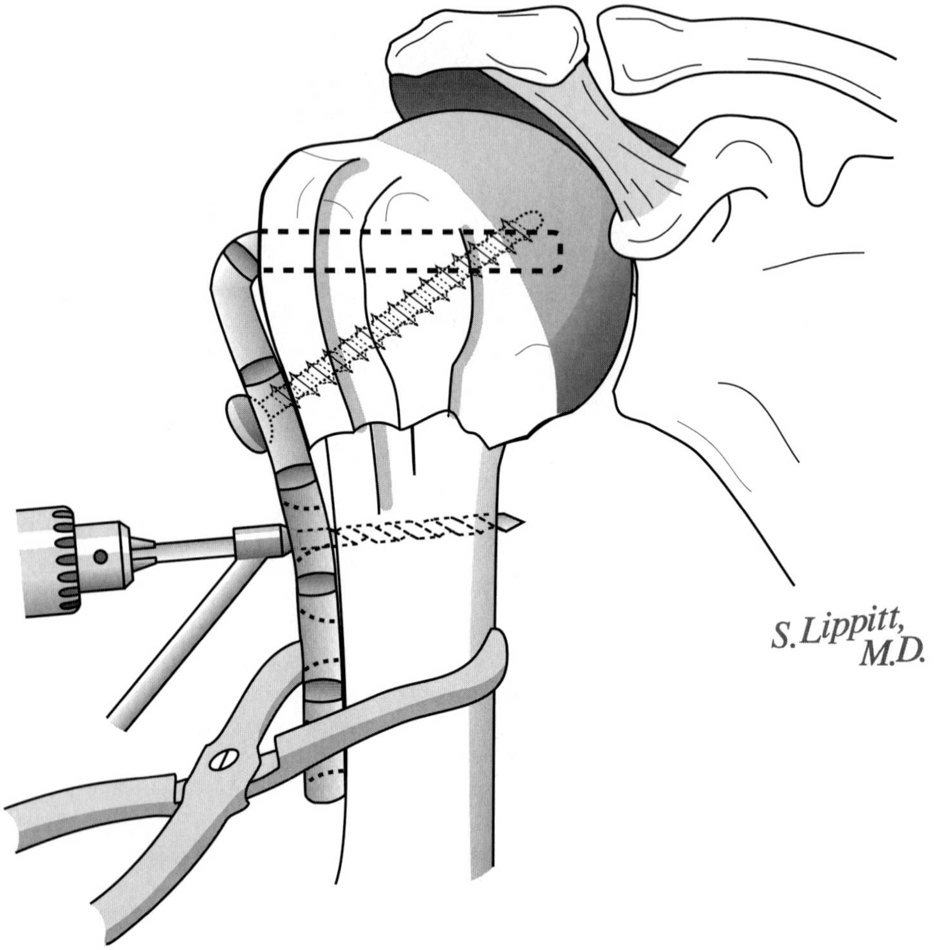


**Figure 35–22. Eccentric drilling**
The shaft is then reduced to the vertical part of the plate, impacted, and held compressed into the proximal fragment with a bone clamp. By placing the screws distally in the holes of the plate, dynamic compression is achieved when the screws are tightened.

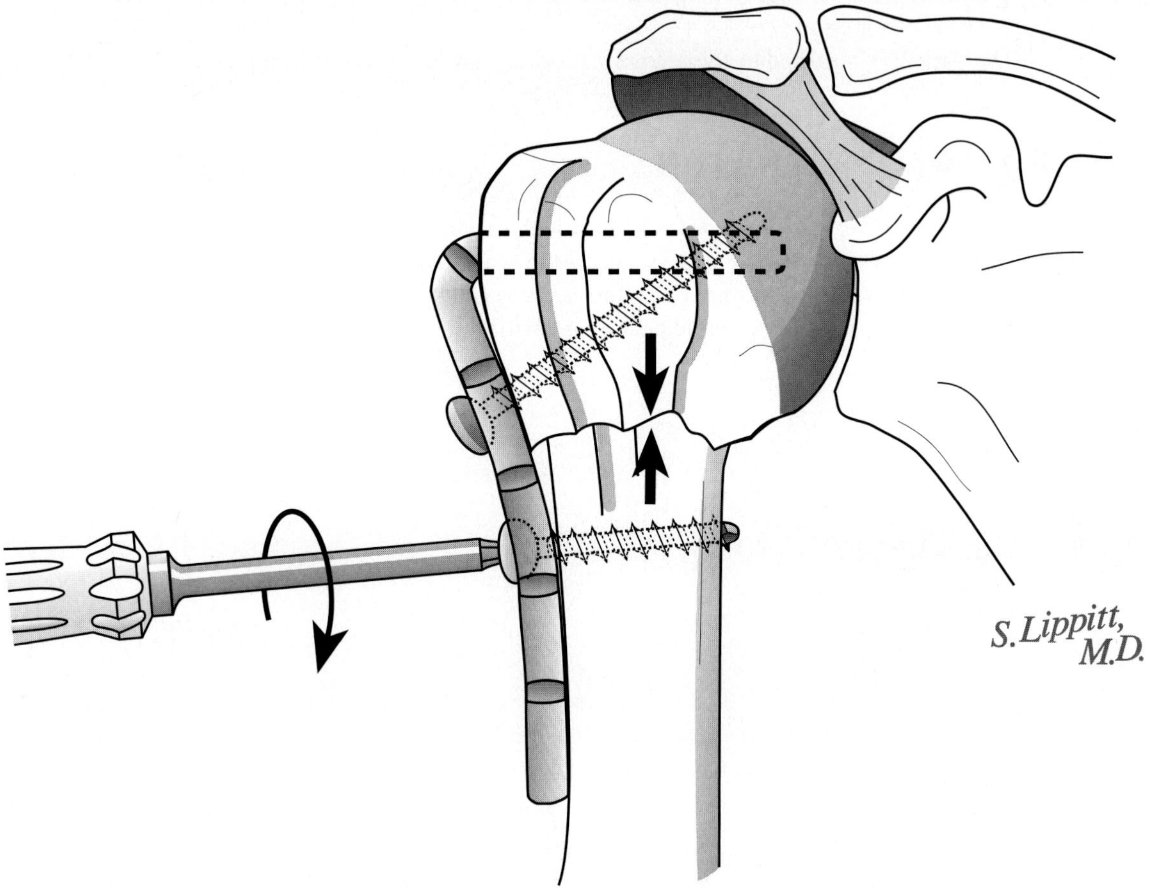


**Figure 35–23. Compressing the fracture**
Tightening these screws compresses the fracture.

Cancellous bone is harvested from the ipsilateral iliac crest in the standard manner through a small skin incision. This incision is closed and dressed after hemostasis and muscle reattachment have been achieved.

The autograft is then packed around the fracture site on a bony bed that has been cleared of soft tissue (**Fig. 35–24**). The security of the screw fixation is verified again.

The wound is thoroughly irrigated and closed in layers. Dry sterile dressings are applied to both incisions.

The patient is returned to the recovery room in satisfactory condition.

## POSTOPERATIVE PLAN

Our postoperative plan is to place the patient on an early mobilization program, encouraging assisted movement throughout the range of motion identified during the intraoperative examination under anesthesia. Care is taken to avoid stressing the fixation in rotation until radiographic healing is verified.

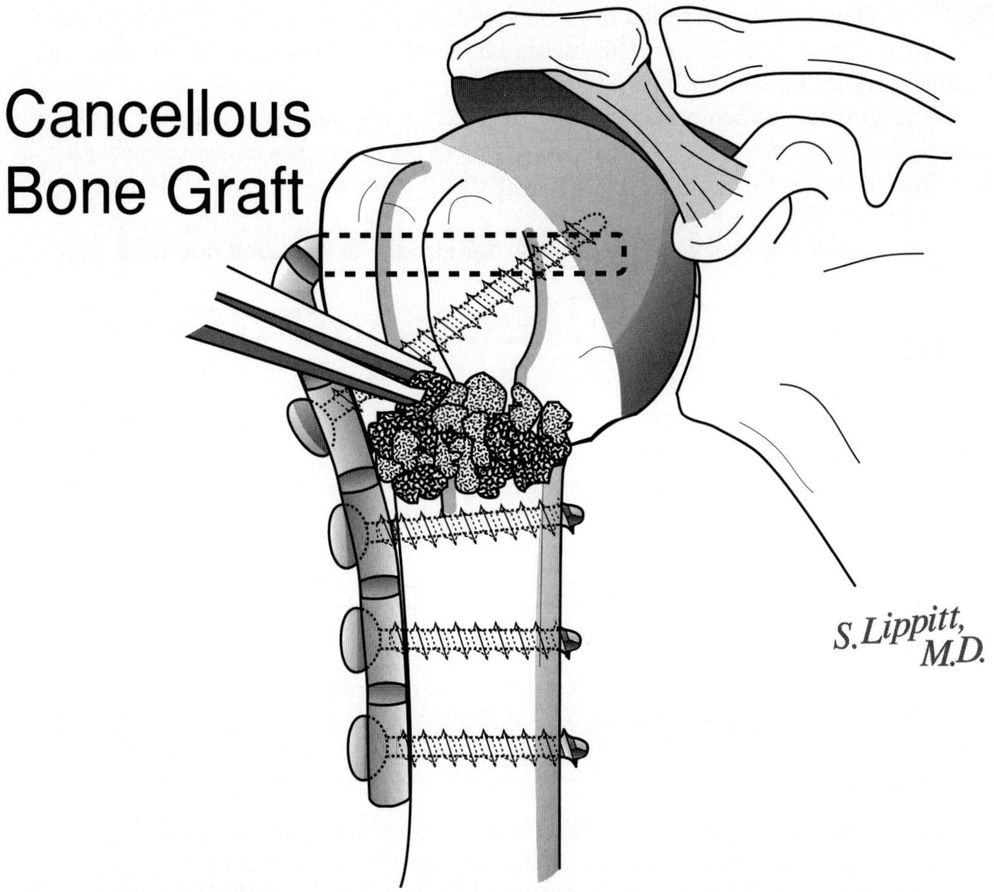


**Figure 35–24. Bone graft**
Iliac crest bone graft is applied around the nonunion site.

CHAPTER 36

# Procedure: Prosthetic Reconstruction for Proximal Humeral Fracture

**Diagnosis**

***Displaced four-segment fracture of the proximal humerus ICD9 CODES 812.00 and 812.03***

**Procedure**

***Proximal humeral reconstruction with proximal humeral prosthesis; bone cement fixation; open reduction, internal fixation of greater and lesser tuberosities; local cancellous autograft CPT CODE 23616***

## INDICATIONS

The patient fell on the outstretched arm, sustaining this fracture. The patient's neurovascular examination findings are normal, but the arm is painful on all movement.

Radiographs, including an anteroposterior view in the plane of the scapula, a scapular lateral view, and an axillary view, reveal that the fracture has resulted in substantial displacement of the humeral articular surface, the lesser tuberosity, the greater tuberosity, and the shaft with respect to each other. The articular surface is pointing superiorly and the greater tuberosity is displaced laterally and somewhat posteriorly (**Fig. 36–1**). There is no evidence of glenohumeral arthritis. The lesser tuberosity is displaced medially. The bone appears somewhat osteopenic. Alternative fracture types that may require prosthetic reconstruction include a three-part proximal humeral fracture (**Fig. 36–2**), a head-splitting fracture (**Fig. 36–3**), and a locked posterior fracture dislocation with loss of more than 50% of the articular surface (**Fig. 36–4**).

Knowing in detail the alternatives as well as the risks of infection, neurovascular injury, excessive stiffness, pain, weakness, fracture, nonunion, component loosening, instability, arthritis, and the need for revision surgery, as well as anesthetic complications, and knowing that this reconstruction cannot be expected to restore the shoulder to its level of comfort and function before the injury, the patient desires to proceed

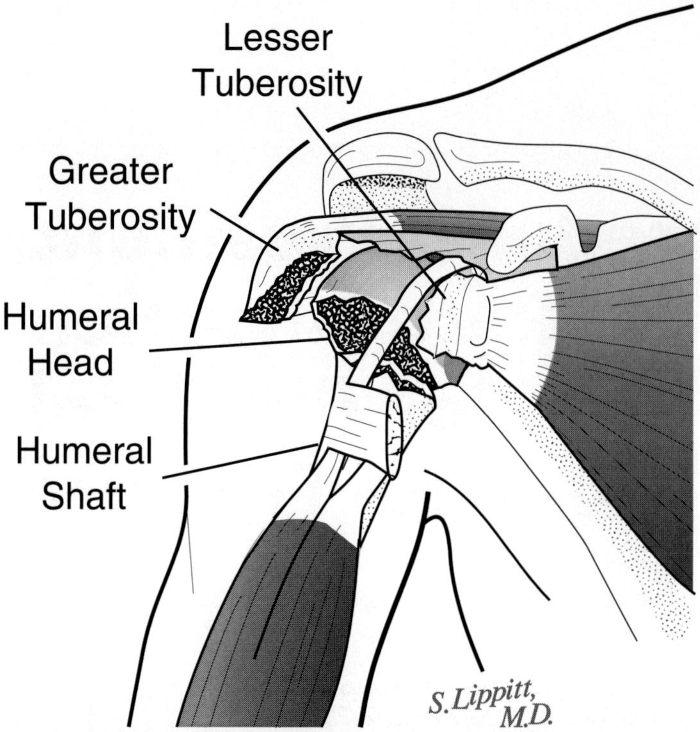


**Figure 36–1. Four-part fracture**
The four displaced parts of the proximal humeral fracture include the greater tuberosity, the lesser tuberosity, the head fragment, and the shaft.

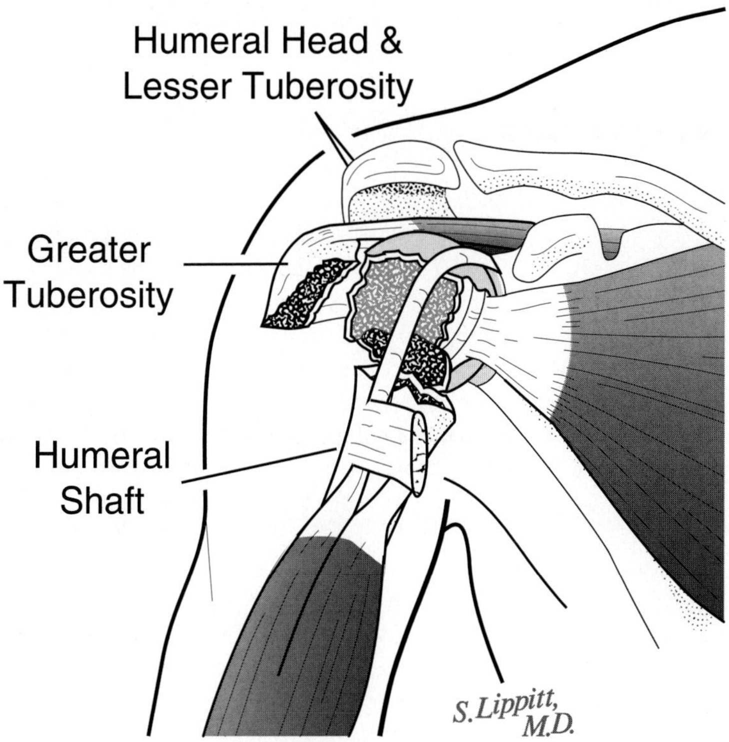


**Figure 36–2. Three-part fracture**
A three-part proximal humeral fracture in which the lesser tuberosity remains intact to the head fragment, pulling it into internal rotation.

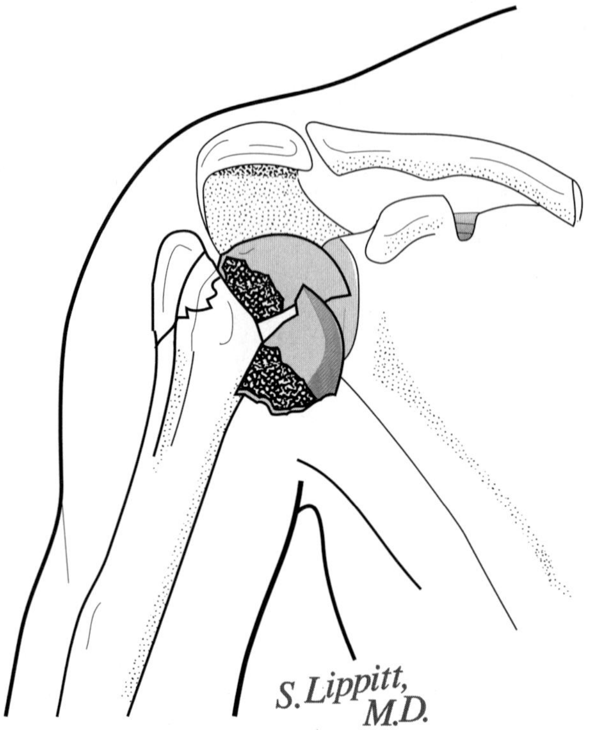


**Figure 36–3. Head split**
The humeral articular surface is split with fragments detached from their vascular supply.

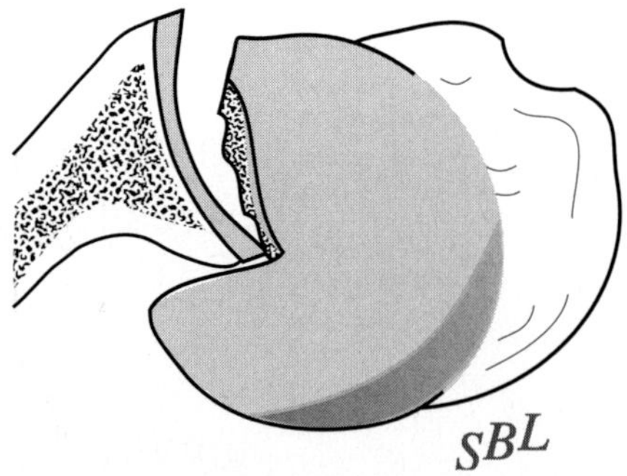


**Figure 36–4. Head impression**
A head impression fracture is seen as a part of a locked posterior fracture dislocation, with loss of more than 50% of the articular surface.

with proximal humeral reconstruction with a cemented prosthesis. The patient understands his or her critical role in the postsurgical rehabilitation.

## FINDINGS

There is bursal thickening in the humeroscapular motion interface. The greater tuberosity fragment is comminuted and pulled posteriorly and superiorly by the pull of the attached supraspinatus and infraspinatus tendons. The subscapularis pulls the lesser tuberosity fragment and the biceps tendon medially. The humeral head, including the articular surface, constitutes a separate fragment with no soft tissue attachment. The proximal end of the shaft is pulled medially by the pectoralis major. The axillary nerve is seen to be intact. The glenoid demonstrates no evidence of arthritis **(Fig. 36–5)**.

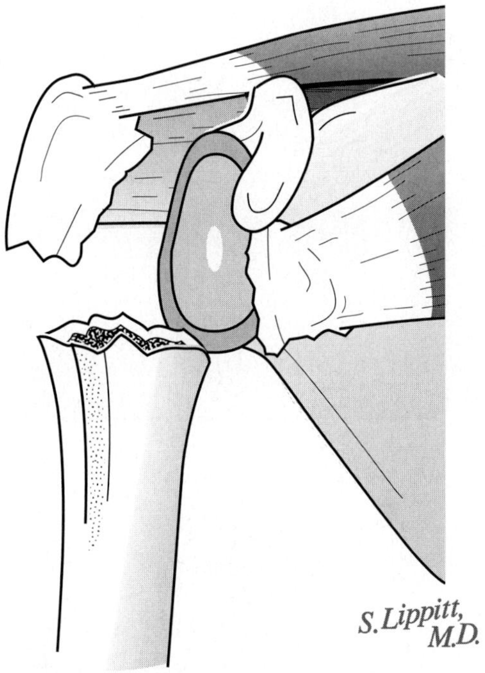


**Figure 36–5. Intact glenoid surface**
The glenoid articular surface is intact.

## SURGICAL PROCEDURE

Under satisfactory anesthesia, the patient is placed in a low beach chair position (**Fig. 36–6**). The entire forequarter is carefully prepped and draped in the usual sterile fashion with the arm free to be moved. Particular attention is paid to preparing the axilla of this shoulder in that it has not been moved in several days.

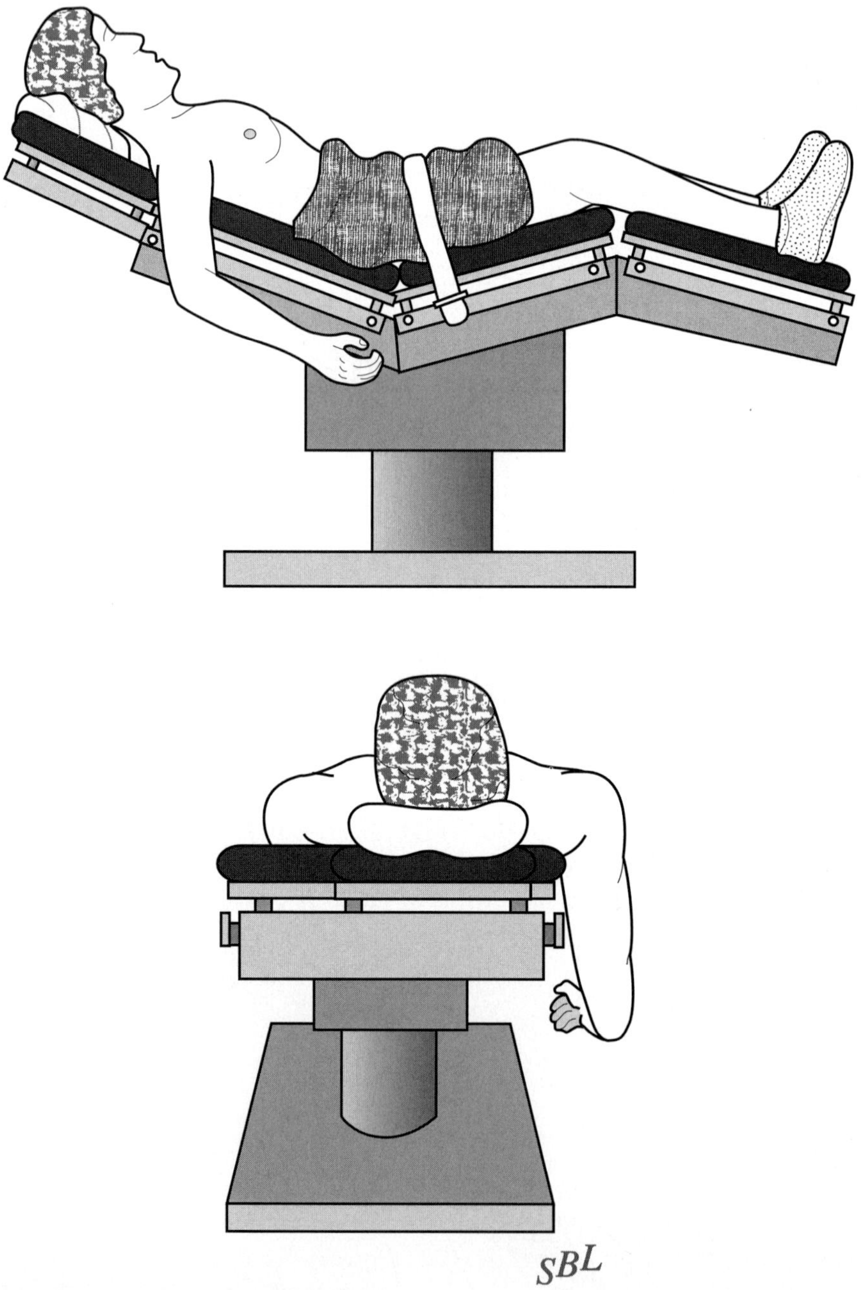


**Figure 36–6. Positioning the patient**
The patient is placed in a comfortable position as in a beach chair with the thorax angled 30 degrees above the horizontal. The neck is in a neutral position. The glenohumeral joint is at the edge of the table and the arm is completely free. Compressive stockings (not shown here) are applied to the legs.

The shoulder is approached through a long anterior deltopectoral incision, avoiding the axillary crease (**Figs. 36–7, 36–8, 36–9,** and **36–10**). The hematoma is evacuated and the bursa is resected to provide excellent visualization of the rotator cuff. A self-retaining retractor is inserted.

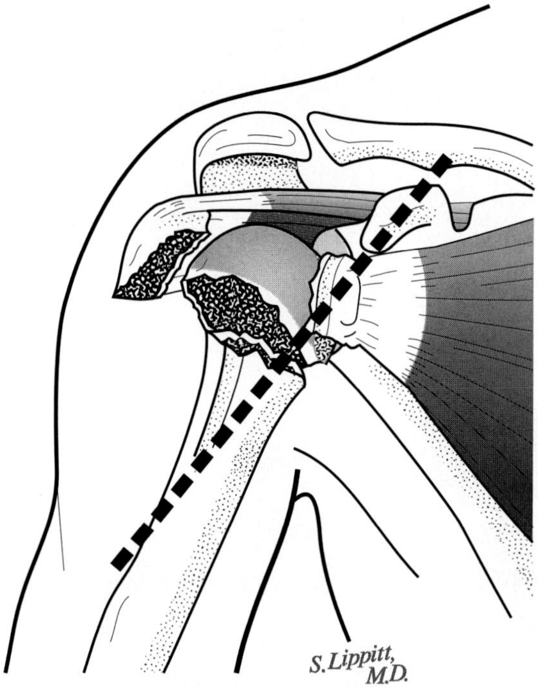


**Figure 36–7. Fracture incision**
The incision is made along a line from mid-clavicle to the deltoid tuberosity at the mid-lateral humerus across the coracoid tip.

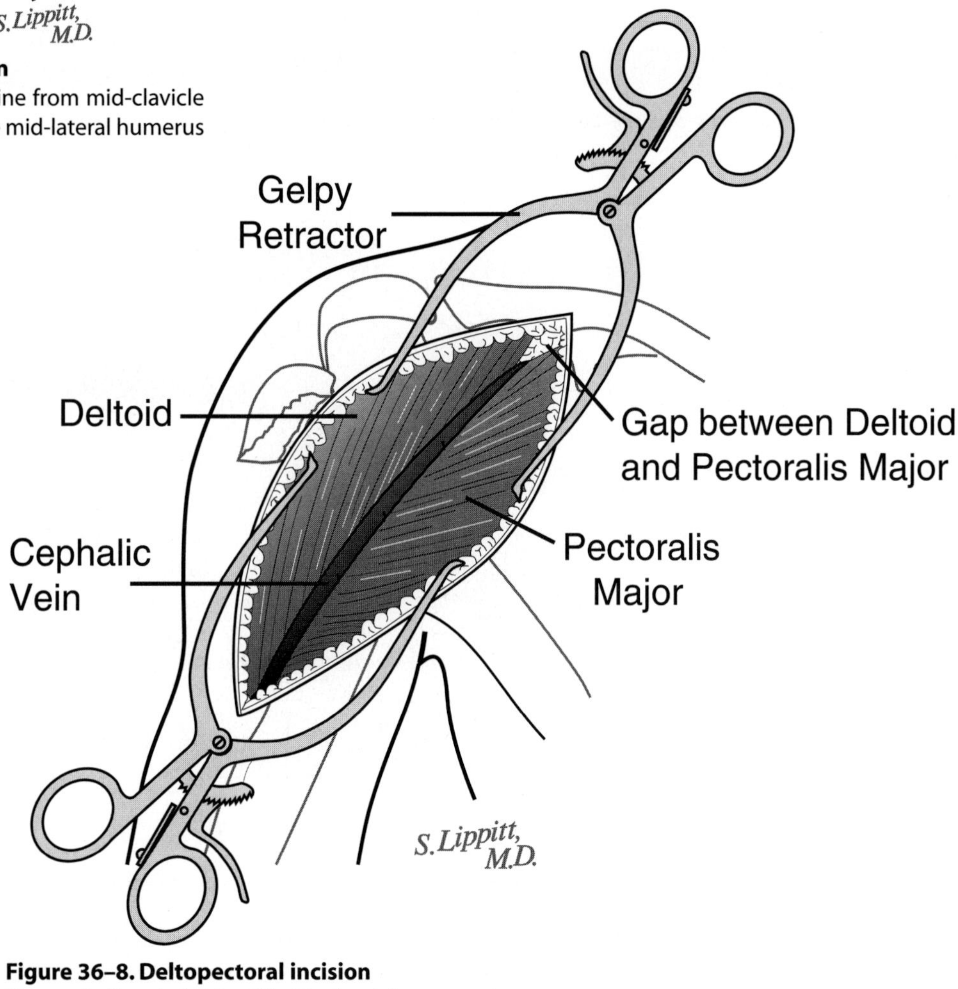


**Figure 36–8. Deltopectoral incision**
The cephalic vein is identified in the deltopectoral groove.

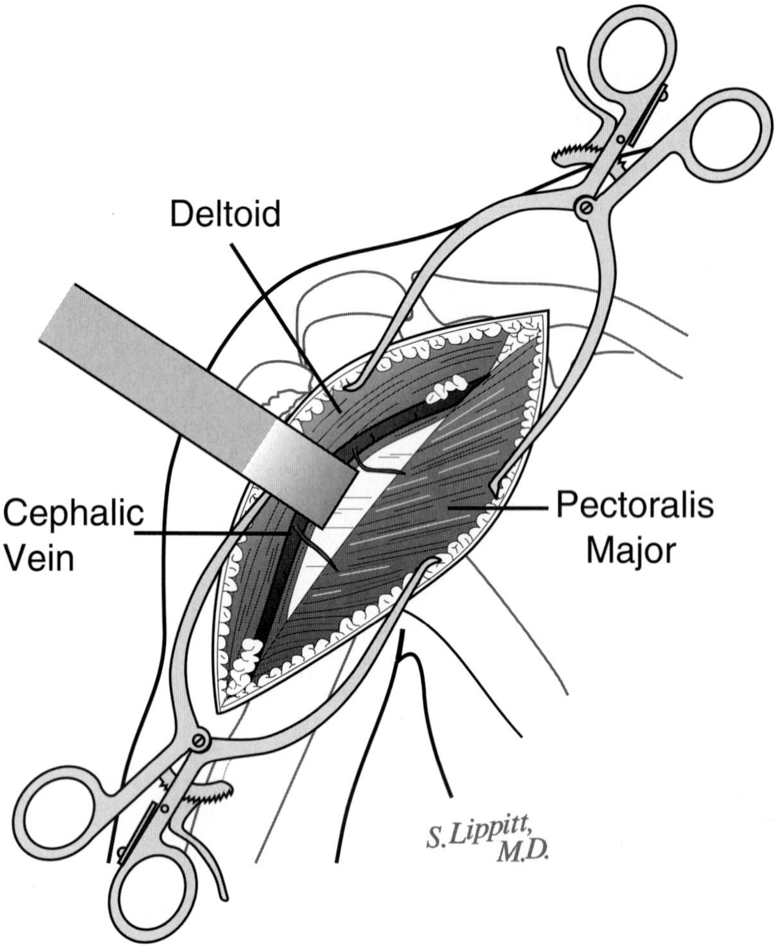


**Figure 36–9. Cephalic vein**
The vein is retracted laterally and the deltopectoral interval is split, revealing the clavipectoral fascia.

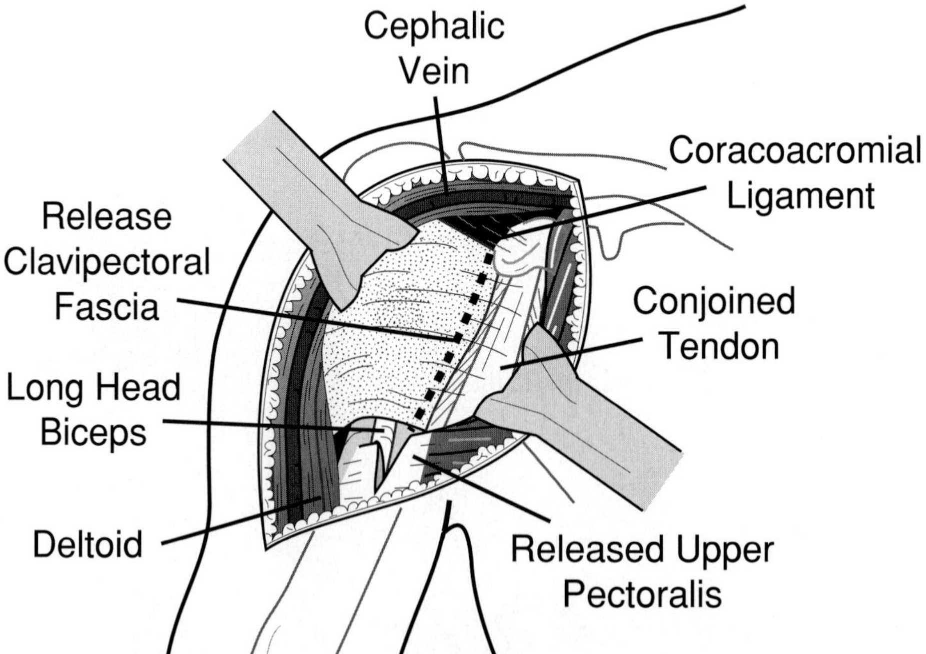


**Figure 36–10. Clavipectoral fascia**
The clavipectoral fascia is split just lateral to the coracoid muscles up to but not through the coracoacromial ligament.

The tendon of the long head of the biceps is identified and used as a guide to the intertubercular groove and the rotator interval, which is then opened (**Fig. 36–11**). The interval fracture line between the greater and lesser tuberosity fragments is found just posterior to the bicipital groove.

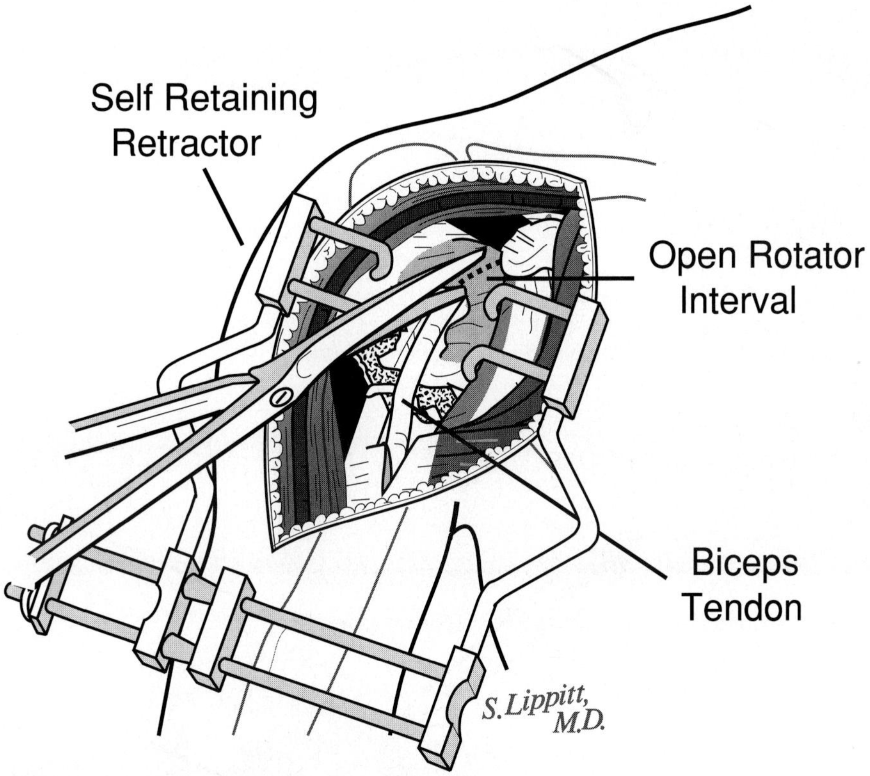


**Figure 36–11. Rotator interval**
The tendon of the long head of the biceps is identified. Dissection is carried along it through the rotator interval capsule to the base of the coracoid process.

Traction sutures are placed around the lesser tuberosity (**Fig. 36–12**). While pulling laterally on these sutures, the surgeon palpates the axillary nerve medially (**Fig. 36–13**).

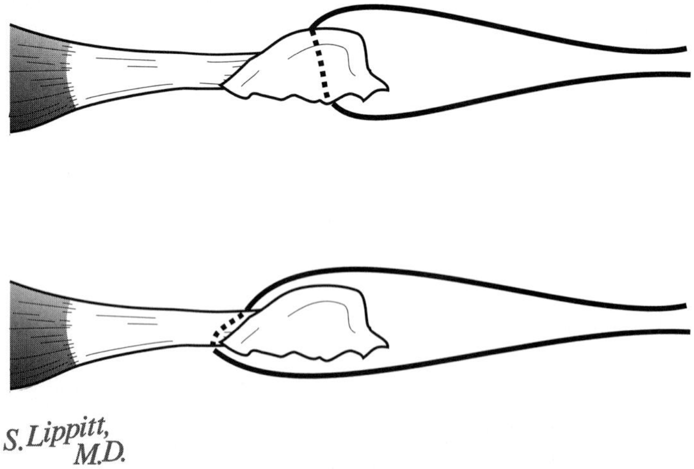


**Figure 36–12. Suturing**
Number 5 braided nonabsorbable traction suture is passed around the lesser tuberosity. Passing sutures *around* the tuberosities provides more secure fixation than passing them *through* osteoporotic bone.

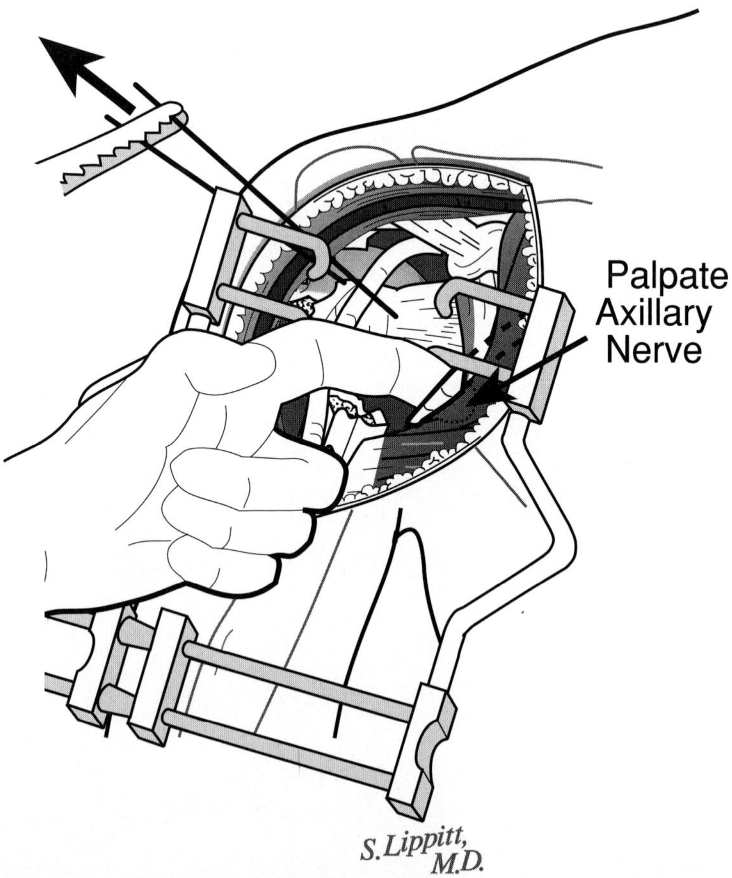


**Figure 36–13. Palpating the axillary nerve**
The axillary nerve is palpated as it runs across the inferior border of the subscapularis and can be palpated as the lesser tuberosity is pulled laterally.

Traction sutures are placed around the greater tuberosity (**Fig. 36–14**). The interval between the tuberosity fragments is opened, revealing the head fragment, which is then removed (**Fig. 36–15**). The diameter of curvature and height of the resected fragment are measured (**Fig. 36–16**) and compared with the available prosthetic head options (**Fig. 36–17**). If the resected head diameter lies between two prosthetic sizes, we tend to

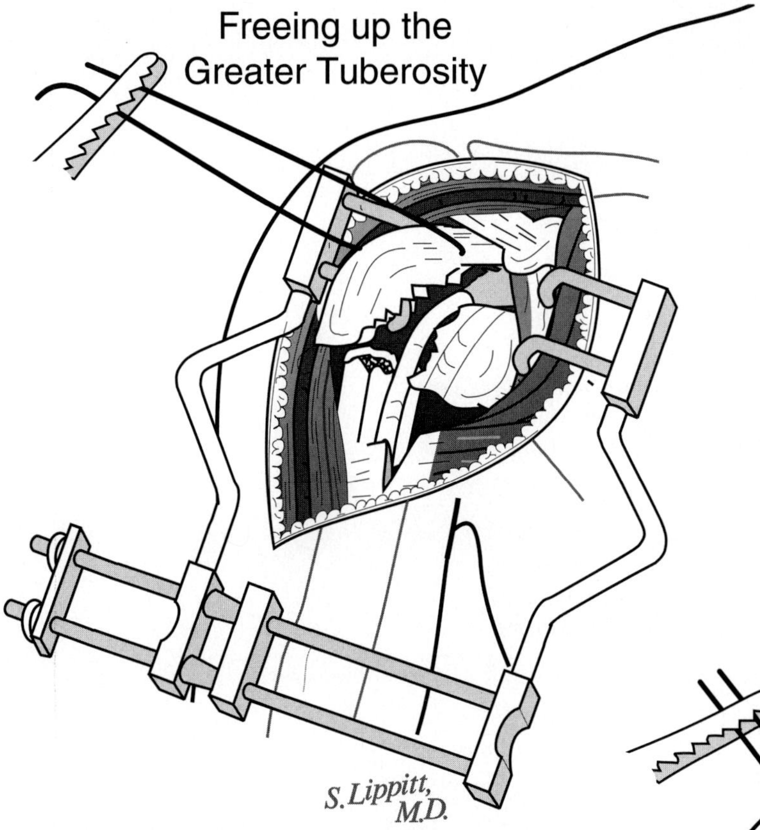


**Figure 36–14. Freeing the greater tuberosity**
Number 5 braided nonabsorbable traction suture is passed around the greater tuberosity and through the cuff tendon. The adhesions around the cuff tendons are lysed while traction is applied to this suture.

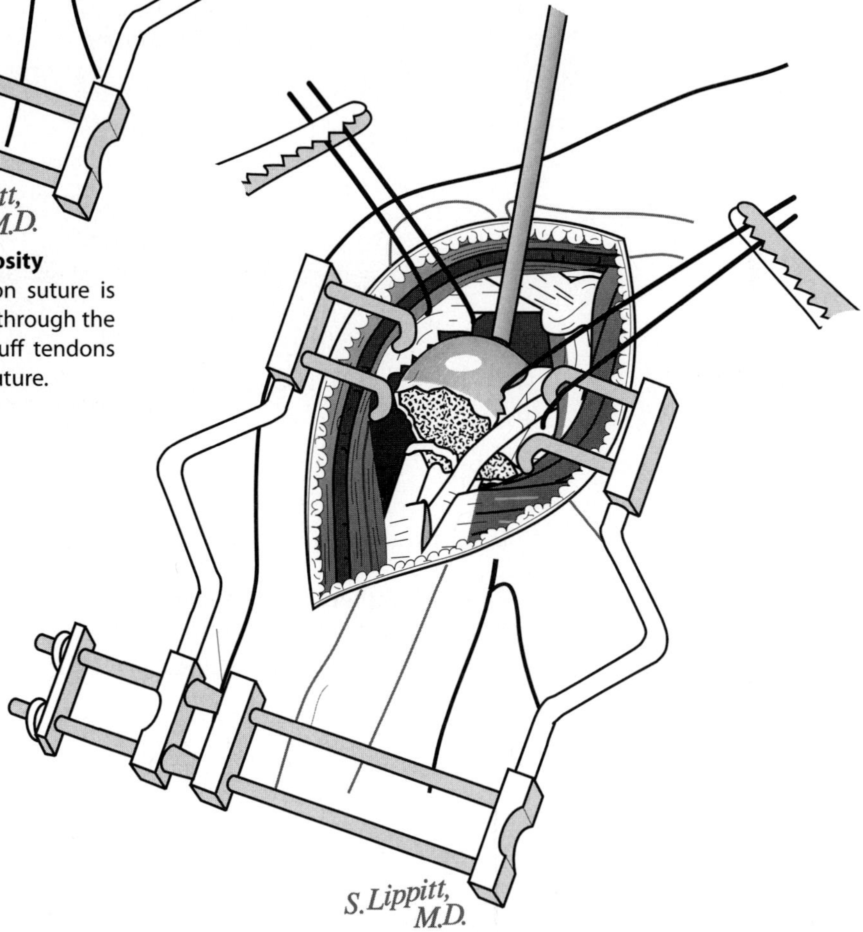


**Figure 36–15. Removing the head fragment**
After traction sutures are placed in the greater tuberosity, the freed humeral head fragment is removed from between the tuberosities.

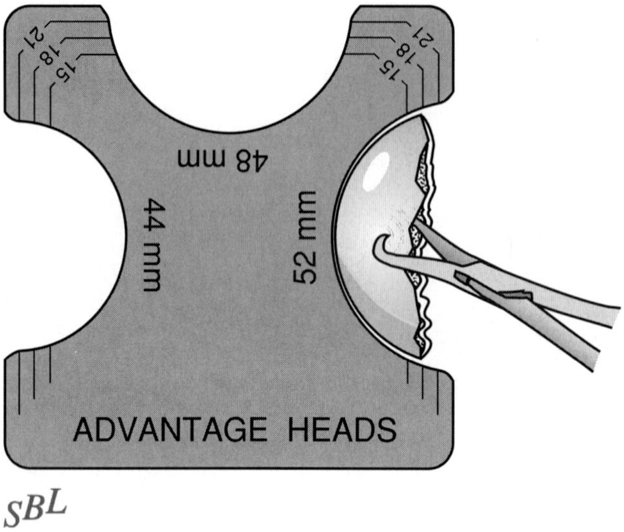


**Figure 36–16. Measuring the head fragment**
The diameter of curvature of the head fragment is measured using a cut-out template. If the exact diameter cannot be matched with a prosthetic head, a slightly too large head diameter is selected.

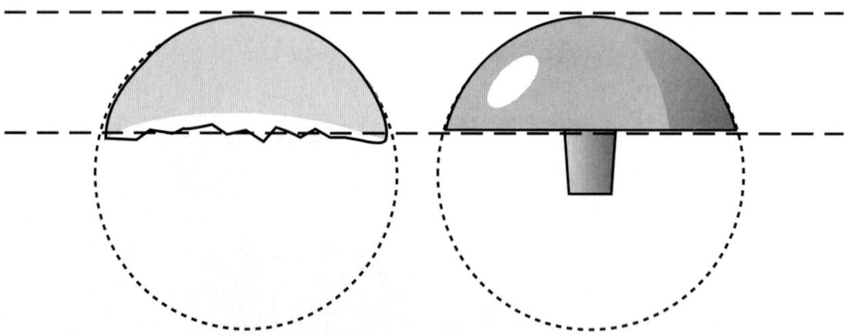

**Figure 36–17. Prosthetic head options**
The resected head is compared to the geometry of the options for prosthetic replacement.

prefer the one that is slightly larger (so that the glenoid is loaded preferentially on its more compliant rim) than the slightly smaller option (which would load the glenoid preferentially on its less compliant center) **(Fig. 36–18)**. The humeral head is then saved for cancellous autograft harvest along with all other bits of bone from the surgery **(Fig. 36–19)**.

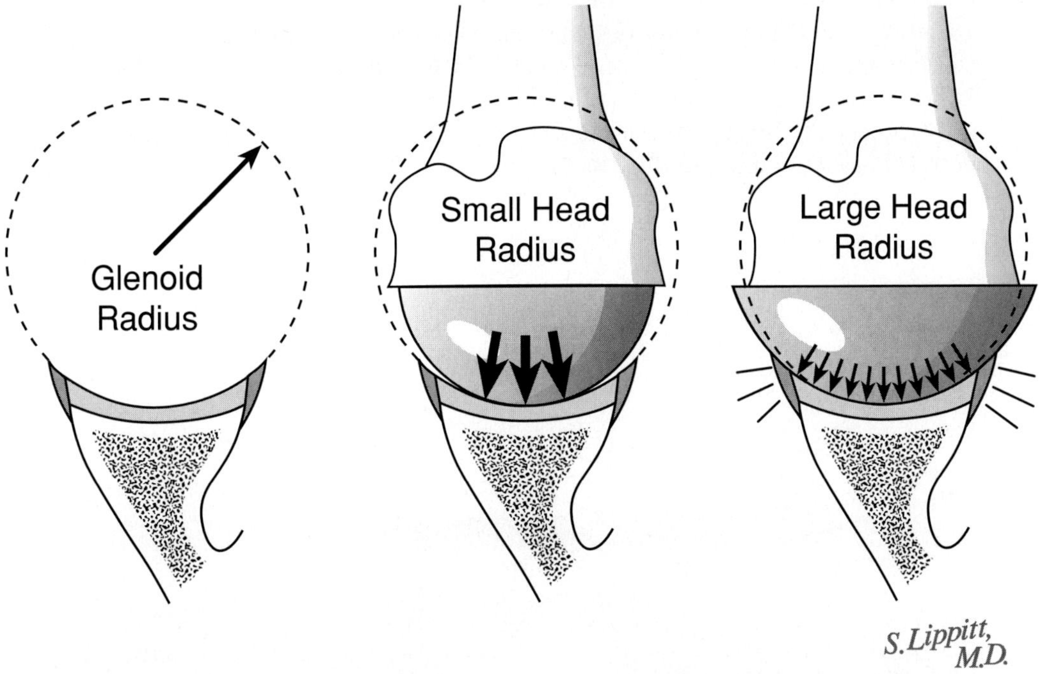


**Figure 36–18. Choosing a humeral component**
A humeral component with a diameter of curvature smaller than that of the glenoid results in high joint pressures in the center of the glenoid. By contrast, a humeral component with a diameter of curvature slightly larger than that of the glenoid can achieve better load distribution owing to the greater compliance of the glenoid periphery.

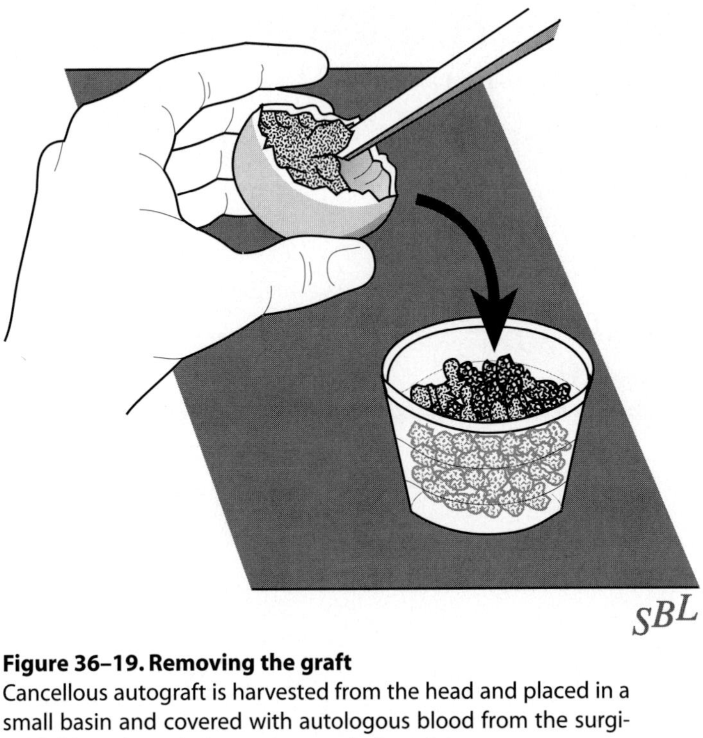


**Figure 36–19. Removing the graft**
Cancellous autograft is harvested from the head and placed in a small basin and covered with autologous blood from the surgical field until needed near the conclusion of the case.

Tag sutures of #5 nonabsorbable braided suture are passed around the lesser tuberosity and through the subscapularis tendon. The subscapularis is released from the coracoid process (**Fig. 36–20**). A 360-degree release is carried out around the subscapularis until a muscular "bounce" is achieved (**Fig. 36–21**).

Similarly, strands of the same type of suture are passed around the comminuted greater tuberosity fragment through the supraspinatus and infraspinatus tendons. The cuff tendons are freed from restricting adhesions.

Looking between the tuberosities, the glenoid is seen to be intact.

The proximal end of the humeral shaft is identified; the proximal centimeter is cleared of soft tissues to optimize bone-to-bone contact. Cylindrical medullary reamers of sequentially larger diameter are passed down the shaft until the first bite in the endosteal surface is obtained (**Fig. 36–22**).

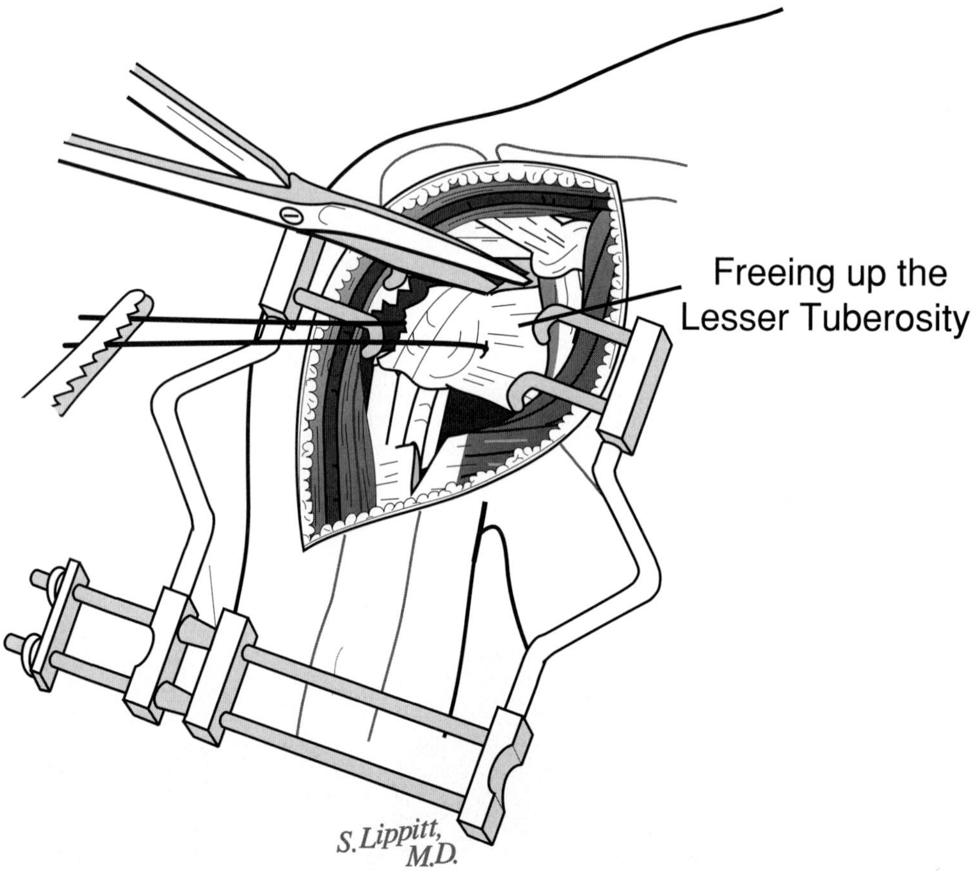


**Figure 36–20. Freeing the subscapularis**

The subscapularis is freed from the coracoid process, and the remnant of the coracohumeral ligament is severed.

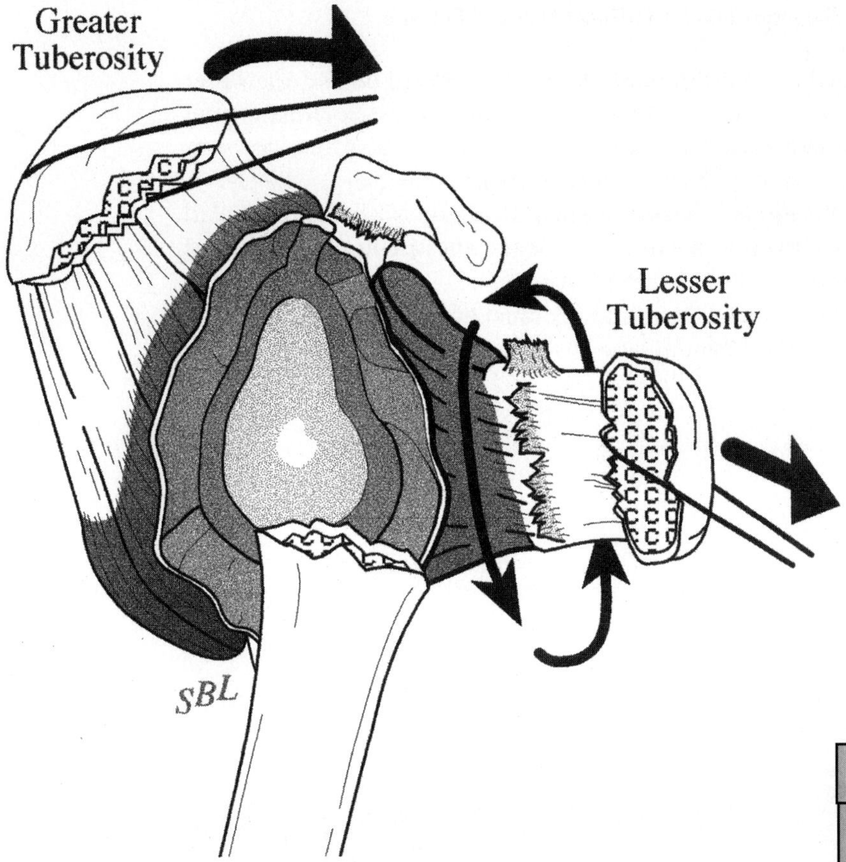


**Figure 36–21. Freeing the subscapularis**
A 360-degree release of the subscapularis is carried out, with care taken to protect the axillary nerve.

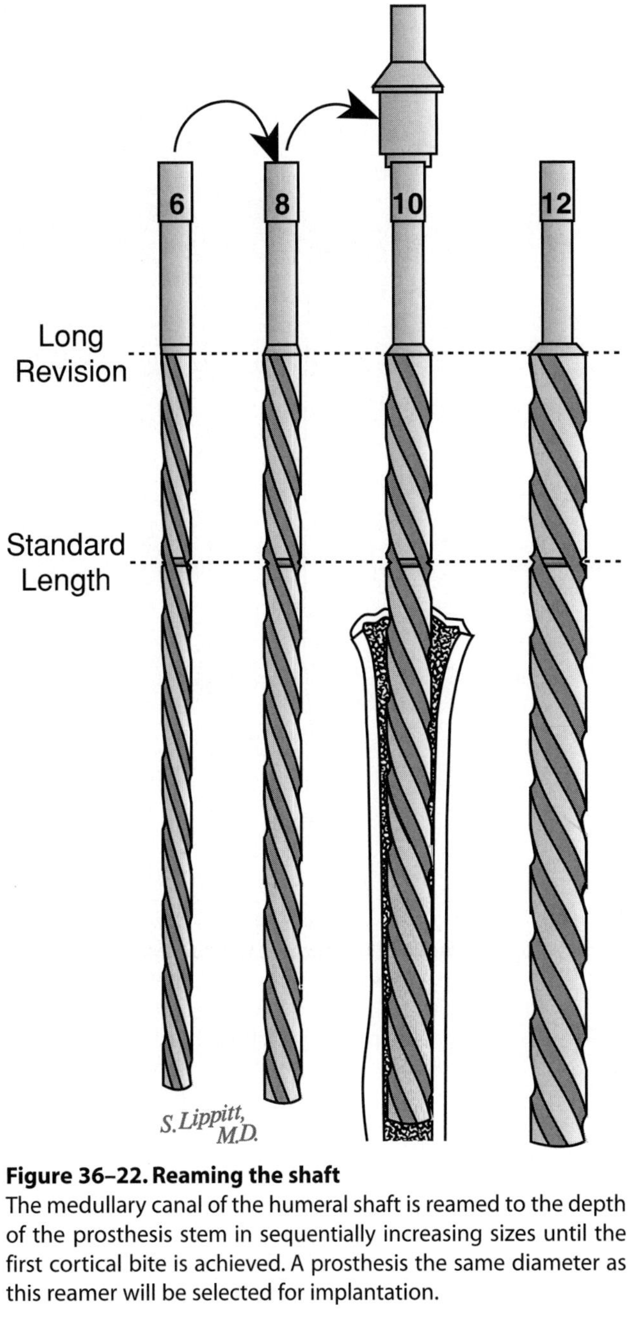


**Figure 36–22. Reaming the shaft**
The medullary canal of the humeral shaft is reamed to the depth of the prosthesis stem in sequentially increasing sizes until the first cortical bite is achieved. A prosthesis the same diameter as this reamer will be selected for implantation.

Reaming is not continued beyond this point, so that the cortical bone stock is preserved. A curette and then a medullary brush are used to remove debris remaining on the inner aspect of the humeral shaft.

A trial prosthesis is selected that has (1) the same shaft diameter as the largest medullary reamer used in the humeral shaft, (2) a head diameter of curvature equal to or slightly larger than that of the resected head, and (3) an effective head height equal to or slightly less than that of the resected head fragment.

The trial prosthesis is inserted into the medullary canal of the shaft. The trial head is oriented in 30 degrees of retroversion; that is, its head points medially, 30 degrees behind the axis of flexion of the elbow (**Fig. 36–23**).

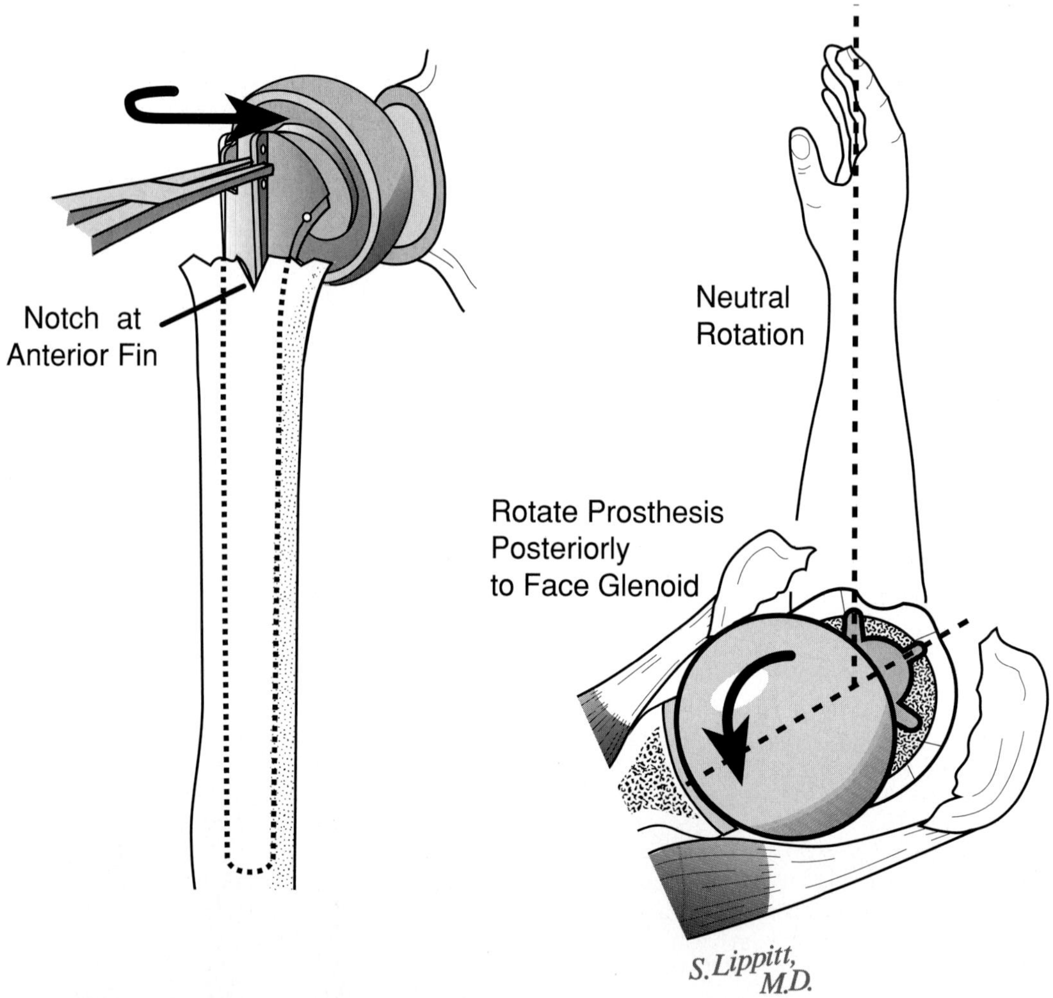


**Figure 36–23. Selecting the version of the prosthesis**
The trial prosthesis is oriented so that the anterior and lateral fins straddle the bicipital groove, the anterior fin points in the direction of the flexed forearm, and the articular surface points 30 degrees posteriorly with the forearm pointing straight ahead. Once the desired version is determined, the location of the anterior fin is marked at the proximal end of the shaft with a notch or electrocautery.

The desired height of the prosthesis is one that allows the upper edge of the tuberosities to fit completely below the edge of the articular aspect of the prosthesis and that allows a few millimeters of overlap of the tuberosities on the shaft to optimize contact for healing **(Fig. 36–24)**.

The height and version of the prosthesis relative to the shaft have now been determined.

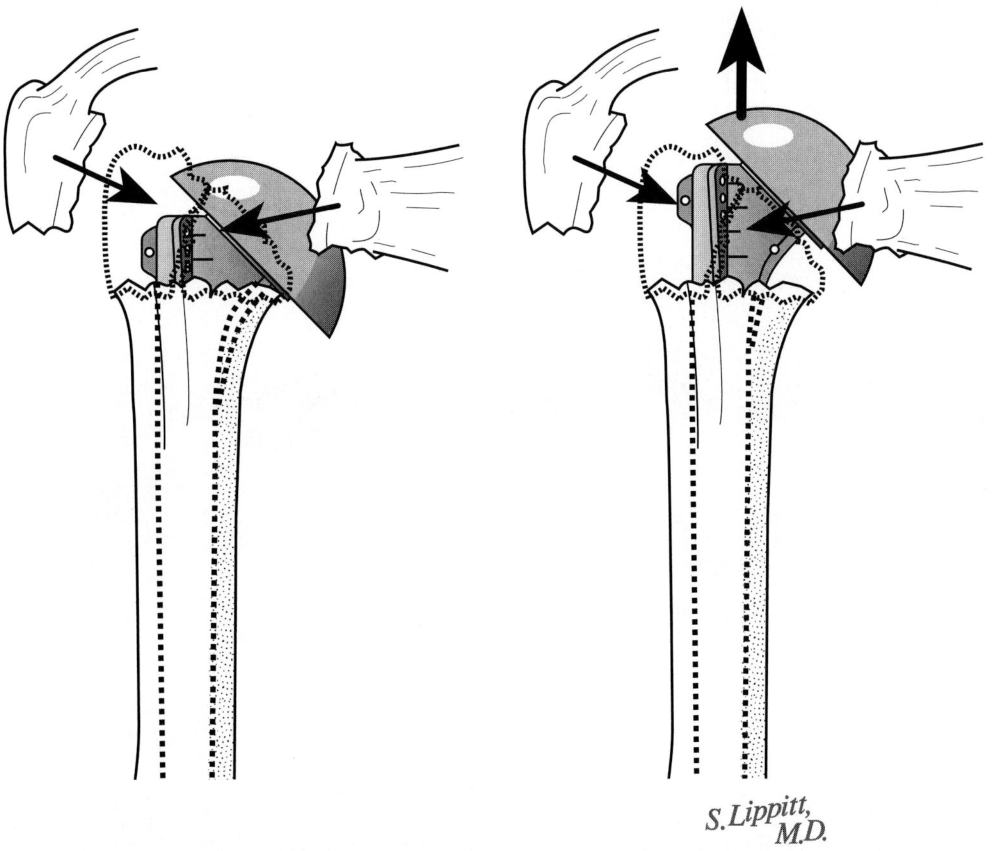


**Figure 36–24. Choosing the prosthesis height**

The desired height of the prosthesis is that which allows the tuberosities to overlap 3 mm with the shaft (*right*). This prosthesis position is often that in which the inferior aspects of the fins on the prosthesis are at the level of the upper end of the shaft. Placing the prosthesis too low (*left*) allows the tuberosities to overlap the articular surface of the humerus and also causes excess slack in the deltoid.

While the trial prosthesis is held at the correct height, the point on it where the stem enters the humerus is marked. A comparable mark will be placed on the definitive prosthesis to serve as a guide at the time of cementing.

The shaft is now prepared for tuberosity attachment. Six drill holes are placed through the proximal humeral shaft around its anterior perimeter. A #5 braided suture is placed through each hole (**Fig. 36–25**). An additional pair of holes is made further distally on the lateral shaft. One long strand of #5 nonabsorbable braided suture is passed through this pair of holes in the lateral shaft (**Fig. 36–26**).

The stem of the prosthesis selected by the trailing process is then marked at the appropriate level of insertion. If the prosthesis is modular, the head and body portions are securely assembled prior to insertion.

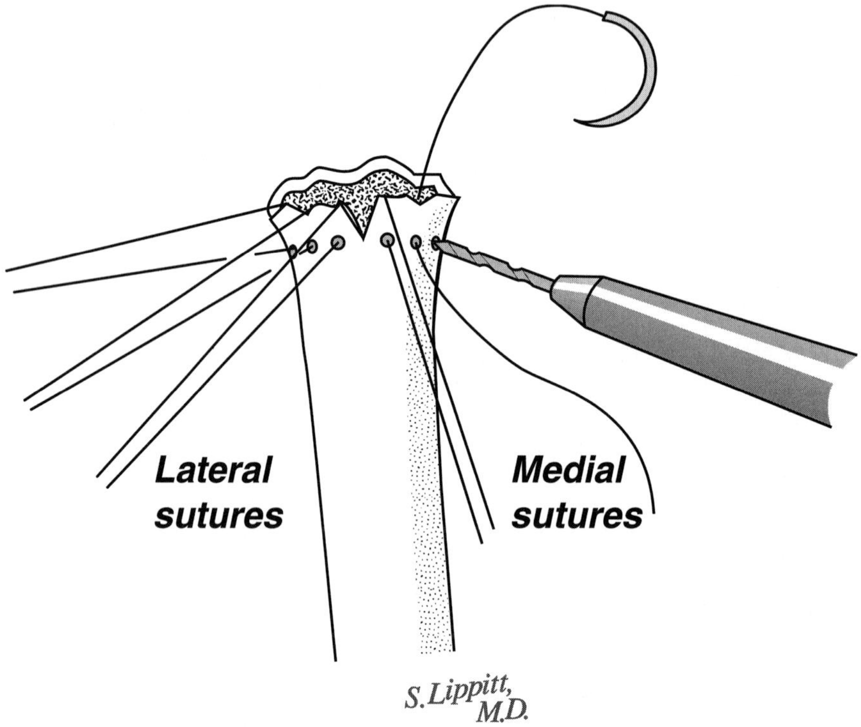


**Figure 36–25. Shaft sutures**
Six drill holes are made around the proximal end of the shaft. Number 5 nonabsorbable braided sutures are passed through these holes.

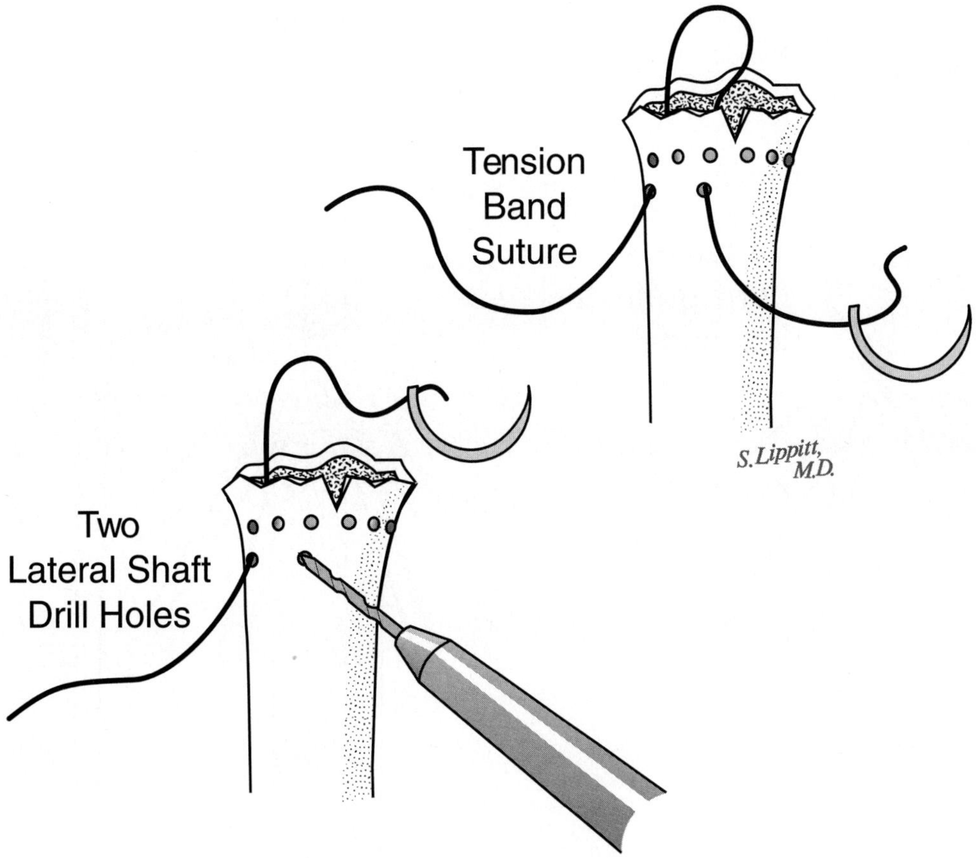


**Figure 36–26. Tension band suture**
A pair of drill holes is made more distally in the lateral shaft and a long strand of #5 braided suture is passed through the holes. This suture will later be used as a tension band.

Cementing of the prosthesis is required to provide secure rotational and height control while the tuberosities are healing. A bone plug is placed at the appropriate depth to accommodate the prosthetic stem and to restrict the flow of cement down the distal shaft (**Fig. 36–27**). After the canal is irrigated and dried, the prosthesis is cemented in the desired height and version. The cement is inserted with finger packing to avoid the risks of pressurization of the often fragile humeral cortex (**Fig. 36–28**).

All excess cement is removed from around the proximal end of the shaft so that it will not interfere with bone-to-bone apposition as the tuberosities are fixed in position (**Fig. 36–29**). The sutures previously placed in the shaft are moved in and out through the holes so that they will slide when tied after the cement has hardened.

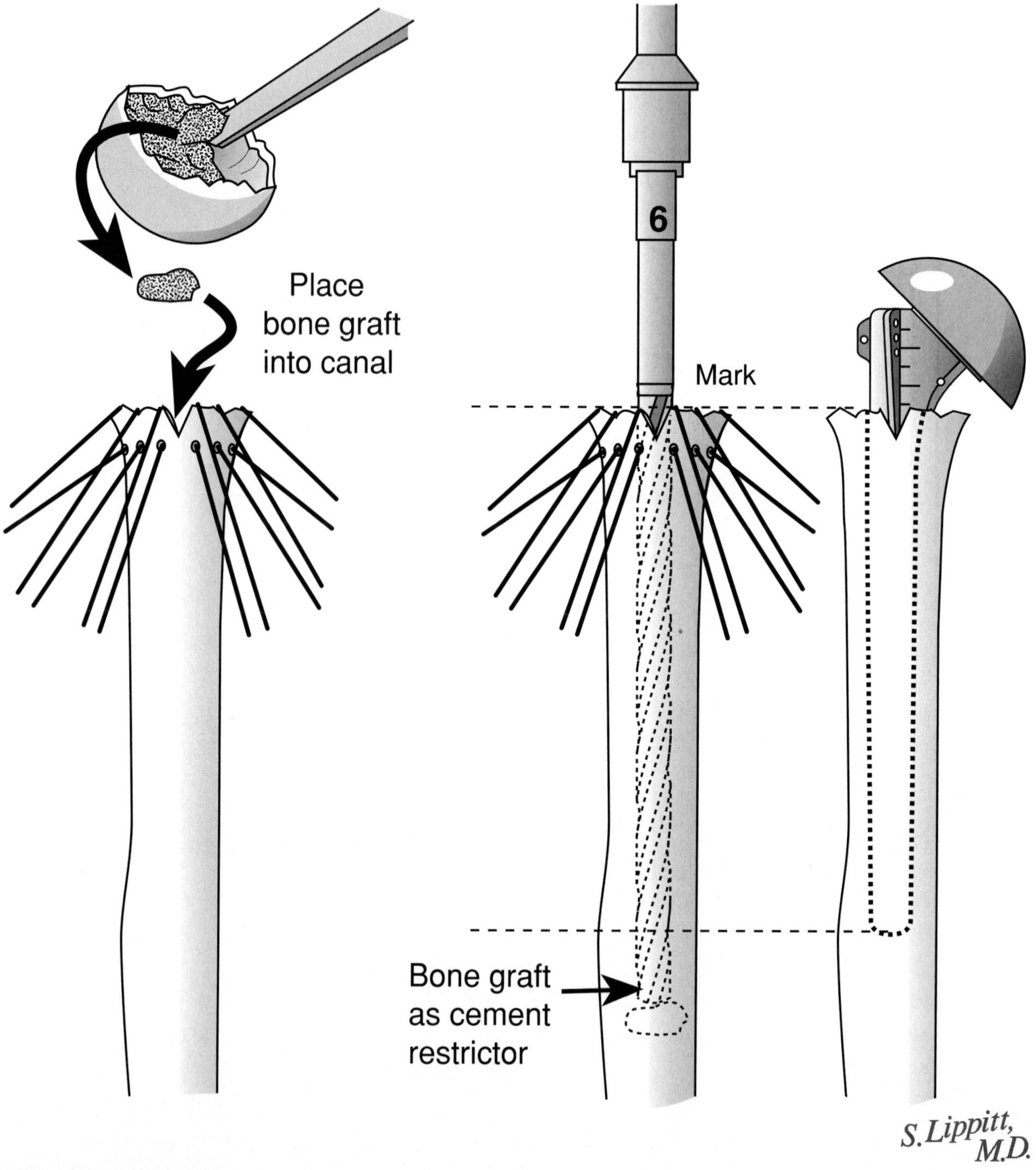


**Figure 36–27. Bone plug**
A plug of cancellous bone harvested from the humeral head is put down the medullary canal. A reamer smaller than the one used to ream the canal is used to tamp the graft down to the level of the tip of the prosthesis.

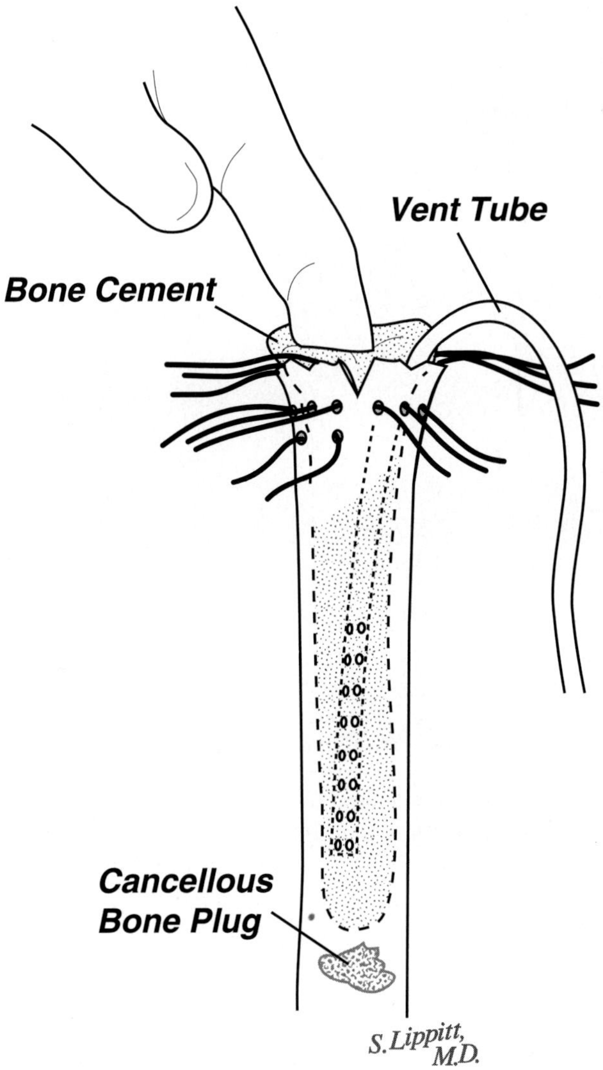


**Figure 36–28. Cementing the canal**
Cement is inserted with moderate pressure against the bone plug using a vent tube as necessary to remove fluid. Major pressurization is avoided to protect the integrity of the shaft.

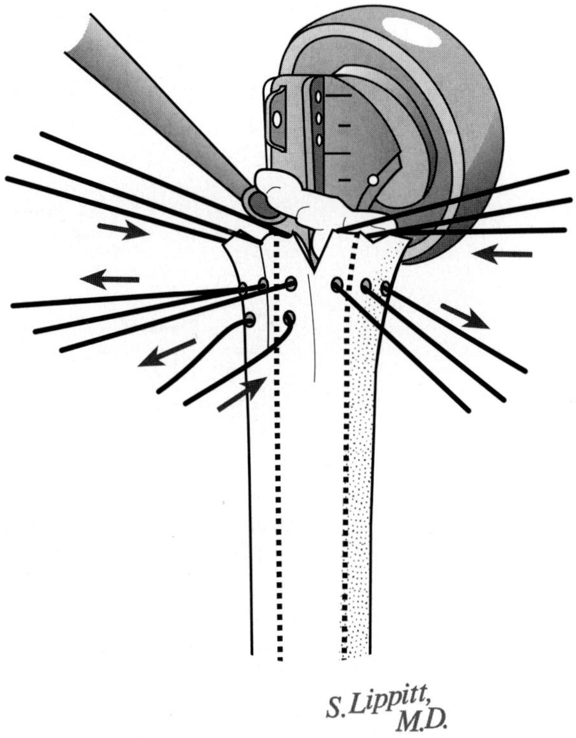


**Figure 36–29. Removal of excess cement**
Excess cement is removed so that it will not interfere with bone graft placement or bone contact. The sutures are moved through the holes back and forth to ensure that the cement does not make them more difficult to tie.

The tension band suture previously passed through the lateral shaft is passed through the supraspinatus, the upper hole in the lateral fin, and the supraspinatus again and clamped to be tied later (**Fig. 36–30**).

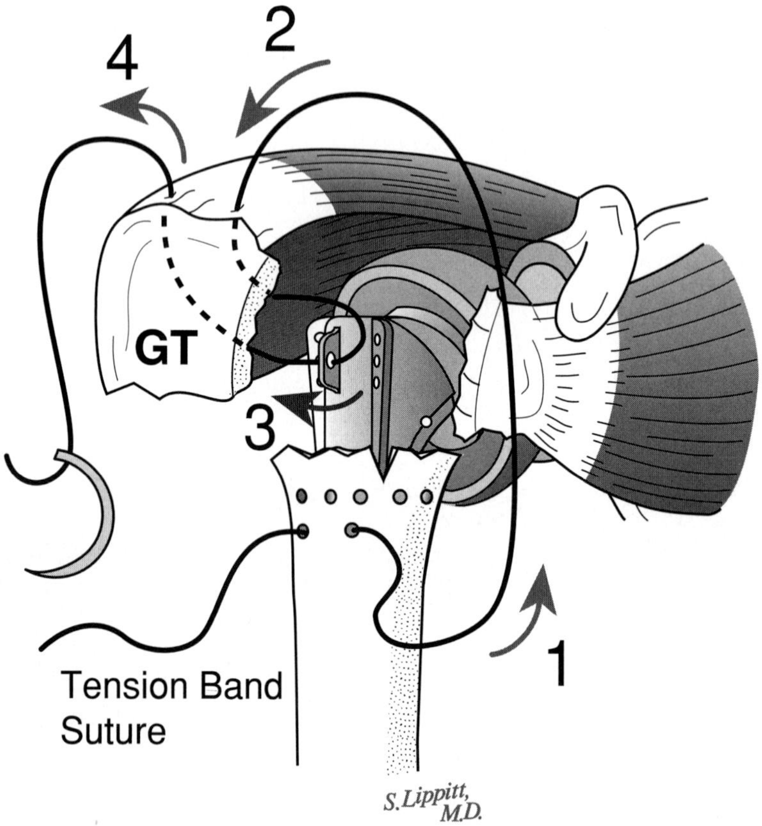


**Figure 36–30. Tension band suture**
One limb of the #5 suture previously passed through the lateral cortex is passed through the supraspinatus tendon near the greater tuberosity, then through the upper hole of the lateral fin, then out through the supraspinatus tendon near the greater tuberosity and clamped with a hemostat for later tying. This is the tension band suture.

The greater tuberosity is placed in the final desired position, overlying the lateral fin of the prosthesis. A notch is sculpted in the deep side of the tuberosity where it contacts the lateral fin of the prosthesis so that the fin acts as a blade sticking into the tuberosity. The tuberosity is further sculpted so that it fits nicely against the side of the shaft that has been freed of all interposed soft tissues. The goal is that impaction of the tuberosity on the fin will provide rotational stability to the tuberosity **(Fig. 36–31)**. A #5 braided nonabsorbable suture is placed in each of the holes of the lateral fin of the prosthesis. These sutures are then passed through drill holes in the greater tuberosity anterior and posterior to the notch in the deep side of the tuberosity so that when these sutures are tied later on in the case, they will compress the notch on the tuberosity on the lateral fin.

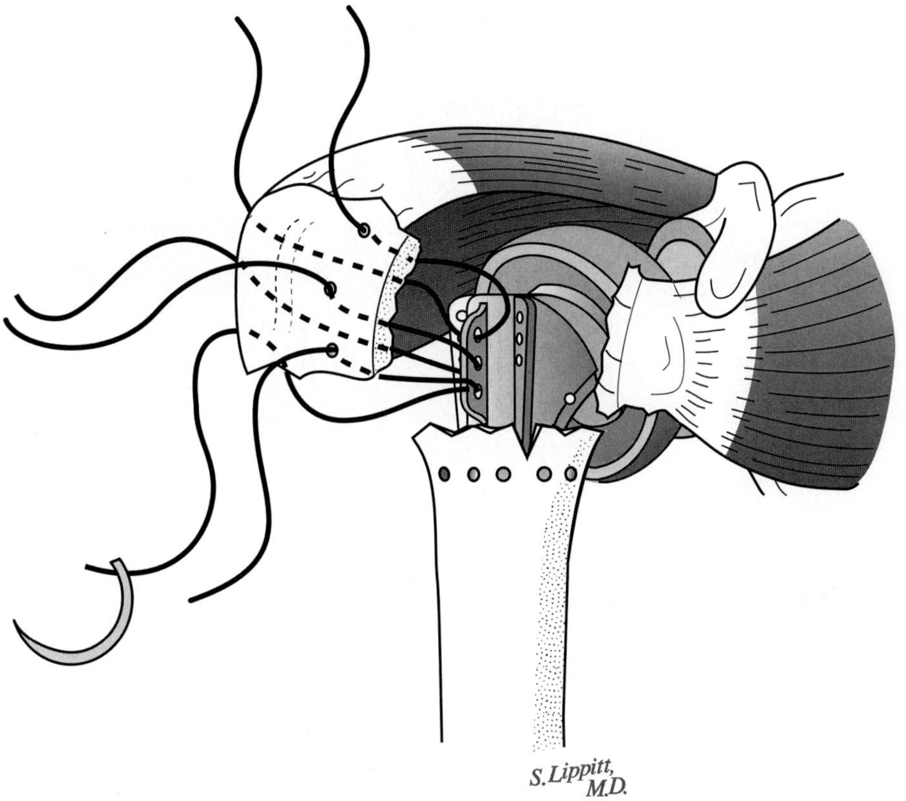


**Figure 36–31. Optimizing rotational control**
Because rotational control of the tuberosities is a premium, we take every advantage to optimize it. Because we know that the lateral fin on the prosthesis should normally lie in the substance of the greater tuberosity, we can construct a notch in the anterior third of the fractured tuberosity that will conform to the side of the prosthesis and incorporate the lateral fin. The #5 sutures passed through the lateral fin holes are brought through drill holes in the greater tuberosity anterior and posterior to the notch that was created in the deep side of the tuberosity to accommodate the lateral fin.

The sutures from the anterior shaft holes are passed around the greater tuberosity (**Fig. 36–32**) and the sutures from the posterior shaft holes are passed around the lesser tuberosity (**Fig. 36–33**).

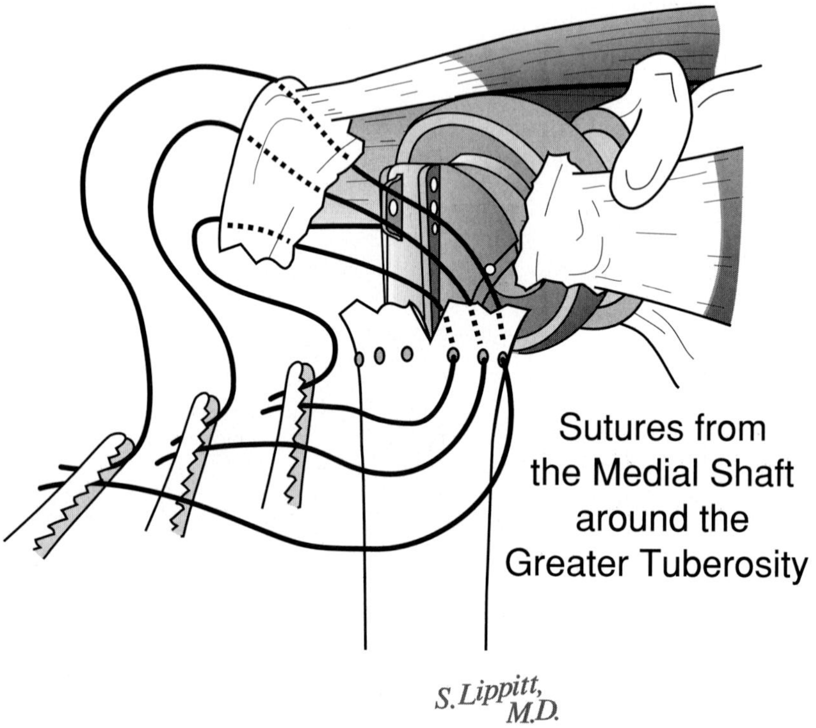


**Figure 36–32. Greater tuberosity sutures**
The #5 sutures from the anterior three holes in the shaft are passed around the greater tuberosity through the cuff tendons.

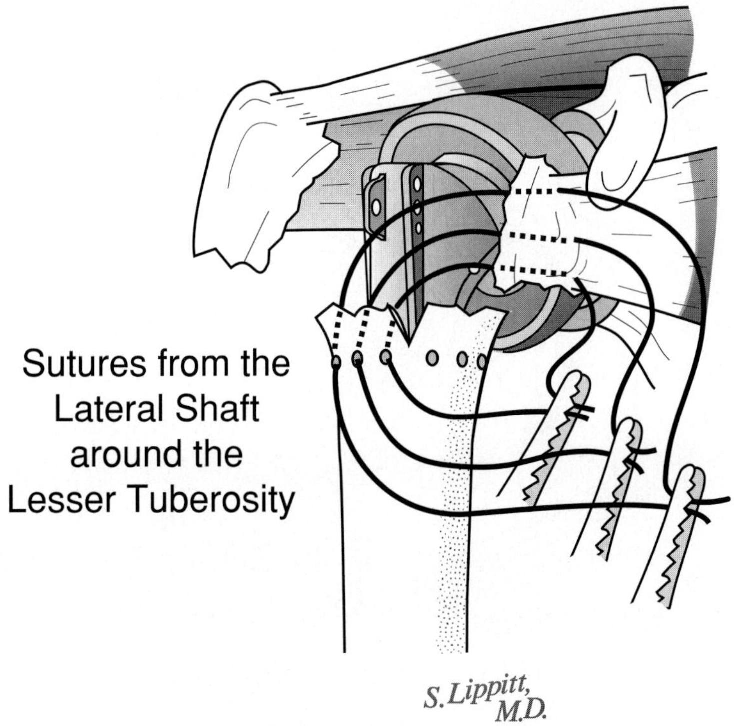


**Figure 36–33. Lesser tuberosity sutures**
The #5 sutures from the posterior three holes in the shaft are passed around the lesser tuberosity through the infraspinatus tendon.

Bone graft is placed around the upper shaft deep to where the tuberosities will lie (**Fig. 36–34**). The sutures on either side of the lateral fin are tied, compressing the notch on the deep side of the tuberosity onto the fin (**Fig. 36–35**). Next, the tension band suture is tied, stabilizing the tuberosity against the upward pull of the

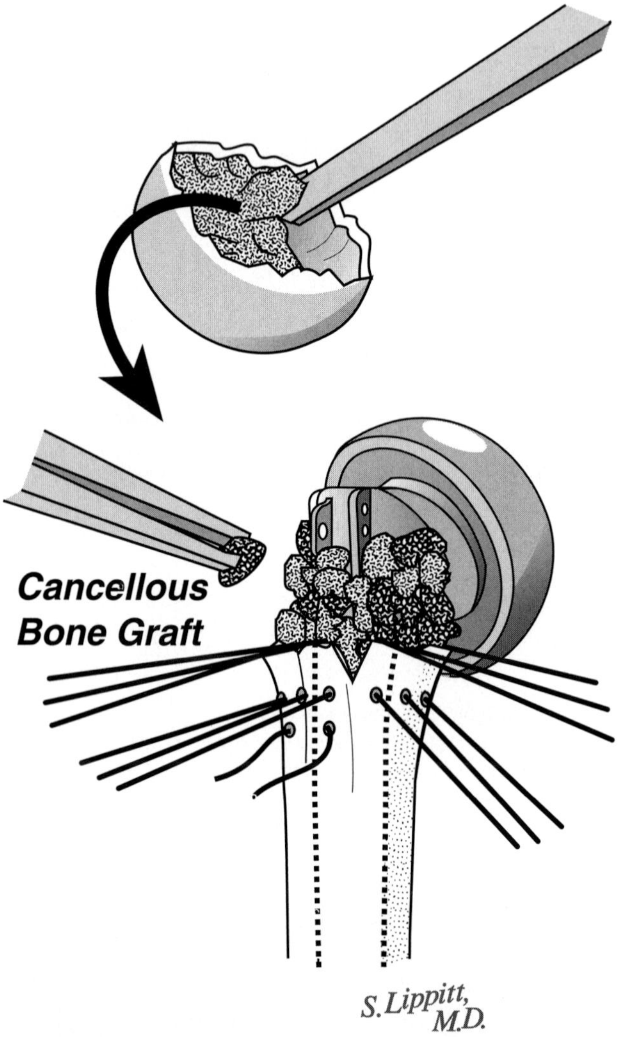


**Figure 36–34. Bone graft**
Bone graft harvested from the humeral head is placed around the prosthesis where the tuberosities will lie.

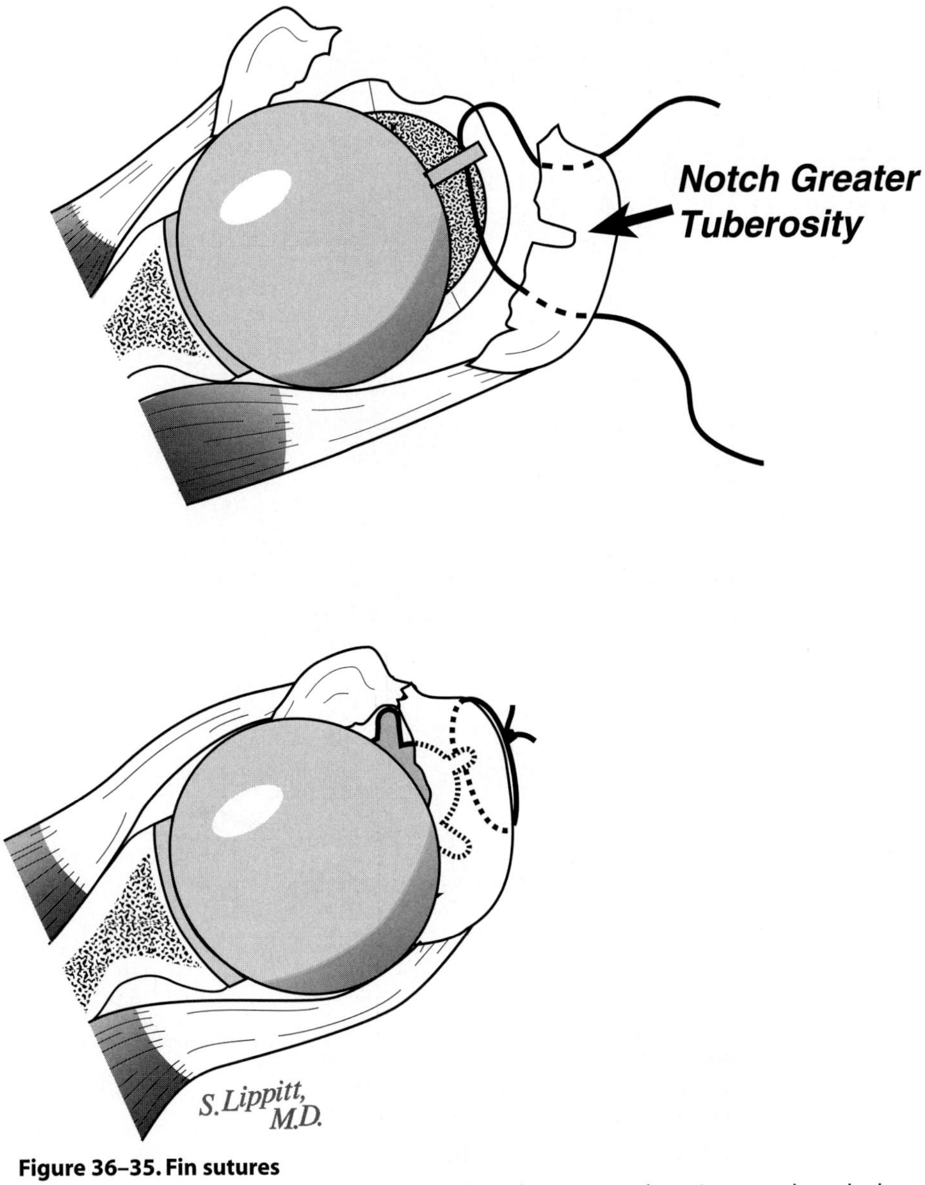


**Figure 36–35. Fin sutures**
Tying the fin sutures securely applies the notch in the greater tuberosity securely to the lateral fin.

supraspinatus (**Figs. 36–36** and **36–37**). Next, the oblique greater tuberosity sutures are tied, managing the posterior pull of the infraspinatus (**Fig. 36–38**). Next, the oblique lesser tuberosity sutures are tied, managing the anterior pull of the subscapularis (**Fig. 36–39**). Additional fixation can be achieved by sutures tied around the greater and lesser tuberosities (**Fig. 36–40**).

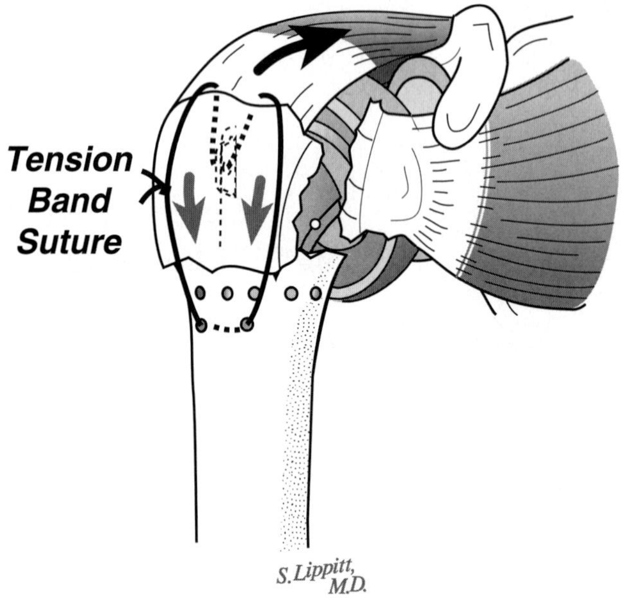


**Figure 36–36. Tension band suture**
The tension band suture is tied resisting the upward pull of the supraspinatus.

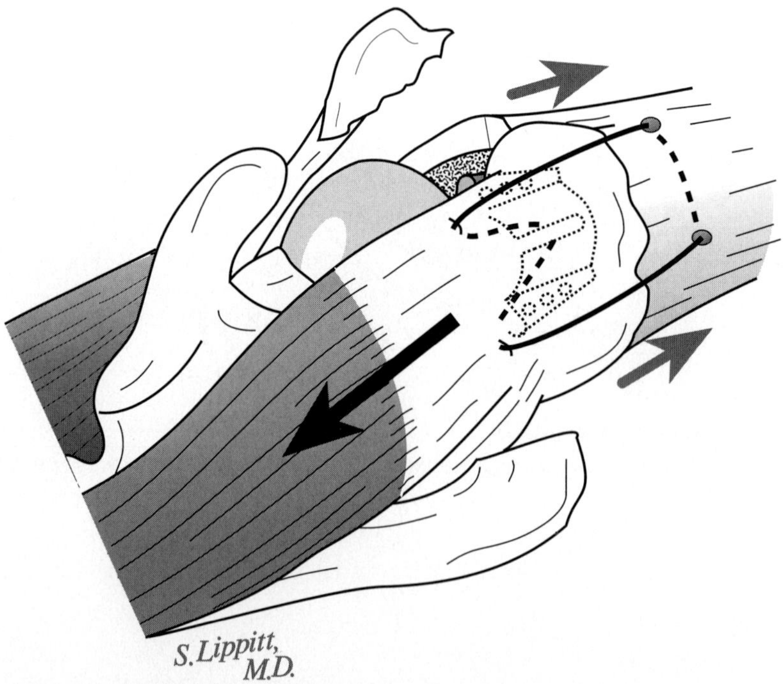


**Figure 36–37. Tension band suture**
The tension band suture effectively manages the supraspinatus force.

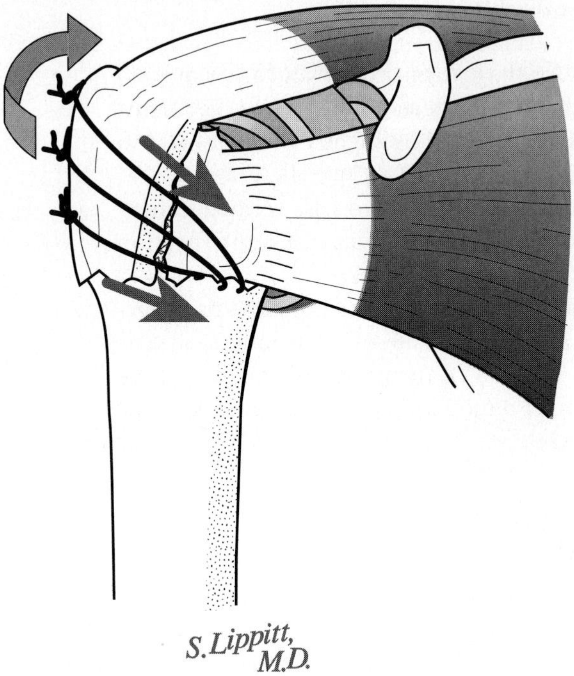


**Figure 36–38. Greater tuberosity sutures**
The oblique placement of the greater tuberosity sutures effectively manages the posterior pull of the infraspinatus.

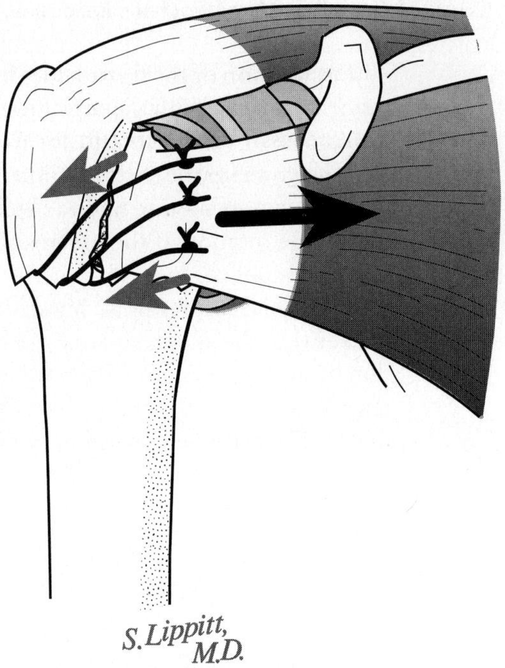


**Figure 36–39. Lesser tuberosity sutures**
The oblique placement of the lesser tuberosity sutures effectively manages the anterior pull of the subscapularis.

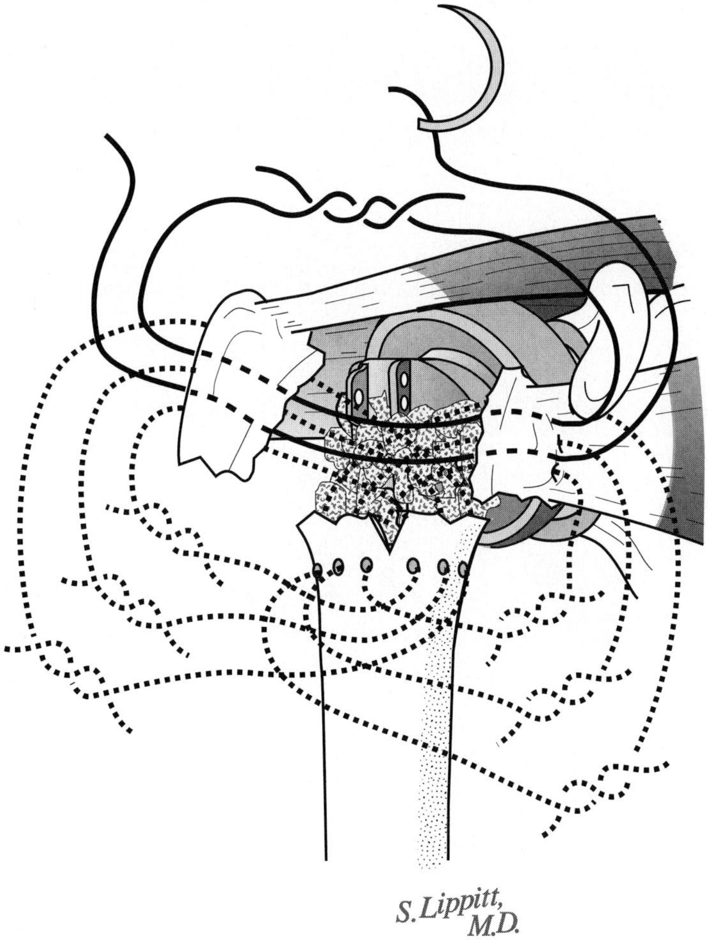


**Figure 36–40. Additional fixation**
Additional fixation can be achieved by sutures passed around the greater and lesser tuberosities.

The position of the tuberosities is checked for the proximal/distal and anterior/posterior relationships to the prosthesis. All of the tuberosity should lie below the articular surface of the prosthesis. Ideally, the tuberosities will be slightly over-reduced so that they overlap the shaft, optimizing the potential for healing.

The range of motion and the security of the tuberosity fixation are verified in flexion and in rotation. If the tuberosities were not stably fixed, additional suture fixation would be applied.

Additional sutures of #2 braided nonabsorbable suture are used to close the interval between the supraspinatus and the subscapularis (**Fig. 36–41**). The long head tendon of the biceps is usually tenodesed in this situation. Care needs to be taken that the tenodesis does not limit the range of glenohumeral motion. If this does occur, the tendon can be sectioned proximal to the tenodesis.

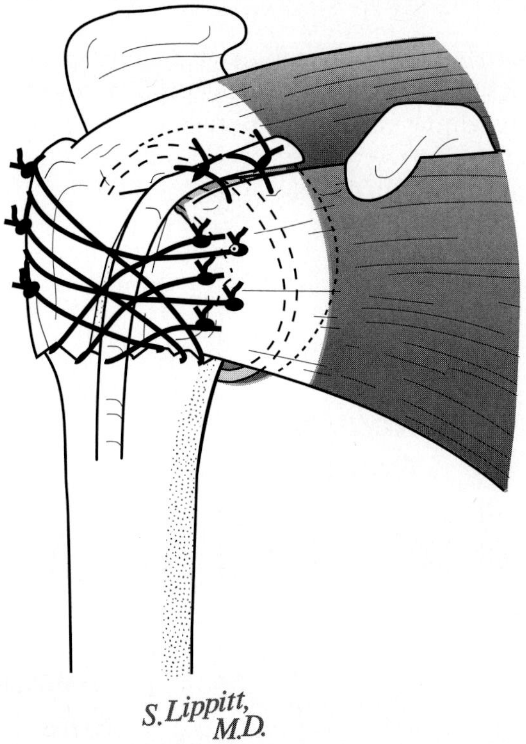


**Figure 36–41. Rotator interval closure**
The rotator interval is closed, making sure that the long head of the biceps is not tenodesed in a position that restricts range of motion.

When all the sutures are tied, there should be no differential motion between the tuberosity fragments and the shaft so that immediate postoperative motion can be implemented (**Figs. 36–42** and **Fig. 36–43**).

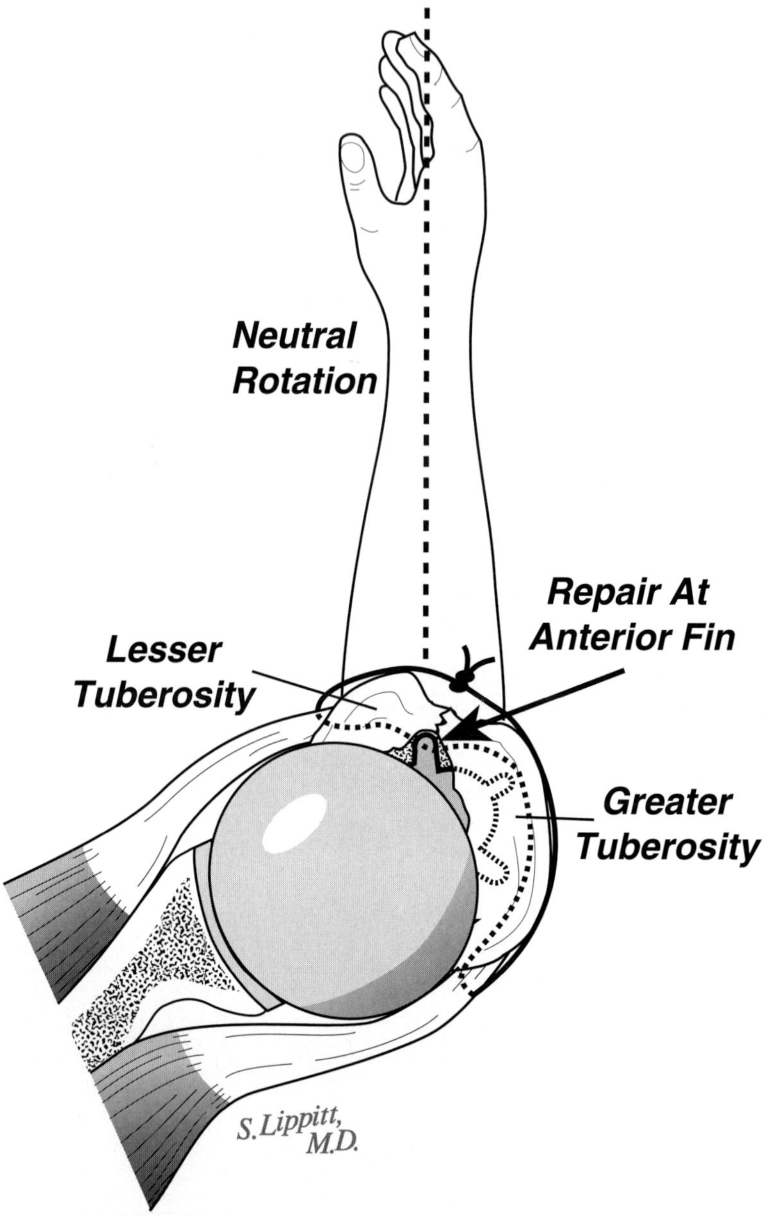


**Figure 36–42. Secure fixation**
Secure fixation is indicated by the lack of motion between the tuberosities and the shaft on humeral rotation.

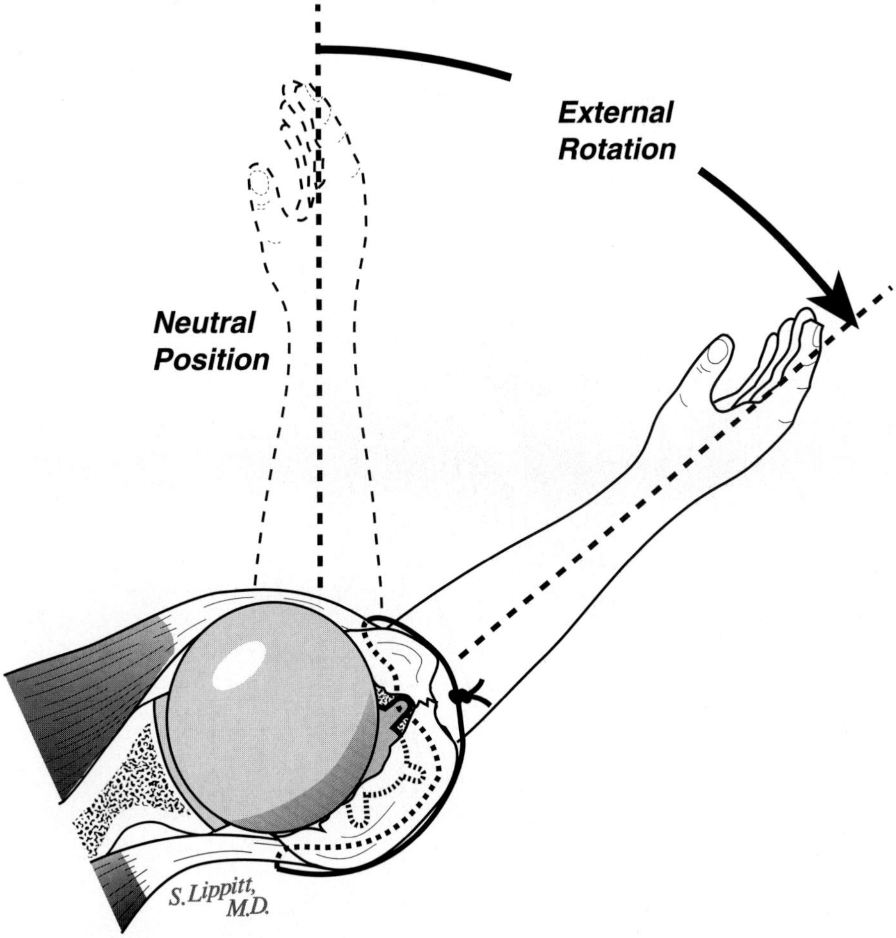


**Figure 36–43. Secure fixation**
It is particularly important to check for security of fixation on maximal external rotation.

The wound is thoroughly irrigated. Additional cancellous bone graft is added at the junction of the tuberosities and shaft. Hemostasis is seen to be excellent.

The deltopectoral incision is closed with absorbable sutures.

The wound is closed with staples after a drain has been placed (**Figs. 36–44 and 36–45**).

Dry sterile dressings are applied.

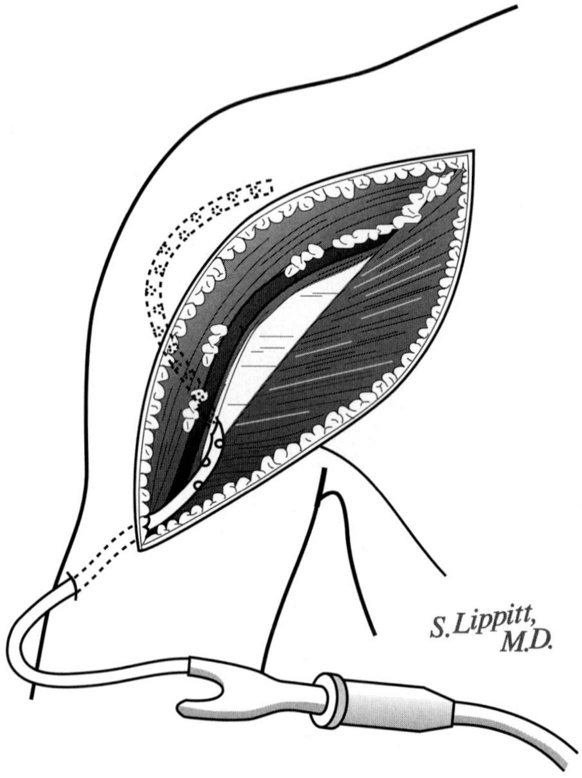


**Figure 36–44. Drain**
A suction drain is used to protect the closure.

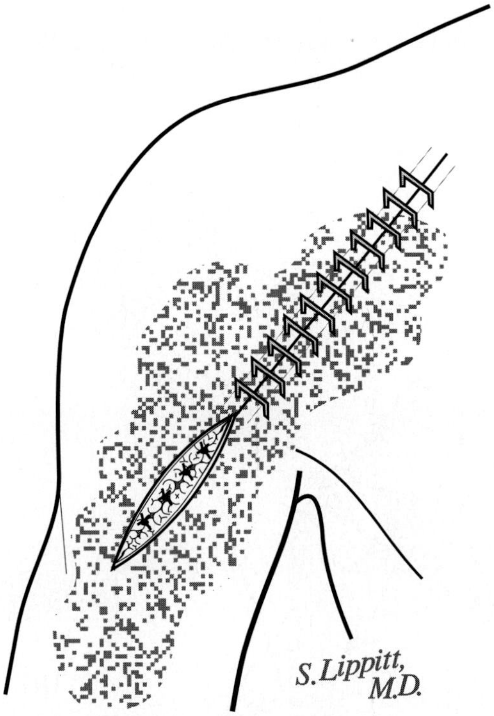


**Figure 36–45. Skin clips**
We prefer interrupted skin closure with staples to allow easy egress of any hematoma.

The patient is returned to the recovery room in satisfactory condition with the arm in continuous passive motion (**Fig. 36–46**).

## POSTOPERATIVE PLAN

Our postoperative plan is for assisted elevation up to 140 degrees and avoidance of active elevation or rotation against resistance for 3 months.

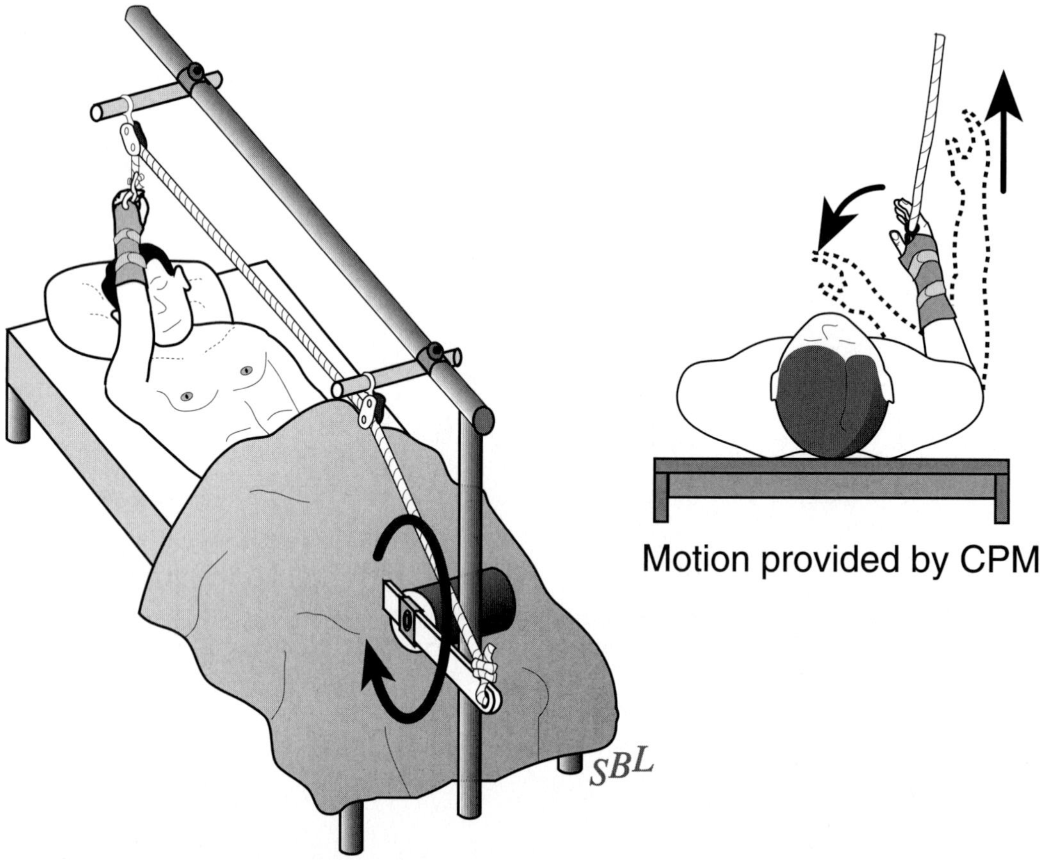


**Figure 36–46. Continuous passive motion**
Because the fixation is secure, continuous passive motion can be started immediately after surgery. (Modified from Matsen FA, Lippitt SB, Sidles JA, et al [eds]: Practical Evaluation and Management of the Shoulder. Philadelphia: WB Saunders, 1994, p. 50.)

# PART VII

# REVISION SURGERY

CHAPTER 37

# Principles of Revision Surgery

## CONCEPTS

### Considering Revision Surgery

Revision shoulder surgery calls on judgment, experience, and technical skills that are an order of magnitude greater than for primary shoulder surgery. There are 10 questions that we ask before taking on a revision case:

1. Do we have sufficient past records on this case?
2. Is the problem a mechanical one that is clearly identified (as opposed to a problem that is manifested as pain or frustration without a clear mechanical cause)?
3. Is there a nonoperative approach to the problem?
4. Is the mechanical problem treatable?
5. Is the patient of sufficient mental and physical health and strength to undergo a revision surgery—are the patient's metabolism and the skin over the shoulder ready for another surgery, has the patient ceased smoking, are alcohol consumption and pain medication use under control?
6. Are the patient's expectations reasonable?
7. Does the patient fully understand the risks and possible outcomes of surgery, including the anticipated incision and the possibility that infection may be encountered?
8. Do we need a consultation to help define the cause and treatment of the problem?
9. Are we the best surgeons to carry out the revision surgery?
10. Do we have the right tools and team to carry out the surgical revision?

To answer these questions, we seek the following information prior to considering a surgical revision:

1. An understanding of the patient's status prior to the index procedure.
2. Previous operative notes, including information on the type, manufacturer, and size of implants.
3. An assessment of the legal and insurance aspects of the case.
4. Knowledge of the medical status of the patient, including the following:
   a. Health conditions that may affect the patient's surgery
   b. Current medications, including pain medications, and dosages
   c. The amount of nicotine and alcohol currently being consumed
   d. The psychological status of the patient
   e. The vocational status of the patient
   f. The social situation and support systems for the patient
   g. Current laboratory values, including complete blood cell count, sedimentation rate, and serum albumin level.

5. High-quality anteroposterior and axillary radiographs as well as an anteroposterior radiograph of the entire humerus.
6. Completed Simple Shoulder Test and Short Form-36 Questionnaires.
7. A physical examination of the neck and shoulder, including the location of skin incisions and the health of the skin in the areas of possible incision.
8. An electromyogram if there is concern about radiculopathy or neuropathy.
9. Consent for bone autograft, tendon autograft, or allograft as necessary.
10. Medicine, anesthesiology, and pain service consults as necessary.
11. Urinalysis to screen for drug, alcohol, and nicotine, if indicated.

## SURGICAL CONSIDERATIONS

### General Principles of Revision Surgery

Before the anesthetic, the patient's consent is checked to make sure it is complete. The instrument and implant inventory are verified for possible variations on the preoperative plan, including the need to modify a prosthesis or to possibly use a special implant (e.g., a long-stemmed humeral implant in case of shaft fracture).

The patient is anesthetized, positioned, prepped, and draped in a manner that anticipates all possible variations on the surgical plan. The entire forequarter is prepped so that incisions can be made anteriorly, posteriorly, or distally as needed. The arm is draped so that it can be moved freely. Ipsilateral iliac crest and hamstring autograft donor sites are prepped if their possible need is anticipated.

Preoperative antibiotics are not administered. Prophylactic antibiotics are administered only after specimens are collected for culture and sensitivity testing.

The incision is made in a manner that provides optimal access to the mechanical problem and, if possible, incorporates or respects previous skin incisions. The possible need for extending the incision is anticipated (**Fig. 37–1**).

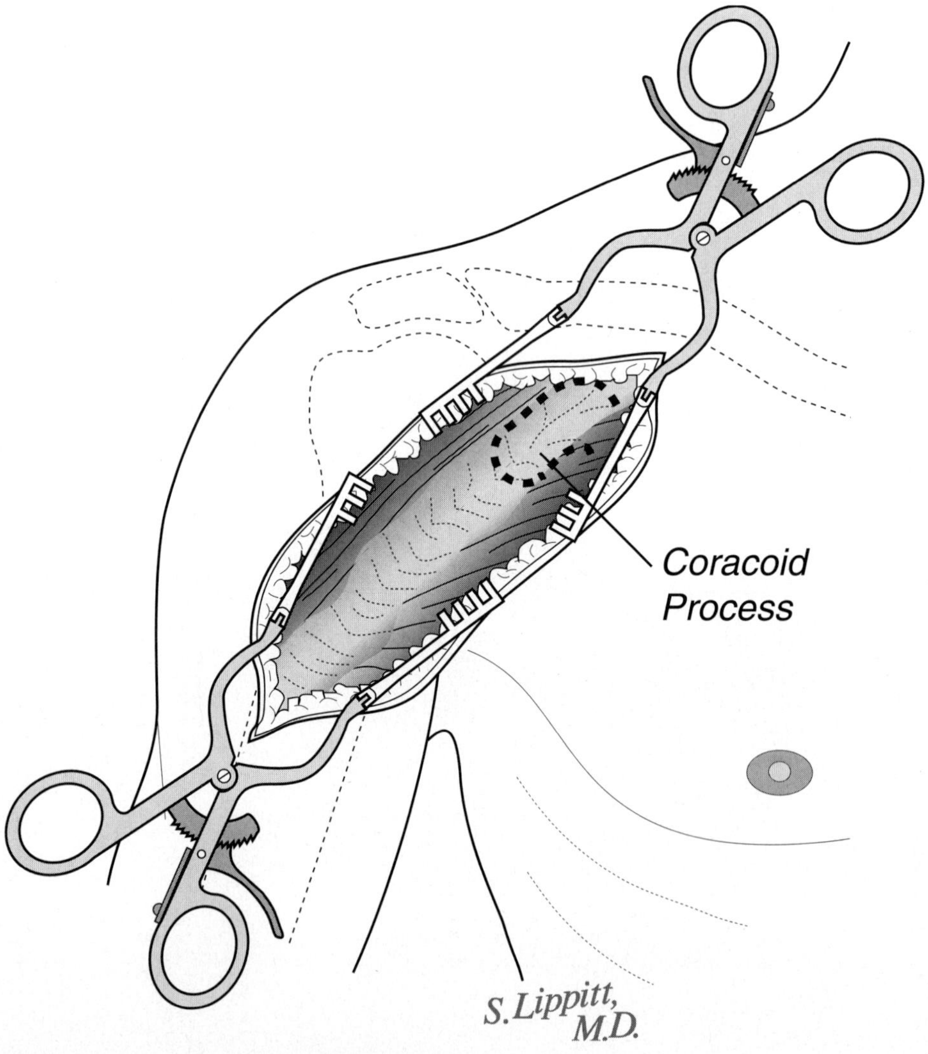


**Figure 37–1. Scarred deltopectoral interval**
The coracoid process is an important landmark when the normal anatomy of the deltopectoral interval is scarred from previous surgery through the anterior approach.

The surgical approach is conducted carefully to protect and preserve the deltoid, the rotator cuff, and the neurovascular structures about the shoulder, each of which may have been altered by previous surgery (**Fig. 37–2**).

The humeroscapular motion interface is entered and all adhesions lysed. Scarring around the coracoid is released. The subscapularis is identified by rotation of the arm. The axillary nerve is identified and protected.

Specimens are collected for aerobic, anaerobic, and fungal culture, sensitivity, and Gram stains. Frozen and permanent sections are obtained of any tissue suspicious for inflammation, infection, or neoplasm. Prophylactic antibiotics are given intravenously at this point.

The specific reconstructive surgery is then carried out. Examples of common revisions are given in the subsequent sections.

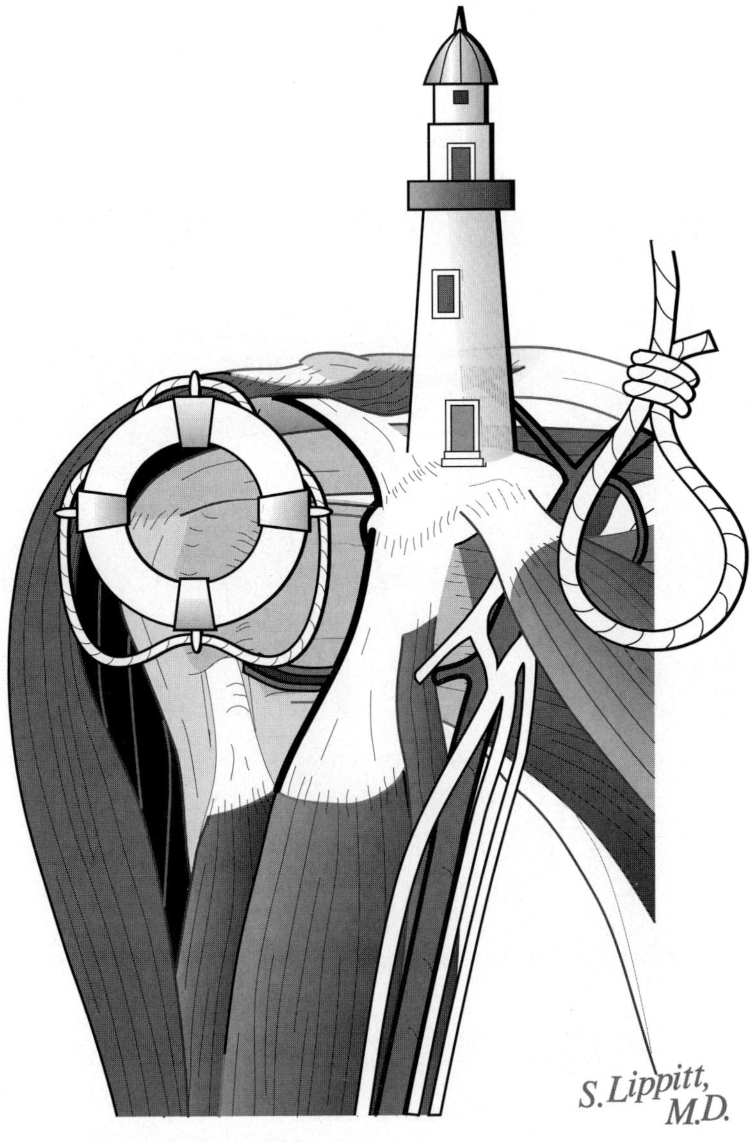


**Figure 37–2. Safe side/suicide**
The coracoid serves as a lighthouse for proper orientation in a scarred shoulder. It divides the lateral (safe side) from the medial side (suicide), where the brachial plexus and vascular structures are located.

## Revision Surgery for Motion (see Chapters 6 and 7)

Before embarking on a surgical revision to restore motion, it is important to determine the cause of the residual stiffness. Previous operative notes are reviewed to discover whether the joint was intentionally tightened and, if so, how this was carried out. Particular note is made of whether the subscapularis was advanced lateral to the bicipital groove and whether thermal or laser capsular cauterization was carried out. Excellent anteroposterior and axillary radiographs are needed to exclude bony or articular causes of shoulder stiffness. The location of hardware and other implants is determined.

Prior to prepping and draping the shoulder, the ranges of flexion, cross-body adduction, internal and external rotation in 90 degrees of abduction, and external rotation at the side as well as the excursion on posterior drawer testing are recorded for both shoulders.

The surgical procedure is performed sequentially, with the range of motion being reexamined after each step of the release. When the desired range is achieved, the procedure can be concluded.

- The initial step is to completely free the humeroscapular motion interface (**Fig. 37–3**). Any prominent suture, suture anchors, hardware, bone, or soft tissue is resected from the proximal humerus to ensure smooth passage within the coracoacromial arch. A nerve-to-nerve release is performed (**Fig. 37–4**).
- The second step is to incise the coracohumeral ligament from around the coracoid process (**Fig. 37–5**).

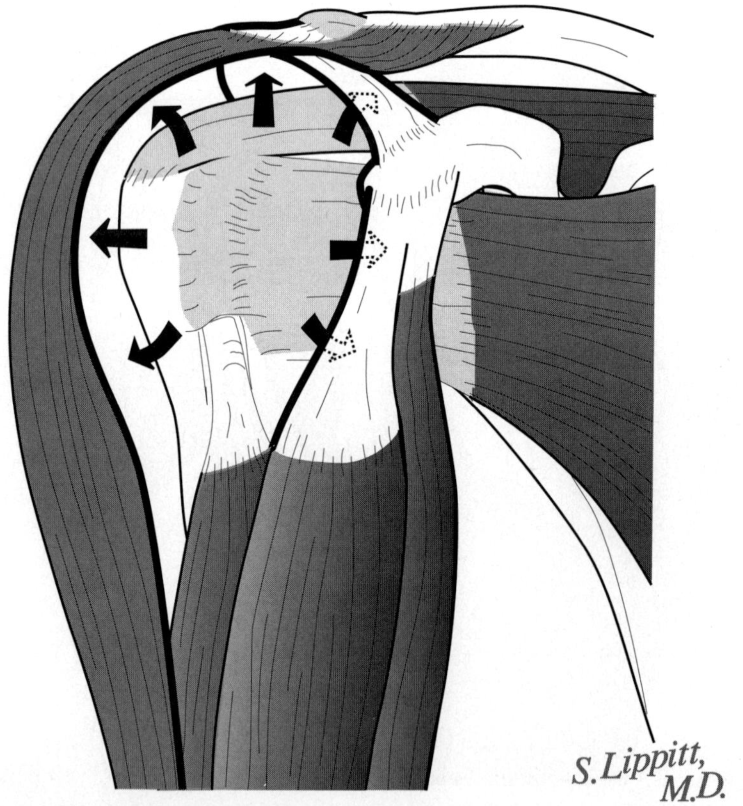


**Figure 37–3. Motion interface**
All scar is freed from the humeroscapular motion interface between the coracoacromial arch and the proximal humeral concavity. (Modified from Matsen FA, Lippitt SB, Sidles JA, et al [eds]: Practical Evaluation and Management of the Shoulder. Philadelphia: WB Saunders, 1994, p. 34.)

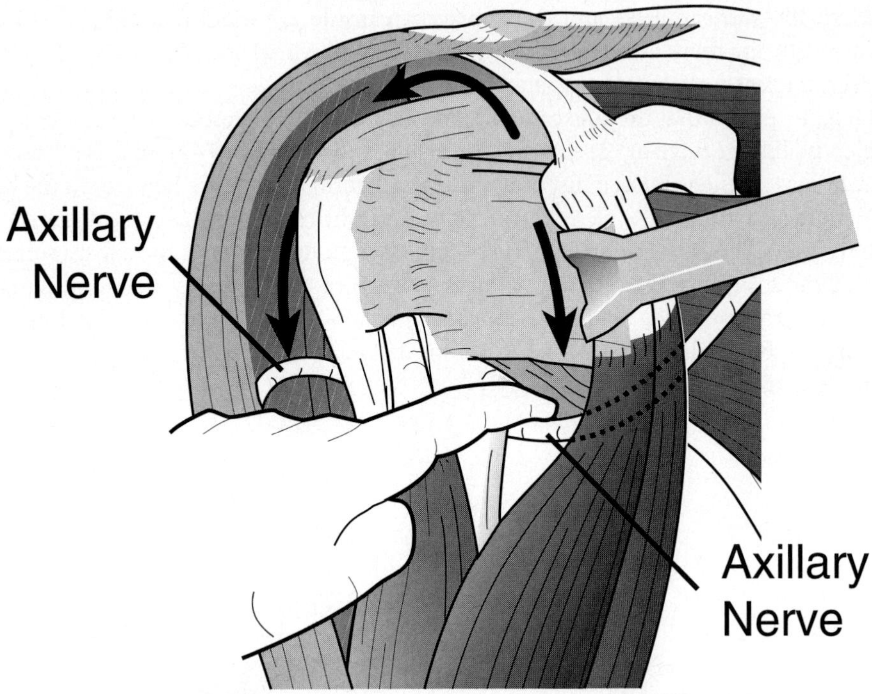


**Figure 37–4. Nerve-to-nerve release**
All scar tissue in the humeroscapular motion interface is released from the axillary nerve medially as it crosses the subscapularis, then under the coracoid, then under the coracoacromial ligament, then under the acromion, and then finally under the deltoid to the axillary nerve posteriorly as it exits the quadrilateral space: the nerve-to-nerve release.

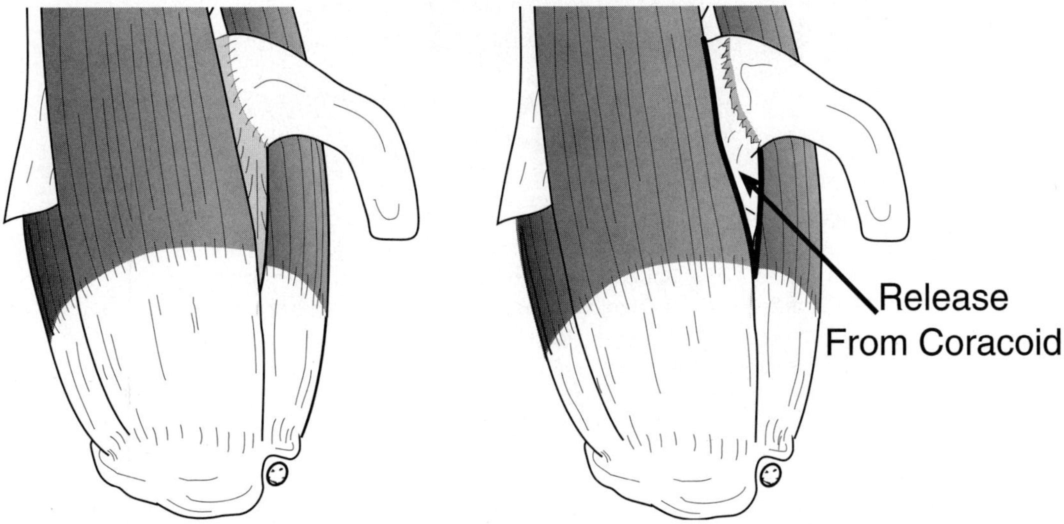


**Figure 37–5. Coracohumeral ligament release**
The supraspinatus and subscapularis tendons are released from the coracoid process, completely incising the coracohumeral ligament from its origin around the coracoid. (Modified from Matsen FA, Lippitt SB, Sidles JA, et al [eds]: Practical Evaluation and Management of the Shoulder. Philadelphia: WB Saunders, 1994, p. 138.)

- Next, the subscapularis and the subjacent capsule are identified (**Fig. 37–6**) and incised from their humeral attachments, with maximal length preserved. A 360-degree release of the subscapularis and anterior capsule is carried out, with care taken to ensure that the subscapularis moves freely with respect to the coracoid, the glenoid lip, the inferior capsule, and the axillary nerve (**Fig. 37–7**). In this release, the anterior capsule is incised just lateral to the labrum, leaving the labrum on the bony glenoid to maintain the glenoid concavity. After the release, the subscapularis should have a nice "bounce" when traction is applied to it. Recall that if the subscapularis is to allow a range of rotation of 115 degrees (two radians) it must have an excursion of twice the radius of the humeral head. Thus, if a humeral head has a radius of 25 mm, a subscapularis excursion of 50 mm will allow a 115-degree range of internal and external rotation (**Fig. 37–8**).

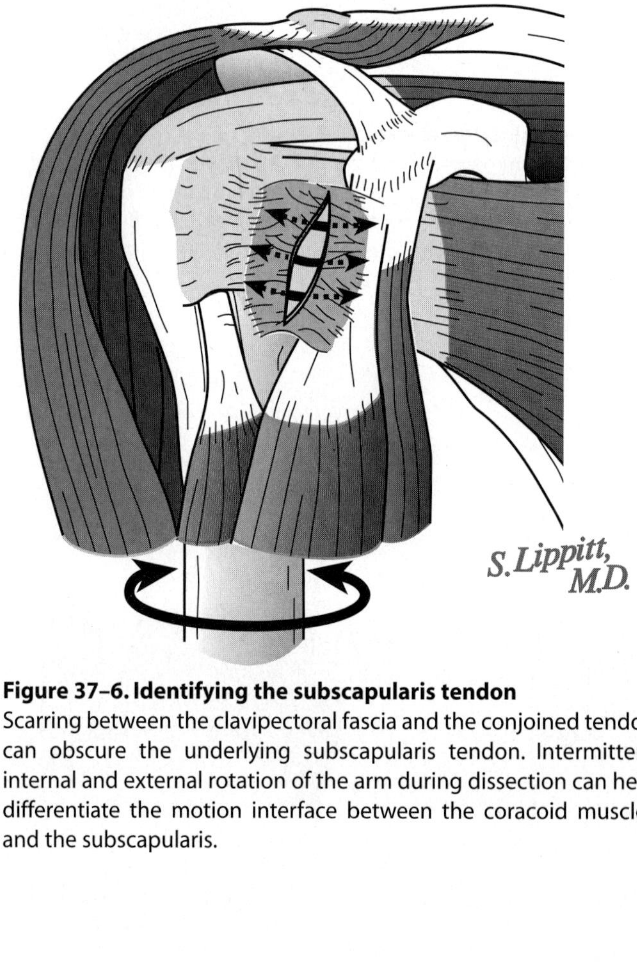


**Figure 37–6. Identifying the subscapularis tendon**
Scarring between the clavipectoral fascia and the conjoined tendon can obscure the underlying subscapularis tendon. Intermittent internal and external rotation of the arm during dissection can help differentiate the motion interface between the coracoid muscles and the subscapularis.

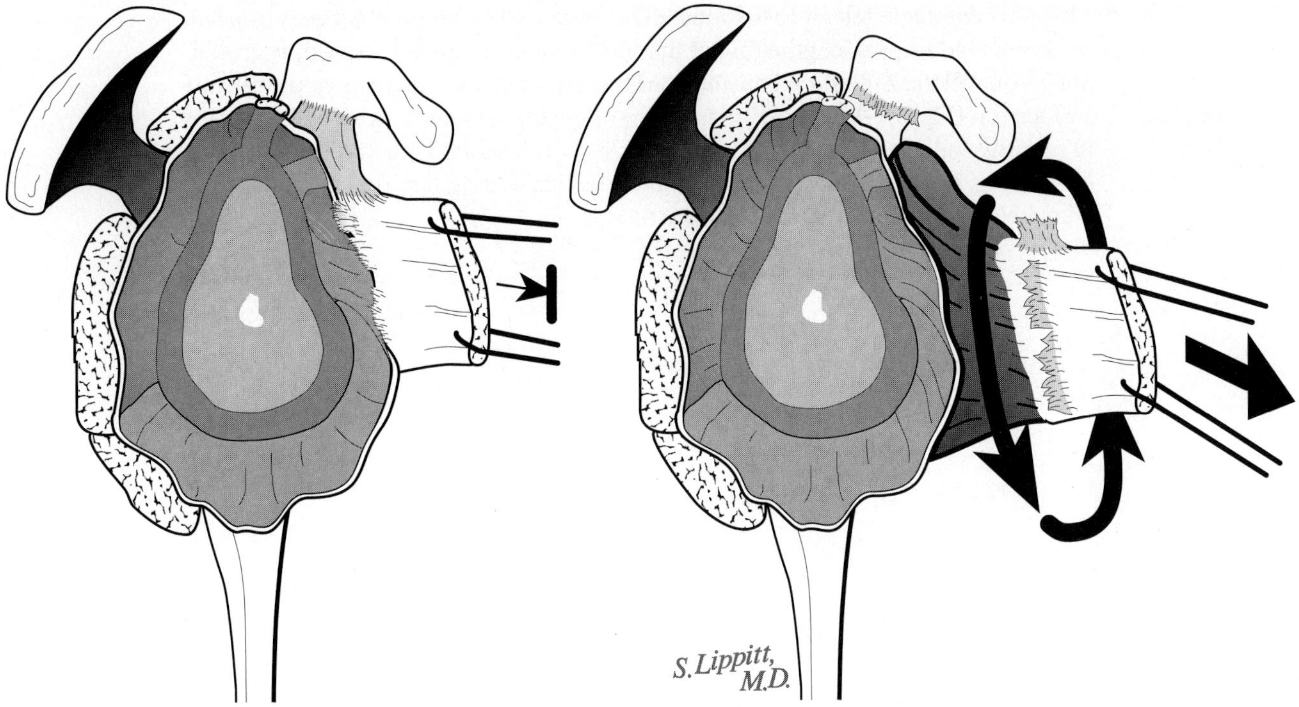


**Figure 37–7. Stiff subscapularis**
Care is taken to ensure that the subscapularis is completely released from the capsule anteriorly and from the coracoid superiorly. After a complete release, the muscle should have an elastic feel when traction is applied to it.

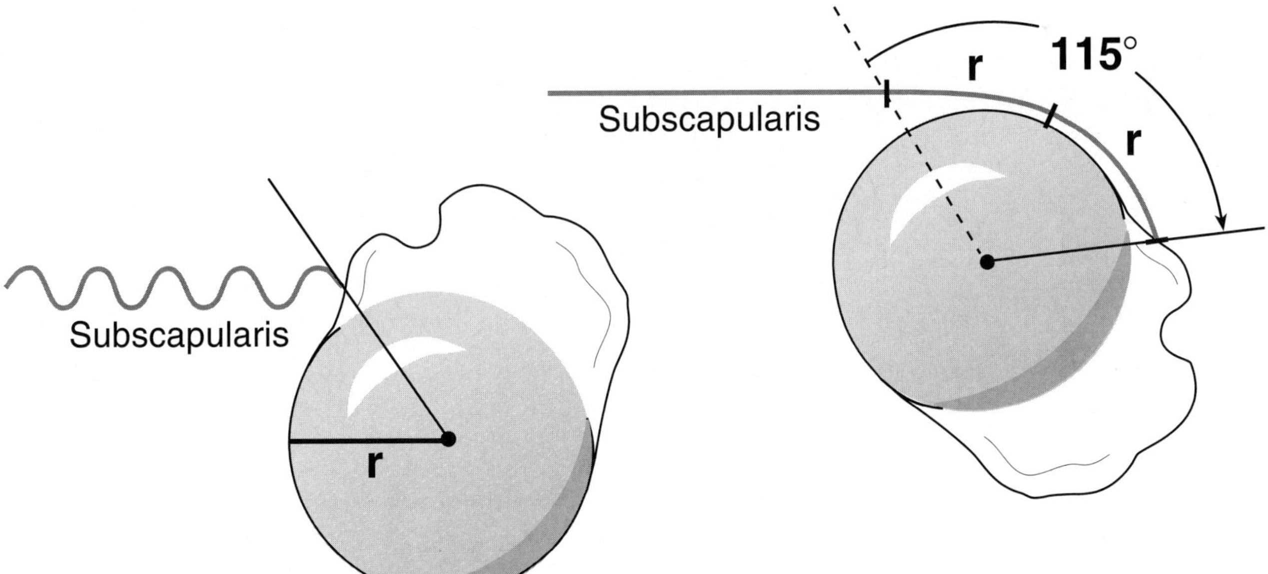


**Figure 37–8. Subscapularis excursion**
Increasing the length of the subscapularis by a distance equal to the radius of the humeral head will increase external rotation by 57.3 degrees. Increasing the length by two radial lengths will increase external rotation by 115 degrees.

- After this complete release, additional subscapularis lengthening is rarely needed. However, if additional lengthening of the subscapularis tendon is needed, an inside-out coronal plane Z-plasty is considered if there is adequate thickness of the capsule and tendon (**Fig. 37–9**). If the Z-plasty is not possible, a hamstring autograft is used to robustly connect the subscapularis to the lesser tuberosity with additional tendon length (**Fig. 37–10**). It must be noted, however, that adding tendon length does not increase the functional excursion of the muscle.

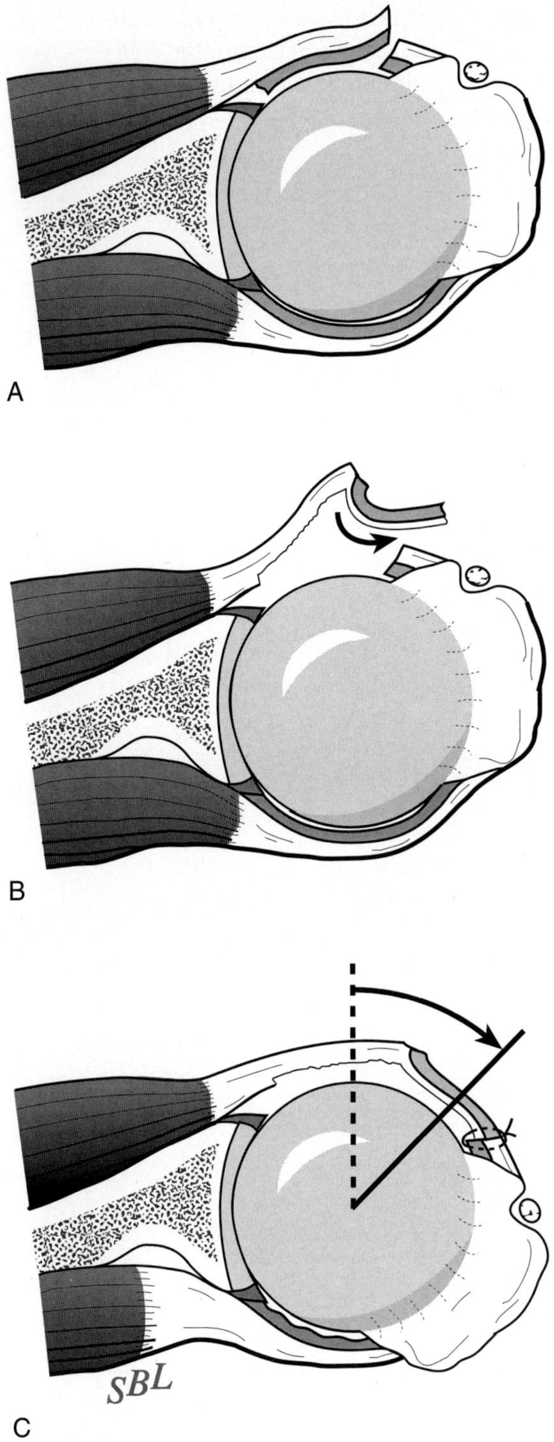


**Figure 37–9. Inside-out subscapularis Z-plasty**
If releases fail to achieve adequate length of the subscapularis, an "inside-out" Z-plasty can be performed, reflecting the medial capsule laterally while preserving its lateral attachment to the subscapularis.

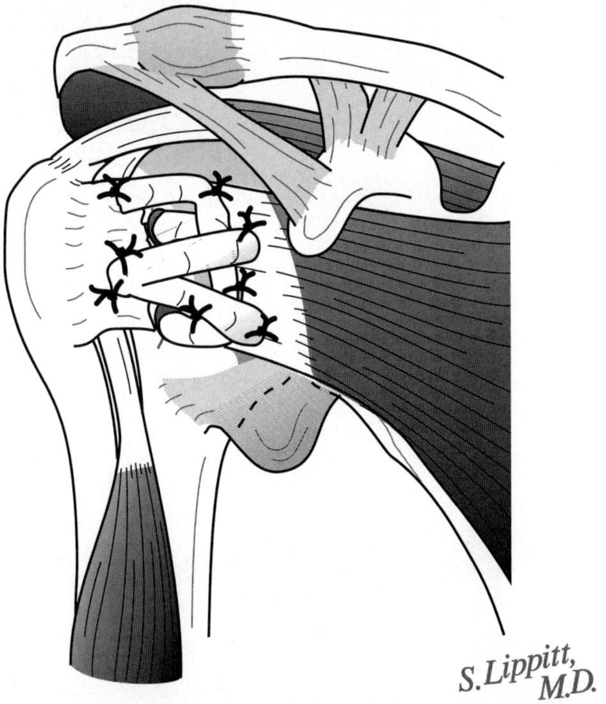


**Figure 37–10. Hamstring graft for subscapularis deficiency**
A deficient subscapularis tendon can be reconstructed using a hamstring autograft woven between the residual tendon and the soft tissue or bone at the lesser tuberosity.

- If the long head tendon of the biceps does not slide freely in the bicipital groove (**Fig. 37–11**), the adhesions in the groove are released (**Fig. 37–12**). If freedom cannot be achieved, the tendon is incised at its insertion to the supraglenoid tubercle and tenodesed to the proximal humerus in its groove (**Figs. 37–13, 37–14, 37–15,** and **37–16**).

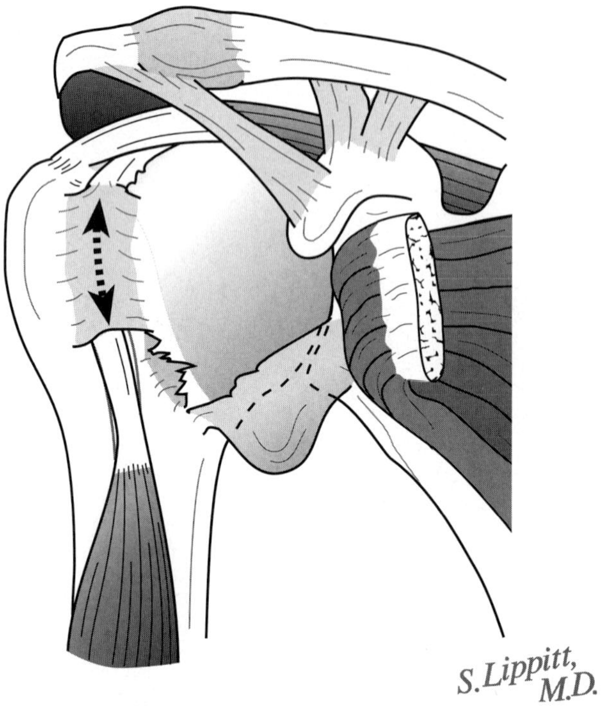


**Figure 37–11. Biceps adhesion**
Adhesion of the biceps tendon to its sheath may impair the range of shoulder motion.

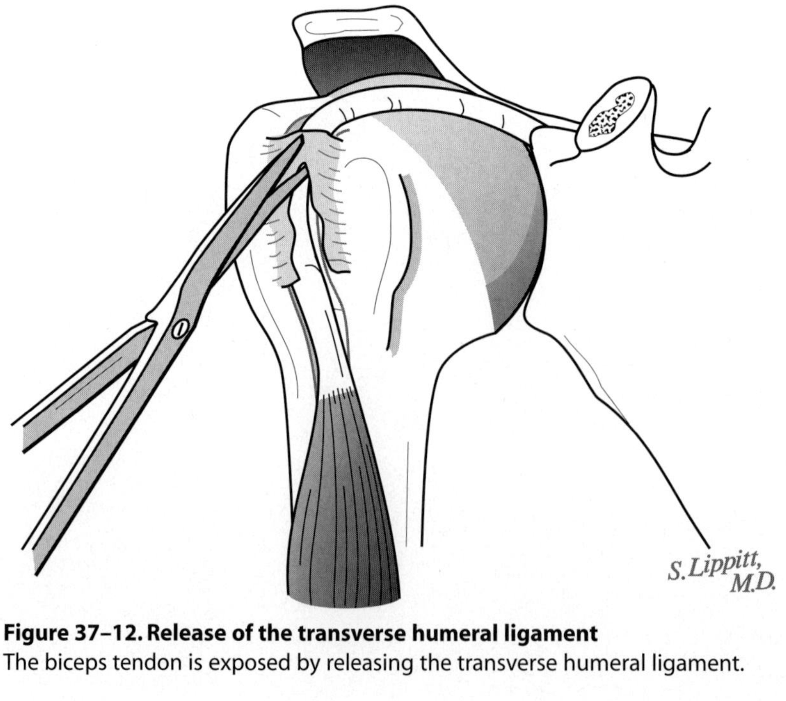


**Figure 37–12. Release of the transverse humeral ligament**
The biceps tendon is exposed by releasing the transverse humeral ligament.

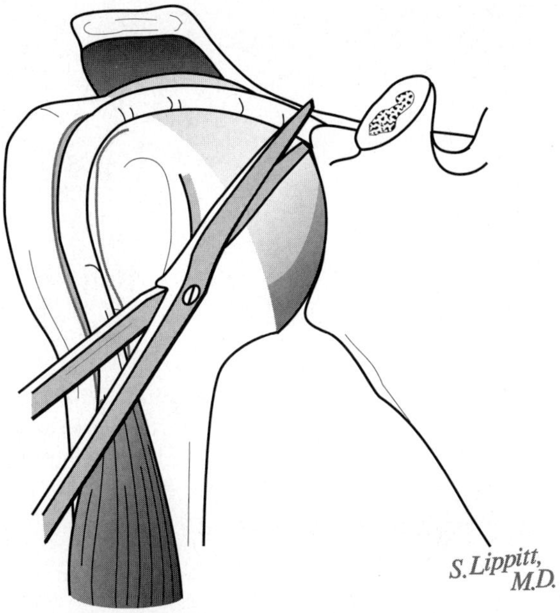


**Figure 37–13. Release of the biceps origin**
The biceps origin can then be released at the supraglenoid tubercle.

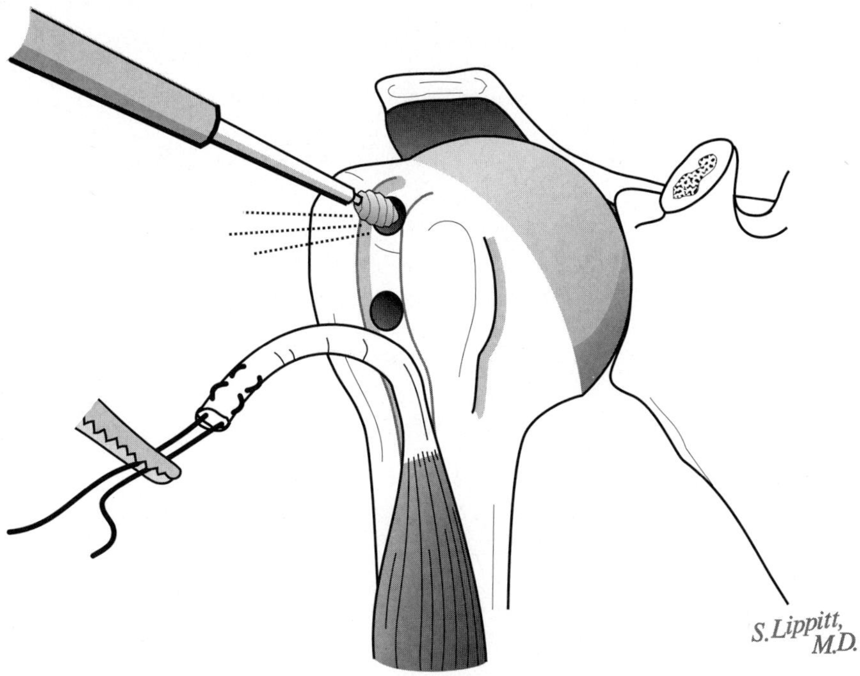


**Figure 37–14. Drill holes**
Two holes are made in the bicipital groove, leaving a 1 cm bridge between them.

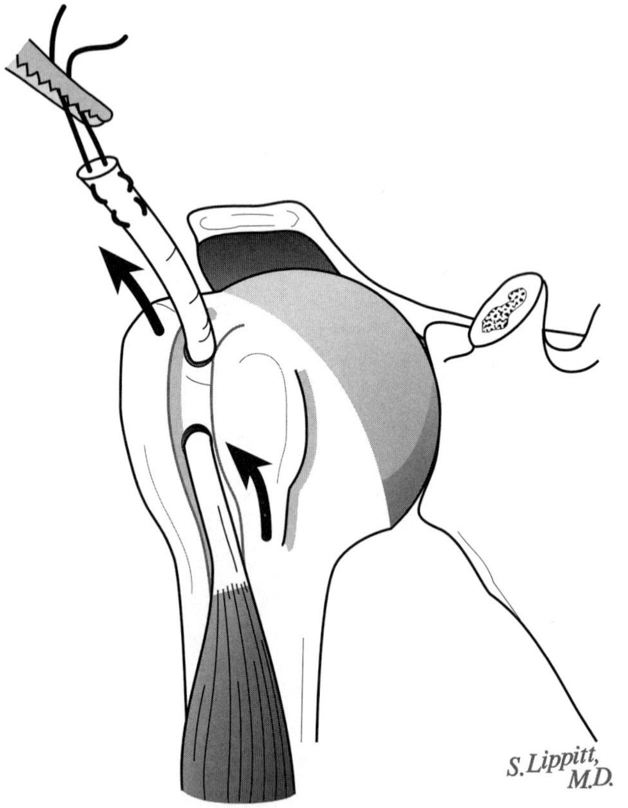


**Figure 37–15. Passing the long tendon**
The long tendon of the biceps is passed into the distal hole and out the proximal hole.

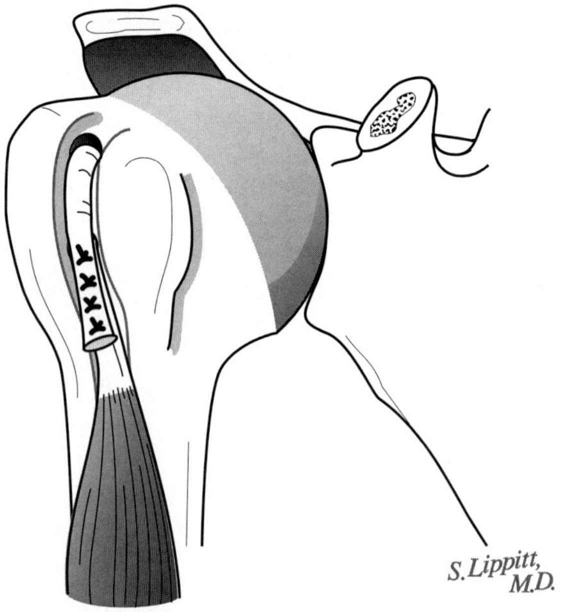


**Figure 37–16. Suturing the tendon**
The tendon exiting the proximal hole is then sutured to the tendon entering the distal hole.

- The next step is, while protecting the axillary nerve with the nondominant index finger, to release the inferior capsule from the inferior glenoid labrum (**Fig. 37–17**). Inserting a humeral head retractor into the joint and rotating its inferior aspect away from the glenoid puts the inferior capsule under tension, facilitating this release. The anterior and posterior bands of the inferior glenohumeral ligament are released. Exposure of the origin of the long head of the triceps signals a complete release (**Fig. 37–18**).
- The articular aspect of the joint is inspected and any bony prominences that potentially block motion are resected. Note is made of the condition of the glenoid and humeral joint surfaces.

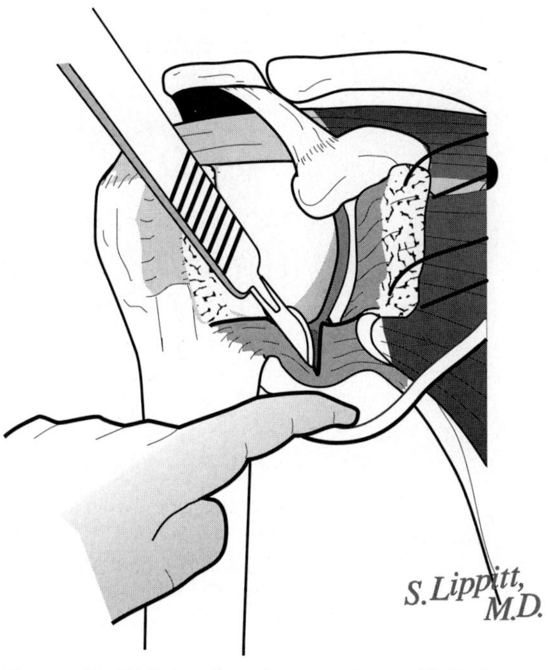


**Figure 37–17. Releasing the anterior and inferior capsule**
The anterior and inferior capsule is released under direct vision, with care taken to identify and protect the axillary nerve. (Modified from Matsen FA, Lippitt SB, Sidles JA, et al [eds]: Practical Evaluation and Management of the Shoulder. Philadelphia: WB Saunders, 1994, p. 205.)

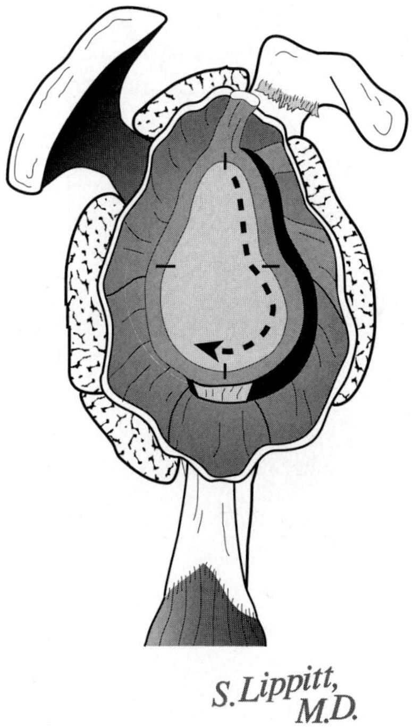


**Figure 37–18. Anterior capsule release**
The capsule is released outside the labrum to preserve the full depth of the glenoid concavity. The release begins at the origin of the long head of the biceps and continues past the origin of the long head of the triceps. This ensures that the anterior and posterior bands of the inferior glenohumeral ligament are released. (Modified from Matsen FA, Lippitt SB, Sidles JA, et al [eds]: Practical Evaluation and Management of the Shoulder. Philadelphia: WB Saunders, 1994, p. 205.)

- Finally, the posterior capsule is released from the posterior glenoid labrum. The capsule is placed under tension by rotating the humeral head retractor away from the glenoid, first inferiorly and then superiorly (**Figs. 37–19** and **37–20**).

At the conclusion of the procedure, the shoulder is put through a full range of motion. The subscapularis tendon is closed robustly to the lesser tuberosity so that immediate, postoperative motion-maintaining exercises can be implemented.

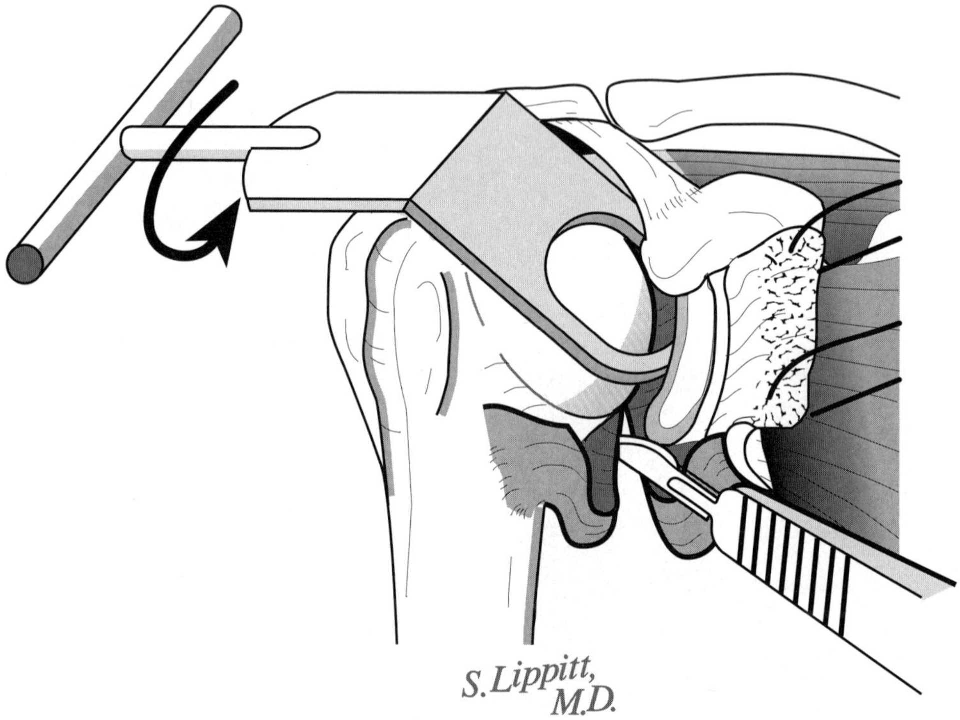


**Figure 37–19. Stiff posterior capsule release**
The posterior capsule is placed under tension by slightly internally rotating the humerus while a twist is applied to the retractor so that the inferior humerus is pushed away from the glenoid. This tensioning facilitates the safe and selective release of the capsule. (From Pearl ML, Lippitt SB: Shoulder arthroplasty with a modular prosthesis. Tech Orthop 8:151–162, 1994.)

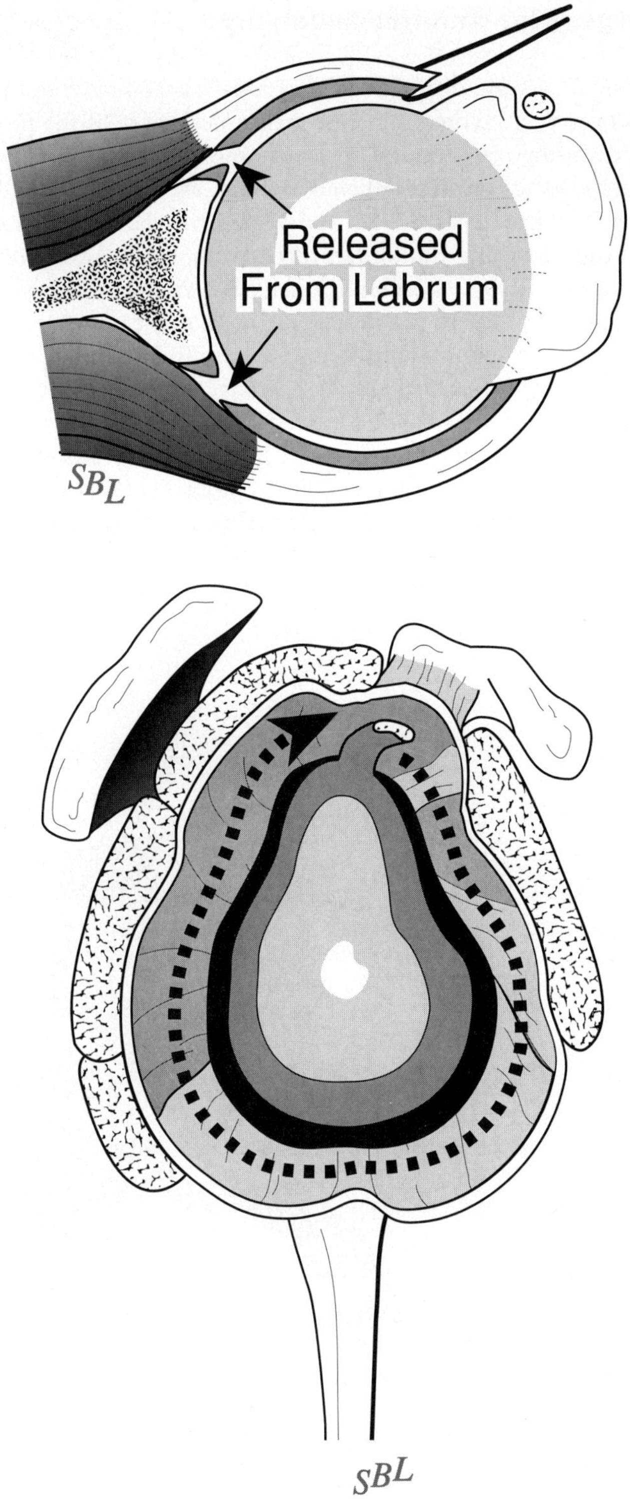


**Figure 37–20. Complete capsule release**
This diagram shows a complete extralabral release of the capsule, 360 degrees around the glenoid. (Modified from Matsen FA, Lippitt SB, Sidles JA, et al [eds]: Practical Evaluation and Management of the Shoulder. Philadelphia: WB Saunders, 1994, p. 138.)

## Revision Surgery for Anterior Instability (see Chapters 8–17)

Before embarking on a surgical revision for residual instability after a previous anterior repair, it is important to determine the mechanical cause of the residual instability. The patient's history is reviewed to learn whether the instability was initially traumatic or atraumatic. Previous operative notes are reviewed to determine the nature of the repair (**Figs. 37–21, 37–22,** and **37–23**). Special note is made of whether thermal or laser capsular cauterization was carried out. Physical examination seeks the presence of (1) an insufficient anterior glenoid lip as revealed by diminished resistance to an anterior load and shift test, (2) subscapularis insufficiency as revealed by diminished torque of internal rotation against the abdomen, and (3) anterior capsular insufficiency as indicated by an abnormally large range of external rotation. Excellent anteroposterior, axillary, and apical oblique radiographs are needed to determine the sufficiency of the anterior bony glenoid and the extent of any posterolateral humeral head defect. The location of suture anchors and other implants is determined. This preoperative evaluation should reveal the potential need for hardware removal instruments, anterior iliac crest graft, hamstring graft, and humeral hemiarthroplasty.

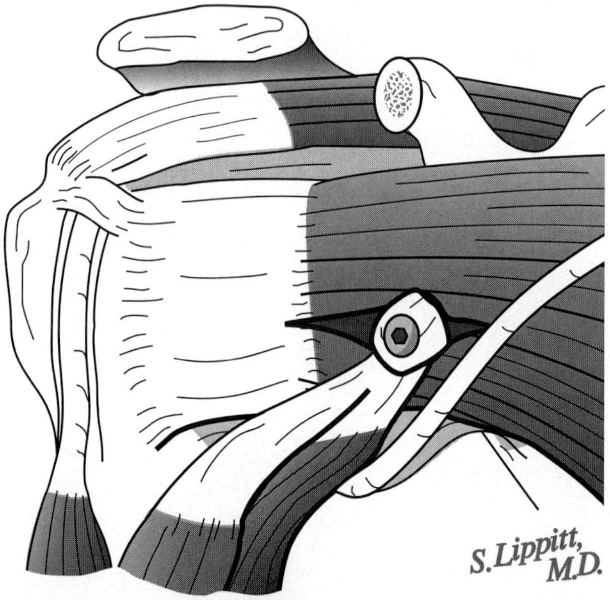


**Figure 37–21. Bristow transfer**
After a Bristow procedure, the subscapularis has been split and often damaged by the coracoid transfer. The axillary nerve may be very difficult to dissect safely.

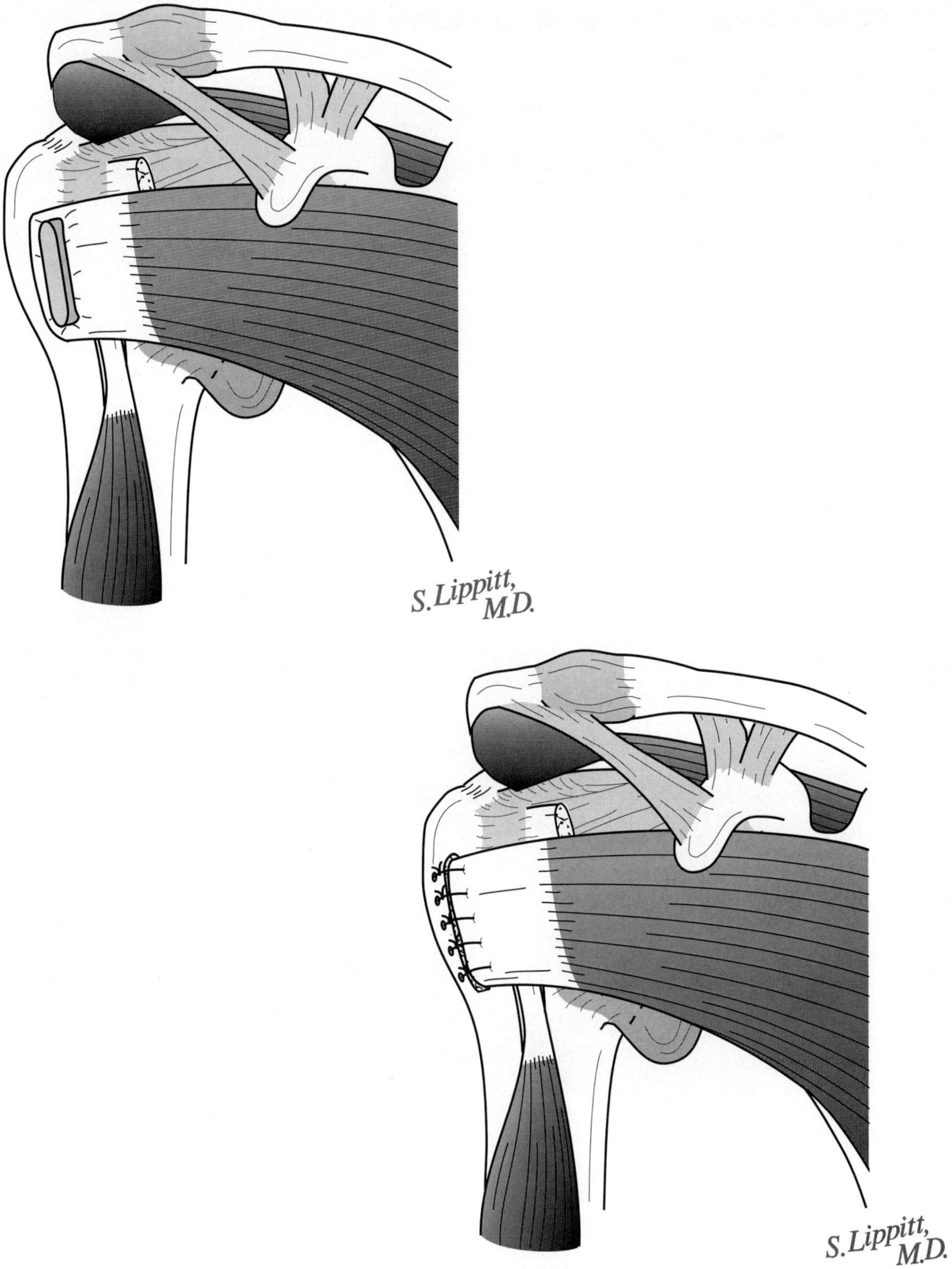


**Figure 37–22. Magnusen-Stack**
In the Magnusen-Stack procedure, the subscapularis tendon may be stapled or sutured lateral to the bicipital groove.

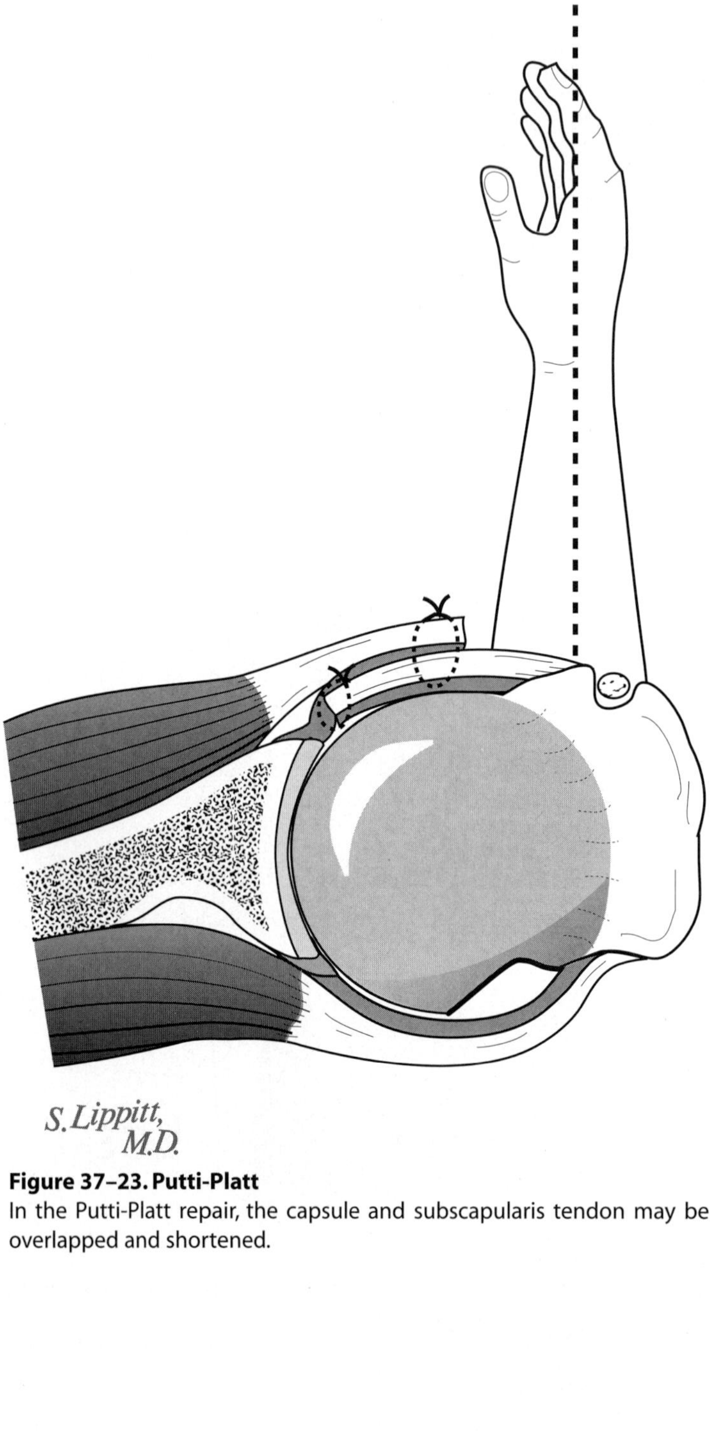


**Figure 37–23. Putti-Platt**
In the Putti-Platt repair, the capsule and subscapularis tendon may be overlapped and shortened.

If appropriate, the shoulder is approached through the previous incisional scar. The humeroscapular motion interface is freed of adhesions and prominent suture. The subscapularis is explored and the axillary nerve identified. The subscapularis is opened through a defect, if present, or incised through its weakest aspect. The capsule is opened through a defect if present, or, if not, it is incised near the lesser tuberosity. The anteroinferior glenoid is explored to verify the mechanical causes of the residual instability. The following is a list of the common findings and how they can be addressed surgically:

1. Failure of healing of the labrum to the glenoid lip (an unhealed Bankart lesion) **(Fig. 37–24)**—repair of the labrum and capsule onto the glenoid lip using drill holes in bone (see Chapter 11).

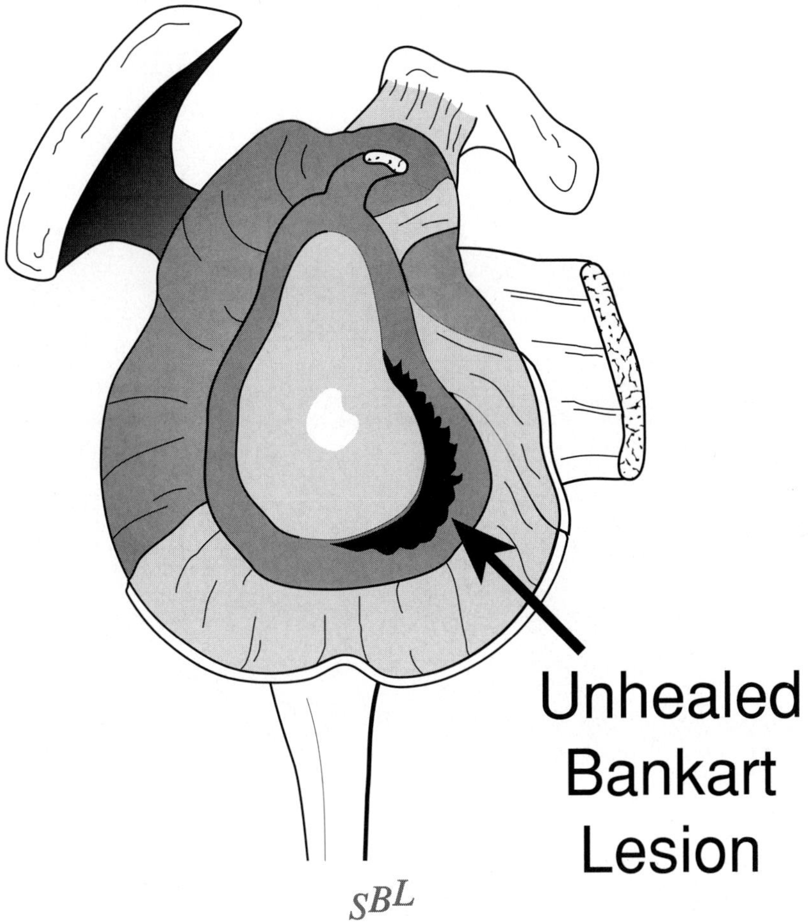


**Figure 37–24. Unhealed Bankart repair**
One of the most common causes of failure of surgical repair for anterior instability is an unhealed Bankart lesion. Persistence of this lesion compromises the attachment of the capsule and ligaments to the glenoid as well as the fossa-deepening effect of the labrum. (Modified from Matsen FA, Lippitt SB, Sidles JA, et al [eds]: Practical Evaluation and Management of the Shoulder. Philadelphia: WB Saunders, 1994, p. 103.)

2. Healing of the labrum to the medial neck of the glenoid rather than the glenoid lip (**Fig. 37–25**)—freeing of the labrum from the neck and repair of the labrum and capsule onto the glenoid lip using drill holes in bone (see Chapter 12).
3. A flattened glenoid labrum that does not deepen the glenoid fossa—a labral augmentation, either by bunching up the labrum and capsule with suture or by injection of autogenous blood into the labrum to fatten it, or both (see Chapter 15).

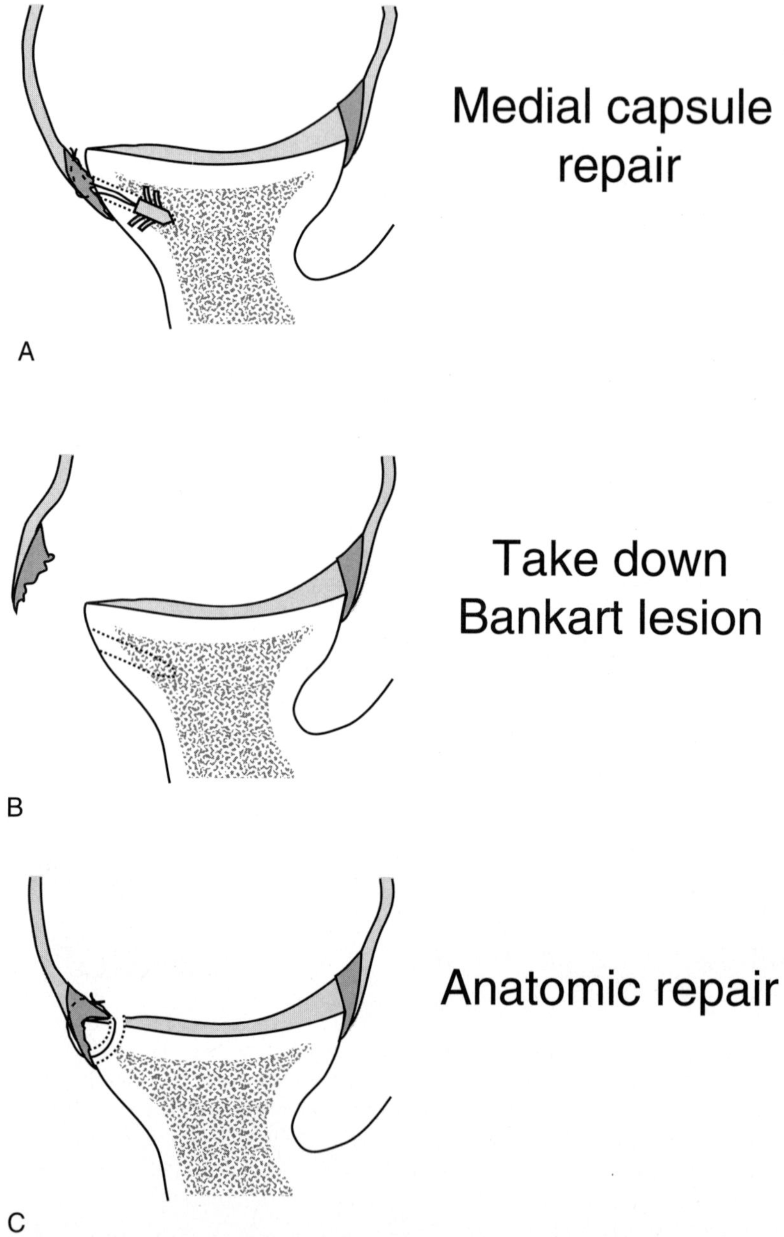


**Figure 37–25. Revision Bankart repair**
When the labrum and capsule heal to the medial glenoid neck, the effective glenoid concavity is not restored. In this situation, it is necessary to take down the previous repair and reattach the labrum and capsule to the glenoid lip using drill holes in bone. (Modified from Matsen FA, Lippitt SB, Sidles JA, et al [eds]: Practical Evaluation and Management of the Shoulder. Philadelphia: WB Saunders, 1994, p. 70.)

4. A bucket handle tear of the labrum (**Fig. 37–26**)—incorporation of the torn labrum into sutures of the capsule to the glenoid lip (see Chapter 11).

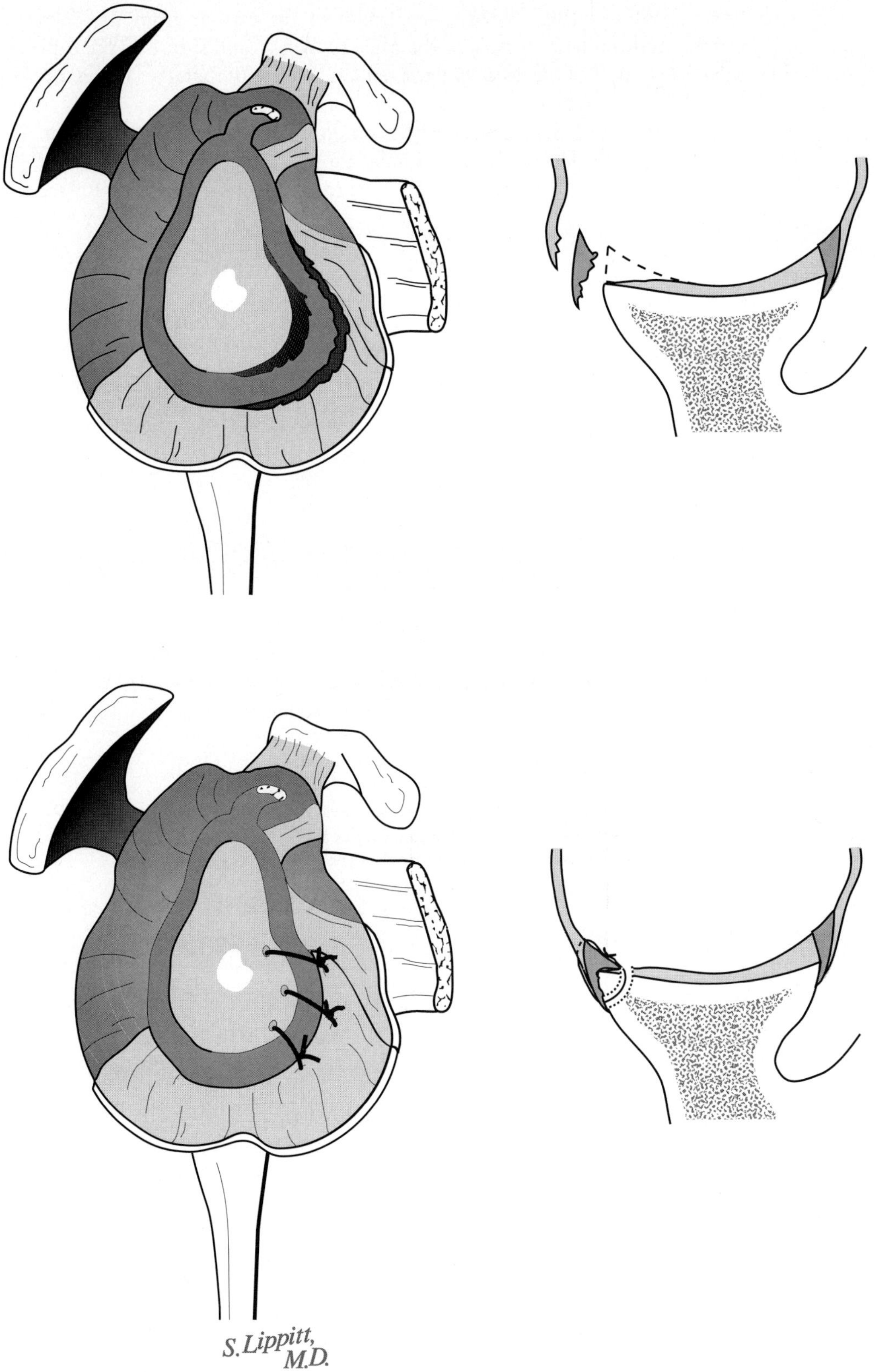


**Figure 37–26. Bucket handle tear**
When there is a bucket handle tear of the labrum, as shown here, the Bankart repair sutures are passed through holes in the glenoid lip, around the bucket handle tear of the labrum, and through the medial edge of the capsule. Tying these sutures incorporates the labrum in reconstituting the depth of the glenoid fossa.

5. Prominent suture anchors (**Fig. 37–27**)—removal, taking care to protect the integrity of the bone and cartilage at the glenoid lip.
6. A capsular defect lateral to the labrum (frequently seen after failed capsular cauterization procedures) (**Fig. 37–28**)—separation of the capsule from the deep aspect of the subscapularis, closure of the capsular defect, and suture of the capsule to the deep aspect of the subscapularis tendon at a length that does not excessively limit external rotation.
7. Significant flattening of the cartilage of the anteroinferior glenoid—restoration of the glenoid lip by repairing the labrum and capsule to the articular surface of the glenoid or an anatomically contoured extracapsular iliac crest graft (see Chapter 12).

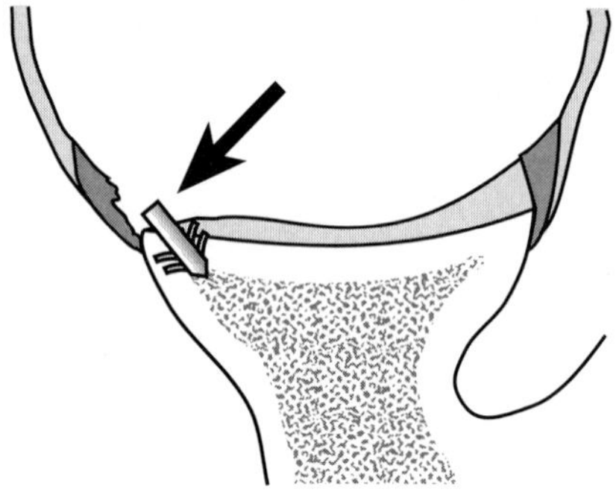

**Figure 37–27. Prominent anchors**
Prominent metal or absorbable suture anchors must be removed, with care taken to preserve as much of the glenoid bone and cartilage as possible. This may require carefully drilling around them with a small drill. A needle holder is often the best tool for suture anchor removal.

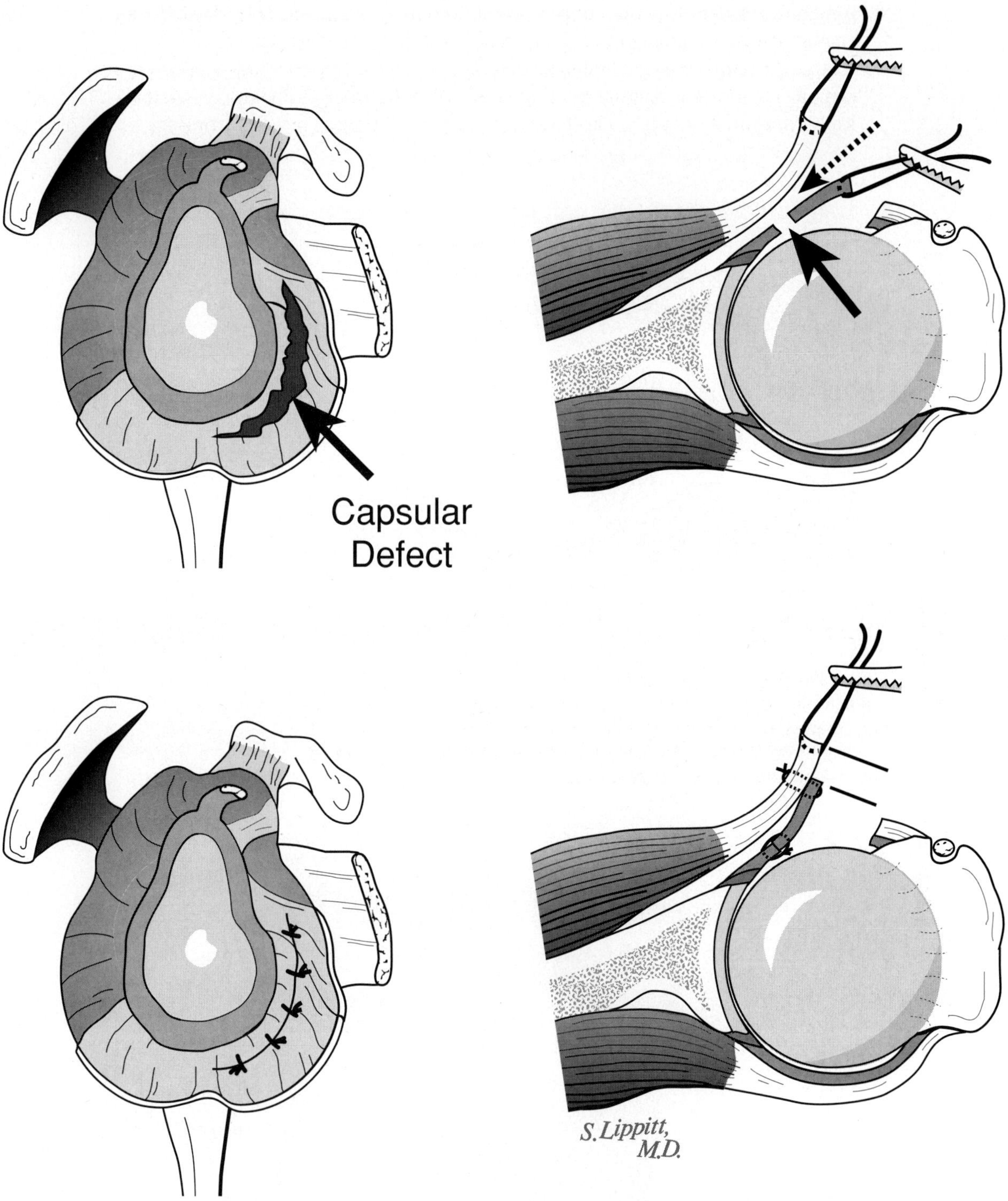


**Figure 37–28. Capsule defect**

Defects in the capsule may be difficult to close, especially after thermal coagulation. Sometimes the capsule can be freed laterally from the subscapularis, the defect closed, and the lateral edge of the capsule closed to the deep side of the subscapularis to avoid limiting external rotation.

8. A significant defect in the bone of the anteroinferior glenoid **(Fig. 37–29)**—an anatomically contoured extracapsular iliac crest graft (see Chapter 12).
9. A large posterolateral humeral head defect (Hill-Sachs) **(Fig. 37–30)**—approaches can include limiting external rotation, beefing up the anterior lip with an anatomically contoured extracapsular iliac crest graft, or a humeral hemiarthroplasty.

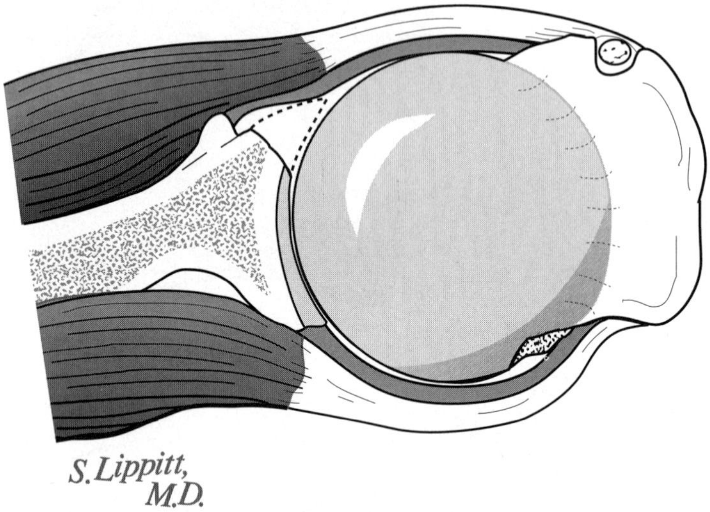


**Figure 37–29. Anterior glenoid rim defect**
A significant defect in the anterior bony lip of the glenoid as shown here may require reconstruction with an extracapsular iliac crest graft. (Modified from Rockwood CA, Matsen FA [eds]: The Shoulder, 2nd ed. Philadelphia: WB Saunders, 1998, p. 615.)

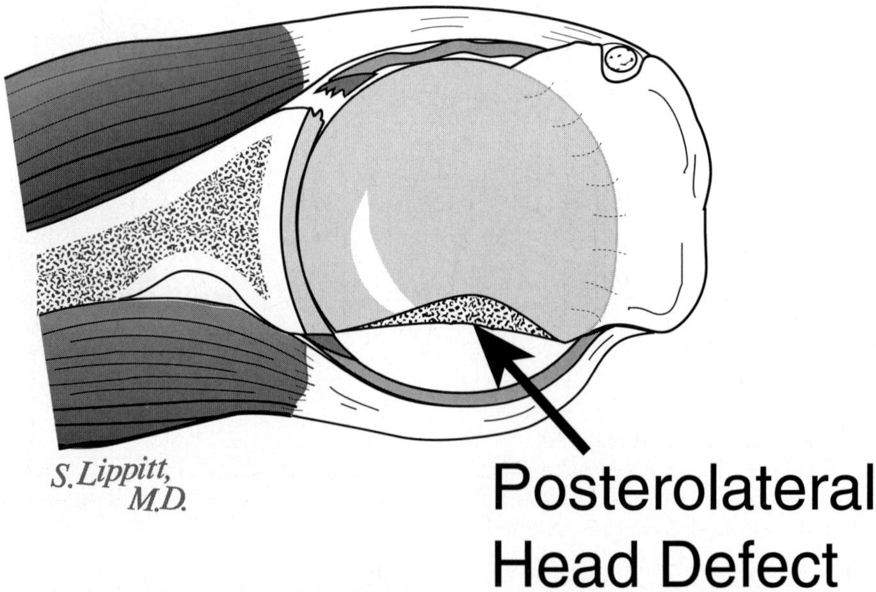


**Figure 37–30. Large Hill-Sachs defect**
In general, the presence of a Hill-Sachs defect (impaction fracture of the posterior-lateral humeral head) does not change the treatment. However, when the lesion is sufficiently large that the glenoid falls into the defect on external rotation of the humerus, special measures such as limitation of external rotation, anterior iliac crest graft, or humeral prosthetic arthroplasty may be necessary.

10. Anterior capsular deficiency allowing excessive external rotation (**Fig. 37–31**)—anterior capsular reconstruction using hamstring autograft through drill holes in the anterior glenoid lip and the lesser tuberosity (see Chapter 16).
11. Subscapularis tendon defect (**Fig. 37–32**)—primary repair if there is sufficient quantity and quality of tendon tissue remaining; hamstring autograft if there is sufficient muscle but insufficient tendon; if muscle is not amenable to reconstruction, a capsular reconstruction (see Chapter 16) to limit external rotation with or without a pectoralis major transfer.

All aspects of the repair should be sufficiently robust that the shoulder can be started on a 90-degree flexion and 0-degree external rotation program immediately after surgery, so that unintended stiffness does not result.

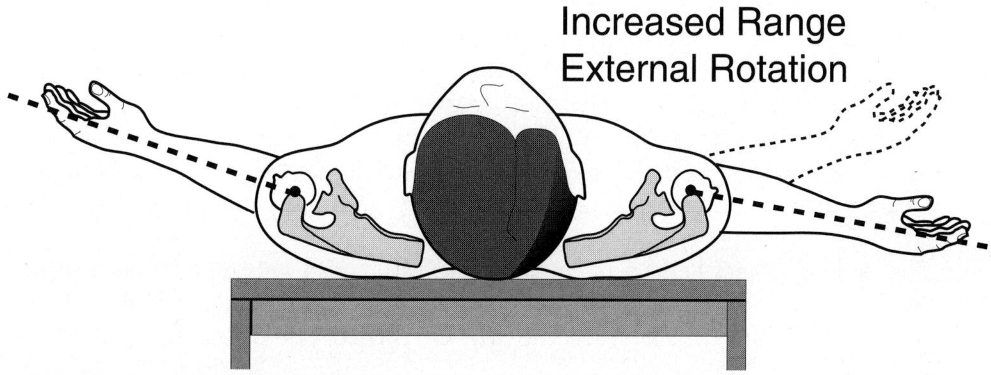


**Figure 37–31. Excess external rotation**
An increase in external rotation suggests failure of the subscapularis and capsule.

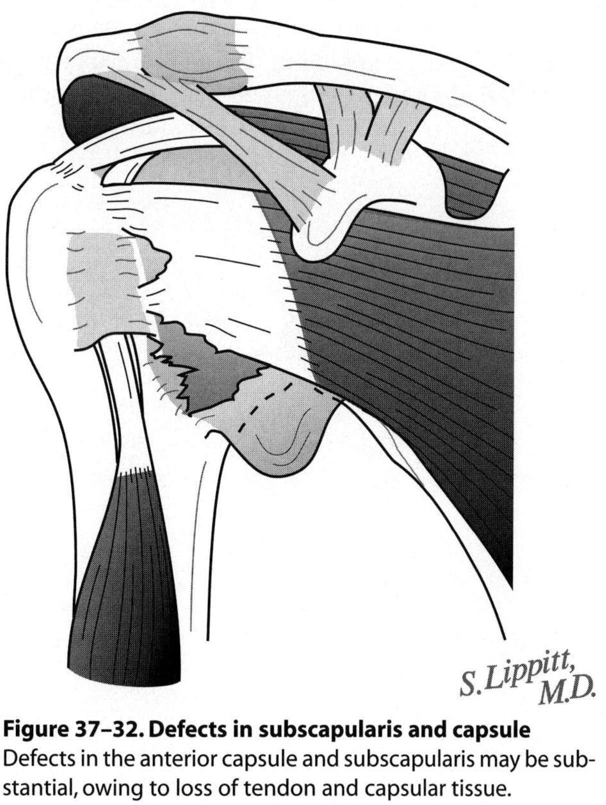


**Figure 37–32. Defects in subscapularis and capsule**
Defects in the anterior capsule and subscapularis may be substantial, owing to loss of tendon and capsular tissue.

## **Revision Surgery for Posterior Instability** (see Chapters 8–17)

Before embarking on a surgical revision for residual instability after a previous posterior repair, it is important to determine the mechanical cause of the residual instability. The history is reviewed to learn whether the instability was initially traumatic or atraumatic. Previous operative notes are reviewed to determine the nature of the repair. Special note is made of whether thermal or laser capsular cauterization was carried out. It is also important to note whether the external rotators were taken down and repaired at the previous surgery.

Physical examination seeks the presence of (1) an insufficient posterior glenoid lip as revealed by diminished resistance to a posterior load and shift test, (2) infraspinatus insufficiency as revealed by diminished external rotation torque, and (3) posterior capsular insufficiency as indicated by an abnormally large range of internal rotation.

Excellent anteroposterior and axillary radiographs are needed to determine the sufficiency of the posterior bony glenoid and the extent of any anteromedial humeral head defect. The location of suture anchors and other implants is determined.

This preoperative evaluation should reveal the potential need for hardware removal instruments, posterior glenoid osteoplasty, posterior iliac crest graft, humeral hemiarthroplasty, or hamstring allograft. If it is determined that the primary mechanical cause of the recurrent posterior glenohumeral instability is the loss of the humeral articular surface, the surgical approach is anterior and the procedure is a humeral hemiarthroplasty.

The patient is anesthetized in the supine position and an examination is performed to confirm the preoperative understanding of the pathomechanics. It is critical to determine which procedure will be carried out before the patient is positioned.

Unless a shoulder arthroplasty is envisioned, the patient is carefully positioned prone with the arm draped free, and the posterior iliac crest is prepped if a posterior iliac crest graft might be needed. Commonly, the mechanical cause for the recurrent instability is a deficient posterior glenoid lip as manifest by diminished resistance to the posterior load and shift test. In that the posterior capsule is often frail, especially after previous surgery, it may not be useful in the revision repair. Study of the preoperative axillary view (and computed tomography scan if necessary) should reveal whether there is sufficient bone for a posterior glenoid osteoplasty **(Fig. 37–33)** or

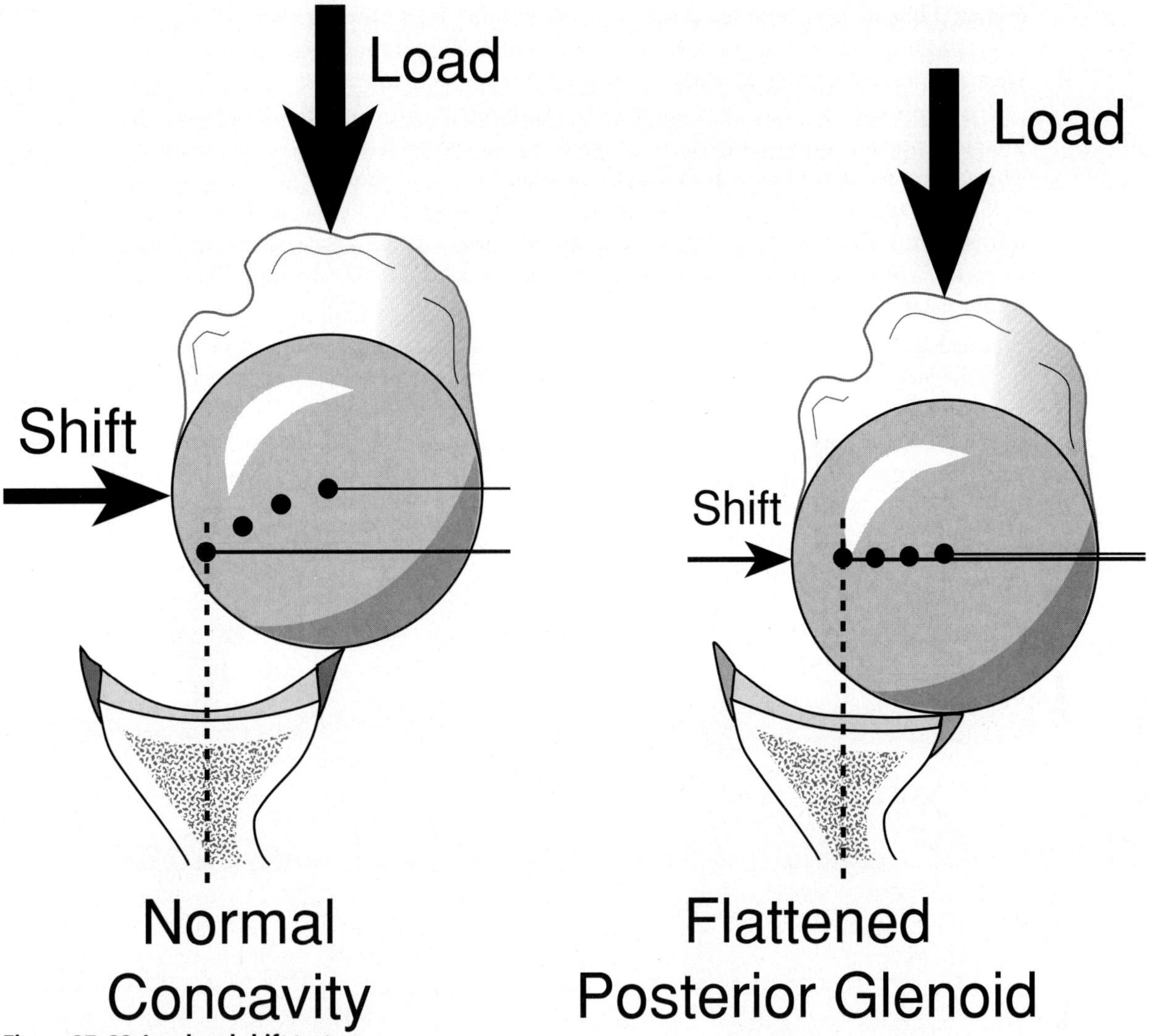


**Figure 37–33. Load and shift test**

When the posterior glenoid lip is insufficient, there is minimal resistance to the load and shift test. The lack of a posterior lip may benefit from a posterior glenoid osteoplasty if there is sufficient posterior glenoid bone.

enough bone deficiency of the posterior glenoid bone stock (for example, after a previous posterior glenoid lip fracture) that an anatomically contoured extracapsular iliac crest graft is needed (**Fig. 37–34**).

If appropriate, the shoulder is approached through the previous incisional scar. The humeroscapular motion interface is freed of adhesions and prominent sutures. The axillary nerve is identified as it exits the quadrilateral space.

The infraspinatus is opened through a defect, if present. If there is no defect in the infraspinatus, this muscle and its tendon are left intact to the greater tuberosity and dissected from the capsule and reflected upward toward the nerve supply. The teres minor is left below, protecting the axillary nerve.

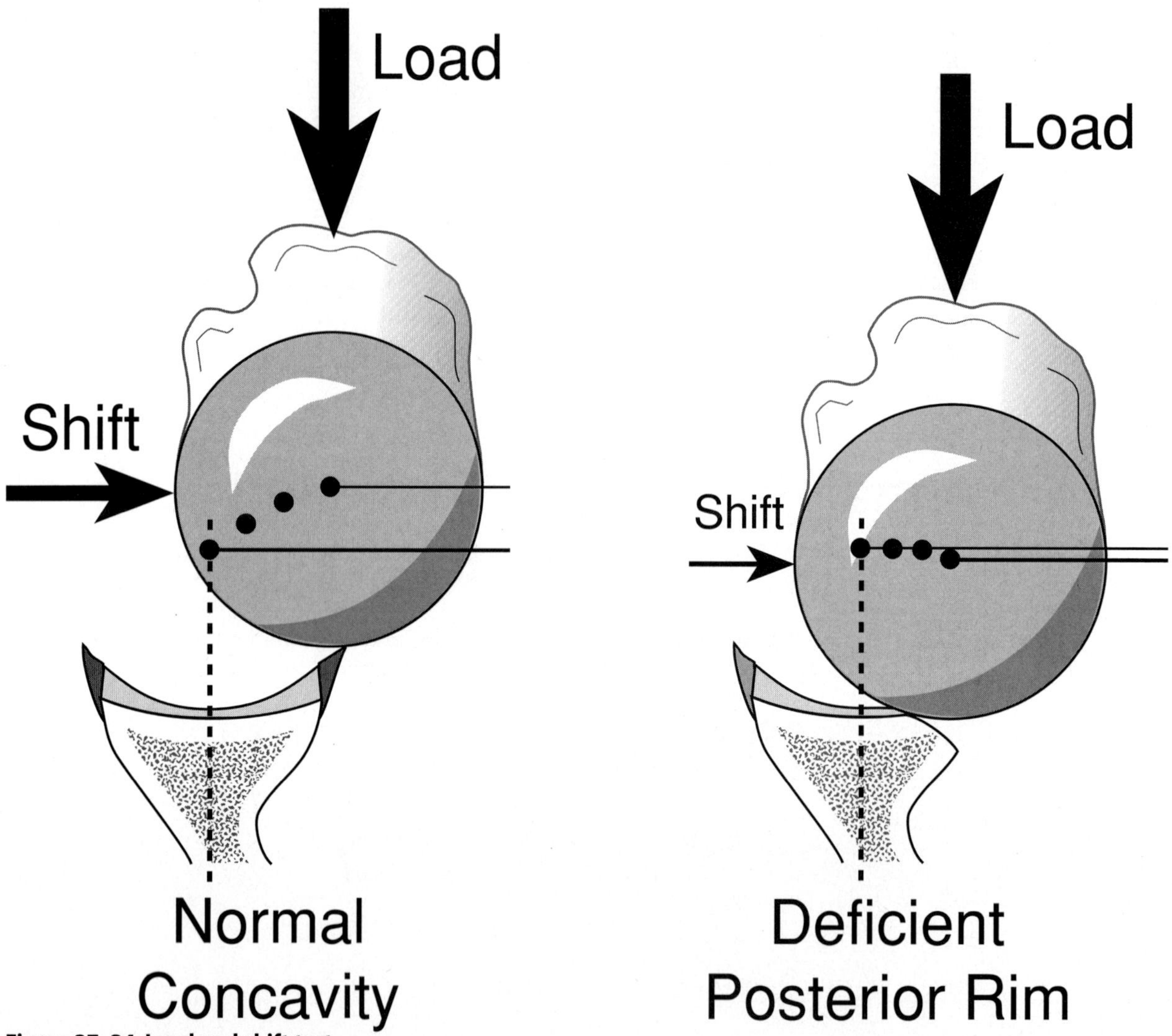


**Figure 37–34. Load and shift test**
When the posterior glenoid lip is insufficient and there is inadequate bone for a posterior glenoid osteoplasty, an extracapsular iliac crest graft may be needed.

The capsule is opened through a defect, if present. If there is no capsular defect and if a posterior glenoid osteoplasty or a posterior glenoid osteotomy is planned, a horizontal capsulotomy is made to monitor the joint surface during the procedure.

The following is a list of the common findings and how they can be addressed surgically:

1. Failure of healing of a previous incision in the posterior rotator cuff—direct repair is usually possible; otherwise, a hamstring allograft may be needed (hamstring autografts are more difficult to harvest with the patient in the prone position) (see Chapter 16).
2. Failure of healing of a previous incision in the posterior capsule—direct repair or autograft reconstruction may be possible, although the tissue may be very flimsy, such that neither reconstruction nor repair is possible. In this situation, we often turn to a bony procedure to augment posterior stability by building up the posterior glenoid lip.
3. Insufficient posterior glenoid lip with adequate posterior bone stock—a posterior glenoid osteoplasty (see Chapter 15).
4. Insufficient posterior glenoid lip without adequate posterior bone stock—an anatomically contoured extracapsular iliac crest graft (see Chapter 13).
5. Insufficient anteromedial humeral articular surface **(Fig. 37–35)**—a humeral hemiarthroplasty with the same diameter of curvature as the biological head and with a neck length sufficient to limit the posterior drawer to no more than 50% of the glenoid width and internal rotation in abduction to no more than 60 degrees to provide stability when the arm is brought forward and across the body (see Chapter 29).

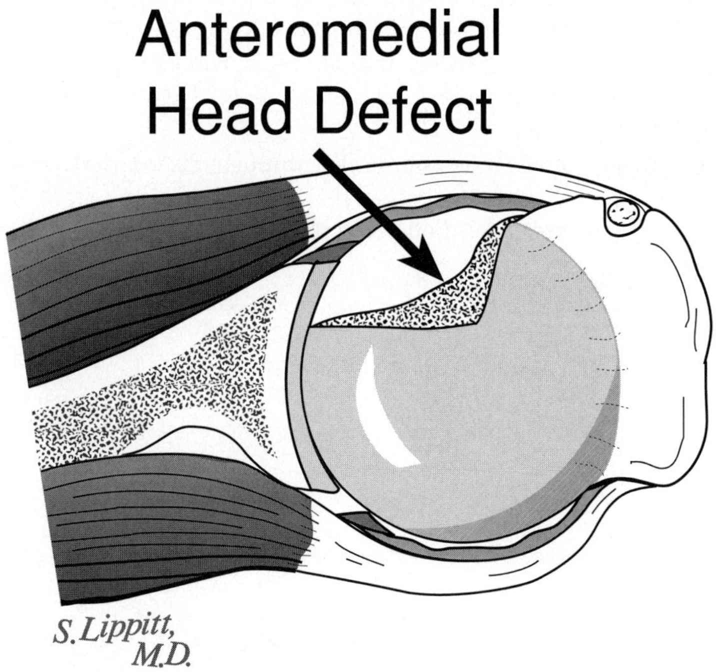


**Figure 37–35. Reversed Hill-Sachs defect**
A major defect in the anterior humeral articular surface may require humeral hemiarthroplasty.

## **Revision Surgery for Strength** (see Chapters 18–24)

Before embarking on a surgical revision for residual weakness after a previous rotator cuff repair, it is important to determine the mechanical cause of the residual weakness. Many of these causes do not have effective surgical treatment: deltoid denervation, deltoid detachment, suprascapular nerve lesions, or insufficient quality and quantity of rotator cuff tissue. The most promising situation is one in which the previous cuff repair was functioning well until the time of a definite re-injury with a force sufficient to disrupt a strong repair. In this situation, a second repair may restore the integrity of the cuff.

We are not convinced that, in our hands, muscle transfers (infraspinatus, subscapularis, deltoid, latissimus, teres major, or others) are effective in improving strength after failed cuff repair. Neither are we convinced that, in our hands, tendon grafts (hamstring, tensor fascia lata, allograft, xenograft, or prosthetic grafts) are helpful in restoring strength to a shoulder after a failed previous cuff surgery.

The patient's history is reviewed to learn whether the original cuff tear was traumatic or atraumatic and whether a major intercurrent injury reproduced the weakness that was present before the index surgery. Previous operative notes are reviewed to determine the technique used in the repair. The history taking, physical examination, and standard radiographic examination are conducted to seek evidence of deltoid detachment, cervical radiculopathy, brachial neuritis, peripheral nerve lesions, cuff tear arthropathy, tuberosity avulsion, prominent or loose suture anchors, supraspinatus and infraspinatus atrophy, or other findings that would affect the treatability of the problem. Expert dynamic sonography is, in our hands, more helpful in evaluating the rotator cuff integrity after previous repairs than magnetic resonance imaging (MRI) or arthrography. Sometimes the cause of failure after cuff surgery is stiffness without loss of cuff integrity. In this case, the shoulder is approached as described at the beginning of this chapter.

The patient is counseled that revision surgery is unlikely to restore the integrity of the rotator cuff unless there was a major reinjury or a primary failure of healing of the initial repair. However, it is possible that shoulder comfort and function can be improved with a "smooth and move" procedure, even if repair is not possible (see Chapters 20, 21, 22).

If appropriate, the shoulder is approached through the previous incisional scar. The deltoid-on approach is used so that the integrity of the deltoid is optimized (**Fig. 37–36**). The humeroscapular motion interface is freed of adhesions and prominent

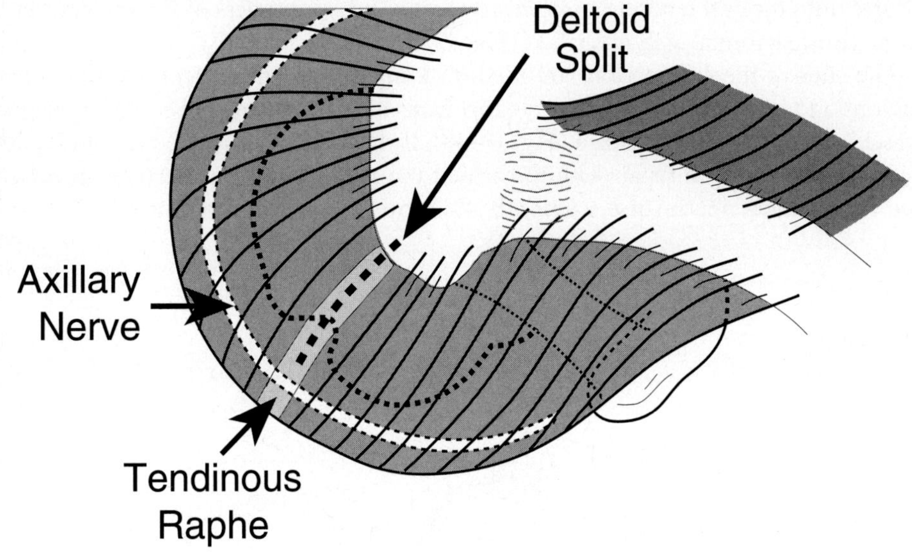


A

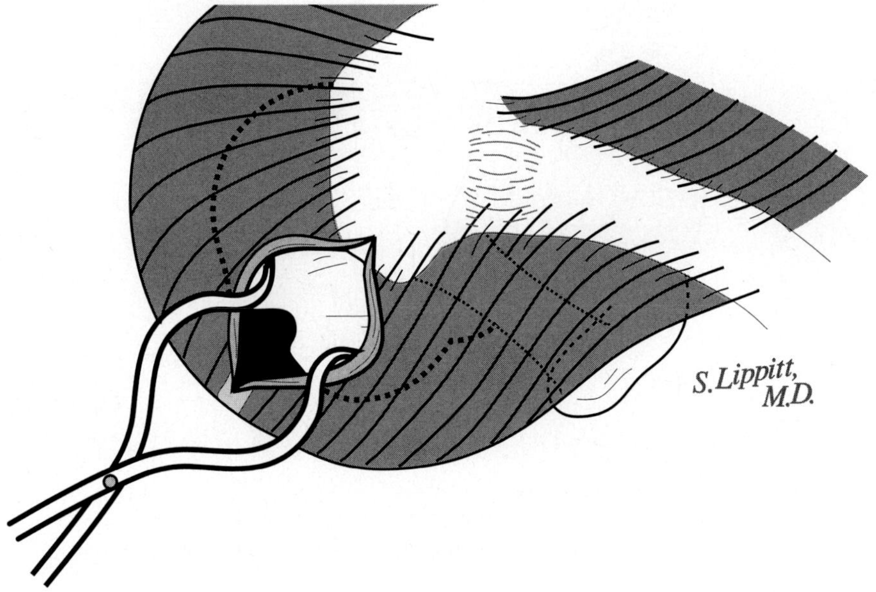


B

**Figure 37–36. Deltoid split**
The deltoid-on approach allows exploration of the subacromial space and the rotator cuff without compromising the deltoid origin. (Modified from Matsen FA, Lippitt SB, Sidles JA, et al [eds]: Practical Evaluation and Management of the Shoulder. Philadelphia: WB Saunders, 1994, p. 135.)

sutures until the cuff tendon can be clearly seen. The smoothness of the undersurface of the coracoacromial arch is verified (**Fig. 37–37**).

The ends of the cuff tendons are identified and tagged with traction sutures. The tendons and subjacent capsule are released from the glenoid labrum so that maximal muscle excursion can be realized (**Fig. 37–38**). If there is sufficient quantity and quality for a secure tendon repair with the arm at the side, a repeat primary repair is carried out. If this is not the case, a smooth and move procedure is conducted.

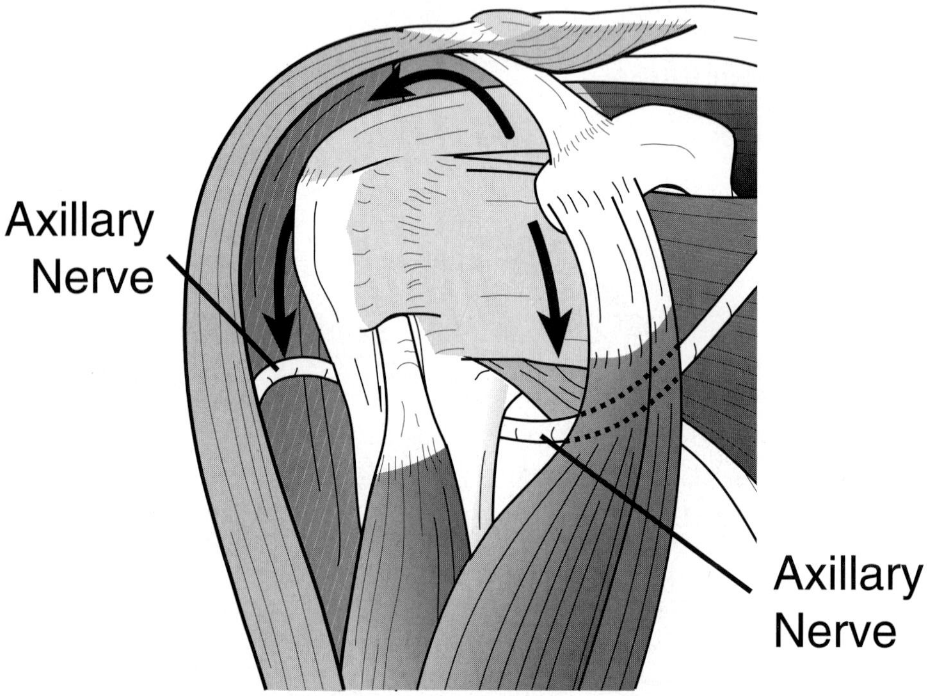


**Figure 37–37. Nerve-to-nerve release**
In revision cuff surgery, it is important to release the humeroscapular motion interface from the axillary nerve medially, under the coracoacromial arch to the axillary nerve laterally.

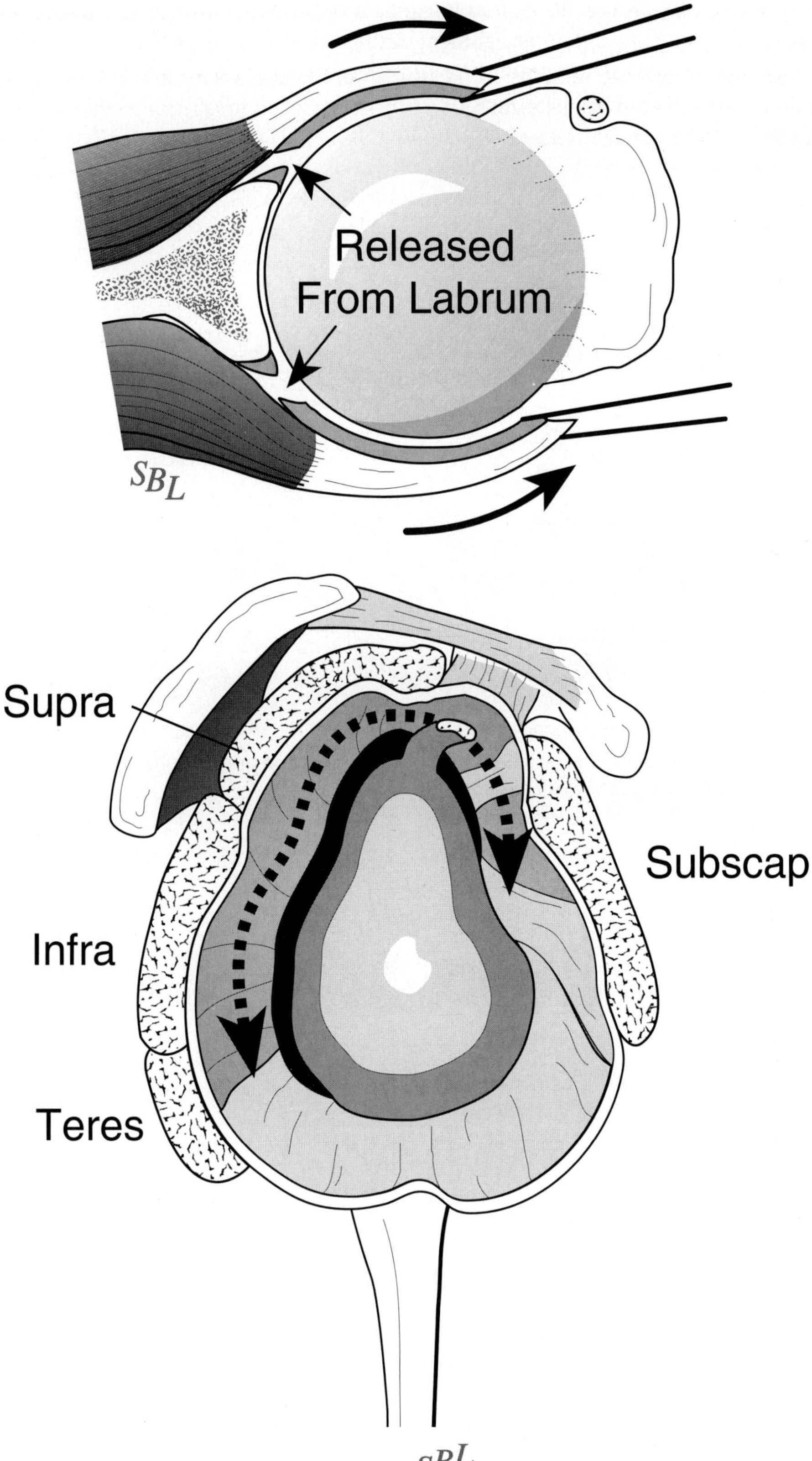


**Figure 37–38. Cuff capsule release**

Releasing the capsule from the labrum around the periphery of the glenoid will help the cuff tendon to be advanced laterally to its insertion on the tuberosities without excessive tension. (Modified from Matsen FA, Lippitt SB, Sidles JA, et al [eds]: Practical Evaluation and Management of the Shoulder. Philadelphia: WB Saunders, 1994, p. 138.)

At the time of closure, the deltoid integrity is optimized; however, it is uncommon to be able to restore a deltoid detachment to the acromion and clavicle (**Fig. 37–39**).

Any repairs carried out should be of sufficient strength to allow early passive motion so that unwanted adhesions are avoided.

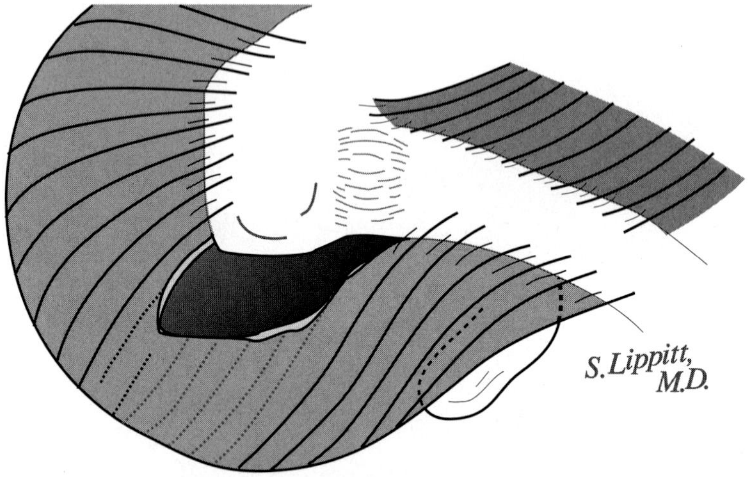


**Figure 37–39. Deficient deltoid origin**
A chronic deltoid detachment may become retracted and atrophic, making anatomic repair difficult or impossible.

## Revision Surgery After a Shoulder Arthroplasty

(see Chapters 25–32)

Before embarking on a surgical revision of a shoulder arthroplasty, it is important to determine the nature of the patient's problems. The following is a list of the common causes of shoulder arthroplasty failure:

- Infection
- Reaction to polyethylene or polymethyl methacrylate
- Fracture
- Stiffness
    - Poor rehabilitation
    - Unwanted bone
    - Tuberosity malunion
    - Overstuffing of the joint
- Instability
    - Anterior
        - Subscapularis deficiency
        - Glenoid component anteversion
        - Tuberosity nonunion
        - Supraspinatus/infraspinatus defect
        - Humeral component anteversion or anterior head offset
        - Insufficient anterior glenoid bone
    - Posterior
        - Glenoid component retroversion
        - Posterior cuff defect
        - Excessive humeral component retroversion or posterior head offset
        - Insufficient posterior glenoid bone
    - Superior
    - Loss of rotator cuff
    - Loss of coracoacromial arch
- Weakness
    - Reduced muscle strength
    - Subscapularis deficiency
    - Supraspinatus/infraspinatus deficiency
    - Tuberosity nonunion or malunion
    - Deltoid detachment
    - Nerve injury
- Humeral component
    - Malpositioned
    - Loose
- Glenoid
    - Bone eroded (hemiarthroplasty)
    - Component malpositioned
    - Component loose

The patient's history and previous records are reviewed to learn the status of the patient and shoulder prior to the index arthroplasty. What were the details of the reconstruction, including the manufacturer, model, and size of the prostheses? How was the rehabilitation conducted? Is there evidence of infection or allergic reaction? Has there been an intercurrent injury? What is the patient's status with respect to nutrition, pain medications, smoking, alcohol, and other concurrent health conditions?

The work-up includes a detailed examination of the motion, stability, strength, and smoothness of the shoulder.

Electromyography and nerve conduction studies, computed tomographic scans, and expert sonography may be useful in evaluating the nerve function, bone, and rotator cuff, respectively.

Laboratory studies include a complete blood cell count and measurement of sedimentation rate and serum albumin level.

Radiographs include an anteroposterior view in the plane of the scapula, an axillary view, and a full humeral view, all of high quality. In cases of instability, examination under fluoroscopy may be useful. The radiographic evaluation must confirm the type and size of components, their position, and the nature of their fixation to bone. The preoperative plan must include a definitive plan for removal of the glenoid and humeral components should this prove necessary, as well as a plan for reconstruction of the humerus and the glenoid after prosthesis removal (see Chapters 29, 30, 31, 32). If removal of a cemented humeral component may be necessary, it is essential to have a full set of cement removal tools, a high-speed saw capable of cutting a prosthetic stem, fluoroscopy, and long-stem prostheses of all possible sizes. The possible need for bone and tendon graft is also anticipated.

The shoulder is doubly prepped and draped as for a primary arthroplasty. Antibiotics are withheld until intraoperative fluid and tissue specimens have been obtained for aerobic, anaerobic, and fungal cultures. The previous incision is used if possible; however, a plan needs to be ready for extending the incision distally in the event of a fracture or the need to osteotomize the humerus for removal of the prosthesis. In these cases, we extend the deltopectoral incision down the lateral aspect of the arm, splitting the brachialis between its lateral quarter and its medial three quarters.

The humeroscapular motion interface is freed of adhesions and prominent suture. The axillary nerve is identified medially as it courses over the subscapularis and laterally as it exits the quadrilateral space. The subscapularis is explored and the axillary nerve identified. The subscapularis is opened through a defect if present or incised through its weakest aspect. If the subscapularis is intact, it is incised from the bone of the lesser tuberosity along with the subjacent capsule.

Tissue and fluid specimens are taken for Gram stain and cultures. Frozen sections are taken of any area of tissue suspicious for inflammation or tumor.

The following is a list of the common findings in failed shoulder arthroplasty and how they can be addressed surgically.

### *Infection*

The diagnosis of infection is made from culture at the time of revision surgery, when multiple samples are taken along with frozen sections. This is why it is so important to avoid administering antibiotics until multiple cultures are obtained to minimize the risk of sampling errors. For this reason, we do not start antibiotics after an aspiration in the office or emergency room because of the possibility that this culture may not yield a representative result (i.e., it may be falsely negative or contaminated by skin flora). If the infection is acute, the organism is sensitive to antibiotics, and the patient is healthy, we may elect a vigorous débridement of soft tissue inflammation, a surgical scrub of the joint surfaces, and irrigation with copious volumes of antibiotic saline solution. If the infection is established, we will usually remove all components and cement and then replace only an uncemented humeral component, smoothing the residual glenoid surface if needed. Culture-specific intravenous antibiotics are used for a minimum of 6 weeks.

*Reaction to Polyethylene or Polymethyl Methacrylate* (**Fig. 37–40**)

The diagnosis is suggested by a persistent inflammatory reaction in the absence of infection. The procedure may include removal of glenoid component, removal of glenoid cement, smoothing of glenoid bone as needed, removal of any humeral cement, humeral canal curettage, and implantation of a press-fit humeral component.

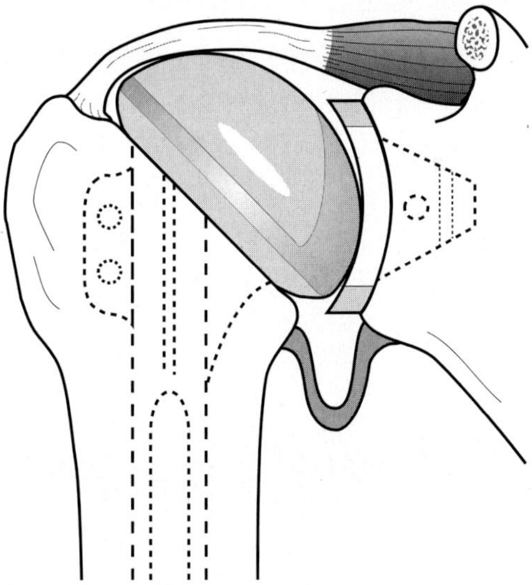

A

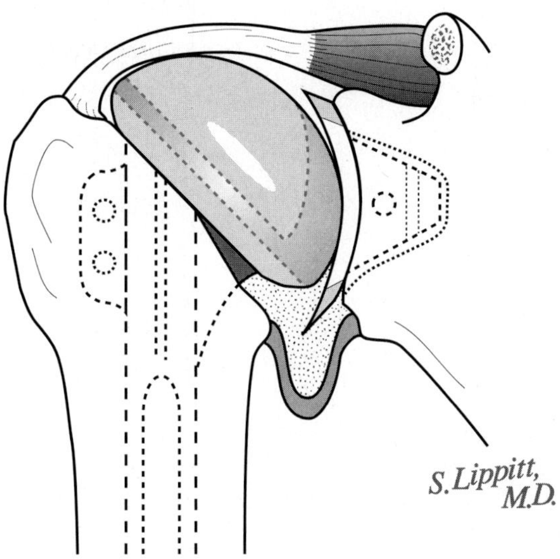


B

**Figure 37–40. Polyethylene wear**
Wear of the glenoid polyethylene results in loss of the normal glenoid shape; the wear particles may cause osteolysis around the glenoid and humeral components.

*Fracture*

The diagnosis is revealed by high-quality anteroposterior and lateral views that span the entire humerus, even if multiple films along the bone are necessary. Spiral fractures are treated with cerclage using a long-stem prosthesis to augment the fixation if necessary (**Fig. 37–41**). Transverse fractures at the distal tip of a well-fixed prosthesis may be managed by a plate with at least three solid screws in the proximal fragment tangential to the prosthesis (**Fig. 37–42**) or by a combination of cerclage and screw fixation of the plate (**Fig. 37–43**). If good fixation cannot be obtained, prosthesis removal and insertion of a long-stem prosthesis may be necessary. Autogenous bone graft is usually preferred.

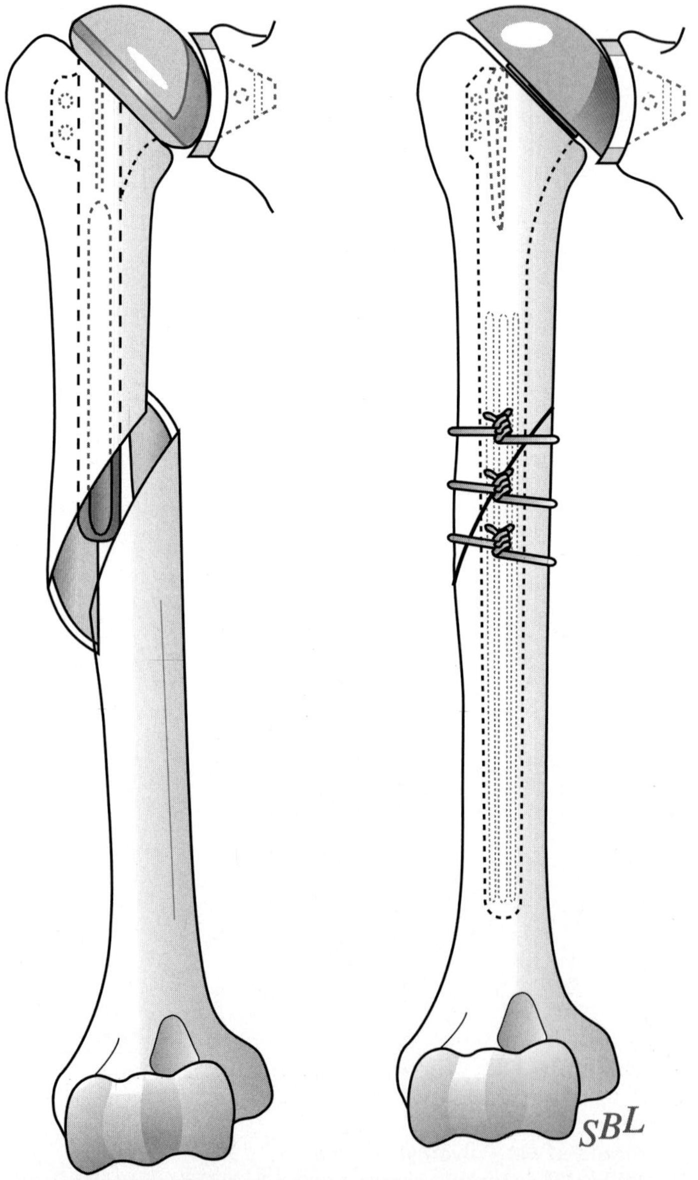


**Figure 37–41. Spiral fracture**
Spiral fractures at the level of the prosthesis tip can be stabilized by removal of the original humeral prosthesis, insertion of a long-stem prosthesis, and cerclage wiring.

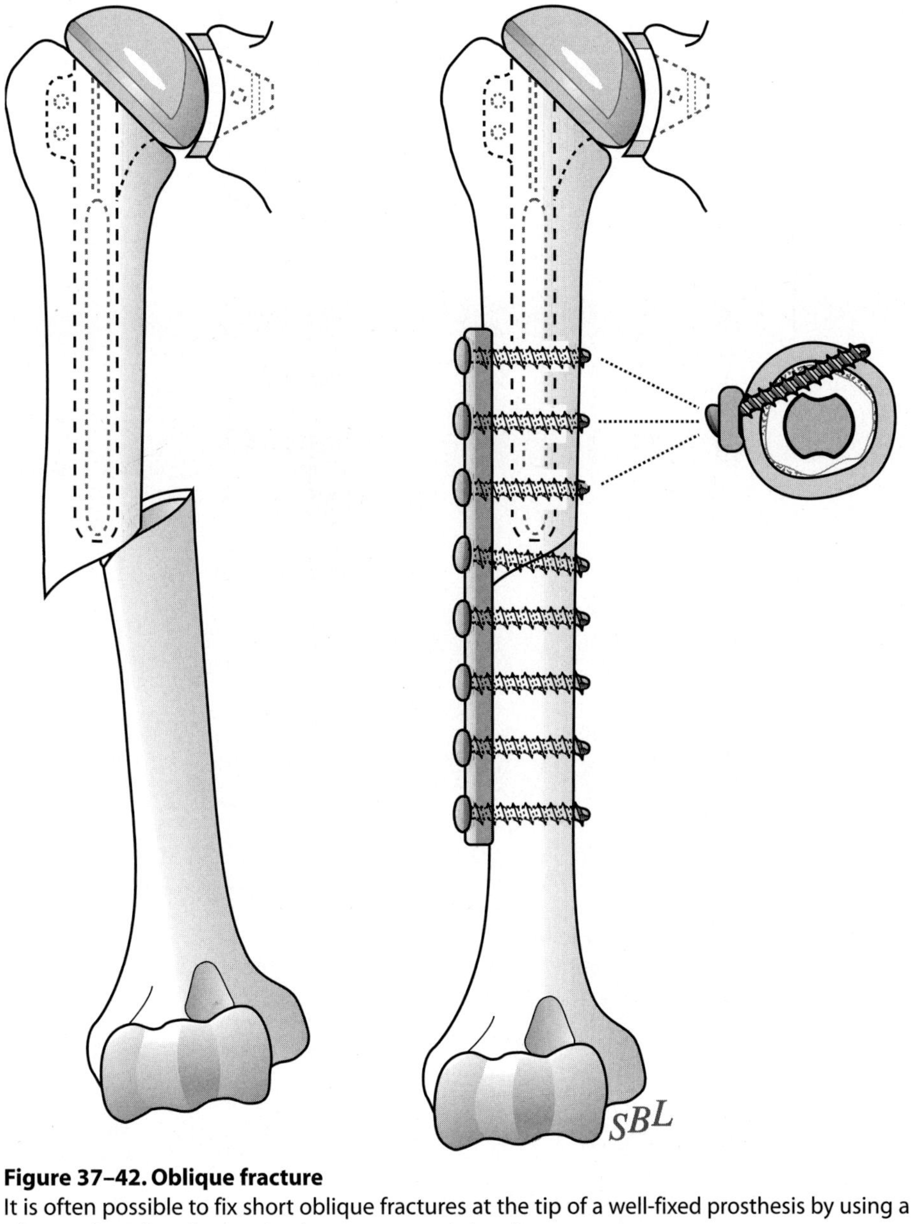


**Figure 37–42. Oblique fracture**
It is often possible to fix short oblique fractures at the tip of a well-fixed prosthesis by using a plate and angling the proximal screws around the plate.

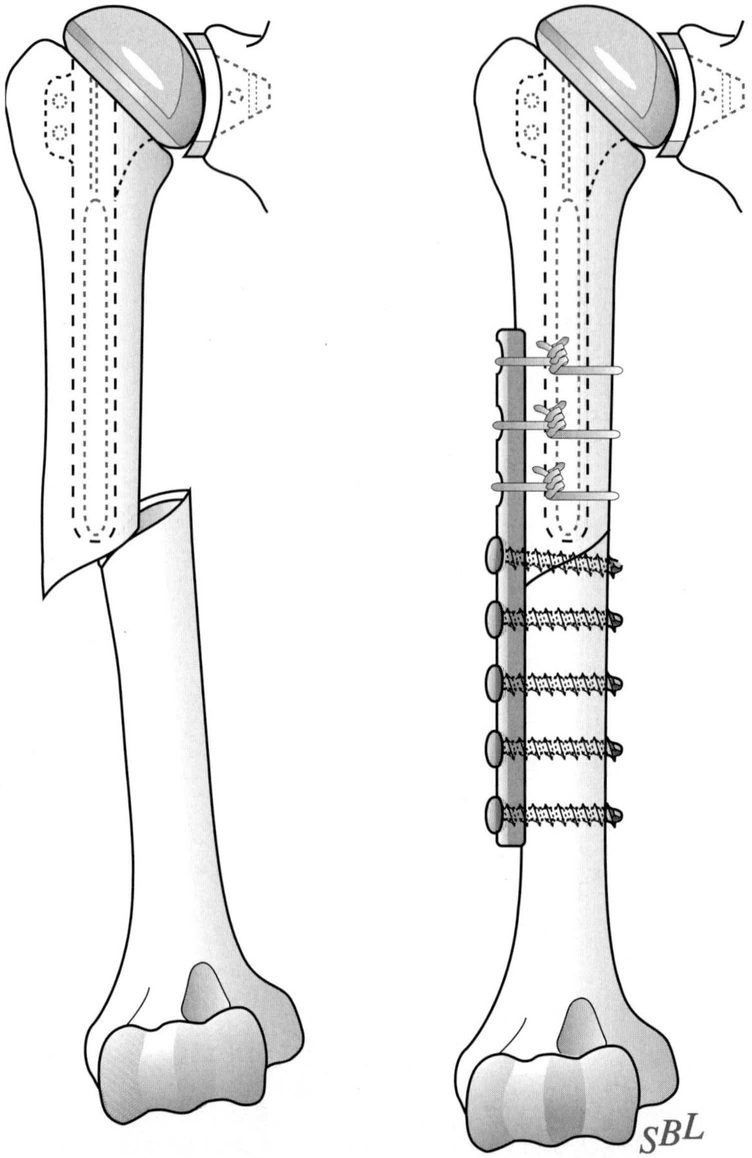


**Figure 37–43. Oblique fracture**
Alternatively, a plate can be screwed to the distal fragment and cerclage applied around the proximal fragment.

*Stiffness*

The diagnosis is made by the finding of reduced humeroscapular rotational laxity in flexion, cross-body adduction, internal and external rotation with the arm at the side, and internal and external rotation with the arm in 90 degrees of abduction. High-quality anteroposterior and axillary radiographs are needed to determine the presence of unwanted bone or displaced tuberosities or other "hard" causes of restriction of motion (**Figs. 37–44** and **37–45**). At surgery, all adhesions in the humeroscapular motion interface are lysed. A 360-degree release of the subscapularis is performed,

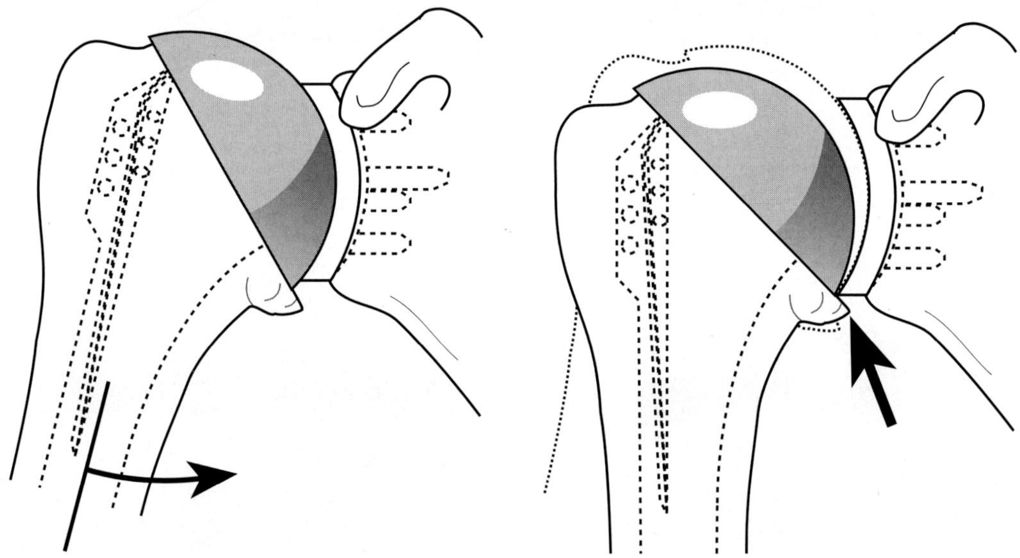

A B

**Figure 37–44. Inferior open book**
Bone extending beyond the curvature of the prosthetic humeral articular surface can abut the inferior glenoid when the arm is adducted.

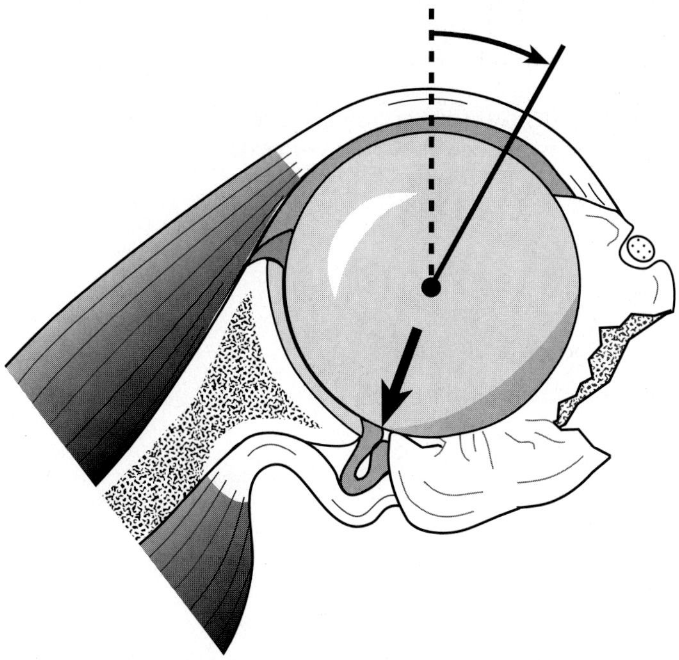

**Figure 37–45. Malunion of the greater tuberosity**
Malunion with posterior displacement of the greater tuberosity allows the tuberosity to abut the glenoid on external rotation.

freeing it from the coracoid, the coracoid muscles, the axillary nerve, and the glenoid lip. The capsule is released around the periphery of the glenoid—360 degrees unless there is posterior instability, in which case the release is stopped at 190 degrees. Unwanted bone, such as residual osteophytes between the medial humerus and inferior glenoid, is removed. If the greater tuberosity is malunited posteriorly, it can block external rotation. We prefer to avoid tuberosity osteotomy unless it is absolutely necessary because of the difficulties of mobilizing the tuberosity and of obtaining a secure tuberosity union to the shaft after a humeral arthroplasty. For this reason, we prefer to resect prominent tuberosity bone, leaving the cuff intact if this is at all possible. If the joint is overstuffed **(Fig. 37–46)**, the intra-articular prosthetic volume may be reduced by removing or revising the glenoid component and by reducing the height or repositioning (i.e., decreasing the varus position) of the humeral head component **(Fig. 37–47)**.

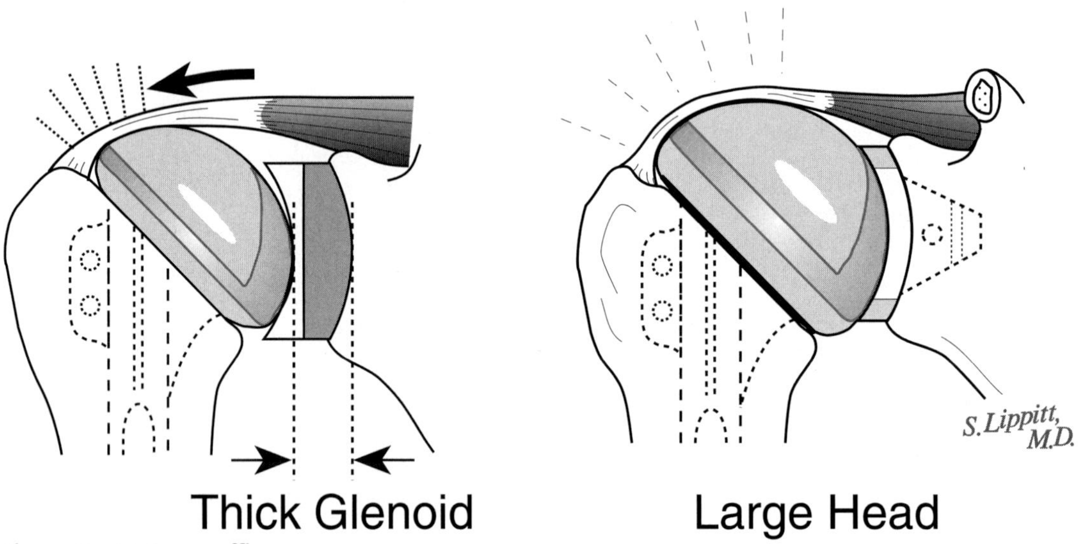


**Figure 37–46. Overstuffing**
Excessive glenoid thickness or excessive height of the humeral articular surface can overstuff the joint and place the rotator cuff under greater tension when the arm is in adduction.

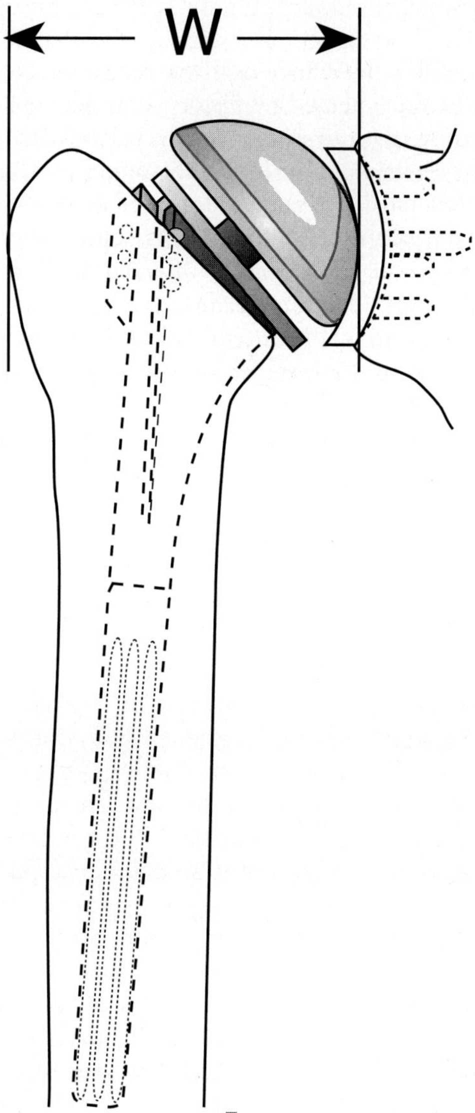


**Figure 37–47. Varus position of the humeral component**

Varus position of the humeral component can increase the distance between the greater tuberosity and the glenoid (W), effectively overstuffing the joint.

### *Instability*

The diagnosis of instability is made by unwanted translation of the humeral head on the glenoid. This can be documented by history, examination, or radiographs. The physical examination of strength in isometric internal rotation with the arm against the abdomen, isometric elevation of the internally rotated arm, and isometric external rotation of the neutrally rotated arm at the side as well as expert shoulder ultrasonography can evaluate the integrity of the subscapularis, supraspinatus, and infraspinatus, respectively. High-quality and appropriately oriented anteroposterior and axillary radiographs will reveal the glenohumeral relationship (including the superior/inferior and anterior/posterior relationship of the center of the humeral head and the center of the glenoid), the integrity of the tuberosities, the orientation of the glenoid, and much about the type and position of the humeral component. If knowledge of the humeral version is essential, it may be necessary to perform an examination under fluoroscopy, noting the rotational position of the arm that places the humeral neck in greatest profile.

*Subscapularis deficiency* may not be reconstructable. If there is good-quality muscle and tendon, a repair may be possible after a complete release of the medial muscle and tendon. A hamstring autograft may be useful for extending the tendon length. A pectoralis major transfer may be helpful.

If the *glenoid component is in excessive anteversion*, its intrinsic balance stability angle does not provide anterior stability because of its misalignment with the net humeral joint reaction force (determined principally by the scapular origin of the scapulohumeral muscles). This cause of anterior instability is suspected when there is minimal resistance to the anterior load and shift test. The diagnosis of glenoid component anteversion can be made by examination of a true axillary view of the joint. The glenoid center line normally projects out the anterior scapular neck at the centering point. In the anteverted glenoid, the glenoid center line projects down the scapular body or behind it. When anterior instability is associated with glenoid anteversion, reorientation of the prosthetic glenoid center line is usually indicated. Because the anterior glenoid lip of a polyethylene component is usually worn by the recurrent instability, the prosthesis often needs to be changed. Thus, the revision is accomplished either by removal of the prosthetic component and performance of a properly oriented nonprosthetic glenoid arthroplasty or by reinsertion of a glenoid component with its center line in proper orientation with the scapula **(Fig. 37–48)**. If the anterior glenoid

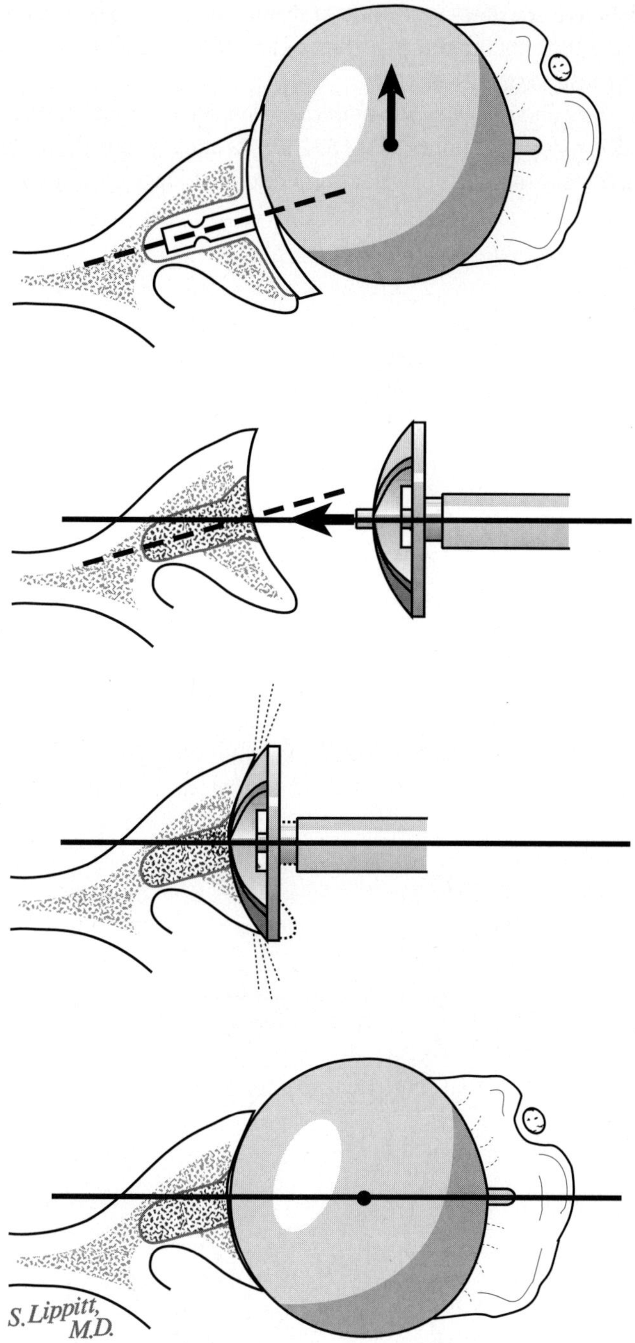


**Figure 37–48. Revising an anteverted glenoid**
When the glenoid is anteverted or anteriorly eroded, its version can often be corrected by reestablishing the normal glenoid center line and reaming along this new axis.

bone stock is deficient, an iliac crest bone graft may be secured to the anterior glenoid and then reamed either for the nonprosthetic glenoid arthroplasty or to fit the back of the glenoid prosthesis (**Fig. 37–49**).

If the *glenoid component is in excessive retroversion*, its intrinsic balance stability angle does not provide posterior stability (**Fig. 37–50**). Clinically, the shoulder will demonstrate diminished resistance to posterior load and shift and instability on cross-body

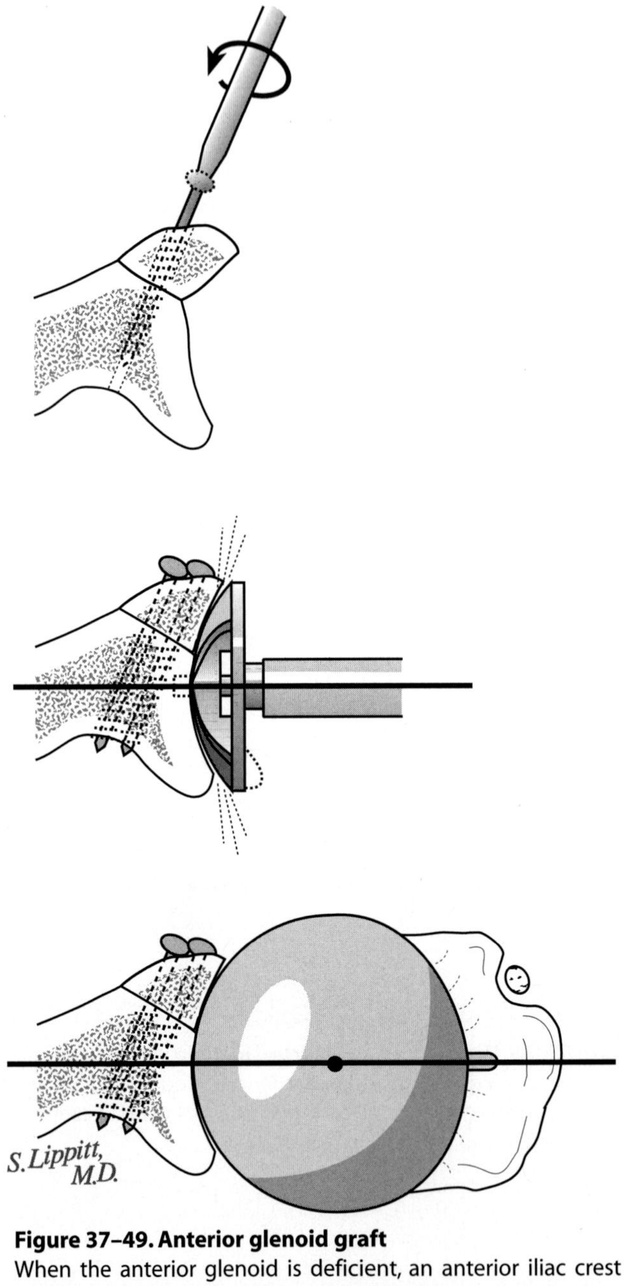


**Figure 37–49. Anterior glenoid graft**
When the anterior glenoid is deficient, an anterior iliac crest graft can be placed, fixed with screws, and then reamed, either for a nonprosthetic or a prosthetic glenoid arthroplasty.

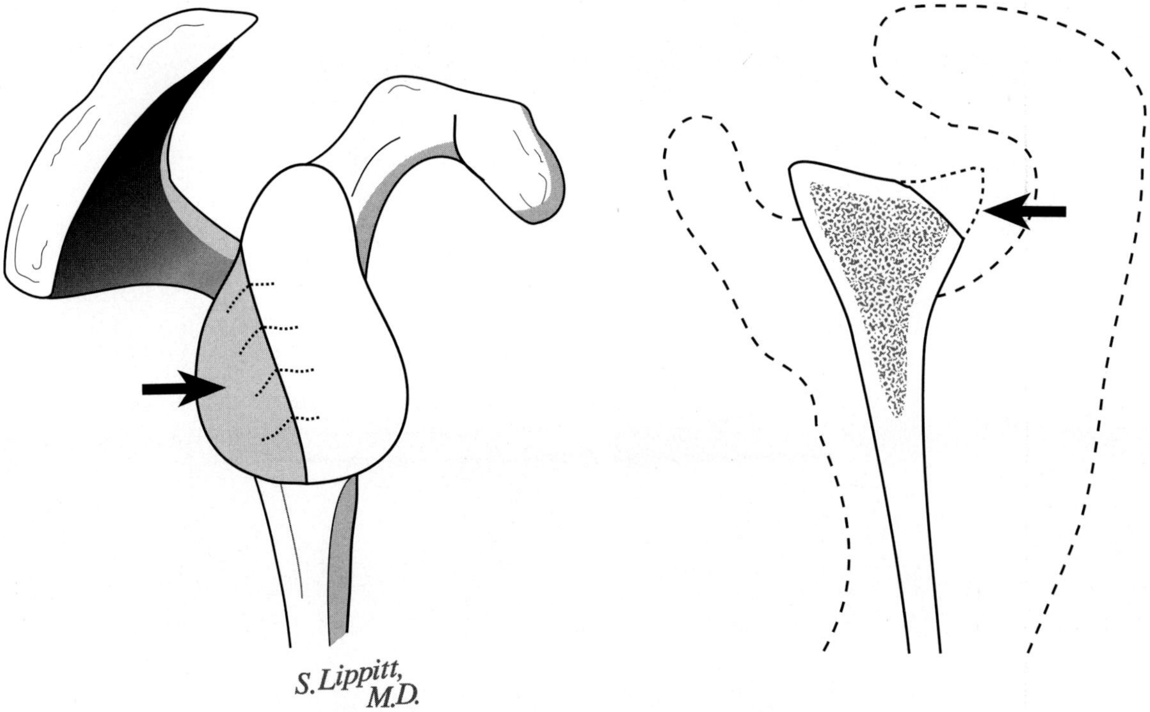


**Figure 37–50. Posterior erosion and rim deficiency**
Posterior glenoid deficiency is a commonly encountered problem in revision arthroplasty.

adduction. On the axillary radiograph, the glenoid center line is seen to project through the bony glenoid more anteriorly than the normal centering point. Correction may include reestablishing the normal glenoid center line and then performing corrective reaming for a nonprosthetic or prosthetic glenoid arthroplasty (**Figs. 37–51, 37–52,** and **37–53**).

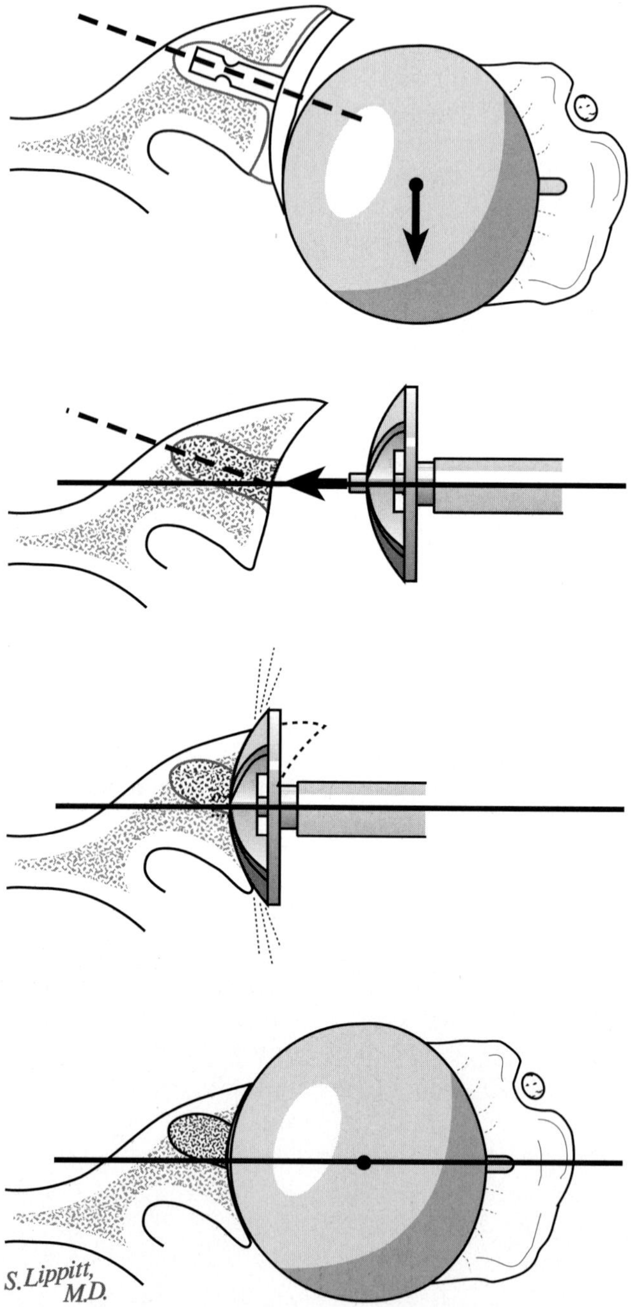


**Figure 37–51. Retroverted glenoid**
When the glenoid is retroverted or posteriorly eroded, its version can often be corrected by reestablishing the normal glenoid center line and reaming along this new axis.

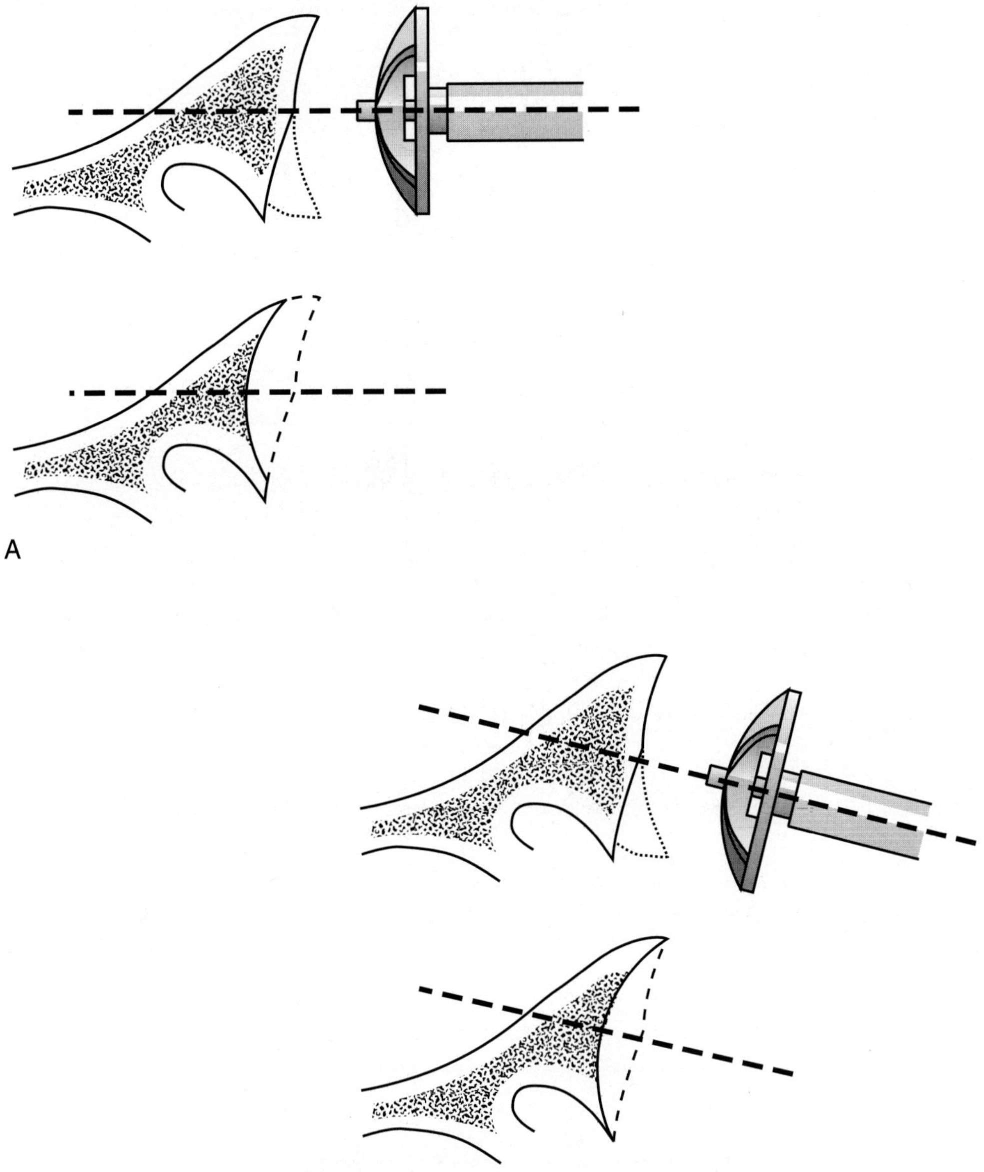

A

B

**Figure 37–52. Corrective glenoid reaming**
It is important that reaming leave a sufficient posterior lip (**A**). A deficient posterior glenoid lip (**B**) may give rise to posterior instability.

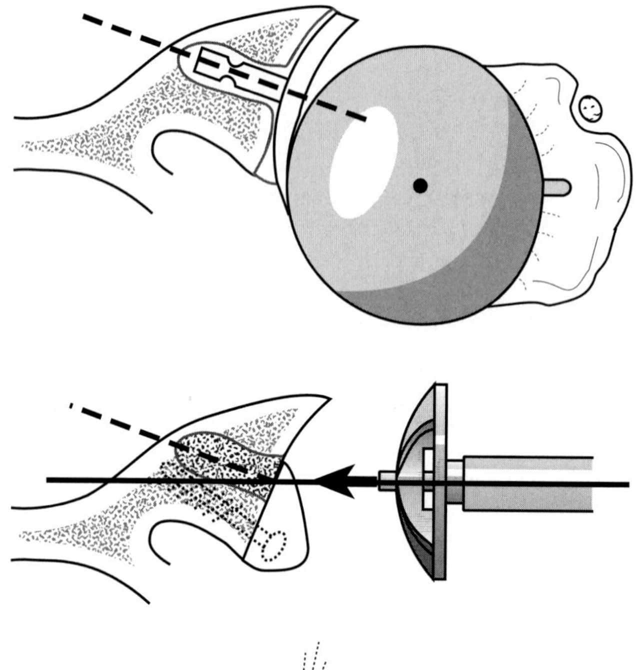


**Figure 37–53. Posterior glenoid graft**
When the posterior glenoid is deficient, a posterior iliac crest graft can be placed. However, rigid fixation of the graft is technically challenging. If the graft can be secured, it can be reamed to the appropriate version and concavity for a nonprosthetic or prosthetic glenoid arthroplasty.

If there is *insufficient glenoid bone* for a reconstruction and if an iliac crest autograft cannot be performed because of insufficient quality bone stock to which it can be anchored, a glenoidectomy can be considered as a salvage procedure (**Fig. 37–54**). In this procedure, the residual glenoid is resected down to the level of the scapular spine. An appropriately sized humeral head prosthesis is inserted to articulate with the glenoid neck, the scapular spine, and the base of the coracoid.

*Nonunion of the greater tuberosity* effectively detaches the superior and posterior rotator cuff from the humeral shaft, allowing the proximal humerus to translate anteriorly with respect to the glenoid (**Fig. 37–55**). Treatment of this nonunion is difficult because the tuberosity is retracted posteromedially and is very difficult to mobilize back to its normal length. If this reconstruction is to be attempted, access to the retracted tendon and the posterior glenoid from which it must be released is greatly facilitated by removal of the humeral prosthesis.

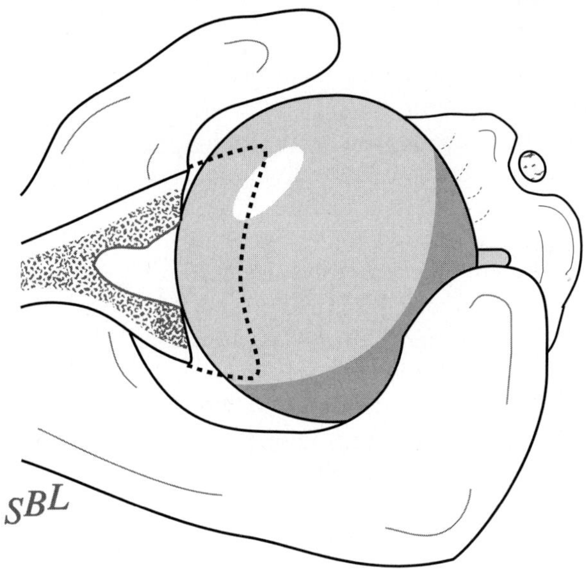


**Figure 37–54. Excising the glenoid**
When there is insufficient bone for reaming to an effective concavity or for grafting, consideration can be given to resecting the glenoid down to the base of the coracoid and scapular spine, leaving a "deep dish" for articulation with a humeral head of relatively large diameter.

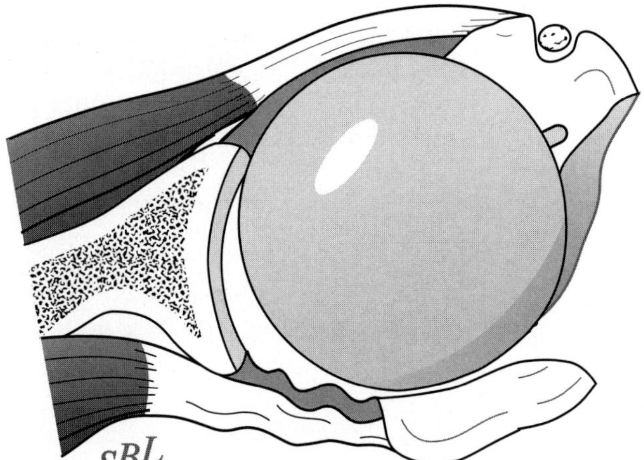


**Figure 37–55. Greater tuberosity nonunion**
Nonunion of the greater tuberosity after a prosthetic arthroplasty creates a difficult situation because the infraspinatus and posterior capsule quickly become contracted and because the amount of bone left on the shaft for healing to the tuberosity is minimal.

*Rotator cuff defects* can be important factors in anterior or posterior instability. These defects may (1) have been present at the time of the initial surgery; (2) have occurred at the time of surgery, for example during the osteotomy of the humeral head; or (3) have occurred due to degeneration or injury after the procedure. Obtaining a strong and durable repair of chronic cuff defects at revision surgery is challenging because of the usually insufficient quantity and quality of the cuff tissue.

*Abnormal humeral component version* may be a factor in glenohumeral instability. Especially if the radius of the head is small and the neck length is large, there can be a substantial offset, and anteverting the prosthesis can move the center of rotation anterior or posterior to the glenoid center. A similar phenomenon can arise with protheses that have an anterior or posterior offset. These factors can be modulated by revising the component diameter, neck length, offset, and version.

*Loss of the integrity of the coracoacromial arch* can be a major problem following shoulder arthroplasty, allowing anterosuperior escape of the proximal humerus from the glenoid (**Fig. 37–56**). It is often coexistent with a rotator cuff defect and with a detachment of the anterolateral origin of the deltoid. We have not found a reconstruction that dependably restores function to shoulders with this problem. On occasion, we have performed a glenoidectomy, allowing an appropriately sized humeral prosthesis to fit quite medially against the glenoid neck, behind the coracoid muscles and in front of the scapular spine.

### *Weakness*

Weakness of the shoulder may be due to reduced muscle strength, tendon defects, tuberosity defects, detachment of the deltoid from its origin, or nerve injuries. The evaluation and management of each of these has been discussed previously. Because of the major challenges in any attempt to restore strength to a chronically weak shoulder after arthroplasty, it is important to be sure that the patient has had the benefit of a protracted effort at shoulder strengthening exercises, especially the progressive tilting supine press. As mentioned previously, robust reattachment of a chronically detached rotator cuff or subscapularis tendons or tuberosities is difficult due to contractures and loss of contractility. This is even more the case with deltoid origin failure—a problem easy to prevent by the deltoid-on or deltopectoral approach and difficult to treat once it has occurred. We have not been impressed with the results of attempts at deltoid reattachment, transfer of the clavicular head of the pectoralis major, or anterior transfer of the lateral or posterior deltoid to restore strength to the anterior deltoid. Injuries to the axillary and suprascapular nerves or upper cervical radiculopathies are important to recognize, so that shoulder weakness will not be attributed to other, more treatable causes.

## **Revision Surgery After Fracture Surgery** (see Chapters 33–36)

Before embarking on a surgical revision of a fracture repair, it is important to determine what combinations of stiffness, weakness, instability, and roughness are compromising the patient's comfort and function. The more common complications include infection, scarring in the humeroscapular motion interface, overstuffing of the joint, overtightening of the cuff, contracture of the subscapularis, rotator cuff failure, nonunited or malunited tuberosities, tuberosity resorption, subtuberous nonunion, subtuberous malunion, prominent hardware, avascular necrosis of the humeral head, suboptimal height or version of a humeral prosthesis, secondary fracture of the shaft, erosion of the glenoid bone, and nerve injuries.

The treatment of each of these problems is highly individualized but is based on the principles of bony union, mobility, stability, and strength.

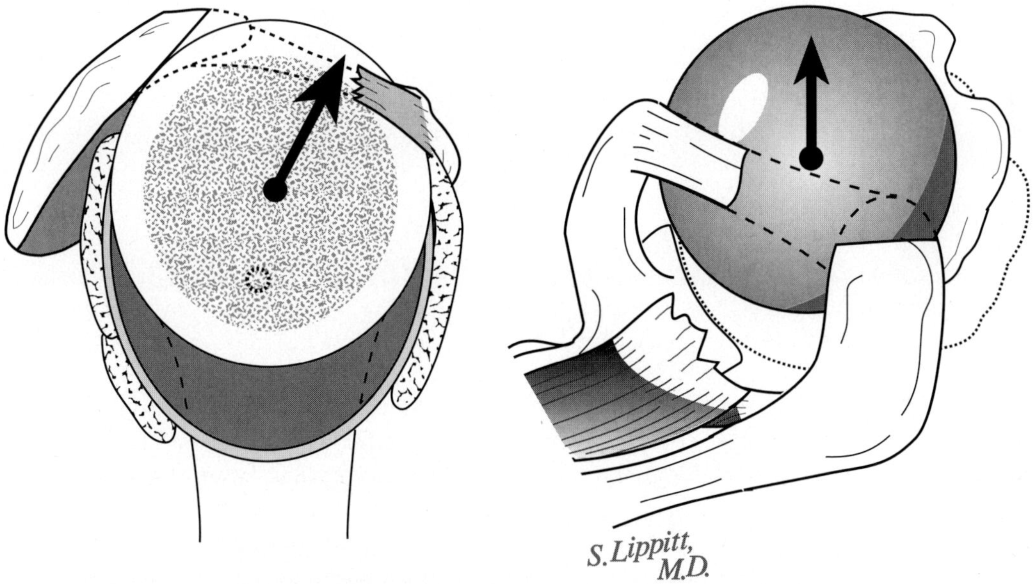


**Figure 37–56. Anterosuperior escape**
When prior surgery has compromised the integrity of the anterior coracoacromial arch, the humeral head may escape anterosuperiorly when the deltoid contracts.

## Removal of a Humeral Implant

In some instances, removal of the head of a modular component is sufficient to accomplish the desired revision (**Figs. 37–57** and **37–58**). Often, however, revision requires removal of the entire humeral component.

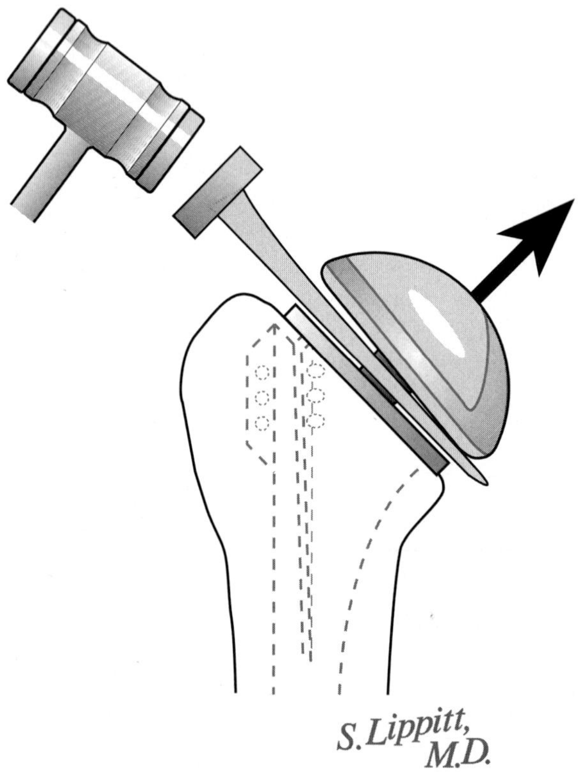


**Figure 37–57. Prosthetic head removal**
Some implant systems have special tools for removing a modular humeral head component, such as the forked wedge shown here.

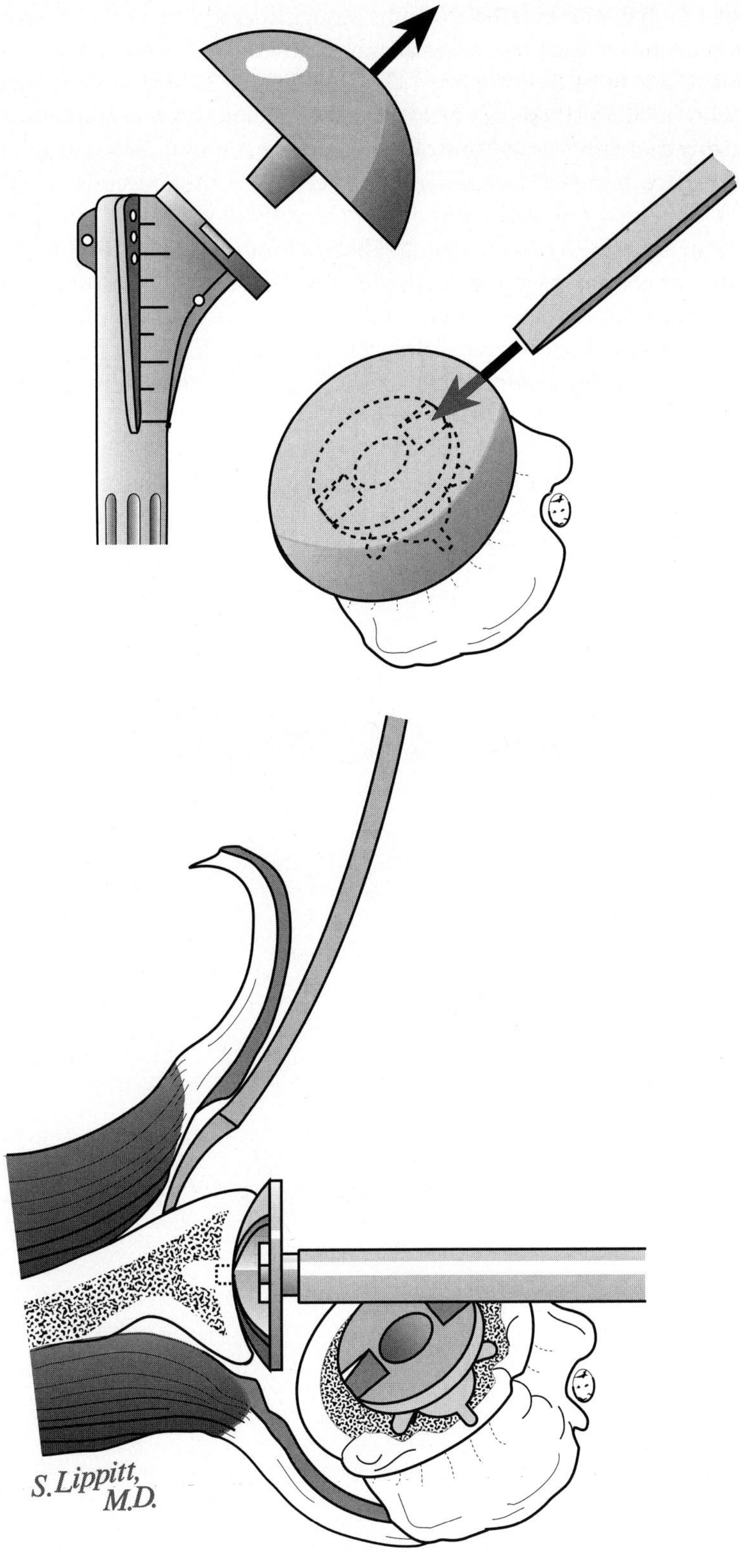


**Figure 37–58. Removing head to access glenoid**
If the stem of a modular component is fixed in the proper position, revision of the glenoid arthroplasty may be accomplished be removing the prosthetic glenoid, thereby gaining necessary access to the glenoid.

Extraction of a humeral prosthesis can be straightforward in a case in which there is a large lucent zone between the humeral endosteum on one hand and the prosthesis and any cement used to fix it on the other (**Figs. 37–59** and **37–60**). On the other hand, removal of a humeral prosthesis can be extremely challenging, for example when it has been thoroughly cemented to the bone of an osteopenic humerus or when an ingrowth or textured surface humeral component has been used. Before embarking on the removal of a cemented humeral component, the difficulty and the necessity of the removal of cement needs to be anticipated. The need for cement removal is influenced by the presence or absence of infection, the requirement to change prosthesis size and position, and the extent of the cementation. In the absence of infection and when the cement is secure to the bone, we will often opt to work within the previous cement mantle (for example, using a component with a smaller diameter stem and recementing within the old cement) rather than running the risk of removing it. The anticipated difficulty and the possibility of fracturing the humeral shaft or tuberosities during the removal are discussed with the patient in detail preoperatively. The surgical inventory is carefully reviewed to ensure that long-stem implants of the appropriate diameters and head sizes are available for the subsequent reconstruction.

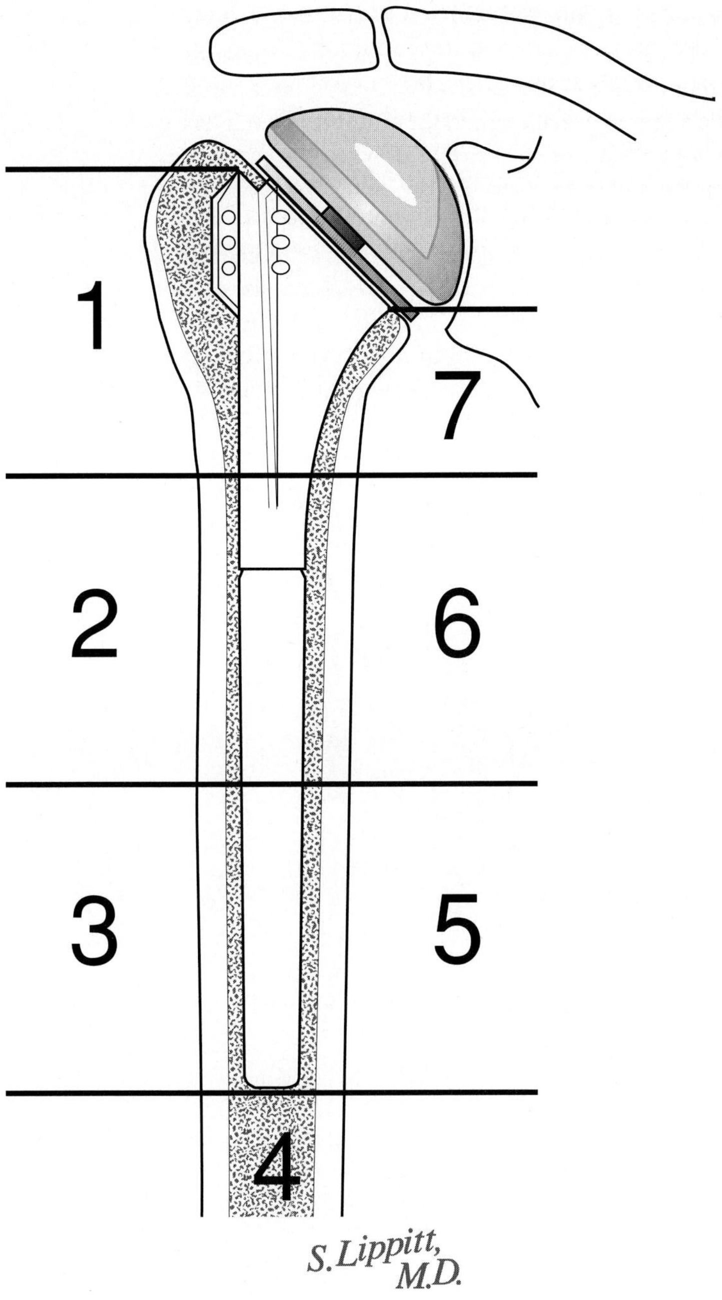


**Figure 37–59. Humeral loosening**
Humeral radiolucent lines can be characterized in terms of seven zones around the humeral component.

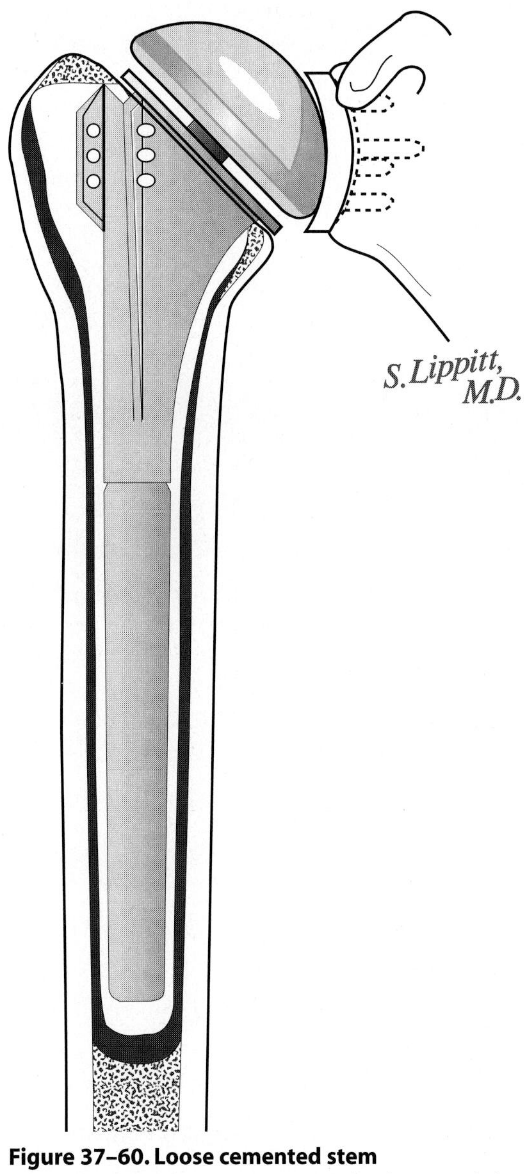


**Figure 37–60. Loose cemented stem**
When there is a lucent zone completely around the humeral component and any cement used for fixation, component removal is usually straightforward.

Our approach to prosthesis removal begins with the removal of soft tissue, bone ingrowth, and cement from around the humeral head or, in the case of a modular prosthesis, from around the collar and from around the fins of the prosthesis (**Fig. 37–61**). If the prosthesis cannot be removed easily at this point, enough bone in the area of the bicipital groove is cut to allow the positioning of a bone tamp parallel to the shaft with one end beneath the collar or head (**Fig. 37–62**). The elbow is flexed to 90 degrees and the arm is stabilized to the thorax while the surgeon strikes the bone tamp so that a longitudinal impact is applied to the proximal prosthesis along the axis

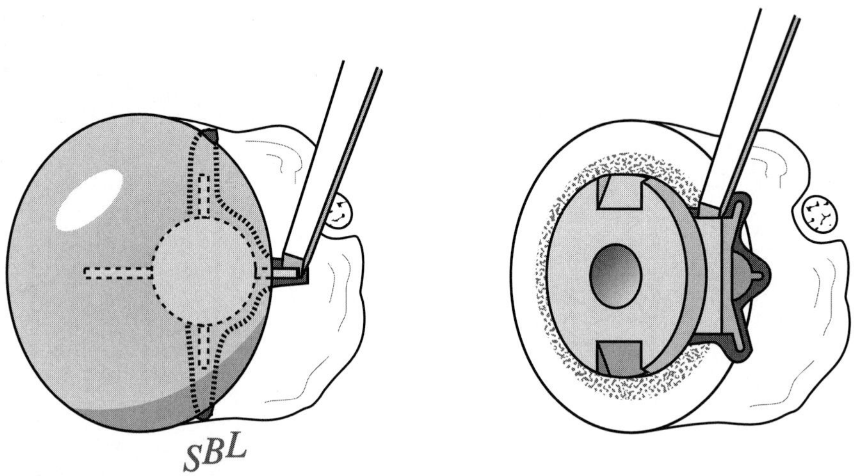


**Figure 37–61. Freeing the fins**
If the stem requires removal, the first step is removing all bone and cement from the path for backing out the fins. Care must be taken to protect the rotator cuff during this dissection.

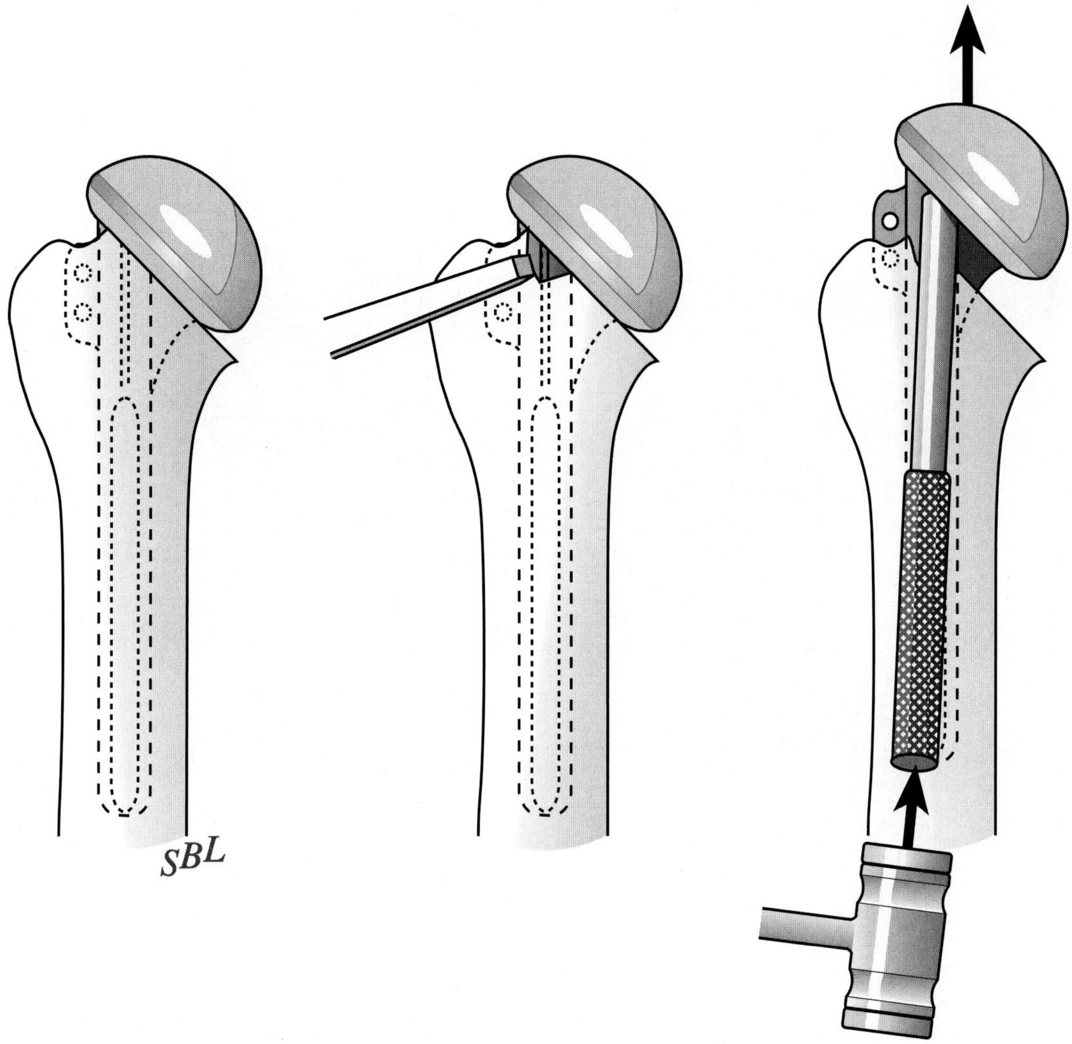


**Figure 37–62. Removing a humeral component**
A simple, effective method for removing a humeral component is to create a notch in the shaft beneath the head of the humeral component. A bone tamp can then be placed in this notch and used to drive the humeral prosthesis out of the shaft with slaps of the hammer in line with the prosthetic stem.

of the humeral shaft. If reasonable impact does not dislodge the prosthesis, a longitudinal humeral osteotomy is started in the bicipital groove (**Fig. 37–63**). When the bone is cut, the osteotome is twisted slightly to open up the endosteal cross section of the humerus. Impact is applied as before with the bone tamp. The linear osteotomy is continued sequentially with the osteotome twisted each time until the prosthesis can be removed.

If cement removal is necessary, this can be performed with the usual cement removal tools inserted down from the canal opening at the proximal humerus or through the humeral osteotomy. In our hands, it seems more safe and effective to monitor the integrity of the bone by extending the incision sufficiently inferiorly so that the bone can be palpated during the cement removal rather than relying on intraoperative fluoroscopy. In any case, burrs and osteotomes tend to cut the often thin and soft bone preferentially to the hard cement; thus, the surgeon must be prepared for bone penetration and its possible consequences (nerve damage, additional fracture, leakage of cement).

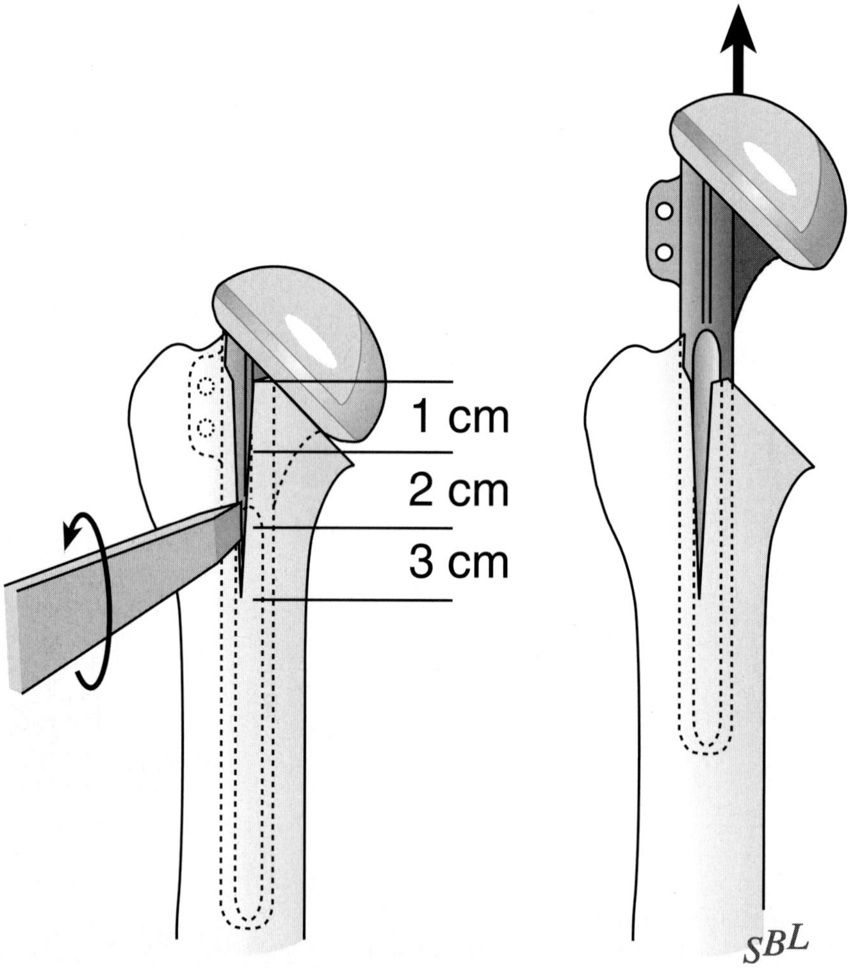


**Figure 37–63. Osteotomy of the humeral shaft**
When the humeral prosthesis cannot be freed from the humerus, an osteotomy is created starting at the upper edge of the bicipital groove. The osteotomy is pried open by turning the osteotome in the bone cut to increase the cross section of the humerus. After each cut, the bone tamp is placed in the osteotomy and a hammer is used to try to drive the prosthesis out proximally. If the component cannot be removed, the osteotomy is extended distally another centimeter and the steps described earlier are repeated until the prosthesis is loose.

If a secure cement mantle remains after humeral component removal, the new humeral component with a smaller diameter can be cemented into the old mantle.

If a cementless reconstruction is desired, the humerus can be reassembled using a long-stem prosthesis press-fit as far down the distal humerus as possible (**Fig. 37–64**). At this point in the case, the medullary canal can be divided into two components—the proximal section that was opened to retrieve the prosthesis and the distal aspect consisting of an intact cylinder. The fixation of the prosthesis depends on this distal segment, especially in the circumstances in which a cementless reconstruction is

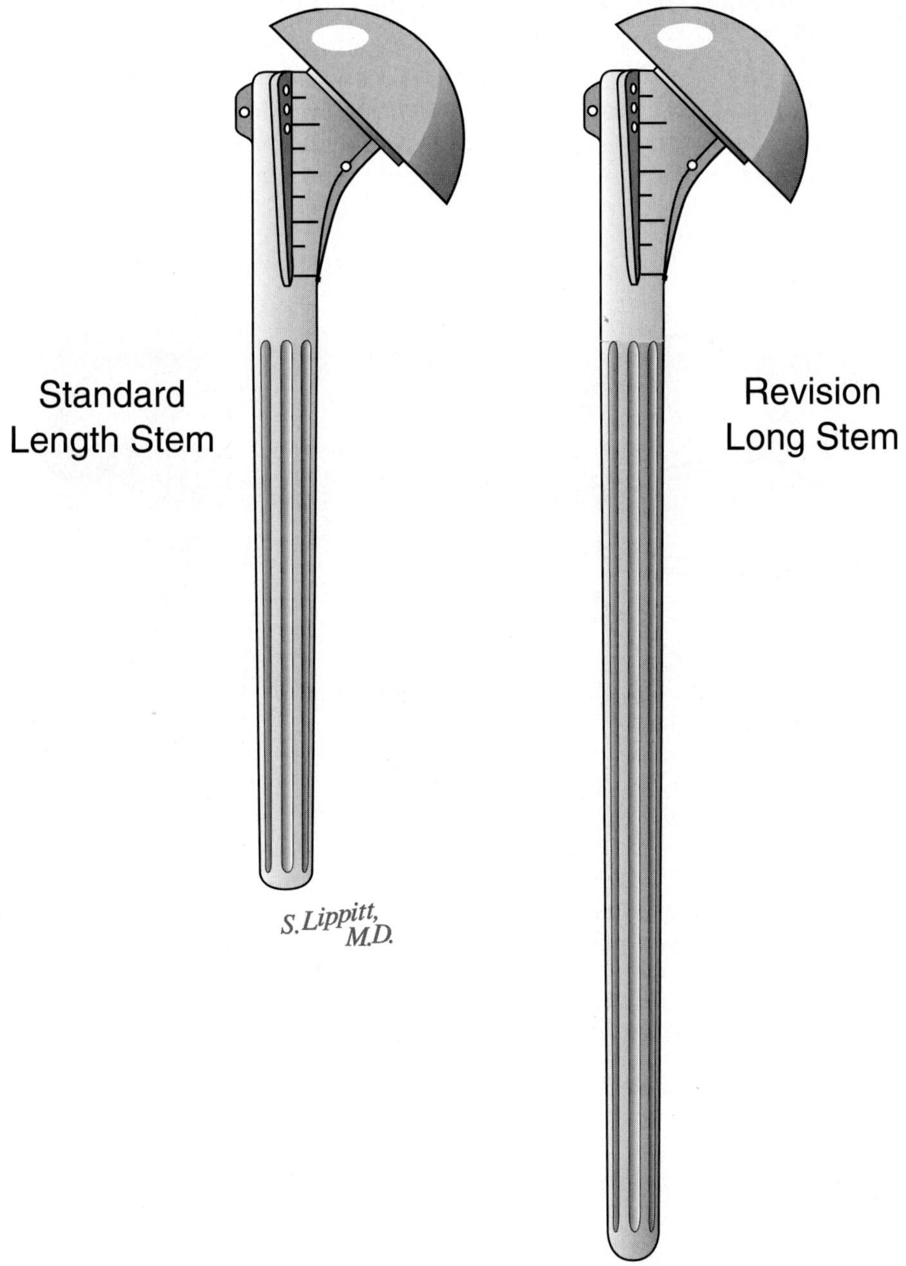


**Figure 37–64. Standard versus long stem**

In preparing for a revision arthroplasty, it is always prudent to have a long-stem prosthesis available. Because it may be difficult to judge the exact prosthetic length and because optimizing the fit in the distal humerus may be critical (for example when there is a fracture of the proximal humerus), we often start with a 300 mm long implant and cut it in the operating room to the desired length.

desired, for example after the débridement of an infected arthroplasty or because of concern regarding an adverse reaction to methylmethacrylate. In this situation, the cylindrical distal humeral segment is reamed with cylindrical reamers until the fit and fill of a cylindrical component stem is optimized. Since the quality of the fit depends on the length of the bone-prosthesis contact, the length of the prosthesis inserted into the cylindrical segment is maximized. This is accomplished by extending the reaming as distally as possible and by maximizing the length of the prosthetic stem. We often start with a 300 mm stem of the proper diameter, insert it fully in the reamed canal and then measure how much of it needs to be trimmed for the articular surface to be in proper register with the glenoid. The stem is then cut with a high-speed motorized disk and smoothed of any burrs remaining from the cut. The prosthesis is then impacted into the distal cylindrical segment, with particular attention paid to the version. The open proximal humeral segment is then folded around the prosthesis. Because the posterior and medial periosteum and muscle attachments have been preserved, the osteotomized bone can be reconstructed by suturing the osteotomy closed using drill holes on either side (**Fig. 37–65**). Cerclage can also be used, but care must be taken to protect the radial nerve, which could be cerclaged in its musculoskeletal groove.

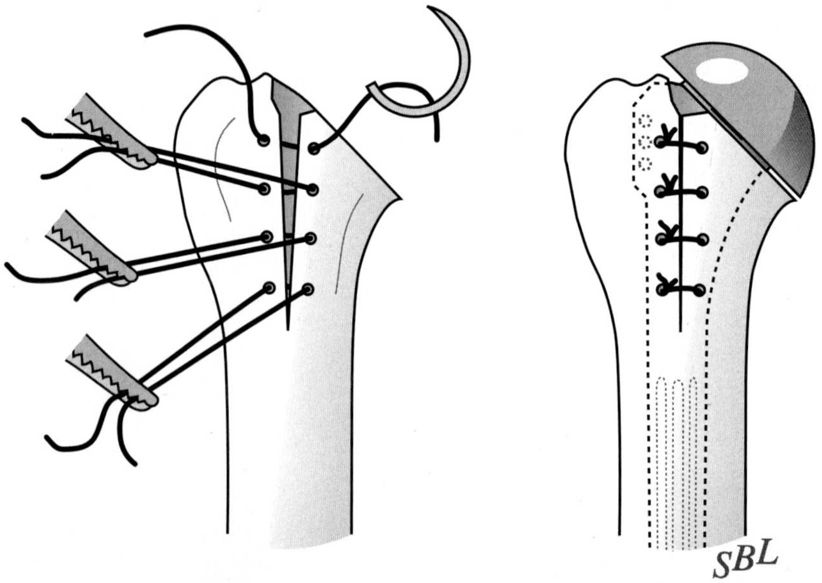


**Figure 37–65. Repairing the shaft**
The osteotomy is repaired by passing #2 braided nonabsorbable sutures through drill holes on either side of the split in the bicipital groove. Tying these sutures reconstitutes the humeral shaft. This repair technique is safer than cerclage, which can endanger the radial nerve posteriorly.

## Removal of Glenoid Implant

The quality of glenoid seating and cement fixation can be evaluated on high-quality preoperative radiographs (**Figs. 37–66** and **37–67**). Most commonly, a glenoid component removal is not followed by a reimplantation, because there is insufficient bone stock, because of concern regarding infection or inflammatory reaction, or because of the lack of interest in subjecting the patient to the even greater risk of loosening of a repeat glenoid insertion. The exception is when there is sufficient bone stock, no suspicion of infection, and a desire on the part of the patient to have another glenoid implant.

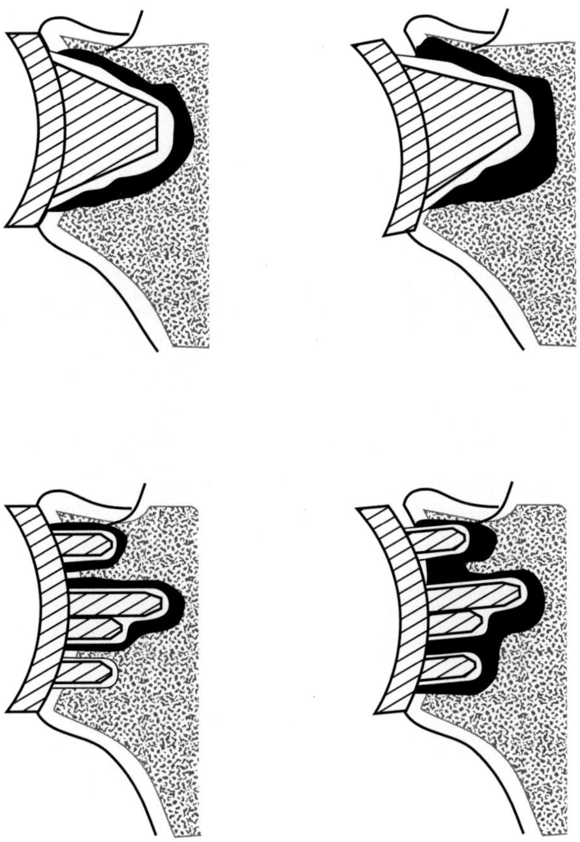

**Figure 37–66. Glenoid lucency**
The radiolucencies around a cemented prosthesis can be characterized using standardized radiographic views, and any progression of the lucency can be documented.

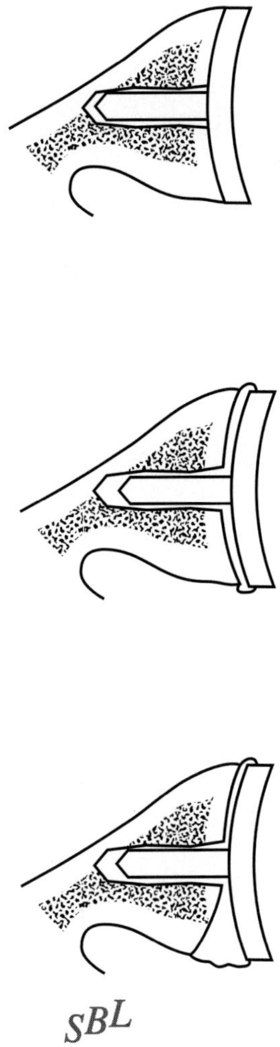


**Figure 37–67. Glenoid seating**
Even if the fixation of the glenoid keel appears solid, the seating of the component onto the bone may be suboptimal.

Removal of a loose glenoid implant is usually quite straightforward and can often be accomplished even without removing the humeral component (**Fig. 37–68**).

If the component is well fixed but requires removal because of damage to it or because of malposition, the goal is to remove the component with minimal damage to the glenoid bone. In an all-polyethylene component, this can be accomplished by passing an osteotome between the glenoid articular surface and the bony glenoid face, transecting the keel or pegs, and then removing them under direct vision (**Fig. 37–69**).

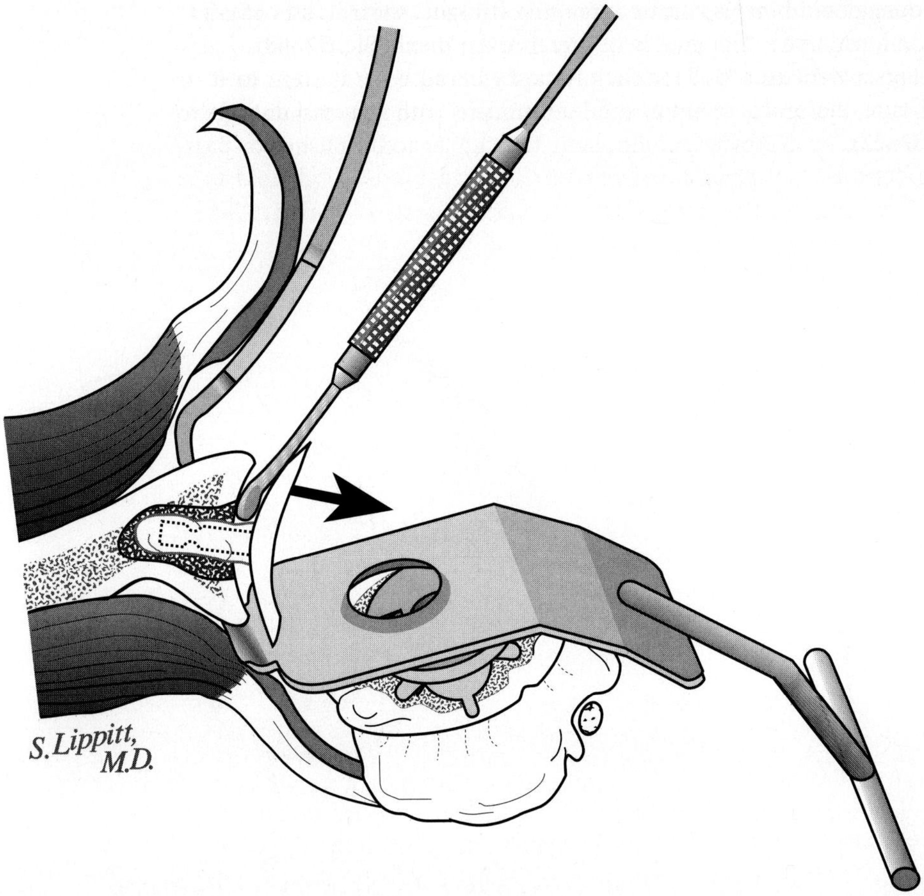


**Figure 37–68. Prying out a loose glenoid component**
When a glenoid component is loose, it can be easily lifted from the glenoid bone.

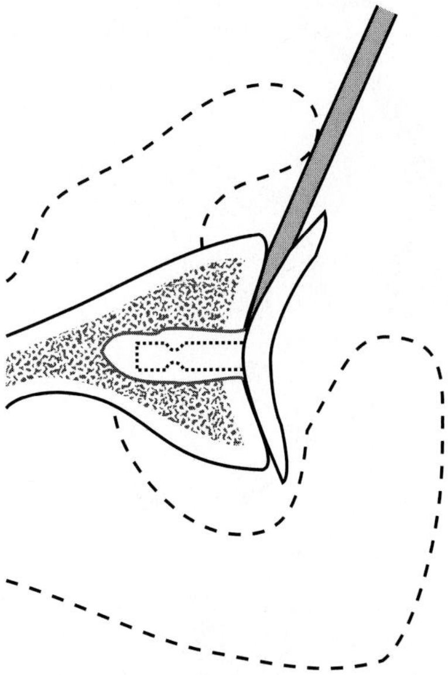

**Figure 37–69. Cutting the glenoid component**
When a polyethylene glenoid component is well fixed, the surface of the component can be cut with an osteotome, allowing access to the pegs or keel and the cement.

After removal, the glenoid bone is curetted free of soft tissue, cement, bits of polyethylene debris, and loose bone. The goal is to preserve the maximal amount of glenoid bone stock (**Figs. 37–70** and **37–71**). The residual glenoid bone is contoured to appropriate shape and version to optimize the load transfer and the stability of the articulation (**Fig. 37–72**).

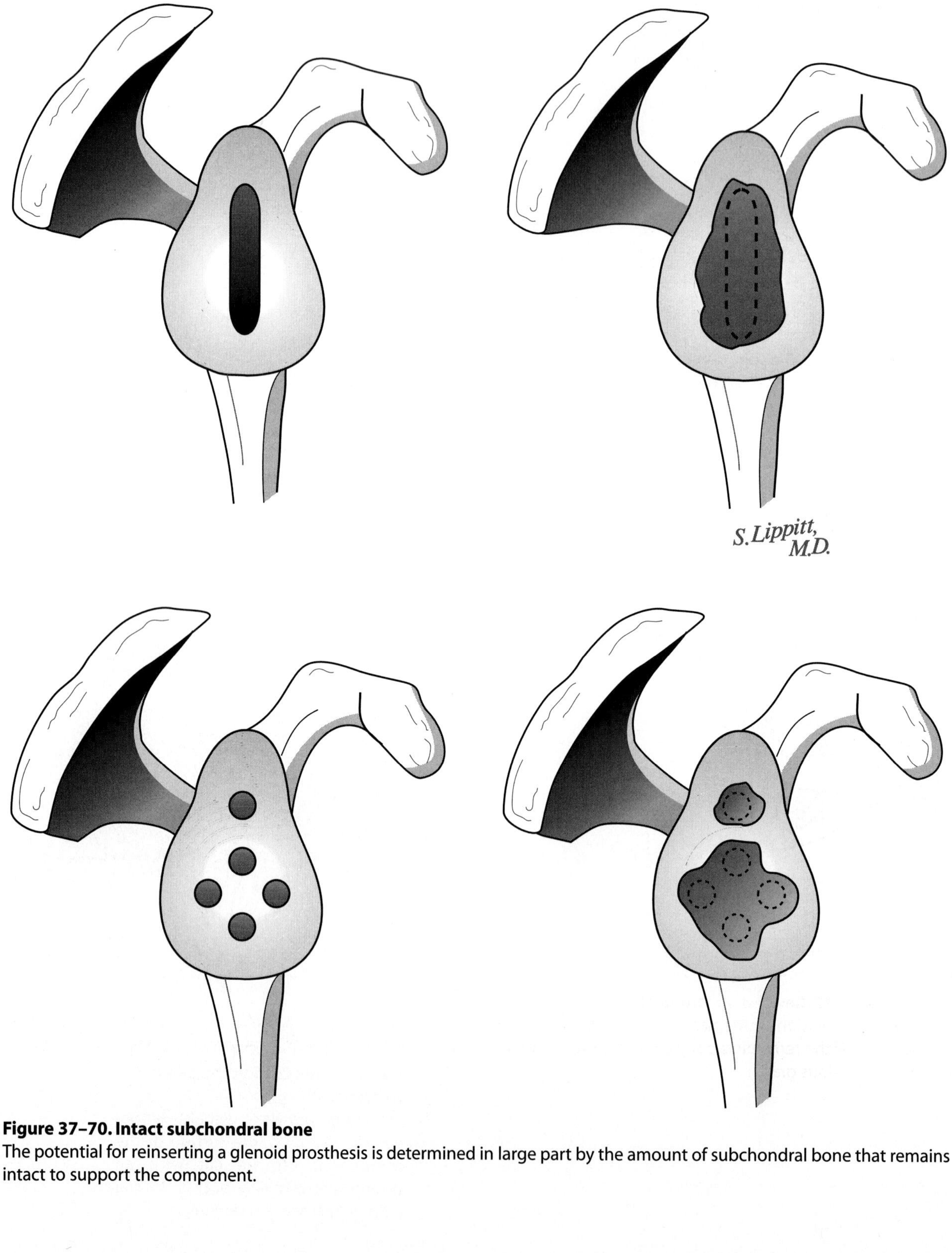


**Figure 37–70. Intact subchondral bone**
The potential for reinserting a glenoid prosthesis is determined in large part by the amount of subchondral bone that remains intact to support the component.

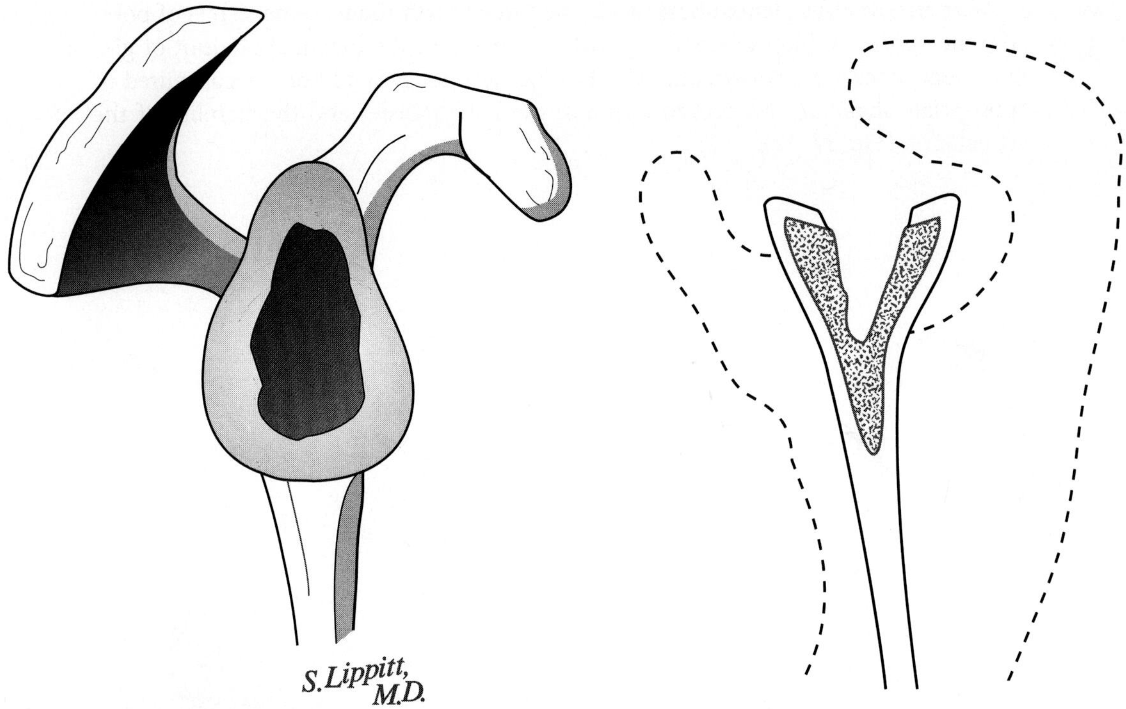


**Figure 37–71. Glenoid defect**
When the defect is large, refixation of a glenoid component may be difficult.

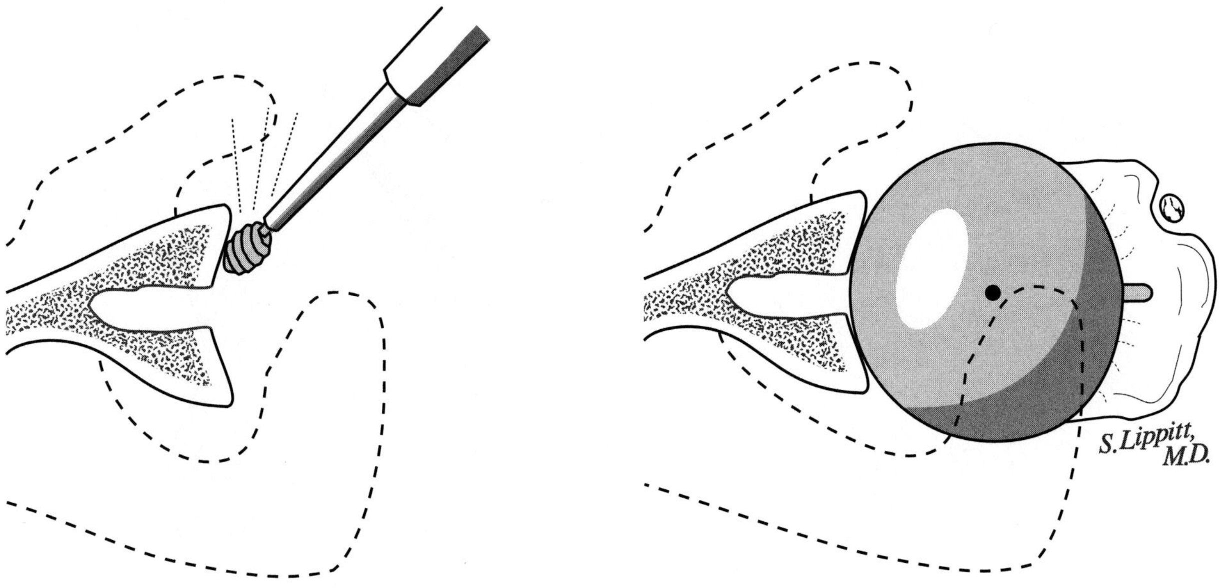


**Figure 37–72. Revision arthroplasty**
When the revision arthroplasty does not allow a secure glenoid component reimplantation, it is usually possible to smooth off the remaining bony glenoid surface with a burr (as shown here) or with a reamer and possibly fill the void with cancellous graft.

# Appendix 1
# Instrument List

| Item | Company | Address and Telephone Number | Part Description |
|---|---|---|---|
| 1. Darrach Retractors | George Tiemann & Co. | 25 Plant Avenue<br>Hauppaugh, NJ 11788<br>1-800-843-6266 | Medium (#80-201)<br>Large (#80-202)<br>X-Large (#80-203) |
| 2. AO Osteotomes | Synthes | 1690 Russell Road<br>Paoli, PA 19301<br>1-800-523-0322 | Handle: #399.54<br>4 Blades: #399.58, 399.57, 399.56, and 399.55 |
| 3. Balfour Retractors | Sklar | 889 S. Matlock<br>West Chester, PA 19380<br>1-800-221-2166 | #60-6670—Non-slip retaining (removing the center blade) |
| 4. Fukuda Retractors | George Tiemann & Co. | 25 Plant Avenue<br>Hauppaugh, NJ 11788<br>1-800-843-6266 | #80-1869L |
| 5. 000 Angled Curette | Codman | Johnson & Johnson<br>425 Hoes Lane<br>Piskataway, NJ 08855<br>1-800-255-2500 | #23-1041 |
| 6. Hohmann Retractors | Synthes | 1690 Russell Road<br>Paoli, PA 19301<br>1-800-523-0322 | Narrow (#399.27): 18 mm width, 235 mm length<br>Wide (#399.22): 43 mm width, 240 mm length |
| 7. Pine Cone/Wire Passer | 3M | 3M Surgical Products<br>17132 Pullman Street<br>Irvine, CA 92714<br>1-800-221-0202 | Pine Cone (#L40B Bur): 4.0 mm cut head<br>Wire passer (#M15W Bur): 1.5 mm cut head |
| 8. Angled Needle Holder | Sklar | 889 S. Matlock<br>West Chester, PA 19380<br>1-800-221-0202 | Heaney (#20-4682) |
| 9. Sofield Retractors | Zimmer | PO Box 708<br>Warsaw, IN 46581<br>1-800-348-2759 | The set: #233-01, 233-02, 233-03, 233-04, 233-05, 233-06<br>The clip: 233-07 |
| 10. Carbojet | Kinamed | 820 Flynn Road<br>Camarillo, CA 93012<br>805-384-2748 | Carbojet handpiece, catalog 25-200-0200<br>Angled tip nozz1e, catalog 25-200-0200<br>Sterilization tray, catalog 25-200-0300 |
| 11. Global Advantage | DePuy, Inc. | 700 Orthopaedic Drive<br>US Highway 30 East<br>Warsaw, IN 46580<br>1-800-366-8143 | |

# Appendix 2 University of Washington Department of Orthopaedics and Sports Medicine Former Shoulder and Elbow ACEs

1/1/88—6/30/89
Craig Arntz, MD
Valley Orthopedic Associates
4011 Talbot Road South, Suite 300
Renton, WA 98055

9/1/88—5/31/89
Douglas T. Harryman II, MD *(Deceased)*
University of Washington
Department of Orthopaedics & Sports Medicine, Box 356500
1959 NE Pacific Street
Seattle, WA 98195

8/1/89—10/31/89
Steven C. Thomas, MD
9499 West Charleston, Suite 200
Las Vegas, NV 89117

1/1/90—6/30/90
David C. Collins, MD
600 South McKinley, Suite 102
Little Rock, AR 72205

7/1/90—6/30/92
Steven B. Lippitt, MD
Akron General Medical Center
224 West Exchange Street, Suite 440
Akron, OH 44302-1718

7/1/91—6/30/92
Michael L. Pearl, MD
Kaiser Permanente Medical Center
4747 Sunset Boulevard
Los Angeles, CA 90027

7/1/92—6/30/93
Anthony A. Romeo, MD
University Orthopaedics Rush Presbyterian St. Luke's Medical Center
1725 West Harrison Street, Suite 1063
Chicago, IL 60612

7/1/93—6/30/94
Mark D. Lazarus, MD
Rothman Institute
925 Chestnut Street
Philadelphia, PA 19107

8/1/94—7/31/95
Dean W. Ziegler, MD
Blount Orthopaedics
625 East St. Paul Avenue
Milwaukee, WI 53202

8/1/95—7/31/96
Kevin L. Smith, MD
University of Washington
Department of Orthopaedics and Sports Medicine, Box 356500
1959 NE Pacific Street
Seattle, WA 98195

8/1/96—7/31/97
David Duckworth, MD
116 Macquarie Street
Parramatta
New South Wales, 2150
Australia

8/1/97—7/31/98
Richard Rozencwaig, MD
Orthopaedic Care and Sports Medicine Center
21000 NE 28th Avenue, Suite 104
Aventura, FL 33180

8/1/98—7/31/99
Benjamin Goldberg, MD
University of Illinois
901 S. Wolcott Avenue M/C 844
Chicago, IL 60612

8/1/98—7/31/99
Marius Scarlat, MD
Service de Chirurgie Orthopedique et Traumatologique
Clinique St. Michel
Place du 4 Septembre, F-83100 Toulon
France

8/1/99—7/31/00
Samer S. Hasan, MD, PhD
Cincinnati Sportsmedicine and Orthopaedic Center
328 Thomas More Parkway
Crestview Hills, KY 41017

8/1/99—7/31/00
Jordan Leith, MD
Allan McGavin Sports Medicine Centre
3055 Wesbrook Mall
Vancouver, BC, Canada, V6T 1Z3

8/1/00—7/31/01
R. Sean Churchill, MD
3003 W Good Hope Road
PO Box 090996
Milwaukee, WI 53209

8/1/00—7/31/01
Edward V. Fehringer, MD
University of Nebraska Medical Center
Department of Orthopaedics & Rehabilitation
981080 Nebraska Medical Center
Omaha, NE 68198

8/1/01—7/31/02
Richard Boorman, MD
50 Royal Oak Point NW
Calgary, Alberta T3G 5C5
Canada

8/1/01—7/31/02
Edward J. Weldon III, MD
Bone and Joint Center
Straub Hospital and Clinic
888 South King Street
Honolulu, HI 96813

8/1/02—7/31/03
Ira M. (Moby) Parsons, MD
Seacoast Orthopaedics and Sports Medicine
237 Route 108
Somersworth, NH 03878

8/1/02—7/31/03
Robert M. Titelman, MD
Resurgens Orthopaedics
5671 Peachtree Dunwoody Road
Suite 900
Atlanta, GA 30342

# Bibliography


1. Arntz, C. T., Jackins, S. E., and Matsen, F. A., III: Prosthetic replacement of the shoulder for the treatment of defects in the rotator cuff and the surface of the glenohumeral joint. *J. Bone Joint Surg.*, 75-A(4):485–491, 1993.
2. Arntz, C. T., and Matsen, F. A., III: Surgical management of complex irreparable rotator cuff deficiencies. *J. Arthroplasty*, 6(4):363–370, 1991.
3. Ballmer, F. T., Lippitt, S. B., Romeo, A. A., and Matsen, F. A., III: Total shoulder arthroplasty: Some considerations related to glenoid surface contact. *J. Shoulder Elbow Surg.*, 3(5):299–306, 1994.
4. Ballmer, F. T., Sidles, J. A., Lippitt, S. B., and Matsen, F. A., III: Humeral head prosthetic arthroplasty: Surgically relevant geometric considerations. *J. Shoulder Elbow Surg.*, 2:296–304, 1993.
5. Barrett, W. P., Franklin, J. L., Jackins, S. E., Wyss, C. R., and Matsen, F. A., III: Total shoulder arthroplasty. *J. Bone Joint Surg.*, 69-A(6):865–872, 1987.
6. Boorman, R., Hacker, S., Lippitt, S. B., and Matsen, F. A., III: A conservative broaching and impaction grafting technique for humeral component placement and fixation in shoulder arthroplasty: The Procrustean method. *Tech. Shoulder Elbow Surg.*, 2:166–175, 2001.
7. Boorman, R., Kopjar, B., Fehringer, E., Churchill, R. S., Smith, K. L., and Matsen, F. A., III: The effect of total shoulder arthroplasty on self-assessed health status is comparable to that of total hip arthroplasty and coronary artery bypass grafting. *J. Shoulder Elbow Surg.*, 12(2):158–163, 2003.
8. Caplan, R. A., Ready, L. B., Oden, R. V., Matsen, F. A., III, Nessly, M. L., and Olsson, G. L.: Transdermal fentanyl for postoperative pain management. A double-blind placebo study. *JAMA*, 261(7):1036–1039, 1989.
9. Castagno, A. A., Shuman, W. P., Kilcoyne, R. F., Haynor, D. R., Morris, M. E., and Matsen, F. A., III: Complex fractures of the proximal humerus: Role of CT in treatment. *Radiology*, 165(3):759–762, 1987.
10. Churchill, R. S., Moskal, M., Lippitt, S. B., and Matsen, F. A., III: Extracapsular anatomically contoured anterior glenoid bone grafting for complex glenohumeral instability. *Tech. Shoulder Elbow Surg.*, 2(3):210–218, 2001.
11. Clark, J. M., Sidles, J. A., and Matsen, F. A., III: The relationship of the glenohumeral joint capsule to the rotator cuff. *Clin. Orthop.*, 254:29–34, 1990.
12. Collins, D. N., Harryman, D. T., II, Lippitt, S. B., Jackins, S. E., and Matsen, F. A., III: The technique of glenohumeral arthroplasty. *Techniques Orthop.*, 6(1):43–59, 1991.
13. Collins, D. N., Tencer, A., Sidles, J. A., and Matsen, F. A., III: Edge displacement and deformation of glenoid components in response to eccentric loading. The effect of preparation of the glenoid bone. *J. Bone Joint Surg.*, 74-A(4):501–507, 1992.
14. Duckworth, D. G., Smith, K. L., Campbell, B., and Matsen, F. A., III: Self-assessment questionnaires document substantial variability in the clinical expression of rotator cuff tears. *J. Shoulder Elbow Surg.*, 8(4):330–333, 1999.
15. Fehringer, E., Schmidt, G., Boorman, R., Churchill, R. S., Smith, K. L., Norman, A., Sidles, J. A., and Matsen, F. A., III: The anteroinferior labrum helps center the humeral head on the glenoid. *J. Shoulder Elbow Surg*, 12(1):53–58, 2003.
16. Fehringer, E. V., Kopjar, B., Boorman, R. S., Churchill, R. S., Smith, K. L., and Matsen, F. A., III: Characterizing the functional improvement after total shoulder arthroplasty for osteoarthritis. *J. Bone Joint Surg.*, 84-A(8):1349–1353, 2002.
17. Franklin, J. L., Barrett, W. P., Jackins, S. E., and Matsen, F. A., III: Glenoid loosening in total shoulder arthroplasty. Association with rotator cuff deficiency. *J. Arthroplasty*, 3(1):39–46, 1988.
18. Gibb, T. D., Sidles, J. A., Harryman, D. T., II, McQuade, K. J., and Matsen, F. A., III: The effect of capsular venting on glenohumeral laxity. *Clin. Orthop.*, 268:120–127, 1991.
19. Goldberg, B. A., Lippitt, S. B., and Matsen, F. A., III: Improvement in comfort and function after cuff repair without acromioplasty. *Clin. Orthop.*, 390:142–150, 2001.
20. Goldberg, B. A., Nowinski, R. J., and Matsen, F. A., III: Outcome of nonoperative management of full-thickness rotator cuff tears. *Clin. Orthop.*, 382:99–107, 2001.
21. Goldberg, B. A., Smith, K. L., Jackins, S. E., Campbell, B., and Matsen, F. A., III: The magnitude and durability of functional improvement after total shoulder arthroplasty for degenerative joint disease. *J. Shoulder Elbow Surg.*, 10(5):464–469, 2001.
22. Harryman, D. T., II, Hettrich, C., Smith, K. L., Campbell, B., Sidles, J. A., and Matsen, F. A., III: A prospective multipractice investigation of patients with full thickness rotator cuff tears: The importance of

co-morbidities, surgeon, and other co-variables on self-assessed shoulder function and health status. *J. Bone Joint Surg.*, 85-A(4):690–696, 2003.

23. Harryman, D. T., II, Lazarus, M. D., Sidles, J. A., and Matsen, F. A., III: Pathophysiology of shoulder instability. *In Operative Arthroscopy.* McGinty, J. B., Caspari, R. B., Jackson, R. W., and Poehling, G. G. (eds.). Lippincott-Raven, Philadelphia, pp. 677–693, 1996.
24. Harryman, D. T., II, Mack, L. A., Wang, K. Y., Jackins, S. E., Richardson, M. L., and Matsen, F. A., III: Repairs of the rotator cuff: Correlation of functional results with integrity of the cuff. *J. Bone Joint Surg.*, 73-A(8):982–989, 1991.
25. Harryman, D. T., II, Sidles, J. A., Clark, J. M., McQuade, K. J., Gibb, T. D., and Matsen, F. A., III: Translation of the humeral head on the glenoid with passive glenohumeral motions. *J. Bone Joint Surg.*, 72-A:1334–1343, 1990.
26. Harryman, D. T., II, Sidles, J. A., Harris, S. L., Lippitt, S. B., and Matsen, F. A., III: The effect of articular conformity and the size of the humeral head component on laxity and motion after glenohumeral arthroplasty. A study in cadavera. *J. Bone Joint Surg.*, 77-A(4):555–563, 1995.
27. Harryman, D. T., II, Sidles, J. A., Harris, S. L., and Matsen, F. A., III: Laxity of the normal glenohumeral joint: A quantitative in vivo assessment. *J. Shoulder Elbow Surg.*, 1:113–118, 1992.
28. Harryman, D. T., II, Sidles, J. A., Harris, S. L., and Matsen, F. A., III: The role of the rotator interval capsule in passive motion and stability of the shoulder. *J. Bone Joint Surg.*, 74-A(1):53–66, 1992.
29. Harryman, D. T., II, Sidles, J. A., and Matsen, F. A., III: The humeral head translates on the glenoid with passive motion. *In Surgery of the Shoulder.* Hawkins, R. J., Morrey, B. F., and Post, M. (eds.). Mosby-Year Book, St. Louis, pp. 186–190, 1990.
30. Harryman, D. T., II, Walker, E. D., Harris, S. L., Sidles, J. A., Jackins, S. E., and Matsen, F. A., III: Residual motion and function after glenohumeral or scapulothoracic arthrodesis. *J. Shoulder Elbow Surg.*, 2(6):275–285, 1993.
31. Hasan, S., Leith, J., Smith, K. L., and Matsen, F. A., III: The distribution of shoulder replacements among surgeons and hospitals is significantly different than that of hip or knee replacements. *J. Shoulder Elbow Surg.*, 12(2):164–169, 2003.
32. Hasan, S. S., Leith, J. M., Campbell, B., Kapil, R., Smith, K. L., and Matsen, F. A., III: Characteristics of unsatisfactory shoulder arthroplasties. *J. Shoulder Elbow Surg.*, 11(5):431–441, 2002.
33. Hawkins, R. J., Bell, R. H., and Lippitt, S. B.: *Atlas of Shoulder Surgery.* Mosby-Year Book, St. Louis, 1996.
34. Hawkins, R. J., Malone, T. R., Matsen, F. A., III, and Savoie, F. H.: Shoulder: Use the low-tech approach. *Patient Care,* 134–174, 1992.
35. Hollister, M. S., Mack, L. A., Patten, R. M., Winter, T. C., III, Matsen, F. A., III, and Veith, R. R.: Association of sonographically detected subacromial/subdeltoid bursal effusion and intraarticular fluid with rotator cuff tear. *Am. J. Roentgenol.*, 165(3):605–608, 1995.
36. Jackins, S., and Matsen, F. A., III: Management of shoulder instability. *J. Hand Ther.*, 7(2):99–106, 1994.
37. Kilcoyne, R. F., and Matsen, F. A., III: Rotator cuff tear measurement by arthropneumotomography. *Am. J. Roentgenol.*, 140(2):315–318, 1983.
38. Kilcoyne, R. F., Shuman, W. P., Matsen, F. A., III, Morris, M., and Rockwood, C. A., Jr.: The Neer classification of displaced proximal humeral fractures: Spectrum of findings on plain radiographs and CT scans (pictorial essay). *Am. J. Roentgenol.*, 154:1029–1033, 1990.
39. Lau, C., Churchill, R. S., Kim, J., Matsen, F. A., III, and Kim, Y.: Asynchronous web-based patient-centered home telemedicine system. *IEEE Trans Biomed Eng,* 49(12):1452–1462, 2002.
40. Lazarus, M. D., Jensen, K. L., Southworth, C., and Matsen, F. A., III: The radiographic evaluation of keeled and pegged glenoid component insertion. *J. Bone Joint Surg.*, 84-A(7):1174–1182, 2002.
41. Lazarus, M. D., Sidles, J. A., Harryman, D. T., II, and Matsen, F. A., III: Effect of a chondral-labral defect on glenoid concavity and glenohumeral stability. A cadaveric model. *J. Bone Joint Surg.*, 78(1):94–102, 1996.
42. Leeson, M. C., and Lippitt, S. B.: Thermal aspects of the use of polymethylmethacrylate in large metaphyseal defects in bone. A clinical review and laboratory study. *Clin. Orthop.*, 295:239–245, 1993.
43. Leeson, M. C., Lippitt, S. B., and Makley, J. T.: Thermal aspects of the use of polymethymethacrylate in large metaphyseal defects in bone. A clinical review and laboratory study. *In New Developments for Limb Salvage in Musculoskeletal Tumors.* Yamamuro, T. (ed.). Springer-Verlag, Tokyo, pp. 277–288, 1989.
44. Lippitt, S. B., Harris, S. L., Harryman, D. T., II, Sidles, J. A., and Matsen, F. A., III: In vivo quantification of the laxity of normal and unstable glenohumeral joints. *J. Shoulder Elbow Surg.*, 3(4):215–223, 1994.
45. Lippitt, S. B., Harryman, D. T., II, and Matsen, F. A., III: A practical tool for evaluating function: The Simple Shoulder Test. *In The Shoulder: A Balance of Mobility and Stability.* Matsen, F. A., III, Fu, F. H., and Hawkins, R. J. (eds.). American Academy of Orthopaedic Surgeons, Rosemont, IL, pp. 501–518, 1993.
46. Lippitt, S. B., Harryman, D. T., II, Sidles, J. A., and Matsen, F. A., III: Diagnosis and management of AMBRI syndrome. *Techniques Orthop.*, 10(1):61–73, 1991.
47. Lippitt, S. B., and Matsen, F. A., III: Mechanisms of glenohumeral joint stability. *Clin. Orthop.*, 291:20–28, 1993.
48. Lippitt, S. B., Vanderhooft, E., Harris, S. L., Sidles, J. A., Harryman, D. T., II, and Matsen, F. A., III: Glenohumeral stability from concavity compression: A quantitative analysis. *J. Shoulder Elbow Surg.*, 2(1):27–35, 1993.
49. Mack, L. A., Gannon, M. K., Kilcoyne, R. F., and Matsen, F. A., III: Sonographic evaluation of the rotator cuff: Accuracy in patients without prior surgery. *Clin. Orthop.*, 234:21–28, 1988.
50. Mack, L. A., and Matsen, F. A., III: Rotator cuff. *Clin. Diagn. Ultrasound,* 30:113–133, 1995.

51. Mack, L. A., Matsen, F. A., III, Kilcoyne, R. F., Davies, P. K., and Sickler, M. E.: Ultrasound: US evaluation of the rotator cuff. *Radiology*, 157(1):205–209, 1985.
52. Mack, L. A., Nyberg, D. A., and Matsen, F. A., III: Sonographic evaluation of the rotator cuff. *Radiol. Clin. North Am.*, 26(1):161–177, 1988.
53. Mack, L. A., Nyberg, D. A., Matsen, F. A., III, Kilcoyne, R. F., and Harvey, D.: Sonography of the postoperative shoulder. *Am. J. Roentgenol.*, 150(5):1089–1093, 1988.
54. Mack, L. A., Rogers, J. V., Winter, T. C., and Matsen, F. A., III: Ultrasound of the rotator cuff. *In Diagnostic Imaging of the Shoulder.* Seeger, L. L. (ed.). Williams & Wilkins, Baltimore, pp. 96–139, 1992.
55. Matsen, F. A., III: Biomechanics of the shoulder. *In Basic Biomechanics of the Skeletal System.* Frankel, V. H., and Nordin, M. (eds.). Lea & Febiger, Philadelphia, pp. 221–242, 1980.
56. Matsen, F. A., III: Glenohumeral instability. *In Surgery of the Musculoskeletal System.* Evarts, C. M. (ed.). Livingston, New York, Vol. 2, pp. 49–75, 1983.
57. Matsen, F. A., III: Capsulorrhaphy with a staple for recurrent posterior subluxation of the shoulder. *J. Bone Joint Surg.*, 73-A(6):950, 1991.
58. Matsen, F. A., III: Presidential address: American Shoulder and Elbow Surgeons, 10th Anniversary Annual Meeting. *J. Shoulder Elbow Surg.*, 1:63, 1992.
59. Matsen, F. A., III: Early effectiveness of shoulder arthroplasty for patients who have primary glenohumeral degenerative joint disease. *J. Bone Joint Surg.*, 78-A(2):260–264, 1996.
60. Matsen, F. A., III: Letters to the editor. *Arthroscopy*, 16(6):673, 2000.
61. Matsen, F. A., III: The biomechanics of glenohumeral stability. *J. Bone Joint Surg.*, 84-A(3):495–496, 2002.
62. Matsen, F. A., III: The relationship of surgical volume to quality of care: Scientific considerations and policy implications. *J. Bone Joint Surg.*, 84-A(8):1482–1483; discussion, 1483–1485, 2002.
63. Matsen, F. A., III, Antoniou, J., Rozencwaig, R., Campbell, B., and Smith, K. L.: Correlates with comfort and function after total shoulder arthroplasty for degenerative joint disease. *J. Shoulder Elbow Surg.*, 9(6):465–469, 2000.
64. Matsen, F. A., III, Arntz, C. A., and Harryman, D. T., II: Rotator cuff tear arthropathy. *In Complications of Shoulder Surgery.* Bigliani, L. U. (ed.). Williams & Wilkins, Baltimore, pp. 44–58, 1993.
65. Matsen, F. A., III, and Arntz, C. T.: Rotator cuff tendon failure. *In The Shoulder.* Rockwood, C. A., Jr., and Matsen, F. A., III (eds.). WB Saunders, Philadelphia, Vol. 2, pp. 647–665, 1990.
66. Matsen, F. A., III, and Arntz, C. T.: Subacromial impingement. *In The Shoulder.* Rockwood, C. A., Jr., and Matsen, F. A., III (eds.). WB Saunders, Philadelphia, Vol. 2, pp. 623–636, 1990.
67. Matsen, F. A., III, Artnz, C. T., and Lippitt, S. B.: Rotator cuff. *In The Shoulder.* Rockwood, C. A., Jr., and Matsen, F. A., III (eds.). WB Saunders, Philadelphia, pp. 755–839, 1998.
68. Matsen, F. A., III, Bonica, J. J., and Franklin, J. L.: Pain in the shoulder, arm, and elbow. *In The Management of Pain.* Bonica, J. J. (ed.). Lea & Febiger, Philadelphia, Vol. 1, pp. 906–923, 1990.
69. Matsen, F. A., III, Fu, F., and Hawkins, R. J. (eds.): *The Shoulder: A Balance of Mobility and Stability.* American Academy of Orthopaedic Surgeons, Rosemont, IL, 1993.
70. Matsen, F. A., III, Harryman, D. T., II, and Sidles, J. A.: Mechanics of glenohumeral instability. *Clin. Sports Med.*, 10(4):783–788, 1991.
71. Matsen, F. A., III, and Kirby, R. M.: Office evaluation and management of shoulder pain. *Orthop. Clin. North Am.*, 13(3):453–475, 1982.
72. Matsen, F. A., III, Lippitt, S. B., Sidles, J. A., and Harryman, D. T., II: *Practical Evaluation and Management of the Shoulder.* WB Saunders, Philadelphia, 1994.
73. Matsen, F. A., III, Rockwood, C. A., Jr., and Iannotti, J.: Humeral fixation by press fit of a tapered metaphyseal stem. A prospective radiograph study. *J. Bone Joint Surg.*, 85-A(2):304–308, 2003.
74. Matsen, F. A., III, Rockwood, C. A., Jr., Wirth, M. A., and Lippitt, S. B.: Glenohumeral arthritis and its management. *In The Shoulder.* Rockwood, C. A., Jr., and Matsen, F. A., III (eds.). WB Saunders, Philadelphia, pp. 840–964, 1998.
75. Matsen, F. A., III, and Smith, K. L.: Effectiveness evaluation and the shoulder. *In The Shoulder.* Rockwood, C. A., Jr., and Matsen, F. A., III (eds.). WB Saunders, Philadelphia, pp. 1313–1340, 1998.
76. Matsen, F. A., III, Smith, K. L., DeBartolo, S. E., and Von Oesen, G.: A comparison of patients with late-stage rheumatoid arthritis and osteoarthritis of the shoulder using self-assessed shoulder function and health status. *Arthritis Care Res.*, 10(1):43–47, 1997.
77. Matsen, F. A., III, Thomas, S. C., and Rockwood, C. A., Jr.: Glenohumeral instability. *In The Shoulder.* Rockwood, C. A., Jr., and Matsen, F. A., III (eds.). WB Saunders, Philadelphia, Vol. 1, pp. 526–569, 1990.
78. Matsen, F. A., III, Thomas, S. C., Rockwood, C. A., and Wirth, M. A.: Glenohumeral instability. *In The Shoulder.* Rockwood, C. A., Jr., and Matsen, F. A., III (eds.). WB Saunders, Philadelphia, pp. 611–754, 1998.
79. Matsen, F. A., III, and Thomas, S. T.: Glenohumeral instability. *In Surgery of the Musculoskeletal System.* Evarts, C. M. (ed.). Churchill Livingstone, New York, Vol. 2, pp. 1439–1469, 1990.
80. Matsen, F. A., III, Ziegler, D. W., and DeBartolo, S. E.: Patient self-assessment of health status and function in glenohumeral degenerative joint disease. *J. Shoulder Elbow Surg.*, 4(5):345–351, 1995.
81. Matsen, F. A., III, and Zuckerman, J. D.: Anterior glenohumeral instability. *Clin. Sports Med.*, 2(2):319–338, 1983.
82. Metcalf, M. H., Duckworth, D. G., Lee, S. B., Sidles, J. A., Smith, K. L., Harryman, D. T., II, and Matsen, F. A., III: Posteroinferior glenoplasty can change glenoid shape and increase the mechanical stability of the shoulder. *J. Shoulder Elbow Surg.*, 8(3):205–213, 1999.

83. Norquist, B. M., Goldberg, B. A., and Matsen, F. A., III: Challenges in evaluating patients lost to follow-up in clinical studies of rotator cuff tears. *J. Bone Joint Surg.*, 82-A(6):838–842, 2000.
84. O'Kane, J. W., Jackins, S., Sidles, J. A., Smith, K. L., and Matsen, F. A., III: Simple home program for frozen shoulder to improve patients' assessment of shoulder function and health status. *J. Am. Board Fam. Pract.*, 12(4):270–277, 1999.
85. Pearl, M. L., Harris, S. L., Lippitt, S. B., Sidles, J. A., Harryman, D. T., II, and Matsen, F. A., III: A system for describing positions of the humerus relative to the thorax and its use in the presentation of several functionally important arm positions. *J. Shoulder Elbow Surg.*, 1:113–118, 1992.
86. Pearl, M. L., Jackins, S. E., Lippitt, S. B., Sidles, J. A., and Matsen, F. A., III: Humero-scapular positions in a shoulder range of motion examination. *J. Shoulder Elbow Surg.*, 1(6):296–305, 1992.
87. Pearl, M. L., and Lippitt, S. B.: Shoulder arthroplasty with a modular prosthesis. *Techniques Orthop.*, 8(3):151–162, 1993.
88. Pearl, M. L., Sidles, J. A., Lippitt, S. B., Harryman, D. T., II, and Matsen, F. A., III: Codman's paradox: 60 years later. *J. Shoulder Elbow Surg.*, 1:219–225, 1992.
89. Rockwood, C. A., Jr., and Matsen, F. A., III (eds.): *The Shoulder.* WB Saunders, Philadelphia, 1990.
90. Rockwood, C. A., Jr., and Matsen, F. A., III (eds.): *The Shoulder.* WB Saunders, Philadelphia, 2nd ed., 1998.
91. Rockwood, C. A., Jr., Matsen, F. A., III, and Lippitt, S. B.: *Global Fx Shoulder Fracture System Surgical Technique (Monograph).* DePuy, Warsaw, IN, 1999.
92. Rockwood, C. A., Jr., Thomas, S. C., and Matsen, F. A., III: Subluxation and dislocations about the glenohumeral joint. *In Rockwood and Green's Fractures in Adults.* Rockwood, C. A., Jr., and Green, D. (eds.). Lippincott, Philadelphia, 1991.
93. Romeo, A. A., Loutzenheiser, T., Rhee, Y. G., Sidles, J. A., Harryman, D. T., II, and Matsen, F. A., III: The humeroscapular motion interface. *Clin. Orthop.*, 350:120–127, 1998.
94. Rozencwaig, R., van Noort, A., Moskal, M. J., Smith, K. L., Sidles, J. A., and Matsen, F. A., III: The correlation of comorbidity with function of the shoulder and health status of patients who have glenohumeral degenerative joint disease. *J. Bone Joint Surg.*, 80-A(8):1146–1153, 1998.
95. Scarlat, M. M., Cuny, C., Goldberg, B. A., Harryman, D. T., II, and Matsen, F. A., III: The lateral impaction of the shoulder. *Int. Orthop.*, 23(5):302–307, 1999.
96. Scarlat, M. M., and Matsen, F. A., III: Observations on retrieved polyethylene glenoid components. *J. Arthroplasty*, 16(6):795–801, 2001.
97. Schiffern, S. C., Rozencwaig, R., Antoniou, J., Richardson, M. L., and Matsen, F. A., III: Anteroposterior centering of the humeral head on the glenoid in vivo. *Am. J. Sports Med.*, 30(3):382–387, 2002.
98. Shuman, W. P., Kilcoyne, R. F., Matsen, F. A., III, Rogers, J. V., and Mack, L. A.: Double-contrast computed tomography of the glenoid labrum. *Am. J. Roentgenol.*, 141(3):581–584, 1983.
99. Smith, K. L., Harryman, D. T., II, Antoniou, J., Campbell, B., Sidles, J. A., and Matsen, F. A., III: A prospective, multipractice study of shoulder function and health status in patients with documented rotator cuff tears. *J. Shoulder Elbow Surg.*, 9(5):395–402, 2000.
100. Smith, K. L., and Matsen, F. A., III: Total shoulder arthroplasty versus hemiarthroplasty. Current trends. *Orthop. Clin. North Am.*, 29(3):491–506, 1998.
101. Thomas, S. C., and Matsen, F. A., III: An approach to the repair of glenohumeral ligament avulsion in the management of traumatic anterior glenohumeral instability. *J. Bone Joint Surg.*, 71-A(4):506–513, 1989.
102. Viola, R. W., Boatright, K. C., Smith, K. L., Sidles, J. A., and Matsen, F. A., III: Do shoulder patients insured by workers' compensation present with worse self-assessed function and health status? *J. Shoulder Elbow Surg.*, 9(5):368–372, 2000.
103. Weldon, E. J., III, Scarlat, M. M., Lee, S. B., and Matsen, F. A., III: Intrinsic stability of unused and retrieved polyethylene glenoid components. *J. Shoulder Elbow Surg.*, 10(5):474–481, 2001.
104. Woodhouse, E., Fehringer, E., Benda, P., and Matsen, F. A., III: Metastatic carcinoma to the acromion in a patient following total shoulder arthroplasty: A case report and review of the literature. *J. Shoulder Elbow Surg.*, 11(6):645–646, 2002.
105. Ziegler, D. W., DeBartolo, S. E., and Matsen, F. A., III: Patient self-assessment of health status and function in glenohumeral degenerative joint disease. *J. Shoulder Elbow Surg.*, 4:345–351, 1995.
106. Zuckerman, J. D., and Matsen, F. A., III: Complications about the glenohumeral joint related to the use of screws and staples. *J. Bone Joint Surg.*, 66-A(2):175–180, 1984.
107. Zuckerman, J. D., and Matsen, F. A., III: Biomechanics of the shoulder. *In Basic Biomechanics of the Skeletal System.* Frankel, V. H. and Nordin, M. (eds.). Lea & Febiger, Philadelphia, pp. 225–247, 1989.

# Index

*Note: Page numbers followed by f indicate figures; page numbers followed by t indicate tables.*

I



J



K



L



M